Interdisciplinary Cancer Research

Volume 24

The “Interdisciplinary Cancer Research” series publishes comprehensive volumes on different cancers and presents the most updated and peer-reviewed articles on human cancers. Over the past decade, increased cancer research has greatly improved our understanding of the nature of cancerous cells which has led to the development of more effective therapeutic strategies to treat cancers. This translational series is of special value to researchers and practitioners working on cell biology, immunology, hematology, biochemistry, genetics, oncology and related fields.

Nima Rezaei
Editor

Cancer Treatment Modalities: An Interdisciplinary Approach

Springer

Editor
Nima Rezaei
Department of Clinical Immunology
Karolinska Institutet
Stockholm, Sweden

Research Center for Immunodeficiencies
Children's Medical Center
Tehran University of Medical Sciences
Tehran, Iran

ISSN 2731-4561 ISSN 2731-457X (electronic)
Interdisciplinary Cancer Research
ISBN 978-3-032-03865-4 ISBN 978-3-032-03866-1 (eBook)
https://doi.org/10.1007/978-3-032-03866-1

This Springer imprint is published by the registered company Springer Nature Switzerland AG
The registered company address is: Gewerbestrasse 11, 6330 Cham, Switzerland

Preface

The Interdisciplinary Cancer Research series publishes comprehensive volumes on different cancers. It plans to present the most updated and peer-reviewed interdisciplinary chapters on cancers. This interdisciplinary book series is of special value to researchers and practitioners working on cell biology, immunology, hematology, biochemistry, genetics, oncology and related fields. This is the main concept of Cancer Immunology Project (CIP) and Network of Immunity in Infection, Malignancy and Autoimmunity (NIIMA), which are two active interest groups of the Universal Scientific Education and Research Network (USERN).

The twenty-fourth volume of the book entitled *Cancer Treatment Modalities: An Interdisciplinary Approach* focuses on cancer treatment. The volume starts with a chapter on an interdisciplinary approach to biomarker discovery for cancer treatment, followed by two other chapters on multidisciplinary approach in cancer management, and the interplay between inflammation and cancer progression. Cancer stem cells and mesenchymal stem cells are discussed in other chapters. RNA epigenetics in cancer diagnosis and treatment and different aspects of telomerase inhibitors in cancer treatment are the subject of subsequent chapters. Relationship between radiation-induced trismus and inflammation and the biological effects of GRID, microbeam, and FLASH radiotherapy are the subjects of other chapters. Then, bioimplants for reconstructive surgery and the interplay of ferroptosis and cuproptosis in cancer are discussed. Liquid biopsy and cancer and mitochondrial transplantation are the subjects of two other chapters. Then, steroids in cancer, surgical treatment, importance of drug interactions during ALK tyrosine kinase inhibitor therapies, and promising anticancer activity of new triazoles and their related compounds, as well as anticancer properties of antipsychotic drugs are explained. Microbial-based therapies in cancer treatment and bacteria-based approach to cancer therapy are the subjects of final chapters of this volume.

I hope that this interdisciplinary book will be comprehensible, cogent, and of special value for those who wish to have an update on cancer treatment modalities.

Stockholm, Sweden Nima Rezaei

Contents

About the Editor

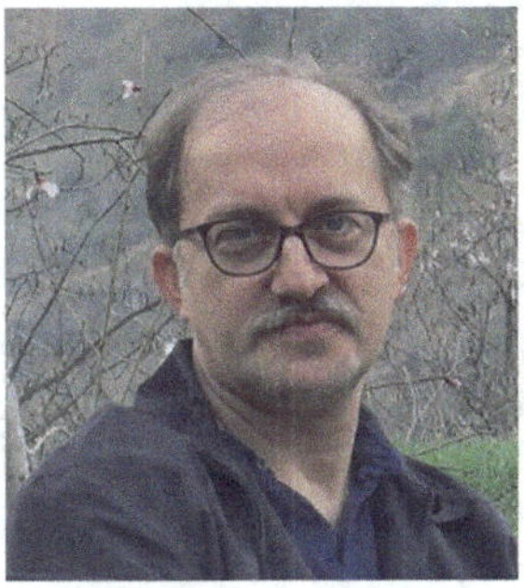

Nima Rezaei, MD, PhD, gained his medical degree (MD) from Tehran University of Medical Sciences and subsequently obtained an MSc in Molecular and Genetic Medicine and a PhD in Clinical Immunology and Human Genetics from the University of Sheffield, UK. He also spent a short-term fellowship of Pediatric Clinical Immunology and Bone Marrow Transplantation in the Newcastle General Hospital. Professor Rezaei is now the Full Professor of Immunology and Vice Dean of Research and Technologies, School of Medicine, Tehran University of Medical Sciences, and the co-founder and Head of the Research Center for Immunodeficiencies. He is also the Founder of Universal Scientific Education and Research Network (USERN). Prof. Rezaei has already been the Director of more than 200 research projects and has designed and participated in several international collaborative projects. Prof. Rezaei is the editor, editorial assistant, or editorial board member of more than 50 international journals. He has edited more than 100 international books, has presented more than 1000 lectures/posters in congresses/meetings, and has published more than 1700 scientific papers in international journals.

Interdisciplinary Approaches to Leverage Biomarker Discovery for Cancer Treatment

Fatemeh Khatami and Nima Rezaei

Abstract

Cancer treatment is a complex process demanding a comprehensive understanding of the disease mechanism, individual differences, and early diagnosis to achieve better therapeutic yield. Biomarker discovery, the core of precision medicine, has revolutionized the field of cancer biology by bridging multiple disciplines to identify the most appropriate targets for arresting or ideally, killing cancer cells. The interdisciplinary approaches have drastically improved the precision and speed of discoveries by integrating the data acquired at various biological levels into unified and explicit output for therapeutic development. This has led to the detection of novel proteins and neoepitopes rooted in an understudied portion of the proteomes called dark proteome or due to genomic mutation or epigenetic modulation of cancer stem cells. Computational models and artificial intelligence offer great opportunities to explore ever-growing datasets to find the most promising candidates, predict their structural configuration, and determine the possible contribution of the candidate biomarkers in the biological alteration of cells. Here, we discuss the necessity of understanding the context and the value of merging experimental techniques with computational models to study intercellular and molecular interactions. The interdisciplinary approaches facilitate the generation of therapeutic drugs with higher efficacy for clinical applications and detection probes for experimental and diagnostic purposes.

F. Khatami · N. Rezaei (✉)
Research Center for Immunodeficiencies, Children's Medical Center, Tehran University of Medical Sciences, Tehran, Iran

Cancer Immunology Project (CIP), Universal Scientific Education and Research Network (USERN), Tehran, Iran
e-mail: rezaei_nima@tums.ac.ir

Interdisciplinary Cancer Research, https://doi.org/10.1007/16833_2025_497
Published online: 13 March 2025

Keywords

AI · Antibody therapeutics · Cancer biomarker · Immune checkpoint · Machine learning · NLM · Proteome

1 Introduction

A cancer biomarker is any endogenous biological molecule such as proteins, RNA, DNA, and metabolites expressed in different quantities or with altered conformation by cells which as a diagnostic tool helps in distinguishing benign from malignant cells. These molecules can be detected in cells or body fluids, and their quantity or configuration can provide beneficial information about the disease onset, progression, and therapeutic response (Henry and Hayes 2012; Passaro et al. 2024). Despite drastic improvements in screening and employing cancer biomarkers, the issues regarding the specificity, timely detection of tumor cells, and therapeutic outcomes in patients with different cancer grades have challenged the traditional strategies for biomarker screening. The malignant transformation of cells (MTC) endows a great level of plasticity to cells ranging from alteration in molecular expression to phenotypic changes (Perez-Gonzalez et al. 2023). Taking into account the dynamics of molecular expression at different stages of cancer development, we require tools and techniques that provide better mechanistic information to identify the most appropriate biomarkers for targeting cancer cells.

The foundation of traditional biomarker discoveries is based upon distinct expression levels of genetic elements or proteins between normal and diseased biological samples. In the traditional approaches, a sample is assigned to a predefined class or disease stage (Duffy 2001; Ludwig and Weinstein 2005). Due to the qualitative nature of such assessments, the diagnostic precision is restricted and prone to bias. However, more advanced strategies in biomarker discovery mainly rely on high-throughput screening methods known as "omics" encompassing various fields including but not limited to genomics, transcriptomics, proteomics, metabolomics, and to a lesser extent liquid biopsies to detect tumor-related circulatory markers such as DNA in the blood (Li et al. 2020; Akhoundova and Rubin 2022; Ulivi and Indraccolo 2022). These strategies correlate the differential expression of a marker to disease activity or sign with higher accuracy than traditional approaches. However, matching the transcriptomic and proteomic findings is sometimes challenging as transcriptomic data is not always an accurate reflection of corresponding proteins due to low expression levels or the turnover rate of the target proteins (Boisvert et al. 2012). This per se, makes the biomarker validation a daunting process. Cross-disciplinary approaches offer the opportunity to look beyond cancer biology by considering the context and the interrelationship between cells and their surrounding environment to extract the most relevant information from these techniques. A clearer insight into the tumor microenvironment helps identify the key molecules that guarantee tumor cell survival. Identifying the right biomarker candidate for therapeutic development ensures the delivery of more effective treatment to patients to mitigate the off-target effect and avoid overtreatment.

2 Context Matters: Immune Cells and Niche Properties

Cells sense and respond to perturbations in their surroundings and distant niches through their receptors and secretory molecules. This cross-talk is crucial for cells to adjust their biological functionality within their immediate niches. Interestingly, compartmentalization in organs like bone marrow (BM) (Passaro et al. 2021), intestine (Hickey et al. 2023), and spleen (Goltsev et al. 2018; Lewis et al. 2019) creates specialized niches with differential cellular and molecular compositions that dictate cell fate. Cancer cells are mainly formed by the process termed "epithelial-mesenchymal transition" (EMT) or from tissue-resident stem cells. (Dongre and Weinberg 2019). A key difference between normal and cancer stem cells is the level of reliance on the niche, as under homeostatic conditions, the proliferation of stem cells is regulated by inhibitory signals from their specialized niches. However, the dysregulated production of niche components such as proliferation-promoting cytokines or accumulation of intrinsic mutations can disrupt the balance between self-renewal and differentiation, leading to tumor development. (Plaks et al. 2015).

The niche components including extracellular matrix (ECM), stromal cells, stem cells, and soluble factors differ based on the organ's specific functionality. This distinction endows unique features to the immune cell profile even in various tissue parts. Understanding the immunological elements of the target tissue and its transformation in response to tumor microenvironment is central to developing immunotherapeutic drugs (Tsagiopoulou et al. 2024) (Fig. 1). Under normal conditions, in the BM niche rich in the chemokine CXCl12, mesenchymal stem cells (MSCs) maintain various populations of cells such as bone-forming cells (e.g., osteoblasts and chondroblasts) and hematopoietic stem cells (HSCs). They also play a pivotal

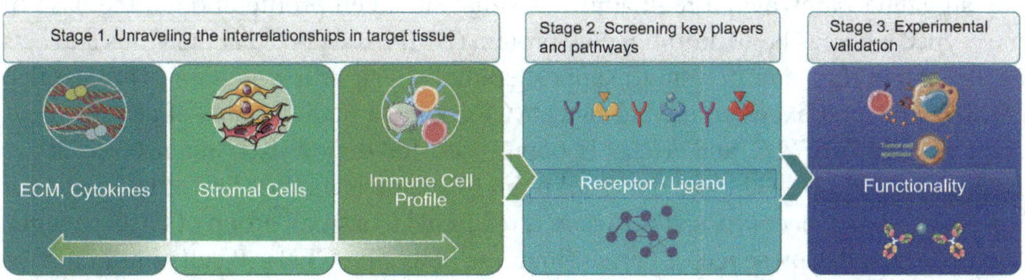

Fig. 1 The key stages for selecting cancer biomarkers. The success of therapeutic development with the potential to specifically target tumor cells largely depends on our knowledge about intercellular interactions and molecular events in their specialized niches that lead to altered biological functionality of the cells. Although there is a bidirectional relationship between technological advances and progress in our understanding of biological events, studying underlying mechanisms using the available tools can significantly influence the methodological design and data interpretation for biomarker screening. Most therapeutic products interact with cell receptors, signaling molecules, or secretory factors, and this renders receptor/ligand as well as pathway analysis a prerequisite. The contribution of biomarker candidates to the biological processes such as proliferation, differentiation, and cancer immune evasion is a determinant factor in developing effective therapeutics and detection tools to impede cancer progression (some elements of the figure adapted from Scidraw.io)

role in immune tolerance through bidirectional interaction with immune cells. However, cells that have escaped the regulatory mechanisms and underwent malignant transformation can remodel the niche components. As such, malignant cells can reduce the production of CXCL12 by MSCs, induce the overexpression of inflammatory cytokines IL-1β, TNF-α, and growth factors and negatively alter the proportion of effector immune cells to support their survival (Mendez-Ferrer et al. 2020). For instance, in the BM of patients with acute lymphoblastic leukemia (ALL), the proportion of effector immune cells like M1 macrophages, CD27+ and CD57+ CD8+ T cells is reduced in favor of tumor-promoting M2 macrophages, and myeloid-derived suppressor cells. The dysregulated niche further supports the upregulation of the coinhibitory molecules T cell immunoglobulin and mucin domain-3 (TIM3), programmed cell death protein 1 (PD1), and cytotoxic T-lymphocyte-associated protein 4 (CTLA-4). The overexpression of coinhibitory markers by T cells in the BM of acute myeloid leukemia (AML) and chronic myeloid leukemia (CML) patients is correlated with a poor survival rate (Brück et al. 2018; Hohtari et al. 2019).

Like the BM, the gastrointestinal (GI) tract has a unique structure and diverse niches at different regions with attributes highly dependent on the anatomical site, microbiota composition, and diet. These attributes greatly impact the diversity of immune cells in different areas of the intestine. Emerging data indicate that stromal cells like fibroblasts but not MSCs have distinct transcriptional profiles that endow them with specialized functions in various areas of the GI tract to support the needs of the local environment (Paerregaard et al. 2023). In this regard, it has been demonstrated that the frequency of plasma cells and CD8+ T cells is lower in the human colon compared to the small intestine, while the number of dendritic cells (DCs) increases (Hickey et al. 2023). In the intestine, Wnt and Notch are among the key signaling pathways in regulating intestinal stem cell proliferation at the base of the crypts, whereas bone morphogenic protein (BMP) is detected at the villus and acts as a negative regulator of Wnt to support epithelial cell differentiation (Thorne et al. 2018). In the context of colorectal cancer (CRC), the mutation status of certain genes such as *KRAS*, *BRAF*, and *NRAS* is being used for diagnosis (Auclin et al. 2017; Bożyk et al. 2022). Although the checkpoint blockade is the first line of treatment for the majority of cancer types, its efficacy is restricted to a small group of CRC patients. Nevertheless, the presence of certain immune cells like CD8+ T cells in the tumor, PD-L1 expression, and pro-inflammatory cytokines IL-4, IL-6, and TNF-α are predictive markers of patients' outcome (Liu et al. 2023; Maryam et al. 2023).

Another niche-associated factor is the composition and spatiotemporal features of ECM that have an immunomodulatory impact on cells. As such, the ECM can modify the expression of classical and nonclassical human leukocyte antigens (HLAs) on the surface of cells. The HLAs are protein molecules that assist the immune system in distinguishing self from nonself (Azizian et al. 2018). In contrast to classical HLA, nonclassical HLA class G proteins are immune inhibitory molecules whose expression is restricted to placental tissue during embryonic development. They are expressed on the surface of trophoblasts or in soluble form to suppress the mother's immunological reactions against the fetus (Jurisicova et al. 1996). Certain tumors use the same strategy to escape antitumor immune response

(Bartolome et al. 2023). Due to growing evidence highlighting the coinhibitory role of HLA-G in various malignancies like CRC and leukemia, this molecule has stood out for developing immunotherapeutic drugs (Rizzo et al. 2014; Gambella et al. 2022). The surface HLA-G can suppress antitumor immunity via a mechanism known as trogocytosis, a process by which immune and nonimmune cells exchange membranous fragments containing receptors and inhibitory molecules. This phenomenon changes the functionality of the recipient immune cells such as NK cells, monocytes, and effector T cells endowing a regulatory phenotype to these cells in the tumor microenvironment (Lin and Yan 2019). This phenomenon further underscores the role of context and cellular interaction in immune modulation.

Due to limited efficacy and varied survival rates in patients receiving current immunotherapeutic drugs, there is a need to identify key biomarkers not only based on their differential expression level but more importantly their impact on the biological behavior of cells to develop more efficacious therapeutics for clinical application. Figure 2 represents a brief overview of biomarker discovery pipeline.

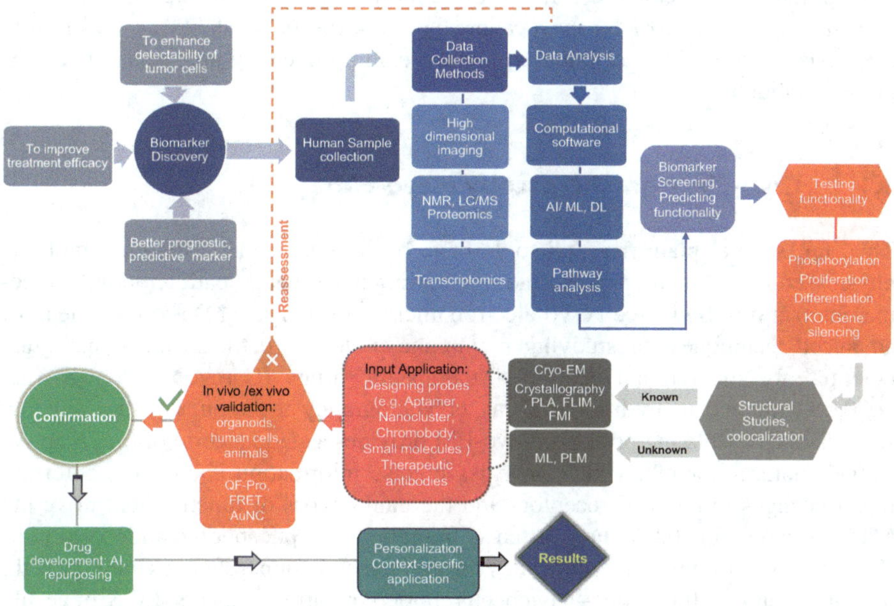

Fig. 2 Schematic representation of biomarker discovery pipeline. The advanced technological tools and computational methods have tremendously impacted biomarker discovery and validation by improving the precision and reliability of the acquired data and circumventing the experimental procedures that in some circumstances are prone to human bias. Given the mechanistic complexity of cancer development, finding the root cause of the disease is something beyond the histological and molecular evaluation of tumor samples. To acquire a better insight, it is necessary to incorporate the information (e.g., dark proteome) that, due to technical limitations, has been overlooked in the screening process, decision-making, and therapeutic drug validation (AI: artificial Intelligence; AuNC: gold nanocluster; DL: deep learning; FLIM: fluorescence-lifetime imaging microscopy; FRET: förster resonance energy transfer: KO: gene knockout; PLA: proximity ligation assay; PLM: protein language models)

3 Current Technologies to Study Biological Behaviors of the Cells

Recent advances in capturing the dynamics of interaction between cells and their niche at the molecular level have profoundly transformed our understanding of the underlying immune mechanisms against cancer. Identifying a biomarker that is a good indication of impaired functionality or cell malignancy relies on the depth of our knowledge about proteins that act as functional units and are the end product of the genes in the form of receptors, enzymes, chemokines, and cytokines in the cells. Despite remarkable progress in the detection of mutated genes using single-cell genomics approaches in various cancer types, the focus of studies on proteins has been far less in part due to their sensitivities to physiological changes and their turnover rate (Sarhadi and Armengol 2022). Nevertheless, this is the receptor-ligand interaction and the nature of the transduced signals that define cell fate (Marchetti et al. 2022). Despite substantial progress in generating therapeutic mAbs against surface biomarkers such as coinhibitory receptors CTLA-4 (ipilimumab) and PD-L1 (durvalumab), the predictive value of these biomarkers for selecting patients histologically is less than 40% for most cancer types (Doroshow et al. 2021). This further emphasizes the need for technical and analytical improvement in biomarker screening and validation.

3.1 Cryo-Electron Microscopy (Cryo-EM)

Thus far, several platforms and tools have been developed by merging biology, physics, computational sciences, and engineering to delineate spatiotemporal molecular interactions. Single-cell cryo-electron microscopy (Cryo-EM) is one of the most advanced techniques for studying membrane protein structures, and it has great potential for the rational design of therapeutic drugs (Garcia-Nafria and Tate 2020). Compared to traditional X-ray crystallography techniques with a shallow success rate of isolating proteins, Cryo-EM provides a static picture of the receptors in their natural context, which provides precise information about the conformational changes in mutated receptors and the gain or loss of function that drive the MTC (Liu et al. 2022). For instance, mutations in phosphoinositide 3-kinases (PI3Ks)—one of the key molecules in cellular functions such as cell growth, migration, and proliferation—have been reported in various cancers. PI3K molecule comprises catalytic (p110α) and regulatory (P85α) subunits. Mutation in p110α endows gain of function to the enzyme by mitigating the inhibitory effect of subunits p85α on p110α. By taking advantage of Cryo-EM technology, Liu et al. demonstrated conformational changes in the p110α subunit, making it a potential drug development option. The findings highlighted the necessity to design more valuable antagonists with lower binding affinity or interaction with unmutated subunits (Liu et al. 2022). The available US Food and Drug Administration (FDA) approved PI3K inhibitors have broad reactivity with both mutated and unmutated molecules (Hassenrück et al. 2023), leading to the disruption of the PI3K signaling pathway in malignant as well as healthy cells.

Using the same technology, Krimmer et al. also investigated the effect of mutation on the configuration of tyrosine kinase receptor KIT. This membrane receptor and its ligand—stem cell factor—play a key part in hematopoiesis and regulating gastrointestinal stromal cell division. In wild type (WT) receptors, the ligand binding enables the interaction between the D4 and D5 domains of the two receptors to form a dimer and activates other signaling cascades. However, in mutant receptors, the computational analysis of Cryo-EM images revealed an asymmetric rearrangement in the D5 domain and more stable D5:D5 contact compared to the WT receptor. The D5 rearrangement renders the D5 a potential target for antagonist development capable of hindering the dimerization of two receptors (Krimmer et al. 2023). The mutation can also modulate the affinity of the receptors for dimerization in the absence of the cognate ligand, resulting in the overactivation of receptors and a change in the equilibrium of monomeric and homo-dimeric receptors. These changes consequently impact the biological output of the cell such as proliferation and differentiation rate. The overexpression of KIT has been linked to colorectal cancer development and the mutated gene has also been detected in a group of AML patients (Hirota et al. 1998; Katagiri et al. 2022; Kucukkose et al. 2022).

3.2 Fluorescence Microscopy Imaging

Despite the drastic shift in our understanding of the molecular mechanisms involved in the aberrant functionality of cells using Cryo-EM technology, the obtained picture is static and does not reflect the dynamics of molecular interaction in live cells. The need to delineate the dynamics of receptor function calls for methods, such as advanced fluorescence microscopy imaging (FMI) technology, that equip us with a better insight into molecular colocalization, interaction, and density in a physiological setting (Wolf et al. 2021). One of the key steps for probing the target molecule is to incorporate a reporter moiety like green fluorescent protein (GFP) into the target molecule without disturbing its functionality. This has a particular value in biomarker selection and evaluating drug mechanisms of action as the application of current monoclonal antibodies conjugated to fluorophore requires several steps of sample fixation, blocking, and washing, which is not optimal for capturing the ephemeral changes in molecular interactions in live cells (Baronaite and Cachat 2024). *Chromobodies* are nanoprobes for visualizing target proteins in living cells. Chromobodies are generated by fusing a nanobody with a fluorescent protein. They are efficient substitutions for mAbs with higher specificity for detecting epitopes and tracking proteins' turnover rate, especially after drug treatment (Moeglin et al. 2021).

Several FMI-based techniques employ the *Förster resonance energy transfer (FRET)* principle. The principle is based on the energy transfer between donors and acceptors labeled with chromophores via intermolecular dipole-dipole coupling (Sekar and Periasamy 2003). The principle can be used to study the interaction of drugs with target molecules and the consequential biological output in cells (Traenkle and Rothbauer 2017). Regarding diagnosis, the traditional approaches have been incapable of quantifying the activation status of biomarkers such as phosphorylation and colocalization of receptors and signaling molecules. However, time-resolved FRET assay has shown promise in improving diagnostic accuracy and predicting therapeutic outcomes in cancer patients. For instance, Veeriah et al. assessed the expression and phosphorylation status of Akt (pAkt) using amplified FRET and IHC in breast cancer tissues. The high throughput FRET analysis revealed that the level of pAKT is a better predictive factor for lower survival rates in patients. The findings highlighted the importance of employing the right strategy and technique for biomarker discovery and data interpretation. According to the authors, compared to the intensity of the signal, which is routinely obtained by IHC analysis, the AKT activation level is a better indication for predicting the survival rate of breast cancer patients (Veeriah et al. 2014). Consistent with the results of this study, Sanchez-Magraner et al. also underscored the necessity for identifying more clinically relevant parameters that reflect the true participation of the biomarker in disease prognosis and the therapeutic effectiveness in different patients. In this study, by exploiting the quantitative functional proteomics [QF-Pro] platform, the interaction of PD-1/PD-L1 was assessed in fixed samples. In QF-Pro bioimaging platform, which is based on the FRET principle, the signals are detected and visualized by fluorescence lifetime imaging microscopy (FLIM). The results indicated that the expression of PD-L1 does not suffice to predict treatment outcomes, while evaluating the level of interaction between PD-1 and PD-L1 is a better predictive factor on patients' survival (Sánchez-Magraner et al. 2023).

3.3 Nanoclusters and Aptamer-Based Cancer Therapy

Nanoclusters are one of the technological advances with paramount potential in cancer diagnosis and treatment. They are made of sub-nanometer scale particles that can be designed and produced with atomic precision. Their structural stability, malleable photonic or fluorescence properties, low toxicity, and biocompatibility make nanoclusters desirable theranostic tools for cancer studies (Zhang et al. 2018). Gold nanoclusters (AuNC) with high tissue penetrability compared to large molecules have emerged as a safe imaging option for in vivo monitoring and thermal elimination of cancer tissues. The AuNC can emit near-infrared (NIR) fluorescence signal with minimal autofluorescence (Liu et al. 2019), and this makes them a valuable carrier for various natural or synthetic molecules such as peptides and aptamers. These molecules can be conjugated to AuNC and act as a ligand or probe for cancer biomarkers by leading the cluster to tumor cells for imaging, inducing apoptosis, or drug delivery. Aptamers are synthetic oligonucleotides designed to recognize a unique structural conformation in known biomarkers in body fluids or cancer cells. To enhance diagnostic precision, they can be designed to target multiple proteins or biomarkers specific to cancer cells simultaneously (Nimjee et al. 2017).

The aptamers' high specificity has paramount value for treating hematopoietic cancers. For instance, Zaimy et al. exploited the aptamer against the CD33 + CD34+ AML cells for targeted delivery of gold nanoparticles functionalized by antisense oligonucleotides. The aim was to silence oncogenes involved in disease progression and induce apoptosis in AML cells in vitro. The results showed that functionalized gold nanoparticles can target AML and induce cell death (Zaimy et al. 2016). The results can be tested further in vivo by taking advantage of NIR-emitting functionalized AuNCs conjugated to aptamer with a binding affinity toward cancer stem cells in the BM. This can facilitate the diagnosis and targeted delivery of the drugs to the malignant cells as explored in other cancer types (Li et al. 2022; Yang et al. 2023a; b).

Chronic lymphoblastic leukemia (CLL) is the most prevalent type of leukemia in adults. Using CLL cells in a coculture system, Hoellenriegel et al. demonstrated that administering NOX-A12, a CXCL12 aptamer inhibitor affects the mobility of CLL cells in the BM and renders them susceptible to chemotherapeutic drugs (Hoellenriegel et al. 2014). The chemokine CXCL12 plays a pivotal role in the retention of hematopoietic cells in the BM by binding to its cognate receptor CXCR4 (Sugiyama et al. 2006). Despite its transitional effect, inhibiting the ligand binding does not solve the root cause of the disease and the influence of unfunctional niches consisting of CXCL12-producing stromal cells and the altered immune profile in the BM niche. It would be more informative to employ trackable ligands against cancer biomarkers to evaluate the sufficiency of the biomarker in diagnosis and delivery of the chemotherapeutic drugs to target cells (Yang et al. 2024).

In solid cancers, an established dialogue between niche components including suppressor immune cells and tumor stem cells promotes cancer cell survival and their metastasis. Targeting the key biomarkers on aberrant cells using multifunctional nanoclusters/-particles improves therapeutic precision. In this regard, Camorani et al. showed that dual targeting of breast cancer and stromal cells using aptamer-conjugated nanoparticles increases the rate of apoptosis in patient-derived cancer organoids. The developed nanoparticles contained Au core, iridium(III) as a luminescent probe, and a surface coated with aptamers. The cognate aptamers were designed against epidermal growth factor receptor (EGFR) and platelet-derived growth factor receptorβ (PDGFRβ) for detecting and photo-induced killing of the target cells (Camorani et al. 2024).

Indeed, the study of molecular dynamics and monitoring the fate of treated cells in the physiological context adds more value to designing, producing, and validating effective therapeutics that eventually will be tested in patients with very complex physiology and individual features.

3.4 Methods to Study Proteins Co-expression and Intercellular Interaction

Protein islands are a cluster of receptors and signaling molecules in close proximity on cell membranes, forming a signaling hub that regulates the intensity of and the duration of transduced signals upon ligand binding (Lillemeier et al. 2006).

Understanding the concept has a particular value in B cell– and T cell–mediated malignancies because modified cluster on adaptive immune cells can affect their capability to detect and generate an effective response against tumor cells (Hui et al. 2017). To gain better insight into the effect of protein islands in cell physiology, some tools and methods have been introduced including proximity ligation assay (PLA), freestanding bilayer microscope (FBM), and phase-separation-based fluorescent reporter (PSFR).

Proximity ligation assay (PLA) is a protein-based technique for detecting biomarkers in biological samples. The method has profoundly enhanced our knowledge about the key interacting proteins and their modification in a cluster using target-specific primary mAbs and secondary mAbs conjugated to oligonucleotides called PLA probes. The connector oligos can only hybridize with the probes and form a circular DNA template when the two probes are nearby. The amplification of the DNA with polymerase forms a concatemeric DNA sequence leading to signal amplification (Bagchi et al. 2015). This allows the localization of the target protein even with a very low expression level. Indeed, PLA offers a valuable platform for target validation as the method principle is based on the functionality of the protein and its contribution to signal transduction. Apart from the specificity, detecting protein biomarkers in plasma and solid tumors by PLA at the onset of disease development when only a scant amount of tumor-specific proteins are available has a substantial impact on treatment efficacy (Salem et al. 2024). Given that cellular phenotypic and functional modulation relies on protein interaction, the PLA is more reliable for selecting and predicting therapeutic outcomes. In patients with melanoma, the assessment of several parameters including the infiltration of CD8+ T cells into the tumor microenvironment, PD-1/PD-L1 expression, and RNA signature of inflammatory cytokines and inhibitory molecules indicated a more meaningful association between the proximity of PD-1 and PD-L1 and patients' survival. The findings showed that patients with higher proximity values respond better to the immune checkpoint therapy. This predictive parameter assists physicians in selecting candidates who are more likely to respond to immune checkpoint inhibitor (ICI) therapy and avoiding unnecessary treatment-related toxicity in nonresponders' patients (Girault et al. 2022).

Of note, protein proximity lacks the potential for deciphering the phenotype and spatiotemporal distribution of interacting cells in the tumor microenvironment. Given PLA probes work at nanoscale radios, studying intercellular interaction and their collective contribution to cell fate decisions is not applicable using this method. To address this limitation, *quinone methide–assisted identification of cell spatial organization (QMID) method and FucoID* have been developed to probe and position the target cells termed "pray" based on their proximity to bait cells. Bait cells are engineered to express enzymes like β-galactosidase or fucosyltransferase. The β-galactosidase catalyzes the liberation of QM and fucosyltransferase promotes fucosyl-biotinylation of the pray cells in a proximal distance (Qiu et al. 2022; Zhang et al. 2023). These methods are particularly interesting for studying B and T cell interaction with antigen-presenting cells (DCs, Mϕ) or cancer cells. One of the promising applications of the FucoID method is for the personalization of adoptive

T cell therapy, where therapeutic efficacy is highly dependent on selecting and enriching tumor-infiltrating T cells harboring specific TCR from a heterogeneous repertoire of cells (Liu et al. 2020).

4 Metabolites as Cancer Biomarkers

Gut microbiota composition serves as a valuable biomarker not only for early diagnosis of CRC (Ternes et al. 2022) but also for some hematological cancers. The modulatory effect of microbiota on immune system development, homeostasis, and malfunction has been evidenced using germ-free mice and human samples (Josefsdottir et al. 2017; Schluter et al. 2020). This modulation is generally through small molecules such as metabolites that can enter the circulation and affect hematopoiesis in the BM (Liu et al. 2024). Eubiosis, which is unique based on an individual's lifestyle, has been indicated as an important factor in the success of immunotherapy in cancer patients. In contrast, dysbiosis can change the bacterial diversity and the metabolites involved in hematopoiesis. This can induce the MTC or promote their proliferation and survival by altering the immune profile in the BM (Calcinotto et al. 2018; Li et al. 2024). Indeed, bacterial metabolites such as short-chain fatty acids (SCFAs), trimethylamine N-oxide (TMAO), and tryptophan-derived metabolites have the potential to be used as predictive biomarkers in various cancers (Gou et al. 2024; Halicki et al. 2024). Apart from bacterial metabolites in the GI tract, a range of metabolites is produced by tumor cells that are detectable in the blood. These metabolites induce immune cell reprogramming and the development of Treg cells in the tumor microenvironment (Song et al. 2023; Zheng et al. 2024).

To probe any deviation, the target metabolites are selected from the metabolic profiles of healthy and cancer patients using techniques such as *time-of-flight mass spectrometry (MSs) and nuclear magnetic resonance (NMR) spectroscopy* (Qiu et al. 2009; Nagana Gowda and Raftery 2021). The combined application of these methods offers high sensitivity and reproducibility for identifying changes in the metabolic profile of cancer patients and discovering new metabolites. Next, the correlation between the target metabolite(s) and the disease manifestation is evaluated, and once proven, the structural configuration of the target molecules is determined for clinical application. Acquiring detailed information about the atomic arrangements of the metabolites using LC/MS and computational modeling is one of the key steps in designing diagnostic tools.

Biosensors and bioreceptors are some of the newly developed tools for detecting metabolites, biomolecules, and cancer cells. The biosensors can measure biological reactions by generating signals proportional to the target molecule concentration in the sample (Bhalla et al. 2016; Lyu et al. 2024). Biosensors offer high specificity and sensitivity for detecting metabolites and compared to MS and NMR techniques are more cost-effective for routine clinical applications. In a recent study, Ueno et al. developed a biosensor to detect 1-methyl nicotinamide (1-MNA), a metabolite produced by nicotinamide N-methyltransferase enzyme, in body fluids like urine. The 1-MNA molecules, which are released by cancer cells, form a complex with

P6AS consisting of 12 sulfonate group (Ueno et al. 2024). The P6As in the photoinduced electron transfer process emit fluorescence following exposure to light. This process is inhibited by 1-MNA and its binding to P6AS, indicating the enzyme's expression level and the patient disease stage.

Various biomolecules such as antibodies, enzymes, and aptamers can be used as bioreceptors in biosensors like *surface enhanced Raman scattering (SERS)* to promote detection specificity. SERS biosensors are analytical tools with extraordinary potential for detecting cancer biomarkers and bacterial metabolites at minute concentrations. The AuNP and silver nanoparticles (AgNP) are routinely used as substrates for examining the analytes and biomolecules in the samples (Lyu et al. 2024). To improve diagnostic accuracy, the NPs can be functionalized by aptamers or antibodies to detect malignant cells as shown by Nguyen et al. for CLL cells (Nguyen et al. 2010). Given the alteration in gut metabolic profile has been linked to hematological cancers (Li et al. 2024), SERS-based analysis of metabolites derived from cancer and bacterial cells can significantly promote the early diagnosis of the disease. The majority of the published studies have employed liquid chromatography and MS analysis to explore the differential production of metabolites between healthy and leukemia patients (Koziol and Pupek 2022; Wang et al. 2022a, b; Xu et al. 2023), which are highly valuable for metabolite screening. However, applying nanoparticles, aptamers, and specific antibodies as probes for key participating metabolites in cancer progression makes biosensors powerful tools for timely diagnosis and monitoring of treatment efficacy in cancer patients (Muhammad et al. 2024).

5 Machine Learning for Leveraging Biomarker Discovery and Drug Design

Our understanding of the molecular mechanisms and intercellular interactions involved in the MTC largely depends on the precision level of our tools and the reagents' specificity. One of the main therapeutic pitfalls is the lack of specific biomarkers for most chronic diseases. To leverage cancer predictive, diagnostic, and monitoring capabilities, we require a comprehensive picture of protein signatures from a large cohort of patients and healthy subjects. Synergizing data acquisition tools like mass spectrometry (MS)-based proteomics, spatial proteomics, and biosensors with computational methods has profoundly revolutionized the field of biomarker discovery (Steyaert et al. 2023; Xiong et al. 2023; Mi et al. 2024).

Machine learning (ML) models are superior tools for analyzing big and highly complex datasets and recognizing patterns, an ability that entails a laborious and sluggish process using traditional approaches. Pattern mining is one of the most important aspects of novel biomarker discovery that is achieved by deep learning approaches. To detect new or slightly deviated patterns in the protein profiles of cancer patients, which can be an indication of cellular malfunctioning, ML algorithms are exposed and learned from large datasets to make a prediction (Mann et al. 2021). Unraveling the features and molecular structure of biomarkers in patients' samples is crucial in drug design and diagnostic applications. The majority of studies utilizing cell lines for cancer biomarkers and drug discovery fail to resemble the complexity of intercellular and architectural properties of the niche as indicated in leukemia patients (Cucchi et al. 2020). This further underscores the pivotal value of ML and DL models for computing, extracting, and integrating information from a large cohort of patients and healthy subjects. The information obtained by different techniques such as high-dimensional imaging, transcriptomics, and MS-based proteomics can be merged to identify the key players in cancer development with higher precision (Steyaert et al. 2023). To make an informed decision, scientists employ DL models for pathway analysis to link the obtained data at various genomics, transcriptomics, and proteomics levels to the biological functionality that causes the disease (Slobodyanyuk et al. 2024). Uncovering the key biomarkers and pathways is of utmost importance in drug design and efficacy assessments.

As mentioned before, the altered expression level of a protein cannot necessarily provide any insight into the likelihood of disease manifestation and therapeutic response. Indeed, the activation level of a protein (e.g., phosphorylation) is the determinant factor influencing the biological functionality of a cell (Veeriah et al. 2014; Kaufman et al. 2023). Determining the activation status of proteins in the context of cancer demands a large sample volume. This can be a limiting factor in the experimental approaches because of the scarcity of patient samples and the allowed volume that can be taken in certain cancer types (Hou et al. 2021). However, the ML-based analysis of phosphoproteins using online resources and algorithms such as PhophoSitePlus, Random Forest and SVM, NetPhos, KSTAR, and KinasePhos has profoundly accelerated the biomarker discovery and prediction of therapeutic outcomes in cancer patients by extracting more information from a small amount of sample (Huang et al. 2021; Crowl et al. 2022; Wang et al. 2022a, b).

Apart from biomarker discovery, the de novo design of cancer drugs has been markedly impacted by computational advancements, allowing the production of molecules with higher binding affinity to target biomarkers. *Convergent motifs for binding sites (COMBS)* is a newly introduced method for designing small molecules with high affinity and specificity to the target proteins. The precision of this method at the atomic level makes it possible to predict and modulate the interaction of amino acids and their chemical groups on the small molecules or ligands with the binding pocket of target proteins. The application of this method combined with Rosetta software for assembling protein backbone substantially shortens the screening procedure and identifying the "hit," which is the most suitable small molecule with therapeutic potential for further processing (Polizzi and DeGrado 2020; Lu et al. 2023).

5.1 ML-Based Protein Language Models (PLMs) for Therapeutic Drug Design

PLMs have emerged as potential tools to analyze the amino acid sequence and predict the interaction between biomarkers/neoantigens with antibodies (Bepler and Berger 2021). This capability largely depends on the quality and size of the data used for training and the depth of our knowledge about the proteins' functionality in a physiological setting. Due to continued technological advancements, the proteins' known functionality, especially those obtained from in vitro or non-humanized animal models, needs reassessment to ensure the data fed into the model is current.

PLMs have already transformed the small molecules' design pipeline and their clinical applications. However, the potential of PLMs for leveraging antibody development is under adaptation. The models can enormously impact the safety and efficacy of therapeutic antibodies by circumventing the possibility of introducing immunogenic epitopes in the structure of antibodies that are routinely developed by traditional methods, structural simplification (e.g., scFv fragments, nanobodies), and predicting the functionality, which per se reduces the need for extensive animal studies and associated costs (Kim et al. 2023). To address this, some models have been developed to leverage antibody specificity similar to the *antibody affinity maturation* process that naturally occurs in B cells following exposure to antigens. Affinity maturation results from somatic hypermutation within the antibody paratope containing three complementary determining regions (CDR1–3) and the selection of antibodies with more specificity toward an antigen. This process can be simulated by language models such as long short-term memory network (LSTM) (Saka et al. 2021), immunoglobulin language model (IgLM) (Shuai et al. 2023), H3OPT (Chen et al. 2024), IgT5, and IgBert (Kenlay et al. 2024). These models promote the specificity of the CDR3—the main binding site of the antibodies paratope with the highest polymorphism—for cancer biomarkers or pathogenic antigens. The PLM-based methods like NeoDisc, NeoPredPipe, and DeepHLAPan and AlphaFold (Schenck et al. 2019; Wu et al. 2019; Yang et al. 2023a, b; Huber et al. 2024) are taking the spotlight to depict the protein landscape and the root cause of defects in cellular machinery. These models can facilitate the discovery of neoantigens for personalizing drug design, refining T cell therapy, and assisting healthcare providers in selecting the best combinatorial treatment based on the patient's cancer features.

5.2 Natural Language Processing Methods (NLM)

In recent years, NLMs have been utilized to leverage the human-computer interface in a more user-friendly manner. NLM enables the conversion of text and voice into amino acid sequences and the design of de novo proteins. NLMs, which have been adopted by several companies and startups such as Generate:Biomedicines, EvolutionaryScale, 310AI, and Profluent have enormous potential for the customization of proteins with desired functionality for therapeutic purposes. ProtGPT2 is one of the recently released models for designing proteins with known structures and also those available in dark proteome with unknown structures and functions (Ferruz et al. 2022). The recent studies using omics data indicated some missing genes (e.g., noncanonical ORFs) with the potential to generate peptides and mini-proteins that are yet to be characterized. It has been experimentally shown that some of these peptides cause MTC either directly by affecting cell survival or indirectly by regulating gene expression in cells. Hence, they can be a potential target for therapeutic drug design (Prensner et al. 2021). This is where the unsupervised training of the language models on billions of parameters available in datasets provides ample opportunities to detect new proteins and generate artificial proteins and peptides. For instance, unnatural amino acids, which are not naturally encoded in humans but can be made artificially through modification of canonical amino acids, can be incorporated into the sequence to purposefully shape the structural stability and pharmacological features of the peptides or proteins (Zhang et al. 2022; Majekodunmi et al. 2024). Predicting incorporation site and product properties by computational methods helps shortcut the laborious experimental validation.

6 Conclusion

This chapter provided an overview of technological advances and the promise of integrating these technologies and experimental tools with AI-based computational models to accelerate cancer biomarker discovery. Among omics-based methods, the quantitative and structural study of proteins is in the spotlight due to their pivotal role in cell biological functionality. Growing evidence highlights the fact that the expression level of a receptor and its binding to a therapeutic ligand does not guarantee the expected therapeutic outcome. The technological advances have shed light on the fact that the activation of receptors and key signaling proteins through phosphorylation or cleavage is a determinant factor in the MTC. The information obtained from the activation state of proteins and their proximity to coreceptors and ligands, which form a signaling hub in the cell membrane, is a valuable predictive parameter for the survival rate of cancer patients after treatment. In addition to the known proteins, the discovery of peptides or mini-proteins expressed by noncanonical ORFs has sparked strong interest in investigating the contribution of these peptides in cancer development (Fox et al. 2023; Posner et al. 2023). In line with progress in our understanding of molecular and intercellular events in cancer development, several language models have been introduced to facilitate data analysis and distill and extract the most relevant information from large datasets that interconnect biological attributes with the transcriptomics and proteomics profile even those available in dark proteome. Such an interdisciplinary approach has already proven beneficial in identifying cancer neoantigens for developing therapeutic antibodies, and more importantly, the underlying mechanistic defect leading to immune modulation and the generation of neoantigens. These models can be tailored for specific diagnostic and therapeutic purposes from engineering antibody fragments to repurposing and refining approved therapeutic drugs as the disease-specific proteome pattern becomes clearer.

Conflict of Interest The authors declare no conflict of interest.

References

Akhoundova D, Rubin MA (2022) Clinical application of advanced multi-omics tumor profiling: shaping precision oncology of the future. Cancer Cell 40:920–938

Auclin E, Zaanan A, Vernerey D, Douard R, Gallois C, Laurent-Puig P, Bonnetain F, Taieb J (2017) Subgroups and prognostication in stage III colon cancer: future perspectives for adjuvant therapy. Ann Oncol 28:958–968

Azizian S, Khatami F, Modaresifar K, Mosaffa N, Peirovi H, Tayebi L, Bahrami S, Redl H, Niknejad H (2018) Immunological compatibility status of placenta-derived stem cells is mediated by scaffold 3D structure. Artif Cells Nanomed Biotechnol 46:876–884

Bagchi S, Fredriksson R, Wallén-Mackenzie Å (2015) In situ proximity ligation assay (PLA). Methods Mol Biol 1318:149–159

Baronaite U, Cachat E (2024) Preparation of chromobodies for the detection of cell surface epitopes. Methods Mol Biol 2774:303–314

Bartolome J, Molto C, Benitez-Fuentes JD, Fernandez-Hinojal G, Manzano A, Perez-Segura P, Mittal A, Tamimi F, Amir E, Ocana A (2023) Prognostic value of human leukocyte antigen G expression in solid tumors: a systematic review and meta-analysis. Front Immunol 14:1165813

Bepler T, Berger B (2021) Learning the protein language: evolution, structure, and function. Cell Syst 12:654–669

Bhalla N, Jolly P, Formisano N, Estrela P (2016) Introduction to biosensors. Essays Biochem 60:1–8

Boisvert FM, Ahmad Y, Gierliński M, Charrière F, Lamont D, Scott M, Barton G, Lamond AI (2012) A quantitative spatial proteomics analysis of proteome turnover in human cells. Mol Cell Proteomics 11:011429

Bożyk A, Krawczyk P, Reszka K, Krukowska K, Kolak A, Mańdziuk S, Wojas-Krawczyk K, Ramlau R, Milanowski J (2022) Correlation between KRAS, NRAS and BRAF mutations and tumor localizations in patients with primary and metastatic colorectal cancer. Arch Med Sci 18: 1221–1230

Brück O, Blom S, Dufva O, Turkki R, Chheda H, Ribeiro A, Kovanen P, Aittokallio T, Koskenvesa P, Kallioniemi O, Porkka K (2018) Immune cell contexture in the bone marrow tumor microenvironment impacts therapy response in CML. Leukemia 32:1643–1656

Calcinotto A, Brevi A, Chesi M, Ferrarese R, Garcia Perez L, Grioni M, Kumar S, Garbitt VM, Sharik ME, Henderson KJ, Tonon G (2018) Microbiota-driven interleukin-17-producing cells and eosinophils synergize to accelerate multiple myeloma progression. Nat Commun 9:4832

Camorani S, Caliendo A, Morrone E, Agnello L, Martini M, Cantile M, Cerrone M, Zannetti A, La Deda M, Fedele M, Ricciardi L (2024) Bispecific aptamer-decorated and light-triggered nanoparticles targeting tumor and stromal cells in breast cancer derived organoids: implications for precision phototherapies. J Exp Clin Cancer Res 43:92

Chen H, Fan X, Zhu S, Pei Y, Zhang X, Zhang X, Liu L, Qian F, Tian B (2024) Accurate prediction of CDR-H3 loop structures of antibodies with deep learning. elife 12

Crowl S, Jordan BT, Ahmed H, Ma CX, Naegle KM (2022) KSTAR: An algorithm to predict patient-specific kinase activities from phosphoproteomic data. Nat Commun 13:4283

Cucchi DG, Groen RW, Janssen JJ, Cloos J (2020) Ex vivo cultures and drug testing of primary acute myeloid leukemia samples: current techniques and implications for experimental design and outcome. Drug Resist Updat 53:100730

Dongre A, Weinberg RA (2019) New insights into the mechanisms of epithelial-mesenchymal transition and implications for cancer. Nat Rev Mol Cell Biol 20:69–84

Doroshow DB, Bhalla S, Beasley MB, Sholl LM, Kerr KM, Gnjatic S, Wistuba II, Rimm DL, Tsao MS, Hirsch FR (2021) PD-L1 as a biomarker of response to immune-checkpoint inhibitors. Nat Rev Clin Oncol 18:345–362

Duffy MJ (2001) Clinical uses of tumor markers: a critical review. Crit Rev Clin Lab Sci 38:225–262

Ferruz N, Schmidt S, Hocker B (2022) ProtGPT2 is a deep unsupervised language model for protein design. Nat Commun 13:4348

Fox BA, Urba WJ, Jensen SM, Page DB, Curti BD, Sanborn RE, Leidner RS (2023) Cancer's dark matter: lighting the abyss unveils universe of new therapies. Clin Cancer Res 29:2173–2175

Gambella A, Scabini S, Zoppoli G, De Silvestri A, Pigozzi S, Paudice M, Campora M, Fiocca R, Grillo F, Mastracci L (2022) HLA-G as a prognostic marker in stage II/III colorectal cancer: not quite there yet. Histochem Cell Biol 158:535–543

Garcia-Nafria J, Tate CG (2020) Cryo-electron microscopy: moving beyond X-ray crystal structures for drug receptors and drug development. Annu Rev Pharmacol Toxicol 60:51–71

Girault I, Adam J, Shen S, Roy S, Brard C, Faouzi S, Routier E, Lupu J, Warren S, Sorg K, Ong S (2022) A PD-1/PD-L1 proximity assay as a theranostic marker for PD-1 blockade in patients with metastatic melanoma. Clin Cancer Res 28:518–525

Goltsev Y, Samusik N, Kennedy-Darling J, Bhate S, Hale M, Vazquez G, Black S, Nolan GP (2018) Deep profiling of mouse splenic architecture with CODEX multiplexed imaging. Cell 174:968–981

Gou H, Zeng R, Lau HCH, Yu J (2024) Gut microbial metabolites: shaping future diagnosis and treatment against gastrointestinal cancer. Pharmacol Res 208:107373

Halicki P, Cieśluk K, Piszcz J (2024) Metabolic profile analysis in hematological malignancies. Acta Haematol Pol 55:22–33

Hassenrück F, Farina-Morillas M, Neumann L, Landini F, Blakemore SJ, Rabipour M, Alvarez-Idaboy JR, Pallasch CP, Hallek M, Rebollido-Rios R, Krause G (2023) Functional impact and molecular binding modes of drugs that target the PI3K isoform p110delta. Commun Biol 6:603

Henry NL, Hayes DF (2012) Cancer biomarkers. Mol Oncol 6:140–146

Hickey JW, Becker WR, Nevins SA, Horning A, Perez AE, Zhu C, Zhu B, Wei B, Chiu R, Chen DC, Cotter DL (2023) Organization of the human intestine at single-cell resolution. Nature 619: 572–584

Hirota S, Isozaki K, Moriyama Y, Hashimoto K, Nishida T, Ishiguro S, Kawano K, Hanada M, Kurata A, Takeda M, Muhammad Tunio G (1998) Gain-of-function mutations of c-kit in human gastrointestinal stromal tumors. Science 279:577–580

Hoellenriegel J, Zboralski D, Maasch C, Rosin NY, Wierda WG, Keating MJ, Kruschinski A, Burger JA (2014) The spiegelmer NOX-A12, a novel CXCL12 inhibitor, interferes with chronic lymphocytic leukemia cell motility and causes chemosensitization. Blood 123:1032–1039

Hohtari H, Brück O, Blom S, Turkki R, Sinisalo M, Kovanen PE, Kallioniemi O, Pellinen T, Porkka K, Mustjoki S (2019) Immune cell constitution in bone marrow microenvironment predicts outcome in adult ALL. Leukemia 33:1570–1582

Hou J, Li X, Xie KP (2021) Coupled liquid biopsy and bioinformatics for pancreatic cancer early detection and precision prognostication. Mol Cancer 20:34

Huang KL, Scott AD, Zhou DC, Wang LB, Weerasinghe A, Elmas A, Liu R, Wu Y, Wendl MC, Wyczalkowski MA, Baral J (2021) Spatially interacting phosphorylation sites and mutations in cancer. Nat Commun 12:2313

Huber F, Arnaud M, Stevenson BJ, Michaux J, Benedetti F, Thevenet J, Bobisse S, Chiffelle J, Gehert T, Müller M, Pak H (2024) A comprehensive proteogenomic pipeline for neoantigen discovery to advance personalized cancer immunotherapy. Nat Biotechnol:1–13

Hui E, Cheung J, Zhu J, Su X, Taylor MJ, Wallweber HA, Sasmal DK, Huang J, Kim JM, Mellman I, Vale RD (2017) T cell costimulatory receptor CD28 is a primary target for PD-1-mediated inhibition. Science 355:1428–1433

Josefsdottir KS, Baldridge MT, Kadmon CS, King KY (2017) Antibiotics impair murine hematopoiesis by depleting the intestinal microbiota. Blood 129:729–739

Jurisicova A, Casper RF, MacLusky NJ, Mills GB, Librach CL (1996) HLA-G expression during preimplantation human embryo development. Proc Natl Acad Sci USA 93:161–165

Katagiri S, Chi S, Minami Y, Fukushima K, Shibayama H, Hosono N, Yamauchi T, Morishita T, Kondo T, Yanada M, Yamamoto K (2022) Mutated KIT tyrosine kinase as a novel molecular target in acute myeloid leukemia. Int J Mol Sci 23

Kaufman B, Abramov O, Ievko A, Apple D, Shlapobersky M, Allon I, Greenshpan Y, Bhattachrya B, Cohen O, Charkovsky T, Gayster A (2023) Functional binding of PD1 ligands predicts response to anti-PD1 treatment in patients with cancer. Sci Adv 9:eadg2809

Kenlay H, Dreyer FA, Kovaltsuk A, Miketa D, Pires D, Deane CM (2024) Large scale paired antibody language models. PLoS Comput Biol 20:e1012646

Kim J, McFee M, Fang Q, Abdin O, Kim PM (2023) Computational and artificial intelligence-based methods for antibody development. Trends Pharmacol Sci 44:175–189

Koziol A, Pupek M (2022) Application of metabolomics in childhood leukemia diagnostics. Arch Immunol Ther Exp 70:28

Krimmer SG, Bertoletti N, Suzuki Y, Katic L, Mohanty J, Shu S, Lee S, Lax I, Mi W, Schlessinger J (2023) Cryo-EM analyses of KIT and oncogenic mutants reveal structural oncogenic plasticity and a target for therapeutic intervention. Proc Natl Acad Sci USA 120:e2300054120

Kucukkose E, Peters NA, Ubink I, van Keulen VAM, Daghighian R, Verheem A, Laoukili J, Kranenburg O (2022) KIT promotes tumor stroma formation and counteracts tumor-suppressive TGFbeta signaling in colorectal cancer. Cell Death Dis 13:617

Lewis SM, Williams A, Eisenbarth SC (2019) Structure and function of the immune system in the spleen. Sci Immunol 4

Li C, Sun YD, Yu GY, Cui JR, Lou Z, Zhang H, Huang Y, Bai CG, Deng LL, Liu P, Zheng K (2020) Integrated omics of metastatic colorectal cancer. Cancer Cell 38:734–747

Li D, Zhao J, Ma J, Yang H, Zhang X, Cao Y, Liu P (2022) GMT8 aptamer conjugated PEGylated Ag@Au core-shell nanoparticles as a novel radiosensitizer for targeted radiotherapy of glioma. Colloids Surf B Biointerfaces 211:112330

Li Y, Zhang B, Jiang L, Cheng T, Cheng H, Qian P (2024) Gut microbiota plays pivotal roles in benign and malignant hematopoiesis. Blood Sci 6:e00200

Lillemeier BF, Pfeiffer JR, Surviladze Z, Wilson BS, Davis MM (2006) Plasma membrane-associated proteins are clustered into islands attached to the cytoskeleton. Proc Natl Acad Sci USA 103:18992–18997

Lin A, Yan WH (2019) Intercellular transfer of HLA-G: its potential in cancer immunology. Clin Trans Immunol 8:e1077

Liu H, Hong G, Luo Z, Chen J, Chang J, Gong M, He H, Yang J, Yuan X, Li L, Mu X (2019) Atomic-precision gold clusters for NIR-II imaging. Adv Mater 31:e1901015

Liu Z, Li JP, Chen M, Wu M, Shi Y, Li W, Teijaro JR, Wu P (2020) Detecting tumor antigen-specific t cells via interaction-dependent fucosyl-biotinylation. Cell 183:1117–1133

Liu X, Zhou Q, Hart JR, Xu Y, Yang S, Yang D, Vogt PK, Wang MW (2022) Cryo-EM structures of cancer-specific helical and kinase domain mutations of PI3Kalpha. Proc Natl Acad Sci USA 119:e2215621119

Liu J, Li J, Luo F, Wu S, Li B, Liu K (2023) The predictive value of CD3+/CD8+ lymphocyte infiltration and PD-L1 expression in colorectal cancer. Curr Oncol 30:9647–9659

Liu X, Zhang H, Shi G, Zheng X, Chang J, Lin Q, Tian Z, Yang H (2024) The impact of gut microbial signals on hematopoietic stem cells and the bone marrow microenvironment. Front Immunol 15:1338178

Lu L, Gou X, Tan SK, Mann SI, Yang H, Zhong X, Gazgalis D, Valdiviezo J, Jo H, Wu Y, Diolaiti ME, Ashworth A, Polizzi NF, DeGrado WF (2023) De novo design of drug-binding proteins with predictable binding energy and specificity. bioRxiv

Ludwig JA, Weinstein JN (2005) Biomarkers in cancer staging, prognosis and treatment selection. Nat Rev Cancer 5:845–856

Lyu N, Hassanzadeh-Barforoushi A, Rey Gomez LM, Zhang W, Wang Y (2024) SERS biosensors for liquid biopsy towards cancer diagnosis by detection of various circulating biomarkers: current progress and perspectives. Nano Converg 11:22

Majekodunmi T, Britton D, Montclare JK (2024) Engineered proteins and materials utilizing residue-specific noncanonical amino acid incorporation. Chem Rev 124:9113–9135

Mann M, Kumar C, Zeng WF, Strauss MT (2021) Artificial intelligence for proteomics and biomarker discovery. Cell Syst 12:759–770

Marchetti L, Porciani D, Mitola S, Giacomelli C (2022) Editorial: molecular insights into ligand-receptor interactions on the cell surface. Front Mol Biosci 9:921677

Maryam S, Krukiewicz K, Haq IU, Khan AA, Yahya G, Cavalu S (2023) Interleukins (Cytokines) as biomarkers in colorectal cancer: progression, detection, and monitoring. J Clin Med 12

Mendez-Ferrer S, Bonnet D, Steensma DP, Hasserjian RP, Ghobrial IM, Gribben JG, Andreeff M, Krause DS (2020) Bone marrow niches in haematological malignancies. Nat Rev Cancer 20: 285–298

Mi H, Sivagnanam S, Ho WJ, Zhang S, Bergman D, Deshpande A, Baras AS, Jaffee EM, Coussens LM, Fertig EJ, Popel AS (2024) Computational methods and biomarker discovery strategies for spatial proteomics: a review in immuno-oncology. Brief Bioinform 25

Moeglin E, Desplancq D, Stoessel A, Massute C, Ranniger J, AG ME, Zeder-Lutz G, Oulad-Abdelghani M, Chiper M, Lafaye P, Di Ventura B, Didier P, Poterszman A, Weiss E (2021) A novel nanobody precisely visualizes phosphorylated histone H2AX in living cancer cells under drug-induced replication stress. Cancers (Basel) 13

Muhammad M, Shao CS, Bashir MA, Yu X, Wu Y, Zhan J, Zhang L, Huang Q (2024) Application of aptamer-SERS nanotags for unveiling the PD-l1 immunomarker progression correlated to the cell metabolic bioprocess. Anal Chem 96:6236–6244

Nagana Gowda GA, Raftery D (2021) NMR-based metabolomics. Adv Exp Med Biol 1280:19–37

Nguyen CT, Nguyen JT, Rutledge S, Zhang J, Wang C, Walker GC (2010) Detection of chronic lymphocytic leukemia cell surface markers using surface enhanced Raman scattering gold nanoparticles. Cancer Lett 292:91–97

Nimjee SM, White RR, Becker RC, Sullenger BA (2017) Aptamers as therapeutics. Annu Rev Pharmacol Toxicol 57:61–79

Paerregaard SI, Wulff L, Schussek S, Niss K, Morbe U, Jendholm J, Wendland K, Andrusaite AT, Brulois KF, Nibbs RJB, Sitnik K, Mowat AM, Butcher EC, Brunak S, Agace WW (2023) The small and large intestine contain related mesenchymal subsets that derive from embryonic Gli1 (+) precursors. Nat Commun 14:2307

Passaro D, Garcia-Albornoz M, Diana G, Chakravarty P, Ariza-McNaughton L, Batsivari A, Borras-Eroles C, Abarrategi A, Waclawiczek A, Ombrato L, Malanchi I, Gribben J, Bonnet D (2021) Integrated OMICs unveil the bone-marrow microenvironment in human leukemia. Cell Rep 35:109119

Passaro A, Al Bakir M, Hamilton EG, Diehn M, Andre F, Roy-Chowdhuri S, Mountzios G, Wistuba II, Swanton C, Peters S (2024) Cancer biomarkers: emerging trends and clinical implications for personalized treatment. Cell 187:1617–1635

Perez-Gonzalez A, Bevant K, Blanpain C (2023) Cancer cell plasticity during tumor progression, metastasis and response to therapy. Nat Cancer 4:1063–1082

Plaks V, Kong N, Werb Z (2015) The cancer stem cell niche: how essential is the niche in regulating stemness of tumor cells? Cell Stem Cell 16:225–238

Polizzi NF, DeGrado WF (2020) A defined structural unit enables de novo design of small-molecule-binding proteins. Science 369:1227–1233

Posner Z, Yannuzzi I, Prensner JR (2023) Shining a light on the dark proteome: non-canonical open reading frames and their encoded miniproteins as a new frontier in cancer biology. Protein Sci 32:e4708

Prensner JR, Enache OM, Luria V, Krug K, Clauser KR, Dempster JM, Karger A, Wang L, Stumbraite K, Wang VM, Botta G, Lyons NJ, Goodale A, Kalani Z, Fritchman B, Brown A, Alan D, Green T, Yang X, Jaffe JD, Roth JA, Piccioni F, Kirschner MW, Ji Z, Root DE, Golub

TR (2021) Noncanonical open reading frames encode functional proteins essential for cancer cell survival. Nat Biotechnol 39:697–704

Qiu Y, Cai G, Su M, Chen T, Zheng X, Xu Y, Ni Y, Zhao A, Xu LX, Cai S, Jia W (2009) Serum metabolite profiling of human colorectal cancer using GC-TOFMS and UPLC-QTOFMS. J Proteome Res 8:4844–4850

Qiu S, Zhao Z, Wu M, Xue Q, Yang Y, Ouyang S, Li W, Zhong L, Wang W, Yang R, Wu P, Li JP (2022) Use of intercellular proximity labeling to quantify and decipher cell-cell interactions directed by diversified molecular pairs. Sci Adv 8:eadd2337

Rizzo R, Audrito V, Vacca P, Rossi D, Brusa D, Stignani M, Bortolotti D, D'Arena G, Coscia M, Laurenti L, Forconi F, Gaidano G, Mingari MC, Moretta L, Malavasi F, Deaglio S (2014) HLA-G is a component of the chronic lymphocytic leukemia escape repertoire to generate immune suppression: impact of the HLA-G 14 base pair (rs66554220) polymorphism. Haematologica 99:888–896

Saka K, Kakuzaki T, Metsugi S, Kashiwagi D, Yoshida K, Wada M, Tsunoda H, Teramoto R (2021) Antibody design using LSTM based deep generative model from phage display library for affinity maturation. Sci Rep 11:5852

Salem DP, Bortolin LT, Gusenleitner D, Grosha J, Zabroski IO, Biette KM, Banerjee S, Sedlak CR, Byrne DM, Hamzeh BF, King MS, Cuoco LT, Santos-Heiman T, Barcaskey GN, Yang KS, Duff PA, Winn-Deen ES, Guettouche T, Mattoon DR, Huang EK, Schekman RW, Couvillon AD, Sedlak JC (2024) Colocalization of cancer-associated biomarkers on single extracellular vesicles for early detection of cancer. J Mol Diagn 26:1109

Sánchez-Magraner L, Gumuzio J, Miles J, Quimi N, Martínez del Prado P, Abad-Villar MT, Pikabea F, Ortega L, Etxezarraga C, Martín-Algarra S, Lozano MD (2023) Functional engagement of the PD-1/PD-L1 complex but not PD-L1 expression is highly predictive of patient response to immunotherapy in non-small-cell lung cancer. J Clin Oncol 41:2561–2570

Sarhadi VK, Armengol G (2022) Molecular biomarkers in cancer. Biomol Ther 12

Schenck RO, Lakatos E, Gatenbee C, Graham TA, Anderson ARA (2019) NeoPredPipe: high-throughput neoantigen prediction and recognition potential pipeline. BMC Bioinformatics 20: 264

Schluter J, Peled JU, Taylor BP, Markey KA, Smith M, Taur Y, Niehus R, Staffas A, Dai A, Fontana E, Amoretti LA, Wright RJ, Morjaria S, Fenelus M, Pessin MS, Chao NJ, Lew M, Bohannon L, Bush A, Sung AD, Hohl TM, Perales MA, van den Brink MRM, Xavier JB (2020) The gut microbiota is associated with immune cell dynamics in humans. Nature 588:303–307

Sekar RB, Periasamy A (2003) Fluorescence resonance energy transfer (FRET) microscopy imaging of live cell protein localizations. J Cell Biol 160:629–633

Shuai RW, Ruffolo JA, Gray JJ (2023) IgLM: infilling language modeling for antibody sequence design. Cell Syst 14:979–989

Slobodyanyuk M, Bahcheli AT, Klein ZP, Bayati M, Strug LJ, Reimand J (2024) Directional integration and pathway enrichment analysis for multi-omics data. Nat Commun 15:5690

Song G, Wang L, Tang J, Li H, Pang S, Li Y, Liu L, Hu J (2023) Circulating metabolites as potential biomarkers for the early detection and prognosis surveillance of gastrointestinal cancers. Metabolomics 19:36

Steyaert S, Pizurica M, Nagaraj D, Khandelwal P, Hernandez-Boussard T, Gentles AJ, Gevaert O (2023) Multimodal data fusion for cancer biomarker discovery with deep learning. Nat Mach Intell 5:351–362

Sugiyama T, Kohara H, Noda M, Nagasawa T (2006) Maintenance of the hematopoietic stem cell pool by CXCL12-CXCR4 chemokine signaling in bone marrow stromal cell niches. Immunity 25:977–988

Ternes D, Tsenkova M, Pozdeev VI, Meyers M, Koncina E, Atatri S, Schmitz M, Karta J, Schmoetten M, Heinken A, Rodriguez F, Delbrouck C, Gaigneaux A, Ginolhac A, TTD N, Grandmougin L, Frachet-Bour A, Martin-Gallausiaux C, Pacheco M, Neuberger-Castillo L, Miranda P, Zuegel N, Ferrand JY, Gantenbein M, Sauter T, Slade DJ, Thiele I, Meiser J, Haan S,

Wilmes P, Letellier E (2022) The gut microbial metabolite formate exacerbates colorectal cancer progression. Nat Metab 4:458–475

Thorne CA, Chen IW, Sanman LE, Cobb MH, Wu LF, Altschuler SJ (2018) Enteroid monolayers reveal an autonomous WNT and BMP circuit controlling intestinal epithelial growth and organization. Dev Cell 44:624–633

Traenkle B, Rothbauer U (2017) Under the microscope: single-domain antibodies for live-cell imaging and super-resolution microscopy. Front Immunol 8:1030

Tsagiopoulou M, Rashmi S, Aguilar-Fernandez S, Nieto J, Gut IG (2024) Multi-organ single-cell transcriptomics of immune cells uncovered organ-specific gene expression and functions. Sci Data 11:316

Ueno M, Sugiyama H, Li F, Nishimura T, Arakawa H, Chen X, Cheng X, Takeuchi S, Takeshita Y, Takamura T, Miyagi S, Toyama T, Soga T, Masuo Y, Kato Y, Nakamura H, Tsujiguchi H, Hara A, Tajima A, Noguchi-Shinohara M, Ono K, Kurayoshi K, Kobayashi M, Tadokoro Y, Kasahara A, Shoulkamy MI, Maeda K, Ogoshi T, Hirao A (2024) A supramolecular biosensor for rapid and high-throughput quantification of a disease-associated niacin metabolite. Anal Chem 96:14499–14507

Ulivi P, Indraccolo S (2022) Liquid biopsies in cancer diagnosis, monitoring and prognosis. Biomedicines 10:2748

Veeriah S, Leboucher P, de Naurois J, Jethwa N, Nye E, Bunting T, Stone R, Stamp G, Calleja V, Jeffrey SS, Parker PJ, Larijani B (2014) High-throughput time-resolved FRET reveals Akt/PKB activation as a poor prognostic marker in breast cancer. Cancer Res 74:4983–4995

Wang R, Yang X, Liu J, Zhong F, Zhang C, Chen Y, Sun T, Ji C, Ma D (2022a) Gut microbiota regulates acute myeloid leukaemia via alteration of intestinal barrier function mediated by butyrate. Nat Commun 13:2522

Wang X, Zhang Z, Zhang C, Meng X, Shi X, Qu P (2022b) TransPhos: a deep-learning model for general phosphorylation site prediction based on transformer-encoder architecture. Int J Mol Sci 23

Wolf P, Gavins G, Beck-Sickinger AG, Seitz O (2021) Strategies for site-specific labeling of receptor proteins on the surfaces of living cells by using genetically encoded peptide tags. Chembiochem 22:1717–1732

Wu J, Wang W, Zhang J, Zhou B, Zhao W, Su Z, Gu X, Wu J, Zhou Z, Chen S (2019) DeepHLApan: a deep learning approach for neoantigen prediction considering both HLA-peptide binding and immunogenicity. Front Immunol 10:2559

Xiong CC, Zhu SS, Yan DH, Yao YD, Zhang Z, Zhang GJ, Chen S (2023) Rapid and precise detection of cancers via label-free SERS and deep learning. Anal Bioanal Chem 415:3449–3462

Xu J, Kang Y, Zhong Y, Ye W, Sheng T, Wang Q, Zheng J, Yang Q, Yi P, Li Z (2023) Alteration of gut microbiome and correlated amino acid metabolism are associated with acute myelocytic leukemia carcinogenesis. Cancer Med 12:16431–16443

Yang G, Pan X, Feng W, Yao Q, Jiang F, Du F, Zhou X, Xie J, Yuan X (2023a) Engineering Au (44) nanoclusters for NIR-II luminescence imaging-guided photoactivatable cancer immunotherapy. ACS Nano 17:15605–15614

Yang Z, Zeng X, Zhao Y, Chen R (2023b) AlphaFold2 and its applications in the fields of biology and medicine. Signal Transduct Target Ther 8:115

Yang S, Wang R, Liu M, Lv Y, Fu H, Cao X, Dong G (2024) Dual-aptamer-decorated reduction-activated dimeric-prodrug nanoparticles for broad-spectrum treatment of leukemia. Biomed Pharmacother 180:117543

Zaimy MA, Jebali A, Bazrafshan B, Mehrtashfar S, Shabani S, Tavakoli A, Hekmatimoghaddam SH, Sarli A, Azizi H, Izadi P, Kazemi B, Shojaei A, Abdalaian A, Tavakkoly-Bazzaz J (2016) Coinhibition of overexpressed genes in acute myeloid leukemia subtype M2 by gold nanoparticles functionalized with five antisense oligonucleotides and one anti-CD33(+)/CD34 (+) aptamer. Cancer Gene Ther 23:315–320

Zhang Q, Yang M, Zhu Y, Mao C (2018) Metallic nanoclusters for cancer imaging and therapy. Curr Med Chem 25:1379–1396

Zhang H, Zheng Z, Dong L, Shi N, Yang Y, Chen H, Shen Y, Xia Q (2022) Rational incorporation of any unnatural amino acid into proteins by machine learning on existing experimental proofs. Comput Struct Biotechnol J 20:4930–4941

Zhang X, Tang Q, Sun J, Guo Y, Zhang S, Liang S, Dai P, Chen X (2023) Cellular-scale proximity labeling for recording cell spatial organization in mouse tissues. Sci Adv 9:eadg6388

Zheng Y, Xu R, Chen X, Lu Y, Zheng J, Lin Y, Lin P, Zhao X, Cui L (2024) Metabolic gatekeepers: harnessing tumor-derived metabolites to optimize T cell-based immunotherapy efficacy in the tumor microenvironment. Cell Death Dis 15:775

Multidisciplinary Approach in Cancer Management

Mohamed El-Kassas and Haytham Abdelkader

Abstract

The management of cancer patients is increasingly becoming a global concern, mostly due to the rapid change of cumulative evidence, the approvals of new medications, and updates in management guidelines. The implementation of the multidisciplinary approach has enabled clinicians to effectively address the increasing demands of cancer patients. One way to accomplish this is by utilizing multidisciplinary clinics, such as breast units, or by convening multidisciplinary tumor boards (MTBs), also referred to as multidisciplinary meetings.

In this chapter, we will explore the multidisciplinary team (MDT) approach from various aspects beginning form its history, implementations, advantages, and limitations.

MDT model in cancer care is defined as cooperation between different specialists aiming for improvement of treatment efficiency for cancer patients with much evidence available regarding its added value.

MDT is a comprehensive healthcare approach where medical and allied health experts engage in discussions about all pertinent treatment choices and jointly develop a personalized treatment plan for each patient. MDT approach can be applied successfully in many cancer types.

Keywords

Cancer care · Multidisciplinary team (MDT) · Multidisciplinary tumor boards (MTB)

M. El-Kassas (✉)
Endemic Medicine Department, Faculty of Medicine, Helwan University, Cairo, Egypt
e-mail: m_elkassas@hq.helwan.edu.eg

H. Abdelkader
Clinical Oncology Department, Faculty of Medicine, Helwan University, Cairo, Egypt

Interdisciplinary Cancer Research, https://doi.org/10.1007/16833_2024_378
Published online: 01 October 2024

Abbreviations

ALBI	Albumin-Bilirubin
BCLC	Barcelona clinic liver cancer
CI	Confidence interval
CRC	Colorectal cancer
CRM	Circumferential resection margin
CT	Computed tomography
GP	General practitioner
HCC	Hepatocellular carcinoma
HR	Hazard ratio
KPI	Key Performance Indicators
MDT	Multidisciplinary team
MDT-FIT	Multidisciplinary Team Feedback for Improving Team-working
MIBC	Muscle invasive bladder cancer
MTB	Molecular tumor board
MTBs	Multidisciplinary tumor boards
NAPRC	National Accredited Programme for Rectal Cancer
NCCCP	National Community Cancer Centers Program
NCCN	National Comprehensive Cancer Network
NGS	Next-generation sequencing
NHS	National Health Service
NSCLC	Non-small cell lung cancer
OS	Overall survival
OSTRiCh	Optimizing the Surgical Treatment of Rectal Cancer
PFS	Progression-free survival
PO	Precision oncology
QOL	Quality of life
RCC	Renal cell carcinoma
SWOG	Southwest Oncology Group
UK	United Kingdom
USA	United States of America

1 Introduction

The implication of a multidisciplinary team (MDT) in treating patients with malignant tumors helped the physicians a lot due to the rapid changes in evidence and recommendations in treatment guidelines, besides the approval of many new medications. All these factors mandate the application of the MDT model in cancer patient management (El Saghir et al. 2014).

MDT in patients with malignant tumors is defined as cooperation between specialists aiming to improve treatment efficiency for cancer patients (Taberna et al. 2020). It is a collaborative model where physicians and all other healthcare providers involved in patient management work together, discuss all the treatment guidelines, and create a plan for each patient according to the latest guidelines. Due to the wide range of specialties involved in cancer patient care, poor communication could be created. MDT represents an ideal model for providing patients with high-quality and updated treatment options based on multiple physicians' opinions and experiences (Silbermann et al. 2013).

MDT was first introduced more than twenty years ago to plan treatment options for patients and improve collaboration between specialists. Since then, the MDT approach has been introduced in many countries and has become recommended by many international treatment guidelines (Cancer Institute New South Wales 2016).

MDT core members include medical oncologists, surgeons, radiation oncologists, pathologists, radiologists, specialized nurses, and administrators. According to the type of cancer, other specialists such as hepatologists, pulmonologists, or others could collaborate on the treatment plan. MDT is usually held once weekly, and the treatment plan should be based on all the clinical data, histopathology, radiology, patient medical history, comorbidities, and patient views (Soukup et al. 2016).

MDT meetings are alternatively referred to as tumor boards, multidisciplinary cancer conferences, multidisciplinary case reviews, or multidisciplinary clinics in various healthcare systems. Different terms may denote the differences in the organizational structure, membership, approach, focus, and decision-making procedures of various gatherings (Fennell et al. 2010).

A recent concept of molecular tumor boards (MTB) was established due to the advances in molecular biology and its implication in treatment decisions. MTB comprises specialties focusing on molecular biology, such as specialists in histopathology, oncology, hematology, basic science, and genetic counseling. MTB could help physicians reach the optimum decision as the genetic profile, and the targetable genetic alterations can play an essential role in the patient's treatment plan (El Saghir et al. 2014).

Tumor boards have existed in the United States for five decades (Berman 1975). Nevertheless, their primary objective has been educating rather than enhancing patient care until recently. During the 1980s, there was a transition toward community-based cancer care in the United States. This shift led to the establishment of tumor boards, which promoted the exchange of information among participating physicians and favorably impacted the quality of care offered (Gross 1987). Over the past twenty years, the primary objective of tumor boards has shifted from education to healthcare provision. The United Kingdom has significantly transformed its cancer services in the past decade, primarily motivated by political and public demands. This was prompted by a series of reports published in the late 1990s, such as the Calman-Hine report (1995), which revealed significant disparities in the quality of care received by cancer patients. Several European countries and Australia promptly embraced the MDT paradigm for cancer care (Van Leeuwen et al. 2004; van Nes and van de Velde 2005).

2 Evolution of MDT

Using a multidisciplinary approach was a logical consequence of the expanding knowledge base and management alternatives. This can be exemplified by examining the progression of breast cancer treatment (Costa 2018). Halsted's groundbreaking proposition of mastectomy in the late 1800s resulted in the adoption of drastic surgery as the primary treatment for breast cancer for several decades. Patients were exclusively managed by surgeons and gynecologists. The pivotal moments in our strategies for treating breast cancer were the identification of hormonal receptors that distinguish hormone-dependent tumors from hormone-independent cancers, the implementation of radiotherapy, the adoption of combined conservative surgery with radiotherapy (Costa 2018; Veronesi et al. 1981), and adopting the "adjuvant chemotherapy" concept (Bonadonna et al. 1977). The ultimate outcome necessitated the recognition that surgeons and gynecologists alone were incapable of treating breast cancer patients.

Consequently, breast cancer has emerged as the primary exemplification of the indispensability and worth of MDTs (Costa 2018). The original core team, consisting of a surgeon, radiation oncologist, and medical oncologist, enlisted the expertise of a pathologist to determine the specific features of the patient's cancer. This includes determining if the disease is hormone-dependent or independent, the rate of growth, the grade of the disease, and whether it is HER2 positive or negative, among other factors. Upon recognizing the necessity of having a team of four specialists instead of a single one to provide the most appropriate treatment for the patient, it is feasible to expand the team to include other specialties like radiology, plastic surgery, and psychology, in addition to a dedicated nurse, resulting in a tumor board, or more accurately, an MDT. This team convenes once a week at a multidisciplinary meeting to deliberate on all new cases (Costa 2018).

3 The Role and Impact of MDT Cancer Care

Over the past years since the introduction of MDT, the literature has supported its application in cancer patient management to ensure commitment to international and national guidelines and improve patient outcomes (Croke and El-Sayed 2012).

3.1 Commitment to Treatment Guidelines

Standard treatment guidelines aid in determining the best treatment plan for each cancer patient, supported explicitly by high-quality evidence, with a commitment to standard guidelines that improve patient outcomes and survival (Kabat et al. 2015).

In the past years, diagnostic and therapeutic choices for malignant tumor patients have been notably developed. This necessitates the implementation of MDT for better collaboration between different specialties and commitment to standard-of-care guidelines (Jury et al. 2010).

3.2 Impact of MDT on Cancer Care Outcomes

The existing body of literature regarding the influence of MDTs on care and outcomes is far-reaching, yet it is characterized by uneven coverage and gaps in knowledge. Numerous studies are of limited size and susceptible to biased case selection. Taplin and his colleagues (Taplin et al. 2015) highlighted the potential for oncologists to gain insights from research on teams in other medical and non-medical fields. To explore this, they conducted a comprehensive evaluation of all published studies on cancer up until 2014. These findings indicated that implementing MDT led to enhanced care processes but did not necessarily result in higher survival rates. Kesson et al. (2012) conducted a comparative analysis to assess the influence of implementing MDTs in a Scottish Health Board located in Glasgow on the survival rates of patients with breast cancer in comparison to the survival rates in neighboring Health Boards that did not implement MDTs. An enhanced survival rate and decreased variability in treatment were observed in the area where MDTs were implemented, involving a total of 13,722 women undergoing treatment for breast cancer. While most studies confirm the importance of MDTs, Munro (2015) highlights the need for MDTs to maintain efficiency to justify the associated costs and staff time. Keeping these costs and time requirements minimal while achieving successful outcomes is crucial. The European Cancer Organization recently published articles on "essential requirements for quality cancer care." These articles emphasize that a multidisciplinary approach should be obligatory for specific types of tumors, such as rare tumors (Andritsch et al. 2017). However, for other types of cancer, such as colorectal cancer (CRC), the multidisciplinary approach may only have an impact on certain subsets of patients (Beets et al. 2017).

3.3 The Influence of Positive Clinical Trials on Extended Patient Outcomes

Southwest Oncology Group (SWOG) conducted an assessment of its trial outcomes on its 60th anniversary. The analysis recognized treatment trials in which the novel experimental medication resulted in a statistically significant overall survival benefit ($p < 0.05$). The newly approved treatments from these trials were presumed to have created new benchmarks for cancer care. The scientists calculated the number of years of life gained by the public from 23 successful treatment trials up until 2015 by applying the impact of the new treatments on the cancer population in the United States. A total of 12,361 patients were registered in the 23 successful studies conducted between 1965 and 2012. The analysis calculated that the application of the outcomes from these 23 trials across the entire population resulted in an estimated gain of 3.34 million life-years (95% CI, 2.39–4.15) by 2015. The ROI was \$125 per life-year gained, as reported by Unger et al. (2017).

3.4 Studies Showing No or Negative Impact of MDT

Survival data was only available from a single randomized controlled trial conducted by Murray et al. The experimental group of the trial utilized a two-step centralized diagnostic technique, which was then reviewed by a multidisciplinary team (MDT). In contrast, the control group followed a standard strategy without MDT review. The selected participants were patients with suspected lung cancer who were considered appropriate candidates for a computed tomography (CT) scan and tissue biopsy. The study revealed no statistically significant discrepancy in the quality of life (QOL) after a period of six weeks and the survival rate after a duration of two years between the intervention and control groups (Murray et al. 2003). Two more observational studies investigating the influence of MDT meetings on high-grade glioma (Back et al. 2007) and non-small cell lung cancer (Martin-Ucar et al. 2004) also discovered no statistically significant difference in survival rates between the MDT and control groups.

Stephens et al. conducted a study to assess the effect of lung cancer MDT meetings on decision-making quality. The study found that the net utility loss resulting from MDT discussions did not significantly differ, and overall, team discussions did not enhance decision-making quality (Stephens et al. 2006).

Overall, a more significant proportion of available data demonstrates a positive impact of cancer MDTs compared to those that did not find any advantages. Nevertheless, the majority of the studies had a subpar design. The studies frequently employed pre- and post-designs, regarded as insufficient evidence for establishing causal relationships due to numerous potential confounding factors. Our understanding of cancer and the range of diagnostic and therapeutic options constantly improves, increasing the likelihood of improved results in the future. Many of these studies employed historical controls, widely recognized for their propensity to introduce substantial biases that can lead to erroneous findings (Patkar et al. 2011). Patients usually feel more confident about their treatment plan when they know that different health professionals are discussing their case and not by a single physician whose decision may be influenced by many factors such as mood, career (risk taker or risk averse), personality (optimistic or pessimistic), financial considerations, and many other reasons that could influence single opinion decision, on the contrary second opinions and MDT meetings offer the benefits of multiple opinions and practically which increase the sense of safety for the patients and their families (NHS 2019).

In order to enhance the effectiveness of MDT, it is imperative to adequately prepare and dispatch cases to team members, allowing sufficient time for the search of supplementary material. Regular MDT meetings should prioritize collaboration rather than competition, with a leader who is acknowledged by the team for their knowledge, skill, and wisdom. Over time, it is expected that every individual should assume accountability for complying with the most recent requirements (NHS 2019).

3.5 Impact of Multidisciplinary Approach on Outcomes of Lung Cancer Patients

Lung cancer needs MDT due to the multiple treatment options employed in management, including surgery, chemotherapy, radiotherapy, immunotherapy, targeted therapies, and others such as palliative care and critical care. Sometimes, these treatment options can be combined or used as single treatment options. Various physician specialties are involved in managing patients with bronchogenic carcinoma, including cardiothoracic surgery, medical oncologists, radiotherapy specialists, radiodiagnosis specialists, pulmonology specialists, nuclear medicine specialists, pathology specialists, palliative care, and specialized nurses. Significantly, patients should be involved in decision-making (Fig. 1). Nowadays, lung cancer management worldwide is made by MDT, which has shown adherence to national and international guidelines and shortened the period between diagnosis and the start of therapy (Bilfinger et al. 2018).

The quality of care and survival in lung cancer patients was assessed in a study comparing patients managed in MDT versus patients managed outside MDT, where National Comprehensive Cancer Network NCCN guidelines (2021) were used as a standard of care. The findings demonstrated a significant enhancement in the median overall survival (36.9 versus 19.3 months; $p < 0.001$) and cancer-specific survival (48 versus 28.1 months; $p < 0.001$) for MDT cases in comparison to the control group. MDT discussions improved NCCN guidelines compliance

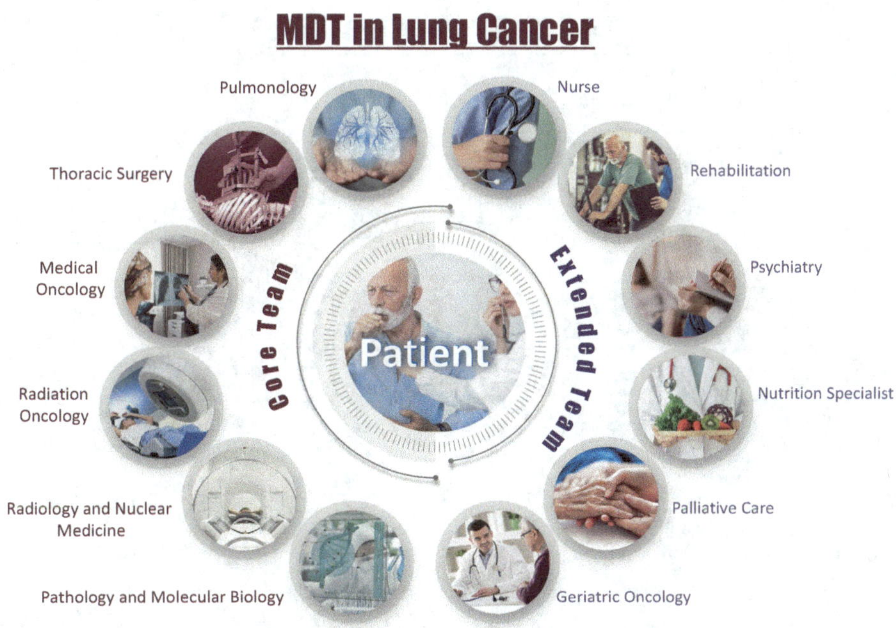

Fig. 1 MDT in lung cancer

from 80% to 94% ($p < 0.001$), and changes in treatment plans following MDT discussions were observed in 41% of cases. All these results showed improvement in survival, necessitating MDT's implication in lung cancer management (Gaudioso et al. 2021).

Another study demonstrated the enhancement in median overall survival in patients with stage III NSCLAC, providing evidence of improvement in NSCLC. The study revealed that patients who underwent treatment after multidisciplinary team (MDT) discussion had a median overall survival of 41.2 months, whereas patients treated without MDT discussion had a median overall survival of 25.7 months ($p = 0.018$). Furthermore, the report demonstrated that MDT had a noteworthy impact on predicting outcomes (Hung et al. 2020).

3.6 MDT Team Approach in Breast Cancer Care

The MDT meetings are usually held once weekly, and the team is composed of one physician from each of those specialties; surgical oncology, medical oncology, radiation oncology, histopathology, and radiodiagnosis beside trainee from those specialties, together with a specialist nurse (Fig. 2), all working together adhering to evidence-based guidelines (Brandão et al. 2021; Kesson et al. 2012).

The effect of MDT on breast cancer management was shown in a study that analyzed impaction of the MDT model on improving the recurrence and mortality

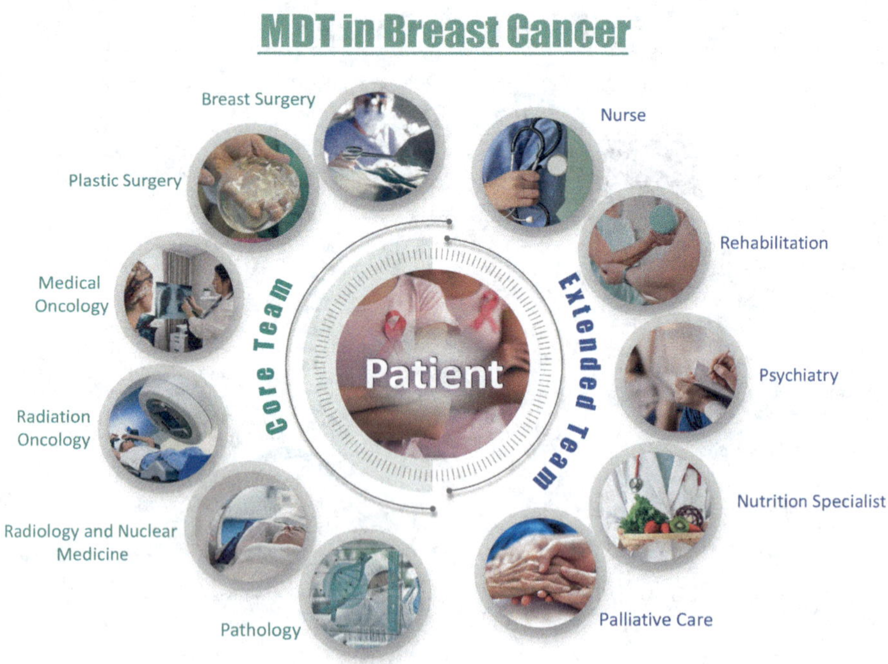

Fig. 2 MDT in breast cancer

in patients with breast cancer. The findings demonstrated a relative risk reduction in recurrence, as shown by a hazard ratio (HR) of 0.84 and a 95% confidence interval (CI) of 0.70–0.99. These data also suggest an impact on mortality. The mortality risk for breast cancer patients who experienced relapse was 8.48 times higher (95% CI, 7.53–9.54) compared to patients who did not have relapse (Tsai et al. 2020).

Also, in rare cases such as breast sarcoma, MDT management is indicated due to the disease rarity, high incidence of local recurrence, and poor prognosis (Duncan and Lautner 2018; Chugh 2021).

3.7 MDT Team Approach in Hepatocellular Carcinoma

Management of hepatocellular carcinoma (HCC) is complex as mortality is an accumulation of malignancy and deteriorated liver function, which mandated the MDT management to improve the outcome of treatment, tailoring the treatment according to the tumor burden and liver dysfunction and other comorbidities (Lhewa et al. 2020).

MDT is typically formed from medical oncology specialists, hepatology specialists, hepatobiliary and liver transplant surgery specialists, radiology specialists, intervention radiology specialists, nurses, and histopathologists. Added to those specialties, general practitioners and supportive care could benefit the MDT. All those specialties collaborate to plan the best therapeutic approach for each patient individually (Gish et al. 2012) (Fig. 3).

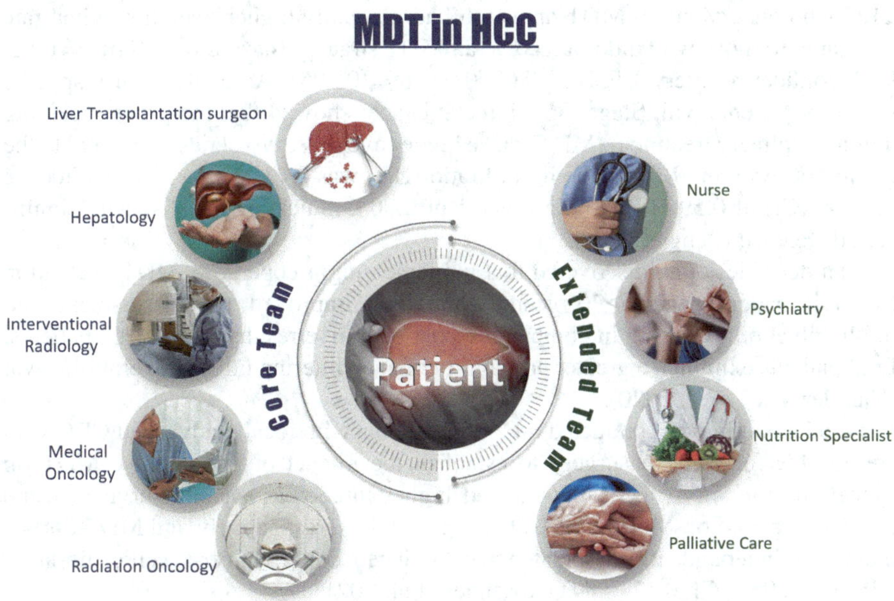

Fig. 3 MDT in HCC

MDT approach is highly recommended to ensure collaboration between different healthcare providers involved in management to improve outcomes (Yang and Heimbach 2020).

MDT management for HCC was associated with improvement in OS, which was proved in a study comparing patients with HCC who were treated in MDT versus patients treated outside MDT where the results showed improvement in 5 years' overall survival in MDT-managed patients versus non-MDT model (71.2% vs. 49.4%, $P < 0.001$), with an adjusted hazard ratio (HR) of 0.47 (95% confidence interval [CI]; 0.41–0.53). The improvement in survival was evident in all patients' subgroups but was remarkably seen in patients with poor liver functions, higher tumor stage, and patients with high alpha-fetoprotein (Sinn et al. 2019).

There are several explanations for improving the outcome of HCC treatment in MDTs, such as an alteration in the direction of care by changes made by imaging interventions, diagnosis revisions, and treatment recommendations (Zhang et al. 2013; Soares et al. 2014). Also, MDT helps shorten the time from diagnosis to treatment (Yopp et al. 2014).

3.8 The Effect of an MDT Approach on Outcomes of Patients with Colorectal Cancer (CRC)

Patients diagnosed with CRC who received treatment through an MDT had a higher overall survival rate compared to those who were treated using a non-MDT method. In a meta-analysis conducted by Peng et al., it was found that patients diagnosed with CRC who underwent an MDT approach had a notably higher overall survival rate compared to those who did not receive an MDT strategy (hazard ratio [HR] = 0.81; 95% confidence interval [CI] = 0.69–0.94; $p = 0.005$). An analysis of a specific subset of patients with Stage IV colorectal cancer showed that the group receiving multidisciplinary treatment (MDT) had a higher overall survival rate compared to the group not receiving MDT. The hazard ratio (HR) was 0.73, with a 95% confidence interval (CI) of 0.59–0.90, and a p-value of 0.004, indicating a statistically significant difference (Peng et al. 2021).

Van der Vlies et al. discovered that implementing preoperative MDT evaluation for frail patients aged ≥70 years with CRC improved risk assessment and pre-habilitation, resulting in comparable post-operative results to non-frail patients. Frail patients exhibited a greater probability of encountering inferior overall survival (Van der Vlies et al. 2020).

Another study was conducted on 2,663 patients with locally advanced CRC who are eligible for elective surgery to establish the impact of preoperative MDT on cancer-specific survival; results showed higher three-year specific survival in the MDT group vs. non-MDT group (80% versus 68%), respectively and MDT assessment was independently associated with reduced colon cancer-specific mortality (HR, 0.70; 95% CI, 0.57–0.84) (Rosander et al. 2021).

3.9 MDT Model in Esophageal and Gastroesophageal Cancer Patients and Impact on Survival and Staging

Multimodality treatment and MDT were reported to be an independent prognostic factor in esophageal cancer patients who were subjected to radiotherapy with (HR, 0.59; 95% CI, 0.38–0.92; p = 0.019), which was most likely due to better patients selection for patients managed in MDT model compared to non-MDT setting (Zhao et al. 2020).

Furthermore, individuals with esophageal cancer who received treatment through an MDT approach exhibited a reduced likelihood of mortality (hazard ratio [HR], 0.73; 95% confidence interval [CI], 0.67–0.79) in comparison to patients who did not receive MDT care. Huang et al. (2021) conducted a subgroup analysis and found that the MDT model significantly decreased the probability of death in stages II, III, and IV. Notably, there was a substantial reduction in stage III (HR, 0.72; 95% CI, 0.67–0.79).

MDT value was also noted in better TNM staging, reflected in survival. A study evaluating the effect of MDT on the staging of gastroesophageal cancer showed that the most precise method for esophageal cancer staging was the endoscopic ultrasound (EUS) (T stage accuracy 78%, N stage accuracy 70%) and also showed that laparoscopic ultrasound was the most precise method for gastric cancer staging with T stage accuracy 91%. The MDT model was more precise in staging than the individual staging model for both gastric and esophageal cancers, with an accuracy range of 88–89% (Davies et al. 2006).

3.10 The Impact of MDT on Pancreatic Cancer, Gastric Cancer, and Biliary System

A retrospective study evaluated the role of MDT in specific gastrointestinal malignancies, including gastric, esophageal, pancreatic, biliary, and colorectal cancer. Results showed improvement in mortality rate where overall mortality rate at two years was 13% (95% CI, 0.06–0.66) in the MDT group versus 38% in (95% CI, 0.10–0.39) non-MDT group (p = 0.08). The study concluded the positive effect of the MDT-managed group and suggested the importance of its inclusion as a standard of care (Basendowah et al. 2021).

Another study analyzed MDT's impact on locally advanced gastric cancer cases. Results for 394 cases that were included in the study revealed a better prognosis of locally advanced gastric cancer for patients with MDT approach versus non-MDT with three years' overall survival 55.6% versus 46.1% with a p-value of 0.005. Also, the analysis revealed that the MDT model could lower mortality (HR = 0.493, $p < 0.001$) (Yuan-Yuan Xiang et al. 2022).

On the contrary, another study concluded that the MDT management approach had a restricted impact on the accuracy of staging and treatment outcomes, such as survival, in patients with resectable gastric cancer. Nevertheless, it was hypothesized that inadequate patient compliance might have influenced the effectiveness of MDT consultation (Chen et al. 2021).

3.11 Multidisciplinary Care in Urological Cancers

The treatment options for prostate cancer, especially advanced cases, continue to evolve; so to ensure the best practice, MDT application is highly recommended (Holmes et al. 2021).

The impact of the MDT approach was shown to have a favorable independent prognostic factor in metastatic hormonal refractory prostate cancer, with an improvement in median overall survival (39.7 versus 27.0 months; HR, 0.549; $p = 0.001$). Furthermore, this survival advantage persisted among patients who received initial treatment (with no specific time limit against 27.0 months; $p = 0.001$) and subsequent treatments (36.7 versus 25.6 months; $p = 0.044$) until the end of the follow-up period (Zhu et al. 2021).

Another study proved MDT's impact in managing cases with metastatic renal cell carcinoma (mRCC). MDT approach improved overall survival regardless of histopathology (OS in MDT group: 94.0 months; non-MDT group: 43.5 months, $p = 0.009$) (Zeng et al. 2023).

Another study defined that MDT management has an effect on managing 38.2% of cases with urogenital malignancies and recommended the use of the MDT approach in all cases with urogenital cancers (Gil et al. 2021).

3.12 The Impact of MDT in the Management of Soft Tissue Sarcoma

Soft tissue sarcomas (STS) are rare, variable, and complex tumors, which necessitates the application of MDT in its management (Nakayama et al. 2020).

A study investigating the effect of MDT on the accuracy of diagnosis and treatment management of bone and (STS) was conducted. Results revealed significant improvement in the accuracy of the new case diagnosis (95.42%) and relapse diagnosis relapse (100%). Also, MDT implication was associated with a high positive pathology rate of 81.2% after the extension of resection margins if the patient was subjected to unplanned resection, which reflects the importance of MDT in the accuracy of diagnosis, relapse, and extension of resection margins after unplanned resection. However, the results were not statistically significant regarding overall survival in patients with osteosarcoma with lung nodules ($p = 0.5751$) (Pang et al. 2022).

Another study in line concluded the importance of MDT in the management of cases with intrathoracic synovial sarcoma with an improved overall survival in patients managed in the MDT model with median OS (46.0 versus 18.0 months, $p = 0.480$) for patients treated in MDT model versus non-MDT respectively (He et al. 2021).

3.13 The Impact of MDT in Managing Central Nervous System Tumors

MDT is an essential treatment strategy in many tumors; however, little has been published about neuro-oncology. A retrospective study of 447 patients with brain tumors was done to evaluate the role of MDT in treatment decisions for cases with brain tumors, focusing on the role of neuroradiologists. The results revealed that revision for diagnostic images was asked in 342 patients; radiotherapists asked for case revision in 58.8%, and neurosurgery specialists in 40.5% were predominantly issued for neuroradiology specialists. The most repeated inquiry was about a treatment plan change (64.4%). Changes in therapeutic policy were seen in 40.5% of patients, depending on neuroradiology revaluation in 76.8% of patients (Gaudino et al. 2022).

Another study evaluated the effect of using MDT in pituitary adenomas management. Research findings provide evidence in favor of Multidisciplinary Team (MDT) approach, showing superior surgical results in patients with clinically functioning tumors. The MDT approach resulted in a higher percentage of improved clinical functioning tumors (42% against 28%, $p = 0.03$), shorter hospital stays (5 versus seven days, $p < 0.001$), and a lower incidence of intrasellar residuals (8% versus 35%, $p < 0.001$) (Grayson et al. 2021).

3.14 MDT and Precision Oncology

Precision oncology (PO) uses molecular profiles for different types of malignancies by next-generation sequencing (NGS) to identify specific genetic alterations that could target specific targeted therapies. The interpretation is best discussed in MDT to decrease the doubt about therapeutic recommendations according to diagnosed specific genetic alteration (Schwartzberg et al. 2018).

Molecular MDTs were established to tailor personalized treatment based on genetic testing results. It was initially recognized with the onset of precision oncology (PO), as many physicians needed to familiarize themselves with interpreting results and incorporating the information into clinical practice. Molecular MDTs have not evolved in the way that PO has evolved, which are integrated into slandered ca. A retrospective review of solid tumor cases that have had NGS evaluating the role of molecular MDTs, where 173 complex cases were discussed in molecular MDTs; results showed changes in decisions of 63 cases which focus on the importance of molecular MDTs (Sadaps et al. 2021).

3.15 MDT and Challenges in Rural Areas

Patients living in rural areas may lack access to high-volume centers where MDT for cancer patients could be held. Developing and implementing communications systems is crucial to improve cross-institutional collaboration and coordination.

Virtual MDTs could be potentially helpful in managing cancer patients in rural areas (DePuccio et al. 2021).

3.16 Possible Key Performance Indicators (KPIs) for Evaluating the Efficiency of the MDT Team

The KPIs used to monitor and evaluate MDTs usually focus on the structure, process, and collaboration between members rather than the outcome. The outcome may be assessed by the number of cancer patients who have received supervision from an MDT before commencing therapy and the average duration from MDT consultation to communication with the general practitioner (White et al. 2021).

3.17 Medicolegal Considerations in the Context of Multidisciplinary Cancer Care

Healthcare personnel involved in MDT cancer discussions may lack awareness of their medicolegal responsibilities. The primary medicolegal concerns associated with MDT care involve patient permission and privacy during MDT meetings, professional liability, formal articulation of differing opinions, and the need to provide care (Karas et al. 2020).

3.18 Effect of the COVID-19 Pandemic on the MDT Approach in Managing Cancer

Challenges have been created for healthcare professionals by the COVID-19 pandemic, which forced the MDT meetings to be held virtually (Labra et al. 2021; Rajasekaran et al. 2021). The shift from physical meetings to virtual ones was mandatory due to the delays in cancer diagnosis and management of cases (Santoro et al. 2021). Holding the MDT virtually increased the opportunity for interaction, participation, communication, and effective coordination (Simpson et al. 2021).

Virtual MDTs could emerge as the predominant method of delivering cancer care in the future. Maximizing efficiency in remote meetings involves leveraging information technology assistance and effectively managing potential distractions (Kerawala et al. 2020).

References

Andritsch E, Beishon M, Bielack S et al (2017) ECCO essential requirements for quality cancer care: soft tissue sarcoma in adults and bone sarcoma. A critical review. Crit Rev Oncol Hematol 110:94–105

Back MF, Ang ELL, Ng WH et al (2007) Improvements in quality of care resulting from a formal multidisciplinary tumour clinic in the management of high-grade glioma. Ann Acad Med Singap 36(5):347–351

Basendowah M et al (2021) Impact of optional multidisciplinary tumour board meeting on the mortality of patients with gastrointestinal cancer: a restrospective observational study. Cancer Rep (Hoboken) 4(4):e1373

Beets G, Sebag-Montefiore D, Andritsch E (2017) ECCO essential requirements for quality cancer care: colorectal cancer. A critical review. Crit Rev Oncol Hematol 110:81–93

Berman HL (1975) The tumor board: is it worth saving? Mil Med 140(8):529–531

Bilfinger TV, Albano D, Perwaiz M et al (2018) Survival outcomes among lung cancer patients treated using a multidisciplinary team approach. Clin Lung Cancer 19:346–351. https://doi.org/10.1016/j.cllc.2018.01.006

Bonadonna G, Rossi A, Valagussa P et al (1977) The CMF program for operable breast cancer with positive axillary nodes. Updated analysis on the disease-free interval, site of relapse and drug tolerance. Cancer 39(suppl):2904–2915

Brandão M, Guisseve A, Bata G et al (2021) Survival impact and cost-effectiveness of a multidisciplinary tumor board for breast cancer in Mozambique. Sub-Saharan Africa Oncol 26: e996–e1008

Calman-Hine Report. Expert Advisory Group on Cancer (1995) A policy framework for commissioning cancer services: a report to the chief medical officers of England and Wales. Department of Health

Cancer Institute New South Wales. NSW cancer plan 2016 [Internet]. Cancer.nsw.gov.au, 2016. Available at: https://www.cancer.nsw.gov.au/getmedia/69ca5241-3620-4898-a32b-e7c7e78cab8b/CancerPlan2016-Web.pdf. Accessed Feb 2021

Chen Y et al (2021) Mutidisciplinary team consultation for resectable gastric cancer: a propensity score matching analysis. J Cancer 12(7):1907–1914

Chugh R (2021) Breast sarcoma: emphasis on the need for a multidisciplinary approach. In: Presentation. ASCO Annual Meeting, 4 June, 2021

Costa A (2018) Multidisciplinary approach to cancer: a true progress. In: Schweizer Krebsbulletin (Swiss Cancer Bulletin), Multidisziplinäre Tumorboards, pp 332–334

Croke JM, El-Sayed S (2012) Multidisciplinary management of cancer patients: chasing a shadow or real value? An overview of the literature. Curr Oncol 19(4):e232–e238. https://doi.org/10.3747/co.19.944

Davies AR, Deans DAC, Penman I, Plevris JN, Fletcher J, Wall L, Phillips H, Gilmour H, Patel D, De Beaux A, Paterson-Brown S (2006) The multidisciplinary team meeting improves staging accuracy and treatment selection for gastro-esophageal cancer. Dis Esophagus 19(6):496–503. https://doi.org/10.1111/j.1442-2050.2006.00629

DePuccio M et al (2021) Clinicians' perspectives on strategies to improve cross-institutional collaboration and coordination of pancreatic cancer care for rural patients. Abstract e13532. J Clin Oncol 39(15 Suppl). https://doi.org/10.1200/JCO.2021.39.15_suppl.e13532

Duncan MA, Lautner MA (2018) Sarcomas of the breast. Surg Clin North Am 98(4):869–876

El Saghir NS, Keating NL, Carlson RW, Khoury KE, Fallowfield L (2014) Tumor boards: optimizing the structure and improving efficiency of multidisciplinary management of patients with cancer worldwide. Am Soc Clin Oncol Educ Book 34:e461–e466. https://doi.org/10.14694/EdBook_AM.2014.34.e461

Fennell ML, Das IP, Clauser S, Petrelli N, Salner A (2010) The organization of multidisciplinary care teams: modeling internal and external influences on cancer care quality. J Natl Cancer Inst Monogr 2010(40):72–80. [PMC free article] [PubMed]

Gaudino S, Giordano C, Magnani F, Cottonaro S, Infante A, Sabatino G, La Rocca G, Della Pepa GM, D'Alessandris QG, Pallini R, Olivi A, Balducci M, Chiesa S, Gessi M, Guadalupi P, Russo R, Schiarelli C, Ausili Cefaro L, Di Lella GM, Colosimo C (2022) Neuro-oncology multidisciplinary tumor board: the point of view of the Neuroradiologist. J Pers Med 12(2):135. https://doi.org/10.3390/jpm12020135. PMID: 35207625; PMCID: PMC8875699

Gaudioso C et al (2021) Impact of a thoracic multidisciplinary conference on lung cancer outcomes. Ann Thorac Surg S0003–4975(21):00523–00523

Gil M et al (2021) The impact of multidisciplinary team conferences in urologic cancer in a tertiary hospital. Int Urol Nephrol 53(1):41–47

Gish RG, Lencioni R, Di Bisceglie AM et al (2012) Role of the multidisciplinary team in the diagnosis and treatment of hepatocellular carcinoma. Expert Rev Gastroenterol Hepatol 6(2): 173–185

Grayson JW et al (2021) Multidisciplinary team care in the surgical management of pituitary adenoma. J Neurol Surg B Skull Base 82(3):295–302

Gross GE (1987) The role of the tumor board in a community hospital. CA Cancer J Clin 37(2): 88–92

He H et al (2021) The value of multidisciplinary team (MDT) management in the diagnosis and treatment of primary intrathoracic synovial sarcomas: a single-Centre experience. J Thorac Dis 13(2):600–612

Holmes A et al (2021) A systematic scoping review of multidisciplinary cancer team and decision-making in the management of men with advanced prostate cancer. World J Urol 39(2):297–306

Huang YC et al (2021) Effect of multidisciplinary team care on survival of oesophageal cancer patients: a retrospective nationwide cohort study. Sci Rep 11(1):13243

Hung HY et al (2020) Multidisciplinary team discussion results in survival benefit for patients with stage III non-small-cell lung cancer. PLoS One 15(10):e0236503

Jury RP, Nadeau L, Wasvary H, Levine R, Robertson J (2010) Implementing a multidisciplinary open-access clinic at a private practice-based community hospital. J Oncol Pract 6(6):e38–e41. https://doi.org/10.1200/JOP.2010.000029

Kabat GC, Matthews CE, Kamensky V, Hollenbeck AR, Rohan TE (2015) Adherence to cancer prevention guidelines and cancer incidence, cancer mortality, and total mortality: a prospective cohort study. Am J Clin Nutr 101(3):558–569. https://doi.org/10.3945/ajcn.114.094854

Karas PL, Rankin NM, Stone E (2020) Medicolegal considerations in multidisciplinary cancer care. JTO Clin Res Rep 1(4):100073. https://doi.org/10.1016/j.jtocrr.2020.100073. Epub 2020 Jul 3. PMID: 33225316; PMCID: PMC7333617

Kerawala C et al (2020) Videoconferencing for multidisciplinary team meetings in the coronavirus disease era- human factors awareness and recognition. J Laryngol Otol 134(12):1118–1119

Kesson EM, Allardice GM, George WD et al (2012) Effects of multidisciplinary team working on breast cancer survival: retrospective, comparative, interventional cohort study of 13722 women. BMJ 344:1–9

Labra L et al (2021) Joven y Fuerte (J&F): multidisciplinary distance care program in Mexico for young women with breast cancer (YWBC) during the COVID-19 pandemic. Abstract e13536. J Clin Oncol 39(15 Suppl). https://doi.org/10.1200/JCO.2021.39.15_suppl.e13536

Lhewa D et al (2020) Multidisciplinary team management of hepatocellular carcinoma is standard of care. Clin Liver Dis 24(4):771–787

Martin-Ucar AE, Waller DA, Atkins JL, Swinson D, O'Byrne KJ, Peake MD (2004) The beneficial effects of specialist thoracic surgery on the resection rate for non-small-cell lung cancer. Lung Cancer 46(2):227–232

Munro AJ (2015) Multidisciplinary team meetings in cancer care: an idea whose time has gone? Clin Oncol (R Coll Radiol) 27:728–731

Murray PV, O'Brien MER, Sayer R et al (2003) The pathway study: results of a pilot feasibility study in patients suspected of having lung carcinoma investigated in a conventional chest clinic setting compared to a centralised two-stop pathway. Lung Cancer 42(3):283–290

Nakayama R et al (2020) A multidisciplinary approach to soft-tissue sarcoma of the extremities. Expert Rev Anticancer Ther 20(10):893–900

National Comprehensive Cancer Network (NCCN) (2021) NCCN guidelines. Available at: https://www.nccn.org/guidelines/category_1. Accessed 24 Aug 2021

NHS National Cancer Action Team. The Characteristics of an Effective Multidisciplinary Team (MDT). www.ncin.org.uk/view?rid=136. Accessed 15 March 2019

Pang K, Guo X, Liu T, Wang L, Chen R, Zhang Z, Li L, He Y, Zhang H, Fan S, Tu C, Li Z (2022) The role of a multidisciplinary team in the diagnosis and treatment of bone and soft tissue sarcomas: a single-center experience. J Pers Med 12(12):2079. https://doi.org/10.3390/jpm12122079. PMID: 36556299; PMCID: PMC9782466

Patkar V, Acosta D, Davidson T, Jones A, Fox J, Keshtgar M (2011) Cancer multidisciplinary team meetings: evidence, challenges, and the role of clinical decision support technology. Int J Breast Cancer 2011:831605. https://doi.org/10.4061/2011/831605

Peng D et al (2021) Improved overall survival of colorectal cancer under multidisciplinary team: a meta-analysis. Biomed Res Int 2021:5541613

Rajasekaran RB et al (2021) Will virtual multidisciplinary team meetings become the norm for musculoskeletal oncology care following the COVID-19 pandemic? Experience from a tertiary sarcoma Centre. BMC Musculoskelet Disord 22(1):18

Rosander E et al (2021) Preoperative multidisciplinary team assessment is associated with improved survival in patients with locally advanced colon cancer; a nationwide cohort study in 3157 patients. Eur J Surg Oncol 47(9):2398–2404

Sadaps M et al (2021) The impact of clinical decision making in a molecular tumour board at a tertiary care Centre. Abstract 3128. J Clin Oncol 39(15 Suppl):3128

Santoro GA et al (2021) DElayed COloRectal cancer care during COVID-19 pandemic (DECOR-19): global perspective from an international survey. Surgery 169(4):796–807

Schwartzberg L, Kim ES, Liu D, Schrag D (2018) Precision oncology: who, how, what, when, and when not? Am Soc Clin Oncol Educ Book 37:160–169. https://doi.org/10.1200/EDBK_174176. PMID: 28561651

Silbermann M, Pitsillides B, Al-Alfi N, Omran S, Al-Jabri K, Elshamy K, Ghrayeb I, Livneh J, Daher M, Charalambous H, Jafferri A, Fink R, El-Shamy M (2013) Multidisciplinary care team for cancer patients and its implementation in several middle eastern countries. Ann Oncol 24 (Suppl 7):vii41–vii47. https://doi.org/10.1093/annonc/mdt265. PMCID: PMC3767159

Simpson L et al (2021) Characteristics of the multidisciplinary cancer conference (tumour boards) in the COVID-19 era. Abstract e13561. J Clin Oncol 39(15 Suppl). https://doi.org/10.1200/JCO.2021.39.15_suppl.e13561

Sinn DH, Choi G-S, Park HC, Kim JM, Kim H, Song KD et al (2019) Multidisciplinary approach is associated with improved survival of hepatocellular carcinoma patients. PLoS One 14(1): e0210730. https://doi.org/10.1371/journal.pone.0210730

Soares KC, Cosgrove DC, Herman JM, Pawlik TM (2014) Multidisciplinary clinic in the management of hepatocellular carcinoma. Ann Surg Oncol 21:1059–1061. https://doi.org/10.1245/s10434-013-3419-2. PMID: 24318097

Soukup T, Petrides K, Lamb BW et al (2016) The anatomy of clinical decision-making in multidisciplinary cancer meetings: a cross-sectional observational study of teams in a natural context. Medicine 95:e3885

Stephens MR, Lewis WG, Brewster AE et al (2006) Multidisciplinary team management is associated with improved outcomes after surgery for esophageal cancer. Dis Esophagus 19(3): 164–171

Taberna M, Moncayo FG, Jané-Salas E, Antonio M, Arribas L, Vilajosana E, Torres EP, Mesía R (2020) The multidisciplinary team (MDT) approach and quality of care. Review article. Front Oncol 10:85. Sec. Head and Neck Cancer. Volume 10–2020. https://doi.org/10.3389/fonc.2020.00085

Taplin SH, Weaver A, Salas E et al (2015) Reviewing cancer care team effectiveness. J Oncol Pract 11:239–246

Tsai CH et al (2020) Effect of multidisciplinary team care on the risk of recurrence in breast cancer patients: a national matched cohort study. Breast 53:68–76

Unger JM, LeBlanc M, Blanke CD (2017) The effect of positive SWOG treatment trials on survival of patients with cancer in the US population. JAMA Oncol 3:1345–1351

Van der Vlies E et al (2020) Implementation of a preoperative multidisciplinary team approach for frail colorectal cancer patients: influence on patient selection, prehabilitation and outcome. J Geriatr Oncol 11(8):1237–1243

Van Leeuwen AF, Voogt E, Visser A, van der Rijt CCD, van der Heide A (2004) Considerations of healthcare professionals in medical decision-making about treatment for clinical end-stage cancer patients. J Pain Symptom Manag 28(4):351–355

van Nes JGH, van de Velde CJH (2005) The multidisciplinary breast cancer care team: promoting better care. Ned Tijdschr Geneeskd 149(35):1929–1931

Veronesi U, Saccozzi R, Del Vecchio M (1981) Comparing radical mastectomy with quadrantectomy, axillary dissection, and radiotherapy in patients with small cancers of the breast. N Engl J Med 305:6–11

White KM et al (2021) Investigating the system effect of reporting multidisciplinary care measures for cancer services in New South Wales, Australia. BMC Health Serv Res 21(1):1044

Xiang Y-Y, Deng C-C, Liu H-Y, Kuo Z-C, Zhang C-H, He Y-L (2022) The prognostic effect of multidisciplinary team intervention in patients with advanced gastric cancer. Curr Oncol 29(2): 1201–1212. https://doi.org/10.3390/curroncol29020102. Published online 2022 Feb 17. PMCID: PMC8871247. PMID: 35200601

Yang JD, Heimbach JK (2020) New advances in the diagnosis and management of hepatocellular carcinoma. BMJ 371:m3544

Yopp AC, Mansour JC, Beg MS et al (2014) Establishment of a multi-disciplinary hepatocellular carcinoma clinic is associated with improved clinical outcome. Ann Surg Oncol 21(04): 1287–1295

Zeng Y, Zhu S, Wang Z, Chen J, Dai J, Liu Z, Sun G, Liang J, Zhang X, Wang Z, Zhao J, Ni Y, Yang J, Wang M, Wei Q, Li X, Chen N, Li Z, Wang X, Shen Y, Yao J, Huang R, Liu J, Cai D, Zeng H, Shen P (2023) Multidisciplinary team (MDT) discussion improves overall survival outcomes for metastatic renal cell carcinoma patients. J Multidiscip Healthc 16:503–513. https://doi.org/10.2147/JMDH.S393457. PMID: 36865786; PMCID: PMC9971520

Zhang J, Mavros MN, Cosgrove D, Hirose K, Herman JM, Smallwood-Massey S et al (2013) Impact of a single-day multidisciplinary clinic on the management of patients with liver tumours. Curr Oncol 20:e123–e131. https://doi.org/10.3747/co.20.1297. PMID: 23559879

Zhao S et al (2020) Role of a multidisciplinary team in administering radiotherapy for oesophageal cancer. BMC Cancer 20(1):974

Zhu S et al (2021) Dynamic multidisciplinary team discussion can improve the prognosis of metastatic castration-resistant prostate cancer patients. Prostate 81(11):721–727

The Interplay Between Inflammation and Cancer Progression: Implications for Therapy

Barka Basharat, Nushrat Jahan, Ashutosh Mishra, Junaid Alam, Yaqoot Taban Khan, Imtaiyaz Md. Hassan, Nadeem Zafar Jilani, and Mohammad "Sufian" Badar

Abstract

Cancer study focuses on the intricate association between aggravation and the growth of cancer, which reveals intricate relationships between malignant cells, cytokines, and pro-inflammatory cells inside the tumor microenvironment (TME). The molecular and cellular processes underpinning this interaction and its consequences for cancer treatment are thoroughly reviewed in this chapter. Inflammation has pro- as well as anti-tumorigenic actions, playing two distinct functions in cancer. Pro-tumorigenic inflammation facilitates the origin, growth,

B. Basharat · N. Jahan
Department of Biotechnology, School of Chemical and Life Sciences, Jamia Hamdard, New Delhi, India

A. Mishra
Department of Surgical Oncology, DR BRA IRCH, All India Institute of Medical Sciences (AIIMS), New Delhi, India

J. Alam
Division of Trauma Surgery and Critical Care, JPN Apex Trauma Centre, All India Institute of Medical Sciences (AIIMS), New Delhi, India

Y. T. Khan
Department of Physiology, Gajara Raja Medical College, Gwalior, Madhya Pradesh, India

I. Md. Hassan
Centre for Interdisciplinary Research in Basic Sciences, Jamia Millia Islamia (JMI), New Delhi, India
e-mail: hassanlab@jmi.ac.in

N. Z. Jilani
Department of Pediatric Emergency, Sidra Medicine, Medical Director Sidra Child Advocacy Program, Doha, Qatar

Pennine Acute Hospitals NHS Trust, Oldham, UK
e-mail: njilani@sidra.org

Interdisciplinary Cancer Research, https://doi.org/10.1007/16833_2024_474
Published online: 10 November 2024

and spread of tumors through processes like inducing genome instability, enhancing blood vessel development, and suppressing tumor-fighting defenses. Inflammatory cells including neutrophils, T lymphocytes, and macrophages as well as signaling pathways like STAT3 and NF-κB are important participants in this mechanism. Furthermore, irritation may stimulate anti-tumorigenic effects by encouraging tissue healing, immunological monitoring, and regression of tumors. Using the immune system's attack against tumors has the potential to lead to the creation of new treatment approaches. Inflammatory management has become an intriguing possibility for cancer treatment. Treatment results may be enhanced by anti-inflammatory medications, immunotherapy procedures, and a combination of treatments that influence the inflammatory TME. But there are still issues to be resolved, like resistance to treatment and variations in inflammation among cancer kinds. Ultimately, comprehending the intricate relationship between inflammation and the advancement of cancer offers new perspectives on methods of therapy and emphasizes the significance of tailored medicines in the fight against cancer. It is highly promising that more studies in this area will help us fight disease and enhance outcomes for patients.

Keywords

Cyclooxygenase · EMT · FGF · Immunotherapy · Mitogen-activated protein kinase · NSAIDs · Nuclear localization signals · Pro-tumorigenic inflammation · TME

1 Introduction

Cancer is the most prevalent cause of fatalities worldwide, marked by rapidly expanding cells and an opportunity to spread to organs that are far away. In recent times, there has been a notable focus on the involvement of prolonged inflammation having a significant impact on malignancy, despite the well-known role of genetic alterations and environmental variables to carcinogenicity (Hanahan and Weinberg 2011). The intricate interaction of immune cells, cytokines, and signaling pathways results in inflammatory processes, a basic reaction to tissue damage and infection. Inflammation over time can promote the genesis, progression, and metastasis of cancer when it is irregular and creates a situation that is favorable to tumor growth

M. S. Badar (✉)
Department of Bioengineering, University of California, Riverside, CA, USA

Universal Scientific Education and Research Network (USERN), Tehran, Iran

SPI Darbhanga, Darbhanga, India

Department of Computer Science and Engineering (Bioinformatics), School of Engineering Sciences and Technology (SEST), Jamia Hamdard University, New Delhi, India
e-mail: msbadar@engr.ucr.edu; msbadar@salfiainstitute.edu.in; msbadar@jamiahamdard.ac.in

(Coussens and Werb 2002). Rudolf Virchow made the initial suggestion that inflammation and cancer are related in the 1800s based on his observation that leukocytes were present in neoplastic tissues. Several methods that explain how chronic inflammation leads to oncogenesis have been clarified by subsequent studies. These consist of the activation of reactive nitrogen species (RNS) and reactive oxygen species (ROS), which in turn lead to genomic instability and damage to DNA, and activation of transcription factors such as signal transducer and activator of transcription 3 (STAT3) and nuclear Factor-kappa B (NF-κB) that encourage the development of genes involved in angiogenesis, their survival, and growth of cells (Hussain and Harris 2007).

Prolonged and chronic inflammation may expose one to carcinogenesis and aid in the growth of cancer. About 15–20% of human tumors are caused by inflammations that are driven by infections. Nevertheless, the existence of a mediator of inflammation in their microenvironment characterizes even tumors that are not epidemiologically associated with infections. The presence of invading leukocytes, cytokines, chemokines, growth hormones, lipid messengers, and matrix-degrading enzymes is the indicator of inflammation linked to cancer (Allavena et al. 2008). Certain cancers can be brought on by chronic inflammation, and solid tumors can start and maintain local inflammatory mechanisms that support tumor growth and metastasis. As a result, efforts to manage cancer have focused on pathways that promote inflammation. The infiltration of circulatory cells as well as antibodies for an adaptive immune reaction to the tissue is facilitated by inflammation, which also serves as a key component of the immune system's innate reaction to tissue harm or infection (Munn 2017) (Fig. 1).

A possible treatment approach is to target inflammatory pathways because of the complex link that exists between cancer and inflammatory diseases. The potential of immune system modulators, cytokine-inhibiting agents, and anti-inflammatory medications to slow the spread of malignancies and enhance patient outcomes is being investigated. Furthermore, new methods like personalized medicine and nanotechnology are being researched to improve the targeted nature and effectiveness of anti-inflammatory cancer therapy. Furthermore, when inflammatory cells like neutrophils, lymphocytes, and macrophages enter the tumor microenvironment, they release chemokines and cytokines that promote the spread and metastasis of the tumor (Nica and Dermitzakis 2013) For example, tumor-associated macrophages (TAMs) can accelerate the growth of tumors by stimulating angiogenesis, reducing defense against the tumor, and assisting with the epithelial-mesenchymal transition (EMT). Similarly, by ensnaring circulating tumor cells and enabling their colonization at distant places, neutrophils and their extracellular barriers (NETs) are linked to metastasis (Qian and Pollard 2010).

Due to their strong influence on carcinogenesis, inflammation and tumors are two related disorders that have generated a great deal of research for cancer studies, the growth of tumors, and treatment results.

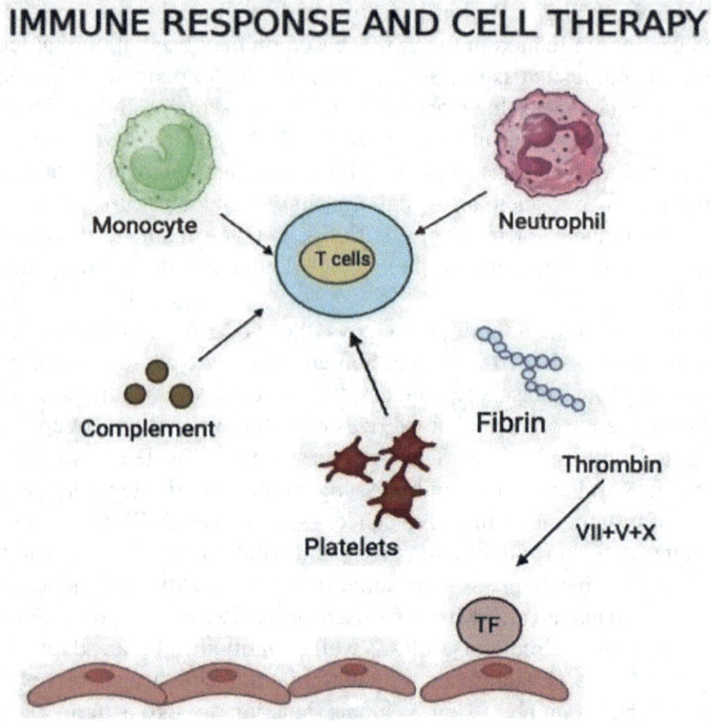

Fig. 1 Overview of immune response and cell therapy

1.1 Inflammation

A medical condition, damage to tissues, or external triggers can all set off an intricate biological reaction known as inflammation. To restore the equilibrium of tissues, it entails the mobilization of immune system cells, the expulsion of pro-inflammatory mediators, and the activation of signals (Munn 2017). However, long-term use of anti-inflammatory medications has been demonstrated to reduce the death rate. Individuals with chronic inflammatory illnesses are more likely to get tumors. Inflammatory processes inevitably serve an essential part in tumor pathogenesis, but the connection between immunity and cancer is very intricate (Hussain and Harris 2007). Inflammation is an essential and protective reaction to damage or infection, but persistent inflammation can have negative consequences, such as accelerating the development of cancer. An elevated risk of acquiring many types of cancer is associated with chronic inflammatory disorders, consisting of chronic hepatitis, chronic obstructive pulmonary disease, and inflammatory bowel disease. An environment that is constantly inflamed fosters alterations in genes, DNA instability, and epigenetic changes, which provide an ideal condition for the development and spread of cancer (Grivennikov et al. 2010) (Fig. 2).

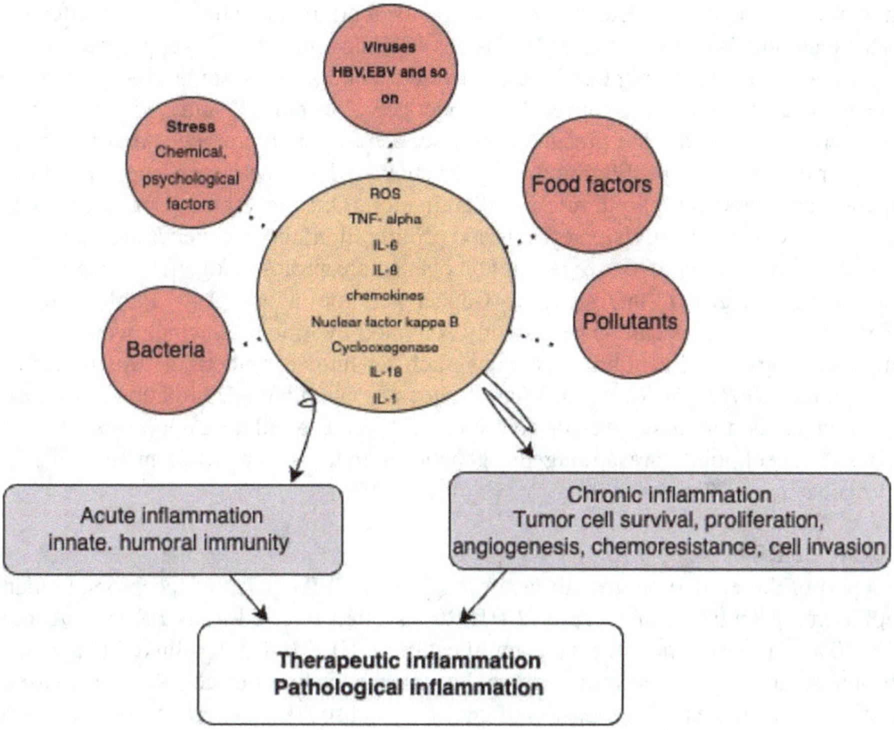

Fig. 2 Different aspects of inflammation and their role in tumorigenesis

The prolonged intake of anti-inflammatory medications, such as nonsteroidal anti-inflammatory medications (NSAIDs), has been demonstrated to lower both the prevalence and mortality of malignancy. The cyclooxygenase (COX) enzymes, which are essential to the inflammatory responses and the production of prostaglandins that promote inflammation, are inhibited by these medications. According to research showing lower rates of colon cancer in people who consistently take NSAIDs, these drugs may be able to reduce irritation and thus the chance of developing cancer(Shavers and Brown 2002). Furthermore, long-term inflammation triggers gene expressions associated with angiogenesis, survival, and growth of cells by activating important transcription factors including signal transducer and activator of transcription 3 and nuclear factor-kappa B (Grivennikov et al. 2010). Long-term inflammation produces ROS and RNS, which may harm DNA and create instability in the genome, which can accelerate the growth of tumors (Hussain and Harris 2007).

1.2 Cancer

The disease is characterized by uncontrolled cell division, invasion of surrounding tissue, and metastasis. The rise in genetic alterations and epigenetic modifications impairs normal cellular functions, leading to aberrant development and lifespan (Hanahan and Weinberg 2011). Variations in oncogenes, tumor suppressor genes, and genes controlling apoptosis and cell cycle checkpoints are some examples of the genetic changes that cause cancer. Proto-oncogenes, or normal genes with mutations or overexpression, are the precursors of oncogenes, which are genes that stimulate cellular division and proliferation. (Fig. 2) shows which factors or faces of inflammation and what can play a role in inflammation. Oncogene precursors are typical genes that control the division of cells and proliferation; the oncogenes are mutant or overproduced forms of these genes. Oncogenes are proto-oncogenes that promote unceasing cell growth and survival (Cancer genome landscapes – PubMed n.d.). These kinds of genes can be persistently activated by mutation, which would result in unceasing cell division. Oncogenes such as human epidermal growth factor receptor 2 (*HER2*), *MYC*, and *RAS* are frequently encountered. Mutation in cancer-causing genes, tumor suppressor genes, and the genes regulating apoptosis and cell division checkpoints are among the genetic alterations that result in malignancy (Vogelstein and Kinzler 2004).

1.2.1 HER2

As part of the epidermal growth factor receptor (EGFR) group of receptors, human epidermal growth factor receptor 2 (HER2) is often referred to as ERBB2. About 15–20% of breast tumors have an amplification of HER2, which is linked to a worse prognosis and a more severe phase of the illness (Slamon et al. 1987). Increased translation or increased expression of genes can cause HER2 overexpression, which increases signaling and promotes tumor survival, growth, and invasion. The primary mode of action for HER2 is heterodimerization of the rest of the EGFR relatives, including HER1, HER3, and HER4. ER2 lacks a recognized ligand. Signaling is more potent and diverse when it is heterodimerized. For example, because HER3 has a significant binding requirement for the p85 subunit of PI3K, HER2/HER3 heterodimers are especially successful in initiating the PI3K/AKT cascade (Graus-Porta et al. 1997). By enhancing the production of vascular endothelial growth factor, HER2 signaling can aid in angiogenesis, the creation of fresh blood vessels. This allows the tumor to develop and metastasize by giving it a sufficient supply of plasma (Konecny et al. 2006).

1.2.2 MYC Oncogene

A crucial modulator of cell division and development, the *MYC* oncogene is implicated in several malignancies, particularly colorectal and Burkitt's lymphoma. As a transcription element, MYC controls the proliferation of a wide range of proteins related to the growth of the cell cycle, metabolism, the production of proteins, and death (Dang 2012). MYC stimulates the synthesis of genes that advance the development of the cell period, including E2F transcription factors such as cyclin D1 and cyclin-dependent kinase (CDKs). MYC aids in the transition of cells into the G1 phase into the phase known as S, promoting replication of DNA and dividing cells by activating those genes (Dang 2012; Stine et al. 2015). By regulating the genes related to the biogenesis of mitochondria, glutaminolysis, and glycolysis, MYC improves the metabolism of cells. This change in metabolism enables the rapidly multiplying cancerous cells to meet their growing energy needs (Oncogenic RUNX3: A Link between p53 Deficiency and MYC Dysregulation – PMC n.d.).

1.2.3 RAS Oncogene

The RAS oncogene relatives, which comprise KRAS, NRAS, and HRAS, are essential for controlling cell division, development, and longevity. Lung, colorectal, and pancreas cancers are among the kinds of human tumors that most frequently include alterations in the *RAS* gene. Because mutant RAS proteins are continuously active, downstream signaling pathways including the PI3K/AKT and MAPK/ERK routes are persistently stimulated (Bos 1989) (Fig. 3).

RAS mechanism of activation

RAS activation starts a chain reaction that includes ERK, MEK, and RAF. ERK that has undergone phosphorylation moves inside the nucleus and stimulates the synthesis of genes known for cell division, survival, and growth (Bos 1989; RAS oncogenes: the first 30 years – PubMed n.d.). Persistently activated RAS mutations cause unchecked cell proliferation and viability by persistently triggering the PI3K/AKT and MAPK/ERK processes. This ongoing signaling encourages neoplastic transformation and interferes with regular cellular processes (Balkwill 2004; Bos 1989).

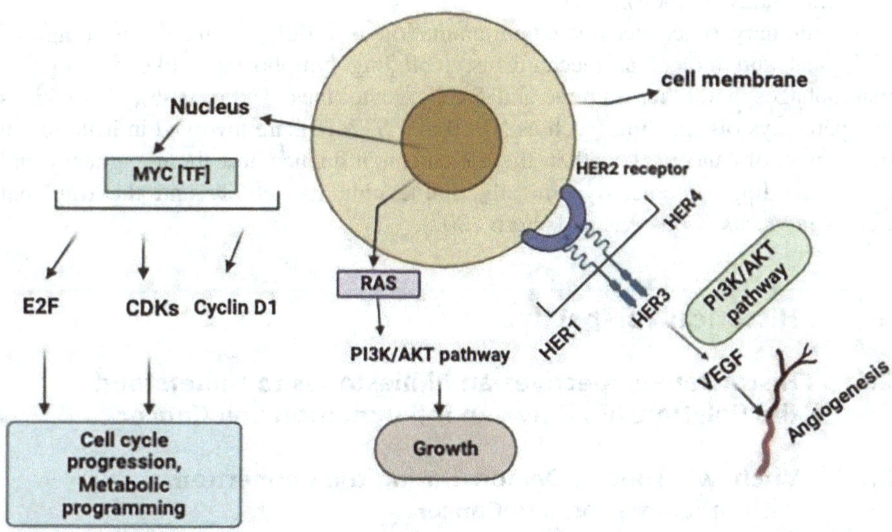

Fig. 3 Pathways of oncogenes in cancer development

1.3 Interaction Among Irritation and Malignancy

It is a complex, reciprocal relationship between cancer and inflammatory processes. By fostering a pro-tumorigenic milieu full of proliferation elements, reactive oxygen compounds, and cytokines that are inflammatory, prolonged inflammation can aid in the growth of tumors (Grivennikov et al. 2010). On the other hand, malignant cells can take advantage of these inflammatory signals to increase their capacity for growth, survival, and metastasis (Balkwill 2004). Epigenetic alterations, which are transmissible adjustments that impact gene expression yet do not modify the sequence of DNA, are involved in the growth of cancer in addition to mutations in the genes. These involve the control of noncoding RNA, histone changes, and DNA methylation. Genes that aid in tumor growth can be activated and safeguard genes silenced because of aberrant patterns of DNA methylation, such as hypomethylation of cancer genes and hypermethylation of tumor-suppressing gene promoters (Jones and Baylin 2002). Furthermore, direct harm to DNA can result in alterations due to inflammatory mediators such as ROS and RNS. The gene involved in angiogenesis, which influences metastasis, growth of cells, and survival are further encouraged to be expressed through the induction of transcription factors like NF-κB and STAT3 in reaction to inflammation signals. For example, the activation of NF-κB may stimulate pro-angiogenic and antiapoptotic DNA, which contribute to tumor growth and durability against cells dying (Karin 2006). On the other hand, cancerous cells can utilize these inflammatory cues to augment their capacity for proliferation, endurance, and metastasis. Inflammatory substances cytokines and chemokines are released by tumor cells to attract antibody-producing cells to the tumor site, hence fostering the growth of cancer. Furthermore, tumors can cause persistent inflammation, which maintains the pro-tumorigenic conditions in the surrounding microenvironment (Balkwill 2004).

A summary of cancer-related inflammation is influenced by a vast range of biological and molecular mechanisms, including lymphocytes (like neutrophils, macrophages, and other immune and T cells), cytokines (TNFα, IL-6), chemokines and pathways of signaling (such as NFκB and STAT3), are involved in irritation in the context of cancers. Together, these elements influence how the malignancy and its surroundings interact dynamically, influencing its activity and the way that treatment works (Coussens and Werb 2002).

2 Historical Perspective

2.1 Historical Perspectives and Milestones to Understand the Relationship Between Inflammation and Cancer

2.1.1 Virchow's Theory: Demonstrating the Connection with Inflammation and Cancer

Renowned German doctor Rudolf Virchow produced an important finding in the middle of the nineteenth century that helped establish the link connecting inflammation and cancer (Turk 1993). His theory, which was first put forth in 1863, suggested that persistent inflammation fosters the growth and development of tumors. Leukocytes are a type of WBCs that Virchow saw in tumor tissues, which served as the basis for his hypothesis. The hypothesis was that the presence of these types of inflammatory cells in neoplastic tissues could suggest that inflammation is crucial in the growth of tumors. Virchow postulated that malignancies may develop as a result of persistent inflammation brought on by an infection, irritation, or other factors. At the time, this was a novel concept since it went against the widely held belief that genetic or inherited elements were the main causes of cancer (Grivennikov et al. 2010). Furthermore, inflammatory cytokines can trigger signaling mechanisms including NF-κB and STAT3 that promote angiogenesis, cell viability, and growth. Examples of these pathways are tumor necrosis factor-alpha (TNFα) and interleukin-6 (IL-6). Additionally, the possible contribution of inflammatory cells to the development and dissemination of tumors was highlighted by Virchow's idea. Tumor-associated macrophages (TAMs), for instance, possess the ability to release growth hormones, proteolytic enzymes, and pro-angiogenic substances that promote the development of new blood vessels (angiogenesis) and the advancement of tumors (Mantovani et al. 2008).

Immune Cells

Researchers saw immune cells, especially macrophages, infiltrating tumor tissues at the beginning of the twentieth century. The hypothesis of inflammation being linked to cancer originated from this observation. According to this notion, immune system cells which are found in the TME have a major impact on the genesis and progression of tumors. Macrophages are multifunctional immune cells that play multiple functions in the tumor environment. They play a part in tissue homeostasis, repair, and defense versus infections. These cells, sometimes referred to as tumor-associated macrophages (TAMs), can manufacture a range of growth factors, cytokines, and proteases that promote the formation of new blood vessels, metastasis, and tumor development TAMs, for example, create vascular endothelial growth factor (VEGF), which encourages angiogenesis, and provide the tumor with both the nutrients and oxygen it requires to keep growing. TAMs can also aid in the extracellular matrix's disintegration, allowing tumor cells to more easily invade adjacent tissues. Additional immune cells that give rise to the inflammatory environment inside tumors include dendritic cells, lymphocytes, and neutrophils. Such cells can secrete chemokines and cytokines that are pro-inflammatory and accelerate the growth of tumors. In particular, cytokines that stimulate pathways of signaling that support the survival of cells, their proliferation, and resisting apoptosis include interleukin-6 (IL-6) and tumor necrosis factor-alpha (TNFα) (Hanahan and Weinberg 2011). In the middle of the twentieth century, epidemiological studies produced strong evidence that some malignancies are more likely to occur in people who had chronic inflammatory disorders. For instance, colitis with ulcers and Crohn's disease, among others, are examples of serious inflammation. Bowel illnesses are connected with an increased risk of of colorectal cancer (Ekbom et al. 1990).

One of the most well-established correlations is that involving colorectal cancer and chronic inflamed bowel illnesses, or IBD. It has been demonstrated that diseases like ulcerative colitis and Crohn's disease, which are characterized by ongoing gastrointestinal tract inflammatory processes, greatly raise the likelihood of colorectal cancer. According to a seminal study, Ekbom people, who had ulcerative colitis, were significantly more likely than people in general to develop colorectal cancer. The research shows the effect of chronic inflammation on the likelihood of cancer by showing that the risk rose as the length and severity of the illness. In a similar vein, additional cancer forms have been connected to ongoing inflammation. For example, there is a substantial correlation between an elevated risk of hepatocellular carcinoma (liver cancer) and infection with hepatitis B and C, which induce persistent inflammation of the liver. A prominent associated risk factor for cervical cancer is human papillomavirus (HPV) infection, which results in ongoing inflammation of the cervical epithelium (Ekbom et al. 1990). These epidemiologic results have played an essential part in drawing attention to the link or association between chronic inflammation and risk for cancer. Additionally, they have sparked more investigation into the cellular mechanisms to which inflammation drives carcinogenesis, which has resulted in the creation of novel treatment approaches that target discomfort to both prevent and treat cancer (Fig. 4).

The discovery of key inflammatory agents, which include cytokines and chemical messengers (chemokines), has greatly expanded our knowledge of how activation contributes to illness, including cancer. Chemokines are tiny signaling factors that are crucial for immune cell attraction and migration to inflammatory areas. Examples of those proteins are CXCL8 (also called IL-8) and CCL2 (MCP-1). These chemicals ensure that immune cells approach and penetrate the tumor environment by directing their migration along the chemotactic gradient; it also activates NF-kappa B factor (Balkwill 2004). The TF known as NF-κB controls the functioning of several genes linked to immunological and inflammatory reactions, cell division, and viability. NF-κB is frequently constitutively active in malignancy, which causes antiapoptotic and proliferating genes to be upregulated and encourages the continued existence and growth of tumor cells. Furthermore, pro-inflammatory cytokines and chemokines can be expressed by NF-κB, which results in a vicious cycle that maintains chronic inflammation in the tumor microenvironment (Karin and Greten 2005). IL-6 is one of the several cytokines and growth variables that stimulate STAT3, a further vital transcription factor. Activation of STAT3 triggers the synthesis of genes in cancer cells that support angiogenesis, immunity evasion, cell viability, and growth. Many malignancies have been linked to persistent STAT3 activation, which is essential for preserving the inflammatory tumor microenvironment (Grivennikov et al. 2010).

The study of molecular processes connecting inflammation and malignancy has greatly improved as a result of developments in genomics and biological sciences. Studies have demonstrated the essential function that inflammatory processes, for example, NF-κB and STAT3, play in the initiation and spread of malignancy (Karin and Greten 2005). A transcription factor called NF-κB controls genes related to immunity, inflammation, cell division, and viability. NF-κB is often active in malignancy, which causes the overexpression of molecules that stop cell death and encourage cell division. Similarly, different cytokines and growth factors, such as

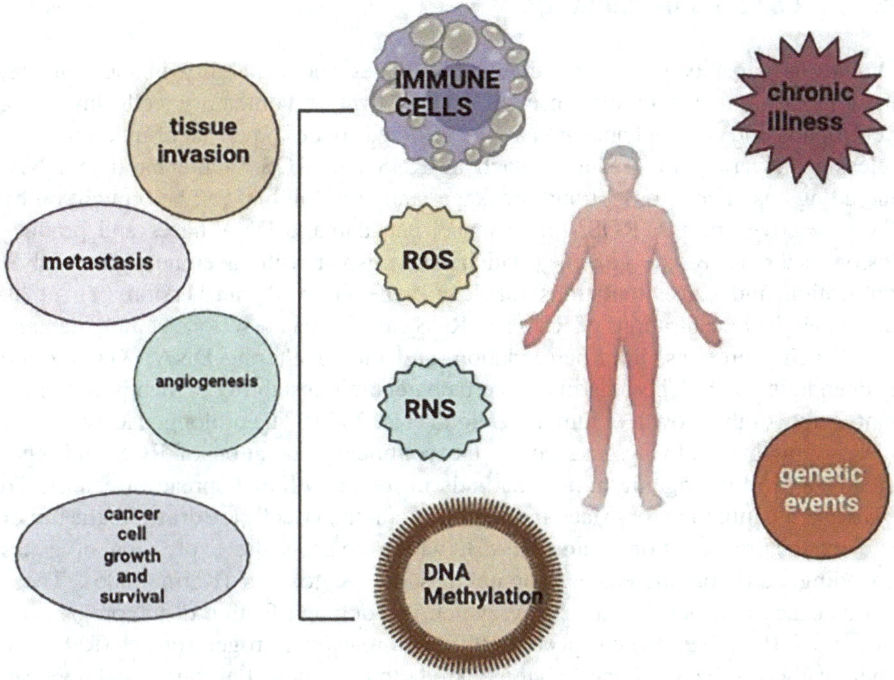

Fig. 4 Chronic inflammation and cancer

IL-6, stimulate STAT3. The stimulation of STAT3 triggers the production of genes in cancer cells that support angiogenesis, resistance to the immune system, cell viability, and growth (Pardoll 2012). STAT3's continuous stimulation has been linked to several cancers. These molecular discoveries identify possible treatment targets and show how chronic inflammation plays a part in the formation of tumors, by comprehending how channels of inflammation function in cancer. Additionally, immunotherapy has become a viable strategy for using the system to combat cancer. Immune checkpoint inhibitors have demonstrated success in reviving the immune system's capacity to combat tumors. Examples of these inhibitors include those that target CTLA-4 and PD-1/PD-L1. Such therapies can combat the suppression of immunity that is frequently present in the tumor microenvironment by modifying the immune response (Pardoll 2012).

3 Mechanism of Linking with ROS and RNS

The processes linking an infection and cancer production of reactive oxygen species and reactive nitrogen species are given below:

3.1 Cancer's Initial Stage

Due to its capacity to foster mutations in genes and instability in the genome, irritation is a factor in the onset of cancer. Anti-inflammatory cells involving neutrophils and macrophages invade the afflicted tissue in persistent inflammation, releasing a variety of mediators such as RNS and ROS. Acute harm to DNA, including base alterations, strand breakage, and crosslinking, can be brought on by these reactive species. ROS, for instance, can damage DNA bases and produce lesions such as 8-oxo guanine, which can mispair with adenine during DNA replication and cause mutations that cause the G to T transversion (Yu et al. 2009). High concentrations of RNS and ROS can also cause serious cellular damage by changing proteins, lipid peroxidation, and further altering DNA (Klaunig and Kamendulis 2004). These harms exacerbate genomic instability, which is an important feature of the growth of tumors (Colotta et al. 2009). The prolonged activation of many signaling pathways caused by the continual generation of ROS and RNS creates a pro-tumorigenic milieu that aids in the growth and spread of cancer. To maintain the inflammatory state, more pro-inflammatory cells are drawn to the tumor site by the transcription factor NF-κB, which controls the expression of genes encoding adhesion molecules, chemokines, and cytokines (Karin 2006). These harms exacerbate genetic instability, which is a defining feature of the progression of tumors. Reactive oxygen species (ROS) and reactive nitrogen species (RNS) are chemically reactive substances that include both oxygen and nitrogen, and they can be produced as a result of long-term illness (Kundu and Surh 2008; Wiseman and Halliwell 1996). A pro-TME is created by the ongoing stimulation of various routes, which facilitates the development and spread of disease. For instance, NF-κB controls the expression of proteins encoding attachment molecules, chemokines, and cytokines that can draw additional pro-inflammatory cells into the tumor site and maintain the state of inflammation (Karin 2006).

3.2 Tumor Progression

Once a tumor starts, it uses cues from inflammation to fuel its expansion and longevity. Tumor growth and development are promoted by inflammatory agents that include chemokines, interleukin-6, and necrosis factor-alpha. (Fig. 5) shows the routes of the immune cell interaction and activating pathways like STAT and cell interaction with ROS and RNS, which lead to the invasion of tumor. These mediators also encourage angiogenesis, which proliferates signaling processes, and the reconstruction of tissues (Coussens and Werb 2002). In addition, these mediators of inflammation aid in the remodeling of the tumor microenvironment and extracellular matrix, which promotes tumor penetration and dissemination. Immune cells are drawn to the tumor site by chemokines like CXCL8 (IL-8), which cause the release of growth stimulants and proteases, which break down the extracellular matrix and facilitate tumor invasion by cells (Waugh and Wilson 2008). Additionally, both the extracellular matrix (ECM) and tumor environment are modified by these mediators

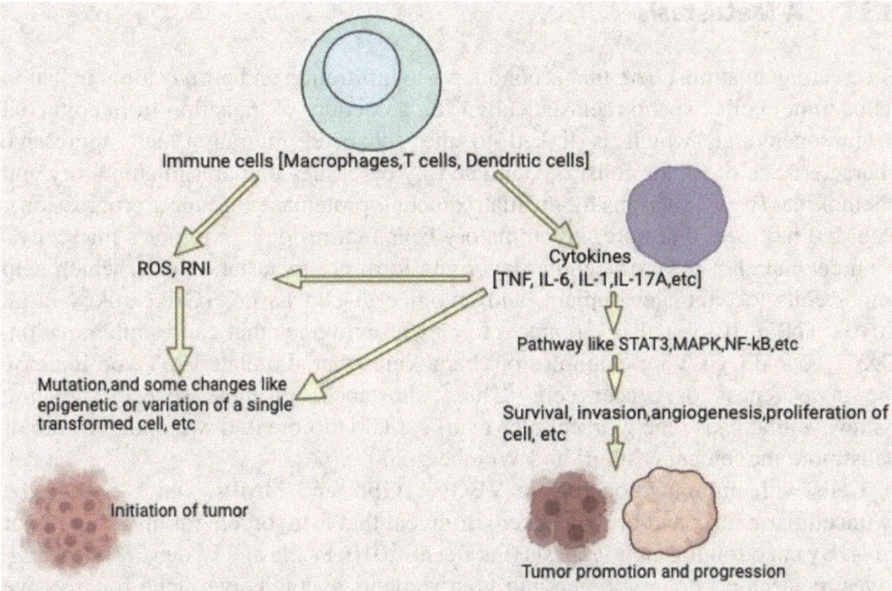

Fig. 5 Overview of the pathway of immune cell interaction with ROS, RNS, and cytokines

of inflammation, facilitating tumor invasion and metastasis. The extracellular matrix (ECM) is an intricate web of protein and additional compounds that supports neighboring cells biochemically and structurally. Enzymes like matrix metalloproteinases (MMPs) alter the extracellular matrix (ECM), promoting the invasion and migration of tumor cells (New functions for the matrix metalloproteinases in cancer progression – PubMed n.d.).

Immune cells that have been drawn to the tumor site by chemokines such as CXCL8 (IL-8) release growth stimulants and proteases that break down the extracellular matrix (ECM) and enable tumor cells to infiltrate neighboring organs (Strieter et al. 2006). Furthermore, IL-8 has a role in the acquisition of immune cells such as neutrophils, which can intensify the inflammation response and advance tumor growth (Waugh and Wilson 2008). Numerous inflammatory substances that are released by neutrophils can promote tumor development and persistence. They generate RNS and ROS, with the potential to harm DNA and encourage mutations in tumor cells. By producing growth factors, cytokines, and proteases, which encourage tumor cell growth, angiogenesis, and assault, neutrophils can aid in the formation of tumors. To help tumor cells migrate, neutrophil-derived elastase, for instance, can break down ECM elements (Infiltrating neutrophils mediate the initial angiogenic switch in a mouse model of multistage carcinogenesis – PubMed n.d.).

3.3 A Metastasis

By creating an atmosphere that is conducive to infiltration and propagation, irritation helps tumor cells expand metastatically. The procedure of transition from epithelial to mesenchymal, which is linked to the enhanced migration and aggressive characteristics of tumor cells, is facilitated by cytokines that are inflammatory and chemokines (New functions for the matrix metalloproteinases in cancer progression – PubMed n.d.). Furthermore, inflammatory cells that reside in a tumor's microenvironment can alter the extracellular layer and form pre-metastatic fields, which help tumor cells to circulate, implant, and colonize distant tissues (Grivennikov et al. 2010). TNFα, IL-6, and IL-1β are examples of cytokines that cause inflammation. CXCL12 and CCL2 are examples of chemokines that stimulate EMT and increase the invasiveness of cancer cells. These substances promote several signaling pathways that cause the extracellular matrix (ECM) to break down and give tumor cells more movement (Kalluri and Weinberg 2009).

Cells with inflammation release VEGF, TGFβ, and MMPs, which change the extracellular matrix and provide an environment that is favorable for invading tumor cells. By encouraging angiogenesis (Park et al. 2010; Psaila and Lyden 2009), VEGF gives metastatic tumors oxygen and nourishment. A conducive niche for invasive tumor cells is created by the substances secreted by inflammatory cells, including VEGF, TGFβ, and MMPs, which alter the extracellular matrix. Additionally, these elements support angiogenesis, which is necessary to supply oxygen to spreading metastatic tumors (Ferrari 2005; Folkman 2002).

4 Transcription Factors (NF-κB and STAT3) and Their Activation

The transcription factors STAT3 and NF-κB play an important part in the development of tumors and inflammation by controlling genes involved for angiogenesis, cell viability, and growth.

4.1 The Canonical NF-κB Regulation in Cancer: The NF-κB Signaling

Pro-inflammatory cytokines like TNFα and IL-1β usually stimulate NF-κB. When these cytokines attach to the specific receptors, IκB kinase (IKK) is recruited and activated, starting the phosphorylation process. IκB proteins are phosphorylated by activated IKK, which marks them to undergo ubiquitination and proteasome destruction. When NF-κB dimers—typically p65/p50—are liberated from this deterioration, they can move to the nuclei and attach to specific DNA sequences to start transcription of targeted genes that regulate inflammatory processes, cell division, and survival (Krajka-Kuźniak et al. 2024; Wu et al. 2011). By encouraging the production of antiapoptotic genes like Bcl-2 and Bcl-xL, which improve cell viability and endure chemotherapy, NF-κB plays a part in malignancy. Additionally, the process increases genes related to angiogenesis (VEGF), metastasis (MMP-9), and cell growth (cyclin D1) (Wu et al. 2011). It has become an important target for treatments for malignancy. It has been demonstrated that NF-κB activation stimulates chemokine receptors such as CXCR4 to facilitate cell migration and metastasis. Breast cancer cells that express CXCR4 have a higher propensity to invade and spread (Helbig et al. 2003). Numerous approaches to prevent the stimulation of NF-B are under consideration, such as the application of peptides, small molecule inhibitors, and naturally occurring substances like chalcones. The goal of these inhibitors is to stop the NF-κB pathway at multiple points, including cytokine-receptor relations, IKK setting up, and the nuclear movement of NF-κB (Aggarwal and Sung 2011) (Fig. 6).

4.2 STAT3 Pathway and Its Activation Mechanism

Among the most important mediators in cellular signaling pathways that are triggered by growth hormones and cytokines, particularly interleukin-6 (IL-6), is signal transducer and activator of transcription 3 (STAT3). As a result of cytokines attaching to particular receptors, like the IL-6 receptor, related Janus kinases (JAKs) become active. JAKs then cause the tyrosine amino acids on the receptor's cytoplasmic tail to become phosphorylated, which opens up docking sites for STAT3 proteins. These phosphorylated locations on the receptor complexes are where STAT3 proteins, which are initially dormant in the cytoplasm, interact.

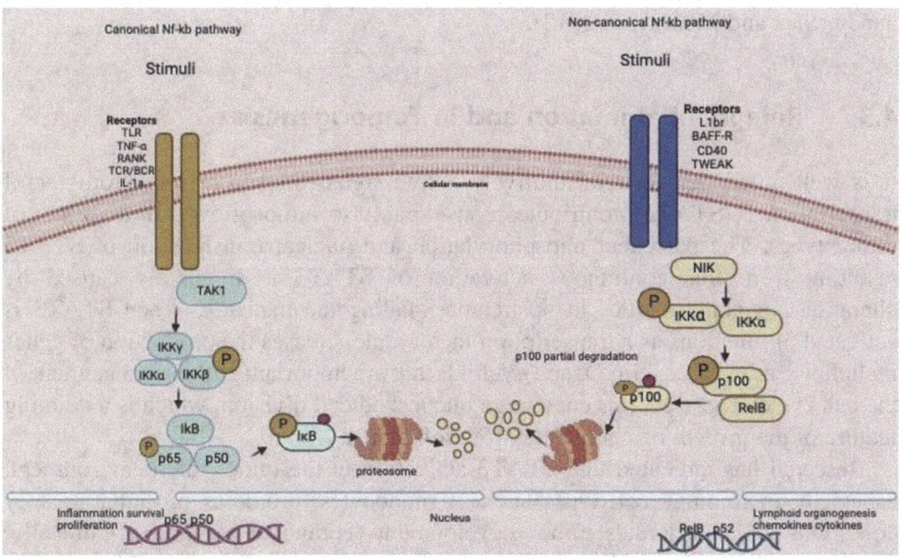

Fig. 6 NF Kappa B mechanism; canonical and non-canonical pathways

JAKs phosphorylate STAT3 at tyrosine 705 (Y705) upon binding. Because of this phosphorylation, STAT3 undergoes a conformational shift that makes it easier for it to dimerize. The dimers can create heterodimers with additional STAT proteins or homodimers (two identical STAT3 receptors) (Darnell 1997). Following phosphorylation, nuclear localization signals (NLS) inside the structure of STAT3 dimers induce their translocation from the cytoplasm to the nucleus. STAT3 dimers attach to specific pieces of DNA in the cytoplasm that are referred to as gamma-activated sequences (GAS) or STAT3-responsive elements (SREs) (Levy and Darnell 2002). By interacting with DNA, STAT3 can operate as a transcription factor and control the expression of target genes that play a role in a variety of biological activities. According to the situation and cellular environment, STAT3's transcriptional processes are capable of stimulating or inhibiting the expression of the genes it targets. STAT3 has a regulating function in many physiological processes, such as immunological reactions, cell viability, division, and growth (Pardoll 2012). Furthermore, STAT3 promotes cell division by activating cyclin D1 and c-Myc, which helps the cell cycles advance from the G1 to the S phase (Yu et al. 2009).

In immunological reactions, STAT3 controls T cell development toward Th17 cells, which are important in autoimmune conditions, and encourages the development of mature B cells and the generation of antibodies (Hirano et al. 2000). Additionally, STAT3 promotes tissue regeneration by macrophage polarization toward the M2 phenotype, yet in tumor situations, it can also promote tumor-promoting circumstances. Through the promotion of angiogenesis through VEGF production and the suppression of antitumor defenses, and prolonged stimulation of STAT3 by inflammatory mediators in the tumor, the microenvironment exacerbates carcinogenesis. Thus, STAT3 combines many signals to coordinate responses from cells that are essential for immune system control and the advancement of malignancy (Sica and Mantovani 2012).

4.3 Role in Inflammation and in Tumorigenesis

It is well noted that the constitutively active signal transducer and promoter of transcription 3 (STAT3) contributes considerably to tumor growth in a variety of tumor types. The persistent phosphorylation and nuclear translocation of STAT3 resulting from this continuous activation of STAT3 is frequently caused by alterations or abnormalities in upstream signaling mechanisms. When STAT3 is activated, it functions as a transcription factor and increases the production of genes including cyclin B1, cyclin D, and cyclin E that are important in the advancement of the cell cycle. These cyclins encourage unchecked cell division, which is a defining feature of the growth of malignancy (Pardoll 2012).

Research has indicated that STAT3 activation in the tumor microenvironment, especially in immune cell types such as monocytes, promotes pro-inflammatory conditions and accelerates tumor development (Hirano et al. 2000). Clinically, focusing on STAT3 signaling mechanisms has been a popular strategy for treating cancer. Blocking upstream kinases like JAKs, which phosphorylate STAT3, or directly inhibiting STAT3 dimerization and the binding of DNA are two methods used to prevent STAT3 stimulation. Interaction and combination in the tumor microenvironment, targeting STAT3 and NF-κB, frequently interact and influence each other's activities. Their mutual influence has a role in maintaining inflammation and advancing malignancy. Simultaneously targeting both mechanisms has demonstrated the potential to improve treatment results. For instance, the capacity of chalcones, a class of naturally occurring chemicals, to block the NF-κB and STAT3 pathways has been investigated. Chalcones and other polyphenols, such as curcumin, have been shown to work synergistically to decrease cellular inflammation and enhance apoptosis in cancer cells (Wu et al. 2011).

4.4 DNA Loss and Instability of the Genome

Numerous pathways allow inflammatory reactions to cause damage to DNA, which in turn leads to genomic instability, a feature of the onset of cancer. Among the crucial procedures involved are two important mechanisms that connect the onset of cancer and persistent inflammation harm to DNA and genomic instability (Fig. 7). The stimulation of ROS and RNS by immune cells amid inflammatory responses is one of these main processes. Reactive elements can directly alter DNA, leading to a variety of lesions such as more serious double-strand breaks (DSBs), base alterations, and single-strand breaks (Helbig et al. 2003). Such harm done to DNA not only jeopardizes the integrity of the genome but also raises the possibility of abnormalities that can lead to neoplastic changes. Apart from the direct harm done to DNA, inflammatory signals also trigger the activation of transcription factors like STAT3 and NF-κB. In addition to being important regulators of immunological responses, these substances can interfere with regular DNA repair processes.

Encouraging the creation of mutations and genomic instability through continuous activation of NF-κB and STAT3 can obstruct DNA repair processes, such as homologous recombination and joining of ends that are not homologous (Grivennikov et al. 2010). Furthermore, genomic instability is further exacerbated by strain on DNA replication brought on by inflammation. Replication stress is brought on by an ongoing inflammatory environment, which makes it difficult for cells to precisely replicate their DNA. Stress can result in chromosome changes, DSBs, and halted replication forks, and all of these raise the risk of tumor development and the advancement of malignancies (He and Karin 2011).

5 Inflammatory Cells in the Tumor Microenvironment

5.1 The Tumor-Associated Macrophages (TAMs)

TAMs are a part of the tumor microenvironment and are involved in the promotion of angiogenesis and also play a part in the suppression of antitumor immunity in the development of malignancy.

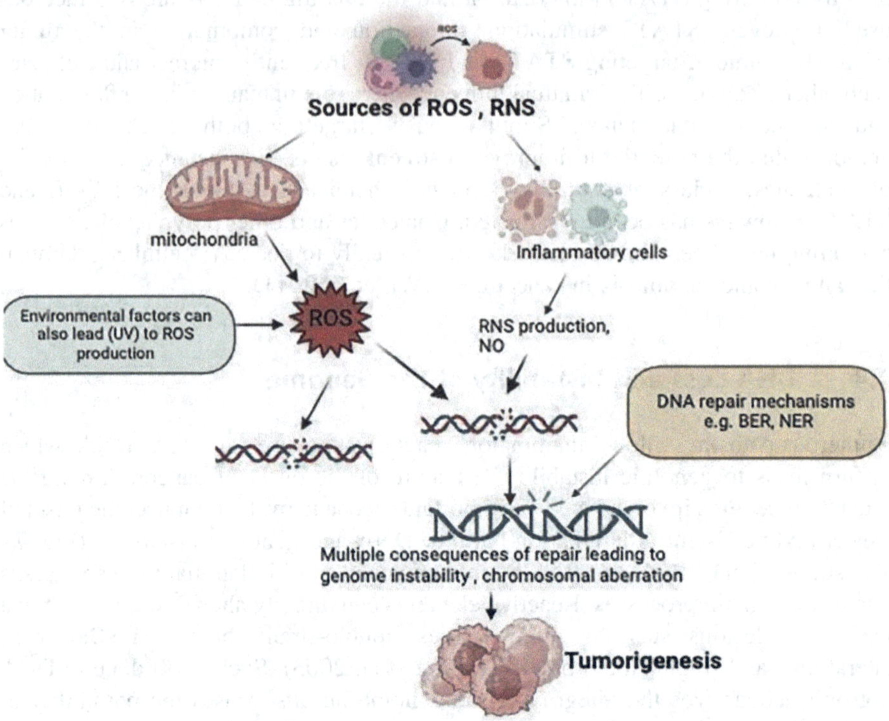

Fig. 7 The pathway depicting sources ROS and RNS production pathway which can lead to genome instability

5.1.1 Role in Formation of Angiogenesis

Angiogenesis, the process of forming new blood vessels to facilitate tumor development and metastases, is greatly aided by TAMs. They release many pro-angiogenic substances, including matrix metalloproteinases (MMPs), fibroblast growth factor (FGF), and vascular endothelial growth factor (VEGF) (Halazonetis et al. 2008). These elements improve the blood flow to the tumor by promoting the migration, growth, and vessel creation of endothelial cells. The tumor's progress and propensity for metastasis are encouraged by this enhanced vascularization, which makes it easier for the tumor to receive oxygen and nutrition. Numerous pro-angiogenic substances secreted by TAMs promote the migration, proliferation, and vessel development of endothelial cells (Fig. 8).

TAMs are an essential component of vascular endothelial growth factor (VEGF), which is a powerful stimulant of angiogenesis. New blood vessels surround the tumor as a result of VEGF's promotion of endothelial cell migration and proliferation (Mantovani et al. 2017). Fibroblast growth factor (FGF): TAMs also release FGF, which encourages angiogenesis by working in concert with VEGF. In the tumor microenvironment, FGF induces endothelial cell proliferation and facilitates

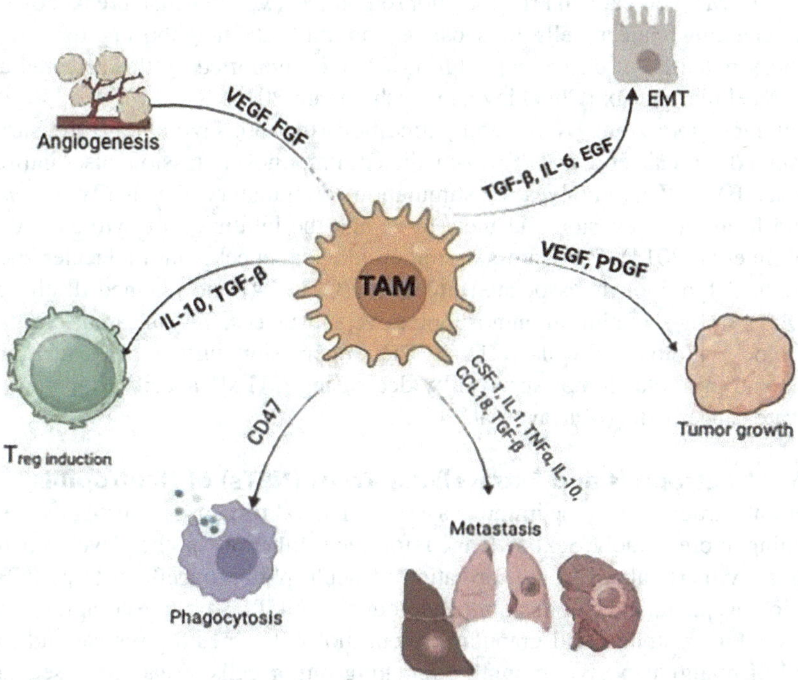

Fig. 8 TAMs' various roles in the tumor microenvironment

the development of capillary-like features (Murdoch et al. 2008). Increased blood flow surrounds the tumor as a result of TAMs' coordinated release of pro-angiogenic substances, which is crucial for providing vital nutrients and oxygen to cancer cells that are growing quickly. Furthermore, increased angiogenesis facilitates the spread of tumor cells to other locations, which aids in metastasis (Mantovani et al. 2008).

5.1.2 Encouragement of the Mesenchymal-to-Epithelial Transition

The natural process known as the "epithelial-mesenchymal transformation" (EMT) causes epithelial cells to lose some of their distinctive features and develop mesenchymal traits, which increases their ability to migrate and invade. This procedure is essential to the development of cancer because it promotes metastasis and treatment resistance.

5.1.3 Support of EMT by TAMs

Cytokines and growth factors are secreted by TAMs, including converting growth factor-beta (TGFβ), IL-6, and the growth factor epidermal (EGF), which is encouraged in nearby tumor cells (Galdiero et al. 2013). These variables lead to the appearance of mesechymal markers such as vimentin, which and N-cadherin to be upregulated, epithelial markers like E-cadherin to be downregulated, which facilitates the change to a more aggressive phenotypic. Remodeling the extracellular matrix: TAMs generate matrix metalloproteinases (MMPs) that break down the ECM, enabling cancer cells to separate and infiltrate neighboring tissues. The migratory potential of cancer cells during EMT is supported by this remodeling of the extracellular matrix (Chockley and Keshamouni 2016).

Immunosuppression: By fostering conditions that are favorable to the survival and spread of cancer cells, TAM-mediated immunosuppression also indirectly promotes EMT. This involves the stimulation of regulatory T cells (Tregs), which can aid in immune evasion and metastasis, and the inhibition of cytotoxic T cells (Franklin et al. 2014). By expressing immunological checkpoint molecules such as cytotoxic B-lymphocyte-associated protein 4 (CTLA-4) and planned death-ligand 1 (PDL1), or by secreting immunosuppressive substances, TAMs can also immediately block cytotoxic T cells (CTLs). This suppression further helps in immune escape and promotes tumor survival by decreasing CTLs' capacity to identify and eradicate cancer cells (Murray et al. 2014).

5.1.4 Neutrophils and Extracellular Traps (NETs) of Neutrophils

Important participants in the immune system's natural response, neutrophils are also becoming more widely acknowledged for their function in the development of malignancy, particularly in the formation of neutrophil extracellular traps (NETs). Function in spread and colonisation: By producing NETs, web-like complexes made of chromatin, histones, and granular protein molecules, neutrophils can aid in the spread of malignancy. By trapping circulating tumor cells, escape into secondary locations and endothelial attachment of cells are facilitated (Cedervall et al. 2015). Immunomodulatory functions: In addition, NETs can influence the tumor microenvironment through the promotion of inflammatory response and the regulation of immune system cell activities (Sangaletti et al. 2012). They have the ability to stimulate immune system cells like dendrite and macrophages which results in the release of chemokines and cytokines which impact the local immunological milieu. Excess NET creation, nevertheless, can also be a factor in long-term suppression and inflammatory processes, which create an environment that is conducive to tumor development and development.

5.1.5 The Role of Lymphocytes in the Development of Tumors

T cells and B cells are two examples of the multiple types of lymphocytes with intricate functions in the tumor microenvironment, influencing the dynamics of cancer growth as well as immunity against tumors. The role in the colonization and metastasis of tumor cells— immunological surveillance regulation: TILs, especially cytotoxic CD8+ T cells, are essential for immunological monitoring of tumor cells that have metastasized. These T cells identify and destroy circulating tumor cells (CTCs) which have entered the bloodstream and made an effort to settle in other organs. Improved clinical results across a range of malignancies are often correlated to an effect on lethal activity from TILs, suggesting that TILs play a role in preventing metastatic dissemination (Fridman et al. 2012). Encouragement of pre-metastatic niche development pre-metastatic niches in distant organs are formed in part by lymphocytes, such as Th17 cells and regulatory T cells (Tregs), which are subtypes of helper T cells. Tregs help in the release of a substance that is inflammatory and immunosuppressive due which promotes the colonization of CTCs by suppressing antitumor immune reactions locally. However, Th17 cells have a knack for increasing vascular permeability and angiogenesis, which makes it easier for CTCs to be recruited and survive at additional sites (Quail and Joyce 2013). Influence on vascular permeability and angiogenesis: Numerous cytokines and chemokines that lymphocytes secrete have an impact on vascular permeability and angiogenesis, two important mechanisms for the propagation of metastatic disease. For example, lymphocytes can release interleukin-8 (IL-8) that increases vascular permeability, which facilitates the extravasation of CTCs from circulation into surrounding tissues. Comparably, lymphocyte-secreted vascular endothelial growth factor (VEGF) encourages angiogenesis, guaranteeing blood supply for the expanding metastatic lesion.

6 Cytokines and Chemokines in Cancer Progression

6.1 Interleukin-6 in Cancer Formation

The pleiotropic cytokine interleukin-6 (IL-6) is essential for the control of allergic reactions and inflammation. Within the framework of cancer, IL-6 plays a role in multiple mechanisms that facilitate the growth and dissemination of tumors. Encouragement of tumor progression: IL-6 increases the growth of tumors by boosting multiple important processes.

Cell Proliferation By activating downstream signaling pathways like the Janus kinase-signal transducer and stimulator of transcription (JAK-STAT) route, IL-6, IL-10, IL-12, and TNF in (Fig. 9) signaling directly promotes the development of cancer cells. This pathway promotes unchecked cell development by controlling the proliferation of genes that regulate the course of the cell cycles (Heinrich et al. 2003).

IL-6 IL-6 is a cytokine that, after interacting with its receptor, IL-6R, activates the JAK-STAT signaling route, which is crucial in the development of malignancy. The phosphorylation of STAT proteins, especially STAT3, results from this stimulation. The STAT proteins then relocate to the nucleus where they control the activity of genes related to cell survival and growth. Inducing cell cycle regulators like cyclin D1 and upregulating antiapoptotic proteins like Bcl-2 and IL-6-mediated STAT3 activation promotes uncontrolled cell proliferation and longevity in a variety of malignancies (Hatano et al. 2020).

IL-10 Although mostly known as an immunosuppressive cytokine, IL-10 has also been linked to the advancement of cancer by affecting the processes that lead to cell survival and development. To control the activity of genes that regulate the advancement of the cell phase and the suppression of apoptosis, IL-10 promotes STAT3 signaling. Through the enhancement of antiapoptotic pathways and the promotion of

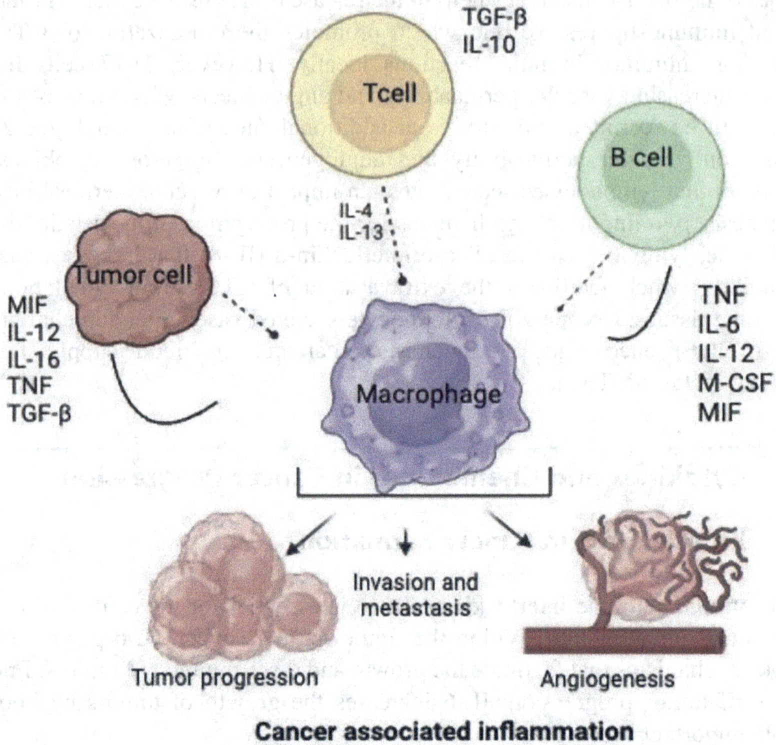

Fig. 9 An overview of the interaction of cells in the progression of tumor, angiogenesis, invasion, and metastasis

cell cycle progression in various kinds of cancer, this stimulation aids in the development and growth of tumor cells (Trinchieri 2003).

IL-12 IL-12 has been demonstrated to regulate the development of tumors by boosting cytotoxic T cell activity and improving antitumor defenses while being mostly known for its function in immune system response. It regulates subsequent processes that impact the advancement of cell cycles and survival, which has an impact on the growth of cells (Trinchieri 2003).

TNF TNF is a strong pro-inflammatory cytokine that triggers the signaling channels of NF-κB and mitogen-activated protein kinase (MAPK), which consequently control genes related to cell survival and development. In the tumor microenvironment, ongoing TNF signaling can promote unregulated cell viability and expansion, which can aid in the growth of malignancy (Balkwill 2009).

Cell Survival By inhibiting apoptotic or programmed cell death, IL-6 promotes the longevity of cancer cells. It increases antiapoptotic signaling and obstructs apoptotic pathways, which increases cancer cell viability in the tumor microenvironment (Helbig et al. 2003).

6.1.1 Role in Angiogenesis

Angiogenesis, the mechanism of forming novel blood vessels from previous vessels, is critical for tumor development and cancer metastases, and IL-6 plays a major role in stimulating this mechanism:

Pro-angiogenic factors, including fibroblast growth factor (FGF), vascular endothelial growth factor (VEGF), and interleukin-8 (IL-8), are expressed within both stromal and cancerous cells when IL-6 is present. These elements promote the expansion, growth, and development of tubes in endothelial cells, which aids in the formation of new blood vessels to provide the expanding tumor mass with both nourishment and oxygen (Rose-John 2012). Increased vascular permeability from IL-6 can facilitate the infiltration of growth stimulants, nutrients, and immune cells into the tumor microenvironment. This mechanism encourages the growth of tumors and makes it easier for malignant tumors to spread metastatically to other locations (Sansone et al. 2007).

6.2 Tumor Necrosis Factor-Alpha (TNFα) in the Advancement of Cancer

Tumor necrosis factor-alpha, or TNFα, is a pro-inflammatory cytokine that affects many facets of tumor development and growth and has an intricate role in the biology of cancer. TNFα stimulates tumor growth through multiple mechanisms.

Promotion of cell survival and proliferation: TNFα triggers signaling pathways that support the survival of cancer cells and growth, such as nuclear factor-kappa B (NF-κB) and mitogen-activated protein kinase (MAPK). Enhanced tumor cell proliferation and aversion to apoptosis result from this (Balkwill and Mantovani 2001).

Increase of angiogenesis: TNFα stimulates the creation of new blood vessels (angiogenesis) surrounding the tumor by inducing the production of angiogenic factors including VEGF and IL-8. This procedure improves the tumor's supply of blood, which promotes the growth and spread of the tumor (Carswell et al. 1975).

Function in the Tumor Microenvironment and Inflammation

Tumor Microenvironment TNFα has a role in fostering the development of a pro-inflammatory microenvironment. Additional cytokines and chemokines that are produced as a result of it attract immune system cells and encourage chronic inflammation; both of them are linked to an improvement in tumor virulence and development (Voronov et al. 2003).

Interactions with Stromal Cells In the tumor microenvironment, TNFα affects how fibroblasts and endothelial cells behave. It increases the synthesis of matrix metalloproteinases (MMPs) and extracellular matrix (ECM) proteins, which promote tumor spread and invasion (Sethi et al. 2008).

6.3 IL-1β in Cancer Development

Interleukin-1-beta, or IL-1β, and the Development of Cancer

A further significant pro-inflammatory factor that plays a major role in the advancement of malignancies is interleukin-1-beta (IL-1β): Encouragement of tumor growth—stimulation of proliferation and survival: By triggering the NF-κB and MAPK routes, IL-1β stimulates the growth of cancer cells. Moreover, it prevents apoptosis, which prolongs the life of malignant cells in the tumor microenvironment (Shanley et al. 1995).

Angiogenesis induction: Like TNFα, IL-1β stimulates the proliferation of angiogenic factors like FGF and VEGF, which encourages the development of new blood vessels surrounding the tumor. This mechanism facilitates the growth of tumors and opens doors for their metastatic spread (Lorentz and Bischoff 2001).

Increased Metastasis and Tumor Invasiveness

ECM Remodeling Tumor cell penetration into adjacent connective tissue and blood vessels is facilitated by IL-1β, which also increases the expression of MMPs along with other proteases. This makes cancer cells more capable of spreading to other organs (Voronov et al. 2003).

Immunological Stimulation In the tumor microenvironment, IL-1β modifies immunological reactions that impact immune system cells' recruiting and functioning. It may encourage immunosuppression mechanisms that let tumors develop and endure while avoiding immune detection (Mantovani et al. 2017). Comprehending the functions of TNFα and IL-1β in the advancement of cancer bears noteworthy consequences for treatment. Using certain inhibitors or antibodies to focus on these messenger molecules or their signaling networks is a potential strategy to stop tumor growth, lessen angiogenesis, and improve the efficacy of current cancer therapy (Galdiero et al. 2013).

6.4 Chemokines and Their Receptors in the Development of Cancer (CXCL12/CXCR4 Axis)

A class of tiny cytokines known as chemokines is involved in tumor biology, immunological reaction, and cell movement. The role of the CXCL12/CXCR4 axis in the advancement of cancer is notably noteworthy among the different chemokine axes.

C-X-C motif chemokine ligand 12, or CXCL12, is a chemokine that binds predominantly to the CXCR4 sensor. It is sometimes referred to as stromal cell–derived factor-1 (SDF-1). It appears in many different tissues, such as the liver, lungs, and bone marrow, and it forms a gradient that directs the movement of the cells which produce CXCR4. C-X-C motif chemokine receptor 4 is known as CXCR4. G-protein-coupled receptor CXCR4 has been identified in a variety of malignancies, including colorectal, lung, breast, and cancers of the prostate. The growth of tumors is aided by the activation of several downstream signaling pathways by the attachment of CXCL12 to CXCR4 (Balkwill 2009).

6.4.1 Part in the Development and Longevity of Tumors

Proliferation and survival: The link between CXCL12 and CXCR4 facilitates the growth and endurance of cancer cells. It triggers channels of signaling that are essential for cell cycle advancement and apoptosis suppression, including PI3K/AKT and MAPK/ERK. This increases the capacity of cancer cells to endure harsh environments, like those brought on by irradiation and chemo (Balkwill 2004). Angiogenesis is the process by which preexisting blood arteries divide into fresh ones, and the CXCL12/CXCR4 axis plays a role in this process. Tumor vascularization is aided by CXCL12, which promotes the migration of endothelial cells and multiplication. Tumors receive more oxygen and nutrients as a result, which supports their development and propensity for metastasis (Sun et al. 2010).

Chemotaxis and Invasion Cancerous cells harboring CXCR4 are drawn to CXCL12-rich tissues like the lungs, liver, and bone marrow by CXCL12, which functions as a chemoattractant. The infiltration of cancer cells onto these far-off locations is facilitated by this motile immigration, which aids in metastasis (Ozga et al. 2021). The procedure that occurs when epithelial cells take on skin, migrating characteristics is known as the epithelial-mesenchymal transition (EMT), and it is also influenced by the CXCL12/CXCR4 axis. In the metastasis cascade, epithelial-mesenchymal transition (EMT) is a crucial stage that allows tumor cells to separate from the main tumor, infiltrate neighboring tissues, and spread to other organs (Müller et al. 2001).

7 Treatment Approaches for Cancer That Aim to Reduce Inflammation

7.1 Anti-inflammatory Medication

NSAIDs or nonsteroidal anti-inflammatory medications are popular drugs that lower high temperature, discomfort, and inflammation. Their main mode of activity is the suppression of the cyclooxygenase (COX) enzymes, which are essential for the production of prostaglandins, which are lipid molecules that cause irritation (Hawkey 1999).

Method of Action

NSAIDs block COX-1 and COX-2 enzymes, which reduce prostaglandin synthesis. Prostaglandins have a role in inflammation or the upkeep of the stomach's protective interior, among other physiological functions. NSAIDs reduce prostaglandin levels, which reduce discomfort and swelling (Simmons et al. 2004; Vane and Botting 1998). A lower incidence of colorectal cancer is being linked to long-term usage of NSAIDs, especially aspirin. According to a systematic review of qualitative research, using aspirin on an ongoing basis could reduce the incidence of colorectal carcinoma by about 20–30%.

7.2 COX-2 Repressors

The gastrointestinal negative consequences of non-select NSAIDs, which inhibit both COX-1 and COX-2, are reduced by inhibitors of COX-2, a category of NSAIDs that specifically block the COX-2 enzyme.

Method of Action

COX-2 inhibitors are designed to precisely locate the COX-2 enzyme, which is elevated in many types of cancer and is triggered during inflammation. These medications lessen discomfort and swelling by specifically blocking COX-2, preserving the beneficial effects of COX-1 on the stomach mucosa (Müller et al. 2001).

Function in the Treatment of Cancer

COX-2 inhibitors can stop tumor growth and metastasis; they have shown promise in the treatment of cancer. Anticancer therapy finds COX-2 to be a desirable target due to its overexpression in numerous tumors (Bertagnolli et al. 2006).

7.3 Cytokine Inhibitors in the Treatment of Tumors

Medicinal substances known as "cytokine inhibitors" are made to prevent the release of particular cytokines, which are important agents in inflammation. The inhibitors address cytokines involved in tumor development and immune escape in the treatment of cancer.

Method of Actions TNFα is bound by anti-TNF treatments, which stop it from binding to receptors found on cell surfaces. This suppression has the potential to lessen angiogenesis and cellular proliferation—two processes that support tumor growth—as well as trigger an inflammatory reaction (Balkwill 2004).

Clinical Uses Infliximab and adalimumab, two anti-TNF medications, are frequently employed to treat autoimmune disorders such as rheumatoid arthritis and bowel inflammation. They are being investigated for use in therapy for cancer, and some research indicates that they can reduce tumor development and migration (Müller et al. 2001).

7.4 IL-1β Inhibition

A pro-inflammatory factor that is linked to a number of malignancies is interleukin-1-beta (IL1β).

Method of Action To inhibit IL-1β action, monoclonal antibodies or channel antagonists are used in IL-1β blocking. This blockade may slow the growth of tumors and lessen inflammation (Bertagnolli et al. 2006).

Clinical Uses The IL-1β inhibiting monoclonal canakinumab has demonstrated potential in reducing inflammation and perhaps the risk of cancer relapse in individuals with cardiovascular disorders, suggesting that it may have advantages in the field of cancer (Dinarello 2011).

7.5 Immune Cell Regulators in the Treatment of Cancer

Immunity cell modulators are treatments intended to modify the function of immune cells and behavior in the microenvironment of tumors to improve antitumor reactions and stop the spread of disease. In this context, leukocyte regulation and macrophage programming are two significant fields of interest.

Stem Cell Reprogramming

Macrophages are multifunctional immune cells that can change their functional state in response to cues from their surroundings. To stop tumor growth and metastasis in the context of cancer, macrophages can be reprogrammed from an antitumor (M1-like) phenotype to a pro-tumor (M2like) phenotype (De Palma and Lewis 2013). The therapeutic effect of transforming monocytes to an M1-like phenotype is enhanced phagocytosis of tumor cells, production of pro-inflammatory cytokines, and presentation of antigens to T cells, all of which contribute to a strong defense against tumors.

Clinical trials for a variety of malignancies are investigating this strategy, which has demonstrated encouraging outcomes in preclinical research (Gordon and Martinez 2010; Jaynes et al. 2020).

Modulation of Neutrophils

A different kind of immune cell involved in malignancy is the neutrophil, which can both stimulate and impede the growth of tumors. One potential treatment approach is to increase the antitumor capabilities of neutrophils by modifying their behavior.

Mechanism of Modulation Within the tumor microenvironment, neutrophils are recruited, activated, and have their structural features altered. This may be accomplished in a number of ways, such as by blocking the creation of extracellular neutrophil traps (NETs), targeting chemokine receptors (such as CXCR2), or using growth variables and cytokines that affect neutrophil behavior (Coffelt et al. 2016; The Multifaceted Roles Neutrophils Play in the Tumor Microenvironment – PubMed n.d.).

Therapeutic Impact Neutrophils can be made more effective in killing tumor cells and supporting other immune responses against tumors by reducing their pro-tumor activities, such as promoting angiogenesis and metastasis, by regulating their behavior. There is active research being done on this strategy in preclinical models and clinical investigations (Origin and Role of a Subset of Tumor-Associated Neutrophils with Antigen-Presenting Cell Features in Early-Stage Human Lung Cancer – PubMed n.d.; Shaul and Fridlender 2019).

8 Novel Techniques and Potential Treatments in the Management of Cancer

8.1 Anti-Inflammatory in Nature Cancer Therapy Using Nanotechnology

Novel methods to address inflammation in cancer treatment are provided by nanotechnology. Anti-inflammatory drugs can be specifically delivered via nanoparticles to the tumor microenvironment, increasing treatment effectiveness and lowering systemic adverse effects.

Tailored Drug Delivery Tumor cells and the inflammatory elements of the tumor's microenvironment can be the precise targets of particles. For instance, anti-inflammatory drugs like NSAIDs or corticosteroids can be put into liposomes as nanoparticles of polymeric material, and gold nanoparticles in order to provide localized therapy and reduce harm to tissues that are healthy (Ferrari 2005; Shaul and Fridlender 2019).

The improved penetration and retention, or EPR, effect occurs when there is a greater accumulation of nanoparticles in the cancerous tissue as opposed to typical tissues because tumors frequently have faulty vasculature. Therapeutic medicines can be delivered to the tumor site more effectively thanks to this increased permeability and retention (EPR) impact (Diverse Applications of Nanomedicine – PubMed n.d.; Tumor vascular permeability and the EPR effect in macromolecular therapeutics: a review – PubMed n.d.).

8.2 Methods in Personalized Medicine

Customizing cancer treatments to each patient's unique tumor's genetic, molecular, and clinical features is known as personalized medicine. This strategy seeks to lessen side effects while increasing treatment efficacy.

Genomic Profiling Cancer specialists can choose tailored medicines that have the best chance of working by examining genetic mutations and alterations present in a patient's tumor. For example, EGFR antagonists may be beneficial for individuals with certain abnormalities in the *EGFR* gene, and trastuzumab may be effective for those with HER2-positive breast cancer (Genomic medicine frontier in human solid tumors: prospects and challenges – PubMed n.d.; Tsimberidou et al. 2012).

Biomarker-Based Treatments The application of immune checkpoint inhibitors can be directed by indicators, such as PD-L1 gene expression rates. Better reactions to anti-PD-1/PD-L1 medicines have been linked to higher levels of PD-L1 protein production in tumors, enabling more individualized therapy regimens (Brauch and Schwab 2014).

Pharmacogenomics Determining the right dose and reducing safety can be aided by knowing how an individual's genetic composition influences drug absorption and reaction. According to CYP2D6 genotyping, pharmacogenomic analysis can direct the administration of medications such as tamoxifen in breast cancer patients (Zitvogel et al. 2006).

8.3 Immunotherapy and Chemotherapy

Chemotherapy plus immunotherapy has demonstrated considerable effectiveness. Chemotherapy can cause immunogenic cell death, which improves how the body's immune system perceives tumor antigen. Consequently, immune checkpoint inhibitors such as PD1/PD-L1 and CTLA-4 blockers become more effective.

Enhanced Immune Response Tumor antigens and damage-related molecular patterns (DAMPs), which activate the body's immune system, can be expressed more frequently during chemo. For example, research has demonstrated that doxorubicin and cyclophosphamide can both boost immune system cell penetration into tumors and enhance the body's reaction to immune checkpoints blockage (Topalian et al. 2012).

Synergistic Effects Individuals with non-small cell cancer of the lungs (NSCLC) have shown better results when pembrolizumab, an anti-PD-1 antibody, is combined with chemotherapy as opposed to chemotherapy alone. Improved clinical outcomes result from this synergy's enhancement of antitumor immune system reactions (Gandhi et al. 2018).

The Synergistic Mechanisms

Medicines for chemotherapy such as taxanes and platinum-based treatments have the ability to cause ICD, or immunogenic cell death, in tumor cells. Damage-associated molecular structures (DAMPs) and tumor proteins are released in response to immunological CD (ICD), which activates dendritic cells and improves the dissemination of antigens. This makes the body's immune system more capable of identifying and eliminating tumor cells (Galluzzi et al. 2017; Gandhi et al. 2018).

An Immune System Checkpoint Blockade Pembrolizumab supports the PD-1/PK-L1 route, which plays a role in reducing T cell activity inside the tumor the surrounding microenvironment pembrolizumab increases T cell activity by inhibiting PD-1, enabling members to identify and destroy tumor cells that have previously eluded immune monitoring. The path of PD-1/PD-L1 and T cell oversight autoimmune checkpoint mechanisms which regulate responses from T cells include the programmed cell death protein 1 (PD-1) receptor and its ligands, PD-L1 and PD-L2. Tumor cells and related immune system cells in malignancy have the ability to increase PD-L1 expression as a means of avoiding immune monitoring. When PD-L1 binds to PD-1 on T cells, it sends signals of inhibition that prevent T cells from activating and performing their functional activities. This encourages tumor cells to evade the immune system's defenses (Pardoll 2012).

Radiation Therapy Personalized medicine and radiation therapy can be used to increase the effectiveness of each therapy. Radiation damages DNA and can increase a tumor's sensitivity to drugs that have the goal of attacking it. A monoclonal antibody called pembrolizumab targets T cells' PD-1 selectively. Pembrolizumab prevents the inhibition of the activation of T cells by adhering to PD-1 and blocking the inhibitory signals that PD-L1 transmits. Because of this inhibition, T cells get reactivated and can identify and destroy tumor cells that would otherwise evade immune recognition and death (Sunshine and Taube 2015).

Radiosensitization Tailored treatments, such cetuximab, an EGFR inhibitory agent, can make tumors more sensitive to radiation. Given the prevalence of EGFR amplification in head and neck malignancies, this combination has been especially successful in treating these diseases. In a considerable number of neck and head malignancies, EGFR is overexpressed or increased, which promotes tumor development, survival, and resistance to treatments like irradiation. A type of monoclonal antibody called cetuximab targets EGFR and disrupts upstream signaling pathways that are important for cell viability and growth. This increases the susceptibility of tumors to radiation therapies (Bonner et al. 2006).

9 Challenges and Future Directions

9.1 Finding a Treatment of Drug Resistance

Drug resistance is still a major therapy challenge for malignancy, as tumors frequently become resistant to treatments that were formerly successful. Genetic mutations, epigenetic modifications, or adaptive processes in the tumor microenvironment can all contribute to this occurrence.

Mechanisms of Resistance It is essential to comprehend the molecular processes underlying drug resistance. Resistance can be caused, for example, by changes in drug targets (EGFR alterations in lung cancer) or stimulation of different survival systems (PI3K/Akt/mTOR pathway in breast cancer) (Stine et al. 2015).

EGFR Changes in Lung Carcinoma Changes or changes in the gene that encodes EGFR frequently result in resistance to certain types of targeted therapy, such as EGFR drugs, in cancers of the lungs. Over time, these modifications may result in modifications to the EGFR drug-binding site, which would decrease therapy efficacy (Yarden and Pines 2012). Enhancing people's quality of life and compliance to therapies depends on minimizing the adverse consequences of chemotherapy for cancer. One strategy is to utilize targeted medicines, which reduce systemic harm by precisely inhibiting tumor cells while preserving functioning organs (Chabner and Roberts 2005). Reducing the side effects of cancer treatments is another problem since they can have a big influence on people's quality of life and compliance with their treatment regimens.

9.2 Precision Medicine

Treatments can be tailored to reduce needless side effects by using biomarkers and genetic analysis. For instance, trastuzumab and other HER2-targeted treatments are beneficial for treating HER2-positive breast cancer, but they can also be harmful to the heart in certain people (Cameron et al. 2013).

9.2.1 HER2-Positive Breast Cancer Treated with Trastuzumab

Targeting HER2, or human epidermal growth factor receptor 2, a protein that is overexpressed in 20–25% of breast cancer cases, is trastuzumab, a sort of monoclonal antibody. Trastuzumab is a very successful treatment for cancers that are HER2 positive, yet certain individuals may have cardiac toxicities as a result of its mode of behavior, which affects the cardiac system (Ewer and Ewer 2015).

Biomarkers and genetic testing are used in targeted therapy to determine individuals who are more likely to experience certain adverse reactions, such as heart toxicity from trastuzumab. Throughout therapy, biomarkers such as natriuretic peptides and troponin are employed to track the condition of the heart. This enables the early identification of cardiotoxicity and the modification of therapies as necessary (Yang et al. 2021).

10 Conclusion

The complex interactions between inflammation and cancer highlight its critical significance at every step of the disease's initiation, spread, and metastasis. Through the generation of reactive molecules, the stimulation of important transcription factors, and the emergence of genetic instability, chronic inflammation creates a situation that is conducive to tumor growth. Tumor-associated macrophages and neutrophils are examples of immune cells that also stimulate angiogenesis, inhibit antitumor immunity, and encourage metastasis. Pro-inflammatory cytokines and chemokines play a part in the course of cancer by promoting tumor formation, angiogenesis, and metastasis. In order to slow the growth of tumors, current treatment approaches, such as immune modulators and anti-inflammatory medications, try to interfere with these inflammatory reactions. Anticipating ahead, personalized medicine will play a significant role in cancer therapy by using proteomic and genetic data to customize therapies based on the unique characteristics of each patient. Combining therapies provides the potential to address the complex character of tumors and enhance treatment outcomes by combining anti-inflammatory drugs with traditional therapies. Targeted delivery systems and innovative innovations like modifying genes and nanotechnology are being driven by the imperative goals of reducing adverse reactions and eliminating drug resistance. We can transform the complex association between inflammation and tumors into effective medicines that improve the likelihood of survival and the standard of life for cancer patients by utilizing these tactics and carrying out extensive studies.

References

Aggarwal BB, Sung B (2011) NF-κB in cancer: a matter of life and death. Cancer Discov 1:469–471. https://doi.org/10.1158/2159-8290.CD-11-0260

Allavena P, Garlanda C, Borrello MG, Sica A, Mantovani A (2008) Pathways connecting inflammation and cancer. Curr Opin Genet Dev 18:3–10. https://doi.org/10.1016/j.gde.2008.01.003

Balkwill F (2004) Cancer and the chemokine network. Nat Rev Cancer 4:540–550. https://doi.org/10.1038/nrc1388

Balkwill F (2009) Tumour necrosis factor and cancer. Nat Rev Cancer 9:361–371. https://doi.org/10.1038/nrc2628

Balkwill F, Mantovani A (2001) Inflammation and cancer: back to Virchow? Lancet Lond Engl 357:539–545. https://doi.org/10.1016/S0140-6736(00)04046-0

Bertagnolli MM, Eagle CJ, Zauber AG, Redston M, Solomon SD, Kim K, Tang J, Rosenstein RB, Wittes J, Corle D, Hess TM, Woloj GM, Boisserie F, Anderson WF, Viner JL, Bagheri D, Burn J, Chung DC, Dewar T, Foley TR, Hoffman N, Macrae F, Pruitt RE, Saltzman JR, Salzberg B, Sylwestrowicz T, Gordon GB, Hawk ET, APC Study Investigators (2006) Celecoxib for the prevention of sporadic colorectal adenomas. N Engl J Med 355:873–884. https://doi.org/10.1056/NEJMoa061355

Bonner JA, Harari PM, Giralt J, Azarnia N, Shin DM, Cohen RB, Jones CU, Sur R, Raben D, Jassem J, Ove R, Kies MS, Baselga J, Youssoufian H, Amellal N, Rowinsky EK, Ang KK (2006) Radiotherapy plus cetuximab for squamous-cell carcinoma of the head and neck. N Engl J Med 354:567–578. https://doi.org/10.1056/NEJMoa053422

Bos JL (1989) Ras oncogenes in human cancer: a review. Cancer Res 49:4682–4689

Brauch H, Schwab M (2014) Prediction of tamoxifen outcome by genetic variation of CYP2D6 in post-menopausal women with early breast cancer. Br J Clin Pharmacol 77:695–703. https://doi.org/10.1111/bcp.12229

Cameron D, Brown J, Dent R, Jackisch C, Mackey J, Pivot X, Steger GG, Suter TM, Toi M, Parmar M, Laeufle R, Im Y-H, Romieu G, Harvey V, Lipatov O, Pienkowski T, Cottu P, Chan A, Im S-A, Hall PS, Bubuteishvili-Pacaud L, Henschel V, Deurloo RJ, Pallaud C, Bell R (2013) Adjuvant bevacizumab-containing therapy in triple-negative breast cancer (BEATRICE): primary results of a randomised, phase 3 trial. Lancet Oncol 14:933–942. https://doi.org/10.1016/S1470-2045(13)70335-8

Cancer genome landscapes – PubMed [WWW Document], (n.d.). URL https://pubmed.ncbi.nlm.nih.gov/23539594/. Accessed 7 June 2024.

Carswell EA, Old LJ, Kassel RL, Green S, Fiore N, Williamson B (1975) An endotoxin-induced serum factor that causes necrosis of tumors. Proc Natl Acad Sci USA 72:3666–3670. https://doi.org/10.1073/pnas.72.9.3666

Cedervall J, Zhang Y, Huang H, Zhang L, Femel J, Dimberg A, Olsson A-K (2015) Neutrophil extracellular traps accumulate in peripheral blood vessels and compromise organ function in tumor-bearing animals. Cancer Res 75:2653–2662. https://doi.org/10.1158/0008-5472.CAN-14-3299

Chabner BA, Roberts TG (2005) Timeline: chemotherapy and the war on cancer. Nat Rev Cancer 5: 65–72. https://doi.org/10.1038/nrc1529

Chockley PJ, Keshamouni VG (2016) Immunological consequences of epithelial-mesenchymal transition in tumor progression. J Immunol Baltim Md 1950(197):691–698. https://doi.org/10.4049/jimmunol.1600458

Coffelt SB, Wellenstein MD, de Visser KE (2016) Neutrophils in cancer: neutral no more. Nat Rev Cancer 16:431–446. https://doi.org/10.1038/nrc.2016.52

Colotta F, Allavena P, Sica A, Garlanda C, Mantovani A (2009) Cancer-related inflammation, the seventh hallmark of cancer: links to genetic instability. Carcinogenesis 30:1073–1081. https://doi.org/10.1093/carcin/bgp127

Coussens LM, Werb Z (2002) Inflammation and cancer. Nature 420:860–867. https://doi.org/10.1038/nature01322

Dang CV (2012) MYC on the path to cancer. Cell 149:22–35. https://doi.org/10.1016/j.cell.2012.03.003

Darnell JE (1997) STATs and gene regulation. Science 277:1630–1635. https://doi.org/10.1126/science.277.5332.1630

De Palma M, Lewis CE (2013) Macrophage regulation of tumor responses to anticancer therapies. Cancer Cell 23:277–286. https://doi.org/10.1016/j.ccr.2013.02.013

Dinarello CA (2011) Interleukin-1 in the pathogenesis and treatment of inflammatory diseases. Blood 117:3720–3732. https://doi.org/10.1182/blood-2010-07-273417

Diverse Applications of Nanomedicine – PubMed [WWW Document] (n.d.). URL https://pubmed.ncbi.nlm.nih.gov/28290206/. Accessed 7 Mar 2024

Ekbom A, Helmick C, Zack M, Adami HO (1990) Ulcerative colitis and colorectal cancer. A population-based study. N Engl J Med 323:1228–1233. https://doi.org/10.1056/NEJM199011013231802

Ewer MS, Ewer SM (2015) Cardiotoxicity of anticancer treatments. Nat Rev Cardiol 12:547–558. https://doi.org/10.1038/nrcardio.2015.65

Ferrari M (2005) Cancer nanotechnology: opportunities and challenges. Nat Rev Cancer 5:161–171. https://doi.org/10.1038/nrc1566

Folkman J (2002) Role of angiogenesis in tumor growth and metastasis. Semin Oncol 29:15–18. https://doi.org/10.1053/sonc.2002.37263

Franklin RA, Liao W, Sarkar A, Kim MV, Bivona MR, Liu K, Pamer EG, Li MO (2014) The cellular and molecular origin of tumor-associated macrophages. Science 344:921–925. https://doi.org/10.1126/science.1252510

Fridman WH, Pagès F, Sautès-Fridman C, Galon J (2012) The immune contexture in human tumours: impact on clinical outcome. Nat Rev Cancer 12:298–306. https://doi.org/10.1038/nrc3245

Galdiero MR, Garlanda C, Jaillon S, Marone G, Mantovani A (2013) Tumor associated macrophages and neutrophils in tumor progression. J Cell Physiol 228:1404–1412. https://doi.org/10.1002/jcp.24260

Galluzzi L, Baehrecke EH, Ballabio A, Boya P, Bravo-San Pedro JM, Cecconi F, Choi AM, Chu CT, Codogno P, Colombo MI, Cuervo AM, Debnath J, Deretic V, Dikic I, Eskelinen E-L, Fimia GM, Fulda S, Gewirtz DA, Green DR, Hansen M, Harper JW, Jäättelä M, Johansen T, Juhasz G, Kimmelman AC, Kraft C, Ktistakis NT, Kumar S, Levine B, Lopez-Otin C, Madeo F, Martens S, Martinez J, Melendez A, Mizushima N, Münz C, Murphy LO, Penninger JM, Piacentini M, Reggiori F, Rubinsztein DC, Ryan KM, Santambrogio L, Scorrano L, Simon AK, Simon H-U, Simonsen A, Tavernarakis N, Tooze SA, Yoshimori T, Yuan J, Yue Z, Zhong Q, Kroemer G (2017) Molecular definitions of autophagy and related processes. EMBO J 36:1811–1836. https://doi.org/10.15252/embj.201796697

Gandhi L, Rodríguez-Abreu D, Gadgeel S, Esteban E, Felip E, De Angelis F, Domine M, Clingan P, Hochmair MJ, Powell SF, Cheng SY-S, Bischoff HG, Peled N, Grossi F, Jennens RR, Reck M, Hui R, Garon EB, Boyer M, Rubio-Viqueira B, Novello S, Kurata T, Gray JE, Vida J, Wei Z, Yang J, Raftopoulos H, Pietanza MC, Garassino MC, KEYNOTE-189 Investigators (2018) Pembrolizumab plus chemotherapy in metastatic non-small-cell lung cancer. N Engl J Med 378:2078–2092. https://doi.org/10.1056/NEJMoa1801005

Genomic medicine frontier in human solid tumors: prospects and challenges – PubMed [WWW Document] (n.d.). URL https://pubmed.ncbi.nlm.nih.gov/23589551/. Accessed 7 Mar 2024

Gordon S, Martinez FO (2010) Alternative activation of macrophages: mechanism and functions. Immunity 32:593–604. https://doi.org/10.1016/j.immuni.2010.05.007

Graus-Porta D, Beerli RR, Daly JM, Hynes NE (1997) ErbB-2, the preferred heterodimerization partner of all ErbB receptors, is a mediator of lateral signaling. EMBO J 16:1647–1655. https://doi.org/10.1093/emboj/16.7.1647

Grivennikov SI, Greten FR, Karin M (2010) Immunity, inflammation, and cancer. Cell 140:883–899. https://doi.org/10.1016/j.cell.2010.01.025

Halazonetis TD, Gorgoulis VG, Bartek J (2008) An oncogene-induced DNA damage model for cancer development. Science 319:1352–1355. https://doi.org/10.1126/science.1140735

Hanahan D, Weinberg RA (2011) Hallmarks of cancer: the next generation. Cell 144:646–674. https://doi.org/10.1016/j.cell.2011.02.013

Hatano K, Fujita K, Nonomura N (2020) Application of anti-inflammatory agents in prostate cancer. J Clin Med 9:2680. https://doi.org/10.3390/jcm9082680

Hawkey CJ (1999) COX-2 inhibitors. Lancet Lond Engl 353:307–314. https://doi.org/10.1016/s0140-6736(98)12154-2

He G, Karin M (2011) NF-κB and STAT3 – key players in liver inflammation and cancer. Cell Res 21:159–168. https://doi.org/10.1038/cr.2010.183

Heinrich PC, Behrmann I, Haan S, Hermanns HM, Müller-Newen G, Schaper F (2003) Principles of interleukin (IL)-6-type cytokine signalling and its regulation. Biochem J 374:1–20. https://doi.org/10.1042/BJ20030407

Helbig G, Christopherson KW, Bhat-Nakshatri P, Kumar S, Kishimoto H, Miller KD, Broxmeyer HE, Nakshatri H (2003) NF-kappaB promotes breast cancer cell migration and metastasis by inducing the expression of the chemokine receptor CXCR4. J Biol Chem 278:21631–21638. https://doi.org/10.1074/jbc.M300609200

Hirano T, Ishihara K, Hibi M (2000) Roles of STAT3 in mediating the cell growth, differentiation and survival signals relayed through the IL-6 family of cytokine receptors. Oncogene 19:2548–2556. https://doi.org/10.1038/sj.onc.1203551

Hussain SP, Harris CC (2007) Inflammation and cancer: an ancient link with novel potentials. Int J Cancer 121:2373–2380. https://doi.org/10.1002/ijc.23173

Infiltrating neutrophils mediate the initial angiogenic switch in a mouse model of multistage carcinogenesis – PubMed [WWW Document] (n.d.). URL https://pubmed.ncbi.nlm.nih.gov/16891410/. Accessed 7 June 2024

Jaynes JM, Sable R, Ronzetti M, Bautista W, Knotts Z, Abisoye-Ogunniyan A, Li D, Calvo R, Dashnyam M, Singh A, Guerin T, White J, Ravichandran S, Kumar P, Talsania K, Chen V, Ghebremedhin A, Karanam B, Bin Salam A, Amin R, Odzorig T, Aiken T, Nguyen V, Bian Y, Zarif JC, de Groot AE, Mehta M, Fan L, Hu X, Simeonov A, Pate N, Abu-Asab M, Ferrer M, Southall N, Ock C-Y, Zhao Y, Lopez H, Kozlov S, de Val N, Yates CC, Baljinnyam B, Marugan J, Rudloff U (2020) Mannose receptor (CD206) activation in tumor-associated macrophages enhances adaptive and innate antitumor immune responses. Sci Transl Med 12: eaax6337. https://doi.org/10.1126/scitranslmed.aax6337

Jones PA, Baylin SB (2002) The fundamental role of epigenetic events in cancer. Nat Rev Genet 3: 415–428. https://doi.org/10.1038/nrg816

Kalluri R, Weinberg RA (2009) The basics of epithelial-mesenchymal transition. J Clin Invest 119: 1420–1428. https://doi.org/10.1172/JCI39104

Karin M (2006) Nuclear factor-kappaB in cancer development and progression. Nature 441:431–436. https://doi.org/10.1038/nature04870

Karin M, Greten FR (2005) NF-kappaB: linking inflammation and immunity to cancer development and progression. Nat Rev Immunol 5:749–759. https://doi.org/10.1038/nri1703

Klaunig JE, Kamendulis LM (2004) The role of oxidative stress in carcinogenesis. Annu Rev Pharmacol Toxicol 44:239–267. https://doi.org/10.1146/annurev.pharmtox.44.101802.121851

Konecny GE, Pegram MD, Venkatesan N, Finn R, Yang G, Rahmeh M, Untch M, Rusnak DW, Spehar G, Mullin RJ, Keith BR, Gilmer TM, Berger M, Podratz KC, Slamon DJ (2006) Activity of the dual kinase inhibitor lapatinib (GW572016) against HER-2-overexpressing and trastuzumab-treated breast cancer cells. Cancer Res 66:1630–1639. https://doi.org/10.1158/0008-5472.CAN-05-1182

Krajka-Kuźniak V, Belka M, Papierska K (2024) Targeting STAT3 and NF-κB signaling pathways in cancer prevention and treatment: the role of Chalcones. Cancers 16:1092. https://doi.org/10.3390/cancers16061092

Kundu JK, Surh Y-J (2008) Inflammation: gearing the journey to cancer. Mutat Res 659:15–30. https://doi.org/10.1016/j.mrrev.2008.03.002

Levy DE, Darnell JE (2002) Stats: transcriptional control and biological impact. Nat Rev Mol Cell Biol 3:651–662. https://doi.org/10.1038/nrm909

Lorentz A, Bischoff SC (2001) Regulation of human intestinal mast cells by stem cell factor and IL-4. Immunol Rev 179:57–60. https://doi.org/10.1034/j.1600-065x.2001.790106.x

Mantovani A, Allavena P, Sica A, Balkwill F (2008) Cancer-related inflammation. Nature 454:436–444. https://doi.org/10.1038/nature07205

Mantovani A, Marchesi F, Malesci A, Laghi L, Allavena P (2017) Tumour-associated macrophages as treatment targets in oncology. Nat Rev Clin Oncol 14:399–416. https://doi.org/10.1038/nrclinonc.2016.217

Müller A, Homey B, Soto H, Ge N, Catron D, Buchanan ME, McClanahan T, Murphy E, Yuan W, Wagner SN, Barrera JL, Mohar A, Verástegui E, Zlotnik A (2001) Involvement of chemokine receptors in breast cancer metastasis. Nature 410:50–56. https://doi.org/10.1038/35065016

Munn LL (2017) Cancer and inflammation. Wiley Interdiscip Rev Syst Biol Med 9. https://doi.org/10.1002/wsbm.1370

Murdoch C, Muthana M, Coffelt SB, Lewis CE (2008) The role of myeloid cells in the promotion of tumour angiogenesis. Nat Rev Cancer 8:618–631. https://doi.org/10.1038/nrc2444

Murray PJ, Allen JE, Biswas SK, Fisher EA, Gilroy DW, Goerdt S, Gordon S, Hamilton JA, Ivashkiv LB, Lawrence T, Locati M, Mantovani A, Martinez FO, Mege J-L, Mosser DM, Natoli G, Saeij JP, Schultze JL, Shirey KA, Sica A, Suttles J, Udalova I, van Ginderachter JA, Vogel SN, Wynn TA (2014) Macrophage activation and polarization: nomenclature and experimental guidelines. Immunity 41:14–20. https://doi.org/10.1016/j.immuni.2014.06.008

New functions for the matrix metalloproteinases in cancer progression – PubMed [WWW Document] (n.d.). URL https://pubmed.ncbi.nlm.nih.gov/11990853/. Accessed 7 May 2024).

Nica AC, Dermitzakis ET (2013) Expression quantitative trait loci: present and future. Philos Trans R Soc Lond Ser B Biol Sci 368:20120362. https://doi.org/10.1098/rstb.2012.0362

Oncogenic RUNX3: A Link between p53 Deficiency and MYC Dysregulation – PMC [WWW Document] (n.d.). URL https://www.ncbi.nlm.nih.gov/pmc/articles/PMC7057839/. Accessed 7 June 24).

Origin and Role of a Subset of Tumor-Associated Neutrophils with Antigen-Presenting Cell Features in Early-Stage Human Lung Cancer – PubMed [WWW Document] (n.d.). URL https://pubmed.ncbi.nlm.nih.gov/27374224/. Accessed 7 Mar 2024).

Ozga AJ, Chow MT, Luster AD (2021) Chemokines and the immune response to cancer. Immunity 54:859–874. https://doi.org/10.1016/j.immuni.2021.01.012

Pardoll DM (2012) The blockade of immune checkpoints in cancer immunotherapy. Nat Rev Cancer 12:252–264. https://doi.org/10.1038/nrc3239

Park EJ, Lee JH, Yu G-Y, He G, Ali SR, Holzer RG, Osterreicher CH, Takahashi H, Karin M (2010) Dietary and genetic obesity promote liver inflammation and tumorigenesis by enhancing IL-6 and TNF expression. Cell 140:197–208. https://doi.org/10.1016/j.cell.2009.12.052

Psaila B, Lyden D (2009) The metastatic niche: adapting the foreign soil. Nat Rev Cancer 9:285–293. https://doi.org/10.1038/nrc2621

Qian B-Z, Pollard JW (2010) Macrophage diversity enhances tumor progression and metastasis. Cell 141:39–51. https://doi.org/10.1016/j.cell.2010.03.014

Quail DF, Joyce JA (2013) Microenvironmental regulation of tumor progression and metastasis. Nat Med 19:1423–1437. https://doi.org/10.1038/nm.3394

RAS oncogenes: the first 30 years – PubMed [WWW Document] (n.d.). URL https://pubmed.ncbi.nlm.nih.gov/12778136/ Accessed 7 June 24).

Rose-John S (2012) IL-6 trans-signaling via the soluble IL-6 receptor: importance for the pro-inflammatory activities of IL-6. Int J Biol Sci 8:1237–1247. https://doi.org/10.7150/ijbs.4989

Sangaletti S, Tripodo C, Chiodoni C, Guarnotta C, Cappetti B, Casalini P, Piconese S, Parenza M, Guiducci C, Vitali C, Colombo MP (2012) Neutrophil extracellular traps mediate transfer of cytoplasmic neutrophil antigens to myeloid dendritic cells toward ANCA induction and associated autoimmunity. Blood 120:3007–3018. https://doi.org/10.1182/blood-2012-03-416156

Sansone P, Storci G, Tavolari S, Guarnieri T, Giovannini C, Taffurelli M, Ceccarelli C, Santini D, Paterini P, Marcu KB, Chieco P, Bonafè M (2007) IL-6 triggers malignant features in mammospheres from human ductal breast carcinoma and normal mammary gland. J Clin Invest 117:3988–4002. https://doi.org/10.1172/JCI32533

Sethi G, Sung B, Aggarwal BB (2008) TNF: a master switch for inflammation to cancer. Front Biosci J Virtual Libr 13:5094–5107. https://doi.org/10.2741/3066

Shanley TP, Schmal H, Friedl HP, Jones ML, Ward PA (1995) Role of macrophage inflammatory protein-1 alpha (MIP-1 alpha) in acute lung injury in rats. J Immunol Baltim Md 1950(154): 4793–4802

Shaul ME, Fridlender ZG (2019) Tumour-associated neutrophils in patients with cancer. Nat Rev Clin Oncol 16:601–620. https://doi.org/10.1038/s41571-019-0222-4

Shavers VL, Brown ML (2002) Racial and ethnic disparities in the receipt of cancer treatment. J Natl Cancer Inst 94:334–357. https://doi.org/10.1093/jnci/94.5.334

Sica A, Mantovani A (2012) Macrophage plasticity and polarization: in vivo veritas. J Clin Invest 122:787–795. https://doi.org/10.1172/JCI59643

Simmons DL, Botting RM, Hla T (2004) Cyclooxygenase isozymes: the biology of prostaglandin synthesis and inhibition. Pharmacol Rev 56:387–437. https://doi.org/10.1124/pr.56.3.3

Slamon DJ, Clark GM, Wong SG, Levin WJ, Ullrich A, McGuire WL (1987) Human breast cancer: correlation of relapse and survival with amplification of the HER-2/neu oncogene. Science 235: 177–182. https://doi.org/10.1126/science.3798106

Stine ZE, Walton ZE, Altman BJ, Hsieh AL, Dang CV (2015) MYC, Metabolism, and Cancer. Cancer Discov 5:1024–1039. https://doi.org/10.1158/2159-8290.CD-15-0507

Strieter RM, Burdick MD, Mestas J, Gomperts B, Keane MP, Belperio JA (2006) Cancer CXC chemokine networks and tumour angiogenesis. Eur J Cancer Oxf Engl 1990(42):768–778. https://doi.org/10.1016/j.ejca.2006.01.006

Sun X, Cheng G, Hao M, Zheng J, Zhou X, Zhang J, Taichman RS, Pienta KJ, Wang J (2010) CXCL12 / CXCR4 / CXCR7 chemokine axis and cancer progression. Cancer Metastasis Rev 29:709–722. https://doi.org/10.1007/s10555-010-9256-x

Sunshine J, Taube JM (2015) PD-1/PD-L1 inhibitors. Curr Opin Pharmacol 23:32–38. https://doi.org/10.1016/j.coph.2015.05.011

The Multifaceted Roles Neutrophils Play in the Tumor Microenvironment – PubMed [WWW Document] (n.d.). URL https://pubmed.ncbi.nlm.nih.gov/24895166/. Accessed 7 Mar 2024).

Topalian SL, Hodi FS, Brahmer JR, Gettinger SN, Smith DC, McDermott DF, Powderly JD, Carvajal RD, Sosman JA, Atkins MB, Leming PD, Spigel DR, Antonia SJ, Horn L, Drake CG, Pardoll DM, Chen L, Sharfman WH, Anders RA, Taube JM, McMiller TL, Xu H, Korman AJ, Jure-Kunkel M, Agrawal S, McDonald D, Kollia GD, Gupta A, Wigginton JM, Sznol M (2012) Safety, activity, and immune correlates of anti-PD-1 antibody in cancer. N Engl J Med 366: 2443–2454. https://doi.org/10.1056/NEJMoa1200690

Trinchieri G (2003) Interleukin-12 and the regulation of innate resistance and adaptive immunity. Nat Rev Immunol 3:133–146. https://doi.org/10.1038/nri1001

Tsimberidou A-M, Iskander NG, Hong DS, Wheler JJ, Falchook GS, Fu S, Piha-Paul S, Naing A, Janku F, Luthra R, Ye Y, Wen S, Berry D, Kurzrock R (2012) Personalized medicine in a phase I clinical trials program: the MD Anderson Cancer Center initiative. Clin Cancer Res Off J Am Assoc Cancer Res 18:6373–6383. https://doi.org/10.1158/1078-0432.CCR-12-1627

Tumor vascular permeability and the EPR effect in macromolecular therapeutics: a review – PubMed [WWW Document] (n.d.). URL https://pubmed.ncbi.nlm.nih.gov/10699287/. Accessed 7 Mar 2024.

Turk JL (1993) Rudolf Virchow–father of cellular pathology. J R Soc Med 86:688–689

Vane JR, Botting RM (1998) Mechanism of action of antiinflammatory drugs. Int J Tissue React 20: 3–15

Vogelstein B, Kinzler KW (2004) Cancer genes and the pathways they control. Nat Med 10:789–799. https://doi.org/10.1038/nm1087

Voronov E, Shouval DS, Krelin Y, Cagnano E, Benharroch D, Iwakura Y, Dinarello CA, Apte RN (2003) IL-1 is required for tumor invasiveness and angiogenesis. Proc Natl Acad Sci USA 100: 2645–2650. https://doi.org/10.1073/pnas.0437939100

Waugh DJJ, Wilson C (2008) The interleukin-8 pathway in cancer. Clin Cancer Res Off J Am Assoc Cancer Res 14:6735–6741. https://doi.org/10.1158/1078-0432.CCR-07-4843

Wiseman H, Halliwell B (1996) Damage to DNA by reactive oxygen and nitrogen species: role in inflammatory disease and progression to cancer. Biochem J 313(Pt 1):17–29. https://doi.org/10.1042/bj3130017

Wu W-Y, Li J, Wu Z-S, Zhang C-L, Meng X-L (2011) STAT3 activation in monocytes accelerates liver cancer progression. BMC Cancer 11:506. https://doi.org/10.1186/1471-2407-11-506

Yang Z, Wang W, Wang X, Qin Z (2021) Cardiotoxicity of epidermal growth factor receptor 2-targeted drugs for breast cancer. Front Pharmacol 12. https://doi.org/10.3389/fphar.2021.741451

Yarden Y, Pines G (2012) The ERBB network: at last, cancer therapy meets systems biology. Nat Rev Cancer 12:553–563. https://doi.org/10.1038/nrc3309

Yu H, Pardoll D, Jove R (2009) STATs in cancer inflammation and immunity: a leading role for STAT3. Nat Rev Cancer 9:798–809. https://doi.org/10.1038/nrc2734

Zitvogel L, Tesniere A, Kroemer G (2006) Cancer despite immunosurveillance: immunoselection and immunosubversion. Nat Rev Immunol 6:715–727. https://doi.org/10.1038/nri1936

Cancer Stem Cells: Robust Features and Therapeutic Targets

Marwa M. Abu-Serie and Eman M. Sarhan

Abstract

Cancer stem cells (CSCs) have considerable pivotal attention in the research field of oncology due to their unique characteristic features that assume their potential as cancer therapeutic targets. Self-renewal, infinite proliferation, and replication are among their stem cell–like features that are responsible for cancer recurrence even after chemotherapy and radiotherapy. Thus, targeting both intrinsic and extrinsic anti-apoptotic pathways for eradicating CSCs is a promising therapeutic approach for decreasing cancer morbidity and mortality. This chapter aims to provide an in-depth summarized exploration of CSCs' robust features and their clinical implications, addressing challenges and future prospects of their therapeutic potential in the most recent context of cancer-targeted therapies.

Keywords

Cancer recurrence and metastasis · Cancer stem cells (CSCs) · Therapeutic resistance · CSC-targeted therapy · Anti-apoptotic pathways · Self-renewal

M. M. Abu-Serie (✉)
Medical Biotechnology Department, Genetic Engineering and Biotechnology Research Institute (GEBRI), City of Scientific Research and Technological Applications (SRTA-City), Alexandria, Egypt
e-mail: mabuserie@srtacity.sci.eg; marwaelhedaia@gmail.com

E. M. Sarhan
Protein Research Department, Genetic Engineering and Biotechnology Research Institute (GEBRI), City of Scientific Research and Technological Applications (SRTA-City), Alexandria, Egypt

Interdisciplinary Cancer Research, https://doi.org/10.1007/16833_2024_366
Published online: 20 September 2024

1 Introduction

To date, cancer is a worldwide major public health concern with high morbidity and mortality rates (de Lima Coutinho et al. 2023). Many cancer patients die, every year, due to disease's resistance to chemo/radiotherapies (Singh et al. 2023), as well as tumor relapse with invasion or metastasis (Bray et al. 2018; Han et al. 2023; Li et al. 2023a). It is now relatively clear that a small subpopulation within the tumor bulk microenvironment, like cancer stem cells (CSCs), circulating tumor cells (CTCs), and cancer-associated fibroblasts (CAFs), is mostly responsible for the mortality of cancer patients. Cancer stem cells (CSCs) are tumor-initiating cells (TICs) with a crucial role in cancer initiation, progression, therapeutic resistance, immune evasion, metastatic potential, and recurrence. The aggressive CSC features are based on their unique self-renewal, multi-differentiation, and tumorigenic capacity by activating Wnt/catenin, Notch, and hedgehog signaling (Aramini et al. 2022; Ibragimova et al. 2022; Lee and Tanggono 2022). These aggressive tumorigenic features of CSCs are currently the major challenges for cancer treatments (Atashzar et al. 2020; Lee and Tanggono 2022). The first compelling evidence of the CSC existence was in human acute myeloid leukemia (Bonnet and Dick 1997). Meanwhile, the presence of CSCs in solid tumor was confirmed in breast cancer since 2003 (Al-Hajj et al. 2003). After that, CSCs have been proven to exist in many other various solid tumor types. The current chapter will discuss the main functional phenotypes of CSCs that confer a more aggressive nature of tumor, where their elusive stemness features are attributed not only to CSC itself but also to its niche (microenvironment), as well as, the most recent advances and future prospects of CSC-targeted therapeutics.

2 Cancer Stem Cells' (CSCs') Robust Features

2.1 CSCs' Stemness Features

One of the basic stem cell properties is the homeostatic balance between self-renewal for maintaining themselves and multi-lineage differentiation potential through symmetric and asymmetric division, respectively (Lathia and Liu 2017; Najafi et al. 2019; Calavul and Özdemİr 2023; Islam and Lam 2023). Asymmetric division occurs by the unequal distribution of cell-fate determinants. Prior to this division, stemness- and differentiation-mediating factors are located at apical and basal sides, respectively, of mother stem cells. Then polarity-determining regulators are enhanced and correlated to the unequal size of two daughter cells. The apical daughter cell which remains as stem cell lineage is larger in size and inherits more maternal DNA and self-renewal promoting factors (e.g., Notch). Meanwhile, a smaller in size basal daughter cell inherits differentiation factors (such as numb "negative inhibitor of Notch") with less maternal DNA (Paul et al. 2019). The mechanisms of self-renewal, proliferation, and asymmetric division are similar between normal stem cells and CSCs (Yoo and Kwon 2015; Ju et al. 2022; Masoudi and Gopalan 2023; Samanta et al. 2023). Hence, the most approved theory for the origin of CSCs is the accumulated oncogenic mutations in normal stem/progenitor cells, rather than differentiated cells, over a long period of time promoting the malignant transformation (De Francesco et al. 2018; Joshi et al. 2022; Derks and van Boxtel 2023).

Adult stem cells (SCs) are quiescent and are only activated upon tissue injury (Brunet et al. 2023; de Morree and Rando 2023; Krauss and Kann 2023). In contrast, CSCs exhibit an uncontrolled self-renewal and differentiate into progenitor cancer cells for generating an unlimited diverse number of new mutated cancer cells, based on the available niche space, leading to tumor formation. In malignancies, self-renewal is overactivated, and multi-lineage differentiation is restricted leading to CSC overpopulation with driving tumor growth (Lathia and Liu 2017; Najafi et al. 2019; Hervieu et al. 2021). Throughout the high-grade cancer progression, CSCs drive a more vigorous undifferentiated stem-like tumor state (Najafi et al. 2019; Gimple et al. 2022; Singh and Dutt 2024). Interestingly, after anticancer drugs' withdrawal, a tumor might relapse where the survived CSCs can propagate and differentiate to replenish all heterogeneous tumor populations (Zhu and Fan 2018; Basu et al. 2022; Paul et al. 2022). All these facts are considered potential reasons for the high cancer incidence and propagation in stem cell–enriched tissues (Najafi et al. 2019).

2.2 Major Cancer Stem Cell (CSC) Signaling Pathways

The main stemness signaling pathways, including wingless-INT (Wnt)/β-catenin, Notch, and Hedgehog (Hh) as well as phosphatidylinositol-3 kinase (PI3K)/AKT/mTOR, are dysregulated in CSCs (Doan et al. 2020; Yanardag and Pugacheva 2021; Vamvoukaki et al. 2023) (Fig. 1).

2.2.1 Wnt/β-Catenin Signaling Pathway

The Wnt signaling might be triggered either through β-catenin-dependent "canonical" or independent "non-canonical" pathways. The canonical Wnt pathway, which is known as Wnt/β-catenin signaling pathway, mainly controls cell proliferation, while the non-canonical Wnt signaling pathway regulates cell polarity and migration (Liu et al. 2022a). Wnt pathway is activated by the binding Wnt-secreted glycoproteins to the N-terminus extracellular cysteine-rich transmembrane domain of Frizzled (FZD) receptor; then β-catenin is released upon degradation of a large protein complex called "destruction complex." This complex is composed of tumor suppressor adenomatous polyposis coli (APC), glycogen synthase kinase-3β (GSK-3β), casein kinase-1α (CK1α) and scaffold protein axin. Both CK1α and GSK3β mediate subsequent phosphorylation at Ser33, Ser37, and Thr41 residues of the β-catenin N-termus. Then the phosphorylated β-catenin is ubiquitinated by beta-transducin repeats–containing E3 ubiquitin ligase "β-TrCP," leading to proteasomal breakdown and release of β-catenin which can then easily translocate into nucleus (Chatterjee et al., 2022). Nuclear β-catenin co-activates with lymphoid

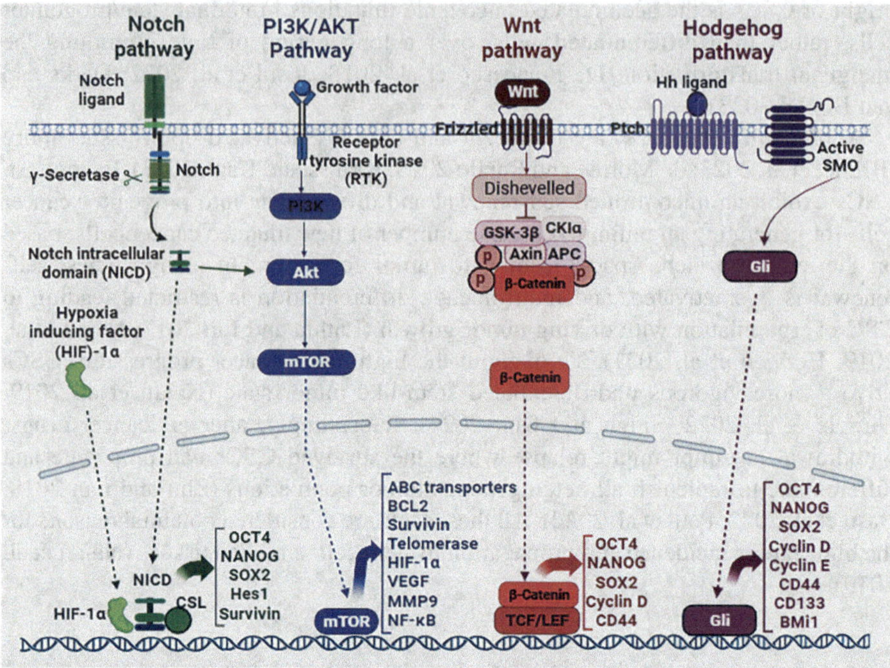

Fig. 1 Schematic representation of the main CSC stemness signaling pathways, including Wnt, Notch, and Hedgehog, as well as PI3K/AKT/mTOR

enhancer factor/T cell factor (LEF/TCF) family complex to initiate transcription of Wnt-target genes, including cyclin-D1 (*CD1*), cellular myelocytomatosis (*C-Myc*), *NANOG*, octamer-binding transcription factor (*OCT4*), and sex-determining region Y-box-2 (*SOX2*) (Wu 2008; Vaz et al. 2014; Hayat et al. 2022; Hiremath et al. 2022; Liu et al. 2022a).

2.2.2 Notch Signaling Pathway

Notch signaling is an evolutionary conserved, intercellular communication pathway that regulates many developmental and cellular processes involving stem cell fate determination, differentiation, and self-renewal in adult tissues and germ layer formation in embryonic development (Kumar et al. 2021). Notch signaling is initiated when a Notch ligand (e.g., Jagged (JAG1-2) and Delta-like (DLL1-4)) binds to the extracellular domain of Notch receptor. Then Notch receptor undergoes two proteolytic cleavages; the first one is an extracellular cleavage, catalyzed by the ADAM family of metalloproteases, while the second is intracellulary, mediated by the γ-secretase enzyme complex (presenilin, nicastrin, PEN2, and APH1). Both types of cleavages provoke the Notch intracellular domain (NICD) release from the membrane and its subsequent nuclear translocation, where it forms a complex with suppressor of hairless (CSL) and hypoxia-inducing factor (HIF) to co-activate and regulate the Notch target gene transcription (Liu et al. 2023; Ordaz-Ramos et al. 2023), including hairy and enhancer of split (*HES*) family genes and *OCT4* (Gao et al. 2014; Zhu and Fan 2018).

2.2.3 Hedgehog (Hh) Signaling Pathway

Hedgehog (Hh) signaling pathway regulates embryogenesis as well as tissue regeneration, homeostasis, and development. Regarding a Hh ligand molecule (e.g., Indian Hedgehog (IHh), Sonic Hedgehog (SHh), and Desert Hedgehog (DHh)) engages with Patched receptor (Ptch1) repressing the transmembrane Smoothened (SMO) receptor and facilitating the release and nuclear translocation of transcriptionally active glioma-associated oncogene (*Gli 1–3*) (Salaritabar et al. 2019; Ordaz-Ramos et al. 2023) Gli1/2 activates the expression of (1) pluripotency genes including *NANOG*, *SOX2*, and B lymphoma Mo-MLV insertion region-1 (*Bmi1*) homolog; (2) feedback loop of Hh genes including *Gli1*, *Ptch1*, and membrane Hh-interacting protein-1 (*Hhip1*); and (3) cell cycle progression genes including cyclin D, cyclin E, and *C-Myc* (Vaz et al. 2014; Cochrane et al. 2015; Zhu and Fan 2018; Montagnani and Stecca 2019).

2.2.4 Crosstalk Between Stemness Wnt, Notch, and Hedgehog Signaling Pathways

The common target genes (*NANOG*, *OCT4*, *SOX2*, and *Bmi1*) of the abovementioned signaling pathways (Wnt, Notch, and Hh) are CSC-specific transcription factors because their expression levels are low in normal stem cells (SCs). These genes are essential to up/downregulate the signature characteristics of CSCs like self-renewal and pluripotency that promote driving the heterogeneous tumor bulk population (Liu et al. 2013; Izadpanah et al. 2023). The uncontrolled expression of NANOG stimulates the overexpression of many CSC-associated molecules (CD44, CD133, and ALDH1A1) with the induction of proliferation via shortening G1/S phase transition (Zhang et al. 2009; Liu et al. 2013; Al-Zubaidi 2022; Fleifel and Cook 2023). Recent studies reported a positive correlation between the expression of *NANOG*, *OCT4*, and *SOX2*, poor differentiation, and advanced stage of tumor (Yang et al. 2018; You et al. 2018; Afroze et al. 2022; Chen et al. 2022; Abdelbary et al. 2023). Also, Bmi1 is co-expressed with CD44 and CD133 (Borah et al. 2015; Xu et al. 2023b). CD133 inhibits caspase 3 and 9, while CD44 increases B cell lymphoma (Bcl)-2 level (Atashzar et al. 2020; Shukla et al. 2023). Bmi-1 is not usually required for the proliferation of all cells, which confirms its preferential need for CSCs (Molofsky et al. 2003; Sahara et al. 2023).

Additionally, the activation of phosphatidylinositol-3 kinase (PI3K)/protein kinase B (AKT)/ mammalian target of rapamycin (mTOR) pathway enhances CSC phenotypes (Fig. 1) (Templeton et al. 2014; Bang et al. 2023; Liao et al. 2023; Guefack et al. 2024). PI3K is activated when an extracellular growth factor like vascular endothelial growth factor (VEGF), epidermal growth factor (EGF), or fibroblast growth factor (FGF) binds to the receptor tyrosine kinase (RTK). This also causes the activation of Ras, integrin-like kinase, and extracellular matrix-integrin-focal adhesion kinase which are important for cell cycle progression and cell invasion. Phosphatidylinositol 3-kinase (PI3K) activates GSK-3, while AKT which is upregulated by the Notch signaling pathway is the main downstream effector of PI3K (Ding et al. 2015; Ghoneum and Said 2019; Tong et al. 2023). AKT can activate nuclear factor kappa-B (NF-κB) which enhances the expression of many genes of stemness (e.g., *SOX2*, *NANOG*, and *Notch*), metastasis (e.g., matrix metalloproteinases (*MMPs*)), and angiogenesis (e.g., *VEGF*) (Martelli et al. 2011; Vazquez-Santillan et al. 2015; Zhang et al. 2023a). AKT Also inhibits caspase-9 and forkhead box-O (FoxO) that stimulates cyclin-dependent kinase (CDK) inhibitors, thus leading to apoptosis prevention and mediating cell cycle progression (Ghoneum and Said 2019; Jha and Arora 2022). The mTOR stimulates mRNA translation of proliferation-promoting genes including *survivin*, *BCL-2*, *C-Myc*, *CD1* and *CDK2*, *VEGF*, *hypoxia-inducing factor-1* (*HIF1*), and *MMP9* (Martelli et al. 2011). Moreover, mTOR enhances translation and posttranslation of telomerase; thus, CSCs have a complete telomere-lengthening mechanism and, in turn, acquire unlimited proliferation ability (immortality) (Dogan and Avci 2018). Otherwise, these stemness pathways, when overactivated, can confer CSCs an innate chemoresistance, immune resistance, and metastatic potential (Kalluri and Weinberg 2009; Gonzalez and Medici 2014; Lathia and Liu 2017; Dogan and Avci 2018; Wu et al. 2023).

3 Cancer Stem Cell Diagnostic Biomarkers

The malignant stem cell (CSC) populations or tumor-initiating cells are characterized by overexpressed stem cell–specific biomarkers like SOX2, OCT4, NANOG, CD133, CD44, and ALDH1 (Lee and Tanggono 2022). Among about 100 up-to-date targets retrieved from STRING Database at a confidence value of 0.4 (Fig. 2), 11 biomarkers, including PROM1, SOX2, CD44, POU5F1, NANOG, CTNNB1, ALDH1A1, CD34, TP53, CD8A, and PSMA7, have the highly text-mining scored evidence in CSC studied and published cases. Also, the most cell adhesion (CD) biomarkers with overexpression evidence in CSCs were CD44, CD34, CD8A, CD24, CD274, CD19, CD4, CD38, CD47, CDH1, PDCD1, CD33, CDK4, and CDH2.

Other evidence-related overexpressed surface cell adhesion biomarkers (CD), as illustrated in Table 1. Although these CDs are similar between CSCs and normal stem cells (SCs) in terms of either self-renewal or the generation of differentiated progeny (pluripotency), only CSCs have tumorigenic activity (Han et al. 2013; Hasanzadeh et al. 2023). This CSC tumorigenicity argued against the stochastic tumor model, which assumed that all cancer cells have an equal potential to propagate malignancy (Rich 2016; Liu et al. 2022b; Valentim et al. 2023).

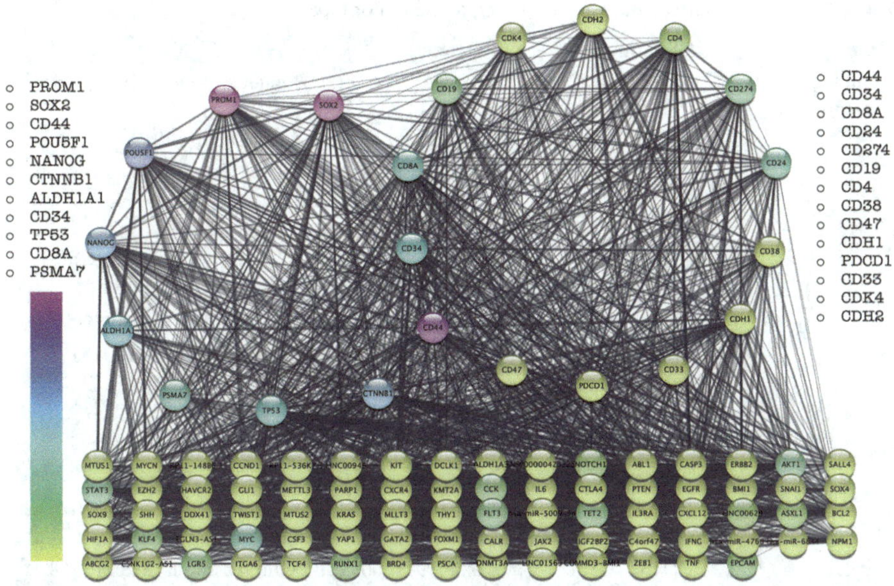

Fig. 2 Network construction of cancer stem cell (CSC) target identification. Mapping color palette starts with pale-yellow color representing low evidence–scored values and ends with purple color representing the high evidence–scored values

4 Challenges In Targeting Cancer Stem Cells

4.1 CSC Therapeutic Multiple Drug Resistance

Multi-drug resistance (MDR) is the phenomenon wherein carcinogenic cells acquire therapeutic resistance against structural analogs of different types of anticancer drug classes (Pote and Gacche 2023). CSCs can escape from drug-induced cellular death by unique overexpression of drug efflux transmembrane proteins (ATP binding cassette (ABC) transporters), quiescence, highly efficient DNA repair, apoptosis resistance, and high ALDH1 activity (Fig. 3).

4.1.1 ABC Transporters (Drug Efflux)

ATP binding cassette (ABC) transporters are one of the many known multi-drug resistance (MDR) mechanisms. These drug efflux pumps play a fundamental role in CSC drug resistance via active transportation, using ATP, against a concentration gradient. It is composed of transmembrane domains (TMD) and nucleotide-binding domains (NBD). The substrate/drug recognition and binding are mediated via TMD which forms a gate that opens up to the extracellular space and spans a large part of the membrane depth. Once a substrate is present, NBD binds and hydrolyzes ATP to ADP. This causes a conformational change in its protein structural folding then the

Table 1 The CSC surface markers according to the tumor type

Tumor type	CSCs marker	References
Acute myeloid leukemia	CD34	Bhatia et al. (1997), Bonnet and Dick (1997), and Blair et al. (1998)
	CD38	Sarry et al. (2011) and Naik et al. (2019)
	CD123	Jin et al. (2009), Busfield et al. (2014), and Espinoza-Gutarra et al. (2021)
	CD47	Jaiswal et al. (2009)
	CD96	Hosen et al. (2007) and Georgiev et al. (2018)
	CD33	Kim et al. (2018) and Fenwarth et al. (2020)
	CD32	Saito et al. (2010) and Heitmann et al. (2020)
	CD25	Saito et al. (2010) and Kageyama et al. (2018)
	CD44	Gutjahr et al. (2015) and Cao et al. (2016)
	CD45RA	Sarry et al. (2011)
	TIM3	Kikushige et al. (2010) and Jan et al. (2011)
	IL1RAP	Askmyr et al. (2013)
	CLL-1/ CLEC12A	Van Rhenen et al. (2007) and Zhao et al. (2010)
Acute lymphoblastic leukemia	CD133	Cox et al. (2009) and Glumac and LeBeau (2018)
Breast cancer	CD44, CD24	Al-Hajj et al. (2003)
Brain cancer	CD90	Zeppernick et al. (2008) and He et al. (2012)
	CD133	Zeppernick et al. (2008), He et al. (2012), and Cheng et al. (2009)
	CD49f	Fukamachi et al. (2013)
	CD15	Son et al. (2009)
	CD44	Jackson et al. (2015)
	CD36	Hale et al. (2014)
	EGFR	Mazzoleni et al. (2010)
	Integrin α6	Lathia et al. (2010)
	A2B5	Ogden et al. (2008)
	L1CAM	Bao et al. (2008)
	LGR5	Parry and Engh (2014)
Pancreatic cancer	CD44, CD24, CD133	Li et al. 2007
Lung cancer	CD44, CD133	MacDonagh et al. (2016)
Colon cancer	CD44, CD24, CD133, CD166	Dalerba et al. (2007) and Vermeulen et al. (2008)
Gastric cancer	CD24	Bekaii-Saab and El-Rayes (2017)
Prostate cancer	CD24, CD166	Moltzahn and Thalmann (2013)
	EpCAM	Deng et al. (2015) and Huang et al. (2018)
	α2β1 integrin	Collins et al. (2005), Hall et al. (2008), and Sottnik et al. (2013)
	ALDH	Moreb et al. (1996), van den Hoogen et al. (2010), and Barclay and Van den Berg (2014)

(continued)

Table 1 (continued)

Tumor type	CSCs marker	References
	EZH2	Ugolkov et al. (2011)
	CXCR4	Darash-Yahana et al. (2004), Domanska et al. (2012), and Dubrovska et al. (2012)
	E-cadherin	Bae et al. (2011)
	ABCG2	Xia et al. (2022)
	CD117	Miettinen and Lasota (2005) and Kerr et al. (2015)
	CD44	Patrawala et al. (2006), Bekaii-Saab and El-Rayes (2017), and Azevedo et al. (2018)
	CD133	Yin et al. (1997), Richardson et al. (2004), Bekaii-Saab and El-Rayes (2017)
Liver cancer	CD44, CD90, CD133	Yang et al. (2008) and Hou et al. (2012)
Melanoma	CD133, CD20, CD271	Klonisch et al. (2008)
Ovarian cancer	CD44, CD117, CD133	Zinzi et al. (2014)
Sarcoma	CD29, CD117, CD133	Adhikari et al. (2010) and Lan et al. (2015)
Esophageal cancer	CD271, CD44, CD24, CD90	Qian et al. (2016)
Cervical cancer	CD13, CD29, CD44, CD105	Yao et al. (2015)
Kidney cancer	CD44, CD105, CD133	Yuan et al. (2016)
Bladder cancer	67LR	Edris et al. (2012)
	CD133	Xia et al. (2022)
	CD47	Chan et al. (2010)
	CD44	Verma et al. (2017)
	ALDH	Su et al. (2010)
	CD44v6	van der Horst et al. (2012)
	EpCAM	Ostrikov et al. (2019)

ABC transporter opens and the substrate is exported out leading to a change in the intracellular and extracellular concentrations of drugs (Pote and Gacche 2023). There are three main members of broad-spectrum ABC transporters (Table 2) including ABCB1/P-gp/MDR1, ABCC1/MRP1, and ABCG2/BCRP (Begicevic and Falasca 2017; Fan et al. 2023). Therefore, a block for a single ABC transporter may not be a good reversal of therapeutic resistance of CSCs (Jiang et al. 2017). Interestingly, previous studies reported that stemness signaling pathways (Wnt, Notch, Hh, and PI3K/AKT/mTOR/NF-κB) play a key role in regulating the expression of ABC transporters (Flahaut et al. 2009; Abdullah and Chow 2013; Chen et al. 2014; Cochrane et al. 2015; Begicevic and Falasca 2017; Lathia and Liu 2017).

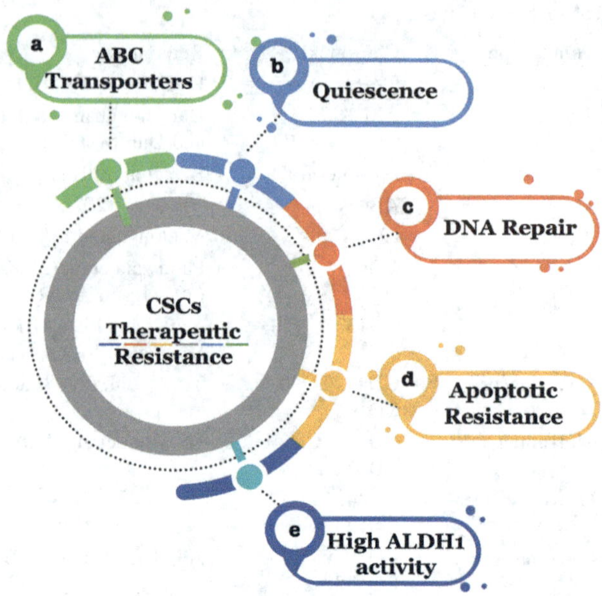

Fig. 3 Schematic illustration of the therapeutic resistance of CSCs. (**a**) ABC transporters, (**b**) quiescence, (**c**) DNA repair "ataxia telangiectasia mutated (ATM)/checkpoint kinase-1 (CHK1) and ATM-Rad3-related checkpoint kinase-2 (ATR/CHK2), (**d**) apoptosis resistance, (**e**) high ALDH1 activity

Table 2 The most studied ABC transporters with their location and substrates (Hipfner et al. 1999; Begicevic and Falasca 2017)

ABC transporters	Expression in CSCs	Chemotherapy
ABCB1/ MDR1/P-gp	Acute myeloid leukemia, brain, kidney, breast, and ovarian	Anthracyclines (e.g., doxorubicin), actinomycin D, colchicine, etoposide, teniposide, methotrexate, mitomycin C, mitoxantrone, taxenes (paclitaxel and docetaxel), vincristine, and vinblastine
ABCC1/ MRP1	Glioblastoma, lung, breast, and prostate	Methotrexate, edatrexate, ZD1694, doxorubicin, daunorubicin, epirubicin, idarubicin, etoposide, vincristine, vinblastine, paclitaxel, irinotecan, SN-38, flutamide, and hydroxyflutamide
ABCG2/ BCRP	Liver, lung, breast, ovarian, and pancreas	Mitoxantrone, imatinib, anthracyclins, doxorubicin, topotecan, flavopiridol, and methotrexate

4.1.2 Quiescence

As mentioned above, CSCs can also develop chemoresistance by spending a long time in a quiescent nonproliferating state (G0 phase). This unique strategy presents as an adaptive response against environmental stress (e.g., chemotherapy) allowing CSC survival and then tumor recurrence that may happen after a very long period (Chen et al. 2021; Garimella et al. 2023). Only proliferating cancer cells are targeted by chemotherapeutic drugs including antimetabolite drugs, mitotic inhibitors, and topoisomerase inhibitors, leaving quiescent CSCs out of the cell cycle with longer time. This reversible quiescence regulates by signaling molecules including inhibitors of CDK (p21, p27, and p57), tumor suppressor p53, retinoblastoma proteins, and p38 mitogen–activated protein kinase (MAPK). In addition to these modulators, the quiescent state can be induced by FoxO and dual-specificity tyrosine phosphorylation-regulated kinase (DYRK) 1 as inhibitors of G1/S transition (Weston and Barr 2023). There are three therapeutic approaches for targeting quiescent CSCs for eradicating and blocking their recurrence. These include the "locked-out" approach in which CSCs are forced to reenter the cell cycle, the "wake-up" strategy for restoring therapeutic sensitivity, and irreversible blocking quiescent CSCs in G0 "locked-in" or targeting quiescent CSCs (Chen et al. 2016).

4.1.3 Efficient DNA Repair and Apoptosis Resistance

One of CSC hallmarks is resistance to chemotherapy-induced DNA damage through both cell cycle arrest at specific checkpoints and DNA repair machine recruitment (Fig. 3c) (Gong et al. 2015; Wang 2015; Chen et al. 2016; Zhang et al. 2021a; Gillespie et al. 2023). This occurs via, first, activation of DNA damage response (DDR) kinases, including ataxia telangiectasia mutated (ATM) and ATM-Rad3-related (ATR). ATM is stimulated upon double-stranded DNA breaks (DSBs) while ATR responds to a wider variety of DNA damages (DNA lesion occurrence during DNA replication and DSBs). Second, ATR and ATM phosphorylate and activate intra-S and G2/M phase checkpoint kinases (CHK) 1 and 2, respectively, and then enhance DNA damage repair as effector response (Chang et al. 2015; Chen et al. 2016; Tabassum et al. 2018; Priya et al. 2023) Additionally, overexpression of DNA repair genes including methyl guanine methyl transferase (*MGMT*) and breast cancer type 1 susceptibility protein (BRCA1) were recorded in CSCs (Mathews et al. 2011; Chen et al. 2016).

Furthermore, the overexpression of key antiapoptotic mediators is another chemoresistance tool of CSCs (Fig. 3d). These mediators include BCL-2, BCL-XL, PI3K/AKT/mTOR, and inhibitor of apoptosis proteins (IAPs) such as survivin (Chen et al. 2016; Safa 2016; Zhou et al. 2023). IAPs play a crucial role in inhibiting apoptotic machinery by binding and ubiquitinating caspases 3, 7, and 9 (Dietz et al. 2023). Also, IAPs can activate NF-κB pathway, by engaging with tumor necrosis factor (TNF) receptor, leading to the upregulation of the expression of BCL-2 (Ramakrishnan et al. 2014; Lambrecht et al. 2023; Shahbaz et al. 2023). BCL-2 inhibits membrane permeabilization by preventing oligomerization of BCL-2 -2-associated X protein (BAX) and BCL-2 antagonist/killer (BAK), thus blocking the release of cytochrome C and caspase activation (Tabassum et al. 2018; Czabotar and Garcia-Saez 2023). Accordingly, high capacity for DNA damage repair and antiapoptosis pathways confer CSC resistance against the cytotoxicity effect of drugs.

4.1.4 Aldehyde Dehydrogenase (ALDH)

Chemo-/radio-resistance of CSCs was further associated with lowering the cellular reactive oxygen species (ROS) by suppressing its production and/or scavenging its already produced contents after therapy using highly efficient free-radical scavenging systems such as ALDH1 (Das et al. 2020). ALDH1 can act as a drug-detoxifying enzyme via the oxidation of the reactive aldehydes into their corresponding carboxylic acids (Pasqualetti et al. 2023). Therefore, ALDH1 confers CSCs a resistance to radiotherapy and to chemotherapeutic drugs, such as cyclophosphamide (Fig. 3), doxorubicin, paclitaxel, cisplatin, gemcitabine, and docetaxel (Han et al. 2013; Chen et al. 2016; Turdo et al. 2019; Pasqualetti et al. 2023). Moreover, ALDH1 serves as a major radiation filter by directly absorbing radiation, scavenging radiation-induced free radicals, and detoxifying radiation-produced aldehydes (Singh et al. 2013).

4.2 Immune Evasion

CSCs have not only an efficient resistance against chemotherapy and radiotherapy but also extensive tools to evade the antitumor immune response (Izadpanah et al. 2023; Verma et al. 2023). CSCs downregulate the expression of both class I and II of human leukocyte antigen (HLA) at a lower extent than that in the differentiated cancer cells (Guo et al. 2023). This impairs antigen presentation and natural killer (NK) activation and halts the susceptibility of CSCs to cytotoxic T lymphocytes (CTL) (McMahon et al. 2023). However, CSCs overexpress neoantigens (e.g., SOX2) that are higher immunogenic than tumor-associated antigens and can mediate an efficient CTL response. To resist this response, CSCs upregulate the expression of immune checkpoints (e.g., CTL antigen-4 and programmed death (PD) receptor 1) that inhibit the survival and proliferation of CTL. CSCs also secrete several immunosuppressive factors, including interleukin (IL)-6, 8, and 10 as well as indolamine 2,3 dioxygenase (IDO), which contributes to the differentiation of regulatory T (Treg) cells and CTL apoptosis (Rouzbahani et al. 2022; Gupta et al. 2023). Additionally, signal transducer and activator of transcription (STAT) 3, which is released by the tumor microenvironment, inhibits the activation of macrophage and NK cells as well as the expression of HLA II and IL-12 in dendritic cells. Collectively, CTL will be unable to initiate the antitumor response (Dogan and Avci 2018; Ravindran et al. 2019; Dianat-Moghadam et al. 2022; Rouzbahani et al. 2022).

To develop more powerful therapeutic resistance properties, CSCs transform from epithelial to mesenchymal phenotypes (Mallini et al. 2014; Tanabe 2022; Garza Treviño et al. 2023). It is important to note that the quiescence nature of CSCs and their transition to the mesenchymal state can be considered as another mechanism of CSC evasion from immunosurveillance (Ravindran et al. 2019; Gupta et al. 2023). There is a positive correlation between expressions of ABC transporter and transcription factors of epithelial-mesenchymal transition (EMT) (Jiang et al. 2017; da Costa et al. 2023).

4.3 Metastasis

4.3.1 Epithelial-Mesenchymal Transition (EMT)

EMT also affects the metastatic ability of CTCs (Huang et al. 2022). CSCs have both high plasticity to regenerate tumor by differentiation into tumorigenic progenitor cells (Nayak et al. 2022; Pérez-González et al. 2023) and an invasion capacity (Marta

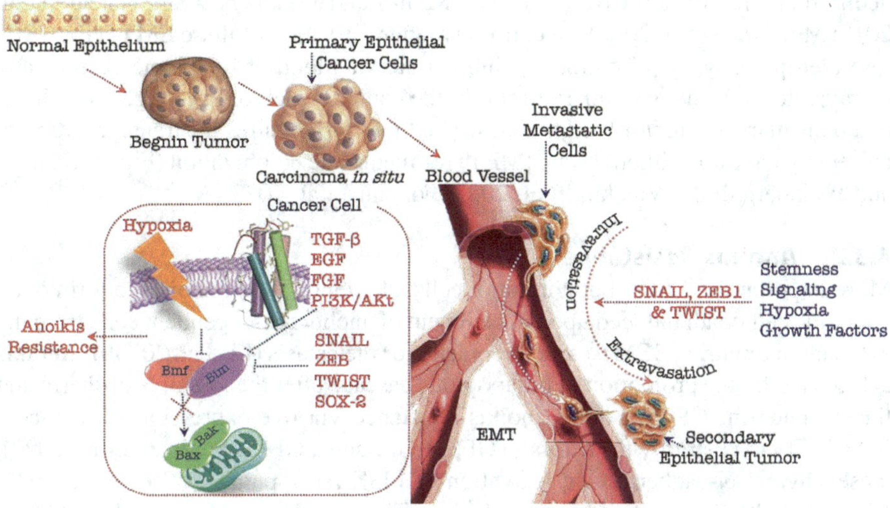

Fig. 4 The metastatic potential of CSCs with their anoikis resistance

Mauro-Lizcano et al. 2022; Peng et al. 2022), which are typical features of malignant tumors but not of benign tumors with a limited proliferative potential (Najafi et al. 2019). The EMT is the critical mechanism for generating invasive and metastatic CSCs (Fig. 4) (Huang et al. 2022). Epithelial-like cells are connected together with an extracellular matrix via specialized adhesion cell-cell junctions including E-cadherin and integrins, while mesenchymal cells lack this phenotype and thus have more ability to move and migrate (Ye and Weinberg 2015; Huang et al. 2022; Pérez-González et al. 2023).

Among the many transcriptional factors of tumor microenvironment signals that can initiate EMT are transforming growth factor-β (TGFβ), hepatocyte growth factor (HGF), platelet-derived growth factor (PDGF), endothelial growth factor (EGF), fibroblast growth factor (FGF), as well as hypoxia-inducible factors (HIFs), especially HIF-1α and HIF-2α (Lindsey and Langhans 2014; Roche 2018; Li et al. 2023b). Stemness-related signaling pathways including Wnt/β-catenin, Notch, Hedgehog, and receptor tyrosine kinases can activate EMT-inducing transcription factors (Kalluri and Weinberg 2009; Gonzalez and Medici 2014; Ervin et al. 2022). These EMT-translational factors (EMT-TFs), including zinc finger E-box binding homeobox (ZEB), Twist, and Snail, trigger the epigenetic silencing of E-cadherin (epithelial cell adhesion protein biomarker). E-cadherin suppression is a critical step toward the loss of epithelial phenotype and EMT initiation (Kalluri and Weinberg 2009; Ervin et al. 2022). Other three EMT-TFs of the SNAIL family (SNAIL1, SNAIL2, and SNAIL3) also can drive EMT by activating the transcription of matrix metalloproteinases (MMPs) including MMP2 and MMP9 which degrade components of the extracellular matrix. Furthermore, Snail upregulates the transcription of other EMT transcription factors (ZEB1/2 and Twist) (Wu et al. 2017; Huang et al. 2022). Moreover, Snail, Twist, and ZEB1 (key regulators of EMT) can induce dedifferentiation of non-CSCs to CSCs (Kalluri and Weinberg 2009; Nakano et al. 2019; Mortezaee et al. 2022). Accordingly, after activation of these EMT-TFs, CSCs lose their polarity, acquire motility, intravasate via blood or lymphatic vessels, and extravasate to form a secondary tumor in the capillary-rich organs (e.g., liver, lung, and bone marrow) and/or lymph nodes. The final step requires the transformation of mesenchymal into epithelial state (MET) for metastatic colonization (Fig. 4) (Kalluri and Weinberg 2009; Valakos et al. 2023; Fontana et al. 2023).

4.3.2 Anoikis Resistance

More importantly, CSCs, but not tumor cells, efficiently evade anoikis, a form of an apoptotic cell death induced upon detachment of anchorage-dependent cells from the extracellular matrix (ECM), as a prerequisite for metastasis (Li et al. 2023b). Anoikis is triggered by the promotion of proapoptotic cascade after the loss of E-cadherin and ligated integrin. CSCs acquire anoikis resistance via overexpression of stemness SOX2, EMT-TFs, growth factors (TGFβ, EGF, and FGF) (Shonibare et al. 2022), mesenchymal N-cadherin, and activation of PI3K/AKT pathway (Lee et al. 2021; Wang et al. 2022) as well as hypoxia (Fig. 4). These mediators downregulate BCL-2-interacting mediator of proanoikis cell death protein (Bim) and BCL-2-modifying factor (Bmf) which are secreted upon the cell-ECM detachment to initiate anoikis by promoting Bax-Bak oligomerization. This oligomerization is requested for the activation of caspase cascade after the release of cytochrome C (Kim et al. 2012; Al Mamun et al. 2020) (Dai et al. 2023). Hence, CSCs of several cancer types, in ultra-low adherent plates and fetal bovine serum-free media, can evade anoikis and propagate into onco-spheres. This tumorsphere formation experiment is widely used to detect CSCs in vitro and investigate the anti-CSC activity of new drugs (Zhu and Fan 2018).

5 Therapeutic Strategies Targeting "CSCs"

CSCs are intractable obstacles that have shown significant resistance and severe limitations with frequent failure to conventional anticancer treatments (Chen et al. 2013b; Guo et al. 2023). Many treatment strategies with insufficient selectivity against CSCs can be toxic to healthy tissues, regardless of the risk of recurrence and metastasis. CSCs' resistance to chemo-/radiotherapies is the most common cause of treatment failure in multiple malignancies. Recently, novel therapeutic approaches targeting the robust CSCs' characteristic features that contribute to their therapeutic resistance have been designed. Alteration in the over-/downexpressed regulatory CSCs' surface biomarkers and cellular signaling pathways are considered among the targeted therapeutic strategies. Recent developments of the monoclonal antibodies (mAb), antibody-drug conjugate (ADC), immunotoxin, bispecific antibodies, chimeric antigen receptor T cell (CAR-T) therapy, phytomedicine, and nanomedicine have promising specificity of the intended cellular target binding with high accuracy. The most frequent therapeutic targeting strategies discussed in the following chapter are (1) targeting surface biomarkers; (2) targeting transcription factors; (3) targeting regulatory signaling pathways (e.g., Notch, Hh, and Wnt/ß-catenin); (4) targeting CSC microenvironment; and (5) targeting ATP-binding cassette transporters. Some of the newly developed therapeutic strategies can successfully kill CSCs, while others are still under preclinical and/or clinical evaluation. Combined therapy of multiple strategies can be much powerful for potential CSCs' selective targeting and tumor eradication

5.1 Targeting Surface Biomarkers and ALDH

Most of the CSC biomarkers are present in both heterogeneous CSCs and normal stem cell populations, for essential regenerative homeostatic functions, making targeted therapy challenging (Zhu and Fan 2018; Walcher et al. 2020). Consequently, CSC targeting should be based on a combination of different surface biomarkers or a combination of surface and intracellular markers (Walcher et al. 2020; Gamage et al. 2023). The most common targeted cellular surface biomarkers such as CD44, CD44v6, CD133, CD123, and EpCAm (Table 1) are considered one of the most effective frequently utilized CSC therapeutic approaches (Chen et al. 2013b) (Zeng et al. 2023). CD123 (IL-3R subunit-α) was one of the most promising surface adhesion targets for leukemic stem cells (LSCs) specific therapy (Jin et al. 2009; Busfield et al. 2014; Espinoza-Gutarra et al. 2021). Although its expression was highly observed in cells surviving chemotherapy (Lane et al. 2021), the development of specific targeted therapy against CD123 has been challenging. Anti-CD123 targeted therapies, including monoclonal antibody "talacotuzumab" (Montesinos et al. 2021), recombinant immunotoxin "tagraxofusp" (TAG, SL-401) (Tandon et al. 2019), and antibody-drug conjugate "IMGN632" (Daver et al. 2021a, b), have been designed and experimentally tested. Some monotherapies and combination therapies were favorably recommended as CD123 targeted therapy, to avoid any noticeable toxicity of few mAb and Ab-drug conjugates, such as TAG with AZA combination (Lane et al. 2021). A bispecific antibody, flotetuzumab (MGD006), has shown a dual-targeting affinity against both CD123 expressing cancer cells and CD3 in T cells (Chichili et al. 2015; Al-Hussaini et al. 2016; Gamage et al. 2023). Ongoing clinical trials on XmAb14045 (NCT02730312), JNJ-63709178 (NCT02715011) (Gaudet et al. 2016), and APVO436 (NCT03647800) (Comeau et al. 2018) are being investigated as potential CD123 x CD3 bispecific antibody-targeted therapies (Gamage et al. 2023). Recent discovery of anti-CD123 CAR-T cell therapy of humanized CSL362-based recombinant mAb has shown potent anticancer activity with minimal toxicity on healthy cells (El Khawanky et al. 2021). CD33 is a surface biomarker expressed in a subset of LSCs and plays a role in its immune invasion. The monoclonal antibody, gemtuzumab ozogamicin (GO), and the monoclonal antibody conjugated with pyrrolobenzodiazepine dimer, vadastuximab talirine (SGN-33A), can target the LSC surface biomarker CD33. A recommended use of GO combined with intensive therapy has proven to improve a 5-year survival rate from 50% to 70% (Borthakur and Kantarjian 2021; Kantarjian et al. 2021). However, its usage is currently restricted to the newly diagnosed or relapsed/refractory (R/R) $CD33^+$ AML cases because of its initially observed toxicity (Goldenson et al. 2021). In 2017, a clinical trial was conducted to investigate the combination of vadastuximab talirine (SGN-33A) with azacitadine or decitabine, in newly diagnosed older patients. However, this trial was terminated because of the infection-related higher death rates (Gamage et al. 2023).

Recent studies have approved the contribution of the C-type lectin-like receptors (CLL-1 or CLEC12A) to increased tumorigenesis (Arima et al. 2020). CLL-1 is a reliable biomarker for minimal residual stem cell disease (MSD), because it is highly quantified on LSCs either after diagnosis or following chemotherapy (Van Rhenen et al. 2005; Daga et al. 2020). Anti-CLL-1 CAR-T therapy has been investigated on small-scale case studies, to be safe and effective for children with R/R AML (Zhang et al. 2021b) and secondary AML (Zhang et al. 2020). However, a recently published phase I study on R/R AML adults revealed the risk of developing severe agranulocytosis where CLL-1 is dominant in granulocytes (Jin et al. 2022). Another transmembrane protein CD44 and its variant CD44v6 have been associated with poor prognosis in AML (Yokota et al. 1998). Promising results had been observed with the use of anti-CD44 including the monoclonal antibody H90 (Jin et al. 2006) and recombinant RG7356 (Vey et al. 2016). While an in vivo recent study has demonstrated that CD44 knockout sensitizes AML cells to venetoclax-based treatment (Yu et al. 2021). CD133/prominin-1 (PROM1) contributes to tumor initiation, metastasis, recurrence, and treatment resistance in hepatocellular carcinoma (HCC) (Liu and Qian 2021). Anti-CD133 CAR-T cell therapy is currently being investigated in HCCs (Gamage et al. 2023). Both in vitro and in vivo animal studies showed an effective anticancer and chemotherapeutic efficacy of the monoclonal antibody CD133mAb (Chen et al. 2013a). In addition, surface marker–targeted therapies against CD44, CD24, CD133, and CD117 for gynecological cancer treatment are being developed (Keyvani et al. 2022). In vitro treatment of hyaluronic acid-paclitaxel (HA-TXL) successfully reduced tumor weight in $CD44^+$ SKOV3 cells (Keyvani et al. 2019). Intraperitoneally administered anti-CD133-targeted toxin was able to selectively reduce the tumor progression in an in vivo mice model (Skubitz et al. 2013). Short hairpin RNA has been suggested to inhibit CD24 causing apoptosis in SKOV3 cells and tumor growth reduction in an in vivo mouse model (Su et al. 2009). Anti-CD117, imatinib mesylate, is used to treat chemoresistant ovarian tumors by inhibiting Wnt/β-catenin-ABCG2 pathway (Raspollini et al. 2004; Chau et al. 2013). Significant in vitro growth inhibition of $CD44^+$ $CD117^+$ CSCs has been demonstrated upon the treatment of metformin (Shank et al. 2012; Zhang et al. 2015) and paclitaxel combined with salinomycin (Chung et al. 2016). A bispecific antibody, catumaxomab (Removab) binds to T cells via CD3 and tumor cells via EpCAM antigen (Linke et al. 2010). A phase II randomized, multicenter clinical trial (NCT00189345) conducted on platinum-resistant epithelial ovarian cancer patients has suggested the modest activity of catumaxomab especially at high doses (Knödler et al. 2018). SPL-108 has shown promise in eradicating $CD44^+$ovarian cancer. Moreover, its combination with weekly paclitaxel was observed to be well tolerated with promising antitumor activity, in a phase I trial of $CD44^+$ advanced ovarian cancer patients (Girda et al.

2022). Salazosulfapyridine (SASP) inhibits xCT subunit of the xc(−) transporter system and thereby suppresses proliferation of CD44v + cancer cells. A combination of SASP with cisplatin-pemetrexed has been proven safe with evidence of increased progression-free survival period in non-small cell lung cancer patients (Otsubo et al. 2017). Also, CD44, CD24, ALDH1, CD113, EpCAM, ABCG2, GD2, and CXCR4 have been identified as key markers of breast cancer stem cells (BCSCs) (Al-Hajj et al. 2003). Anti-CD44 monoclonal antibody, P245, is known to inhibit the basal-like triple-negative breast cancer (TNBC) proliferation and prevents tumor recurrence, in vivo (Marangoni et al. 2009). Many evidence proved that BCSC tumorigenicity has been reduced using CD44 binding peptide (CD44BP) (Yang et al. 2013), fk506 binding protein-like (FKBPL) and its peptide derivative AD-01 (McClements et al. 2013) as well as biocompatible nanoplatform of multi-functionalized iron oxide magnetic nanoparticles (MNPs) with anti-CD44 antibody and gemcitabine derivatives (Aires et al. 2016). In vitro and in vivo preclinical studies on monoclonal antibody–based KMP1 have revealed its antitumor activity against CD44+ bladder cancer cells (Chen et al. 2018). The effectiveness of Oncofid-P-B, an anti-CD44 receptor binder, has been revealed as safe with 75% effectiveness against Bacillus Calmette-Guérin (BCG) unresponsive in situ bladder carcinoma (Hurle et al. 2022). Anti-CD113 monoclonal antibody (CD133NPs) combined with paclitaxel has been shown to reduce the formation and local recurrence of BCSCs than using paclitaxel alone (Swaminathan et al. 2013). Adecatumumab, an EpCAM-specific antibody, was shown to have great clinical potential in patients with hormone-resistant prostate cancer (Oberneder et al. 2006).

Quercetin, a naturally occurring substance, has been investigated to inhibit BCSCs' proliferation, self-renewal, and invasiveness by targeting ALDH1 (Wang et al. 2018). Also, synthetic curcumin analogs targeting ALDH1 have shown promising potential in reducing the chemotherapy resistance (Kesharwani et al. 2015). In addition, using nanoparticles in combination with low doses of decitabine (NPDAC) and doxorubicin (NPDOX) has shown a significant reduction in the ALDH1+BCSC population and increases sensitivity to the drugs administered (Li et al. 2015). Several in vitro and in vivo studies have shown the potent inhibitory effect of nanoformulations of disulfiram or diethyldithiocarbamate with metal oxide NPs on ALDH1 and ALDH2 in suppressing CSC-mediated aggressive growth and metastasis of several cancer types (Abu-Serie and Eltarahony 2021a, b; Abu-Serie and Abdelfattah 2022; Abu-Serie and Abdelfattah 2023; Abu-Serie 2023; Abu-Serie et al. 2024a, b; Abu-Serie 2024).

5.2 Targeting Transcription Factors

Various CSC-associated transcription factors (TFs), including OCT4, SOX2, c-Myc, KLF4, NANOG, and PBX1, have been considered as potential CSC therapeutic targets (Zeng et al. 2023). Preclinical studies on some TF inhibitors have significantly revealed that statins can downregulate KLF4 (Li et al. 2017), while D347–2761 would block c-Myc (Yao et al. 2022) in CSCs derived from osteosarcoma. Ivermectin, a polycyclic lactone pesticide, has been examined to have an inhibitory effect on CSCs by targeting *OCT4*, *SOX2*, and *NANOG* (Dominguez-Gomez et al. 2018). ZF-5985KD and the peptide aptamer P42 have been proven to inhibit CSC by targeting *SOX2* (Stolzenburg et al. 2012). Moreover, T417 is a novel potential agent that targets PBX1-TF, thereby inhibiting CSCs in ovarian carcinoma (Shen et al. 2021).

5.3 Targeting Regulatory Signaling Pathways

Currently, among the main targeted CSC-related signaling pathways for cancer therapy are Notch, WNT/β-catenin, and Hh signaling pathways (Zeng et al. 2023).

5.3.1 Targeting Notch Signaling Pathway

Notch-targeted cancer therapies could be categorized into three major classes of Notch-signaling pathway inhibitors, including Notch receptor antibodies, Notch ligand antibodies, and γ-secretase inhibitors (GSIs) (Zeng et al. 2023). Among the γ-secretase inhibitors are MK-0752 (Schott et al. 2013), RO4929097 (Wu et al. 2012), and PF-03084014 (Punnasseril et al. 2023), which have well-tolerated antitumor activity against CSCs in different cancer tissue types, while others including LY3039478 (NCT02836600), AL101 (NCT03691207), and BMS-906024 (NCT01292655) are still under clinical investigation. To date, over 30 clinical trials have investigated the antitumor activity of RO4929097 in various solid tumors (NCT01131234), sarcoma (NCT01154452), and melanoma (NCT01196416) (Tolcher et al. 2012; Huang et al. 2021; Zeng et al. 2023). Inhibition of Notch receptors and ligands is another strategy for blocking Notch signaling pathway. Brontictuzumab (OMP-52 M51), an anti-Notch1 mAb, has notable clinical benefits by inhibiting Notch signaling pathway in Notch1-mutated adenoid cystic carcinoma (ACC) patients (Ferrarotto et al. 2018). Clinical evidence has reported the antitumor efficacy of anti-DLL4 mAb, demcizumab (OMP-21 M18), on advanced tumors (Smith et al. 2014; Zhang et al. 2023b). Another prominent Notch ligand is the anti-DLL4 bispecific antibody ABL001 that impedes angiogenesis in gastric and colon cancers, while also reducing the CSC population (Kim et al. 2020; Yeom et al. 2021).

Various phytomedicines have been studied targeting the components of Notch signaling pathway (Punnasseril et al. 2023). Among them, Chinese multiple herbs formula, including Qingyihuaji formula (QYHJ) (Yanli et al. 2015), Pien Tze Huang (Qi et al. 2016), and Xiaotan Sanjie (XTSJ) (Yan et al. 2014), have shown effectiveness on different CSC tissue types including pancreatic, colorectal, and gastric, respectively. Psoralidin, a natural phenolic compound derived from *Psoralea corylifolia* seeds, has also proven to inhibit Notch1 signaling in breast CSCs, and subsequently, inhibits tumor growth and induces apoptosis (Suman et al. 2013; Punnasseril et al. 2023)

5.3.2 Targeting Hedgehog (Hh) Signaling Pathway

Sonic hedgehog (Shh) signaling has been proven in various cancer tissue types. SMO, a transmembrane protein, is a main transduction component in the Shh signaling pathway that mediates TF transfer and maintains CSC stemness (Merchant and Matsui 2010; Zeng et al. 2023). Inhibitors targeting SMO have noticed to exhibit greater effectiveness in treating basal cell carcinoma (BCC) and medulloblastoma compared to other cancer types (Justilien and Fields 2015; Zeng et al. 2023). A clinical trial (NCT00833417) on an FDA-approved SMO inhibitor named Vismodegib has indicated that 73% of the enrolled BCC patients had tumor shrinkage after vismodegib treatment (Sekulic et al. 2012). However, vismodegib's therapeutic effect was not satisfactory in other solid tumors (NCT01064622 and NCT01209143) (Zeng et al. 2023). Increasing evidence (NCT01546038) has demonstrated the promising therapeutic effect of glasdegib on AML by inhibiting Shh signaling (Cortes et al. 2019; Sarkaria and Heaney 2021). Other Shh inhibitors, including BMS-833923, LDE225, and LEQ506, are under ongoing clinical trial investigations (Zeng et al. 2023).

There are a variety of phytomedicines, either as multiple herbal preparations or naturally isolated active ingredients, that have been found to target the Hh pathway. A Korean herbal preparation, MSC500, has proven to modulate SHh, Notch, and Wnt/β-catenin pathways, thus suppressing CSC markers in glioblastoma (GBM) 8,401 cancer cells (Yao et al. 2014). Also, BRM270, a preparation of seven medicinal plants, inhibits metastasis and stemness of PDAC cells (Huynh et al. 2019). Evidence revealed the potential of several natural bioactive ingredients to block the SHh signaling and subsequently decrease cell proliferation, reduce tumor growth, and induce apoptosis, including curcumin in bladder CSCs (Wang et al. 2017), as well as sulforaphane (Li et al. 2013) and baicalein in pancreatic CSCs (Punnasseril et al. 2023).

5.3.3 Targeting WNT/ß-Catenin Signaling Pathway

WNT/β-catenin signaling pathway activation contributes to the maintenance of CSC characteristics, tumor propagation, and poor patient prognosis (Zeng et al. 2023). Until recently, agents targeting the WNT/β-catenin signaling components have been under clinical trial investigations. A novel β-catenin inhibitor small molecule named CWP232291 aims to suppress β-catenin and potentially achieve clinical remission in prostatic carcinoma (Pak et al. 2019). Phase I clinical studies have shown its effectiveness on acute myeloid leukemia (NCT03055286) (Cortes et al. 2015), as well as recurrent or refractory myeloma (NCT02426723) (Min et al. 2019). Both vantictumab (OMP-18R5) and ipafricept have shown effective antitumor activity in breast, ovarian, and pancreatic cancers through targeting and blocking frizzled receptors (Fischer et al. 2017). Ongoing clinical trials are conducted to investigate effectiveness of other various WNT/β-catenin signaling inhibitors including ETC-1922159 (NCT02521844), OMP-54F28 (NCT01608867 and NCT02092363), PRI-724 (NCT01606579), and LGK974 (NCT01351103) (Zeng et al. 2023).

Currently, phytomedicines targeting the Wnt/β-catenin signaling components are being investigated (Punnasseril et al. 2023). Diallyl trisulfide (DATS), a predominant organosulfur-active ingredient in garlic, was effectively able to reduce β-catenin, and suppress Wnt/β-catenin pathway in colorectal CSCs (Antony and Singh 2011; Zhang et al. 2018, 2023b; He et al. 2020). Koenimbin, derived from curry tree plant, was found to reduce β-catenin and cyclin-D1 expression in an in vitro study on CSCs of MCF7, a breast cancer cell line (Ahmadipour et al. 2015). Also, sulforaphane, derived from cruciferous vegetables, inhibited the CSC nasopharyngeal spheroid tumor formation (Chen et al. 2019). Other effective naturally occurring active ingredients include gomisin M2 for breast CSCs (Yang et al. 2019), chelerythrine chloride and sanguinarine for lung cancer (Yang et al. 2016; Heng and Cheah 2020), ginsenoside-Rb1 for ovarian CSCs (Deng et al. 2017), and evodiamine for colon CSCs (Kim et al. 2019) and gastric CSCs (Wen et al. 2015).

5.4 Targeting CSC Microenvironment

Therapies targeting the CSC microenvironment may be useful in evading treatment resistance (Xu et al. 2023a). Chen et al. indicated that orally administered erlotinib was efficiently able to normalize the tumor vascular system, improve perfusion and oxygenation, as well as enhance the nanodrug chemotherapeutic effects in an in vivo mouse model of BC (Chen et al. 2017). Several drugs targeting metalloproteinases (MMPs) have been developed to control CSC invasion and metastasis (Roma-Rodrigues et al. 2019). For instance, incyclinide, also known as CMT-3 or COL-3, is an MMP inhibitor that went through several clinical trial investigations for advanced carcinomas (NCT00004147, NCT00003721, NCT00001683, and NCT00020683) (Fingleton 2003; Gu et al. 2005; Chu et al. 2007). Other MMP inhibitors include JNJ0966, with a high selectivity toward MMP-9 (Scannevin et al. 2017), and the antibody Fab 3,369 that targets MMP-14 (Ling et al. 2017). Therapies designed to tackle hypoxia-induced factor-1 (HIF-1) or its targets can also avoid tumor progression (Paolicchi et al. 2016; Yu et al. 2017; Roma-Rodrigues et al. 2019). Among these, topotecan, an FDA-approved topoisomerase-1 inhibitor, is used as second-line treatment for both ovarian and small cell lung cancer. A clinical trial (NCT00117013) studied the use of topotecan for the treatment of refractory advanced solid neoplasms expressing HIF-1α (Duffy et al. 2010). Other clinical trials were conducted to evaluate the metformin effect in tissue oxygenation of neck and head squamous cell carcinoma (NCT03510390); everolimus (RAD001) effect in phase IV trial (NCT01206764) on patients with advanced renal cell carcinoma; everolimus (RAD001) conjugated with lenvatinib effect in phase II study (NCT03324373) on renal cell carcinoma; and digoxin (DIG-HIF1) pharmacodynamics in phase II study (NCT01763931) of newly diagnosed operable breast cancer (Roma-Rodrigues et al. 2019). Tumor microenvironment (TME) acidification seems to protect tumor cells from chemotherapy (Kolosenko et al. 2017). Thus, current clinical trial investigations propose the use of combined therapies targeting carbonic anhydrase and tumor cells to ensure efficient drug delivery in the acidic TME. Among them are the use of acetazolamide and radiotherapy (NCT03467360) for small cell lung cancer (SCLC) treatment, using SLC-0111 and gemcitabine (NCT03450018) for carbonic anhydrase-IX positive pancreatic ductal cancer treatment, and combination of acetazolamide and temozolomide (NCT03011671) for brain malignant glioma treatment cancer (Roma-Rodrigues et al. 2019). In addition, AzCDF, a small molecule drug, has been reported to target a hypoxic BCSC microenvironment, blocking its tumor growth and lowering tumorigenesis rates (Kim et al. 2021).

A few TME-targeted nanomedicines are already under clinical trials, with only one already approved. Liposomal mifamurtide, the one already approved nanoformula only in Europe, targets specifically the immune system by activating monocytes and macrophages (Siegler et al. 2016). Two more ongoing clinical trials on mifamurtide, including an observational study (NCT03737435) analyzing TME in localized osteosarcoma patients treated with mifamurtide, and a phase II trial evaluating the mifarmutide efficacy as add-on treatment to the postoperative chemotherapy in high-risk osteosarcoma patients. Another two recruiting clinical trials using CRLX101, a polymeric nanoparticle with camptothecin targeting HIF-1, are conducted to investigate its efficacy in combination with enzalutamide for prostate cancer treatment (NCT03531827) or with olaparib for relapsed/refractory small cell lung cancer treatment (NCT02769962). Also, phase I clinical trials (NCT00356980 and NCT00436410) use CYT-6091, gold nanoparticles with TNFα, for targeting the immune system (Roma-Rodrigues et al. 2019).

5.5 Targeting ATP-Binding Cassette Transporters

Apatinib, also known as rivoceranib, can significantly inhibit BCSC proliferation by downregulating the ABCG2 expression (Jiang et al. 2022). Progesterone has been demonstrated to increase BCSC sensitivity to the drug treatment by modulating ABCG2 transcriptional activity, leading to decreased drug efflux (Wu et al. 2013). Also, lapatinib was found to block ABCG2-mediated efflux in an in vitro study on HER2-positive BC cells (Vannini et al. 2009). Another ABCG2-transporter inhibitor, elacridar, has been reported to enhance the lapatinib therapeutic effect on HER2-positive advanced and metastatic BC (Karbownik et al. 2020). Yi et al. indicated that pyrotinib was able to inhibit ABCG2 expression to restore the sensitivity of drug-resistant HER2-positive BC cells (Yi et al. 2020; Xu et al. 2023a). Nutrition supplement of a vitamin B derivative named fursultiamine, also known as thiamine tetrahydrofurfuryl disulfide (TTFD), has efficiently suppressed ABCB1 and ABCG2 expression in CSC tumor spheres of esophageal carcinoma (Bighetti-Trevisan et al. 2019).

6 Conclusion and Future Perspectives

Many obstacles are frequently encountered while developing a new CSC targeted remedy. A better understanding of CSC's robust characteristic features, cellular signaling mechanisms, and diagnostic biomarkers could open the road to new targeted therapeutic strategies and improve patient survival in the near future. The underpinning mediators of aggressive CSC phenotypes including self-renewal, chemo-/immune-resistance, metastasis, and metabolic plasticity are critical for developing true cancer-fighting approaches. As it was declared, these unique features are mediated not only by CSC itself but also its niche. It is worth noting that hypoxic niche and TGFβ, which is secreted by cancer-associated fibroblasts (CAFs) and tumor-associated macrophages (TAMs), induce dedifferentiation of cancer cells to CSCs and EMT. This indicates conventional chemotherapy that only combats non-CSCs or CSC-targeted therapy cannot efficiently eradicate the tumor. Because, in the case of chemotherapy, chemoresistant CSCs can regenerate heterogeneous populations of the tumor. Regarding CSC-targeted drugs, the survived differentiated cancer cells can dedifferentiate into CSCs in order to maintain the proper dynamic balance between them. Consequently, this switch between non-CSCs and CSCs confirms the importance of combining traditional therapy with CSC-targeted drugs. It also implies that targeting niche will offer successful outcomes for both suppressing stemness and dedifferentiating non-CSCs. In this context, due to CSCs' metabolic flexibility, dual inhibition of anaerobic glycolysis and OxPhos may be an effective antimetabolite therapy for eliminating both CSCs and non-CSCs.

The CSCs' overexpression of ABC transports represents a huge obstacle for cancer therapy; hence, nanoparticles that cannot be recognized by these drug efflux pumps could be promising to overcome therapeutic resistance. Future challenges should, therefore, include the loading of chemotherapeutic drug with CSC inhibitor in single nanocarrier, increasing drug retention, and improving the specificity and effectiveness of this nanodrug against tumor with the lowest toxicity on normal tissues. Also, when designing a new anticancer drug, attention should be paid to targeting the niche.

Accordingly, it is urgently required to develop a new nanodrug loading with a safe compound which has a dual inhibitory potential against CSC stemness and their niche along with conventional chemotherapeutic compound. This nanodrug may be considered a promising ideal strategy for cancer eradication without relapse.

Acknowledgments Not applicable.

Declarations

Compliance with Ethical Standards Not applicable.

Funding Not applicable.

Consent for Publication Not applicable.

Competing Interests The authors declare that they have no competing interests.

References

Abdelbary AM, Atwa HA, Elfarargy OM et al (2023) Prognostic Implications of CD24, SOX2, and Nanog Expression in Invasive Urothelial Carcinoma. Appl Immunohistochem Mol Morphol 31: 421

Abdullah LN, Chow EK-H (2013) Mechanisms of chemoresistance in cancer stem cells. Clin Transl Med 2:3. https://doi.org/10.1186/2001-1326-2-3

Abu-Serie, MM (2023) Targeted ferroptotic potency of ferrous oxide nanoparticles-diethyldithiocarbamate nanocomplex on the metastatic liver cancer. Front Pharmacol 13: 1089667.

Abu-Serie, MM (2024) Synergistic eradicating impact of 5-fluouracil with FeO nanoparticles-diethyldithiocarbamate in colon cancer spheroids. Nanomedicine (Lond). 19(11):979–994.

Abu-Serie, MM, Eltarahony M (2021a) Novel nanoformulation of disulfiram with bacterially synthesized copper oxide nanoparticles for augmenting anticancer activity: An in vitro study. Cancer Nanotechnol 12:25.

Abu-Serie MM, Eltarahony M (2021b) Novel nanoformulated diethyldithiocarbamate complexes with biosynthesized or green chemosynthesized copper oxide nanoparticles: An in vitro comparative anticancer study. Int J Pharm 609:121130.

Abu-Serie MM, Abdelfattah EZ A (2022) Anti-metastatic breast cancer potential of novel nanocomplexes of diethyldithiocarbamate and green chemically synthesized iron oxide nanoparticles. Int J Pharm 627:122208.

Abu-Serie MM, Abdelfattah EZ A (2023) A comparative study of smart nanoformulations of diethyldithiocarbamate with Cu_4O_3 nanoparticles or zinc oxide nanoparticles for efficient eradication of metastatic breast cancer. Sci Rep 13:3529.

Abu-Serie MM, Barakat A, Ramadan S, Habashy NH (2024a) Superior cuproptotic efficacy of diethyldithiocarbamate-Cu_4O_3 nanoparticles over diethyldithiocarbamate-Cu_2O nanoparticles in metastatic hepatocellular carcinoma. Front Pharmacol 15:1388038.

Abu-Serie MM, Osuka S, Heikal LA, Teleb M, Barakat A, Dudeja V (2024b) Diethyldithiocarbamate-ferrous oxide nanoparticles inhibit human and mouse glioblastoma stemness: aldehyde dehydrogenase 1A1 suppression and ferroptosis induction. Front Pharmacol 15:1363511.

Adhikari AS, Agarwal N, Wood BM et al (2010) CD117 and Stro-1 identify osteosarcoma tumor-initiating cells associated with metastasis and drug resistance. Cancer Res 70:4602–4612. https://doi.org/10.1158/0008-5472.CAN-09-3463

Afroze SN, Rao GV, Suri S (2022) Elucidating the immunohistochemistry of Nanog: A transcription marker in the oral squamous cell carcinoma with emphasis on its origin as embryonic stem cell. J Oral Maxillofac Pathol 26:476–482. https://doi.org/10.4103/jomfp.jomfp_347_22

Ahmadipour F, Noordin MI, Mohan S et al (2015) Koenimbin, a natural dietary compound of murraya koenigii (L) spreng: Inhibition of MCF7 breast cancer cells and targeting of derived MCF7 breast cancer stem cells (CD44+/CD24−/low): An in vitro study. Drug Des Devel Ther 9:1193–1208

Aires A, Ocampo SM, Simões BM et al (2016) Multifunctionalized iron oxide nanoparticles for selective drug delivery to CD44-positive cancer cells. Nanotechnology 27:65103

Al Mamun M, Mannoor K, Cao J et al (2020) SOX2 in cancer stemness: tumor malignancy and therapeutic potentials. J Mol Cell Biol 12:85–98. https://doi.org/10.1093/JMCB/MJY080

Al-Hajj M, Wicha MS, Benito-Hernandez A et al (2003) Prospective identification of tumorigenic breast cancer cells. Proc Natl Acad Sci USA 100:3983–3988. https://doi.org/10.1073/pnas.0530291100

Al-Hussaini M, Rettig MP, Ritchey JK et al (2016) Targeting CD123 in acute myeloid leukemia using a T-cell–directed dual-affinity retargeting platform. Blood 127:122–131. https://doi.org/10.1182/blood-2014-05-575704

Al-Zubaidi MA (2022) Analysis of protein-protein interaction network based on transcriptome profiling of human induced pluripotent stem cellsidentifies candidate genes. J Pharm Negat Results 13:66–73. https://doi.org/10.47750/pnr.2022.13.03.010

Antony ML, Singh SV (2011) Molecular mechanisms and targets of cancer chemoprevention by garlic-derived bioactive compound diallyl trisulfide. Indian J Exp Biol 49:805

Aramini B, Masciale V, Arienti C et al (2022) Cancer stem cells (CSCs), circulating tumor cells (CTCs) and their interplay with cancer associated fibroblasts (CAFs): a new world of targets and treatments. Cancers (Basel) 14:1–20

Arima Y, Nobusue H, Saya H (2020) Targeting of cancer stem cells by differentiation therapy. Cancer Sci 111:2689–2695. https://doi.org/10.1111/cas.14504

Askmyr M, Ågerstam H, Hansen N et al (2013) Selective killing of candidate AML stem cells by antibody targeting of IL1RAP. Blood J Am Soc Hematol 121:3709–3713

Atashzar MR, Baharlou R, Karami J et al (2020) Cancer stem cells: A review from origin to therapeutic implications. J Cell Physiol 235:790–803. https://doi.org/10.1002/jcp.29044

Azevedo R, Gaiteiro C, Peixoto A et al (2018) CD44 glycoprotein in cancer: a molecular conundrum hampering clinical applications. Clin Proteomics 15:1–5

Bae K-M, Parker NN, Dai Y et al (2011) E-cadherin plasticity in prostate cancer stem cell invasion. Am J Cancer Res 1:71

Bang J, Jun M, Lee S et al (2023) Targeting EGFR/PI3K/AKT/mTOR Signaling in Hepatocellular Carcinoma. Pharmaceutics 15. https://doi.org/10.3390/pharmaceutics15082130

Bao S, Wu Q, Li Z et al (2008) Targeting cancer stem cells through L1CAM suppresses glioma growth. Cancer Res 68:6043–6048

Barclay AN, Van den Berg TK (2014) The interaction between signal regulatory protein alpha (SIRPα) and CD47: structure, function, and therapeutic target. Annu Rev Immunol 32:25–50

Basu S, Dong Y, Kumar R et al (2022) Slow-cycling (dormant) cancer cells in therapy resistance, cancer relapse and metastasis. Semin Cancer Biol 78:90–103. https://doi.org/10.1016/j.semcancer.2021.04.021

Begicevic RR, Falasca M (2017) ABC transporters in cancer stem cells: Beyond chemoresistance. Int J Mol Sci 18. https://doi.org/10.3390/ijms18112362

Bekaii-Saab T, El-Rayes B (2017) Identifying and targeting cancer stem cells in the treatment of gastric cancer. Cancer 123:1303–1312. https://doi.org/10.1002/cncr.30538

Bhatia M, Wang JCY, Kapp U et al (1997) Purification of primitive human hematopoietic cells capable of repopulating immune-deficient mice. Proc Natl Acad Sci 94:5320–5325

Bighetti-Trevisan RL, Sousa LO, Castilho RM, Almeida LO (2019) Cancer stem cells: powerful targets to improve current anticancer therapeutics. Stem Cells Int 2019:1. https://doi.org/10.1155/2019/9618065

Blair A, Hogge DE, Sutherland HJ (1998) Most acute myeloid leukemia progenitor cells with long-term proliferative ability in vitro and in vivo have the phenotype CD34+/CD71−/HLA-DR−. Blood, J Am Soc Hematol 92:4325–4335

Bonnet D, Dick JE (1997) Human acute myeloid leukemia is organized as a hierarchy that originates from a primitive hematopoietic cell. Nat Med 3:730–737. https://doi.org/10.1038/nm0797-730

Borah A, Raveendran S, Rochani A et al (2015) Targeting self-renewal pathways in cancer stem cells: clinical implications for cancer therapy. Oncogenesis 4:e177. https://doi.org/10.1038/oncsis.2015.35

Borthakur G, Kantarjian H (2021) Core binding factor acute myelogenous leukemia-2021 treatment algorithm. Blood Cancer J 11:114. https://doi.org/10.1038/s41408-021-00503-6

Bray F, Ferlay J, Soerjomataram I et al (2018) Global cancer statistics 2018: GLOBOCAN estimates of incidence and mortality worldwide for 36 cancers in 185 countries. CA Cancer J Clin 68:394–424. https://doi.org/10.3322/caac.21492

Brunet A, Goodell MA, Rando TA (2023) Ageing and rejuvenation of tissue stem cells and their niches. Nat Rev Mol Cell Biol 24:45–62. https://doi.org/10.1038/s41580-022-00510-w

Busfield SJ, Biondo M, Wong M et al (2014) Targeting of acute myeloid leukemia in vitro and in vivo with an anti-CD123 mAb engineered for optimal ADCC. Leukemia 28:2213–2221

Calavul A, Özdemİr İ (2023) The role of stem cell in plastic reconstructive and aesthetic surgery. IKSAD Publishing House

Cao H, Heazlewood SY, Williams B et al (2016) The role of CD44 in fetal and adult hematopoietic stem cell regulation. Haematologica 101:26

Chan KS, Volkmer J-P, Weissman I (2010) Cancer stem cells in bladder cancer: a revisited and evolving concept. Curr Opin Urol 20:393

Chang CH, Zhang M, Rajapakshe K et al (2015) Mammary stem cells and tumor-initiating cells are more resistant to apoptosis and exhibit increased DNA repair activity in response to DNA damage. Stem Cell Reports 5:378–391. https://doi.org/10.1016/j.stemcr.2015.07.009

Chatterjee A, Paul S, Bisht B et al (2022) Advances in targeting the WNT/β-catenin signaling pathway in cancer. Drug Discov Today 27:82–101. https://doi.org/10.1016/j.drudis.2021.07.007

Chau WK, Ip CK, Mak ASC et al (2013) c-Kit mediates chemoresistance and tumor-initiating capacity of ovarian cancer cells through activation of Wnt/β-catenin–ATP-binding cassette G2 signaling. Oncogene 32:2767–2781

Chen H, Luo Z, Sun W et al (2013a) Low glucose promotes CD133mAb-elicited cell death via inhibition of autophagy in hepatocarcinoma cells. Cancer Lett 336:204–212. https://doi.org/10.1016/j.canlet.2013.04.031

Chen K, Huang YH, Chen JL (2013b) Understanding and targeting cancer stem cells: Therapeutic implications and challenges. Acta Pharmacol Sin 34:732–740. https://doi.org/10.1038/aps.2013.27

Chen Y, Bieber MM, Teng NNH (2014) Hedgehog signaling regulates drug sensitivity by targeting ABC transporters ABCB1 and ABCG2 in epithelial ovarian cancer. Mol Carcinog 53:625–634. https://doi.org/10.1002/mc.22015

Chen W, Dong J, Haiech J et al (2016) Cancer stem cell quiescence and plasticity as major challenges in cancer therapy. Stem Cells Int 2016:1

Chen Q, Xu L, Chen J et al (2017) Tumor vasculature normalization by orally fed erlotinib to modulate the tumor microenvironment for enhanced cancer nanomedicine and immunotherapy. Biomaterials 148:69–80

Chen Y, Wang H, Zuo Y et al (2018) A novel monoclonal antibody KMP1 has potential antitumor activity of bladder cancer by blocking CD44 in vivo and in vitro. Cancer Med 7:2064–2077. https://doi.org/10.1002/cam4.1446

Chen L, Chan LS, Lung HL et al (2019) Crucifera sulforaphane (SFN) inhibits the growth of nasopharyngeal carcinoma through DNA methyltransferase 1 (DNMT1)/Wnt inhibitory factor 1 (WIF1) axis. Phytomedicine 63:153058. https://doi.org/10.1016/j.phymed.2019.153058

Chen K, Zhang C, Ling S et al (2021) The metabolic flexibility of quiescent CSC: implications for chemotherapy resistance. Cell Death Dis 12:835. https://doi.org/10.1038/s41419-021-04116-6

Chen YA, Lu CY, Cheng WF et al (2022) An experimental model for ovarian cancer: propagation of ovarian cancer initiating cells and generation of ovarian cancer organoids. BMC Cancer 22: 1–21. https://doi.org/10.1186/s12885-022-10042-3

Cheng J-X, Liu B-L, Zhang X (2009) How powerful is CD133 as a cancer stem cell marker in brain tumors? Cancer Treat Rev 35:403–408

Chichili GR, Huang L, Li H, et al (2015) A CD3xCD123 bispecific DART for redirecting host T cells to myelogenous leukemia: Preclinical activity and safety in nonhuman primates. Sci Transl Med 7:289ra82-289ra82. https://doi.org/10.1126/scitranslmed.aaa5693

Chu QSC, Forouzesh B, Syed S et al (2007) A phase II and pharmacological study of the matrix metalloproteinase inhibitor (MMPI) COL-3 in patients with advanced soft tissue sarcomas. Investig New Drugs 25:359–367

Chung H, Kim Y-H, Kwon M et al (2016) The effect of salinomycin on ovarian cancer stem-like cells. Obstet Gynecol Sci 59:261. https://doi.org/10.5468/ogs.2016.59.4.261

Cochrane CR, Szczepny A, Watkins DN, Cain JE (2015) Hedgehog signaling in the maintenance of cancer stem cells. Cancers (Basel) 7:1554–1585. https://doi.org/10.3390/cancers7030851

Collins AT, Berry PA, Hyde C et al (2005) Prospective identification of tumorigenic prostate cancer stem cells. Cancer Res 65:10946–10951

Comeau MR, Miller RE, Bader R et al (2018) Abstract 1786: APVO436, a bispecific anti-CD123 x anti-CD3 ADAPTIR™ molecule for redirected T-cell cytotoxicity, induces potent T-cell activation, proliferation and cytotoxicity with limited cytokine release. Cancer Res 78:1786. https://doi.org/10.1158/1538-7445.AM2018-1786

Cortes JE, Faderl S, Pagel J et al (2015) Phase 1 study of CWP232291 in relapsed/refractory acute myeloid leukemia (AML) and myelodysplastic syndrome (MDS). J Clin Oncol 33:7044. https://doi.org/10.1200/jco.2015.33.15_suppl.7044

Cortes JE, Heidel FH, Hellmann A et al (2019) Randomized comparison of low dose cytarabine with or without glasdegib in patients with newly diagnosed acute myeloid leukemia or high-risk myelodysplastic syndrome. Leukemia 33:379–389. https://doi.org/10.1038/s41375-018-0312-9

Cox CV, Diamanti P, Evely RS et al (2009) Expression of CD133 on leukemia-initiating cells in childhood ALL. Blood J Am Soc Hematol 113:3287–3296

Czabotar PE, Garcia-Saez AJ (2023) Mechanisms of BCL-2 family proteins in mitochondrial apoptosis. Nat Rev Mol Cell Biol 24:732–748. https://doi.org/10.1038/s41580-023-00629-4

da Costa KM, Freire-de-Lima L, da Fonseca LM et al (2023) ABCB1 and ABCC1 function during TGF-β-induced epithelial-mesenchymal transition: relationship between multidrug resistance and tumor progression. Int J Mol Sci 24:1–18. https://doi.org/10.3390/ijms24076046

Daga S, Rosenberger A, Kashofer K et al (2020) Sensitive and broadly applicable residual disease detection in acute myeloid leukemia using flow cytometry-based leukemic cell enrichment followed by mutational profiling. Am J Hematol 95:1148–1157. https://doi.org/10.1002/ajh.25918

Dai Y, Zhang X, Ou Y et al (2023) Anoikis resistance—protagonists of breast cancer cells survive and metastasize after ECM detachment. Cell Commun Signal 21:1–24

Dalerba P, Dylla SJ, Park IK et al (2007) Phenotypic characterization of human colorectal cancer stem cells. Proc Natl Acad Sci USA 104:10158–10163. https://doi.org/10.1073/pnas.0703478104

Darash-Yahana M, Pikarsky E, Abramovitch R et al (2004) Role of high expression levels of CXCR4 in tumor growth, vascularization, and metastasis. FASEB J 18:1240–1242

Das PK, Islam F, Lam AK (2020) The roles of cancer stem cells and therapy resistance in colorectal carcinoma. Cells 9:1–21. https://doi.org/10.3390/cells9061392

Daver N, Aribi A, Montesinos P et al (2021a) Safety and efficacy from a phase 1b/2 study of IMGN632 in combination with azacitidine and venetoclax for patients with CD123-positive acute myeloid leukemia. Blood 138:372. https://doi.org/10.1182/blood-2021-146503

Daver N, Aribi A, Montesinos P et al (2021b) A phase 1b/2 Study of the CD123-targeting antibody-drug conjugate IMGN632 as monotherapy or in combination with Venetoclax and Azacitidine for patients with CD123-positive acute myeloid leukemia. Blood 138:4440. https://doi.org/10.1182/blood-2021-146585

De Francesco EM, Sotgia F, Lisanti MP (2018) Cancer stem cells (CSCs): metabolic strategies for their identification and eradication. Biochem J 475:1611–1634. https://doi.org/10.1042/BCJ20170164

de Lima Coutinho L, Junior TCT, Rangel MC (2023) Sulforaphane: An emergent anti-cancer stem cell agent. Front Oncol 13:1–10. https://doi.org/10.3389/fonc.2023.1089115

de Morree A, Rando TA (2023) Regulation of adult stem cell quiescence and its functions in the maintenance of tissue integrity. Nat Rev Mol Cell Biol 24:334–354. https://doi.org/10.1038/s41580-022-00568-6

Deng Z, Wu Y, Ma W et al (2015) Adoptive T-cell therapy of prostate cancer targeting the cancer stem cell antigen EpCAM. BMC Immunol 16:1–9

Deng S, Wong CKC, Lai HC, Wong AST (2017) Ginsenoside-Rb1 targets chemotherapy-resistant ovarian cancer stem cells via simultaneous inhibition of Wnt/β-catenin signaling and epithelial-to-mesenchymal transition. Oncotarget 8:25897–25914. https://doi.org/10.18632/oncotarget.13071

Derks LLM, van Boxtel R (2023) Stem cell mutations, associated cancer risk, and consequences for regenerative medicine. Cell Stem Cell 30:1421–1433. https://doi.org/10.1016/j.stem.2023.09.008

Dianat-Moghadam H, Mahari A, Salahlou R et al (2022) Immune evader cancer stem cells direct the perspective approaches to cancer immunotherapy. Stem Cell Res Ther 13:1–12. https://doi.org/10.1186/s13287-022-02829-9

Dietz L, Ellison CJ, Riechmann C et al (2023) Structural basis for SMAC-mediated antagonism of caspase inhibition by the giant ubiquitin ligase BIRC6. Science (80-) 379:1112–1117. https://doi.org/10.1126/science.ade8840

Ding S, Li C, Cheng N et al (2015) Redox regulation in cancer stem cells. Oxid Med Cell Longev 2015

Doan P, Musa A, Murugesan A et al (2020) Glioblastoma multiforme stem cell cycle arrest by alkylaminophenol through the modulation of EGFR and CSC signaling pathways. Cells 9. https://doi.org/10.3390/cells9030681

Dogan F, Avci CB (2018) Correlation between telomerase and mTOR pathway in cancer stem cells. Gene 641:235–239. https://doi.org/10.1016/j.gene.2017.09.072

Domanska UM, Timmer-Bosscha H, Nagengast WB et al (2012) CXCR4 inhibition with AMD3100 sensitizes prostate cancer to docetaxel chemotherapy. Neoplasia 14:709–718

Dominguez-Gomez G, Chavez-Blanco A, Medina-Franco JL et al (2018) Ivermectin as an inhibitor of cancer stem-like cells. Mol Med Rep 17:3397–3403. https://doi.org/10.3892/mmr.2017.8231

Dubrovska A, Elliott J, Salamone RJ et al (2012) CXCR4 expression in prostate cancer progenitor cells. PLoS One 7:e31226

Duffy AG, Melillo G, Turkbey B et al (2010) A pilot trial of oral topotecan (TPT) in patients with refractory advanced solid neoplasms expressing HIF-1α. J Clin Oncol 28:e13518–e13518

Edris B, Weiskopf K, Volkmer AK et al (2012) Antibody therapy targeting the CD47 protein is effective in a model of aggressive metastatic leiomyosarcoma. Proc Natl Acad Sci 109:6656–6661

El Khawanky N, Hughes A, Yu W et al (2021) Demethylating therapy increases anti-CD123 CAR T cell cytotoxicity against acute myeloid leukemia. Nat Commun 12:6436. https://doi.org/10.1038/s41467-021-26683-0

Ervin EH, French R, Chang CH, Pauklin S (2022) Inside the stemness engine: mechanistic links between deregulated transcription factors and stemness in cancer. Semin Cancer Biol 87:48–83. https://doi.org/10.1016/j.semcancer.2022.11.001

Espinoza-Gutarra MR, Green SD, Zeidner JF, Konig H (2021) CD123-targeted therapy in acute myeloid leukemia. Expert Rev Hematol 14:561–576. https://doi.org/10.1080/17474086.2021.1935855

Fan J, To KKW, Chen ZS, Fu L (2023) ABC transporters affects tumor immune microenvironment to regulate cancer immunotherapy and multidrug resistance. Drug Resist Updat 66:100905. https://doi.org/10.1016/j.drup.2022.100905

Fenwarth L, Fournier E, Cheok M et al (2020) Biomarkers of gemtuzumab ozogamicin response for acute myeloid leukemia treatment. Int J Mol Sci 21:5626

Ferrarotto R, Eckhardt G, Patnaik A et al (2018) A phase I dose-escalation and dose-expansion study of brontictuzumab in subjects with selected solid tumors. Ann Oncol 29:1561–1568. https://doi.org/10.1093/annonc/mdy171

Fingleton B (2003) CMT-3. CollaGenex. Curr Opin Investig Drugs 4:1460–1467

Fischer MM, Cancilla B, Yeung VP et al (2017) WNT antagonists exhibit unique combinatorial antitumor activity with taxanes by potentiating mitotic cell death. Sci Adv 3:e1700090. https://doi.org/10.1126/sciadv.1700090

Flahaut M, Meier R, Coulon A et al (2009) The Wnt receptor FZD1 mediates chemoresistance in neuroblastoma through activation of the Wnt/β-catenin pathway. Oncogene 28:2245–2256. https://doi.org/10.1038/onc.2009.80

Fleifel D, Cook JG (2023) G1 dynamics at the crossroads of pluripotency and cancer. Cancers (Basel) 15:1–17. https://doi.org/10.3390/cancers15184559

Fontana R, Mestre-Farrera A, Yang J (2023) Update on epithelial-mesenchymal plasticity in cancer progression. Annu Rev Pathol Mech Dis 19:133. https://doi.org/10.1146/annurev-pathmechdis-051222-122423

Fukamachi H, Seol HS, Shimada S et al (2013) CD49fhigh cells retain sphere-forming and tumor-initiating activities in human gastric tumors. PLoS One 8:e72438

Gamage SK, Ranaweera CD, Maduwage KP et al (2023) Novel therapeutics targeting cancer stem cell surface markers BT – cancer stem cells: basic concept and therapeutic implications. In: Islam F, Lam AK (eds) . Springer Nature, Singapore, pp 167–198

Gao F, Zhang Y, Wang S et al (2014) Hes1 is involved in the self-renewal and tumourigenicity of stem-like cancer cells in colon cancer. Sci Rep 4. https://doi.org/10.1038/srep03963

Garimella SV, Gampa SC, Chaturvedi P (2023) Mitochondria in cancer stem cells: from an innocent bystander to a central player in therapy resistance. Stem Cells Cloning Adv Appl 16:19–41. https://doi.org/10.2147/SCCAA.S417842

Garza Treviño EN, Quiroz Reyes AG, Rojas Murillo JA et al (2023) Cell therapy as target therapy against colon cancer stem cells. Int J Mol Sci 24:1–21. https://doi.org/10.3390/ijms24098163

Gaudet F, Nemeth JF, McDaid R et al (2016) Development of a CD123xCD3 bispecific antibody (JNJ-63709178) for the treatment of acute myeloid leukemia (AML). Blood 128:2824. https://doi.org/10.1182/blood.V128.22.2824.2824

Georgiev H, Ravens I, Papadogianni G, Bernhardt G (2018) Coming of age: CD96 emerges as modulator of immune responses. Front Immunol 9:1072

Ghoneum A, Said N (2019) PI3K-AKT-mTOR and NFkB pathways in ovarian cancer: Implications for targeted therapeutics. Cancers (Basel) 11. https://doi.org/10.3390/cancers11070949

Gillespie MS, Ward CM, Davies CC (2023) DNA repair and therapeutic strategies in cancer stem cells. Cancers (Basel) 15. https://doi.org/10.3390/cancers15061897

Gimple RC, Yang K, Halbert ME et al (2022) Brain cancer stem cells: resilience through adaptive plasticity and hierarchical heterogeneity. Nat Rev Cancer 22:497–514. https://doi.org/10.1038/s41568-022-00486-x

Girda E, Hou J, Nelson D et al (2022) Phase I trial of daily subcutaneous SPL-108 injections in combination with paclitaxel in patients with platinum resistant CD44+ advanced ovarian epithelial cancer. Int J Gynecol Cancer 32:1032

Glumac PM, LeBeau AM (2018) The role of CD133 in cancer: a concise review. Clin Transl Med 7:1–14

Goldenson BH, Goodman AM, Ball ED (2021) Gemtuzumab ozogamicin for the treatment of acute myeloid leukemia in adults. Expert Opin Biol Ther 21:849–862. https://doi.org/10.1080/14712598.2021.1825678

Gong C, Liu B, Yao Y et al (2015) Potentiated DNA damage response in circulating breast tumor cells confers resistance to chemotherapy. J Biol Chem 290:14811–14825. https://doi.org/10.1074/jbc.M115.652628

Gonzalez DM, Medici D (2014) Signaling mechanisms of the epithelial-mesenchymal transition. Sci Signal 7:re8–re8. https://doi.org/10.1126/scisignal.2005189

Gu Y, Lee H, Golub LM et al (2005) Inhibition of breast cancer cell extracellular matrix degradative activity by chemically modified tetracyclines. Ann Med 37:450–460

Guefack M-GF, Talukdar D, Mukherjee R et al (2024) Hypericum roeperianum bark extract suppresses breast cancer proliferation via induction of apoptosis, downregulation of PI3K/

Akt/mTOR signaling cascade and reversal of EMT. J Ethnopharmacol 319:117093. https://doi.org/10.1016/j.jep.2023.117093

Guo F, Zhang Y, Bai L, Cui J (2023) Natural killer cell therapy targeting cancer stem cells: Old wine in a new bottle. Cancer Lett 570:216328. https://doi.org/10.1016/j.canlet.2023.216328

Gupta I, Hussein O, Sastry KS et al (2023) Deciphering the complexities of cancer cell immune evasion: Mechanisms and therapeutic implications. Adv Cancer Biol Metastasis 8:100107. https://doi.org/10.1016/j.adcanc.2023.100107

Gutjahr JC, Greil R, Hartmann TN (2015) The role of CD44 in the pathophysiology of chronic lymphocytic leukemia. Front Immunol 6:177

Hale JS, Otvos B, Sinyuk M et al (2014) Cancer stem cell-specific scavenger receptor CD36 drives glioblastoma progression. Stem Cells 32:1746–1758

Hall CL, Dubyk CW, Riesenberger TA et al (2008) Type I collagen receptor (α2β1) signaling promotes prostate cancer invasion through RhoC GTPase. Neoplasia 10:797–803

Han L, Shi S, Gong T et al (2013) Cancer stem cells: therapeutic implications and perspectives in cancer therapy. Acta Pharm Sin B 3:65–75. https://doi.org/10.1016/j.apsb.2013.02.006

Han Q, Qiu S, Hu H et al (2023) The relationship between the Hippo signaling pathway and bone metastasis of breast cancer. Front Oncol 13:1–10. https://doi.org/10.3389/fonc.2023.1188310

Hasanzadeh A, Ebadati A, Dastanpour L et al (2023) Applications of innovation technologies for personalized cancer medicine: stem cells and gene-editing tools. ACS Pharmacol Transl Sci 6:1758. https://doi.org/10.1021/acsptsci.3c00102

Hayat R, Manzoor M, Hussain A (2022) Wnt signaling pathway: a comprehensive review. Cell Biol Int 46:863–877. https://doi.org/10.1002/cbin.11797

He J, Liu Y, Zhu T et al (2012) CD90 is identified as a candidate marker for cancer stem cells in primary high-grade gliomas using tissue microarrays. Mol Cell Proteomics 11(M111):010744. https://doi.org/10.1074/mcp.M111.010744

He P, Wang Z, Sheng B et al (2020) Diallyl trisulfide regulates cell apoptosis and invasion in human osteosarcoma U2OS cells through regulating PI3K/AKT/GSK3β signaling pathway. Histol Histopathol 35:1511–1520

Heitmann JS, Hagelstein I, Hinterleitner C et al (2020) Fc gamma receptor expression serves as prognostic and diagnostic factor in AML. Leuk Lymphoma 61:2466–2474

Heng WS, Cheah S-C (2020) Chelerythrine chloride downregulates β-catenin and inhibits stem cell properties of non-small cell lung carcinoma. Molecules 25:224

Hervieu C, Christou N, Battu S, Mathonnet M (2021) The role of cancer stem cells in colorectal cancer: From the basics to novel clinical trials. Cancers (Basel) 13:1–26. https://doi.org/10.3390/cancers13051092

Hipfner DR, Deeley RG, Cole SPC (1999) Structural, mechanistic and clinical aspects of MRP1. Biochim Biophys Acta Biomembr 1461:359–376. https://doi.org/10.1016/S0005-2736(99)00168-6

Hiremath IS, Goel A, Warrier S et al (2022) The multidimensional role of the Wnt/β-catenin signaling pathway in human malignancies. J Cell Physiol 237:199–238. https://doi.org/10.1002/jcp.30561

Hosen N, Park CY, Tatsumi N et al (2007) CD96 is a leukemic stem cell-specific marker in human acute myeloid leukemia. Proc Natl Acad Sci 104:11008–11013

Hou Y, Zou Q, Ge R et al (2012) The critical role of CD133 + CD44 +/high tumor cells in hematogenous metastasis of liver cancers. Cell Res 22:259–272. https://doi.org/10.1038/cr.2011.139

Huang L, Yang Y, Yang F et al (2018) Functions of EpCAM in physiological processes and diseases. Int J Mol Med 42:1771–1785

Huang T, Zhao C, Zhao Y et al (2021) RO4929097 regulates RANKL-induced osteoclast formation and LPS-mediated bone resorption. Aging (Albany NY) 13:12526

Huang Y, Hong W, Wei X (2022) The molecular mechanisms and therapeutic strategies of EMT in tumor progression and metastasis. J Hematol Oncol 15:1–27. https://doi.org/10.1186/s13045-022-01347-8

Hurle R, Guazzoni G, Colombo P, et al (2022) Oncofid-PB: a novel treatment for BCG unresponsive carcinoma in situ (CIS) of the bladder: results of a prospective European Multicentre study at 15 months from treatment start. In: Urologic oncology: seminars and original investigations. Elsevier, pp 11-e9

Huynh DL, Koh H, Chandimali N et al (2019) Brm270 inhibits the proliferation of cd44 positive pancreatic ductal adenocarcinoma cells via downregulation of sonic hedgehog signaling. Evid Complem Altern Med 2019:1. https://doi.org/10.1155/2019/8620469

Ibragimova M, Tsyganov M, Litviakov N (2022) Tumour stem cells in breast cancer. Int J Mol Sci 23:1–21. https://doi.org/10.3390/ijms23095058

Islam F, Lam AK (2023) Cancer stem cells: basic concept and therapeutic implications. Springer Nature

Izadpanah A, Mohammadkhani N, Masoudnia M et al (2023) Update on immune-based therapy strategies targeting cancer stem cells. Cancer Med 12:18960–18980. https://doi.org/10.1002/cam4.6520

Jackson M, Hassiotou F, Nowak A (2015) Glioblastoma stem-like cells: at the root of tumor recurrence and a therapeutic target. Carcinogenesis 36:177–185

Jaiswal S, Jamieson CHM, Pang WW et al (2009) CD47 is upregulated on circulating hematopoietic stem cells and leukemia cells to avoid phagocytosis. Cell 138:271–285

Jan M, Chao MP, Cha AC et al (2011) Prospective separation of normal and leukemic stem cells based on differential expression of TIM3, a human acute myeloid leukemia stem cell marker. Proc Natl Acad Sci 108:5009–5014

Jha H, Arora R (2022) In: Shukla D, Vishvakarma NK, Nagaraju GP (eds) Cytotoxic and chemopreventive activity of polyphenols and their derivatives in colon cancer BT – colon cancer diagnosis and therapy, vol 3. Springer, Cham, pp 241–275

Jiang ZS, Sun YZ, Wang SM, Ruan JS (2017) Epithelial-mesenchymal transition: Potential regulator of ABC transporters in tumor progression. J Cancer 8:2319–2327. https://doi.org/10.7150/jca.19079

Jiang B, Zhu H, Tang L et al (2022) Apatinib inhibits stem properties and malignant biological behaviors of breast cancer stem cells by blocking Wnt/β-catenin signal pathway through downregulating LncRNA ROR. Anti-Cancer Agents Med Chem (Formerly Curr Med Chem Agents) 22:1723–1734

Jin L, Hope KJ, Zhai Q et al (2006) Targeting of CD44 eradicates human acute myeloid leukemic stem cells. Nat Med 12:1167–1174. https://doi.org/10.1038/nm1483

Jin L, Lee EM, Ramshaw HS et al (2009) Monoclonal antibody-mediated targeting of CD123, IL-3 receptor α chain, eliminates human acute myeloid leukemic stem cells. Cell Stem Cell 5:31–42

Jin X, Zhang M, Sun R et al (2022) First-in-human phase I study of CLL-1 CAR-T cells in adults with relapsed/refractory acute myeloid leukemia. J Hematol Oncol 15:1–5. https://doi.org/10.1186/s13045-022-01308-1

Joshi K, Zhang L, Breslin S.J P, et al (2022) Role of TET dioxygenases in the regulation of both normal and pathological hematopoiesis. J Exp Clin Cancer Res 41:. https://doi.org/10.1186/s13046-022-02496-x, 294

Ju F, Atyah MM, Horstmann N et al (2022) Characteristics of the cancer stem cell niche and therapeutic strategies. Stem Cell Res Ther 13:1–17. https://doi.org/10.1186/s13287-022-02904-1

Justilien V, Fields AP (2015) Molecular pathways: Novel approaches for improved therapeutic targeting of hedgehog signaling in cancer stem cells. Clin Cancer Res 21:505–513. https://doi.org/10.1158/1078-0432.CCR-14-0507

Kageyama Y, Miwa H, Arakawa R et al (2018) Expression of CD25 fluctuates in the leukemia-initiating cell population of CD25-positive AML. PLoS One 13:e0209295

Kalluri R, Weinberg RA (2009) The basics of epithelial-mesenchymal transition. J Clin Invest 119:1420–1428

Kantarjian HM, Kadia TM, DiNardo CD et al (2021) Acute myeloid leukemia: treatment and research outlook for 2021 and the MD Anderson approach. Cancer 127:1186–1207. https://doi.org/10.1002/cncr.33477

Karbownik A, Sobańska K, Płotek W et al (2020) The influence of the coadministration of the p-glycoprotein modulator elacridar on the pharmacokinetics of lapatinib and its distribution in the brain and cerebrospinal fluid. Investig New Drugs 38:574–583

Kerr BA, Miocinovic R, Smith AK et al (2015) CD117+ cells in the circulation are predictive of advanced prostate cancer. Oncotarget 6:1889

Kesharwani RK, Srivastava V, Singh P et al (2015) A novel approach for overcoming drug resistance in breast cancer chemotherapy by targeting new synthetic curcumin analogues against aldehyde dehydrogenase 1 (ALDH1A1) and glycogen synthase kinase-3 β (GSK-3β). Appl Biochem Biotechnol 176:1996–2017

Keyvani V, Farshchian M, Esmaeili S-A et al (2019) Ovarian cancer stem cells and targeted therapy. J Ovarian Res 12:1–11

Keyvani V, Riahi E, Yousefi M et al (2022) Gynecologic Cancer, Cancer Stem Cells, and Possible Targeted Therapies. Front Pharmacol 13:823572

Kikushige Y, Shima T, Takayanagi S et al (2010) TIM-3 is a promising target to selectively kill acute myeloid leukemia stem cells. Cell Stem Cell 7:708–717

Kim Y-N, Koo KH, Sung JY et al (2012) Anoikis resistance: an essential prerequisite for tumor metastasis. Int J Cell Biol 2012:1

Kim MY, Yu K-R, Kenderian SS et al (2018) Genetic inactivation of CD33 in hematopoietic stem cells to enable CAR T cell immunotherapy for acute myeloid leukemia. Cell 173:1439–1453

Kim H, Yu Y, Choi SG et al (2019) Evodiamine eliminates colon cancer stem cells via suppressing Notch and Wnt signaling. Molecules 24. https://doi.org/10.3390/molecules24244520

Kim DH, Lee S, Kang HG et al (2020) Synergistic antitumor activity of a DLL4/VEGF bispecific therapeutic antibody in combination with irinotecan in gastric cancer. BMB Rep 53:533–538. https://doi.org/10.5483/BMBRep.2020.53.10.103

Kim JH, Verwilst P, Won M et al (2021) A small molecule strategy for targeting cancer stem cells in hypoxic microenvironments and preventing tumorigenesis. J Am Chem Soc 143:14115–14124

Klonisch T, Wiechec E, Hombach-Klonisch S et al (2008) Cancer stem cell markers in common cancers – therapeutic implications. Trends Mol Med 14:450–460. https://doi.org/10.1016/j.molmed.2008.08.003

Knödler M, Körfer J, Kunzmann V et al (2018) Randomised phase II trial to investigate catumaxomab (anti-EpCAM× anti-CD3) for treatment of peritoneal carcinomatosis in patients with gastric cancer. Br J Cancer 119:296–302

Kolosenko I, Avnet S, Baldini N, et al (2017) Therapeutic implications of tumor interstitial acidification. In: Seminars in cancer biology. Elsevier, pp 119–133

Krauss RS, Kann AP (2023) Muscle stem cells get a new look: dynamic cellular projections as sensors of the stem cell niche. BioEssays 45:2200249. https://doi.org/10.1002/bies.202200249

Kumar V, Vashishta M, Kong L et al (2021) The role of Notch, Hedgehog, and Wnt signaling pathways in the resistance of tumors to anticancer therapies. Front Cell Dev Biol 9:1–24. https://doi.org/10.3389/fcell.2021.650772

Lambrecht R, Delgado ME, Gloe V et al (2023) Liver receptor homolog-1 (NR5A2) orchestrates hepatic inflammation and TNF-induced cell death. Cell Rep 42:113513. https://doi.org/10.1016/j.celrep.2023.113513

Lan J, Liu R, Ju X et al (2015) Expression of cancer stem cell markers and their correlation with pathogenesis in vascular tumors. Int J Clin Exp Pathol 8:12621–12633

Lane AA, Stein AS, Garcia JS et al (2021) Safety and efficacy of combining Tagraxofusp (SL-401) with Azacitidine or Azacitidine and Venetoclax in a phase 1b study for CD123 positive AML, MDS, or BPDCN. Blood 138:2346. https://doi.org/10.1182/blood-2021-147486

Lathia JD, Liu H (2017) Overview of cancer stem cells and stemness for community oncologists. Target Oncol 12:387–399. https://doi.org/10.1007/s11523-017-0508-3

Lathia JD, Gallagher J, Heddleston JM et al (2010) Integrin alpha 6 regulates glioblastoma stem cells. Cell Stem Cell 6:421–432

Lee Y, Tanggono AS (2022) Potential role of the circadian clock in the regulation of cancer stem cells and cancer therapy. Int J Mol Sci 23. https://doi.org/10.3390/ijms232214181

Lee Y, Yoon J, Ko D et al (2021) TMPRSS4 promotes cancer stem–like properties in prostate cancer cells through upregulation of SOX2 by SLUG and TWIST1. J Exp Clin Cancer Res 40: 1–19. https://doi.org/10.1186/s13046-021-02147-7

Li C, Heidt DG, Dalerba P et al (2007) Identification of pancreatic cancer stem cells. Cancer Res 67: 1030–1037. https://doi.org/10.1158/0008-5472.CAN-06-2030

Li SH, Fu J, Watkins DN et al (2013) Sulforaphane regulates self-renewal of pancreatic cancer stem cells through the modulation of Sonic hedgehog-GLI pathway. Mol Cell Biochem 373:217–227. https://doi.org/10.1007/s11010-012-1493-6

Li S-Y, Sun R, Wang H-X et al (2015) Combination therapy with epigenetic-targeted and chemotherapeutic drugs delivered by nanoparticles to enhance the chemotherapy response and overcome resistance by breast cancer stem cells. J Control Release 205:7–14. https://doi.org/10.1016/j.jconrel.2014.11.011

Li Y, Xian M, Yang B et al (2017) Inhibition of KLF4 by statins reverses adriamycin-induced metastasis and cancer stemness in osteosarcoma cells. Stem Cell Reports 8:1617–1629. https://doi.org/10.1016/j.stemcr.2017.04.025

Li Y, Yu W, Li L et al (2023a) Oncology nursing on the move: a contemporary issue on Chinese oncology nursing in cancer care. Front Public Heal 11:1–11. https://doi.org/10.3389/fpubh.2023.1061572

Li YR, Fang Y, Lyu Z et al (2023b) Exploring the dynamic interplay between cancer stem cells and the tumor microenvironment: implications for novel therapeutic strategies. J Transl Med 21:1–23. https://doi.org/10.1186/s12967-023-04575-9

Liao W, Zhang L, Chen X et al (2023) Targeting cancer stem cells and signalling pathways through phytochemicals: A promising approach against colorectal cancer. Phytomedicine 108:154524. https://doi.org/10.1016/j.phymed.2022.154524

Lindsey S, Langhans SA (2014) Crosstalk of oncogenic signaling pathways during epithelial-mesenchymal transition. Front Oncol 4:1–10. https://doi.org/10.3389/fonc.2014.00358

Ling B, Watt K, Banerjee S et al (2017) A novel immunotherapy targeting MMP-14 limits hypoxia, immune suppression and metastasis in triple-negative breast cancer models. Oncotarget 8:58372

Linke R, Klein A, Seimetz D (2010) Catumaxomab: clinical development and future directions. In: MAbs, vol 2. Taylor & Francis, pp 129–136

Liu F, Qian Y (2021) The role of CD133 in hepatocellular carcinoma. Cancer Biol Ther 22:291–300. https://doi.org/10.1080/15384047.2021.1916381

Liu A, Yu X, Liu S (2013) Pluripotency transcription factors and cancer stem cells: Small genes make a big difference. Chin J Cancer 32:483–487. https://doi.org/10.5732/cjc.012.10282

Liu J, Xiao Q, Xiao J et al (2022a) Wnt/β-catenin signalling: function, biological mechanisms, and therapeutic opportunities. Signal Transduct Target Ther 7:3. https://doi.org/10.1038/s41392-021-00762-6

Liu Y, Feng C, Zhou Y et al (2022b) Simulating the dynamic intra-tumor heterogeneity and therapeutic responses. Cancers (Basel) 14. https://doi.org/10.3390/cancers14071645

Liu G, Wei J, Xiao W et al (2023) Insights into the Notch signaling pathway in degenerative musculoskeletal disorders: Mechanisms and perspectives. Biomed Pharmacother 169:115884. https://doi.org/10.1016/j.biopha.2023.115884

MacDonagh L, Gray SG, Breen E et al (2016) Lung cancer stem cells: the root of resistance. Cancer Lett 372:147–156. https://doi.org/10.1016/j.canlet.2016.01.012

Mallini P, Lennard T, Kirby J, Meeson A (2014) Epithelial-to-mesenchymal transition: What is the impact on breast cancer stem cells and drug resistance. Cancer Treat Rev 40:341–348. https://doi.org/10.1016/j.ctrv.2013.09.008

Marangoni E, Lecomte N, Durand L et al (2009) CD44 targeting reduces tumour growth and prevents post-chemotherapy relapse of human breast cancers xenografts. Br J Cancer 100:918–922

Marta Mauro-Lizcano, Sotgia F, Lisanti MP (2022) SOX2-high cancer cells exhibit an aggressive phenotype, with increases in stemness, proliferation and invasion, as well as higher metabolic activity and ATP production. Aging (Albany NY) 14:9877–9889

Martelli AM, Evangelisti C, Follo MY et al (2011) Targeting the phosphatidylinositol 3-kinase/Akt/mammalian target of rapamycin signaling network in cancer stem cells. Curr Med Chem 18: 2715–2726

Masoudi R, Gopalan V (2023) Cancer stem cells in cancer initiation and progression BT – cancer stem cells: basic concept and therapeutic implications. In: Islam F, Lam AK (eds) . Springer Nature Singapore, Singapore, pp 119–133

Mathews LA, Cabarcas SM, Hurt EM et al (2011) Increased expression of DNA repair genes in invasive human pancreatic cancer cells. Pancreas 40:730–739. https://doi.org/10.1097/MPA.0b013e31821ae25b

Mazzoleni S, Politi LS, Pala M et al (2010) Epidermal growth factor receptor expression identifies functionally and molecularly distinct tumor-initiating cells in human glioblastoma multiforme and is required for gliomagenesis. Cancer Res 70:7500–7513

McClements L, Yakkundi A, Papaspyropoulos A et al (2013) Targeting treatment-resistant breast cancer stem cells with FKBPL and its peptide derivative, AD-01, via the CD44 pathway. Clin Cancer Res 19:3881–3893

McMahon RA, D'Souza C, Neeson PJ, Siva S (2023) Innate immunity: Looking beyond T-cells in radiation and immunotherapy combinations. Neoplasia (United States) 46:100940. https://doi.org/10.1016/j.neo.2023.100940

Merchant AA, Matsui W (2010) Targeting Hedgehog – a cancer stem cell pathway. Clin Cancer Res 16:3130–3140. https://doi.org/10.1158/1078-0432.CCR-09-2846

Miettinen M, Lasota J (2005) KIT (CD117): a review on expression in normal and neoplastic tissues, and mutations and their clinicopathologic correlation. Appl Immunohistochem Mol Morphol 13:205–220

Min C-K, Sung-Soo Yoon, Kim JS, Manasanch E (2019) Clinical study of CWP232291 in relapsed or refractory myeloma patients Texas, United States

Molofsky AV, Pardal R, Iwashita T et al (2003) Bmi-1 dependence distinguishes neural stem cell self-renewal from progenitor proliferation. Nature 425:962–967. https://doi.org/10.1038/nature02060

Moltzahn F, Thalmann GN (2013) Cancer stem cells in prostate cancer. Transl Androl Urol 2:242–253. https://doi.org/10.3978/j.issn.2223-4683.2013.09.06

Montagnani V, Stecca B (2019) Role of protein kinases in hedgehog pathway control and implications for cancer therapy. Cancers (Basel) 11. https://doi.org/10.3390/cancers11040449

Montesinos P, Roboz GJ, Bulabois C-E et al (2021) Safety and efficacy of talacotuzumab plus decitabine or decitabine alone in patients with acute myeloid leukemia not eligible for chemotherapy: results from a multicenter, randomized, phase 2/3 study. Leukemia 35:62–74. https://doi.org/10.1038/s41375-020-0773-5

Moreb J, Schweder M, Suresh A, Zucali JR (1996) Overexpression of the human aldehyde dehydrogenase class I results in increased resistance to 4-hydroperoxycyclophosphamide. Cancer Gene Ther 3:24–30

Mortezaee K, Majidpoor J, Kharazinejad E (2022) Epithelial-mesenchymal transition in cancer stemness and heterogeneity: updated. Med Oncol 39:193. https://doi.org/10.1007/s12032-022-01801-0

Naik J, Themeli M, de Jong-Korlaar R et al (2019) CD38 as a therapeutic target for adult acute myeloid leukemia and T-cell acute lymphoblastic leukemia. Haematologica 104:e100

Najafi M, Farhood B, Mortezaee K (2019) Cancer stem cells (CSCs) in cancer progression and therapy. J Cell Physiol 234:8381–8395. https://doi.org/10.1002/jcp.27740

Nakano M, Kikushige Y, Miyawaki K et al (2019) Dedifferentiation process driven by TGF-beta signaling enhances stem cell properties in human colorectal cancer. Oncogene 38:780–793. https://doi.org/10.1038/s41388-018-0480-0

Nayak A, Warrier NM, Kumar P (2022) Cancer stem cells and the tumor microenvironment: targeting the critical crosstalk through nanocarrier systems. Stem Cell Rev Reports 18:2209–2233. https://doi.org/10.1007/s12015-022-10426-9

Oberneder R, Weckermann D, Ebner B et al (2006) A phase I study with adecatumumab, a human antibody directed against epithelial cell adhesion molecule, in hormone refractory prostate cancer patients. Eur J Cancer 42:2530–2538

Ogden AT, Waziri AE, Lochhead RA et al (2008) Identification of A2B5+ CD133− tumor-initiating cells in adult human gliomas. Neurosurgery 62:505–515

Ordaz-Ramos A, Tellez-Jimenez O, Vazquez-Santillan K (2023) Signaling pathways governing the maintenance of breast cancer stem cells and their therapeutic implications. Front Cell Dev Biol 11:1–17. https://doi.org/10.3389/fcell.2023.1221175

Ostrikov K, Michl T, MacGregor M, Vasilev K (2019) Bladder cancer cell capture: Elucidating the effect of sample storage conditions on capturing bladder cancer cells via surface immobilized EpCAM antibody. ACS Appl Bio Mater 2:3730–3736

Otsubo K, Nosaki K, Imamura CK et al (2017) Phase I study of salazosulfapyridine in combination with cisplatin and pemetrexed for advanced non-small-cell lung cancer. Cancer Sci 108:1843–1849

Pak S, Park S, Kim Y et al (2019) The small molecule WNT/β-catenin inhibitor CWP232291 blocks the growth of castration-resistant prostate cancer by activating the endoplasmic reticulum stress pathway. J Exp Clin Cancer Res 38:1–13. https://doi.org/10.1186/s13046-019-1342-5

Paolicchi E, Gemignani F, Krstic-Demonacos M et al (2016) Targeting hypoxic response for cancer therapy. Oncotarget 7:13464

Parry PV, Engh JA (2014) Knockdown of LGR5 suppresses the proliferation of glioma cells in vitro and in vivo. Neurosurgery 74:N14–N15

Pasqualetti F, Miniati M, Gonnelli A et al (2023) Cancer stem cells and glioblastoma: time for innovative biomarkers of radio-resistance? Biology (Basel) 12:1295. https://doi.org/10.3390/biology12101295

Patrawala L, Calhoun T, Schneider-Broussard R et al (2006) Highly purified CD44+ prostate cancer cells from xenograft human tumors are enriched in tumorigenic and metastatic progenitor cells. Oncogene 25:1696–1708

Paul S, Dutta A, Basak U et al (2019) Cancer stem cell fate determination: a nuclear phenomenon. The Nucleus 62:109–118. https://doi.org/10.1007/s13237-019-00281-4

Paul R, Dorsey JF, Fan Y (2022) Cell plasticity, senescence, and quiescence in cancer stem cells: Biological and therapeutic implications. Pharmacol Ther 231:107985. https://doi.org/10.1016/j.pharmthera.2021.107985

Peng CY, Yu CC, Huang CC et al (2022) Magnolol inhibits cancer stemness and IL-6/Stat3 signaling in oral carcinomas. J Formos Med Assoc 121:51–57. https://doi.org/10.1016/j.jfma.2021.01.009

Pérez-González A, Bévant K, Blanpain C (2023) Cancer cell plasticity during tumor progression, metastasis and response to therapy. Nat Cancer 4:1063–1082. https://doi.org/10.1038/s43018-023-00595-y

Pote MS, Gacche RN (2023) ATP-binding cassette efflux transporters and MDR in cancer. Drug Discov Today 28:103537. https://doi.org/10.1016/j.drudis.2023.103537

Priya B, Ravi S, Kirubakaran S (2023) Targeting ATM and ATR for cancer therapeutics: Inhibitors in clinic. Drug Discov Today 28:103662. https://doi.org/10.1016/j.drudis.2023.103662

Punnasseril JMJ, Gopalan V, Islam F (2023) Therapeutics targeting cancer stem cell signalling pathways BT – cancer stem cells: basic concept and therapeutic implications. In: Lam AK (ed) Islam F. Springer Nature Singapore, Singapore, pp 199–219

Qi F, Wei L, Shen A et al (2016) Pien Tze Huang inhibits the proliferation, and induces the apoptosis and differentiation of colorectal cancer stem cells via suppression of the Notch1 pathway. Oncol Rep 35:511–517. https://doi.org/10.3892/or.2015.4378

Qian X, Tan C, Wang F et al (2016) Esophageal cancer stem cells and implications for future therapeutics. Onco Targets Ther 9:2247–2254. https://doi.org/10.2147/OTT.S103179

Ramakrishnan V, Painuly U, Kimlinger T et al (2014) Inhibitor of apoptosis proteins as therapeutic targets in multiple myeloma. Leukemia 28:1519–1528. https://doi.org/10.1038/leu.2014.2

Raspollini MR, Amunni G, Villanucci A et al (2004) c-KIT expression and correlation with chemotherapy resistance in ovarian carcinoma: an immunocytochemical study. Ann Oncol 15:594–597

Ravindran S, Rasool S, Maccalli C (2019) The cross talk between cancer stem cells/cancer initiating cells and tumor microenvironment: the missing piece of the puzzle for the efficient targeting of these cells with immunotherapy. Cancer Microenviron 12:133–148. https://doi.org/10.1007/s12307-019-00233-1

Rich JN (2016) Cancer stem cells: understanding tumor hierarchy and heterogeneity. Medicine (Baltimore) 95:S2–S7. https://doi.org/10.1097/MD.0000000000004764

Richardson GD, Robson CN, Lang SH et al (2004) CD133, a novel marker for human prostatic epithelial stem cells. J Cell Sci 117:3539–3545

Roche J (2018) The epithelial-to-mesenchymal transition in cancer. Cancers (Basel) 10:9–12. https://doi.org/10.3390/cancers10020052

Roma-Rodrigues C, Mendes R, Baptista PV, Fernandes AR (2019) Targeting tumor microenvironment for cancer therapy. Int J Mol Sci 20. https://doi.org/10.3390/ijms20040840

Rouzbahani E, Majidpoor J, Najafi S, Mortezaee K (2022) Cancer stem cells in immunoregulation and bypassing anti-checkpoint therapy. Biomed Pharmacother 156:113906. https://doi.org/10.1016/j.biopha.2022.113906

Safa AR (2016) Resistance to cell death and its modulation in cancer stem cells. Crit Rev Oncog 21:203

Sahara S, Warner KA, Herzog AE et al (2023) Therapeutic inhibition of Bmi-1 ablates chemoresistant cancer stem cells in adenoid cystic carcinoma. Oral Oncol 142:106437. https://doi.org/10.1016/j.oraloncology.2023.106437

Saito Y, Kitamura H, Hijikata A et al (2010) Identification of therapeutic targets for quiescent, chemotherapy-resistant human leukemia stem cells. Sci Transl Med. 2:17ra9-17ra9 2:17ra9

Salaritabar A, Berindan-Neagoe I, Darvish B et al (2019) Targeting Hedgehog signaling pathway: paving the road for cancer therapy. Pharmacol Res 141:466–480. https://doi.org/10.1016/j.phrs.2019.01.014

Samanta P, Bhowmik A, Biswas S et al (2023) Therapeutic effectiveness of anticancer agents targeting different signaling molecules involved in asymmetric division of cancer stem cell. Stem Cell Rev Reports 19:1283–1306. https://doi.org/10.1007/s12015-023-10523-3

Sarkaria SM, Heaney ML (2021) Glasdegib in newly diagnosed acute myeloid leukemia. Expert Rev Anticancer Ther 21:573–581. https://doi.org/10.1080/14737140.2021.1891885

Sarry J-E, Murphy K, Perry R et al (2011) Human acute myelogenous leukemia stem cells are rare and heterogeneous when assayed in NOD/SCID/IL2Rγc-deficient mice. J Clin Invest 121:384–395

Scannevin RH, Alexander R, Haarlander TM et al (2017) Discovery of a highly selective chemical inhibitor of matrix metalloproteinase-9 (MMP-9) that allosterically inhibits zymogen activation. J Biol Chem 292:17963–17974

Schott AF, Landis MD, Dontu G et al (2013) Preclinical and clinical studies of gamma secretase inhibitors with docetaxel on human breast tumors. Clin Cancer Res 19:1512–1524. https://doi.org/10.1158/1078-0432.CCR-11-3326

Sekulic A, Migden MR, Oro AE et al (2012) efficacy and safety of vismodegib in advanced basal-cell carcinoma. N Engl J Med 366:2171–2179. https://doi.org/10.1056/nejmoa1113713

Shahbaz M, Imran M, Hussain M et al (2023) Curcumin: a bioactive compound with molecular targets for human malignancies. Food Agric Immunol 34. https://doi.org/10.1080/09540105.2023.2280524

Shank JJ, Yang K, Ghannam J et al (2012) Metformin targets ovarian cancer stem cells in vitro and in vivo. Gynecol Oncol 127:390–397

Shen YA, Jung J, Shimberg GD, et al (2021) Development of small molecule inhibitors targeting PBX1 transcription signaling as a novel cancer therapeutic strategy. iScience 24. https://doi.org/10.1016/j.isci.2021.103297, 24

Shonibare Z, Monavarian M, O'Connell K et al (2022) Reciprocal SOX2 regulation by SMAD1-SMAD3 is critical for anoikis resistance and metastasis in cancer. Cell Rep 40:111066. https://doi.org/10.1016/j.celrep.2022.111066

Shukla KK, Choudhary GR, Sankanagoudar S et al (2023) Deregulation of miR-10b and miR-21 correlate with cancer stem cells expansion through the apoptotic pathway in prostate cancer. Asian Pacific J Cancer Prev 24:2105–2119. https://doi.org/10.31557/APJCP.2023.24.6.2105

Siegler EL, Kim YJ, Wang P (2016) Nanomedicine targeting the tumor microenvironment: Therapeutic strategies to inhibit angiogenesis, remodel matrix, and modulate immune responses. J Cell Immunother 2:69–78

Singh B, Dutt S (2024) Chapter 9 – role of cancer stem cells in maintenance of tumor heterogeneity in brain tumors. In: Pathak S, Banerjee ABT-CSC, SP (eds). Academic, pp 165–184

Singh S, Brocker C, Koppaka V et al (2013) Aldehyde dehydrogenases in cellular responses to oxidative/electrophilicstress. Free Radic Biol Med 56:89–101. https://doi.org/10.1016/j.freeradbiomed.2012.11.010

Singh AK, Jingjing L, Rishabha M (2023) Prediction of cancer treatment using advancements in machine learning. Recent Patents Anti-Cancer Drug Discov Bentham Sci Publ 18:364. https://doi.org/10.2174/1574892818666221018091415

Skubitz APN, Taras EP, Boylan KLM et al (2013) Targeting CD133 in an in vivo ovarian cancer model reduces ovarian cancer progression. Gynecol Oncol 130:579–587

Smith DC, Eisenberg PD, Manikhas G et al (2014) A phase I dose escalation and expansion study of the anticancer stem cell agent demcizumab (Anti-DLL4) in patients with previously treated solid tumors. Clin Cancer Res 20:6295–6303. https://doi.org/10.1158/1078-0432.CCR-14-1373

Son MJ, Woolard K, Nam D-H et al (2009) SSEA-1 is an enrichment marker for tumor-initiating cells in human glioblastoma. Cell Stem Cell 4:440–452

Sottnik JL, Daignault-Newton S, Zhang X et al (2013) Integrin alpha 2 beta 1 (α 2 β 1) promotes prostate cancer skeletal metastasis. Clin Exp Metastasis 30:569–578

Stolzenburg S, Rots MG, Beltran AS et al (2012) Targeted silencing of the oncogenic transcription factor SOX2 in breast cancer. Nucleic Acids Res 40:6725–6740. https://doi.org/10.1093/nar/gks360

Su D, Deng H, Zhao X et al (2009) Targeting CD24 for treatment of ovarian cancer by short hairpin RNA. Cytotherapy 11:642–652

Su Y, Qiu Q, Zhang X et al (2010) Aldehyde dehydrogenase 1 A1–positive cell population is enriched in tumor-initiating cells and associated with progression of bladder cancer. Cancer Epidemiol Biomarkers Prev 19:327–337

Suman S, Das TP, Damodaran C (2013) Silencing NOTCH signaling causes growth arrest in both breast cancer stem cells and breast cancer cells. Br J Cancer 109:2587–2596. https://doi.org/10.1038/bjc.2013.642

Swaminathan SK, Roger E, Toti U et al (2013) CD133-targeted paclitaxel delivery inhibits local tumor recurrence in a mouse model of breast cancer. J Control Release 171:280–287

Tabassum N, Verma V, Kumar M et al (2018) Nanomedicine in cancer stem cell therapy: from fringe to forefront. Cell Tissue Res 374:427–438. https://doi.org/10.1007/s00441-018-2928-5

Tanabe S (2022) Epithelial–mesenchymal transition and cancer stem cells BT – cancer stem cell markers and related network pathways. In: Tanabe S (ed). Springer, Cham, pp 1–49

Tandon A, Zhang Y, Sokol L (2019) Tagraxofusp, a novel CD123-directed cytotoxin to treat blastic plasmacytoid dendritic cell neoplasm. Drugs of Today 55:735–742. https://doi.org/10.1358/dot.2019.55.12.3058917

Templeton AK, Miyamoto S, Babu A et al (2014) Cancer stem cells: progress and challenges in lung cancer. Stem Cell Investig 2014:1–18. https://doi.org/10.3978/j.issn.2306-9759.2014.03.06

Tolcher AW, Messersmith WA, Mikulski SM et al (2012) Phase I study of RO4929097, a gamma secretase inhibitor of notch signaling, in patients with refractory metastatic or locally advanced solid tumors. J Clin Oncol 30:2348–2353. https://doi.org/10.1200/JCO.2011.36.8282

Tong H, Liu X, Peng C et al (2023) Silencing of KNTC1 inhibits hepatocellular carcinoma cells progression via suppressing PI3K/Akt pathway. Cell Signal 101:110498. https://doi.org/10.1016/j.cellsig.2022.110498

Turdo A, Veschi V, Gaggianesi M et al (2019) Meeting the challenge of targeting cancer stem cells. Front Cell Dev Biol 7:1–16. https://doi.org/10.3389/fcell.2019.00016

Ugolkov AV, Eisengart LJ, Luan C, Yang XJ (2011) Expression analysis of putative stem cell markers in human benign and malignant prostate. Prostate 71:18–25

Valakos D, Klagkou E, Kokkalis A et al (2023) Combinatorial targeting of a specific EMT/MET network by macroH2A variants safeguards mesenchymal identity. PLoS One 18:1–21. https://doi.org/10.1371/journal.pone.0288005

Valentim CA, Rabi JA, David SA (2023) Cellular-automaton model for tumor growth dynamics: Virtualization of different scenarios. Comput Biol Med 153:106481. https://doi.org/10.1016/j.compbiomed.2022.106481

Vamvoukaki R, Chrysoulaki M, Betsi G, Xekouki P (2023) Pituitary tumorigenesis – implications for management

van den Hoogen C, van der Horst G, Cheung H et al (2010) High aldehyde dehydrogenase activity identifies tumor-initiating and metastasis-initiating cells in human prostate cancer. Cancer Res 70:5163–5173

van der Horst G, Bos L, van der Pluijm G (2012) Epithelial plasticity, cancer stem cells, and the tumor-supportive stroma in bladder carcinoma. Mol Cancer Res 10:995–1009

Van Rhenen A, Feller N, Kelder A et al (2005) High stem cell frequency in acute myeloid leukemia at diagnosis predicts high minimal residual disease and poor survival. Clin Cancer Res 11:6520–6527. https://doi.org/10.1158/1078-0432.CCR-05-0468

Van Rhenen A, Van Dongen GAMS, Kelder A et al (2007) The novel AML stem cell–associated antigen CLL-1 aids in discrimination between normal and leukemic stem cells. Blood, J Am Soc Hematol 110:2659–2666

Vannini I, Zoli W, Fabbri F et al (2009) Role of efflux pump activity in lapatinib/caelyx combination in breast cancer cell lines. Anti-Cancer Drugs 20:918–925

Vaz AP, Ponnusamy MP, Seshacharyulu P, Batra SK (2014) A concise review on the current understanding of pancreatic cancer stem cells. J Cancer Stem Cell Res 2:1. https://doi.org/10.14343/jcscr.2014.2e1004

Vazquez-Santillan K, Melendez-Zajgla J, Jimenez-Hernandez L et al (2015) NF-κB signaling in cancer stem cells: a promising therapeutic target? Cell Oncol 38:327–339. https://doi.org/10.1007/s13402-015-0236-6

Verma A, Kapoor R, Mittal RD (2017) Cluster of differentiation 44 (CD44) gene variants: a putative cancer stem cell marker in risk prediction of bladder cancer in North Indian population. Indian J Clin Biochem 32:74–83

Verma C, Pawar VA, Srivastava S et al (2023) Cancer vaccines in the immunotherapy era: promise and potential. Vaccines 11(12):1783.

Vermeulen L, Todaro M, De Sousa MF et al (2008) Single-cell cloning of colon cancer stem cells reveals a multi-lineage differentiation capacity. Proc Natl Acad Sci USA 105:13427–13432. https://doi.org/10.1073/pnas.0805706105

Vey N, Delaunay J, Martinelli G et al (2016) Phase I clinical study of RG7356, an anti-CD44 humanized antibody, in patients with acute myeloid leukemia. Oncotarget 7:32532–32542. https://doi.org/10.18632/oncotarget.8687

Walcher L, Kistenmacher A-K, Suo H et al (2020) Cancer stem cells – origins and biomarkers: perspectives for targeted personalized therapies. Front Immunol 11:1280

Wang Q-E (2015) DNA damage responses in cancer stem cells: Implications for cancer therapeutic strategies. World J Biol Chem 6:57–64. https://doi.org/10.4331/wjbc.v6.i3.57
Wang D, Kong X, Li Y et al (2017) Curcumin inhibits bladder cancer stem cells by suppressing Sonic Hedgehog pathway. Biochem Biophys Res Commun 493:521–527. https://doi.org/10.1016/j.bbrc.2017.08.158
Wang R, Yang L, Li S et al (2018) Quercetin inhibits breast cancer stem cells via downregulation of aldehyde dehydrogenase 1A1 (ALDH1A1), chemokine receptor type 4 (CXCR4), mucin 1 (MUC1), and epithelial cell adhesion molecule (EpCAM). Med Sci Monit Int Med J Exp Clin Res 24:412
Wang Z, Xie D, Lu A, Liang C (2022) Anoikis resistance and tumor metastasis BT – handbook of cancer and immunology. In: Rezaei N (ed). Springer, Cham, pp 1–25
Wen Z, Feng S, Wei L et al (2015) Evodiamine, a novel inhibitor of the Wnt pathway, inhibits the self-renewal of gastric cancer stem cells. Int J Mol Med 36:1657–1663. https://doi.org/10.3892/ijmm.2015.2383
Weston WA, Barr AR (2023) A cell cycle centric view of tumour dormancy. Br J Cancer 129:1535. https://doi.org/10.1038/s41416-023-02401-z
Wu X-Z (2008) Origin of Cancer Stem Cells: The Role of Self-Renewal and Differentiation. Ann Surg Oncol 15:407–414. https://doi.org/10.1245/s10434-007-9695-y
Wu J, LoRusso PM, Matherly LH, Li J (2012) Implications of plasma protein binding for pharmacokinetics and pharmacodynamics of the γ-secretase inhibitor RO4929097. Clin Cancer Res 18:2066–2079. https://doi.org/10.1158/1078-0432.CCR-11-2684
Wu X, Zhang X, Sun L et al (2013) Progesterone negatively regulates BCRP in progesterone receptor-positive human breast cancer cells. Cell Physiol Biochem 32:344–354
Wu WS, You RI, Cheng CC et al (2017) Snail collaborates with EGR-1 and SP-1 to directly activate transcription of MMP 9 and ZEB1. Sci Rep 7:1–13. https://doi.org/10.1038/s41598-017-18101-7
Wu B, Shi X, Jiang M, Liu H (2023) Cross-talk between cancer stem cells and immune cells: potential therapeutic targets in the tumor immune microenvironment. Mol Cancer 22:1–22. https://doi.org/10.1186/s12943-023-01748-4
Xia P, Liu D-H, Xu Z-J, Ren F (2022) Cancer stem cell markers for urinary carcinoma. Stem Cells Int 2022:1
Xu L, Han F, Zhu L et al (2023a) Advances in understanding the role and mechanisms of tumor stem cells in HER2-positive breast cancer treatment resistance (Review). Int J Oncol 62:1–11. https://doi.org/10.3892/ijo.2023.5496
Xu LB, Qin YF, Su L et al (2023b) Cathepsin-facilitated invasion of BMI1-high hepatocellular carcinoma cells drives bile duct tumor thrombi formation. Nat Commun 14:7033. https://doi.org/10.1038/s41467-023-42930-y
Yan B, Liu L, Zhao Y et al (2014) Xiaotan Sanjie decoction attenuates tumor angiogenesis by manipulating Notch-1-regulated proliferation of gastric cancer stem-like cells. World J Gastroenterol 20:13105–13118. https://doi.org/10.3748/wjg.v20.i36.13105
Yanardag S, Pugacheva EN (2021) Primary cilium is involved in stem cell differentiation and renewal through the regulation of multiple signaling pathways. Cells 10. https://doi.org/10.3390/cells10061428
Yang ZF, Ho DW, Ng MN et al (2008) Significance of CD90+ Cancer Stem Cells in Human Liver Cancer. Cancer Cell 13:153–166. https://doi.org/10.1016/j.ccr.2008.01.013
Yang X, Sarvestani SK, Moeinzadeh S et al (2013) Effect of CD44 binding peptide conjugated to an engineered inert matrix on maintenance of breast cancer stem cells and tumorsphere formation. PLoS One 8:1–15. https://doi.org/10.1371/journal.pone.0059147
Yang J, Fang Z, Wu J et al (2016) Construction and application of a lung cancer stem cell model: antitumor drug screening and molecular mechanism of the inhibitory effects of sanguinarine. Tumour Biol 37:13871–13883. https://doi.org/10.1007/s13277-016-5152-5

Yang F, Zhang J, Yang H (2018) OCT4, SOX2, and NANOG positive expression correlates with poor differentiation, advanced disease stages, and worse overall survival in HER2+ breast cancer patients. Onco Targets Ther 11:7873–7881. https://doi.org/10.2147/OTT.S173522

Yang Y, Hao E, Pan X et al (2019) Gomisin M2 from Baizuan suppresses breast cancer stem cell proliferation in a zebrafish xenograft model. Aging (Albany NY) 11:8347–8361. https://doi.org/10.18632/aging.102323

Yanli X, Feiye Z, Shan X, Luming L (2015) Anti-tumor effect of the extract from Qingyihuaji formula on pancreatic cancer by down-regulating Notch-4 and Jagged-1. J Tradit Chinese Med 35:77–83. https://doi.org/10.1016/S0254-6272(15)30012-1

Yao CJ, Han TY, Shih PH et al (2014) Elimination of cancer stem-like side population in human glioblastoma cells accompanied with stemness gene suppression by Korean herbal recipe MSC500. Integr Cancer Ther 13:541–554. https://doi.org/10.1177/1534735414549623

Yao T, Lu R, Zhang Y et al (2015) Cervical cancer stem cells. Cell Prolif 48:611–625. https://doi.org/10.1111/cpr.12216

Yao R, Zhang M, Zhou J et al (2022) Novel dual-targeting c-Myc inhibitor D347-2761 represses myeloma growth via blocking c-Myc/Max heterodimerization and disturbing its stability. Cell Commun Signal 20:1–16. https://doi.org/10.1186/s12964-022-00868-6

Ye X, Weinberg RA (2015) Epithelial-mesenchymal plasticity: a central regulator of cancer progression. Trends Cell Biol 25:675–686. https://doi.org/10.1016/j.tcb.2015.07.012

Yeom DH, Lee YS, Ryu I et al (2021) Abl001, a bispecific antibody targeting vegf and dll4, with chemotherapy, synergistically inhibits tumor progression in xenograft models. Int J Mol Sci 22:1–14. https://doi.org/10.3390/ijms22010241

Yi J, Chen S, Yi P et al (2020) Pyrotinib sensitizes 5-fluorouracil-resistant HER2+ breast cancer cells to 5-fluorouracil. Oncol Res 28:519

Yin AH, Miraglia S, Zanjani ED et al (1997) AC133, a novel marker for human hematopoietic stem and progenitor cells. Blood, J Am Soc Hematol 90:5002–5012

Yokota A, Ishii G, Sugaya Y et al (1998) Expression of exon v6-containing CD44 isoforms is related to poor prognosis of acute myelocytic leukemia. Hematol Oncol 16:131–141. https://doi.org/10.1002/(SICI)1099-1069(199812)16:4<131::AID-HON631>3.0.CO;2-K

Yoo YD, Kwon YT (2015) Molecular mechanisms controlling asymmetric and symmetric self-renewal of cancer stem cells. J Anal Sci Technol 6:28. https://doi.org/10.1186/s40543-015-0071-4

You L, Guo X, Huang Y (2018) Correlation of cancer stem-cell markers OCT4, SOX2, and NANOG with clinicopathological features and prognosis in operative patients with rectal cancer. Yonsei Med J 59:35–42. https://doi.org/10.3349/ymj.2018.59.1.35

Yu T, Tang B, Sun X (2017) Development of inhibitors targeting hypoxia-inducible factor 1 and 2 for cancer therapy. Yonsei Med J 58:489–496

Yu X, Munoz-Sagredo L, Streule K et al (2021) CD44 loss of function sensitizes AML cells to the BCL-2 inhibitor venetoclax by decreasing CXCL12-driven survival cues. Blood 138:1067–1080. https://doi.org/10.1182/blood.2020006343

Yuan ZX, Mo J, Zhao G et al (2016) Targeting strategies for renal cell carcinoma: From renal cancer cells to renal cancer stem cells. Front Pharmacol 7:1–15. https://doi.org/10.3389/fphar.2016.00423

Zeng Z, Fu M, Hu Y et al (2023) Regulation and signaling pathways in cancer stem cells: implications for targeted therapy for cancer. Mol Cancer 22:1–31. https://doi.org/10.1186/s12943-023-01877-w

Zeppernick F, Ahmadi R, Campos B et al (2008) Stem cell marker CD133 affects clinical outcome in glioma patients. Clin Cancer Res 14:123–129. https://doi.org/10.1158/1078-0432.CCR-07-0932

Zhang X, Neganova I, Przyborski S et al (2009) A role for NANOG in G1 to S transition in human embryonic stem cells through direct binding of CDK6 and CDC25A. J Cell Biol 184:67–82. https://doi.org/10.1083/jcb.200801009

Zhang R, Zhang P, Wang H et al (2015) Inhibitory effects of metformin at low concentration on epithelial-mesenchymal transition of CD44+CD117+ ovarian cancer stem cells. Stem Cell Res Ther 6:1–12. https://doi.org/10.1186/s13287-015-0249-0

Zhang Q, Li XT, Chen Y et al (2018) Wnt/β-catenin signaling mediates the suppressive effects of diallyl trisulfide on colorectal cancer stem cells. Cancer Chemother Pharmacol 81:969–977. https://doi.org/10.1007/s00280-018-3565-0

Zhang H, Gan W-T, Hao W-G et al (2020) Successful anti-CLL1 CAR T-cell therapy in secondary acute myeloid leukemia. Front Oncol 10:685

Zhang H, Steed A, Co M, Chen X (2021a) Cancer stem cells, epithelial-mesenchymal transition, ATP and their roles in drug resistance in cancer. Cancer Drug Resist 4:684–709. https://doi.org/10.20517/cdr.2021.32

Zhang H, Wang P, Li Z et al (2021b) Anti-CLL1 chimeric antigen receptor T-cell therapy in children with relapsed/refractory acute myeloid leukemia. Clin Cancer Res 27:3549–3555. https://doi.org/10.1158/1078-0432.CCR-20-4543

Zhang G, Zhang Y, Jing L, Zhao H (2023a) Lead exposure induced developmental nephrotoxicity in Japanese quail (Coturnix japonica) via oxidative stress-based PI3K/AKT pathway inhibition and NF-κB pathway activation. Comp Biochem Physiol Part C Toxicol Pharmacol 268:109599. https://doi.org/10.1016/j.cbpc.2023.109599

Zhang Z, Wu W, Shao Z (2023b) NOTCH signaling in osteosarcoma. Curr Issues Mol Biol 45: 2266–2283. https://doi.org/10.3390/cimb45030146

Zhao X, Singh S, Pardoux C et al (2010) Targeting C-type lectin-like molecule-1 for antibody-mediated immunotherapy in acute myeloid leukemia. Haematologica 95:71

Zhou X, Zeng Y, Zheng R et al (2023) Natural products modulate cell apoptosis: a promising way for treating endometrial cancer. Front Pharmacol 14:1–20. https://doi.org/10.3389/fphar.2023.1209412

Zhu P, Fan Z (2018) Cancer stem cells and tumorigenesis. Biophys Rep 4:178–188. https://doi.org/10.1007/s41048-018-0062-2

Zinzi L, Contino M, Cantore M et al (2014) ABC transporters in CSCs membranes as a novel target for treating tumor relapse. Front Pharmacol 5 JUL:1–13. https://doi.org/10.3389/fphar.2014.00163

Stem Cell-Derived Cell Therapy for Cancer

Matthew Wilson, Zibai Lyu, Ying Fang, and Yan-Ruide Li

Abstract

The advent of genetic engineering strategies has transformed the landscape of cancer immunotherapy, leading to the development and adoption of CAR-T cell therapy. However, the current autologous CAR-T cell platform is hindered by several factors including limited potency against solid tumors and limited scalability across multiple patients, placing a heavy cost burden on patients. The development of stem-cell-based technologies is poised to provide an alternative "off-the-shelf" platform to the current CAR-T model, which can help overcome these issues. In this review, we examine the current state of stem-cell-based therapies encompassing potential stem-cell sources, engineering approaches, clinical implementations, and prevailing challenges facing the field.

Keywords

Allogeneic cancer therapy · Cancer genetic engineering · Cancer immunotherapy · Chimeric antigen receptor (CAR) · CRISPR-Cas9 · Graft-versus-host disease (GvHD) · Natural killer T (NKT) cell · Stem cell

1 Introduction

Cancer poses a significant challenge in contemporary medicine, comprising a diverse group of diseases with a global impact. Traditional treatments, encompassing surgery, chemotherapy, and radiation therapy, have made considerable advancements, offering improved survival rates to patients. However, the complexity of cancer demands

---

M. Wilson · Z. Lyu · Y. Fang · Y.-R. Li (✉)
Department of Microbiology, Immunology & Molecular Genetics, University of California, Los Angeles, Los Angeles, CA, USA
e-mail: charlie.li@ucla.edu

Interdisciplinary Cancer Research, https://doi.org/10.1007/16833_2023_196
Published online: 08 November 2023

innovative strategies to augment existing therapeutic options. One promising avenue lies in the realm of stem cell-derived cell therapy for cancer.

Stem cells, renowned for their unique ability to self-renew and differentiate into diverse cell types, have captivated the scientific and clinical communities for their regenerative potential (Wilson 2009). Stem cell applications have extended to various medical conditions, ranging from cardiac and neurological disorders to autoimmune diseases (Wilson 2009). Currently, researchers are exploring the transformative potential of stem cells in revolutionizing cancer treatment strategies.

The emerging field of stem cell-derived cell therapy for cancer holds promise in overcoming pivotal challenges in oncology (Li et al. 2023). Engineered stem cells present an opportunity for developing standardized cellular products, eliminating the need for personalized and patient-specific approaches (Hermanson et al. 2016; Li et al. 2018, 2021c; Shankar et al. 2020; Zhang et al. 2020; Frank et al. 2020; Euchner et al. 2021; Zhou et al. 2022). By performing gene engineering or gene editing on a limited pool of stem cells, the consumption of gene-engineering materials, such as lentivectors and CRISPR/Cas9/gRNA, could be minimized. This approach enhances cost-efficiency while maximizing the effectiveness of gene engineering/editing, a characteristic inherited by subsequent cell divisions and final cell products (Xu et al. 2019; Gerew et al. 2021; Li et al. 2021b). Additionally, the evolution of stem cell-engineered cellular therapy facilitates the potential for large-scale manufacturing and stockpiling of products.

This chapter delves into the dynamic field of stem cell-derived cell therapy for cancer. We explore various stem cell types under investigation, including mesenchymal stem cells (MSCs), hematopoietic stem cells (HSCs), and induced pluripotent stem cells (iPSCs), elucidating their therapeutic applications. We evaluate promising findings from preclinical and clinical studies while addressing imminent challenges, ranging from safety optimization to enhancing the scalability of these innovative therapies.

2 Stem Cell Sources for Cell Therapy

The pursuit of innovative cancer therapies and stem cells has emerged as a promising avenue of exploration. This section delves into the various types of stem cells—embryonic stem cells (ESCs), induced pluripotent stem cells (iPSCs), mesenchymal stem cells (MSCs), and hematopoietic stem cells (HSCs)—as potential cell sources for advancing cancer treatment (Sagar et al. 2007). Each stem cell type possesses unique attributes and faces distinct challenges within the context of cancer therapy. ESCs represent a unique class of pluripotent cells derived from embryos fertilized in vitro. The process of ESC cultivation involves the development of these embryos into blastocysts, from which the undifferentiated inner cell mass (ICM) can be isolated. The hallmark characteristic of ESCs is their pluripotency, enabling them to self-renew indefinitely and differentiate into all cell types except for placenta (Hochedlinger and Jaenisch 2003; Wobus and Boheler 2005). This inherent versatility positions ESCs as an attractive candidate for cancer treatment and development of tumor models. ESCs can be programmed into therapeutic cells, particularly T and natural killer (NK) cells, which can be genetically modified to express tumor-suppressing proteins, immunostimulatory molecules, and chimeric antigen receptors (CARs), enabling targeted cancer therapy and immune cell recruitment to tumor sites (Hochedlinger and Jaenisch 2003; Wobus and Boheler 2005; Zeng et al. 2012). These customized cells can effectively target cancer cells or recruit other immune elements to the tumor microenvironment, fostering a multifaceted approach to cancer treatment. However, the extensive proliferative and differentiating capabilities of ESCs present potential drawbacks. Their propensity for unlimited division mirrors cancer behavior, raising concerns about tumorigenic potential, especially following genetic modifications. Ethical dilemmas also loom over ESCs, as their generation involves the destruction of in vitro-fertilized embryos, sparking regulatory variations across countries and affecting ESC research (Tam et al. 2023; Iltis et al. 2023). Overall, the complex signaling pathways governing ESC behavior remain incompletely understood, and overcoming immune rejection and generating safe, heterogeneous cell lines pose ongoing challenges in ESC-based therapies (Fig. 1).

iPSCs share functional similarities with ESCs while diverging in their origin, derived through reprogramming adult somatic cells, such as dermal fibroblasts, peripheral blood cells, or adipose tissue cells. This reprogramming process involves

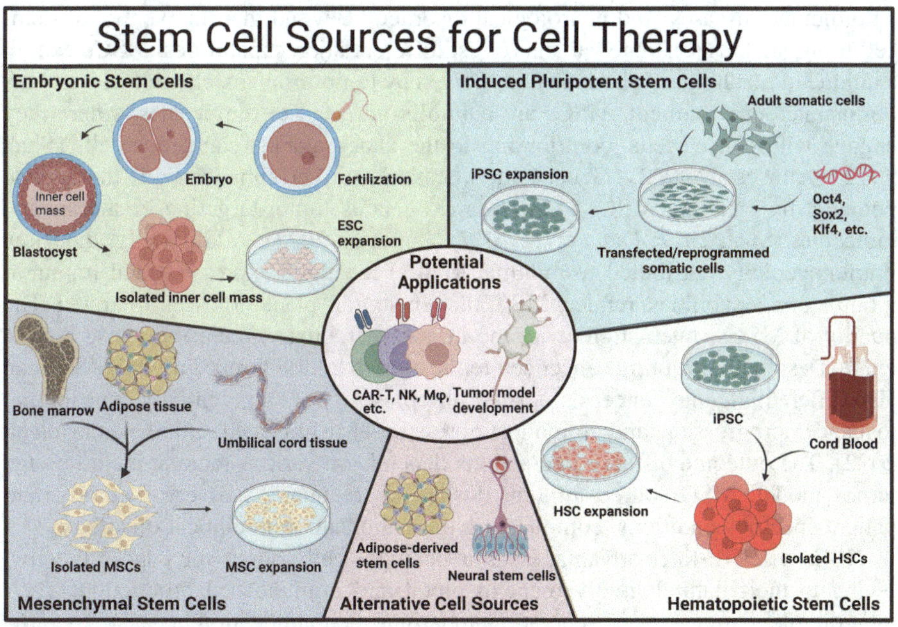

Fig. 1 Stem cell sources for cell therapy. A diverse array of stem cell sources suitable for cell therapy is shown, encompassing embryonic stem cells, induced pluripotent stem cells, mesenchymal stem cells, and hematopoietic stem cells, among others.

the activation of key pluripotency factors like Oct4, Sox2, and Klf4 (Sharkis et al. 2012; Hansen et al. 2018). iPSCs closely mimic ESCs in research settings, providing an ethical advantage by utilizing cells sourced from consenting adult donors. This ethical consideration facilitates their transition into clinical trials, where iPSCs exhibit potential in cancer therapy, particularly in cell-based immunotherapy (Li et al. 2018; Gutbier et al. 2020; Frank et al. 2020; Iriguchi et al. 2021; Aoki et al. 2023). They can be reprogrammed into T lymphocytes, retaining T-cell receptor genes for subsequent differentiation into T cells. These reprogrammed T cells can be engineered to express CARs and other molecules for targeted cancer therapy (Li et al. 2018; Allen et al. 2021). iPSCs' ability to differentiate into various tissue and cell types offers opportunities for tissue regeneration and disease modeling, aiding diagnostics, and advancing therapeutics. Nevertheless, the development of effective differentiation protocols for desired cell types from iPSCs remains labor-intensive due to their diverse sources and potential differentiations. The absence of Good Manufacturing Practice (GMP)-compliant protocols raises safety concerns during iPSC generation, expansion, and differentiation, emphasizing the need for standardized procedures to ensure consistency within clinical practice.

Another promising source for cancer therapy resides in MSCs, originating from bone marrow, adipose tissue, and umbilical cord tissue. MSCs possess the ability to differentiate into bone, cartilage, and fat tissues, and they are noted for their regenerative and immunomodulatory properties (Hmadcha et al. 2020). These attributes render MSCs suitable for clinical trials spanning orthopedic injuries, autoimmune diseases, and neurological disorders. Beyond their conventional stem-cell traits, such as self-renewal and robust differentiation capabilities, MSCs exhibit a unique tumor-homing phenomenon. Driven by tumor tropism, chemotaxis, and the tumor microenvironment, MSCs are naturally attracted to tumor sites, where they engage with cancer cells, contributing to the attack against cancerous cells (Shah 2012; Datta et al. 2022). Genetic modifications further enhance their therapeutic potential by enabling MSCs to express exogenous tumor-targeting or therapeutic molecules (Shah 2012; Datta et al. 2022; Yan et al. 2023). Additionally, their low immunogenicity, attributed to minimal MHC-I molecule expression and immunomodulatory capabilities, renders MSC allogeneic transplantation well-tolerated. The duality of MSCs' interactions with the tumor microenvironment may pose a challenge. Despite interrupting cancer cell replication to inhibit tumor growth, MSCs can also differentiate into cancer-associated fibroblasts (CAFs), potentially contributing to cancer progression and immunosuppression (Mishra et al. 2009; Datta et al. 2022). The outcome of these interactions depends on various factors, including the tumor model, MSC source, timing, dosage of treatment, delivery methods, and patient-specific conditions, complicating their application in clinical oncology.

HSCs offer distinct advantages as a potential cell source for cancer therapy, owing to their natural involvement in blood and immune cell production. Their integral role in immune cell generation underpins their application in cancer therapy, notably in HSC transplantation (HSCT). HSCT facilitates reconstruction of a patient's immune system, providing a valuable tool for treating hematological malignancies such as leukemia and lymphoma (Rowe et al. 2016; Ng and Alexander

2017). HSCs can be genetically engineered to generate specialized immune cells, including T cells and NK cells, which can express CARs and other tumor-targeting molecules (Gschweng et al. 2014; Rowe et al. 2016). These modified immune cells have demonstrated promise in enhancing the patient's immune response against cancer cells. However, one of the primary limitations of HSCs is their propensity for the onset of graft-versus-host disease (GvHD), where HSC-derived immune target the recipient's healthy tissues, potentially leading to severe complications. Stringent donor-recipient matching and immunosuppressive treatments are essential to mitigate this risk in HSCT or HSC-derived cell therapy, strongly limiting usage (Montoro et al. 2023). Furthermore, while HSC-based therapies have exhibited success in certain blood-related cancers, their application in solid tumors is more nebulous, demanding further research to unlock their full potential in these contexts. Nevertheless, HSCs remain a valuable asset in cancer therapy, particularly in the management of hematological malignancies and as a foundation for advancing innovative immunotherapies.

Beyond the well-explored stem cell types mentioned above, several other cell sources hold potential for cell therapy applications. One such source is the adipose-derived stem cells (ASCs), isolated from fat tissue. ASCs exhibit regenerative properties and have shown promise in tissue repair and regeneration, making them valuable in treating conditions like skin injuries and degenerative joint diseases. Another cell type, neural stem cells (NSCs), derived from the nervous system, possess the ability to differentiate into various neural cell types. These cells hold potential for addressing neurological disorders and injuries, offering avenues for neural tissue repair and restoration (Stuckey and Shah 2014). Research into harnessing the therapeutic potential of ASCs and NSCs continues to expand, highlighting the dynamic landscape of stem cell-based therapies in diverse medical fields.

3 Differentiated Cell Types for Therapy

Stem cells possess the potential for genetic modifications and the ability to replicate in a clonal manner, resulting in the generation of exceptionally pure effector cells. Advancements in stem cell culture and differentiation techniques have broadened the spectrum of stem cell-derived cellular candidates. This now encompasses conventional T cells, non-conventional T cells, NK cells, dendritic cells (DCs), macrophages, and myeloid cells, all of which can be further engineered to acquire anticancer properties (Fig. 2).

The groundbreaking achievements of immune checkpoint inhibitors and CAR-T cell therapies, exemplified by the FDA-approved anti-CD19 CAR-T cell therapy for B-cell malignancies, have underscored the critical role of T cells in immunotherapy (Sterner and Sterner 2021). Accordingly, conventional αβ T cells have emerged as a pivotal component of the investigation of stem cell engineering. In alignment with established T-cell genetic engineering techniques, stem cell-derived αβ T cells can be modified to express physiological TCRs or synthetic CARs to acquire specificity

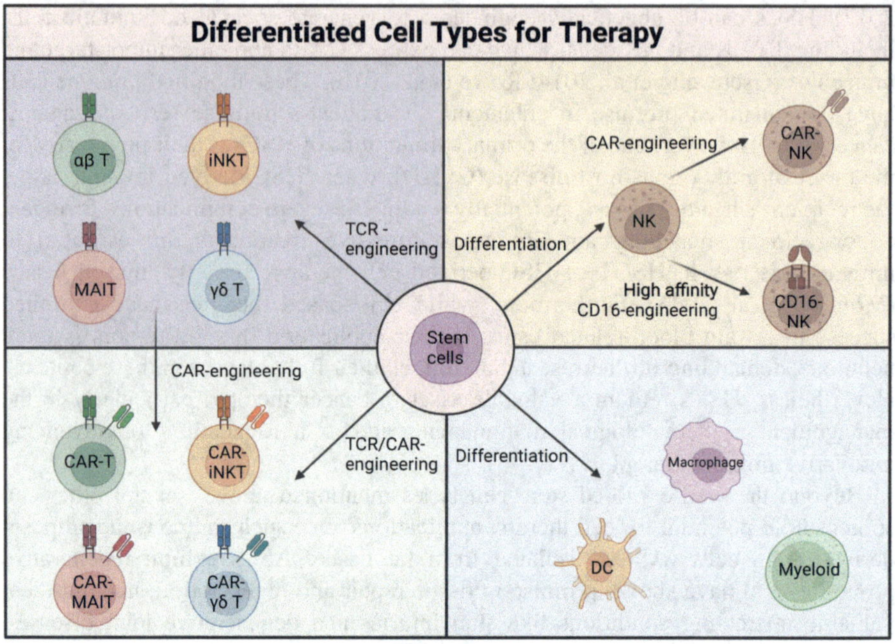

Fig. 2 Differentiated cell types for therapy. The figure shows various types of differentiated cells that can be derived from stem cells for cancer therapy and how these differentiated cells can be engineered to possess anticancer properties. *iNKT* invariant natural killer T cell, *MAIT* mucosal-associated invariant T cell, *NK* natural killer cell, *DC* dendritic cell

for tumor antigens (Sadelain et al. 2017). For example, TCR-engineered T cells such as NY-ESO-1-specific TCR-engineered T cells have propelled advancements in the treatment for myeloma, lung cancer, melanoma, and sarcoma (Rapoport et al. 2015; Zhang et al. 2022b). In addition to anti-CD19 CAR-T cell therapy, B-cell maturation antigen (BCMA) CAR-T cell therapy has also gained approval for the treatment of multiple myeloma and various B-cell malignancies (Raje et al. 2019; D'Agostino and Raje 2020; Li et al. 2023). Stem cell-derived αβ T cells can further mitigate the limitations of current CAR-T cell therapy, particularly cytokine release syndrome (CRS), owing to their different cytokine patterns (Themeli et al. 2013; Li et al. 2023). Moreover, considering the clinical significance of the CD4+:CD8+ ratio in therapeutic outcomes, allogeneic αβ T cells derived from induced pluripotent stem cells (iPSCs) or hematopoietic stem cells (HSCs) can circumvent the challenges posed by unstable or unfavorable T-cell compositions through precise gene editing techniques (Themeli et al. 2015; Turtle et al. 2016).

NK cells distinguish target cells through a combination of activating and inhibitory receptors, independently of MHC recognition, thereby mitigating the risk of GvHD, a concern often associated with conventional CAR-T cell therapy (Ruggeri et al. 2007; Fang et al. 2017; Rezvani et al. 2017; Abel et al. 2018). Similar to NK cells derived from other sources ranging from autologous patients to allogeneic donors, stem cell-derived NK cells can be enhanced via multiple approaches (Hermanson et al. 2016; Li et al. 2018). Promising modifications on NK cells, validated through preclinical studies, encompass the incorporation of CARs, engineering non-cleavable, high-affinity Fc receptors CD16 to optimize antibody-dependent cellular cytotoxicity (ADCC), the introduction of IL-15 or IL-2 to augment NK cell persistence and cytotoxicity, as well as the blockade of inhibitory receptors such as killer cell immunoglobulin-like receptor (KIR) or NKG2A (Cany et al. 2015; Rezvani et al. 2017; Mehta and Rezvani 2018; Liu et al. 2018; Li et al. 2018; Zhu et al. 2020a).

Unlike conventional αβ T cells, innate-like T cells such as γδ T cells, invariant natural killer T (iNKT) cells, and mucosal-associated invariant T (MAIT) cells employ a distinct recognition mechanism. They identify target cells through a combination of NK receptors and TCRs without binding to peptide-MHC complexes, thereby reducing the risk of GvHD (Li et al. 2022a). Remarkably, these unconventional T-cell populations can also be derived from iPSCs or HSCs engineered with specific TCRs and exhibit effective cytotoxicity against multiple myeloma, leukemia, and solid tumors (Wakao and Fujita 2013; Zhu et al. 2019; Wakao 2020). This progress underscores the potential for additional genetic modifications on innate-like T cells, such as CAR-iNKT cells or CAR-MAIT cells, providing a foundation for future off-the-shelf cancer immunotherapy initiatives (Dogan et al. 2022; Rowan et al. 2023). Besides, preclinical studies have demonstrated the successful generation of other innate immune cell types including DCs, macrophages, and myeloid cells from iPSCs (Hansen et al. 2018; Horton et al. 2020; Zhang et al. 2020). These iPSC-derived innate immune cells are highly immunostimulatory and therefore can be further modified to enhance cytokine secretion, facilitate phagocytosis of target tumor cells, and develop into an antitumor state (Horton et al. 2020; Zhang et al. 2020).

4 Mechanisms of Action

Stem cell-derived cell therapies have revolutionized cancer treatment by involving a wide range of adaptive immune cells and innate immune cells as mentioned in the previous section, each with unique mechanisms. In this section, major mechanisms by which these therapies exert their anticancer effects, along with examples of studies that demonstrate these mechanisms in action, will be elucidated.

Stem cell-derived conventional T cells are often armed with specific TCRs or CARs designed to recognize corresponding antigens on tumor cell surfaces. When these engineered stem cell-derived T cells are activated, either through CAR binding to tumor surface antigens or TCR interaction with peptide-MHC complexes, intracellular signaling pathways that trigger direct cytotoxicity are initiated (Eshhar et al. 1993; Jensen and Riddell 2015; Benmebarek et al. 2019). Consequently, these activated engineered T cells release perforin and granzyme, launching an attack on target cells. This process leads to rapid and highly specific T-cell-mediated lysis of tumor cells, complemented by the activation of the Fas-FasL pathway, which triggers apoptotic pathways in cancer cells (Kägi et al. 1994; Lowin et al. 1994).

Stem cell-derived NK cells mediate tumor cell killing via two pathways. Upon interaction between NK cell activating receptors and stress-induced ligands on tumor cell surface under hypoxia or DNA damage, NK cells initiate direct cell killing through degranulation (Paul and Lal 2017; Zhou et al. 2022). Moreover, NK cells can also initiate apoptosis of opsonized cells via Fc receptors through ADCC (Paul and Lal 2017; Goldenson et al. 2020; Bagheri et al. 2021). It is noteworthy that preclinical studies have confirmed the robust cytotoxicity exerted by iPSC-derived NK cells against a wide range of hematologic and solid tumors and their compatibility with traditional T cell and immune checkpoint inhibitor therapies (Cichocki et al. 2020). Multiple off-the-shelf iPSC-derived NK cell products, such as FT576, that undergo clinical trials have also demonstrated superior cytotoxicity compared to peripheral blood NK cells, alongside enhanced persistence (Zhou et al. 2022).

Stem cells also serve as an infinite and renewable source for innate-like T cells, such as MR1-restricted MAIT cells, CD1d-restricted iNKT cells, and γδ T cells, and their CAR-engineered counterparts. These cells, in addition to utilizing NK activating receptors for direct cell killing, elicit cytotoxicity through their TCRs independently of MHC molecules present on tumor cells (Beckman et al. 1994; Dias et al. 2018). Given the capacity for macrophages to infiltrate solid tumors, CAR-macrophages (CAR-Ms) have been generated to target both hematologic malignancies and solid tumors, and iPSC-derived macrophages have further enlarged the pool for stable and large-scale CAR-Ms production. Human anti-CD19- and anti-HER2-CAR-Ms, generated by Klichinsky et al., display a pro-inflammatory (M1) phenotype and accelerate the transition from pro-tumor M2 macrophages into antitumor M1 macrophages when targeting myelogenous leukemia and ovarian cancer respectively. They also play a critical role in recruiting and activating cytotoxic T lymphocytes (CTL), thereby constructing a pro-inflammatory tumor microenvironment (Klichinsky et al. 2020).

Playing a crucial tool in the initiation of immune responses, DC-based immunotherapy can also be enhanced by stem cells considering the extremely low number of circulating DCs in human peripheral blood (<1.0%) (Oba et al. 2021). Oba et al. stated that compared with bone marrow-derived DCs, iPSC-derived DCs express similar levels of surface DC markers and possess comparable antigen-presenting ability, and these DCs, in combination with traditional radiotherapy, can expedite the sensitization of tumor-specific CD8+ T cells (Senju et al. 2003, 2009; Oba et al. 2021). Additionally, Cai et al. highlighted the contributions made by iPSC-derived regulatory DCs (DCregs) with regard to immune modulation. These DCregs can suppress allograft rejection by facilitating the maturation of alloantigen-specific regulatory T cells, emphasizing their significance in immune regulation (Cai et al. 2017).

Bridging the innate and adaptive immune systems, iNKT cells have taken a prominent position in cancer immunotherapy. Although the low quantity of iNKT cells in human peripheral blood poses a challenge, their large-scale generation can be augmented through HSCs or iPSCs (Zhu et al. 2019; Li et al. 2021c). Notably,

Watarai et al. demonstrated that upon α-GalCer stimulation, iPSC-iNKT cells can expand in number, facilitate DC maturation, and activate CTLs and NK cells by releasing IFN-γ (Watarai et al. 2010). In addition to IFN-γ secreted by iPSC-iNKT, other pro-inflammatory/antitumor cytokines may be supplemented with a diverse array of stem cell-derived immune cells in cancer immunotherapy. Upon TCR-dependent activation, γδ T cells possess the capacity to release abundant pro-inflammatory cytokines including IL-2, IL-12, IL-15, and IL-18, therefore improving rapid, direct cell killing (Kabelitz et al. 2020). Similarly, MAIT cells, characterized by their high expression of pro-inflammatory cytokine receptors such as IL-12R and IL-18R, reciprocally secrete antitumor cytokines including IFN-γ and TNF-α, which can be further complemented by stem cell-derived MAIT cells (Petley et al. 2021). Moreover, stem cell-derived immune cells can be genetically modified to express antitumor cytokines. For instance, Mizuhashi et al. reported that mouse iPSC-derived proliferating MCs (iPSC-pMCs), genetically engineered to produce IL-15 and IL-15/Rα, can augment the NK-mediated cytotoxicity in mice, improving the treatment for mouse melanoma with major histocompatibility complex (MHC) class I loss (Mizuhashi et al. 2021).

5 Engineering Approaches

Through a multitude of approaches to genetic engineering, the therapeutic persistence, anticancer homing, and tumor-killing efficacy of stem-cell-derived immunotherapy are open to further enhancement. The earliest methods of gene editing, including zinc-finger nucleases (ZFNs) and transcription activation-like effector nucleases (TALENs), have largely fallen out of favor in lieu of CRISPR-Cas9 mediated editing on account of its greater editing versatility, site specificity, and reduced off-target binding (Ding et al. 2013; Wright et al. 2014; Ul Ain et al. 2015; Lanigan et al. 2020; Boti et al. 2023). Editing of the genome alone can enhance therapeutic cell efficacy and longevity through site-specific knockouts of TCR genes (e.g., TRAC and TRBC) (Morton et al. 2020; Kagoya et al. 2020; Zhang et al. 2022a; Ottaviano et al. 2022; Lamothe et al. 2023) to avoid onset of graft vs. host disease (GvHD) in conventional αβ T-cell therapy, MHC-class genes (e.g., B2M and CIITA) to reduce host allorejection (Liu and Zhao 2018; Kagoya et al. 2020; Naeem et al. 2023) and immune checkpoint genes (e.g., PD-1, CTLA-4, LAG-3, TIM3) regulating activation state (Rupp et al. 2017; Dötsch et al. 2023; Zhu et al. 2020b; Beane et al. 2015; Agarwal et al. 2023; Shi et al. 2017; Zhang et al. 2017). During the early stages of stem cell culture, engineered expression of transcription factors driving lineage differentiation may be incorporated to further enhance immune cell maturity and purity (Ng et al. 2021). Within the clinic, CRISPR-Cas9 modifications have demonstrated a safe platform for the implementation of a universal, allogeneic CD19-CAR T-cell therapy that could help reduce individual patient costs following the current autologous model (Hu et al. 2021; Ottaviano et al. 2022).

In cancer immunotherapy, one of the most well-established methods of enhancing tumor recognition is through engineered expression of tumor-specific CARs recognizing cancer antigens. Expression of synthetic CARs has been most-extensively adopted and implemented in conventional αβ T cells, with 6 treatments utilizing CD19- or BCMA-targeting CARs having been FDA-approved for the treatment of B-cell lymphoma and multiple myeloma (Shohdy et al. 2023; Gordon et al. 2023; Dhaliwal and Ravi 2023; Awasthi et al. 2023). Currently, broad applications for CAR-based therapies are being explored against different cancers: the viability of alternative CAR antigens, such as mesothelin (MSLN) (Ding et al. 2023; Zhu et al. 2023; Yang et al. 2023a), glypican-3 (GPC3) (Shi et al. 2020; Sun et al. 2022a, b), and CD70 (Sauer et al. 2021; Panowski et al. 2022) for respective treatment of ovarian cancer, hepatocellular carcinoma, and acute myeloid leukemia (AML). Furthermore, the potency of arming other immune cells is currently being explored in innate immune cell types to produce CAR-Ms (Zhang et al. 2020; Chen et al. 2023; Duan et al. 2023) and CAR-NK cells (Golubovskaya et al. 2023; Yang et al. 2023a) displaying potent antitumor targeting as well as adjuvant stimulation of endogenous immune cells. The benefits of both innate and adaptive immune recognition pathways may be harnessed through CAR-engineering of unconventional innate-like iNKT and MAIT cells for the production of CAR-iNKT and CAR-MAIT cell therapy. Our group has particularly explored the potential of allogeneic CAR-iNKT cell therapy on account of their tripartite recognition of tumor cells and immunosuppressive cells through the CAR domain, lineage-restricted invariant TCR, and activating NK markers (Zhu et al. 2019; Li et al. 2022b). As an alternative to CAR-T cell therapy, the aforementioned cell types do not engage with classic MHC-I and MHC-II markers, providing an ideal allogeneic alternative to traditional CAR-T cell therapy without the risk of inducing GvHD (Li et al. 2022b; Sadowski et al. 2022). While limited preclinical success has been observed for non-T cell-based cancer immunotherapies, there still remains a need to verify safety and success within the clinic.

The engineering of autonomous cytokine expression has also demonstrated the potential to significantly enhance the efficacy and persistence of therapeutic cells administered to patients, including IL-15, IL-2, IL-12, and IL-18 (Yeku and Brentjens 2016). Secretion of IL-15 in particular is vital for supporting NK and innate-like T cells, enhancing antitumor targeting and in vivo persistence (Liu et al. 2018; Makkouk et al. 2021; Ruixin et al. 2023; Bodden et al. 2023). Furthermore, IL-15 secretion could potentially aid in the remediation of the tumor environment through the reprogramming of immunosuppressive cells (Zannikou et al. 2023). Similar effects have also been observed in vivo on account of recombinant secretion of IL-2 and IL-12 to enhance CAR-T cell infiltration and proliferation, though they have been explored to a lesser degree (Becknell and Caligiuri 2005; Yang et al. 2023b; Fang et al. 2023). Recent advances in CAR engineering have seen the incorporation of such genes encoding IL-2 or IL-15 within the CAR construct itself, providing continuous cytokine support (Liu et al. 2018). Cytokine stimulation has been implemented in various forms, including secretion of either soluble or membrane-bound cytokines or downstream activation (Allen et al. 2021; Christodoulou et al. 2021).

6 Preclinical and Clinical Manufacturing

Within the field of cancer treatment, cell-based therapeutics hold great potential, but are limited by several factors, including high variability, protracted manufacturing, high sensitivity and low stability, and product heterogeneity (Taefehshokr et al. 2022; Blache et al. 2022). Stringent GMP regulations may abate variability between batches of cell products by standardizing cell characterization, including testing of yield, purity, and tumorigenicity (Bedford et al. 2018). Additionally, external aspects to the manufacturing process itself may impact efficacy in the clinic, including stem cell origin, administration route, dosing, and combination with other products, to name a few.

The preclinical applications of these cell products have yielded promising results in the treatment of a wide range of cancers across various models. Among the most well-explored preclinically are DCs produced from stem cells as a vaccine to stimulate an immune response through cancer antigen presentation. Engineering can further facilitate DC enhancement either through self-expression of target cancer antigens or overexpression of presenting molecules (i.e., MHC-I and II, CD1d, MR1, etc.) to promote stimulation of endogenous lymphocytes (Zeng et al. 2012; Tominaga et al. 2023). Regarding cytotoxic cell types, NK and T cells have been the most extensively stem cell-derived therapeutic cells. Belonging to opposite arms of innate and adaptive immunity, both employ unique recognition and killing pathways that may be homed to tumor cells using CAR engineering (Huang et al. 2022; Klaihmon et al. 2023). Through innate-like T cells, which simultaneously express NK activating markers and a lineage-specific TCR, the antitumor potential of both cell types may be synergized within a single model. In our hands, we have developed a malleable platform for engineering CAR-iNKT cells against a variety of tumor-specific antigens, showing strong suppression of cancer growth with limited GvHD onset in mice (Li et al. 2021c, 2022b). The potency of innate-like T cells has yet to be fully explored in the preclinical setting, providing potential opportunities to expand upon the established success of CAR-T cell therapy. Although therapies encompassing other unconventional T cells, such as MAIT and γδ T cells, have not yet broken through to clinical trials, they still show great promise within the preclinical setting (Wakao et al. 2013; Watanabe et al. 2018; Zeng et al. 2019). Through a stem cell-based platform, rare immune cell subtypes such as these may be more easily generated for stockpiling of "off-the-shelf" therapeutic doses for cancer patients.

Expanding on this preclinical success, several clinical trials have been established to examine the safety and potency of stem cell-based therapies in cancer patients (Table 1). While the majority of these studies are still recruiting or remain ongoing, those that have concluded have shown promising results for patient remission. In particular, Fate Therapeutics has established several therapeutic CAR-NK cell products derived from a human clonal master iPSC line, providing both a highly malleable and controlled platform for generating therapeutic cells. FT500, their earliest CAR-NK cell product, has demonstrated strong preclinical potency, engaging in innate cytotoxicity, producing adjuvant stimulation of endogenous T cells, and augmenting the efficacy of anti-PD-1 combination therapy (Cichocki

Table 1 Current stem cell-derived cell therapies in preclinical or clinical trials

Cell therapy	Phase	Clinical trial identifier	Description	Results
NK	Clinical	NCT05182073	FT576 in Subjects with Multiple Myeloma	Phase I: Recruiting
		NCT05336409	CNTY-101 in Participants with CD19^{+} B-Cell Malignancies	Phase I: Recruiting
		NCT04630769 NCT04551885 NCT04023071	FT516 and IL2 with Enoblituzumab for Ovarian Cancer; Solid Tumors; Hematologic Malignancies	Phase I: Completed—Limited adverse systemic effects reported in all individuals; Phase I: Active; Phase I: Active
		NCT05950334	FT522 With Rituximab in Relapsed B-Cell Lymphoma	Phase I: Not Yet Recruiting
		NCT05069935; NCT04714372; NCT04614636; NCT05708924	FT538 in Combination with mAb in Advanced Solid Tumors; Acute Myeloid Leukemia; Advanced Hematologic Malignancies; Recurrent Ovarian, Fallopian Tube, Primary Peritoneal Cancer	Phase I: Active; Phase I: Recruiting; Phase I: Active; Phase I: Recruiting
		NCT05395052	FT536 Monotherapy and Combination with mAb in Advanced Solid Tumors	Phase I: Active
		NCT04245722; NCT04555811	FT596 as Monotherapy and Combination with anti-CD20 mAb; Combination with Rituximab for Relapse Prevention in Non-Hodgkin Lymphoma	Phase I: Active; Phase I: Active
		NCT03841110; NCT04106167	FT500 as Monotherapy and Combination with Immune Checkpoint Inhibitors in Solid Tumor; Long-term, Observational Study Post-Treatment	Phase I: Results not yet reported; Ongoing
	Preclinical	iPSC-CD19CAR NK cells show selective targeting of CD19^{+} hematologic cancers in vitro and elevated NK activation marker levels post-exposure (Klaihmon et al. 2023; Chang et al. 2023) iPSC-MCAR NK cells display enhanced cytotoxicity against solid TNBC in vitro and in vivo (Yang et al. 2023a)		

DC	Clinical	Not Available	Therapeutic DC Vaccination with IL-2 as Consolidation Therapy for Ovarian Cancer Patients	Phase I/II Trial: Autologous HSC-derived DCs secrete IL-12, reduce inhibitory $CD4^+CD25^+$ T cell subsets, and enhance proportion of $CD8^+$ IFNγ-secreting T cells (Baek et al. 2011)
	Preclinical	Embryoid bodies form mixed $CD11c^+$ DC populations, which can be enriched for cross-presentation specialized $CD141^+$ DCs through $CD1c^+$ depletion (Sachamitr et al. 2017) iPSCs (Horton et al. 2020; Oba et al. 2021; Tominaga et al. 2023), ESCs (Zeng et al. 2012), and CBSCs (Chang et al. 2012) are viable input for generation of stem-cell-derived DCs, which show strong adjuvant stimulation and cytokine profile Adjuvant effects can be further enhanced through genetic engineering of tumor antigens expression (e.g., MSLN) (Tominaga et al. 2023) or overexpression of antigen-presenting markers (e.g., CD1d) (Zeng et al. 2012)		
Macrophage	Preclinical	iPSC-macrophages show proper function and polarization compared to primary macrophages (Gutbier et al. 2020) iPSC-CD19CAR macrophages display durable suppression of K562 leukemia cells in vitro and in vivo (Zhang et al. 2020)		
T	Clinical	NCT04629729	FT819 in Subjects with B-Cell Malignancies	Phase I: Recruiting
	Preclinical	iPSC-T cells display normal differentiation into single-positive lineages (Nishimura and Nakauchi 2019; Iriguchi et al. 2021) CD8 αβ T cells demonstrate transient ability to suppress H226 hepatocarcinoma growth in vitro and in vivo (Iriguchi et al. 2021) Anti-EGFRvIII iPSC-CAR T cells demonstrate extravasation across the blood-brain barrier and significantly reduce within GBM burden in vitro (Huang et al. 2022)		
iNKT	Clinical	jRCT2033200116	Phase I Study of iPS-NKT in Patients with Recurrent or Advanced Head and Neck Cancer	Phase I: Ongoing
	Preclinical	iPSC-NKT cells display adjuvant effects for endogenous DCs and NK cells (Kitayama et al. 2016; Yamada et al. 2016; Aoki et al. 2023) IL-15 stimulation drives phenotypic maturity of iPSC-NKT cells, with Th1-like phenotype bias, that show tumor cell killing in vitro (Kitayama et al. 2016) and in vivo (Yamada et al. 2016)		
MAIT	Preclinical	iPSC-MAIT cells exhibit appropriate lineage-specific TCR, appropriate chemokine and cytokine response profiles in vitro, and population of bone marrow, liver, spleen niches in NSG mice (Wakao et al. 2013)		
γδ T	Preclinical	iPSC-derived γδ T cells can be produced from whole blood PBMC input (Watanabe et al. 2018) Mimetic CD19CAR γδ T cells, expressing Vγ9Vδ2TCR and high level of NK markers, but no/low phenotypic γδ markers, show broad in vitro tumor killing (Zeng et al. 2019)		

et al. 2020). Within human patients, FT500 administered in weekly doses, both as monotherapy and in concert with immune checkpoint blockade, has shown tumor suppression in patients resistant to blockade therapy alone, with limited adverse reactions (Hong et al. 2020). Furthermore, more elaborately engineered products such as FT516, a CAR-NK cell line expressing non-cleavable CD16 for enhanced antibody-dependent cellular cytotoxicity, has shown similar success for combination therapy against liquid and solid tumors (Strati et al. 2021). These trials underscore the preliminary efficacy of such therapies against a broad range of cancers, particularly as a course of therapy for patients resistant to first-line interventions. As clinical trials continue to establish the efficacy of stem cell-derived lymphocytes, the foundation for introducing such therapies into clinical practice draws nearer to becoming a reality.

7 Challenges and Future Directions

Despite the success achieved through the current autologous model of CAR-T cell therapy, its clinical utility is limited by its lack of efficacy against solid tumors, limited scalability for multiple patients, and financial burden placed on cancer patients. The development of an "off-the-shelf" therapy will reduce the weight of these expenses by circumventing the need to develop a tailored immunotherapy for each patient receiving therapy. While other immune cell subtypes, including NK cells and innate-like T cells, avoid onset of GvHD on account of their intrinsic recognition mechanisms, necessary steps in isolation, expansion, and genetic engineering present a challenge to maximizing cell product yield. Especially for innate-like T cells, which represent an extremely low proportion of lymphocytes in peripheral blood, producing a sufficient number of cells for multiple doses precludes direct harvest as a cost-effective method.

These barriers to development can be overcome through stem-cell engineering, which provides a highly scalable and malleable platform that can produce cell products with limited heterogeneity. The scalability of NK, iNKT, MAIT, and γδ T cell-based therapies derive from their MHC-independent recognition of tumor cells, abrogating the onset of GvHD. Among potential sources for stem cell engineering, currently the greatest interest lies in iPSCs due to ease of collection of more common, terminally differentiated cells for reprogramming. Selecting a lineage closely related to the desired iPSC-derived lymphocyte can help mitigate functional variability arising from epigenetic modifications associated with the origin cell type for iPSCs (Polo et al. 2010; Zhou et al. 2022). Additional variation may arise from differences in manufacturing protocol, even among products of the same cell subtype. Additionally, it is necessary to further explore the mechanisms underlying stem-cell-based therapies. It remains unclear whether there are any discrepancies between the maturity and cytotoxic capacity of stem cell-derived products versus their endogenous counterparts. The extensive stem cell manufacturing and engineering process itself may also lend to differences in therapeutic potency. It is also yet to be determined if there are any long-term implications associated with the administration of stem cell-derived products to patients.

Although more comprehensive analysis of stem cell-based therapies is necessary to fully understand their capabilities, it is undeniable that the platform has already achieved significant successes in both preclinical and clinical settings. Particularly in combination with immune checkpoint blockade, these products may provide a durable alternative for cancer immunotherapy enabling treatment of resistant cancers. As further advancements in cell engineering continue to progress and become integrated into the workflow of the stem cell platform, it holds the promise of producing more ambitious and efficacious cell products for cancer immunotherapy.

8 Discussion

Stem cells, including MSCs, HSCs, ESCs, and iPSCs, represent compelling candidates for cancer immunotherapy. The current body of research and early-stage clinical trials provide substantiated evidence supporting the feasibility of engineered stem cells as a means to generate potent effector cells and bolster antitumor immune responses for the eradication of cancer. Stem cell engineering and differentiation confer not only an inexhaustible supply of therapeutic cellular products but also establish a versatile and adaptable platform for further modifications aimed at enhancing the antitumor efficacy of resultant cellular products.

The realization of whether stem cell-engineered approaches manifest additional efficacy in comparison to those employing mature human periphery blood mononuclear cell (PBMC)-derived immune cells as therapeutic targets hinges upon clinical trials. It is conceivable that the two approaches may, in some instances, complement each other. Ongoing development of clinical trials is poised to provide preliminary insights.

Given the intricate nature of diseases like cancer, it is probable that the attainment of enduring therapeutic benefits will necessitate combination therapies. Engineered stem cell products, characterized by their "off-the-shelf" availability, hold promise as constituents of treatment regimens that encompass established cancer therapies, such as surgery, radiation, chemotherapy, and targeted interventions, as well as emerging cancer immunotherapies, including immune checkpoint inhibitors, oncolytic viruses, cancer vaccines, and adoptive cellular therapies (Depil et al. 2020; Li et al. 2021a). The adaptability of engineered stem cell products, their suitability for customization, and scalability to cater to specific cancer types render them a promising addition to the oncological arsenal, poised to enhance treatment outcomes and ameliorate patients' quality of life (Li et al. 2023). As the field continues to evolve, a methodical and prudent approach is imperative to ensure the safe and efficient translation of stem cell-based therapies into clinical settings.

Acknowledgments We thank Dr. Lili Yang from the University of California, Los Angeles (UCLA) for her insightful discussion. Y.-R.L. is supported by a UCLA MIMG M. John Pickett Post-Doctoral Fellow Award, and a CIRM-BSCRC Postdoctoral Fellowship.

Declaration of Interests The authors declare no competing interests.

References

Abel AM, Yang C, Thakar MS, Malarkannan S (2018) Natural killer cells: development, maturation, and clinical utilization. Front Immunol 9:1869

Agarwal S, Aznar MA, Rech AJ et al (2023) Deletion of the inhibitory co-receptor CTLA4 enhances and invigorates chimeric antigen receptor T cells. Immunity S1074-7613(23): 00407–00407. https://doi.org/10.1016/j.immuni.2023.09.001

Allen AG, Pattali R, Izzo KM et al (2021) A bicistronic vector expressing CD16 and a membrane bound IL-15 construct in iPSC derived NK cells increased cytotoxicity and persistence. Blood 138:4809. https://doi.org/10.1182/blood-2021-153258

Aoki T, Motohashi S, Koseki H (2023) Regeneration of invariant natural killer T (iNKT) cells: application of iPSC technology for iNKT cell-targeted tumor immunotherapy. Inflamm Regen 43:27. https://doi.org/10.1186/s41232-023-00275-5

Awasthi R, Maier HJ, Zhang J, Lim S (2023) Kymriah® (tisagenlecleucel)—an overview of the clinical development journey of the first approved CAR-T therapy. Hum Vaccines Immunother 19:2210046. https://doi.org/10.1080/21645515.2023.2210046

Baek S, Kim C-S, Kim S-B et al (2011) Combination therapy of renal cell carcinoma or breast cancer patients with dendritic cell vaccine and IL-2: results from a phase I/II trial. J Transl Med 9:178. https://doi.org/10.1186/1479-5876-9-178

Bagheri Y, Barati A, Aghebati-Maleki A et al (2021) Current progress in cancer immunotherapy based on natural killer cells. Cell Biol Int 45:2–17. https://doi.org/10.1002/cbin.11465

Beane JD, Lee G, Zheng Z et al (2015) Clinical scale zinc finger nuclease-mediated gene editing of PD-1 in tumor infiltrating lymphocytes for the treatment of metastatic melanoma. Mol Ther J Am Soc Gene Ther 23:1380–1390. https://doi.org/10.1038/mt.2015.71

Beckman EM, Porcelli SA, Morita CT et al (1994) Recognition of a lipid antigen by CD1-restricted αβ+ T cells. Nature 372:691–694. https://doi.org/10.1038/372691a0

Becknell B, Caligiuri MA (2005) Interleukin-2, interleukin-15, and their roles in human natural killer cells. Adv Immunol 86:209–239. https://doi.org/10.1016/S0065-2776(04)86006-1

Bedford P, Jy J, Collins L, Keizer S (2018) Considering cell therapy product "good manufacturing practice" status. Front Med 5:118. https://doi.org/10.3389/fmed.2018.00118

Benmebarek M-R, Karches CH, Cadilha BL et al (2019) Killing mechanisms of chimeric antigen receptor (CAR) T cells. Int J Mol Sci 20:1283. https://doi.org/10.3390/ijms20061283

Blache U, Popp G, Dünkel A et al (2022) Potential solutions for manufacture of CAR T cells in cancer immunotherapy. Nat Commun 13:5225. https://doi.org/10.1038/s41467-022-32866-0

Bodden M, Häcker A, Röder J et al (2023) Co-expression of an IL-15 superagonist facilitates self-enrichment of GD2-Targeted CAR-NK cells and mediates potent cell killing in the absence of IL-2. Cancer 15:4310. https://doi.org/10.3390/cancers15174310

Boti MA, Athanasopoulou K, Adamopoulos PG et al (2023) Recent advances in genome-engineering strategies. Genes 14:129. https://doi.org/10.3390/genes14010129

Cai S, Hou J, Fujino M et al (2017) iPSC-derived regulatory dendritic cells inhibit allograft rejection by generating alloantigen-specific regulatory T cells. Stem Cell Rep 8:1174–1189. https://doi.org/10.1016/j.stemcr.2017.03.020

Cany J, van der Waart AB, Spanholtz J et al (2015) Combined IL-15 and IL-12 drives the generation of CD34+-derived natural killer cells with superior maturation and alloreactivity potential following adoptive transfer. Onco Targets Ther 4:e1017701. https://doi.org/10.1080/2162402X.2015.1017701

Chang M-C, Lee C-N, Chen Y-L et al (2012) Cord blood stem-cell-derived dendritic cells generate potent antigen-specific immune responses and anti-tumour effects. Clin Sci Lond Engl 1979 123:347–360. https://doi.org/10.1042/CS20110272

Chang Y, Jin G, Luo W et al (2023) Engineered human pluripotent stem cell-derived natural killer cells with PD-L1 responsive immunological memory for enhanced immunotherapeutic efficacy. Bioact Mater 27:168–180. https://doi.org/10.1016/j.bioactmat.2023.03.018

Chen Y, Zhu X, Liu H et al (2023) The application of HER2 and CD47 CAR-macrophage in ovarian cancer. J Transl Med 21:654. https://doi.org/10.1186/s12967-023-04479-8

Christodoulou I, Koldobskiy M, Ho WJ et al (2021) Engineered interleukin-15 autocrine signaling invigorates anti-CD123 CAR-NK cells. Blood 138:2806. https://doi.org/10.1182/blood-2021-146609

Cichocki F, Bjordahl R, Gaidarova S et al (2020) iPSC-derived NK cells maintain high cytotoxicity and enhance in vivo tumor control in concert with T cells and anti–PD-1 therapy. Sci Transl Med 12:eaaz5618. https://doi.org/10.1126/scitranslmed.aaz5618

D'Agostino M, Raje N (2020) Anti-BCMA CAR T-cell therapy in multiple myeloma: can we do better? Leukemia 34:21–34. https://doi.org/10.1038/s41375-019-0669-4

Datta J, Dai X, Bianchi A et al (2022) Combined MEK and STAT3 inhibition uncovers stromal plasticity by enriching for cancer-associated fibroblasts with mesenchymal stem cell-like features to overcome immunotherapy resistance in pancreatic cancer. Gastroenterology 163: 1593–1612. https://doi.org/10.1053/j.gastro.2022.07.076

Depil S, Duchateau P, Grupp SA et al (2020) "Off-the-shelf" allogeneic CAR T cells: development and challenges. Nat Rev Drug Discov 19:185–199. https://doi.org/10.1038/s41573-019-0051-2

Dhaliwal A, Ravi S (2023) Myelodysplastic syndrome after anti-CD19 chimeric antigen receptor T-cell therapy: a case series. Cureus 15:e44677. https://doi.org/10.7759/cureus.44677

Dias J, Boulouis C, Gorin J-B et al (2018) The CD4−CD8− MAIT cell subpopulation is a functionally distinct subset developmentally related to the main CD8+ MAIT cell pool. Proc Natl Acad Sci 115:E11513–E11522. https://doi.org/10.1073/pnas.1812273115

Ding Q, Regan SN, Xia Y et al (2013) Enhanced efficiency of human pluripotent stem cell genome editing through replacing TALENs with CRISPRs. Cell Stem Cell 12:393–394. https://doi.org/10.1016/j.stem.2013.03.006

Ding J, Guyette S, Schrand B et al (2023) Mesothelin-targeting T cells bearing a novel T cell receptor fusion construct (TRuC) exhibit potent antitumor efficacy against solid tumors. Onco Targets Ther 12:2182058. https://doi.org/10.1080/2162402X.2023.2182058

Dogan M, Karhan E, Kozhaya L et al (2022) Engineering human MAIT cells with chimeric antigen receptors for cancer immunotherapy. J Immunol 209:1523–1531. https://doi.org/10.4049/jimmunol.2100856

Dötsch S, Svec M, Schober K et al (2023) Long-term persistence and functionality of adoptively transferred antigen-specific T cells with genetically ablated PD-1 expression. Proc Natl Acad Sci U S A 120:e2200626120. https://doi.org/10.1073/pnas.2200626120

Duan Z, Li Z, Wang Z et al (2023) Chimeric antigen receptor macrophages activated through TLR4 or IFN-γ receptors suppress breast cancer growth by targeting VEGFR2. Cancer Immunol Immunother 72:3243–3257. https://doi.org/10.1007/s00262-023-03490-8

Eshhar Z, Waks T, Gross G, Schindler DG (1993) Specific activation and targeting of cytotoxic lymphocytes through chimeric single chains consisting of antibody-binding domains and the gamma or zeta subunits of the immunoglobulin and T-cell receptors. Proc Natl Acad Sci 90: 720–724. https://doi.org/10.1073/pnas.90.2.720

Euchner J, Sprissler J, Cathomen T et al (2021) Natural killer cells generated from human induced pluripotent stem cells mature to CD56(bright)CD16(+)NKp80(+/-) in-vitro and express KIR2DL2/DL3 and KIR3DL1. Front Immunol 12:640672. https://doi.org/10.3389/fimmu.2021.640672

Fang F, Xiao W, Tian Z (2017) NK cell-based immunotherapy for cancer. Semin Immunol 31:37–54. https://doi.org/10.1016/j.smim.2017.07.009

Fang L, Yuan S, Wang M et al (2023) Recombinant oncolytic adenovirus armed with CCL5, IL-12, and IFN-γ promotes CAR-T infiltration and proliferation in vivo to eradicate local and distal tumors. Cell Death Dis 9:328. https://doi.org/10.1038/s41420-023-01626-4

Frank C, Ryan B, Svetlana G et al (2020) iPSC-derived NK cells maintain high cytotoxicity and enhance in vivo tumor control in concert with T cells and anti–PD-1 therapy. Sci Transl Med 12: eaaz5618. https://doi.org/10.1126/scitranslmed.aaz5618

Gerew A, Sexton S, Wasko KM et al (2021) Deletion of CISH and TGFβR2 in iPSC-derived NK cells promotes high cytotoxicity and enhances in vivo tumor killing. Blood 138:2780. https://doi.org/10.1182/blood-2021-150731

Goldenson BH, Zhu H, Wang YM et al (2020) Umbilical cord blood and iPSC-derived natural killer cells demonstrate key differences in cytotoxic activity and KIR profiles. Front Immunol 11

Golubovskaya V, Sienkiewicz J, Sun J et al (2023) CAR-NK cells generated with mRNA-LNPs kill tumor target cells in vitro and in vivo. Int J Mol Sci 24:13364. https://doi.org/10.3390/ijms241713364

Gordon LI, Liu FF, Braverman J et al (2023) Lisocabtagene maraleucel for second-line relapsed or refractory large B-cell lymphoma: patient-reported outcomes from the PILOT study. Haematologica. https://doi.org/10.3324/haematol.2023.283162

Gschweng E, De Oliveira S, Kohn DB (2014) Hematopoietic stem cells for cancer immunotherapy. Immunol Rev 257:237–249. https://doi.org/10.1111/imr.12128

Gutbier S, Wanke F, Dahm N et al (2020) Large-scale production of human iPSC-derived macrophages for drug screening. Int J Mol Sci 21:4808. https://doi.org/10.3390/ijms21134808

Hansen M, Varga E, Aarts C et al (2018) Efficient production of erythroid, megakaryocytic and myeloid cells, using single cell-derived iPSC colony differentiation. Stem Cell Res 29:232–244. https://doi.org/10.1016/j.scr.2018.04.016

Hermanson DL, Bendzick L, Pribyl L et al (2016) Induced pluripotent stem cell-derived natural killer cells for treatment of ovarian cancer. Stem Cells 34:93–101. https://doi.org/10.1002/stem.2230

Hmadcha A, Martin-Montalvo A, Gauthier BR et al (2020) Therapeutic potential of mesenchymal stem cells for cancer therapy. Front Bioeng Biotechnol 8:43. https://doi.org/10.3389/fbioe.2020.00043

Hochedlinger K, Jaenisch R (2003) Nuclear transplantation, embryonic stem cells, and the potential for cell therapy. N Engl J Med 349:275–286. https://doi.org/10.1056/NEJMra035397

Hong D, Patel S, Patel M et al (2020) 380 Preliminary results of an ongoing phase I trial of FT500, a first-in-class, off-the-shelf, induced pluripotent stem cell (iPSC) derived natural killer (NK) cell therapy in advanced solid tumors. J Immunother Cancer 8. https://doi.org/10.1136/jitc-2020-SITC2020.0380

Horton C, Davies TJ, Lahiri P et al (2020) Induced pluripotent stem cells reprogrammed from primary dendritic cells provide an abundant source of immunostimulatory dendritic cells for use in immunotherapy. Stem Cells Dayt Ohio 38:67–79. https://doi.org/10.1002/stem.3095

Hu Y, Zhou Y, Zhang M et al (2021) CRISPR/Cas9-engineered universal CD19/CD22 dual-targeted CAR-T cell therapy for relapsed/refractory B-cell acute lymphoblastic leukemia. Clin Cancer Res 27:2764–2772. https://doi.org/10.1158/1078-0432.CCR-20-3863

Huang J, Li YB, Charlebois C et al (2022) Application of blood brain barrier models in pre-clinical assessment of glioblastoma-targeting CAR-T based immunotherapies. Fluids Barriers CNS 19:38. https://doi.org/10.1186/s12987-022-00342-y

Iltis AS, Koster G, Reeves E, Matthews KRW (2023) Ethical, legal, regulatory, and policy issues concerning embryoids: a systematic review of the literature. Stem Cell Res Ther 14:209. https://doi.org/10.1186/s13287-023-03448-8

Iriguchi S, Yasui Y, Kawai Y et al (2021) A clinically applicable and scalable method to regenerate T-cells from iPSCs for off-the-shelf T-cell immunotherapy. Nat Commun 12:430. https://doi.org/10.1038/s41467-020-20658-3

Jensen MC, Riddell SR (2015) Designing chimeric antigen receptors to effectively and safely target tumors. Curr Opin Immunol 33:9–15. https://doi.org/10.1016/j.coi.2015.01.002

Kabelitz D, Serrano R, Kouakanou L et al (2020) Cancer immunotherapy with γδ T cells: many paths ahead of us. Cell Mol Immunol 17:925–939. https://doi.org/10.1038/s41423-020-0504-x

Kägi D, Vignaux F, Ledermann B et al (1994) Fas and perforin pathways as major mechanisms of T cell-mediated cytotoxicity. Science 265:528–530. https://doi.org/10.1126/science.7518614

Kagoya Y, Guo T, Yeung B et al (2020) Genetic ablation of HLA class I, class II, and the T-cell receptor enables allogeneic T cells to be used for adoptive T-cell therapy. Cancer Immunol Res 8:926–936. https://doi.org/10.1158/2326-6066.CIR-18-0508

Kitayama S, Zhang R, Liu T-Y et al (2016) Cellular adjuvant properties, direct cytotoxicity of re-differentiated Vα24 invariant NKT-like cells from human induced pluripotent stem cells. Stem Cell Rep 6:213–227. https://doi.org/10.1016/j.stemcr.2016.01.005

Klaihmon P, Kang X, Issaragrisil S, Luanpitpong S (2023) Generation and functional characterization of anti-CD19 chimeric antigen receptor-natural killer cells from human induced pluripotent stem cells. Int J Mol Sci 24:10508. https://doi.org/10.3390/ijms241310508

Klichinsky M, Ruella M, Shestova O et al (2020) Human chimeric antigen receptor macrophages for cancer immunotherapy. Nat Biotechnol 38:947–953. https://doi.org/10.1038/s41587-020-0462-y

Lamothe RC, Storlie MD, Espinosa DA et al (2023) Novel CRISPR-associated gene-editing systems discovered in metagenomic samples enable efficient and specific genome engineering. CRISPR J 6:243–260. https://doi.org/10.1089/crispr.2022.0089

Lanigan TM, Kopera HC, Saunders TL (2020) Principles of genetic engineering. Genes 11:291. https://doi.org/10.3390/genes11030291

Li Y, Hermanson DL, Moriarity BS, Kaufman DS (2018) Human iPSC-derived natural killer cells engineered with chimeric antigen receptors enhance anti-tumor activity. Cell Stem Cell 23:181–192.e5. https://doi.org/10.1016/j.stem.2018.06.002

Li Y-R, Dunn ZS, Zhou Y et al (2021a) Development of stem cell-derived immune cells for off-the-shelf cancer immunotherapies. Cell 10. https://doi.org/10.3390/cells10123497

Li Y-R, Zhou Y, Kim YJ et al (2021b) Development of allogeneic HSC-engineered iNKT cells for off-the-shelf cancer immunotherapy. Cell Rep Med 2:100449. https://doi.org/10.1016/j.xcrm.2021.100449

Li Y-R, Zhou Y, Kramer A, Yang L (2021c) Engineering stem cells for cancer immunotherapy. Trends Cancer. https://doi.org/10.1016/j.trecan.2021.08.004

Li Y-R, Dunn ZS, Garcia G et al (2022a) Development of off-the-shelf hematopoietic stem cell-engineered invariant natural killer T cells for COVID-19 therapeutic intervention. Stem Cell Res Ther 13:112. https://doi.org/10.1186/s13287-022-02787-2

Li Y-R, Zeng S, Dunn ZS et al (2022b) Off-the-shelf third-party HSC-engineered iNKT cells for ameliorating GvHD while preserving GvL effect in the treatment of blood cancers. iScience 25: 104859. https://doi.org/10.1016/j.isci.2022.104859

Li Y-R, Dunn ZS, Yu Y et al (2023) Advancing cell-based cancer immunotherapy through stem cell engineering. Cell Stem Cell. https://doi.org/10.1016/j.stem.2023.02.009

Liu X, Zhao Y (2018) CRISPR/Cas9 genome editing: fueling the revolution in cancer immunotherapy. Curr Res Transl Med 66:39–42. https://doi.org/10.1016/j.retram.2018.04.003

Liu E, Tong Y, Dotti G et al (2018) Cord blood NK cells engineered to express IL-15 and a CD19-targeted CAR show long-term persistence and potent antitumor activity. Leukemia 32:520–531. https://doi.org/10.1038/leu.2017.226

Lowin B, Hahne M, Mattmann C, Tschopp J (1994) Cytolytic T-cell cytotoxicity is mediated through perforin and Fas lytic pathways. Nature 370:650–652. https://doi.org/10.1038/370650a0

Makkouk A, Yang XC, Barca T et al (2021) Off-the-shelf Vδ1 gamma delta T cells engineered with glypican-3 (GPC-3)-specific chimeric antigen receptor (CAR) and soluble IL-15 display robust antitumor efficacy against hepatocellular carcinoma. J Immunother Cancer 9:e003441. https://doi.org/10.1136/jitc-2021-003441

Mehta RS, Rezvani K (2018) Chimeric antigen receptor expressing natural killer cells for the immunotherapy of cancer. Front Immunol 9

Mishra PJ, Mishra PJ, Glod JW, Banerjee D (2009) Mesenchymal stem cells: flip side of the coin. Cancer Res 69:1255–1258. https://doi.org/10.1158/0008-5472.CAN-08-3562

Mizuhashi S, Kubo Y, Fukushima S et al (2021) Immune cell therapy against disseminated melanoma by utilizing induced pluripotent stem cell-derived myeloid cell lines producing interferon-beta or interleukin-15/interleukin-15 receptor alpha. J Dermatol Sci 102:133–136. https://doi.org/10.1016/j.jdermsci.2021.03.005

Montoro J, Balaguer-Roselló A, Sanz J (2023) Recent advances in allogeneic transplantation for acute myeloid leukemia. Curr Opin Oncol 35:564–573. https://doi.org/10.1097/CCO.0000000000000992

Morton LT, Reijmers RM, Wouters AK et al (2020) Simultaneous deletion of endogenous TCRαβ for TCR gene therapy creates an improved and safe cellular therapeutic. Mol Ther J Am Soc Gene Ther 28:64–74. https://doi.org/10.1016/j.ymthe.2019.10.001

Naeem M, Hazafa A, Bano N et al (2023) Explorations of CRISPR/Cas9 for improving the long-term efficacy of universal CAR-T cells in tumor immunotherapy. Life Sci 316:121409. https://doi.org/10.1016/j.lfs.2023.121409

Ng AP, Alexander WS (2017) Haematopoietic stem cells: past, present and future. Cell Death Dis 3: 17002. https://doi.org/10.1038/cddiscovery.2017.2

Ng AHM, Khoshakhlagh P, Arias JER et al (2021) A comprehensive library of human transcription factors for cell fate engineering. Nat Biotechnol 39:510–519. https://doi.org/10.1038/s41587-020-0742-6

Nishimura T, Nakauchi H (2019) Generation of Antigen-Specific T Cells from Human Induced Pluripotent Stem Cells. Methods Mol Biol Clifton NJ 1899:25–40. https://doi.org/10.1007/978-1-4939-8938-6_3

Oba T, Makino K, Kajihara R et al (2021) In situ delivery of iPSC-derived dendritic cells with local radiotherapy generates systemic antitumor immunity and potentiates PD-L1 blockade in pre-clinical poorly immunogenic tumor models. J Immunother Cancer 9:e002432. https://doi.org/10.1136/jitc-2021-002432

Ottaviano G, Georgiadis C, Gkazi SA et al (2022) Phase 1 clinical trial of CRISPR-engineered CAR19 universal T cells for treatment of children with refractory B cell leukemia. Sci Transl Med 14:eabq3010. https://doi.org/10.1126/scitranslmed.abq3010

Panowski SH, Srinivasan S, Tan N et al (2022) Preclinical development and evaluation of allogeneic CAR T cells targeting CD70 for the treatment of renal cell carcinoma. Cancer Res 82:2610–2624. https://doi.org/10.1158/0008-5472.CAN-21-2931

Paul S, Lal G (2017) The molecular mechanism of natural killer cells function and its importance in cancer immunotherapy. Front Immunol 8

Petley EV, Koay H-F, Henderson MA et al (2021) MAIT cells regulate NK cell-mediated tumor immunity. Nat Commun 12:4746. https://doi.org/10.1038/s41467-021-25009-4

Polo JM, Liu S, Figueroa ME et al (2010) Cell type of origin influences the molecular and functional properties of mouse induced pluripotent stem cells. Nat Biotechnol 28:848–855. https://doi.org/10.1038/nbt.1667

Raje N, Berdeja J, Lin Y et al (2019) Anti-BCMA CAR T-cell therapy bb2121 in relapsed or refractory multiple myeloma. N Engl J Med 380:1726–1737. https://doi.org/10.1056/NEJMoa1817226

Rapoport AP, Stadtmauer EA, Binder-Scholl GK et al (2015) NY-ESO-1–specific TCR–engineered T cells mediate sustained antigen-specific antitumor effects in myeloma. Nat Med 21:914–921. https://doi.org/10.1038/nm.3910

Rezvani K, Rouce R, Liu E, Shpall E (2017) Engineering natural killer cells for cancer immunotherapy. Mol Ther 25:1769–1781. https://doi.org/10.1016/j.ymthe.2017.06.012

Rowan AG, Ponnusamy K, Ren H et al (2023) CAR-iNKT cells targeting clonal TCRVβ chains as a precise strategy to treat T cell lymphoma. Front Immunol 14

Rowe RG, Mandelbaum J, Zon LI, Daley GQ (2016) Engineering hematopoietic stem cells: lessons from development. Cell Stem Cell 18:707–720. https://doi.org/10.1016/j.stem.2016.05.016

Ruggeri L, Mancusi A, Capanni M et al (2007) Donor natural killer cell allorecognition of missing self in haploidentical hematopoietic transplantation for acute myeloid leukemia: challenging its predictive value. Blood 110:433–440. https://doi.org/10.1182/blood-2006-07-038687

Ruixin S, Yifan L, Chuanlong W et al (2023) Expressing IL-15/IL-18 and CXCR2 improve infiltration and survival of EGFRvIII-targeting CAR-T cells in breast cancer. Biochem Pharmacol 212:115536. https://doi.org/10.1016/j.bcp.2023.115536

Rupp LJ, Schumann K, Roybal KT et al (2017) CRISPR/Cas9-mediated PD-1 disruption enhances anti-tumor efficacy of human chimeric antigen receptor T cells. Sci Rep 7:737. https://doi.org/10.1038/s41598-017-00462-8

Sachamitr P, Leishman AJ, Davies TJ, Fairchild PJ (2017) Directed differentiation of human induced pluripotent stem cells into dendritic cells displaying tolerogenic properties and resembling the CD141+ subset. Front Immunol 8:1935. https://doi.org/10.3389/fimmu.2017.01935

Sadelain M, Rivière I, Riddell S (2017) Therapeutic T cell engineering. Nature 545:423–431. https://doi.org/10.1038/nature22395

Sadowski K, Olejarz W, Basak G (2022) Modern advances in CARs therapy and creating a new approach to future treatment. Int J Mol Sci 23:15006. https://doi.org/10.3390/ijms232315006

Sagar J, Chaib B, Sales K et al (2007) Role of stem cells in cancer therapy and cancer stem cells: a review. Cancer Cell Int 7:9. https://doi.org/10.1186/1475-2867-7-9

Sauer T, Parikh K, Sharma S et al (2021) CD70-specific CAR T cells have potent activity against acute myeloid leukemia without HSC toxicity. Blood 138:318–330. https://doi.org/10.1182/blood.2020008221

Senju S, Hirata S, Matsuyoshi H et al (2003) Generation and genetic modification of dendritic cells derived from mouse embryonic stem cells. Blood 101:3501–3508. https://doi.org/10.1182/blood-2002-07-2254

Senju S, Haruta M, Matsunaga Y et al (2009) Characterization of dendritic cells and macrophages generated by directed differentiation from mouse induced pluripotent stem cells. Stem Cells 27:1021–1031. https://doi.org/10.1002/stem.33

Shah K (2012) Mesenchymal stem cells engineered for cancer therapy. Adv Drug Deliv Rev 64:739–748. https://doi.org/10.1016/j.addr.2011.06.010

Shankar K, Capitini CM, Saha K (2020) Genome engineering of induced pluripotent stem cells to manufacture natural killer cell therapies. Stem Cell Res Ther 11:234. https://doi.org/10.1186/s13287-020-01741-4

Sharkis SJ, Jones RJ, Civin C, Jang Y-Y (2012) Pluripotent stem cell-based cancer therapy: promise and challenges. Sci Transl Med 4:127ps9. https://doi.org/10.1126/scitranslmed.3003920

Shi L, Meng T, Zhao Z et al (2017) CRISPR knock out CTLA-4 enhances the anti-tumor activity of cytotoxic T lymphocytes. Gene 636:36–41. https://doi.org/10.1016/j.gene.2017.09.010

Shi D, Shi Y, Kaseb AO et al (2020) Chimeric antigen receptor-glypican-3 T-cell therapy for advanced hepatocellular carcinoma: results of phase I trials. Clin Cancer Res 26:3979–3989. https://doi.org/10.1158/1078-0432.CCR-19-3259

Shohdy KS, Pillai M, Guest R et al (2023) Evidence of clinical efficacy of a first generation CD19 CAR T cell in B cell malignancies. EJHaem 4:882–885. https://doi.org/10.1002/jha2.731

Sterner RC, Sterner RM (2021) CAR-T cell therapy: current limitations and potential strategies. Blood Cancer J 11:1–11. https://doi.org/10.1038/s41408-021-00459-7

Strati P, Bachanova V, Goodman A et al (2021) Preliminary results of a phase I trial of FT516, an off-the-shelf natural killer (NK) cell therapy derived from a clonal master induced pluripotent stem cell (iPSC) line expressing high-affinity, non-cleavable CD16 (hnCD16), in patients (pts) with relapsed/refractory (R/R) B-cell lymphoma (BCL). J Clin Oncol 39:7541–7541. https://doi.org/10.1200/JCO.2021.39.15_suppl.7541

Stuckey DW, Shah K (2014) Stem cell-based therapies for cancer treatment: separating hope from hype. Nat Rev Cancer 14:683–691. https://doi.org/10.1038/nrc3798

Sun H, Xing C, Jiang S et al (2022a) Long term complete response of advanced hepatocellular carcinoma to glypican-3 specific chimeric antigen receptor T-cells plus sorafenib, a case report. Front Immunol 13:963031. https://doi.org/10.3389/fimmu.2022.963031

Sun Y, Dong Y, Sun R et al (2022b) Chimeric anti-GPC3 sFv-CD3ε receptor-modified T cells with IL7 co-expression for the treatment of solid tumors. Mol Ther Oncolytics 25:160–173. https://doi.org/10.1016/j.omto.2022.04.003

Taefehshokr S, Parhizkar A, Hayati S et al (2022) Cancer immunotherapy: challenges and limitations. Pathol Res Pract 229:153723. https://doi.org/10.1016/j.prp.2021.153723

Tam TTKK, Xu S, Liu P, De Los Angeles A (2023) Dawn of development: exploring early human embryogenesis using stem cells. Cell Stem Cell 30:1006–1007. https://doi.org/10.1016/j.stem.2023.07.009

Themeli M, Kloss CC, Ciriello G et al (2013) Generation of tumor-targeted human T lymphocytes from induced pluripotent stem cells for cancer therapy. Nat Biotechnol 31:928–933. https://doi.org/10.1038/nbt.2678

Themeli M, Rivière I, Sadelain M (2015) New cell sources for T cell engineering and adoptive immunotherapy. Cell Stem Cell 16:357–366. https://doi.org/10.1016/j.stem.2015.03.011

Tominaga S, Ojima T, Miyazawa M et al (2023) Induced pluripotent stem cell-derived dendritic cell vaccine therapy genetically modified on the ubiquitin-proteasome system. Gene Ther 30:552–559. https://doi.org/10.1038/s41434-023-00388-z

Turtle CJ, Hanafi L-A, Berger C et al (2016) CD19 CAR–T cells of defined $CD4^+$: $CD8^+$ composition in adult B cell ALL patients. J Clin Invest 126:2123–2138. https://doi.org/10.1172/JCI85309

Ul Ain Q, Chung JY, Kim Y-H (2015) Current and future delivery systems for engineered nucleases: ZFN, TALEN and RGEN. J Control Release 205:120–127. https://doi.org/10.1016/j.jconrel.2014.12.036

Wakao H (2020) Reprogramming of MAIT cells to pluripotency and redifferentiation. In: Kaipe H, Magalhaes I (eds) MAIT cells: methods and protocols. Springer, New York, pp 237–257

Wakao H, Fujita H (2013) Toward the realization of cell therapy. Cell Cycle 12:2341–2342. https://doi.org/10.4161/cc.25706

Wakao H, Yoshikiyo K, Koshimizu U et al (2013) Expansion of functional human mucosal-associated invariant T cells via reprogramming to pluripotency and redifferentiation. Cell Stem Cell 12:546–558. https://doi.org/10.1016/j.stem.2013.03.001

Watanabe D, Koyanagi-Aoi M, Taniguchi-Ikeda M et al (2018) The generation of human γδT cell-derived induced pluripotent stem cells from whole peripheral blood mononuclear cell culture. Stem Cells Transl Med 7:34–44. https://doi.org/10.1002/sctm.17-0021

Watarai H, Fujii S, Koseki H, Taniguchi M (2010) P84. Murine induced pluripotent stem cells can be derived from and differentiate into natural killer T cells. Differentiation 80:S45. https://doi.org/10.1016/j.diff.2010.09.090

Wilson JM (2009) A history lesson for stem cells. Science 324:727–728. https://doi.org/10.1126/science.1174935

Wobus AM, Boheler KR (2005) Embryonic stem cells: prospects for developmental biology and cell therapy. Physiol Rev 85:635–678. https://doi.org/10.1152/physrev.00054.2003

Wright DA, Li T, Yang B, Spalding MH (2014) TALEN-mediated genome editing: prospects and perspectives. Biochem J 462:15–24. https://doi.org/10.1042/BJ20140295

Xu H, Wang B, Ono M et al (2019) Targeted disruption of HLA genes via CRISPR-Cas9 generates iPSCs with enhanced immune compatibility. Cell Stem Cell 24:566–578.e7. https://doi.org/10.1016/j.stem.2019.02.005

Yamada D, Iyoda T, Vizcardo R et al (2016) Efficient regeneration of human Vα24+ invariant natural killer T cells and their anti-tumor activity in vivo. Stem Cells Dayt Ohio 34:2852–2860. https://doi.org/10.1002/stem.2465

Yan L, Li J, Zhang C (2023) The role of MSCs and CAR-MSCs in cellular immunotherapy. Cell Commun Signal 21:187. https://doi.org/10.1186/s12964-023-01191-4

Yang M, Guan T, Chen C-F et al (2023a) Mesothelin-targeted CAR-NK cells derived from induced pluripotent stem cells have a high efficacy in killing triple-negative breast cancer cells as shown in several preclinical models. J Immunother Hagerstown Md 1997 46:285–294. https://doi.org/10.1097/CJI.0000000000000483

Yang Y, Yang H, Alcaina Y et al (2023b) Inducible expression of interleukin-12 augments the efficacy of affinity-tuned chimeric antigen receptors in murine solid tumor models. Nat Commun 14:2068. https://doi.org/10.1038/s41467-023-37646-y

Yeku OO, Brentjens RJ (2016) Armored CAR T-cells: utilizing cytokines and pro-inflammatory ligands to enhance CAR T-cell anti-tumour efficacy. Biochem Soc Trans 44:412–418. https://doi.org/10.1042/BST20150291

Zannikou M, Duffy JT, Levine RN et al (2023) IL15 modification enables CAR T cells to act as a dual targeting agent against tumor cells and myeloid-derived suppressor cells in GBM. J Immunother Cancer 11:e006239. https://doi.org/10.1136/jitc-2022-006239

Zeng J, Shahbazi M, Wu C et al (2012) Enhancing immunostimulatory function of human embryonic stem cell-derived dendritic cells by CD1d overexpression. J Immunol Baltim Md 1950 188:4297–4304. https://doi.org/10.4049/jimmunol.1102343

Zeng J, Tang SY, Wang S (2019) Derivation of mimetic γδ T cells endowed with cancer recognition receptors from reprogrammed γδ T cell. PLoS One 14:e0216815. https://doi.org/10.1371/journal.pone.0216815

Zhang Y, Zhang X, Cheng C et al (2017) CRISPR-Cas9 mediated LAG-3 disruption in CAR-T cells. Front Med 11:554–562. https://doi.org/10.1007/s11684-017-0543-6

Zhang L, Tian L, Dai X et al (2020) Pluripotent stem cell-derived CAR-macrophage cells with antigen-dependent anti-cancer cell functions. J Hematol Oncol 13:153. https://doi.org/10.1186/s13045-020-00983-2

Zhang Q, Yang J, Manoharan ENEA et al (2022a) CRISPR/Cas9-mediated gene knockout followed by negative selection leads to a complete TCR depletion in ortho CAR19 T cells. Bio-Protocol 12:e4485. https://doi.org/10.21769/BioProtoc.4485

Zhang Y, Liu Z, Wei W, Li Y (2022b) TCR engineered T cells for solid tumor immunotherapy. Exp Hematol Oncol 11:38. https://doi.org/10.1186/s40164-022-00291-0

Zhou Y, Li M, Zhou K et al (2022) Engineering induced pluripotent stem cells for cancer immunotherapy. Cancer 14:2266. https://doi.org/10.3390/cancers14092266

Zhu Y, Smith DJ, Zhou Y et al (2019) Development of hematopoietic stem cell-engineered invariant natural killer T cell therapy for cancer. Cell Stem Cell 25:542–557.e9. https://doi.org/10.1016/j.stem.2019.08.004

Zhu H, Blum RH, Bjordahl R et al (2020a) Pluripotent stem cell–derived NK cells with high-affinity noncleavable CD16a mediate improved antitumor activity. Blood 135:399–410. https://doi.org/10.1182/blood.2019000621

Zhu H, You Y, Shen Z, Shi L (2020b) EGFRvIII-CAR-T cells with PD-1 knockout have improved anti-glioma activity. Pathol Oncol Res 26:2135–2141. https://doi.org/10.1007/s12253-019-00759-1

Zhu Y, Zuo D, Wang K et al (2023) Mesothelin-targeted CAR-T therapy combined with irinotecan for the treatment of solid cancer. J Cancer Res Clin Oncol. https://doi.org/10.1007/s00432-023-05279-9

Mesenchymal Stem Cells in Cancer Therapy: A Road to the Future or Exaggerated Expectations

Mikhail V. Kiselevskiy, Irina Zh. Shubina, Raymonda J. Vlasenko, Natalia Yu. Anisimova, Ramil R. Fatkhullin, and Kirill I. Kirgizov

Abstract

Allogeneic (haploidentical) hematopoietic blood stem cell transplantation (allo-HSCT) is one of the main therapies for patients with malignant diseases of the blood system in children and adults with poor prognosis. The indications for allo-HSCT could not be extended due to a high risk of complications that are still associated with transplantation of hematopoietic stem cells. Non-engraftment of the hematopoietic stem cells leads to high morbidity and mortality as a result of infectious complications along with long-term neutropenia and organ dysfunctions resulting from the toxicity of the drugs used in the conditioning regimen. Graft-versus-host disease (GVHD) is one of the common, and in some cases fatal, complications of allo-HSCT. Current medicinal methods of treatment and prevention of graft failure and GVHD do not always achieve a clinical effect. One of the promising strategies for reducing the severity of GVHD is the use of mesenchymal stem cells (MSCs), which have tolerogenic characteristics. In addition, the ability of MSCs to stimulate hematopoiesis by producing a number of growth factors makes the basis for their use in case of graft failure. In general, numerous clinical studies have shown the effectiveness of this strategy. However, contradictory results and lack of standard conditions for MSC culture and the need for therapeutic regimens are the main reasons why the researchers cannot make a final conclusion about the MSC perspectives in the treatment and prevention of transplant failure and GVHD.

M. V. Kiselevskiy (✉) · I. Z. Shubina · R. J. Vlasenko · N. Y. Anisimova · R. R. Fatkhullin
K. I. Kirgizov
N.N. Blokhin National Medical Research Center of Oncology (N.N. Blokhin NMRCO) of the Ministry of Health of the Russian Federation, Moscow, Russia
e-mail: kiselevskii.mv@misis.ru

Interdisciplinary Cancer Research, https://doi.org/10.1007/16833_2024_376
Published online: 27 September 2024

Keywords

Graft-versus-host disease · Hematopoietic stem cell transplantation · Mesenchymal stem cells

1 Introduction

Mesenchymal stem cells (MSC) were first described by Friedenstein in 1968 (Friedenstein et al. 1968). Since then, numerous studies have been performed that described various types of MSC functions. MSCs are a heterogeneous population of stromal stem cells that can be isolated from many tissues; MSCs can proliferate effectively and differentiate into specific cells of mesodermal origin (Uccelli et al. 2008) (Fig. 1).

MSCs differentiate into stromal cells, osteocytes, osteoblasts, preadipocytes, and endothelial cells in the bone marrow (BM). MSCs and their derivatives in this microenvironment provide a scaffold for hematopoiesis and a complex network of cytokines, adhesion molecules, and bioactive molecules, forming hematopoietic niches (Muguruma et al. 2006; Kiel and Morrison 2008) (Fig. 2).

Therefore, MSCs regulate the survival, proliferation, growth, and differentiation of hematopoietic stem cells (HSCs), and enhance their engraftment (Zhu et al. 2003; Li et al. 2009). In addition to supporting hematopoiesis, MSCs can modulate immune responses via intercellular contacts between MSCs and target cells and production of soluble immunosuppressive factors (Allan et al. 2020). These immunomodulating effects of MSCs have found clinical application in the treatment of graft-versus-host disease (GVHD) after allogeneic hematopoietic stem cell transplantation (allo-HSCT) (Hashmi et al. 2016; Ringden et al. 2018). MSCs express mesenchymal markers (CD105 and CD73) and adhesion molecules (CD29, CD44, CD106, and CD90) on their surface and have no surface hematopoietic cell antigens (CD45, CD14, CD11b, CD19 and CD79α) (Yagi et al. 2010). MSC authenticity is proved by their special aptitude to provide trilineage mesenchymal differentiation, including osteoblasts, adipocytes, and chondroblasts (Dominici et al. 2006). Besides

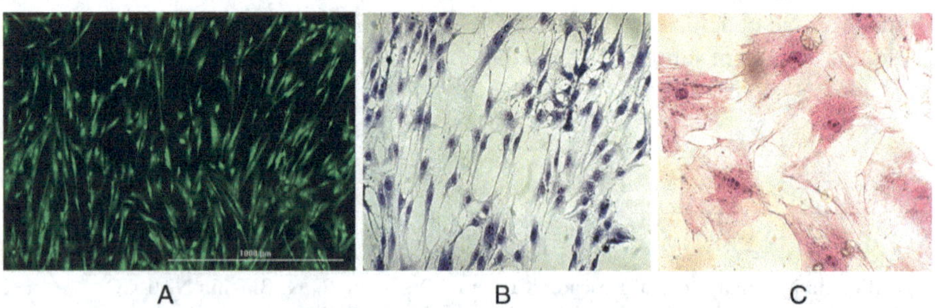

Fig. 1 Morphology of MSCs derived from bone marrow: (**a**) calcein AM staining, x100, (**b**) methylene blue staining, x200, (**c**) azur II – eosin staining, x900

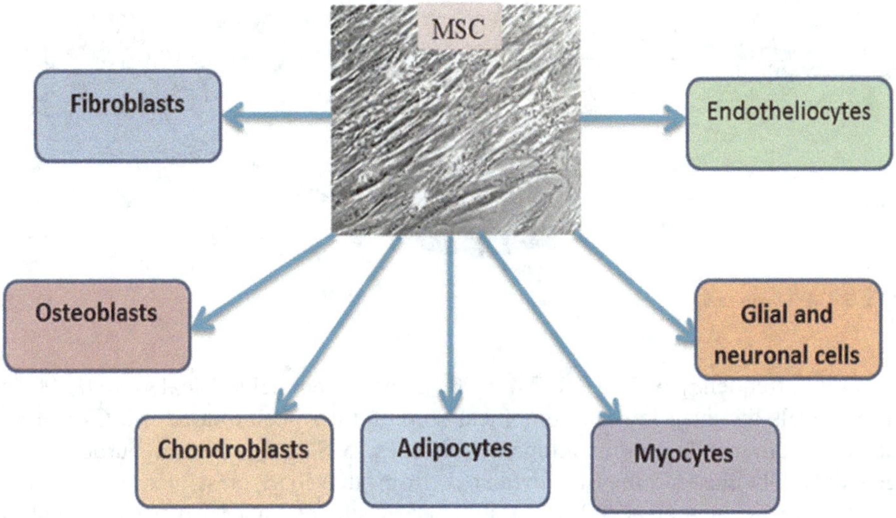

Fig. 2 Directions of MSC differentiations

that, MSCs have a wider differentiation potential and can differentiate into myocytes, tendinocytes, cardiomyocytes, neurons, and other cell types. MSCs express low levels of HLA class I and II, co-stimulatory molecules such as CD80, CD86, and CD40 and, therefore, they are able to avoid allogeneic rejection. Moreover, MSCs are effectively cultured for expansion and cryopreservation. Thus, donor's MSCs can be expanded ex vivo and cryopreserved for clinical use, particularly for the enhancement of HSC engraftment and GVHD prevention after allo-HSCT.

2 MSC Sources

MSCs can be isolated from various sources: adipose tissue, bone marrow, peripheral blood, dental pulp, umbilical cord blood and placenta, as well as from fetal tissues (O'Donoghue and Fisk 2004; Tolouei et al. 2023). Adult bone marrow-derived MSCs (BM-MSCs) are the most widely used in clinical research; however, MSCs from fetal tissues have additional biological characteristics, such as high proliferative capacity, longer lifespan, and higher differentiation potential (Hass et al. 2011). MSCs obtained from different sources have similar functions. The researchers prefer MSCs generated from adipose tissue due to their availability and the potential for expansion in sufficient quantity. These cells have the ability to respond to inflammation and interact with immune cells in damaged areas, regulating the local immune response through the secretion of chemokines and cytokines (Dai et al. 2016). MSCs in bone marrow (BM) are reported to be a very rare population (0.01–0.001%). Wexlel et al. have shown that MSCs in bone marrow

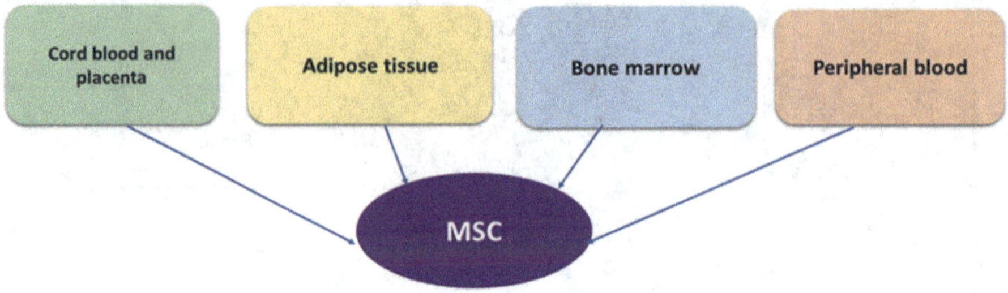

Fig. 3 MSC sources

occur at a frequency of 1 in 3.1–3.4 × 10^4 mononuclear cells (Wexler et al. 2003). Their levels are even lower in umbilical cord and peripheral blood. MSCs can be derived from autologous or allogeneic sources. MSCs for clinical purposes are generally obtained from BM extracted from the iliac crest, femur, or tibia (Rodríguez-Fuentes et al. 2021). A number of studies have also used placental-derived MSCs (PMSCs). The results showed that placenta produced large amounts of highly plastic MSCs that could differentiate into both mesodermal and non-mesodermal lineages (Alviano et al. 2008). PMSCs have several advantages over BM-extracted MSCs (BM-MSCs). For instance, a cell-based therapy requires infusion of a large number of MSCs, but the amount of donor's BM is obviously limited. Moreover, collection of donor's BM is an invasive procedure. Besides, the BM-MSCs may be contaminated with malignant cells in case of purposes for autologous antitumor therapies. Thus, PMSCs may be an ideal successor to BM-MSCs. However, additional studies are needed to confirm the effectiveness and safety of using MSCs of fetal origin (Fig. 3).

3 Methods for MSC Culturing

The MSC-based therapies require generation of a large number of cells. A single injection of MSCs at a dose of 0.5–3.0 million/kg requires 20 million - 100 million cells determined by the patient's weight. Such abundant amount of cells for clinical use is available due to the MSC potential for ex vivo expansion and is based on particular characteristics of MSCs such as adhesion to plastic and subsequent intensive proliferation in the passage cycles. The process of culturing primary isolated heterogeneous cells involves removal of the impurity of non-adherent cells when the culture medium is regularly replaced and expansion of the MSCs, which makes it possible to obtain a large amount of MSCs with no admixture of foreign cells. This approach is universal and can be used to generate MSCs from mononuclear cells of the bone marrow, adipose tissue, umbilical cord, placenta, and other sources.

The preparation of therapeutic MSCs includes several stages:

1. Isolation of mononuclear cells from target tissue (from BM, adipose tissuc, umbilical cord, etc.).
2. Culturing the cells in culture medium for a certain number of passages (expansion in the passage cycle).
3. Identification of cell characteristics and cell delivery to the clinic or cryopreservation if needed.
4. Thawing MSCs and delivery of freshly thawed cells to the clinic or after reculturing for 3–5 days in order to restore their functions.

MSCs isolated from BM (syngeneic, haploidentical, or allogeneic), being the most studied and safe, are mainly used in clinical trials of MSCs for steroid-resistant GVHD and hematopoietic depression after BM transplantation. The approximate volume of BM aspirate necessary to obtain the required dose of MSCs (0.5 million/kg) depends on the patient's weight. In case of generating the required MSC numbers at the end of the third or fourth passages, BM aspirate should be obtained approximately at 10 ml for 35 kg of weight; 15 ml – for a weight from 35 to 50 kg and 20 ml for a weight of more than 50 kg (Goto et al. 2018).

Despite a long history of research and clinical trials, no standard protocol for clinical MSC culture has been adopted, yet. The protocols of different research centers vary in the composition of culture medium and culturing conditions. Generally, researchers use classical media such as MEM, DMEM–LG, DMEM/F-12, or alpha-MEM that are proved to be the most appropriate for the isolation and expansion of MSCs of therapeutic quality (Sotiropoulou et al. 2006).

Basic media are enriched with the addition of L-glutamine (alanyl-glutamine), antibiotics (penicillin/streptomycin, gentamicin), antimycotics, HEPES (10–20 mM), and the most important component, a growth additive. Preclinical and early clinical trials (Lazarus et al. 1995) used 10–15% fetal bovine serum (FBS) as a growth supplement. Later, it was rejected due to the risk of transmitting zoonotic infections and possible immune reaction to residual xenogeneic proteins, because the culture cells internalized the serum components which intensive washing could not help eliminate (Spees et al. 2004). Avoiding animal products in growth media is an important requirement for MSCs of clinical quality. In 2005, Doucet et al. proposed a safe replacement of FBS with human platelet lysate (PL), a natural source of platelet-derived growth factor (PDGF), which supported MSC proliferation (Doucet et al. 2005). In addition to PDGF, PL contained basic fibroblast growth factor (bFGF), transforming growth factor (TGF-β), and insulin-like growth factor-1 (IGF-1). BM-derived MSCs cultured in a medium with PL had the same morphology, phenotype, and plasticity (ability for trilinear differentiation) as MSCs from a culture with FBS, but their colonies of clonogenic cells were 1.5–2 times larger in size and their proliferation rate was 1.5–2 times higher (Capelli et al. 2007). MSCs maintained genetic stability during long-term culture in the presence of PL similar to the MSCs in culture with FBS. A comparison of the immunoregulatory functions of MSCs showed a similar suppression of cytotoxic activity of T-reg and enhanced early production of

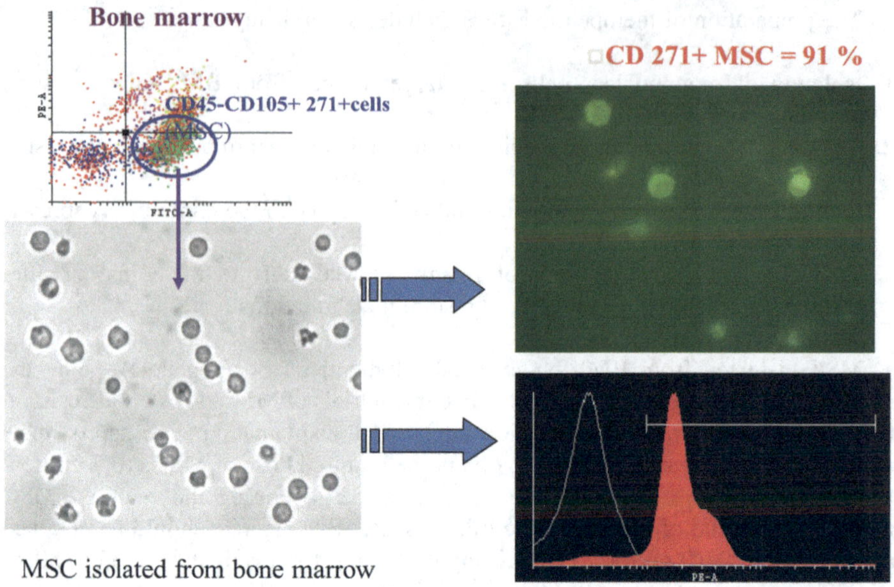

Fig. 4 Immunomagnetic separation of MSCs from bone marrow cells

IL-10 compared with that of MSCs cultured with FBS (Bernardo et al. 2007). The content of growth factors in PL (PDGF-AB, TGF-β1, bFGF, or IGF-1) is significantly higher in young donors (<35 years) compared to older donors (>45 years), which influenced the proliferation of MSCs in culture (Lohmann et al. 2012). Taking into account the individual characteristics of donors, pooled PL from several donors is used to standardize the growth additive, and its optimal concentration (4–10%) in the growth medium is determined for each new batch (Kuçi et al. 2016). Heparin (2–3 UI/ml of medium) should be added along with PL to the growth medium to stabilize viscosity. The most popular method for isolating mononuclear cells from BM aspirate is centrifugation on a density gradient of 1.077 g/ml or 1.073 g/ml at 450 g - 800 g for 20–30 min (Grisendi et al. 2010). This approach provides good clearance of red blood cells and granulocytes, but the release of mononuclear cells ranges from 25% to 50% determined by the gradient type (Pösel et al. 2012). A more effective method for isolating MSCs is immunomagnetic separation, which, however, is not widely used for expansion of clinical MSCs (Fig. 4).

Clinical experience and experimental data on MSC aging have demonstrated that the expansion cycle is usually limited to 4 passages. The problem of achieving the required number of cells is resolved by combining MSCs from several donors. This approach has shown that MSCs in the treatment of (aGvHD) are safe and effective and it helps overcome MSC donor-to-donor variability. Importantly, the clinical end products had significantly higher allosuppressive potential than the average allosuppressive potential of MSCs obtained from the same donors individually (Kuçi et al. 2016).

Oxygen levels are an important regulator of stem cell behavior. Currently, MSCs are usually cultured in an incubator at an oxygen level of 20% O_2, while MSCs in BM are in the conditions of reduced oxygen. Therefore, culturing MSCs under hypoxic conditions can maintain the MSC stemness as well as influence their proliferation and differentiation (Mohyeldin et al. 2010). Long-term in vitro culture is required to generate a sufficient number of MSCs for clinical use. However, numerous passages lead to aging of MSCs, making them similar to MSCs from older people. Senescent MSCs have reduced therapeutic potential and can even produce suppressive factors that affect young MSCs (Rasouli et al. 2024). The reduced functional activity of aging MSCs is associated with a decrease in proliferation, colony formation, telomere length, differentiation ability, and secretion of bioactive molecules. A research showed that the clonogenicity of MSCs declined significantly after the twelfth passage, which indicated the senescence of MSCs (Wilson et al. 2019). BM-MSCs of late passages become senescent and have an altered immunophenotype and morphology (Kundrotas et al. 2016). MSCs derived from adipose tissue expressed a low percentage of aneuploid cells at early passages 0–4, while long-term cultures at passages 5–16 were characterized by a significantly high percentage of aneuploidy with no malignant transformations (Roemeling-van Rhijn et al. 2013). Aging of MSCs in vitro or in vivo is a serious problem in cell-based therapy, since senescent MSCs change their therapeutic potential (Rasouli et al. 2024). Therefore, overcoming early aging of MSCs has become major interest in MSC studies aimed at maintaining optimal immunoregulatory capacity of MSCs. Senescent MSCs are characterized by a loss of DNA repair and antioxidant functions, thereby they become more susceptible to tumorigenesis (Uruski et al. 2021). Since MSC senescence develops with increased number of passages, which is demonstrated by a gradual loss of stem cell characteristics, MSCs for cell-based therapy should be used only at the early stages of in vitro culture (Bonab et al. 2006). The researchers proposed that MSCs for clinical use should be collected within six culture passages (Troyer and Weiss 2008). Donor's age also affects the rate of MSC senescence in vitro and therefore it should be considered as well (Stenderup et al. 2003).

4 Prevention and Treatment of Graft Failure

Allogeneic (haploidentical) HSC transplantation (allo/haplo-HSCT) is a method of radical treatment of various benign and malignant hematopoietic diseases. Thus, allo-HSCT is a standard therapeutic option for patients with acute myeloid leukemia (Zhang et al. 2021). Successful transplantation depends on the establishment of the engraftment with the donor's cells being safely integrated into the recipient's cell population. Although allo-HSCT is an effective treatment for various malignant and benign diseases, it is still complicated by graft failure and mortality. Unsatisfactory engraftment of transplanted HSCs increases the risk of worsening pancytopenia and the development of serious complications of bacterial, viral, and fungal infections. Treatment of graft failure usually involves administration of hematopoietic growth factors such as granulocyte colony-stimulating factor (G-CSF) or requires retransplantation. However, these methods are associated with short-term effects and a significant risk of developing GVHD, which requires treatment by immunosuppressive agents that inevitably affect hematopoiesis (Yoshida et al. 2014; Im et al. 2015). MSCs induce a variety of growth factors that stimulate hematopoiesis, prepare hematopoietic niches, protect primitive progenitor cells, supporting both erythroid and myeloid lineage, and can produce a range of cytokines that improve hematopoietic stem cell engraftment and reduce the incidence and severity of GVHD (Le Blanc et al. 2007; Wang et al. 2013). MSCs induce polarization of T cells toward a regulatory phenotype, which may help reduce inflammation, prevent GVHD, and improve the BM niche. MSCs also increase the expression of many hematopoietic factors and inhibit apoptosis, allowing HSCs to survive and proliferate in the stroma (Diehl et al. 2017). MSCs can directly influence HSCs by releasing soluble compounds such as IDO, prostaglandin E2, nitric oxide, transforming growth factor, interferon, and interleukin 1, although the net interactions between cells are unknown. Optimization of HSC self-renewal and proliferation depends on the HSC survival and homing to the BM. The use of MSCs improves homing and hematopoietic reconstitution and provides higher chimerism than that with traditional transplantation (Yin et al. 2020). Postnatal HSCs are mainly localized in special BM niches and are necessary to maintain HSC homeostasis (Acar et al. 2015). HSC transplantation typically involves preconditioning with radiation or chemotherapy to ablate host stem cells and provide implantation of donor's HSCs. However, the likelihood of developing the donor's chimerism is very low without preconditioning (Bhattacharya et al. 2009). On the other hand, conditioning not only depletes recipient's HSCs, but also impairs the function of hematopoietic niches, damaging sinusoidal blood vessels and stromal cells (Kopp et al. 2005). MSCs play an important role in maintaining tissue homeostasis and are an essential component of hematopoietic niches (Mendelson and Frenette 2014). Immunodeficient mice show poor engraftment of human HSCs, which may be due to the lack of a humanized microenvironment to support hematopoiesis after transplantation. These data confirm the importance of the microenvironment that shapes the hematopoietic niche for the regulation of hemopoiesis. Conditioning regimens of high-dose chemotherapy or radiation therapy before transplantation damage both hematopoietic cells and mesenchymal cells of the BM niches, resulting in the decreased production of factors that contribute to the restoration of hematopoiesis, since the host microenvironment cannot provide sufficient support for transplanted donor's HSCs. Thus, hematopoietic niches are an important factor limiting the effective restoration of hematopoiesis. Hematopoietic niches include MSCs and their differentiation products: endothelial cells, preadipocytes, osteoblasts, chondrocytes, and fibroblasts (Figs. 5 and 6) (Fröbel et al. 2021). Therefore, a promising approach to enhance HSC engraftment is the transplantation of MSCs, which can speed up the restoration of hematopoietic niches (Yin et al. 2020). Overall, preclinical results indicate the ability of MSCs to mediate HSC engraftment in both xenogeneic and allogeneic hematopoietic cell transplantation animal models. And the study results show no toxicity of MSC-based therapy (Garrigós et al. 2022).

Fig. 5 The hematopoietic niche is formed by MSCs and the cells of MSC differentiation, osteoblasts, preadipocytes, and fibroblasts

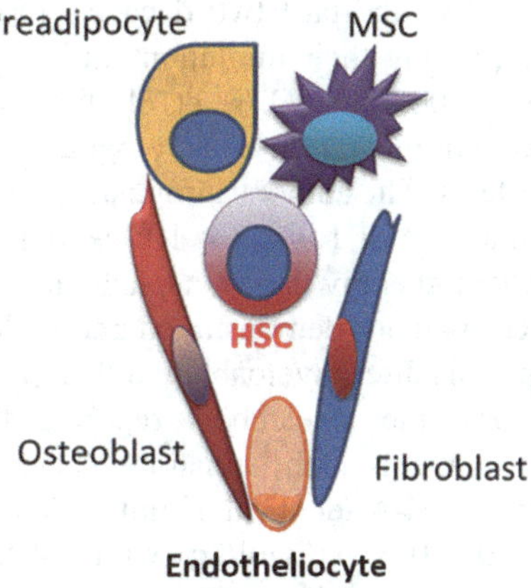

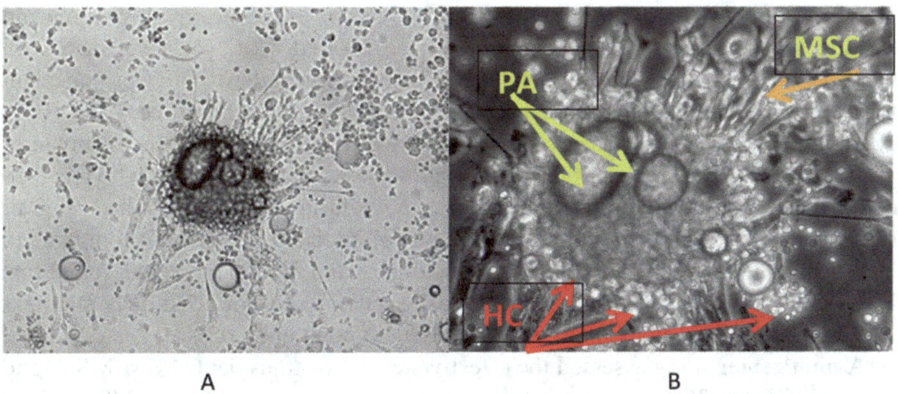

Fig. 6 In vitro model of the hematopoietic niche: proliferation of hematopoietic cells (HC) on a substrate of MSCs and preadipocytes (PA) of bone marrow. (**a**) ×100, (**b**) ×400, phase contrast

Therefore, the use of MSCs is considered as a promising approach for the treatment of graft hypofunction and GVHD. Due to the small numbers of mesenchymal progenitor cells in human bone marrow (0.001%–0.01% of mononuclear cells), ex vivo expansion of MSCs is necessary to generate sufficient cell numbers for clinical use (Polchert et al. 2008).

MSCs have a high proliferative potential along with their multipotency, and the use of allogeneic MSCs in clinical practice will require production of significant amount of a biomedical cell product and creation of cell banks (Pittenger et al. 2019). Studies have shown that MSCs secrete cytokines and growth factors that have beneficial effects on target cells, enhancing tissue repair and regeneration, cell survival, anti-apoptosis, proliferation, differentiation, hematopoiesis, angiogenesis, and myogenesis, as well as slowing down the immune response (Wilson and Trumpp 2006).

Over the past two decades, more than 1,000 clinical studies have used MSCs exploiting their immunomodulatory properties and ability to differentiate in vitro. In 2000, Koc O.N. et al. first reported rapid recovery of hematopoiesis after co-administration of autologous MSCs during allo-HSCT with no significant side effects. The authors administered intravenous donor's BM-MSCs after 2–6 passages at a dose of 1.0–2.2 × 10^6 cell/kg to 28 patients with breast cancer after high-dose chemotherapy and transplantation of autologous peripheral-blood progenitor-cells. The patients demonstrated good tolerance of MSCs and rapid restoration of hematopoiesis after myeloablative therapy under these conditions (Koc et al. 2000). Afterward, the researchers reported the data from a multicenter study involving 46 patients with hematological malignancies who received allo-HSCs and MSCs from HLA-identical siblings. The patients had intravenous infusions of MSCs (1.0–5.0 × 10^6 cell/kg) within 4 h before infusion of bone marrow or peripheral blood stem cells, and the researchers observed rapid restoration of hematopoiesis in most cases (Lazarus et al. 2005).

In addition to promoting engraftment, MSCs are effective in preventing and treating graft failure. In 2007, Le Blanc et al. reported MSC cotransplantation in three patients with previous graft failure or rejection in order to prevent transplant rejection. All three patients achieved neutrophil and platelet engraftment and 100% donor chimerism, which demonstrated a potential role for MSCs in the treatment of graft failure (Le Blanc et al. 2007). Ball et al. showed that 14 children who received cotransplantation of MSCs from the same donors during haplo-HSCT had no graft rejection; and the authors reported fewer cases of infection and GVHD compared to historical controls (Ball et al. 2007). On the other hand, Bacigalupo et al. found that BM-MSCs from patients with severe aplastic anemia did not effectively suppress T cell proliferation and cytokine release (Bacigalupo et al. 2005).

A multicenter study assessed the effectiveness of co-transplanted BM-MSCs and haplo-HSCT in 35 children with severe aplastic anemia (SAA). MSCs were cryopreserved after the second passage of culture. The freshly cultured BM-MSCs of the third passage were administered at a dose of 1 × 10^6 cells/kg. The first BM-MSC infusion was performed 6 h before the bone marrow stem cell infusion. The second BM-MSC infusion was on day 14 after stem cell transplantation. All 35 patients achieved restoration of hematopoiesis and persistent complete donor chimerism. However, the study had no control group and no final conclusion could be made about the effectiveness of MSC cotransplantation in allo-HSCT (Wang et al. 2019).

Since obtaining BM-MSCs is an invasive and painful procedure, a number of studies used fetal-type MSCs. Fetal-type MSCs can proliferate faster than BM-MSCs, reducing the time required for expansion of sufficient cell quantity for clinical use. These advantages imply that fetal-type MSCs may become an alternative source of MSCs in clinical treatment. However, many studies have shown that infusion of BM-MSCs in humans is safe and does not cause the development of ectopic tissue and other serious adverse events (Lazarus et al. 2005; Lucchini et al. 2010; Macmillan et al. 2009). However, unlike BM-MSCs, the safety of fetal-type

MSCs remains uncertain given the limited experience with their clinical use (Yagi et al. 2010).

Despite numerous studies, the optimal dose of cells has not yet been established and it is unclear whether the therapeutic effect increases with the infusion of higher doses of MSCs. In addition, there is no consensus on the frequency of MSC administrations (Nauta et al. 2006). Besides, it should be noted that a number of clinical studies reported ambiguous results regarding the MSC effectiveness in stimulating hematopoiesis after HSCT.

5 Intrabone Transplantation

The typical approach to the use of MSCs in allo-HSCT is the intravenous infusion of HSCs and MSCs, which, as a result of homing, populate the hematopoietic niches in the BM. Following common intravenous injection, most MSCs are retained in the lungs and liver and do not reach the bone marrow (Panoskaltsis-Mortari et al. 2004).

According to some estimates, more than 99% of these cells remain in the lungs, liver, and spleen, while those that reach the target tissue have a short survival period and, in case of their aggregation, can contribute to the development of thrombosis (Lai et al. 2012). When administered intravenously, MSCs are retained in the lungs and liver and are quickly eliminated by the recipient's immune cells (Morikawa et al. 2009). As a result, only a low number of intravenously infused MSCs reach BM (Mabuchi et al. 2013).

Experimental studies showed that intrabone injection of MSCs could improve the engraftment of transplanted HSCs as compared with intravenous injection. Preclinical studies showed that injection of MSCs into the bone marrow was safe and stimulated of hematopoiesis (Yuan et al. 2016a, b). In addition, the results showed a significantly higher engraftment of transplanted HSCs both in the injection site of the bone marrow and in the contralateral area without direct injection of MSCs.

Over the recent years different methods for direct injection of MSCs into bone marrow have been intensively developed on the base of the experimental data, which may improve the engraftment of transplanted HSCs more effectively than their intravenous injection. Clinical studies have shown the feasibility and safety of intravenous cotransplantation of MSCs with cord blood cells in pediatric patients, but not in adult patients, who are at a greater risk of graft rejection. Regarding the route of MSC administration, it is assumed that direct intraosseous injection of MSCs leads to a higher cord blood cell engraftment as compared with intravenous injection. On the base of the obtained results, a clinical trial was designed to develop a new strategy to improve engraftment and prevent GVHD development after HSC transplantation (Goto et al. 2018). A phase I clinical trial included the target group of 5 patients aged $\geq$20 years with hematological diseases who received HSCT. All patients reported recovery of neutrophils, reticulocytes, and platelets, and there were no side effects associated with intraosseous injection of BM-MSCs. Acute grade II-IV GVHD developed in three patients from the control group, but not in patients of the target group. These results suggest that enhanced engraftment of transplanted

HSCs is achieved to a large extent by direct injection of MSCs into the bone marrow. Combining intraosseous injection of MSCs with HSCT is a safe and feasible therapeutic strategy. In addition, these data suggest that intraosseous injection of MSCs can prevent the development of GVHD along with decreased levels of certain inflammatory cytokines without inhibiting HSC engraftment. The strategy may be applicable to prevent severe GVHD, especially in the setting of HLA mismatch, and will reduce the burden on HSC donors by fewer numbers of stem cells required (Goto et al. 2018).

6 MSCs and Cytokine Storm

Inflammatory mediators play an important role in the pathogenesis of GVHD (Ferrara 1993). Cytokine release syndrome and cytokine storm are life-threatening complications observed after allo-HSCT and require urgent intervention with supportive treatment in the intensive care unit and administration of tocilizumab (Agarwal et al. 2023). MSCs are capable of altering the profile of cytokine secretion by macrophages, dendritic cells, naive and effector T cells (T helper types 1 and 2), as well as natural killer (NK) cells, thus inducing an anti-inflammatory or tolerant phenotype. In particular, MSCs inhibited the secretion of proinflammatory cytokines (TNF-α and IFN-γ) by mature dendritic cells (DCs) and increased the secretion of anti-inflammatory cytokines IL-10 and IL-4. MSCs increased the suppressor subpopulation of T-regulatory cells (T-reg) in the blood as well (Heinrichs et al. 2016; Keto et al. 2018). MSCs demonstrated promising effects in experimental acute respiratory distress syndrome (ARDS), reversing the effects of alveolar collapse, collagen accumulation, and cell apoptosis in lung tissue. Several randomized phase 1 clinical trials confirmed the safety of MSCs obtained from various sources at a single dose of one million cells/kg to ten million cells/kg in patients with non-viral ARDS (Wilson et al. 2015; Zheng et al. 2014; Chang et al. 2014). MSCs are considered as a promising therapeutic strategy for the treatment of steroid-resistant forms of macrophage activation syndrome (MAS) in juvenile idiopathic arthritis (Swart et al. 2019). The clinical efficacy of peripheral blood MSCs was demonstrated in influenza A (H7N9) patients with ARDS. In particular, the study showed that mortality in the group of patients who received MSCs was 17.6% versus 54.5% in the control group. The authors suggested that the data provided the ground for using MSCs in patients with COVID-19, given the similarity of complications caused by these viruses (Chen et al. 2020). Another recent pilot study involving 7 patients with COVID-19 pneumonia showed that clinical symptoms in all patients improved significantly within 2 days of MSC transplantation. Besides, the results showed an increase of peripheral blood lymphocytes and the disappearance of activated subpopulations secreting cytokines, such as CXCR3+/CD4 + T cells, CXCR3+/CD8 + T cells, and CXCR3+ NK cells. In addition, the content of CD14+/CD11c+/CD11b^{mid} DC regulatory subpopulations increased. TNF-α levels decreased significantly, while IL-10 levels increased in patients receiving MSCs compared to patients receiving standard therapy (Leng et al. 2020). However, despite a large number of clinical studies of the effectiveness of MSCs in various pathological conditions associated with the induction of pro-inflammatory factors, no clear recommendations are available to regulate MSC use, and the results of various trials are quite contradictory (Kiselevskiy et al. 2021; Li et al. 2021; Kiselevskiy et al. 2020). The tolerogenic functions of MSCs in the regulation of the immune response are mainly mediated by a range of secreted bioregulators that suppress the proliferation, activation and effector activity of dendritic cells, macrophages, lymphocytes, and neutrophils (Kyurkchiev et al. 2014; Siegel et al. 2009). On the other hand, MSCs can present not only immunosuppressive, but also pro-inflammatory phenotype, which depends on the microenvironment, and thus promote the activation of neutrophils and T cells and enhance the immune response (Gazdic et al. 2015). MSCs produce anti-inflammatory factors such as IL-10, prostaglandin E2, and indoleamine dioxygenase (IDO). At the same time, MSCs can secrete a range of proinflammatory cytokines, such as monocyte chemoattractant protein-1 (MCP-1), IL-6, IL-8, TNFα, and IL-1β. These data indicate that MSCs do not exhibit immunosuppressive activity in all cases. Probably, the involvement of MSC-expressed Toll-like receptors may determine MSC pro- or anti-inflammatory effects (Ma et al. 2014). In addition, the duration of MSC culturing is important for their immunomodulatory functions; it is assumed that no more than 3 passages of MSC culture should be acquired for the clinical use of MSCs (Connard et al. 2021). Our data showed that BM-derived MSCs cultured for 4 passages express a pronounced pro-inflammatory phenotype. In particular, MSCs secrete significant amounts of IL-6, IL-8, and MCP-1, while anti-inflammatory cytokines IL-10 and IL-4 were practically not detected (Kiselevskii et al. 2021). The results are confirmed by other researchers who have shown no significant change in the production of IL-6, IL-8, and MCP-1 after 9 culture passages, except for the increased level of IL-8 at passages 6–9 (Connard et al. 2021). Importantly, IL-6, IL-8, and MCP-1 are considered to be the most important factors in the development of the proinflammatory cascade and GVHD (Wu et al. 2015; Gu et al. 2000). Moreover, the studies established that the severity of hyperthermia in GVHD correlates with the levels of IL-6 and IL-8 (Ferrà et al. 1998), and current trends in the treatment of cytokine storm, both in COVID19 and in GVHD, involve IL-6 receptor inhibitors to block IL-6 –signaling (Drobyski et al. 2011). Yet, MSC natural function includes IL-6 production and probably, secretion of other pro-inflammatory biomolecules, that helps maintain MSCs in an undifferentiated state, MSC proliferative activity, prevents apoptosis, and inhibits adipogenic, osteogenic, and chondrogenic differentiation of MSCs (Pricola et al. 2009). The seeming controversy in the spectrum of pro-inflammatory cytokines and the immunosuppressive functions of MSCs could be explained by the fact that IL-6 has both pro-inflammatory and anti-inflammatory activity. The studies have demonstrated that IL-6 suppresses the secretion of many pro-inflammatory cytokines, such as IL-1, TNFα, GM-CSF, INFγ, and induces the production of glucocorticoids, IL-10, IL-1 receptor antagonist, and soluble receptor for TNFα McElvaney (McElvaney et al. 2021; Steensberg et al. 2003). These data are supported by the results showing that IL-6 levels correlate with the immunosuppressive effects of MSCs (Chan et al. 2012). Besides immunomodulatory functions,

MSCs can stimulate hematopoiesis through the production of growth and colony-stimulating factors. According to our studies, BM-MSCs could secrete G-CSF, GM-CSF, and IL-3, but the levels of these factors were insignificant and were not observed in all cases. MSCs also produce IL-7, which is involved in lymphopoiesis and differentiation of T and B lymphocytes. However, researchers have found that IL-7 level increases under the stimulation of IL-6 high concentrations and supports the pro-inflammatory cascade (Coppin et al. 2021; Ponchel et al. 2021). Numerous clinical studies involving MSCs have demonstrated their effectiveness in the treatment of COVID-19 and related complications. At present, more than 100 registered clinical trials are investigating MSC application in the treatment of COVID-19. Most of these studies have focused on patients with severe grade of COVID-19. Patients treated with cord blood MSCs showed improvement in clinical symptoms such as weakness, fatigue, shortness of breath, as well as an improvement in oxygenation index as early as the third day of treatment (Shu et al. 2020). A multicenter, randomized, double-blind study of patients with ARDS in course of COVID-19 found significant increase in PaO_2/FiO_2 ratio in cord blood MSC group compared with placebo group (Monsel et al. 2022). Another clinical trial studied mesenchymal stromal cells derived from human menstrual blood for the treatment of patients with COVID-19 at severe and critical stage of the disease and reported significant improvement in dyspnea and SpO_2 and PaO_2 after MSC infusion. Additionally, patients in the MSC group had significantly lower mortality (7.69% in the study group vs. 33.33% in the control group; $p = 0.048$) (Xu et al. 2021). Thus, the clinical results of the MSC use for patients with COVID-19 at critical stage showed the effectiveness of MSCs for the treatment of cytokine storm (Guo et al. 2023).

Obviously, the reason for the ambiguity of the results of MSC clinical studies is the MSC dual effect on the immune response, which depends on the conditions of cell culture and the state of reactivity of patients, as well as on the modes of MSC administration.

7 Potential Use of MSCs for the Treatment and Prevention of GVHD

One of the main complications of allo-HSCT is developing GVHD where donor immune cells, especially T-lymphocytes, attack recipient's organs (D'Souza et al. 2020).

Corticosteroids are still the main therapy for GVHD, while steroid-resistant GVHD remains a leading cause of morbidity and mortality (El Jurdi et al. 2021). MSCs are used for the treatment and prevention of GVHD in order to inhibit the production of proinflammatory cytokines, which play an important role in the pathogenesis of GVHD (Li et al. 2016). A number of clinical studies have confirmed the effectiveness of intravenous infusion of MSCs in patients after HSC transplantation. The first report demonstrating the clinical effectiveness of treating GVHD with MSCS infusion was published in 2004 (Le Blanc et al. 2004). Since then, numerous clinical trials have been performed to study this technology and researchers reported contradictory data. A recent meta-analysis of allogeneic MSCs used for the prevention or treatment of acute patients ($n = 654$) or chronic patients ($n = 76$) with GVHD after HSCT showed that MSCs enhanced overall survival by 17% compared with the control group. At the same time, significantly fewer cases of grade IV acute GVHD (aGVHD) and chronic GVHD (cGVHD) were recorded in the group of patients receiving preventive MSC regimens. On the base of the analysis, the authors recommended to use MSCs as adjuvant therapy from the onset of the disease (Morata-Tarifa et al. 2020).

A clinical trial involving 11 patients with hemablastosis aged <12 years who received autologous MSCs (4 weekly infusions at a dose of $2x10^6$/kg) demonstrated the effectiveness of this strategy in GVHD treatment. A complete or partial response was observed in three out of four patients with aGVHD. After 3 months, five of the seven patients with cGVHD had a partial response, one had stabilization, and only one patient had cGVHD progression. No significant differences were observed between dose levels in peripheral blood lymphocyte subpopulations; however, it was noted that autologous MSCs were hardly feasible as treatment beyond four doses (Stenger et al. 2022). A meta-analysis of 13 non-randomized studies including a total of 336 patients with aGVHD showed that MSC treatment increased the 6-month survival of patients with steroid-refractory aGVHD, but had no impact on overall survival. The results of the analysis showed no differences of MSC effects related to age, cell culture, or doses (Hashmi et al. 2016). The first randomized, placebo-controlled trial included 260 patients aged 6 months - 70 years who received 8 intravenous infusions of commercial MSCs (remestemcel-L) or placebo over 4 weeks. Similar to the previous clinical trial, remestemcel-L was well tolerated but did not result in a significant benefit compared with placebo (Kebriaei et al. 2020). However, a phase 3 clinical trial that included 54 children with primary aGVHD who had no previous immunosuppressive therapy showed that MSC-based remestemcel-L infused at a dose of 2×10^6 cells/kg twice a week for 4 weeks significantly improved 28-day overall response rate (ORR) compared with the prespecified control. A statistically significant ORR (70.4% versus 45%) persisted for 100 days. Remestemcel-L was well tolerated with no signs of therapy-related toxicity (Kurtzberg et al. 2020).

Although most studies have reported the effectiveness of MSCs for the treatment and prevention of GVHD, other studies have resulted in the lack of effectiveness of this therapeutic strategy. An Australian clinical trial evaluating the effectiveness of MSCs in 87 children with allo-HCT found that MSC treatment showed neither improved survival nor any significant clinical benefit (Australian Public Assessment Report 2015). The results of more recent studies also did not demonstrate a significant improvement in the survival of patients with GVHD after MSC therapy. However, it should be noted that MSCs were obtained from different donors, and MSC cell products were generated ex vivo under different culture conditions, which significantly affected the activity of MSCs (Dotoli et al. 2017). To increase the therapeutic effectiveness of MSCs, they were used in combination with basiliximab, a calcineurin inhibitor. An open-label, randomized phase 3 study, demonstrated that the combination resulted in significantly improved efficacy with higher ORR at days

28 and 56 in patients with steroid-refractory GVHD (SR-GVHD) (Kiselevskiy et al. 2021; Zhao et al. 2022).

The controversial data of the studies with MSCs for the treatment of GVHD are associated with the lack of standardized methods for generating MSCs, the doses used, the frequency of injections, and the patient's age. The low clinical efficacy of commercial MSC products may be associated with the procedures where cells are cryopreserved and administered to the patient immediately after thawing. Preclinical studies have shown that MSCs are functionally "paralyzed" after thawing compared to the culture-reconstituted cells (Francois et al. 2012; Chinnadurai et al. 2016; Cottle et al. 2022). Restoration of MSC functions after cryopreservation and thawing requires additional cell culturing. Besides, MSC products, especially commercial ones, involve long-term cell expansion ex vivo, which can lead to the "senescence" of MSCs and loss of their functional characteristics. The suggestion is supported by clinical data indicating that late passages of MSCs had low efficacy in the treatment of aGVHD (von Bahr et al. 2012).

Macías-Sánchez et al. (2022) studied MSCs from BM and adipose tissue generated in GMP setting. The analysis included 62 patients (adults and children) with steroid-resistant aGVHD and cGVHD. Patients received MSC intravenously. The administration of MSCs was generally well tolerated and showed no increase in the incidence of infectious complications. However, four patients developed MSC therapy-related adverse events: one patient had temporary cardiac arrest, and another patient had syncope during the MSC infusion. A patient who received 4 doses of MSCs developed chest pain and tachycardia during the third infusion. One patient had induration and pain at the infusion site. All described manifestations were successfully cured. No other side effects were reported. None of the adverse events was observed in the pediatric population. Overall, 58.7% of patients with aGVHD and 62.5% of patients with cGVHD responded to MSC therapy. The aGVHD treatment outcomes were observed in patients refractory to steroids and other immunosuppressants. Overall survival was higher in responders and very poor in nonresponders. Two-year survival rates for acute and chronic GVHD of responders accounted for 51.85% (14 of 27) and 70% (7 of 10 patients), respectively.

Despite theoretical and experimental basis for the beneficial use of MSCs to reduce the severity of GVHD and improve the engraftment of HSCs, the results of clinical trials are ambiguous. Primarily, that is due to different methods of MSC generation, routes of MSC administration, and MSC doses. On the other hand, researchers have not reached a consensus on the standard conditioning regimen before HSC transplantation, which is classified as myeloablative or nonmyeloablative, and is necessary to prevent graft rejection and reduce tumor burden (Gyurkocza and Sandmaier 2014). Conditioning regimens facilitate remission of hematologic disease but they have various grades of toxicity, and therefore individual differences in chemotherapy regimens may have important implications for subsequent HSC transplantation. Another factor that adds variability between studies is the rate of HSC donor compatibility (Zeiser and Blazar 2017).

Although MSCs are used in clinical setting for the treatment and prevention of GVHD, as well as for the improvement of the engraftment of allogeneic HSCs, there are currently no approved routes of administration and doses of MSCs for treatment of steroid-resistant GVHD in children with poor prognosis (MacMillan et al. 2020). National Health Service, England concluded that MSCs may have a role in third-line treatment options but recognize that this is an area of active research and that MSCs may have a greater role in the management of aGvHD in the future (NHS England Specialised Services 2017).

Therefore, it is necessary to standardize generation and evaluation of the MSC authenticity, the routes of administration and effective doses, and develop a biomedical cell product based on these standards.

8 Promising Approaches for Increasing the Efficiency and Viability of MSCs

8.1 3D Culture

In recent years, increasing data have appeared about the advantages of MSC 3D culture compared to the standard 2D monolayer cultures. Transplantation of a suspension of MSCs generated in 2D culture could be less effective as a result of the rapid death of the cells entering the microenvironment of target tissues and prompt passage into the systemic circulation, even in case of local injection. In tissue engineering, biomimetic 3D matrices populated with MSCs are effectively used to restore defects in bone, cartilage, and other tissues (Kiselevskiy et al. 2023; Wang et al. 2016). Another method of 3D culture uses spheroids, which present dense cellular structures that form cell aggregates. Spheroids build their own intercellular matrix that contributes to cell expansion. Due to the endogenous matrix and improved cell-cell interactions, spheroids better mimic the microenvironment of the native tissue. 3D spheroid MSCs are characterized by immunomodulatory activity with anti-inflammatory effects caused by the secretion of pro-inflammatory factors such as prostaglandin E2 (PGE2) and the suppression of inflammatory cytokines such as tumor necrosis factor-α (TNF-α) (Hsu et al. 2011). Moreover, a number of researchers have reported that MSC 3D spheroids have more pronounced immunomodulatory activity than MSC 2D culture (Cheng et al. 2012; Petrenko et al. 2017; Ohori-Morita et al. 2022). Studies in mouse models of inflammation have also demonstrated higher anti-inflammatory activity of MSC 3D spheroids compared to MSC 2D cultures (Jiang et al. 2017; Shimazawa et al. 2022). A recent study examining the safety profile of intravenous infusion of human 3D spheroid MSCs in healthy monkeys registered no physiological changes and no evidence of small vessel embolism. On the base of the experimental results, the authors made a conclusion that the procedure was safe with less lung damage and better survival of 3D spheroid MSCs compared to 2D cultured MSC suspension (Yeung et al. 2022).

The accumulated data suggest the high potential of MSC 3D spheroids for clinical use in a wide range of medical indications (Griffin et al. 2022; Yen et al. 2023). One of the promising applications for 3D spheroid MSCs, given their increased viability and immunomodulatory activity, may include the treatment and prevention of

GVHD. In addition, this technology can be used to stimulate hematopoiesis and improve graft survival after allo-HSCT.

9 CAR-T Technologies and MSCs

One of the promising and rapidly developing areas is genetic engineering technologies that are employed to increase the efficiency and viability of MSCs introduced into the body. Numerous studies aimed at the development of MSC-based genetically modified products and early stages of clinical trials have started their programs. These studies were encouraged by recent achievements in immunotherapy of patients with hematologic malignancies by genetically modified chimeric antigen receptor T cells (CAR-T). The development of MSC-based gene therapy might solve the problem of the short life of MSCs in the body and their inability to produce the required bioregulators (Muhammad et al. 2017). Genetically modified MSCs are considered a potential cell-based therapy for solid tumors, vascular diseases and a number of critical conditions, including sepsis, systemic inflammatory response, and cytokine storm (Yuan et al. 2016a, b). Genetic modification can improve the natural function of MSCs by reprogramming MSCs, activating or suppressing their native genes, leading to controlled production of their own natural specific products, such as pro/anti-inflammatory mediators and cytokines (Hodgkinson et al. 2010).

The technologies used for generation of CAR-T cells, including lenti- and adenoviral vectors, as well as non-viral delivery systems, such as plasmid DNA, nanoplasmids, liposomes, and polymers were proposed for MSC genetic modification. However, MSCs introduced into the body in the form of a suspension have limited therapeutic efficacy due to their poor survival and low production of bioregulators in vivo. Therefore, genetic modification of cells was suggested in order to improve engraftment and augment the functionality of the cell product. Like that for CAR-T cells, genetic modification of MSCs includes both viral vectors (including retroviruses, adenoviruses, lentiviruses, and adeno-associated viruses) and non-viral vectors, such as lipids or polymers, etc. (Naso et al. 2017). Studies on mice have shown that implantation of MSCs overexpressing growth factor led to increased remodeling of affected areas of the heart muscle, decreased neurological function, and improved liver function (Chen et al. 2018). MSCs engineered to overexpress VEGF increased cell viability under hypoxic conditions in vitro and promoted capillary formation in animal models of myocardial infarction, hindlimb ischemia, and skin defects (Han et al. 2014). G-CSF is widely used in clinical practice due to its various effects along with its stimulating activity of neutropoiesis. Since MSCs produce G-CSF, the researchers suggested that MSCs overexpressing G-CSF (MSC-G-CSF) could enhance therapeutic effects. Genetically engineered MSCs overexpressing G-CSF were studied in a rat model of angiotensin II-mediated cardiac injury. The authors demonstrated a more essential reduction in inflammation, fibrosis, and cytokine modulation with MSC-G-CSF compared to conventional MSCs. The achieved effect was associated with an increased ability to recruit populations of suppressor cells such as Tregs and myeloid cells (Pinto et al. 2013). At the same time, MSC-based genetic engineering technologies are just emerging and are focused mainly on the treatment of oncological, metabolic, and inflammatory diseases, and on stimulating the repair of damaged tissues (Sage et al. 2016). The described approaches were proposed to ensure MSC localization in the body since it was unclear where modified MSCs migrated after intravenous infusion and previous studies showed MSC limited effectiveness due to rapid clearance from the circulation.

10 Conclusion

Allo-HSCT is one of the main therapies for children and adults with malignant diseases of the blood system with a poor prognosis. Despite significant achievements in hematopoietic cell transplantation, the most severe specific complication and one of the main causes of death during allogeneic transplantations is graft failure and GVHD. The use of MSCs for GVHD treatment and prevention, as well as for the improvement of HSC engraftment and stimulation of hematopoiesis after allo-HSCT is a promising therapeutic strategy. However, so far, numerous clinical studies have demonstrated conflicting results regarding MSC effectiveness for GVHD prevention after allo-HSCT. No definite data can support the assumption that MSCs stimulate the engraftment of transplanted HSCs. Probably, the lack of MSC effectiveness is a result of just a small number of the intravenously infused cells that reach BM, which cannot significantly determine the engraftment of transplanted HSCs. Intraosseous injection of MSCs can probably increase their effectiveness for engrafting HSCs and stimulating hematopoiesis.

It is important to take into account not only immunosuppressive MSC functions, but also MSC capability to enhance immune responses. The dual role of MSCs in modulating immunity may be associated with recipient's pro-inflammatory cytokines. Probably, the profile of pro-inflammatory/anti-inflammatory cytokines depends largely on the conditions of culturing MSCs in vitro, the number of passages of cell culture, etc. Therefore, it is necessary to standardize methods for generating and validating MSCs, as well as routes of administration, and establish effective MSC doses. It is also possible to enhance the effectiveness of the use of MSCs in patients who have undergone allo-HSCT by increasing their viability in 3D culture and the use of MSCs in the form of cell spheroids.

References

Acar M, Kocherlakota KS, Murphy MM, Peyer JG, Oguro H, Inra CN, Jaiyeola C, Zhao Z, Luby-Phelps K, Morrison SJ (2015) Deep imaging of bone marrow shows non-dividing stem cells are mainly perisinusoidal. Nature 526(7571):126–130. https://doi.org/10.1038/nature15250/

Agarwal N, Rotz S, Hanna R (2023) Medical emergencies in pediatric blood & marrow transplant and cellular therapies. Front Pediatr 11:1075e644. https://doi.org/10.3389/fped.2023.1075644

Allan D, Tieu A, Lalu M, Burger D (2020) Mesenchymal stromal cell-derived extracellular vesicles for regenerative therapy and immune modulation: progress and challenges toward clinical application. Stem Cells Transl Med 9:39–46. https://doi.org/10.1002/sctm.19-0114

Alviano F, Bagnara GP, Bilic G, Bühring HJ, Evangelista M, Hennerbichler S, Liu B, Magatti M, Mao N, Miki T, Marongiu F, Nakajima H, Nikaido T, Portmann-Lanz CB, Sankar V, Soncini M, Stadler G, Surbek D, Takahashi TA, Redl H, Sakuragawa N, Wolbank S, Zeisberger S, Zisch A, Strom SC (2008) Concise review: isolation and characterization of cells from human term placenta: outcome of the first international workshop on placenta derived stem cells. Stem Cells 26(2):300–311. https://doi.org/10.1634/stemcells.2007-0594

Australian Public Assessment Report for Remestemcel-L, ex vivo adult human mesenchymal stem cells (2015) TGA. Australia 74 p. https://www.tga.gov.au/sites/default/files/auspar-remestemcel-l-150315.pdf

Bacigalupo A, Valle M, Podesta M, Pitto A, Zocchi E, De Flora A, Pozzi S, Luchetti S, Frassoni F, Van Lint MT, Piaggio G (2005) T-cell suppression mediated by mesenchymal stem cells is deficient in patients with severe aplastic anemia. Exp Hematol 33:819–827. https://doi.org/10.1016/j.exphem.2005.05.006

Ball LM, Bernardo ME, Roelofs H, Lankester A, Cometa A, Egeler RM, Locatelli F, Fibbe WE (2007) Cotransplantation of ex vivo expanded mesenchymal stem cells accelerates lymphocyte recovery and may reduce the risk of graft failure in haploidentical hematopoietic stem-cell transplantation. Blood 110:2764–2767. https://doi.org/10.1182/blood-2007-04-087056

Bernardo ME, Avanzini MA, Perotti C, Cometa AM, Moretta A, Lenta E, Del Fante C, Novara F, de Silvestri A, Amendola G, Zuffardi O, Maccario R, Locatelli F (2007) Optimization of in vitro expansion of human multipotent mesenchymal stromal cells for cell-therapy approaches: further insights in the search for a fetal calf serum substitute. J Cell Physiol 211(1):121–130. https://doi.org/10.1002/jcp.20911

Bhattacharya D, Czechowicz A, Ooi AG, Rossi DJ, Bryder D, Weissman IL (2009) Niche recycling through division-independent egress of hematopoietic stem cells. J Exp Med 206:2837–2850. https://doi.org/10.1084/jem.20090778

Bonab MM, Alimoghaddam K, Talebian F, Ghaffari SH, Ghavamzadeh A, Nikbin B (2006) Aging of mesenchymal stem cell in vitro. BMC Cell Biol 7:14. https://doi.org/10.1186/1471-2121-7-14

Capelli C, Domenghini M, Borleri G, Bellavita P, Poma R, Carobbio A, Micò C, Rambaldi A, Golay J, Introna M (2007) Human platelet lysate allows expansion and clinical grade production of mesenchymal stromal cells from small samples of bone marrow aspirates or marrow filter washouts. Bone Marrow Transplant 40(8):785–791. https://doi.org/10.1038/sj.bmt.1705798

Chan C-K, Wu K-H, Lee Y-S, Hwang S-M, Lee M-S, Liao S-K, Cheng E-H, See L-C, Tsai C-N, Kuo M-L, Huang J-L (2012) The comparison of interleukin 6-associated immunosuppressive effects of human ESCs, fetal-type MSCs, and adult-type MSCs. Transplantation 94(2):132–138. https://doi.org/10.1097/TP.0b013e31825940a4

Chang YS, Ahn SY, Yoo HS, Sung SI, Choi SJ, Oh WI, Park WS (2014) Mesenchymal stem cells for bronchopulmonary dysplasia: phase 1 dose-escalation clinical trial. J Pediatr 164:966–972

Chen X, Nomani A, Patel N, Nouri FS, Hatefi A (2018) Bioengineering a non-genotoxic vector for genetic modification of mesenchymal stem cells. Biomaterials 152:1–14. https://doi.org/10.1016/j.biomaterials.2017.10.02

Chen J, Hu C, Chen L, Tang L, Zhu Y, Xu X, Chen L, Gao H, Lu X, Yu L, Dai X, Xiang C, Li L (2020) Clinical study of mesenchymal stem cell treating acute respiratory distress syndrome induced by epidemic Influenza A (H7N9) infection, a hint for COVID-19 treatment. Engineering (Beijing) 6(10):1153–1161. https://doi.org/10.1016/j.eng.2020.02.006

Cheng NC, Wang S, Young TH (2012) The influence of spheroid formation of human adipose-derived stem cells on chitosan films on sternness and differentiation capabilities. Biomaterials 33(6):1748–1758. https://doi.org/10.1016/j.biomaterials.2011.11.049

Chinnadurai R, Copland IB, Garcia MA, Petersen CT, Lewis CN, Waller EK et al (2016) Cryopreserved mesenchymal stromal cells are susceptible to T-cell mediated apoptosis which is partly rescued by IFNγ licensing. Stem Cells 34(9):2429–2442. https://doi.org/10.1002/stem.2415

Connard SS, Linardi RL, Even KM, Berglund AK, Schnabel LV, Ortved KF (2021) Effects of continuous passage on the immunomodulatory properties of equine bone marrow-derived mesenchymal stem cells in vitro. Vet Immunol Immunopathol 234:110203. https://doi.org/10.1016/j.vetimm.2021.110203

Coppin E, Sundarasetty BS, Rahmig S, Blume J, Verheyden NA, Bahlmann F, Ravens S, Schubert U, Schmid J, Ludwig S, Geissler K, Guntinas-Lichius O, von Kaisenberg C, Groten T, Platz A, Naumann R, Ludwig B, Prinz I, Waskow C, Krueger A (2021) Enhanced differentiation of functional human T cells in NSGW41 mice with tissue-specific expression of human interleukin-7. Leukemia 35(12):3561–3567. https://doi.org/10.1038/s41375-021-01259-5

Cottle C, Porter AP, Lipat A, Turner-Lyles C, Nguyen J, Moll G et al (2022) Impact of cryopreservation and freeze-thawing on therapeutic properties of mesenchymal Stromal/Stem cells and other common cellular therapeutics. Curr Stem Cell Rep 8(2):72–92. https://doi.org/10.1007/s40778-022-00212-1

D'Souza A, Fretham C, Lee SJ, Arora M, Brunner J, Chhabra S et al (2020) Current use of and trends in hematopoietic cell transplantation in the United States. Biol Blood Marrow Transplant 26(8):e177–e182. https://doi.org/10.1016/j.bbmt.2020.04.013

Dai R, Wang Z, Samanipour R, Koo KI, Kim K (2016) Adipose-derived stem cells for tissue engineering and regenerative medicine applications. Stem Cells Int 2016:6737345. https://doi.org/10.1155/2016/6737345

Diehl R, Ferrara F, Müller C, Dreyer AY, McLeod DD, Fricke S, Boltze J (2017) Immunosuppression for in vivo research: state-of-the-art protocols and experimental approaches. Cell Mol Immunol 14:146–179. https://doi.org/10.1038/cmi.2016.39

Dominici M, Le Blanc K, Mueller I, Slaper-Cortenbach I, Marini F, Krause D, Deans R, Keating A, Prockop D (2006) Minimal criteria for defining multipotent mesenchymal stromal cells. The International Society for Cellular Therapy position statement. Cytotherapy 8:315–317. https://doi.org/10.1080/14653240600855905

Dotoli GM, De Santis GC, Orellana MD, de Lima PK, Caruso SR, Fernandes TR, Rensi Colturato VA, Kondo AT, Hamerschlak N, Simões BP, Covas DT (2017) Mesenchymal stromal cell infusion to treat steroid-refractory acute GvHD III/IV after hematopoietic stem cell transplantation. Bone Marrow Transplant 52(6):859–862. https://doi.org/10.1038/bmt.2017.35

Doucet C, Ernou I, Zhang Y, Llense JR, Begot L, Holy X, Lataillade JJ (2005) Platelet lysates promote mesenchymal stem cell expansion: a safety substitute for animal serum in cell-based therapy applications. J Cell Physiol 205(2):228–236. https://doi.org/10.1002/jcp.20391

Drobyski WR, Pasquini M, Kovatovic K, Palmer J, Douglas Rizzo J, Saad A, Saber W, Hari P (2011) Tocilizumab for the treatment of steroid refractory graft-versus-host disease. Biol Blood Marrow Transplant 17:1862–1868. https://doi.org/10.1016/j.bbmt.2011.07.001

El Jurdi N, Rayes A, MacMillan ML, Holtan SG, DeFor TE, Witte J et al (2021) Steroid-dependent acute GVHD after allogeneic hematopoietic cell transplantation: risk factors and clinical outcomes. Blood Adv 5(5):1352–1359. https://doi.org/10.1182/bloodadvances.202000393

Ferrà C, de Sanjosé S, Gallardo D, Berlanga JJ, Rueda F, Marìn D, de la Banda E, Ancìn I, Peris J, Garcìa J, Grañena A (1998) IL-6 and IL-8 levels in plasma during hematopoietic progenitor transplantation. Haematologica 83(12):1082–1087

Ferrara JL (1993) Cytokine dysregulation as a mechanism of graft versus host disease. Curr Opin Immunol 5(5):794–799. https://doi.org/10.1016/0952-7915(93)90139-j

Francois M, Copland IB, Yuan S, Romieu-Mourez R, Waller EK, Galipeau J (2012) Cryopreserved mesenchymal stromal cells display impaired immunosuppressive properties as a result of heat-shock response and impaired interferon-gamma licensing. Cytotherapy 14(2):147–152. https://doi.org/10.3109/14653249.2011.623691

Friedenstein AJ, Petrakova KV, Kurolesova AI, Frolova GP (1968) Heterotopic of bone marrow. Analysis of precursor cells for osteogenic and hematopoietic tissues. Transplantation 6:230–247

Fröbel J, Landspersky T, Percin G, Schreck C, Rahmig S, Ori A, Nowak D, Essers M, Waskow C, Oostendorp RAJ (2021) The hematopoietic bone marrow niche ecosystem. Front Cell Dev Biol 9:705410. https://doi.org/10.3389/fcell.2021.705410

Garrigós MM, de Oliveira FA, Nucci MP, Nucci LP, Alves ADH, Dias OFM, Gamarra LF (2022) How mesenchymal stem cell cotransplantation with hematopoietic stem cells can improve engraftment in animal models. World J Stem Cells 14(8):658–679. https://doi.org/10.4252/wjsc.v14.i8.658

Gazdic M, Volarevic V, Arsenijevic N, Stojkovic M (2015) Mesenchymal stem cells: a friend or foe in immune-mediated diseases. Stem Cell Rev Rep 11(2):280–287. https://doi.org/10.1007/s12015-014-9583-3

Goto T, Murata M, Terakura S, Nishida T, Adachi Y, Ushijima Y, Shimada K, Ishikawa Y, Hayakawa F, Nishio N, Nishiwaki S, Hirakawa A, Kato K, Takahashi Y, Kiyoi H (2018) Phase I study of cord blood transplantation with intrabone marrow injection of mesenchymal stem cells: a clinical study protocol. Medicine (Baltimore) 97(17):e0449. https://doi.org/10.1097/MD.0000000000010449

Griffin KH, Fok SW, Kent Leach J (2022) Strategies to capitalize on cell spheroid therapeutic potential for tissue repair and disease modeling. NPJ Regen Med 7(1):70. https://doi.org/10.1038/s41536-022-00266-z

Grisendi G, Annerén C, Cafarelli L, Sternieri R, Veronesi E, Cervo GL, Luminari S, Maur M, Frassoldati A, Palazzi G, Otsuru S, Bambi F, Paolucci P, Pierfranco C, Horwitz E, Dominici M (2010) GMP-manufactured density gradient media for optimized mesenchymal stromal/stem cell isolation and expansion. Cytotherapy 12(4):466–477. https://doi.org/10.3109/14653241003649510

Gu L, Tseng S, Horner RM, Tam C, Loda M, Rollins BJ (2000) Control of TH2 polarization by the chemokine monocyte chemoattractant protein-1. Nature 404:407–411

Guo BC, Wu KH, Chen CY, Lin WY, Chang YJ, Lee TA, Lin MJ, Wu HP (2023) Mesenchymal stem cells in the treatment of COVID-19. Int J Mol Sci 24(19):14800. https://doi.org/10.3390/ijms241914800

Gyurkocza B, Sandmaier BM (2014) Conditioning regimens for hematopoietic cell transplantation: one size does not fit all. Blood 124:344–353. https://doi.org/10.1182/blood-2014-02-5147

Han Y, Tao R, Han Y, Sun T, Chai J, Xu G, Liu J (2014) Microencapsulated VEGF gene-modified umbilical cord mesenchymal stromal cells promote the vascularization of tissue-engineered dermis: an experimental study. Cytotherapy 16(2):160–169. https://doi.org/10.1016/j.jcyt.2013.10.014

Hashmi S, Ahmed M, Murad MH et al (2016) Survival after mesenchymal stromal cell therapy in steroid-refractory acute graft-versus-host disease: systematic review and meta-analysis. Lancet Haematol 3:e45–e52. https://doi.org/10.1016/S2352-3026(15)00224-0

Hass R, Kasper C, Böhm S, Jacobs R (2011) Different populations and sources of human mesenchymal stem cells (MSC): a comparison of adult and neonatal tissue-derived MSC. Cell Commun Signal 9:12. https://doi.org/10.1186/1478-811X-9-12

Heinrichs J, Bastian D, Veerapathran A, Anasetti C, Betts B, Yu XZ (2016) Regulatory T-cell therapy for graft-versus-host disease. J Immunol Res Ther 1:1–14

Hodgkinson CP, Gomez JA, Mirotsou M, Dzau VJ (2010) Genetic engineering of mesenchymal stem cells and its application in human disease therapy. Hum Gene Ther 21(11):1513–1526. https://doi.org/10.1089/hum.2010.16

Hsu SH, Huang TB, Cheng SJ, Weng SY, Tsai CL, Tseng CS, Chen DC, Liu TY, Fu KY, Yen BL (2011) Chondrogenesis from human placenta-derived mesenchymal stem cells in three-dimensional scaffolds for cartilage tissue engineering. Tissue Eng Part A 17(11–12):1549–1560. https://doi.org/10.1089/ten.TEA.2010.0419

Im HJ, Koh KN, Seo JJ (2015) Haploidentical hematopoietic stem cell transplantation in children and adolescents with acquired severe aplastic anemia. Korean J Ped 58:199–205. https://doi.org/10.3345/kjp.2015.58.6.199

Jiang B, Yan L, Miao Z et al (2017) Spheroidal formation preserves human stem cells for prolonged time under ambient conditions for facile storage and transportation. Biomaterials 133:275–286. https://doi.org/10.1016/j.biomaterials.2017.03.050

Kebriaei P, Hayes J, Daly A, Uberti J, Marks DI, Soiffer R, Waller EK, Burke E, Skerrett D, Shpall E, Martin PJ (2020) A phase 3 randomized study of remestemcel-l versus placebo added to second-line therapy in patients with steroid-refractory acute graft-versus-host disease. Biol Blood Marrow Transplant 26(5):835–844. https://doi.org/10.1016/j.bbmt.2019.08.029

Keto J, Kaartinen T, Salmenniemi U, Castrén J, Partanen J, Hänninen A, Korhonen M, Lähteenmäki K, Itälä-Remes M, Nystedt J (2018) Immunomonitoring of MCK-treated GvHD patients reveals only moderate potential for response prediction but indicates treatment safety. Mol Ther Methods Clin Dev 9:109–118. https://doi.org/10.1016/j.omtm.2018.02.001

Kiel MJ, Morrison SJ (2008) Uncertainty in the niches that maintain haematopoietic stem cells. Nat Rev Immunol 8:290–301. https://doi.org/10.1038/nri2279

Kiselevskii MV, Vlasenko RY, Stepanyan NG, Shubina IZ, Sitdikova SM, Kirgizov KI, Varfolomeeva SR (2021) Secretome of mesenchymal bone marrow stem cells: is it immunosuppressive or proinflammatory? Bull Exp Biol Med 172(2):250–253. https://doi.org/10.1007/s10517-021-05371-5

Kiselevskiy M, Shubina I, Chikileva I, Sitdikova S, Samoylenko I, Anisimova N, Kirgizov K, Suleimanova A, Gorbunova T, Varfolomeeva S (2020) Immune pathogenesis of COVID-19 intoxication: storm or silence? Pharmaceuticals (Basel) 13(8):166. https://doi.org/10.3390/ph130801

Kiselevskiy M, Vlasenko R, Reshetnikova V, Chikileva I, Shubina I, Osmanov E, Valiev T, Sidorova N, Batmanova N, Stepanyan N, Kirgizov K, Varfolomeeva S (2021) Potential use of mesenchymal multipotent cells for hemopoietic stem cell transplantation: pro and contra. J Pediatr Hematol Oncol 43(3):90–94. https://doi.org/10.1097/MPH.0000000000002065

Kiselevskiy MV, Anisimova NY, Kapustin AV, Ryzhkin AA, Kuznetsova DN, Polyakova VV, Enikeev NA (2023) Development of bioactive scaffolds for orthopedic applications by designing additively manufactured titanium porous structures: a critical review. Biomimetics 8:546. https://doi.org/10.3390/biomimetics8070546

Koc ON, Gerson SL, Cooper BW, Dyhouse SM, Haynesworth SE, Caplan AI, Lazarus HM (2000) Rapid hematopoietic recovery after coinfusion of autologous-blood stem cells and culture-expanded marrow mesenchymal stem cells in advanced breast cancer patients receiving high-dose chemotherapy. J Clin Oncol 18:307–316. https://doi.org/10.1200/JCO.2000.18.2.307

Kopp HG, Avecilla ST, Hooper AT, Shmelkov SV, Ramos CA, Zhang F, Rafii S (2005) Tie2 activation contributes to hemangiogenic regeneration after myelosuppression. Blood 106(2):505–513. https://doi.org/10.1182/blood-2004-11-4269

Kuçi Z, Bönig H, Kreyenberg H, Bunos M, Jauch A, Janssen JW, Škifić M, Michel K, Eising B, Lucchini G, Bakhtiar S, Greil J, Lang P, Basu O, von Luettichau I, Schulz A, Sykora KW, Jarisch A, Soerensen J, Salzmann-Manrique E, Seifried E, Klingebiel T, Bader P, Kuçi S (2016) Mesenchymal stromal cells from pooled mononuclear cells of multiple bone marrow donors as rescue therapy in pediatric severe steroid-refractory graft-versus-host disease: a multicenter survey. Haematologica 101(8):985–994. https://doi.org/10.3324/haematol.2015.140368

Kundrotas G, Gasperskaja E, Slapsyte G, Gudleviciene Z, Krasko J, Stumbryte A et al (2016) Identity, proliferation capacity,genomic stability and novel senescence markers of mesenchymal stem cells isolated from low volume of humanbone marrow. Oncotarget 7(10):10788–10802. https://doi.org/10.18632/oncotarget.7456

Kurtzberg J, Abdel-Azim H, Carpenter P, Chaudhury S, Horn B, Mahadeo K, Nemecek E, Neudorf S, Prasad V, Prockop S, Quigg T, Satwani P, Cheng A, Burke E, Hayes J, Skerrett D (2020) MSB-GVHD001/002 study group. A phase 3, single-arm, prospective study of remestemcel-L, ex vivo culture-expanded adult human mesenchymal stromal cells for the treatment of pediatric patients who failed to respond to steroid treatment for acute graft-versus-host disease. Biol Blood Marrow Transplant 26(5):845–854. https://doi.org/10.1016/j.bbmt.2020.01.018

Kyurkchiev D, Bochev I, Ivanova-Todorova E, Mourdjeva M, Oreshkova T, Belemezova K, Kyurkchiev S (2014) Secretion of immunoregulatory cytokines by mesenchymal stem cells. World J Stem Cells 6(5):552–570. https://doi.org/10.4252/wjsc.v6.i5.552

Lai RC, Tan SS, Teh BJ, Sze SK, Arslan F, de Kleijn DP, Choo A, Lim SK (2012) Proteolytic potential of the MSC exosome proteome: implications for an exosome-mediated delivery of therapeutic proteasome. Int J Proteom 2012:971907. https://doi.org/10.1155/2012/971907

Lazarus HM, Haynesworth SE, Gerson SL, Rosenthal NS, Caplan AI (1995) Ex vivo expansion and subsequent infusion of human bone marrow-derived stromal progenitor cells (mesenchymal progenitor cells): implications for therapeutic use. Bone Marrow Transplant 16(4):557–564

Lazarus HM, Koc O, Devine SM, Curtin P, Maziarz RT, Holland HK, Shpall EJ, McCarthy P, Atkinson K, Cooper BW, Gerson SL, Laughlin MJ, Loberiza FR Jr, Moseley AB, Bacigalupo A (2005) Cotransplantation of HLA-identical sibling culture-expanded mesenchymal stem cells and hematopoietic stem cells in hematologic malignancy patients. Biol Blood Marrow Trans Plant 11:389–398. https://doi.org/10.1016/j.bbmt.2005.02.001

Le Blanc K, Rasmusson I, Sundberg B, Götherström C, Hassan M, Uzunel M et al (2004) Treatment of severe acute graft-versus-host disease with third party haploidentical mesenchymal stem cells. Lancet 393:1439–1441. https://doi.org/10.1016/S0140-6736(04)16104-7

Le Blanc K, Samuelsson H, Gustafsson B, Remberger M, Sundberg B, Arvidson J, Ljungman P, Lönnies H, Nava S, Ringdén O (2007) Transplantation of mesenchymal stem cells to enhance engraftment of hematopoietic stem cells. Leukemia 21:1733–1738

Leng Z, Zhu R, Hou W, Feng Y, Yang Y, Han Q, Zhao RC (2020) Transplantation of $ACE2^-$ mesenchymal stem cells improves the outcome of patients with COVID-19 pneumonia. Aging Dis 11(2):216. https://doi.org/10.14336/ad.2020.0228

Li Y, Chen S, Yuan J, Yang Y, Li J, Ma J, Wu X, Freund M, Pollok K, Hanenberg H et al (2009) Mesenchymal stem/progenitor cells promote the reconstitution of exogenous hematopoietic stem cells in Fancg−/− mice in vivo. Blood 113:2342–2351. https://doi.org/10.1182/blood-2008-07-168138

Li H, Ghazanfari R, Zacharaki D, Lim HC, Scheding S (2016) Isolation and characterization of primary bone marrow mesenchymal stromal cells. Ann N Y Acad Sci 1370:109–118. https://doi.org/10.1111/nyas.13102

Li T, Luo C, Zhang J, Wei L, Sun W, Xie Q, Liu Y, Zhao Y, Xu S, Wang L (2021) Efficacy and safety of mesenchymal stem cells co-infusion in allogeneic hematopoietic stem cell transplantation: a systematic review and meta-analysis. Stem Cell Res Ther 12(1):246. https://doi.org/10.1186/s13287-021-02304-x

Lohmann M, Walenda G, Hemeda H, Joussen S, Drescher W, Jockenhoevel S, Hutschenreuter G, Zenke M, Wagner W (2012) Donor age of human platelet lysate affects proliferation and differentiation of mesenchymal stem cells. PLoS One 7(5):e37839. https://doi.org/10.1371/journal.pone.0037839

Lucchini G, Introna M, Dander E, Rovelli A, Balduzzi A, Bonanomi S, Salvade A, Capelli C, Belotti D, Gaipa G, Perseghin P, Vinci P, Lanino E, Chiusolo P, Orofino MG, Marktel S, Golay J, Rambaldi A, Biondi A, D'Amico G, Biagi E (2010) Platelet-lysate-expanded mesenchymal stromal cells as a salvage therapy for severe resistant graft-versus-host disease in a pediatric population. Biol Blood Marrow Transplant 16:1293–1301. https://doi.org/10.1016/j.bbmt.2010.03.017

Ma S, Xie N, Li W, Yuan B, Shi Y, Wang Y (2014) Immunobiology of mesenchymal stem cells. Cell Death Differ 21:216–225. https://doi.org/10.1038/cdd.2013.158

Mabuchi Y, Morikawa S, Harada S et al (2013) LNGFR+THY-1+VCAM-1hi+ cells reveal functionally distinct subpopulations in mesenchymal stem cells. Stem Cell Reports 1:152–165. https://doi.org/10.1016/j.stemcr.2013.06.001. Noort WA, Kruisselbrink AB, in't Anker PS et al (2002) Mesenchymal stem cells promote engraftment of human umbilical cord blood-derived CD34+ cells in NOD/SCID mice. Exp Hematol 30:870–878. https://doi.org/10.1016/s0301-472x(02)00820-2

Macías-Sánchez MDM, Morata-Tarifa C, Cuende N, Cardesa-Gil A, Cuesta-Casas MÁ, Pascual-Cascon MJ, Pascual A, Martín-Calvo C, Jurado M, Perez-Simón JA, Espigado I, Garzón López S, Carmona Sánchez G, Mata-Alcázar-Caballero R, Sánchez-Pernaute R (2022) Mesenchymal stromal cells for treating steroid-resistant acute and chronic graft versus host disease: a multicenter compassionate use experience. Stem Cells Transl Med 11(4):343–355. https://doi.org/10.1093/stcltm/szac003

Macmillan ML, Blazar BR, DeFor T, Wagner JE (2009) Transplantation of ex vivo culture-expanded parental haploidentical mesenchymal stem cells to promote engraftment in pediatric recipients of unrelated donor umbilical cord blood: results of a phase I–II clinical trial. Bone Marrow Transplant 43:447–454. https://doi.org/10.1038/bmt.2008.348

MacMillan ML, Holtan SG, Rashidi A, DeFor TE, Blazar BR, Weisdorf DJ (2020) Pediatric acute GVHD: clinical phenotype and response to upfront steroids. Bone Marrow Transplant 55(1):165–171. https://doi.org/10.1038/s41409-019-0651-9

McElvaney OJ, Curley GF, Rose-John S, McElvaney NG (2021) Interleukin-6: obstacles to targeting a complex cytokine in critical illness. Lancet Respir Med 16:S2213–S2600. https://doi.org/10.1016/S2213-2600(21)00103-X

Mendelson A, Frenette PS (2014) Hematopoietic stem cell niche maintenance during homeostasis and regeneration. Nat Med 20:833–846. https://doi.org/10.1038/nm.3647

Mohyeldin A, Garzón-Muvdi T, Quiñones-Hinojosa A (2010) Oxygen in stem cell biology: a critical component of the stem cell niche. Cell Stem Cell 7(2):150–161. https://doi.org/10.1016/j.stem.2010.07.007

Monsel A, Hauw-Berlemont C, Mebarki M, Heming N, Mayaux J, Nguekap TO, Diehl J-L, Demoule A, Annane D, Marois C (2022) Treatment of COVID-19-associated ARDS with mesenchymal stromal cells: a multicenter randomized double-blind trial. Crit Care 26:48. https://doi.org/10.1186/s13054-022-03930-4

Morata-Tarifa C, Macías-Sánchez MDM, Gutiérrez-Pizarraya A, Sanchez-Pernaute R (2020) Mesenchymal stromal cells for the prophylaxis and treatment of graft-versus-host disease-a meta-analysis. Stem Cell Res Ther 11(1):64. https://doi.org/10.1186/s13287-020-01592-z

Morikawa S, Mabuchi Y, Kubota Y, Nagai Y, Niibe K, Hiratsu E, Suzuki S, Miyauchi-Hara C, Nagoshi N, Sunabori T (2009) Prospective identification, isolation, and systemic transplantation of multipotent mesenchymal stem cells in murine bone marrow. J Exp Med 206:2483–2496. https://doi.org/10.1084/jem.20091046

Muguruma Y, Yahata T, Miyatake H, Sato T, Uno T, Itoh J, Kato S, Ito M, Hotta T, Ando K (2006) Reconstitution of the functional human hematopoietic microenvironment derived from human mesenchymal stem cells in the murine bone marrow compartment. Blood 107:1878–1887

Muhammad G, Xu J, Bulte JWM, Jablonska A, Walczak P, Janowski M (2017) Transplanted adipose-derived stem cells can be short-lived yet accelerate healing of acid-burn skin wounds: a multimodal imaging study. Sci Rep 7(1):4644. https://doi.org/10.1038/s41598-017-04484-0

Naso MF, Tomkowicz B, Perry WL, Strohl WR (2017) Adeno-associated virus (AAV) as a vector for gene therapy. Bio Drugs 31(4):317–334. https://doi.org/10.1007/s40259-017-0234

Nauta AJ, Westerhuis G, Kruisselbrink AB, Lurvink EGA, Willemze R, Fibbe WE (2006) Donor-derived mesenchymal stem cells are immunogenic in an allogeneic host and stimulate donor graft rejection in a nonmyeloablative setting. Blood 108:2114–2120. https://doi.org/10.1182/blood-2005-11-011650

NHS England Specialised Services Clinical Reference Group for Blood and Marrow Transplantation (2017) Clinical commissioning policy: treatments for graft versus host disease (GvHD) following haematopoietic stem cell transplantation, p 20. https://www.england.nhs.uk/wp-content/uploads/2017/03/gvhd-heamatopoietic-stem-cell.pdf

O'Donoghue K, Fisk NM (2004) Fetal stem cells. Best Pract Res Clin Obstet Gynaecol 18:853–875. https://doi.org/10.1016/j.bpobgyn.2004.06.010

Ohori-Morita Y, Niibe K, Limraksasin P, Nattasit P, Miao X, Yamada M, Mabuchi Y, Matsuzaki Y, Egusa H (2022) Novel mesenchymal stem cell spheroids with enhanced stem cell characteristics and bone regeneration ability. Stem Cells Transl Med 11(4):434–449. https://doi.org/10.1093/stcltm/szab030

Panoskaltsis-Mortari A, Price A, Hermanson JR, Taras E, Lees C, Serody JS, Blazar BR (2004) In vivo imaging of graft-versus-hostdisease in mice. Blood 103:3590–3598. https://doi.org/10.1182/blood-2003-08-2827

Petrenko Y, Sykova E, Kubinova S (2017) The therapeutic potential of three-dimensional multipotent mesenchymal stromal cell spheroids. Stem Cell Res Ther 8(1):94. https://doi.org/10.1186/s13287-017-0558-6

Pinto ARAR, Chandran A, Rosenthal NANA, Godwin JWJW (2013) Isolation and analysis of single cells from the mouse heart. J Immunol Methods 393:74–80. https://doi.org/10.1016/j.jim.2013.03.012

Pittenger MF, Discher DE, Peault BM, Phinney DG, Hare JM, Caplan AI (2019) Mesenchymal stem cell perspective: cell biology to clinical progress. NPJ Regen Med 4:22. https://doi.org/10.1038/s41536-019-0083-6

Polchert D, Sobinsky J, Douglas G, Kidd M, Moadsiri A, Reina E, Genrich K, Mehrotra S, Setty S, Smith B, Bartholomew A (2008) IFN-gamma activation of mesenchymal stem cells for treatment and prevention of graft versus host disease. Eur J Immunol 38(6):1745–1755. https://doi.org/10.1002/eji.200738129

Ponchel F, Churchman S, El-Jawhari JJ, Burska AN, Chambers P, Vital EM, El-Sherbiny YM, Jones E, Conaghan PG, Goeb V, Emery P (2021) Interleukin-7: a potential factor supporting B-cell maturation in the rheumatoid arthritis synovium. Clin Exp Rheumatol 39(2):253–262

Pösel C, Möller K, Fröhlich W, Schulz I, Boltze J, Wagner D-C (2012) Density gradient centrifugation compromises bone marrow mononuclear cell yield. PLoS One 7(12):e50293. https://doi.org/10.1371/journal.pone.0050293

Pricola KL, Kuhn NZ, Haleem-Smith H, Song Y, Tuan RS (2009) Interleukin-6 maintains bone marrow-derived mesenchymal stem cell stemness by an ERK1/2-dependent mechanism. J Cell Biochem 108(3):577–588. https://doi.org/10.1002/jcb.22289

Rasouli M, Naeimzadeh Y, Hashemi N, Hosseinzadeh S (2024) Age-related alterations in mesenchymal stem cell function: understanding mechanisms and seeking opportunities to bypass the cellular aging. Curr Stem Cell Res Ther 19(1):15–32. https://doi.org/10.2174/1574888X18666230113144016

Ringden O, Baygan A, Remberger M, Gustafsson B, Winiarski J, Khoein B, Moll G, Klingspor L, Westgren M, Sadeghi B (2018) Placenta derived decidua stromal cells for treatment of severe acute graft versus host disease. Stem Cells Transl Med 7:325–331. https://doi.org/10.1002/sctm.17-0167

Rodríguez-Fuentes DE, Fernández-Garza LE, Samia-Meza JA, Barrera-Barrera SA, Caplan AI, Barrera-Saldaña HA (2021) Mesenchymal stem cells current clinical applications: a systematic review. Arch Med Res 52:93–101. https://doi.org/10.1016/j.arcmed.2020.08.006

Roemeling-van Rhijn M, de Klein A, Douben H, Pan Q, van der Laan LJ, Ijzermans JN, Betjes MG, Baan CC, Weimar W, Hoogduijn MJ (2013) Culture expansioninduces non-tumorigenic aneuploidy in adipose tissue derived mesenchymal stromal cells. Cytotherapy 15(11):1352–1361. https://doi.org/10.1016/j.jcyt.2013.07.004

Sage EK, Thakrar RM, Janes SM (2016) Genetically modified mesenchymal stromal cells in cancer therapy. Cytotherapy 18(11):1435–1445. https://doi.org/10.1016/j.jcyt.2016.09.003

Shimazawa Y, Kusamori K, Tsujimura M, Shimomura A, Takasaki R, Takayama Y, Shimizu K, Konishi S, Nishikawa M (2022) Intravenous injection of mesenchymal stem cell spheroids improves the pulmonary delivery and prolongs in vivo survival. Biotechnol J 17(1):e2100137. https://doi.org/10.1002/biot.202100137

Shu L, Niu C, Li R, Huang T, Wang Y, Huang M, Ji N, Zheng Y, Chen X, Shi L (2020) Treatment of severe COVID-19 with human umbilical cord mesenchymal stem cells. Stem Cell Res Ther 11(1):361. https://doi.org/10.1186/s13287-020-01875-5

Siegel G, Schäfer R, Dazzi F (2009) The immunosuppressive properties of mesenchymal stem cells. Transplantation 87:S45–S49. https://doi.org/10.1097/TP.0b013e3181a285b0

Sotiropoulou PA, Perez SA, Salagianni M, Baxevanis CN, Papamichail M (2006) Characterization of the optimal culture conditions for clinical scale production of human mesenchymal stem cells. Stem Cells 24(2):462–471. https://doi.org/10.1634/stemcells.2004-0331

Spees JL, Gregory CA, Singh H, Tucker HA, Peister A, Lynch PJ, Hsu SC, Smith J, Prockop DJ (2004) Internalized antigens must be removed to prepare hypoimmunogenic mesenchymal stem cells for cell and gene therapy. Mol Ther 9(5):747–756. https://doi.org/10.1016/j.ymthe.2004.02.012

Steensberg A, Fischer CP, Keller C, Møller K, Pedersen BK (2003) IL-6 enhances plasma IL-1ra, IL-10, and cortisol in humans. Am J Physiol Endocrinol Metab 285(2):E433–E437

Stenderup K, Justesen J, Clausen C, Kassem M (2003) Aging is associated with decreased maximal life span and accelerated senescence of bone marrow stromal cells. Bone 33:919–926. https://doi.org/10.1016/j.bone.2003.07.005

Stenger E, Giver CR, Langston A, Kota D, Das PK, Chinnadurai R, Galipeau J, Waller EK, Qayed M (2022) Safety of autologous freshly expanded mesenchymal stromal cells for the treatment of graft-versus-host disease. Front Immunol 13:959658. https://doi.org/10.3389/fimmu.2022.959658

Swart JF, de Roock S, Nievelstein RAJ, Slaper-Cortenbach ICM, Boelens JJ, Wulffraat NM (2019) Bone-marrow derived mesenchymal stromal cells infusion in therapy refractory juvenile idiopathic arthritis patients. Rheumatology (Oxford) 58(10):1812–1817. https://doi.org/10.1093/rheumatology/kez157

Tolouei AE, Oruji F, Tehrani S, Rezaei S, Mozaffari A, Jahri M, Nasiri K (2023) Gingival mesenchymal stem cell therapy, immune cells, and immunoinflammatory application. Mol Biol Rep 50(12):10461–10469. https://doi.org/10.1007/s11033-023-08826-2

Troyer DL, Weiss ML (2008) Wharton's jelly-derived cells are a primitive stromal cell population. Stem Cells 26:591–599. https://doi.org/10.1634/stemcells.2007-0439

Uccelli A, Moretta L, Pistoia V (2008) Mesenchymal stem cells in health and disease. Nat Rev Immunol 8:726–736

Uruski P, Sepetowska A, Konieczna C, Pakuła M, Wyrwa M, Tussupkaliyev A, Tykarski A, Mikuła-Pietrasik J, Książek K (2021) Primary high-grade serousovarian cancer cells are sensitive to senescence induced by carboplatin and paclitaxel in vitro. Cell Mol Biol Lett 26(1):44–53. https://doi.org/10.1186/s11658-021-00287-4

von Bahr L, Sundberg B, Lönnies L, Sander B, Karbach H, Hägglund H, Ljungman P, Gustafsson B, Karlsson H, Le Blanc K, Ringdén O (2012) Long-term complications, immunologic effects, and role of passage for outcome in mesenchymal stromal cell therapy. Biol Blood Marrow Transplant 18(4):557–564. https://doi.org/10.1016/j.bbmt.2011.07.023

Wang ZH, Wu XX, Cao YB, Liu ZY, Xu LX, Li XH, Wu YM, Liu B, Yan B, Da WM (2013) Clinical analysis of high risk and refractory malignant hematologic diseases treated with haploidentical hematopoietic stem cell transplantation combined with umbilical cord mesenchymal stem cells using modified conditioning regimen. Zhongguo Shi Yan Xue Ye Xue Za Zhi 21:1224–1227. https://doi.org/10.7534/j.issn.1009-2137.2013.05.028

Wang Z, Samanipour R, Kim K, Wang Z (2016) Organ-on-a-chip platforms for drug screening and tissue engineering. In: Biomedical engineering: frontier research and converging technologies, vol 9. Springer, Berlin, Germany, pp 209–233

Wang Z-K, Yu H-J, Cao F-L, Liu Z-H, Liu Z-U, Feng W-J, Liu X-L, Yu Y-Y, Xiao Y, Li L-M, Zhou J (2019) Donor-derived marrow mesenchymal stromal cell co-transplantation following a haploidentical hematopoietic stem cell transplantation trail to treat severe aplastic anemia in children. Ann Hematol 98(2):473–479. https://doi.org/10.1007/s00277-018-3523-2

Wexler SA, Donaldson C, Denning-Kendall P, Rice C, Bradley B, Hows JM (2003) Adult bone marrow is a rich source of human mesenchymal 'stem' cells but umbilical cord and mobilized adult blood are not. Br J Haematol 121:368–374. https://doi.org/10.1046/j.1365-2141.2003.04284.x

Wilson A, Trumpp A (2006) Bone-marrow haematopoietic-stem-cell niches. Nat Rev Immunol 6(2):93–106. https://doi.org/10.1038/nri1779

Wilson JG, Liu KD, Zhuo H, Caballero L, McMillan M, Fang X, Cosgrove K, Vojnik R, Calfee CS, Lee JW, Rogers AJ, Levitt J, Wiener-Kronish J, Bajwa EK, Leavitt A, McKenna D, Thompson BT, Matthay MA (2015) Mesenchymal stem (stromal) cells for treatment of ARDS: a phase 1 clinical trial. Lancet Respir Med 3(1):24–32. https://doi.org/10.1016/S2213-2600(14)70291-7

Wilson A, Hodgson-Garms M, Frith JE, Genever P (2019) Multiplicity of mesenchymal stromal cells: finding the right route to therapy. Front Immunol 10:1112. https://doi.org/10.3389/fimmu.2019.01112

Wu X, Chen L, Xu Y, Wen J, Ruan Y, He Y, Li C (2015) The relationship between some cytokines and graft versus host disease after allogeneic hematopoietic stem cell transplantation in thalassemia major patients. Blood 126(23):5471. https://doi.org/10.1182/blood.V126.23.5471.5471

Xu X, Jiang W, Chen L, Xu Z, Zhang Q, Zhu M, Ye P, Li H, Yu L, Zhou X (2021) Evaluation of the safety and efficacy of using human menstrual blood-derived mesenchymal stromal cells in treating severe and critically ill COVID-19 patients: an exploratory clinical trial. Clin Transl Med 11:e297. https://doi.org/10.1002/ctm2.297

Yagi H, Soto-Gutierrez A, Parekkadan B, Kitagawa Y, Tompkins RG, Kobayashi N, Yarmush ML (2010) Mesenchymal stem cells: mechanisms of immunomodulation and homing. Cell Transplant 19:667–679. https://doi.org/10.3727/096368910X508762

Yen BL, Hsieh CC, Hsu PJ, Chang CC, Wang LT, Yen ML (2023) Three-dimensional spheroid culture of human mesenchymal stem cells: offering therapeutic advantages and in vitro glimpses of the in vivo state. Stem Cells Transl Med 12(5):235–244. https://doi.org/10.1093/stcltm/szad01

Yeung CK, Yan Y, Yan L, Duan Y, Li E, Huang B, Lu K, Li K, Zhou M, Zhang L, Wu Y, Luo KQ, Ji W, Xu RH, Si W (2022) Preclinical safety evaluation and tracing of human mesenchymal stromal cell spheroids following intravenous injection into cynomolgus monkeys. Biomaterials 289:121759. https://doi.org/10.1016/j.biomaterials.2022.121759

Yin X, Hu L, Zhang Y, Zhu C, Cheng H, Xie X, Shi M, Zhu P, Zhao X, Chen W, Zhang L, Arakaki C, Hao S, Wang M, Cao W, Ma S, Zhang XB, Cheng T (2020) PDGFB-expressing mesenchymal stem cells improve human hematopoietic stem cell engraftment in immunodeficient mice. Bone Marrow Transplant 55(6):1029–1040. https://doi.org/10.1038/s41409-019-0766-z

Yoshida N, Kobayashi R, Yabe H, Kosaka Y, Yagasaki H, Watanabe K, Kudo K, Morimoto A, Ohga S, Muramatsu H, Takahashi Y, Kato K, Suzuki R, Ohara A, Kojima S (2014) First-line treatment for severe aplastic anemia in children: bone marrow transplantation from a matched family donor versus immunosuppressive therapy. Haematologica 99:1784–1791. https://doi.org/10.3324/haematol.2014.109355

Yuan YH, Zhou CF, Lu ZY et al (2016a) Intrabone marrow injection enhances placental mesenchymal stem cell mediated support of hematopoiesis in mice. Turk J Med Sci 46:174–184. https://doi.org/10.3906/sag-1411-161

Yuan Z, Lourenco SDS, Sage EK, Kolluri KK, Lowdell MW, Janes SM (2016b) Cryopreservation of human mesenchymal stromal cells expressing TRAIL for human anti-cancer therapy. Cytotherapy 18:860–869. https://doi.org/10.1016/j.jcyt.2016.04.005

Zeiser R, Blazar BR (2017) Acute graft-versus-host disease – biologic process, prevention, and therapy. N Engl J Med 377:2167–2179. https://doi.org/10.1056/NEJMra1609337

Zhang XH, Chen J, Han MZ, Huang H, Jiang EL, Jiang M, Lai YR, Liu DH, Liu QF, Liu T, Ren HY, Song YP, Sun ZM, Tang XW, Wang JM, Wu DP, Xu LP, Zhang X, Zhou DB, Huang XJ (2021) The consensus from the Chinese society of hematology on indications, conditioning regimens and donor selection for allogeneic hematopoietic stem cell transplantation: 2021 update. J Hematol Oncol 14(1):145. https://doi.org/10.1186/s13045-021-01159-2

Zhao K, Lin R, Fan Z, Chen X, Wang Y, Huang F, Xu N, Zhang X, Zhang X, Xuan L, Wang S, Lin D, Deng L, Nie D, Weng J, Li Y, Zhang X, Li Y, Xiang AP, Liu Q (2022) Mesenchymal stromal cells plus basiliximab, calcineurin inhibitor as treatment of steroid-resistant acute graft-versus-host disease: a multicenter, randomized, phase 3, open-label trial. J Hematol Oncol 15(1):22. https://doi.org/10.1186/s13045-022-01240-4

Zheng G, Huang L, Tong H, Shu Q, Hu Y, Ge M, Deng K, Zhang L, Zou B, Cheng B, Xu J (2014) Treatment of acute respiratory distress syndrome with allogeneic adipose-derived mesenchymal stem cells: a randomized, placebo-controlled pilot study. Respir Res 15:39. https://doi.org/10.1186/1465-9921-15-39

Zhu GR, Zhou XY, Lu H, Zhou JW, Li AP, Xu W, Li JY, Wang CY (2003) Human bone marrow mesenchymal stem cells express multiple hematopoietic growth factors. Zhongguo Shi Yan Xue Ye Xue Za Zhi 11(2):115–119

From Modification Maps to Clinical Impact: RNA Epigenetics in Cancer Diagnosis and Treatment

Osama Sweef, Malek Asfar, Eun-Seok Choi, Yalitza Lopez Corcino, Venetia D. Thomas, Ali Albowaidy, and Saori Furuta

Abstract

The intricacy of RNA modifications has emerged as a focal topic of cancer research, accounting for the multifaceted roles of epitranscriptomic modifications in tumor initiation, progression, and therapeutic responses. In particular, dysregulated RNA modifications, exemplified by aberrant N6-methyladenosine (m6A), 5-methylcytosine (m5C), have been closely linked to oncogenic transformation, tumor progression, and therapeutic resistance across various cancer types. Thus, the use of certain RNA modification profiles as diagnostic biomarkers holds promise for precision medicine interventions. Moreover, targeting enzymes responsible for RNA modification dynamics has emerged as a new cancer therapeutic strategy. This chapter provides a comprehensive review

O. Sweef (✉)
Division of Cancer Biology, Department of Medicine, MetroHealth Medical Center, Case Western Reserve University School of Medicine, Cleveland, OH, USA

Department of Zoology, Faculty of Science, Tanta University, Tanta, Egypt
e-mail: oas38@case.edu; osama.sweef@case.edu

M. Asfar
Department of Pathology, MetroHealth Medical Center, Case Western Reserve University School of Medicine, Cleveland, OH, USA
e-mail: malassfar@metrohealth.org

E.-S. Choi · Y. L. Corcino · V. D. Thomas · S. Furuta (✉)
Division of Cancer Biology, Department of Medicine, MetroHealth Medical Center, Case Western Reserve University School of Medicine, Cleveland, OH, USA
e-mail: sxf494@case.edu

A. Albowaidy
Department of Microbiology, Immunology, and Cell Biology, School of Medicine, West Virginia University, Morgantown, WV, USA

The Ragon Institute, Mass General, MIT, and Harvard, Cambridge, MA, USA

Interdisciplinary Cancer Research, https://doi.org/10.1007/16833_2024_460
Published online: 07 November 2024

of RNA modifications, including m6A and m5C, and pseudouridine (Ψ), highlighting their functional implications, diagnostic potentials, and therapeutic significance within the context of cancer. Through a detailed examination of recent studies, the review describes the dynamic regulatory mechanisms of diverse RNA modifications and their contributions to altered gene expression, splicing pattern, and translation efficiency. Lastly, the chapter describes the transformative potential of RNA-based diagnostics and therapeutics in reshaping cancer research and treatment modalities.

Keywords

Biomarker · Cancer · Diagnosis · Epitranscriptomics · RNA modification · Therapeutic target

Abbreviations

3′-UTR	3′-untranslated region
5′-UTR	5′-untranslated region
ARID	autosomal recessive forms of intellectual disabilities
CDS	coding sequence
DS	Dubowitz syndrome
eRNA	enhancer RNA
HCC	hepatocellular carcinoma
lincRNA	long intergenic noncoding RNA
lncRNA	long noncoding RNA
MERFF	myoclonic epilepsy with ragged red fibers
MiRNA	microRNA
mRNA	messenger RNA
Mt-tRNA	mitochondrial tRNA
NA	information not found
PAD	peripheral arterial disease
rRNA	ribosomal RNA
scaRNA	small Cajal body-specific RNA
snoRNA	small nucleolar RNA
snRNA	small nuclear RNA
tRNA	transfer RNA

1 Introduction

Recently, regulatory roles of RNA modifications have garnered increasing attention due to their intricate involvements in tumor initiation, progression, and therapeutic response. RNAs are no longer regarded as mere intermediaries between DNAs and proteins; instead, they emerge as dynamic entities susceptible to a myriad of chemical alterations that impact their structures, stabilities, and functions (Wu et al. 2023). These RNA modifications have shed light on a new dimension of the molecular complexity of cancer, serving as novel diagnostic biomarkers and therapeutic targets. Emerging evidence supports the pivotal contributions of various RNA modifications, such as m6A, m5C, 2′-O-methylation, inosine (I), N1-methyladenosine (m1A), 5-hydroxymethylcytosine (hm5C), N7-methylguanosine (m7G), ribose 2′-O-methylation, methylations of ribose, and pseudouridine (Ψ), in modulating RNA stability, localization, translation efficiency, and splicing patterns. Dysregulation of these modifications has been linked to oncogenic transformation, tumor metastasis, and therapeutic resistance in a wide spectrum of cancer types (Barbieri and Kouzarides 2020). As our understanding of these intricate molecular mechanisms expands, the potential to harness RNA modifications for diagnostic and therapeutic purposes becomes increasingly tangible.

The identification of RNA modifications as potential diagnostic biomarkers holds significant promise in the realm of precision medicine (Sun et al. 2019). The distinct patterns of RNA modifications that arise in cancer cells can serve as fingerprints that differentiate them from normal counterparts, offering a novel avenue for non-invasive early detection and accurate classification of malignancies (Jin et al. 2023). Moreover, the dynamic nature of RNA modifications enables real-time monitoring of disease progression and treatment response, presenting an opportunity to tailor therapeutic interventions to individual patient profiles. Beyond diagnostics, RNA modifications also unveil a trove of therapeutic targets that can be exploited to rewire cancer cell behavior. Targeting enzymes responsible for installing or erasing specific modifications emerges as a novel strategy to disrupt oncogenic signaling pathways, restore tumor suppressor functions, and sensitize cancer cells to existing treatments (Liu and Su 2021). By understanding the precise roles of individual RNA modifications within various cellular contexts, the development of selective and efficacious therapies can be advanced.

In this review, we comprehensively explore the intricate landscape of RNA modifications in cancer, elucidating their functional implications, diagnostic potential, and therapeutic significance. By delving into recent advancements and studies that unravel the interplay between RNA modifications and cancer biology, we aim to provide a comprehensive overview of the evolving field and highlight its potential to revolutionize cancer diagnosis and treatment strategies.

2 RNA Modification Landscape in Cancer

RNA modifications constitute a vital layer of gene expression regulation that extends beyond the DNA code. Emerging evidence attests to their critical involvement in cancer pathogenesis, underscoring the need for a better understanding of the RNA modification landscape in malignancies (Deng et al. 2018). This review serves as an exhaustive exploration of the current state of knowledge regarding RNA modifications in the cancer context, offering insights into their mechanisms and significance.

2.1 Various Types of RNA Modifications Dysregulated in Cancer

RNA modifications are key regulators of cellular processes, impacting RNA stability, structure, and function. m6A, one of the most abundant RNA modifications, is controlled by writer, eraser, and reader proteins, influencing messenger RNA (mRNA) stability, splicing, translation, and localization. Its dysregulation is linked to cancer progression, suggesting potential therapeutic targets (Yu et al. 2022). Similarly, m5C plays a role in RNA stability and is implicated in cancer, with a complex role in tumor-suppressive and oncogenic pathways. Pseudouridine (Ψ) is another significant modification that contributes to RNA stability and function, affecting ribosome assembly and splicing. The impact of 2′-O-methylation on RNA-protein interactions and translation efficiency also underscores its importance in cellular processes and its potential role in cancer (Zhang et al. 2021). Inosine allows for flexible codon-anticodon interactions, with a noted influence on RNA editing and miRNA targeting in cancer contexts. N1-Methyladenosine (m1A) influences translation and RNA structure, suggesting a role in gene regulation. 5-Hydroxymethylcytosine (hm5C), though less understood, has implications for RNA stability and translation, with emerging links to cancer. Additionally, N7-methylguanosine (m7G) plays a crucial role in ribosome function and stability, impacting translational efficiency (Stockert et al. 2019). Other modifications, such as N6-threonylcarbamoyladenosine (t6A) and 2-thiocytidine (s2C), are also of interest due to their impact on translational fidelity and tRNA function. The variety and complexity of these RNA modifications highlight their significance in both normal cellular functions and disease mechanisms, particularly in oncogenesis. Dysregulation in these modifications can contribute to cancer progression, underscoring the need for further exploration to understand their therapeutic potential (Dominissini et al. 2011). These contents are briefly summarized in Fig. 1 and Table 1.

3 RNA Modifications as Diagnostic Biomarkers

RNA modifications have garnered increasing attention as potential diagnostic biomarkers in various diseases, including cancer. These modifications, such as m6A, m5C, and Ψ, exhibit dynamic alterations in disease states, reflecting underlying changes in gene expression and cellular processes. Dysregulated m6A modification has been implicated in cancer progression and drug resistance. While aberrant m5C levels are associated with cancer subtype classification. Ψ modification, known to impact tRNA stability and translation efficiency, may serve as a diagnostic marker for cancer subtyping and prognosis prediction (Qiu et al. 2023). The integration of RNA modification profiles as diagnostic indicators holds promise for enhancing disease detection and facilitating tailored therapeutic interventions.

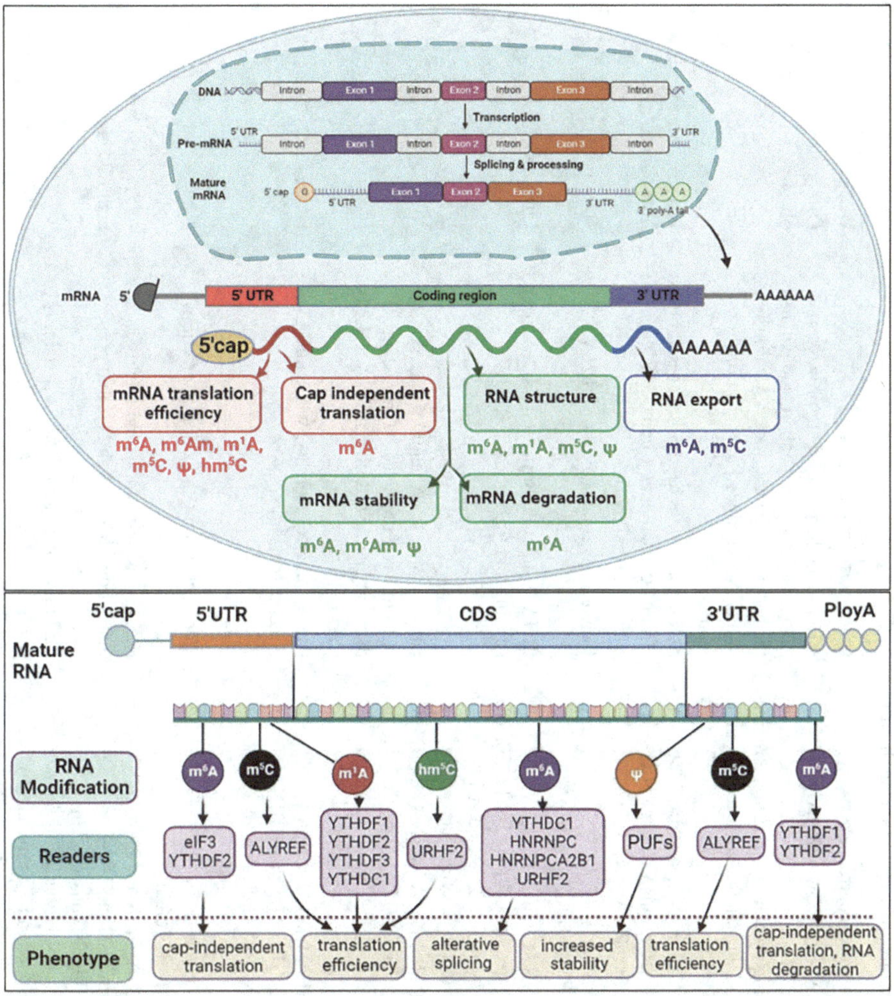

Fig. 1 A diagram illustrating representative RNA maturation and modification types. (**a**) The impact of mRNA base modifications on post-transcriptional gene regulation. Within the nucleus, these modifications play crucial roles in (1) pre-mRNA processing, (2) pri-miRNA maturation, and (3) facilitating the export of these molecules from the nucleus. Once in the cytoplasm, RNA base modifications continue to exert influence by regulating (4) mRNA degradation, (5) mRNA stability, (6) RNA structure, and (7) mRNA translation efficiency. (**b**) The diagram portrays potential chemical alterations occurring at distinct nitrogen bases within mRNA. It meticulously highlights the favored positions of each modification along the mRNA sequence and provides insight into the associated reader proteins. Notably, the modifications featured include m6A, pseudouridine (Ψ), m5C, 5-hydroxymethylcytidine (hm5C), and N1-methyladenosine (m1A)

Table 1 Varieties of RNA modifications: functions and implications in disease

Modification type	RNA types with occurrence	Role and function	Diseases
N6-methyladenosine	(rRNA, tRNA, mRNA, miRNA, lncRNA, circRN, snRNA) mRNA is highly concentrated in the regions of 5′-UTRs, surrounding stop codons, and within 3′ UTRs	mRNA: modulates splicing processes, triggers mRNA degradation, and enhances translation efficiency; lncRNA: contributes to lncRNA-mediated transcriptional repression	Osteoporosis, HCC, obesity
Pseudouridine	(rRNA, tRNA, mRNA, snRNA, Mt-tRNA, scaRNA, snoRN, miRNA, lincRNA) tRNA: p. 55; mRNA: 5′UTR, 3′UTR, CDS	rRNA contributes to ribosome assembly and ensures translational accuracy. tRNA enhances stability	Prostate, breast, and lung cancers; HCC
Archaeosine	(tRNA) tRNA: p. 15 (always), p.13	Increases thermal stability of tRNA	NA
Dihydrouridine	(tRNA, mRNA, snoRNA) tRNA: Located at positions 16, 17, 20, 20a, 20b, and 47. mRNA: Detected at 130 sites in 112 transcripts in S. cerevisiae	tRNA destabilizes structure; mRNA impacts splicing and translation	Lung cancer
2′-O-methylation	(rRNA, tRNA, mRNA, snRNA, snoRNA) mRNA: 5′UTR, 3′UTR, CDS; tRNA: p. 4	Nm enhances RNA stability and promotes A-form RNA duplexes by increasing thermodynamic stability in RNA:RNA base pairs	Asthma, Alzheimer's
7-methylguanosine	(miRNA, rRNA, mRNA, tRNA,) RNA: SSU G1639 (human); tRNA: p. 46; mRNA: 4522 clusters in 2318 mRNAs	tRNA enhances stability, while mRNA governs translation	HCC, PAD, lung cancer
Wybutosine	(tRNA) tRNAPhe: p. 37 (often)	Stabilizes codon–anticodon interactions	NA
5-methylcytidine	(rRNA, tRNA, mRNA, eRNA, miRNA, lncRNA, snRNA, snoRNA) rRNA: are highly conserved in eukaryotes. tRNA: Variability in the loop, anticodon loop, and T stem. mRNA: Abundantly enriched in the 5′UTR region.	rRNA: Ensures folding and fidelity in translation. tRNA: Stability, and proper codon-anticodon interactions, maintaining reading frame. mRNA: Impacts stability and translation speed. lncRNA: Influences stability	ARID, DS, lactic acidosis, breast cancer

N2,N2-dimethylguanosine	(tRNA, mRNA) tRNA: p. 10, p. 26 (always); mRNA (0.00051% G in S. cerevisiae)	tRNA ensures correct folding and prevents misfolding. mRNA decreases translation accuracy based on position and codon	NA
5-methyluridine	(rRNA, tRNA) tRNA: p. 54	tRNA translation accuracy, folding, and stability	Breast cancer
5-methylaminomethyl-2-thiouridine	(tRNA) tRNALys3UUU: p. 34 (always)	Required for decoding of the lysine codons AAA and AAG by tRNALys3UUU	NA
N4-acetylcytidine	(rRNA, tRNA, mRNA) tRNA: Consistently found at position 12. rRNA: Located in helix 34 and 45. mRNA: in 5′UTR and CDS regions	tRNA enhances translation precision and speed. mRNA boosts stability	NA
N1-methyladenosine	(rRNA, tRNA, mRNA, lncRNA) rRNA: p.1322 in 28S; tRNA: p. 9, 14, 16, 22, 57, 58; mRNA: rare	rRNA: ensures proper folding; tRNA: ensures stability and proper folding	HCC, pancreatic, breast cancer
5-formylcytidine	(tRNA) mt-tRNAMet: p.C34 (always)	Essential for AUA codon decoding in mitochondria	NA
3-methyluridine	(rRNA, tRNA) rRNA: U1498 (always in E. coli 16S), U2634 U2843 (in S. cerevisiae 25S)	Unknown	NA
Wyosine	(tRNA) tRNAPhe: p. 37 (often)	Enhances codon-anticodon stability	NA
1-methylinosine	(tRNA) tRNAAla: p. 37 (eukaryotes); tRNA: p. 57 (archaea)	Unknown	NA
3-methylcytidine	(tRNA) tRNA: p. 32 (30–90%, depending on tRNA)	Unknown	Many cancer
Queuosine	(tRNA) tRNATyr, tRNAHis, tRNAAsn, tRNAAsp: p. 34 (humans)	Enhances tRNA's coding potential, shielding it from ribonuclease cleavage	T-cell lymphoma, colon cancer

(continued)

Table 1 (continued)

Modification type	RNA types with occurrence	Role and function	Diseases
5-methoxycarbonylmethyl-2-thiouridine	(tRNA) tRNALysUUU, tRNAGluUUC, tRNAGlnUUG: p. 34 (always)	Enhances tRNA decoding efficacy	NA
1-methylguanosine	(tRNA, mRNA) tRNALeuCUN, tRNAProCCN, tRNAArgCGG: p. 37 (always); tRNA: p. 9 (always in S. cerevisiae); mRNA (0.00046% G in S. cerevisiae)	tRNA prevents frameshifting, while mRNA reduces translation fidelity in a codon-dependent manner	NA
2-thiocytidine	(tRNA) tRNAArg, tRNASer2GCU: p. 32 (always)	Limits recognition of specific wobble codons	NA
N6-threonylcarbamoyladenosine	(tRNA) tRNAANN: p. A37 (always)	Enhances codon-anticodon pairing and prevents frameshifts during protein synthesis	MERFF, neurodegeneration, diabetes
N6-isopentenyladenosine	(tRNA) tRNAUNN: p. A37 (always)	Enhances fidelity and efficiency of translation for specific codons	NA
Inosine	(tRNA, mRNA, miRNA) tRNA: p. 34, 37, 57; mRNA: dsRNA regions	tRNA is essential for recognizing wobble codons, while mRNA influences stability, localization, and alters the protein sequence	HCC; gastric, colorectal, glioblastoma, and lung cancers

3.1 Identification of RNA Modifications as Potential Cancer Biomarkers

Post-transcriptional RNA modifications have gained prominence as potential cancer biomarkers due to their dynamic roles in gene expression regulation. The diverse landscape of RNA modifications, including m6A, m5C, Ψ, and others, exhibits aberrant patterns in cancer cells that can be leveraged for diagnostic and prognostic purposes (Deng et al. 2023). These modifications influence various aspects of RNA processing, stability, and translation, impacting cancer-related pathways. The identification of specific RNA modification signatures holds promise for cancer subtype classification, prognosis prediction, and therapeutic stratification. A comprehensive table listing these RNA modifications and their associated cancer implications is provided in Table 2.

3.2 Detection Methods and Technologies for Assessing RNA Modifications

Recent strides in cancer research have spotlighted the crucial role of RNA modifications in gene expression and cancer progression. These modifications,

Table 2 RNA modifications as potential cancer biomarkers

RNA modification	Cancer type	Cancer implications	References
N6-methyladenosine	Glioblastoma, gastric, leukemia, breast	Stemness, drug resistance, metastasis	Li et al. (2022b)
5-Methylcytosine	Lung, colorectal, leukemia	mRNA stability, translational efficiency, oncogenesis	Huang et al. (2023)
Pseudouridine	Lung, prostate	Altered tRNA stability, translational control	Stockert et al. (2021)
Inosine	Multiple	miRNA binding, RNA structure modulation, immune response	Lee et al. (2017)
N1-methyladenosine	Uterus, ovarian	tRNA stability, translation regulation, cell growth	Zhao et al. (2023)
5-Hydroxymethylcytosine	Brain, blood, liver	Epitranscriptomic modulation, DNA methylation	Li et al. (2017)
N7-methylguanosine	Breast, liver, colon	tRNA and rRNA modification, translation regulation	Li et al. (2023a)
Ribose 2′-O-methylation	Colorectal, breast	RNA structure and function, splicing regulation	Tusup et al. (2018)
Methylations of ribose	Glioblastoma, ovarian	rRNA processing, protein synthesis, ribosome biogenesis	Majd et al. (2020)

including m6A, m5C, and Ψ, regulate key cellular processes like mRNA stability and translation, affecting cancer growth, metastasis, and drug resistance (Orsolic et al. 2023). Notably, their dysregulation has been linked to various cancers, such as breast, lung, and leukemia, suggesting their potential as diagnostic, prognostic, and therapeutic targets. For instance, aberrant m6A patterns in breast cancer correlate with tumor development, while m5C changes in lung cancer align with chemotherapy resistance, highlighting the clinical relevance of RNA modifications (Wang et al. 2023). The rise of high-throughput sequencing and bioinformatics has enabled more detailed profiling of these modifications, aiding in the discovery of novel biomarkers and advancing precision medicine.

High-performance liquid chromatography-mass spectrometry (HPLC-MS) is a popular technique for analyzing RNA modifications, combining liquid chromatography's separation ability with mass spectrometry's precision to identify and quantify various modified nucleosides like m6A, pseudouridine, and 5-methylcytosine. Despite its high sensitivity and accuracy, HPLC-MS demands extensive sample preparation, which can limit throughput (Gregorova et al. 2021). Antibody-based approaches, such as enzyme-linked immunosorbent assay (ELISA) and MeRIP-seq, utilize antibodies to capture modified RNA, with MeRIP-seq gaining traction for mapping m6A modifications across entire transcriptomes. However, these methods can suffer from antibody cross-reactivity and require high-quality antibodies (Körtel et al. 2021). Chemical labeling and sequencing involve using modified nucleotide analogs or chemical probes to detect specific RNA modifications, offering valuable insights but sometimes introducing artifacts during preparation (Peng et al. 2022). Emerging techniques like single-molecule real-time sequencing (SMRT-seq) and nanopore sequencing show promise for direct, long-read detection of RNA modifications without PCR amplification, although they still face challenges such as higher error rates and lower throughput (Boo and Kim 2020). As technology progresses, researchers can choose from a variety of methods to study RNA modifications, each with unique strengths and limitations, leading to a better understanding of these crucial biological processes.

3.3 Case Studies of Specific RNA Modifications as Diagnostic Indicators

Recent high-throughput sequencing technologies have revolutionized the profiling of RNA modifications, revealing their diagnostic and prognostic potential in cancer. This review highlights the role of specific RNA modifications, such as m6A, m5C, and Ψ, in cancer detection and prognosis, with case studies illustrating their clinical relevance (Meng et al. 2023). m6A is one of the most common RNA modifications in eukaryotes, dynamically regulated by writers, erasers, and readers, and is linked to tumorigenesis, metastasis, and drug resistance. In HCC, m6A modifications in the 3′ UTR of the KIAA1429 gene have been shown to promote cancer progression, indicating its potential as a diagnostic marker. Similarly, m5C plays a role in gene expression and has been associated with cancer progression and therapy response. In breast cancer, high levels of m5C in tRNA-derived fragments (tRFs) were correlated with poor survival, suggesting m5C as a prognostic indicator (Huang et al. 2021). Pseudouridine (Ψ), the most abundant RNA modification, is involved in various cellular processes. Though its diagnostic utility is less explored, targeting Ψ has therapeutic potential. For example, pseudouridine synthase 1 (PUS1) inhibitors have shown promise in treating acute myeloid leukemia (AML). These findings suggest that exploring RNA modifications could lead to new diagnostic and therapeutic strategies in cancer (He et al. 2022). Overall, these examples demonstrate that RNA modifications hold promise as diagnostic and prognostic markers, as well as therapeutic targets in cancer. Further research could lead to their clinical translation and broaden the scope of personalized cancer treatments.

4 Functional Roles of RNA Modifications in Cancer

The intricate regulatory landscape of cancer biology has recently expanded to encompass RNA modifications as pivotal players in shaping the pathogenesis of this multifaceted disease. This comprehensive review delves into the evolving understanding of the functional roles of RNA modifications in cancer, with a keen focus on their impact on gene expression, splicing, translation, and RNA stability (Teng et al. 2021). In addition, we explore the cellular pathways influenced by dysregulated RNA modifications that contribute to the complex tapestry of cancer progression. As we embark on this exploration, we incorporate the most up-to-date references, providing a contemporary perspective on the significance of RNA modifications in cancer, and highlighting their potential as targets for innovative therapeutic strategies.

4.1 Impact of RNA Modifications on Gene Expression and RNA Processing

Gene Expression RNA modifications, particularly m6A, have gained attention for their profound influence on gene expression in cancer. Recent studies have revealed that m6A modifications can either promote or suppress oncogene expression, thereby modulating cellular processes critical to cancer progression. Additionally, m6A modifications have been implicated in the regulation of tumor suppressor genes, exemplifying the multifaceted role of RNA modifications in cancer (Han et al. 2019).

Splicing RNA modifications, such as m6A and m5C, have been linked to alternative splicing events in cancer. These modifications can impact the splicing machinery, leading to aberrant isoform expression patterns in cancer cells. Dysregulated splicing, in turn, contributes to the generation of cancer-specific transcript variants with functional consequences for tumor development and progression (Kasowitz et al. 2018).

Translation M1A and Ψ modifications have been implicated in the regulation of translation efficiency and fidelity. Dysregulation of these modifications can result in the selective translation of cancer-associated transcripts, further emphasizing their role in cancer biology (Elliott and Holley 2021).

RNA Stability RNA modifications, such as 2′-O-methylation (2′-O-Me), have been shown to influence RNA stability. These modifications can affect the susceptibility of RNA molecules to degradation, impacting the turnover rates of transcripts involved in cancer-related processes (Yang et al. 2023).

4.2 Cellular Pathways Influenced by Dysregulated RNA Modifications in Cancer Progression

Dysregulated RNA modifications including perturbed m6A modification patterns have a significant impact on cellular pathways in cancer progression. It affects signaling pathways by disrupting mRNA stability, translation efficiency, and splicing events of key oncogenes and tumor suppressor genes (Liu et al. 2022). These alterations contribute to enhanced cell survival, proliferation, and epithelial-mesenchymal transition (EMT), fostering tumor aggressiveness. Furthermore, disrupted m6A dynamics have been associated with compromised DNA damage response pathways, potentially promoting genomic instability and therapeutic resistance (Liu and Su 2021). Understanding the intricate interplay between dysregulated RNA modifications and these cellular pathways is vital for identifying potential targets for precision cancer therapies.

4.2.1 RNA Modification-Mediated Signaling Pathways

Proliferation and Growth Signaling Pathways Aberrant RNA modifications can disrupt vital pathways like Wnt/β-catenin, PI3K/AKT, and MAPK/ERK, leading to uncontrolled cell division and tumor growth. This imbalance promotes oncogenesis and underscores the importance of understanding these modifications for therapeutic targeting (Liu et al. 2021a).

Apoptosis and Cell Death Pathways Altered RNA modifications can affect the balance between pro-apoptotic and anti-apoptotic genes, impeding programmed cell death and promoting tumor survival. This disruption often leads to unchecked growth and metastasis, highlighting the need for strategies to restore apoptosis and curb tumor progression (Xu et al. 2022).

DNA Damage Response Pathways RNA modifications can influence DNA repair mechanisms, with dysregulation leading to impaired responses to genotoxic stress and genomic instability. This contributes to the accumulation of genetic aberrations, driving malignant transformation and tumor progression. Understanding these processes is critical for developing therapies to restore DNA repair integrity (Xiang et al. 2017).

Epithelial-Mesenchymal Transition (EMT) Pathway Dysregulated RNA modifications can drive the transition from an epithelial to a mesenchymal phenotype, promoting tumor cell invasion and metastasis. This transition, facilitated by changes in EMT-associated gene expression, underscores the significance of RNA modifications in cancer metastasis (Alemu et al. 2016).

Angiogenesis Pathway RNA modifications can influence the expression of pro-angiogenic factors, promoting the formation of new blood vessels that support tumor growth and metastasis (Yang et al. 2020). Dysregulation in this pathway contributes to the vascularization of tumors, emphasizing the need for targeted approaches to control angiogenesis and impede tumor expansion.

4.2.2 Immune Evasion and RNA Modifications

Cancer cells use various mechanisms to evade the immune system, promoting tumor growth and progression. Recent research has revealed that RNA modifications, particularly m6A and m5C, play a key role in these immune evasion strategies. By altering RNA modification patterns, cancer cells can modulate immune-related gene expression, which impacts the production of immune checkpoint molecules, cytokines, and chemokines. These changes create an immunosuppressive tumor microenvironment that helps cancer cells avoid detection and destruction by the immune system (Li et al. 2022a, b). RNA modifications like m6A can affect the stability and translation of mRNA-encoding enzymes involved in cellular metabolism, such as glycolysis, the tricarboxylic acid (TCA) cycle, fatty acid metabolism, and amino acid metabolism. These pathways are crucial for immune cell activation and function, influencing how immune cells respond to pathogens and tumors. Additionally, m6A modifications regulate the expression of immune checkpoint molecules like PD-1 and CTLA-4, which are central to immune tolerance and activation (Yang et al. 2022).

By regulating cytokines and chemokines, RNA modifications also impact immune cell trafficking, inflammation, and effector functions, which are vital for effective immune responses. Understanding how RNA modifications interact with immune evasion mechanisms is critical for developing novel cancer therapies and targeting other immune-related diseases. This complex interplay between RNA modifications and immune evasion underscores the importance of further research to identify new therapeutic targets and strategies to combat cancer's ability to evade immune surveillance (Li et al. 2020).

4.2.3 RNA Modifications in Immune Recognition of Pathogens

The immune system's ability to detect foreign invaders like bacteria and viruses is heavily influenced by RNA modifications, which help distinguish self from non-self and guide appropriate immune responses. This concept is also crucial in cancer immunotherapy, where understanding how the immune system recognizes various RNA signatures can inform effective treatment strategies (Liu et al. 2021a, b).

Pattern recognition receptors (PRRs) in the innate immune system, such as Toll-like receptors (TLRs), are key to identifying microbial RNA. TLR7, for example, detects uridine-rich sequences in viral RNA, triggering immune responses through proinflammatory cytokines and type I interferons. Another significant recognition mechanism involves cytoplasmic RNA sensors like retinoic acid-inducible gene I (RIG-I) and melanoma differentiation-associated protein 5 (MDA5), which identify viral RNA by its 5′-triphosphate (5′-ppp) ends, in contrast to the 5′-monophosphate (5′-p) cap structure of host RNA (Wei et al. 2021). RNA editing enzymes, like adenosine deaminases acting on RNA (ADARs), also play a role in immune recognition by converting adenosine to inosine, potentially impacting viral RNA structure and its detection by RIG-I and MDA5. In cancer immunotherapy, understanding these mechanisms can lead to new treatments that leverage the immune system's ability to recognize unique RNA profiles in cancer cells, improving patient outcomes and advancing cancer therapies (Fritzell et al. 2018).

4.2.4 Epitranscriptomic Targeted Therapies

The dysregulation of RNA modifications in cancer has led to the development of epitranscriptomic targeted therapies. Recent advancements in this area include the design of small molecules and CRISPR-based approaches to modulate specific RNA modifications, offering new avenues for cancer treatment (Huang et al. 2020). In cancer, dysregulated RNA modifications contribute to tumor initiation, progression, and therapeutic resistance. By understanding the interplay between RNA modifications and cancer biology, researchers can develop innovative therapies to selectively modulate oncogenic pathways or sensitize tumors to conventional treatments. Moreover, RNA modifications play pivotal roles in neurological disorders, viral infections, and autoimmune diseases (Lennox and Behlke 2020). Harnessing the power of epitranscriptomics enables the design of RNA-targeted therapies tailored to specific disease signatures and patient populations. For instance, small molecules, antisense oligonucleotides (ASOs), and RNA-targeting enzymes offer versatile platforms for modulating RNA modifications and restoring cellular homeostasis. The development of epitranscriptomic targeted therapies presents both opportunities and challenges (Zhu et al. 2020). While the precise manipulation of RNA modifications holds immense therapeutic potential, deciphering the complex regulatory networks governing epitranscriptomic landscapes remains a daunting task.

5 RNA Modifications and Therapeutic Targets

The dynamic and reversible nature of RNA modifications, such as m6A, m5C, and Ψ, has positioned them as promising candidates for the development of novel therapeutic interventions. Targeting specific enzymes and regulatory proteins involved in RNA modification processes has shown considerable potential in modulating gene expression, splicing patterns, and RNA stability, thereby influencing critical cellular pathways implicated in disease progression (Cayir 2022).

Notably, the dysregulation of RNA modification writers, erasers, and readers has been linked to the pathogenesis of numerous cancers, highlighting the therapeutic relevance of manipulating these enzymes to restore normal RNA modification patterns and, consequently, mitigate oncogenic processes. Strategies aimed at modulating RNA modification machinery, either through small molecule inhibitors, RNA-based therapeutics, or gene editing technologies, offer exciting prospects for precision medicine approaches that can effectively target the molecular vulnerabilities of cancer cells while minimizing off-target effects (Mathis and Le Masson 2018). Consequently, a comprehensive understanding of the intricate interplay between RNA modifications and disease pathology is imperative for the development of targeted and efficacious therapeutic modalities aimed at combating the complexities of various diseases, including cancer.

5.1 RNA Modification-Related Enzymes as Therapeutic Targets

In cancer, aberrant expression and activity of RNA modification-related enzymes contribute to tumor initiation, progression, and therapeutic resistance. For instance, alterations in the expression levels of m6A methyltransferases, such as METTL3 and METTL14, have been observed in multiple cancer types and are associated with poor prognosis. Conversely, overexpression of m6A demethylases, including FTO and ALKBH5, has been linked to enhanced tumor growth and metastasis (Yang et al. 2021). These findings underscore the potential of RNA modification-related enzymes as attractive targets for cancer therapy. Controlling the activities of RNA modification-related enzymes through small molecule inhibitors, gene editing, and RNA-based therapeutics is a promising area for novel cancer therapeutic strategies. In recent years, significant progress has been made in identifying and optimizing small-molecule inhibitors targeting m6A writers and erasers, some of which have shown promising anticancer effects in preclinical studies (Hu et al. 2023).

Additionally, emerging strategies, such as CRISPR-based genome editing, offer precise control over the expression and activity of RNA modification-related enzymes, providing new avenues for therapeutic intervention in cancer. Pseudouridine (Ψ), a prevalent RNA modification, has garnered significant attention in the context of cancer research. Dysregulation of pseudouridine synthases, such as DKC1, is frequently observed in malignancies, indicating their potential as therapeutic targets. Recent studies have demonstrated the efficacy of small molecule inhibitors targeting these enzymes in restoring normal RNA pseudouridylation patterns (Elsharawy et al. 2020). This highlights the therapeutic potential of modulating pseudouridine (Ψ) modification pathways in cancer treatment. Moreover, emerging RNA-targeted therapeutic modalities offer novel approaches to selectively target pseudouridine-modified transcripts. Antisense oligonucleotides (ASOs), for instance, have shown promise in selectively depleting specific RNA targets, including pseudouridine-modified transcripts. ASOs provide a versatile platform for modulating gene expression at the RNA level, offering potential therapeutic benefits in cancer therapy. The development of small molecule inhibitors and RNA-targeted therapeutic modalities represents promising avenues for targeting pseudouridine (Ψ) modification pathways in cancer (El Dirani-Diab et al. 1997). By selectively modulating pseudouridine (Ψ) levels and restoring normal RNA pseudouridylation patterns, these approaches hold potential for overcoming dysregulated RNA modification dynamics associated with cancer progression.

5.2 Strategies for Modulating RNA Modifications

Strategies for modulating RNA modifications involve cutting-edge approaches such as RNA editing technologies, which enable precise manipulation of RNA to alter gene expression. RNA-based therapies, including RNA interference and antisense oligonucleotides, offer targeted degradation of disease-associated RNA. Advances in small molecule inhibitors and RNA-based therapies selectively target enzymes involved in RNA regulation, providing a means to disrupt aberrant RNA modification patterns and attenuate cancer progression (Zhang and Zhang 2023). These strategies collectively demonstrate the transformative potential of RNA-focused interventions in precision oncology and therapeutic.

5.2.1 RNA Editing Technologies

RNA editing technologies, such as CRISPR-based systems, have become invaluable for precise manipulation of RNA sequences, with significant potential for understanding and treating various diseases. These tools enable targeted RNA modifications, offering promising applications in addressing genetic disorders and cancer. In diseases like cystic fibrosis, where mutations in the CFTR gene disrupt chloride ion transport, CRISPR-based RNA editing can correct these defects at the transcript level, potentially restoring protein function and mitigating disease symptoms. Similarly, in oncology, RNA editing allows for the targeted alteration of oncogenic transcripts, aiming to inhibit tumor growth and metastasis. This precision opens the door to personalized treatment strategies tailored to an individual's unique genetic profile, fostering the development of precision medicine (Chiavetta et al. 2023). As RNA editing technologies continue to advance, their clinical applications are likely to grow, presenting innovative solutions for a wide range of genetic and oncological conditions.

5.2.2 RNA-Based Cancer Therapies

RNA-based therapies are an exciting and innovative approach to cancer treatment, utilizing synthetic RNA molecules like small interfering RNAs (siRNAs), miRNAs, and messenger RNAs (mRNAs) to target specific genes and pathways involved in cancer progression. These therapies offer a range of strategies for precision medicine and personalized cancer treatment. For instance, siRNAs can silence specific oncogenes, as seen with the BCR-ABL gene in chronic myeloid leukemia, which, when inhibited, disrupts the signaling pathway responsible for the uncontrolled growth of leukemic cells, resulting in decreased tumor growth and improved outcomes. Similarly, mRNA-based vaccines have transformed cancer immunotherapy by stimulating the immune system to recognize and attack tumor cells (Khan et al. 2021). The success of mRNA vaccines in targeting neoantigens in melanoma and other solid tumors has demonstrated their ability to induce strong and lasting antitumor immune responses. Additionally, miRNA-based therapies offer another layer of regulation by targeting miRNAs that play key roles in cancer development (Yang et al. 2016). For example, anti-miRNA oligonucleotides targeting miR-21, an oncomiR associated with several cancers, have shown promise in reducing tumor growth, invasion, and metastasis. With advancements in RNA delivery methods and formulation techniques, these therapies could become a cornerstone of modern oncology, providing more targeted and personalized options for cancer treatment (Bautista-Sánchez et al. 2020). The ongoing development and integration of these RNA-based therapies hold the potential to meet the complex challenges of diverse cancer types, indicating a shift toward more refined and patient-specific therapeutic approaches in oncology.

5.3 Advances in Small Molecule Inhibitors and RNA-Based Therapies

Small molecule inhibitors targeting RNA modifications have become a key focus in the search for new therapeutic strategies, particularly in cancer treatment. These inhibitors can modulate RNA modification pathways, impacting gene expression and cellular processes crucial for disease progression. A significant area of interest is targeting the m6A modification, with several small molecule inhibitors showing promise in modulating RNA metabolism and exerting anticancer effects (Kara et al. 2022). One such inhibitor is YTHDF3-AS1, which targets the m6A reader protein YTHDF3, disrupting its interaction with m6A-modified transcripts in colorectal cancer. This disruption hampers oncogenic gene expression, reducing tumor growth and metastasis. Additionally, small molecule inhibitors targeting m6A methyltransferase METTL3 have shown potential in influencing the m6A landscape, affecting key oncogenes and tumor suppressor genes in hepatocellular carcinoma. These inhibitors, by targeting the m6A pathways, offer a promising approach to suppressing tumor proliferation and promoting apoptosis (Somasekharan et al. 2022).

These developments in small molecule inhibitors for RNA modification-based therapies mark a significant advancement in precision medicine, allowing for targeted modulation of disease-associated RNA modification patterns. This approach holds potential not only for innovative anticancer treatments but also for broader therapeutic applications in other RNA modification-related disorders. The growing interest in this field is evident in the development of selective METTL3 and FTO inhibitors, along with several RNA-based therapies entering clinical trials. These advances suggest a promising future for translating RNA modification research into effective therapeutic strategies (Li et al. 2023a, b).

6 RNA Editing in Cancer Therapy

Certainly, RNA editing has emerged as a promising avenue in cancer therapy, offering a novel approach to manipulate RNA sequences and gene expression patterns, thereby modulating critical cellular processes implicated in cancer development and progression. A notable strategy involves harnessing the power of adenosine deaminases acting on RNA (ADARs) enzymes to catalyze site-specific conversions of adenosine to inosine within RNA transcripts (Pfaller et al. 2021). This process, known as A-to-I RNA editing, can alter the coding potential and functional properties of cancer-associated genes, thereby impacting various oncogenic pathways. Recent preclinical studies have demonstrated the therapeutic potential of targeting aberrant RNA editing events in specific cancer types, highlighting the feasibility of using RNA editing modulators as precision medicine tools to restore normal cellular functions and suppress tumorigenesis. While challenges such as off-target effects and delivery mechanisms remain to be addressed, the emerging landscape of RNA editing in cancer therapy holds great promise in the development of innovative, tailored treatment approaches aimed at improving patient outcomes and overcoming drug resistance mechanisms prevalent in various malignancies (Wen et al. 2021).

6.1 A-to-I RNA Editing as a Therapeutic Avenue for Targeted Mutagenesis

A-to-I RNA editing is a crucial post-transcriptional modification mechanism that introduces adenosine-to-inosine substitutions in RNA molecules, thereby altering their coding potential and functional properties. Orchestrated by the adenosine deaminase acting on RNA (ADAR) family of enzymes, which includes ADAR1, ADAR2, and ADAR3 in mammals, this process is implicated in the fine-tuning of gene expression, maintenance of RNA stability, and generation of proteome diversity (Raghava Kurup et al. 2022). Through the precise deamination of adenosine bases, A-to-I RNA editing serves as a regulatory mechanism that modulates neurotransmission, ion channel function, and immune response, thereby impacting various physiological and pathological processes (Gatsiou et al. 2018). Understanding the intricate interplay between A-to-I RNA editing and disease pathogenesis holds promise for the development of innovative therapeutic strategies, paving the way for targeted interventions in various genetic disorders and malignancies.

6.1.1 Biological Significance and Mechanisms of A-to-I RNA Editing

A-to-I RNA editing is a key regulatory process in which adenosine (A) residues in double-stranded RNA (dsRNA) are converted to inosine (I) by adenosine deaminases acting on RNA (ADAR) enzymes. This alteration changes the RNA sequence, affecting gene expression and protein translation, as inosine is interpreted as guanosine (G), leading to different amino acid incorporations (Booth et al. 2023). This process has broad implications in various biological contexts, including neurotransmitter receptor modulation, impacting synaptic transmission and neuronal excitability, and aiding in immune response regulation by affecting antiviral defense and inflammatory signaling. Dysregulation of A-to-I RNA editing is linked to neurological disorders like epilepsy and ALS, as well as certain cancers where it can affect tumor progression and treatment resistance. Understanding this process is crucial for precision medicine, as manipulating RNA editing could provide new therapeutic avenues for a range of diseases (Hwang et al. 2019).

6.1.2 A-to-I RNA Editing as a Therapeutic Tool

A-to-I RNA editing, facilitated by ADAR enzymes, offers a promising therapeutic approach for treating neurological disorders and cancer. By altering RNA sequences without changing DNA, this technology affects protein expression, showing potential in addressing conditions like ALS, Parkinson's disease, and even treatment resistance in cancer. Recent advances in CRISPR and engineered ADAR enzymes have made precise RNA editing more feasible, though challenges like off-target effects and delivery methods persist. This technique could also be used to correct genetic mutations at the RNA level, with applications in cystic fibrosis, muscular dystrophies, and neurodegenerative disorders. Despite its promise, the technology faces hurdles, including potential side effects, inefficient editing, and delivery difficulties. Continued research and rigorous testing are essential to ensure safety and effectiveness in clinical applications (Gupta et al. 2019).

6.2 Potential for Correcting Cancer-Associated Mutations Using RNA Editing technologies

The emergence of RNA editing technologies has opened new avenues for the correction of cancer-associated mutations. This topic provides a comprehensive examination of the potential and challenges associated with utilizing RNA editing tools, such as CRISPR-Cas systems and base editors, to rectify genetic anomalies linked to cancer (Han et al. 2022).

6.2.1 RNA Editing Technologies: Mechanisms and Tools

CRISPR-Cas Systems The Clustered Regularly Interspaced Short Palindromic Repeats (CRISPR)-associated (Cas) systems have revolutionized genetic engineering. By utilizing guide RNAs to target specific genomic loci, these systems offer a versatile platform for precise RNA editing. Recent advancements in CRISPR-Cas technologies, such as the development of prime editing and RNA-targeting Cas proteins, have expanded the range of editable RNA sequences, thus enhancing the potential for cancer mutation correction.

Base Editors Base editing, a groundbreaking innovation, enables the direct conversion of one DNA base pair into another without causing double-strand breaks. The adaptation of base editing techniques for RNA editing (REPAIR) holds immense promise in correcting cancer-associated mutations at the RNA level (Elliott et al.

2021). The versatility of base editors in mediating transitions and transversions broadens their applicability in addressing diverse cancer mutations.

6.2.2 Strategies for Correcting Cancer-Associated Mutations

Precision Medicine RNA editing technologies offer a highly personalized approach to cancer therapy. By tailoring RNA-targeting sequences to individual patient profiles, precise correction of disease-causing mutations can be achieved. This personalized medicine approach minimizes off-target effects and maximizes therapeutic efficacy (Hu and Ke 2022).

Therapeutic Targets Identification of suitable therapeutic targets is pivotal in RNA editing for cancer correction. Tumor-specific mutations, such as those in oncogenes or tumor suppressor genes, can be selectively edited to mitigate the oncogenic potential or restore tumor-suppressive functions. The study of tumor genomics and molecular pathways informs target selection. Exploring the potential of RNA editing in non-coding RNAs, such as miRNAs and long non-coding RNAs, could unveil novel therapeutic strategies for cancer. These regulatory RNAs play crucial roles in oncogenesis and can be targeted for therapeutic intervention (Medina-Munoz et al. 2023). Combining RNA editing technologies with existing cancer therapies, such as immunotherapy or chemotherapy, may yield synergistic effects. This approach could enhance treatment outcomes and overcome resistance mechanisms.

7 RNA Modifications and Cancer Immunotherapy

At the heart of cancer immunotherapy lies the endeavor to harness the body's immune system to recognize and eliminate cancer cells effectively. RNA modifications, particularly those in non-coding RNAs such as miRNAs, lncRNAs, and circular RNAs (ciRNAs), exert multifaceted effects on gene expression and cellular processes, including immune response modulation. One of the primary mechanisms through which RNA modifications influence cancer immunotherapy is by regulating immune checkpoint pathways. Post-transcriptional modifications in immune-related genes can alter their expression levels, thereby modulating the activity of checkpoint proteins like PD-1, PD-L1, CTLA-4, and others. For instance, dysregulated miRNAs in cancer cells can disrupt the expression of checkpoint molecules leading to immune evasion and tumor progression (Platt et al. 2014). Moreover, RNA modifications contribute to the tumor microenvironment's immunosuppressive milieu. Alterations in RNA methylation patterns, such as m6A, influence the stability and translation efficiency of mRNAs encoding immune regulatory factors and cytokines. Consequently, aberrant RNA modifications can skew the balance toward immune tolerance, hindering the effectiveness of immunotherapies like immune checkpoint blockade and adoptive cell therapy.

Nevertheless, the dynamic nature of RNA modifications also presents opportunities for therapeutic intervention in cancer immunotherapy. Recent advances in RNA editing technologies, such as CRISPR-based RNA editing and small molecule inhibitors targeting RNA modifiers, offer innovative strategies to manipulate RNA modifications selectively. By modulating the expression and activity of key immune-related genes, these approaches hold promise for enhancing the efficacy and durability of immunotherapeutic responses. Furthermore, RNA modifications serve as potential biomarkers for patient stratification and treatment selection in cancer immunotherapy. Profiling RNA modification patterns in tumor samples can provide valuable insights into the tumor's immunogenicity and susceptibility to immunotherapy. Integrating RNA modification signatures with other omics data enables comprehensive molecular characterization of tumors, facilitating personalized treatment strategies tailored to individual patients (Qu et al. 2019).

RNA modifications exert profound influences on cancer immunotherapy outcomes by regulating immune checkpoint pathways, shaping the tumor microenvironment, and serving as therapeutic targets and biomarkers. Understanding the intricate interplay between RNA modifications and the immune response is crucial for developing more effective and personalized immunotherapeutic approaches in the fight against cancer (Wang et al. 2020). As research in this field progresses, harnessing the potential of RNA modifications holds immense promise for transforming cancer treatment paradigms and improving patient outcomes.

8 Clinical Deployment and Future Landscapes

Clinical deployment of RNA modification analysis holds significant promise in shaping the future landscapes of cancer therapy. As we delve deeper into the intricate world of RNA modifications, their clinical integration stands poised to revolutionize cancer treatment paradigms.

8.1 Clinical Integration and Anticipated Developments

RNA modifications have significant clinical implications, influencing key cellular processes like mRNA splicing, translation, and degradation. Dysregulation of these processes is linked to diseases such as cancer, neurodegenerative disorders, and viral infections, suggesting that understanding RNA modifications can reveal new therapeutic targets and diagnostic biomarkers. Recent success with modified RNA molecules, especially mRNA vaccines used during the COVID-19 pandemic, has highlighted the potential of RNA-based therapies. These modifications can improve RNA stability, translation, and immunogenicity, enabling innovative approaches in gene therapy and cancer immunotherapy. To maximize the therapeutic benefits of RNA modifications, researchers are exploring advanced sequencing technologies, bioinformatics, and structural biology to understand these processes better. The development of small molecule inhibitors and CRISPR-based RNA editing further expands the potential for targeted therapeutic interventions (Marsh et al. 2020).

8.2 Translational Potential of Targeting RNA Modifications in Cancer Diagnosis and Therapy

Targeting RNA modifications in cancer diagnosis and therapy has the potential to transform oncology. These modifications play a crucial role in regulating gene expression in cancer cells, where dysregulation can lead to the production of oncogenic or tumor-suppressive RNA isoforms, affecting cancer development and treatment response. Identifying and quantifying specific RNA modifications in cancer can offer new diagnostic tools, aiding in subtype classification, prognosis prediction, and therapy stratification. Abnormal RNA modification profiles have been found in several cancer types, including glioblastoma and acute myeloid leukemia, pointing to their utility as diagnostic biomarkers. Therapeutically, targeting RNA modifications opens up promising avenues for cancer treatment. Manipulating these modifications, such as correcting A-to-I editing patterns or selectively altering other modifications, can inhibit tumor growth and sensitize cancer cells to other therapies. Preclinical studies show that these approaches can even lead to synthetic lethality in some cases, suggesting a potential for significant anticancer effects (Schlegel et al. 2022).

To fully realize the potential of targeting RNA modifications in cancer, researchers must address issues of specificity, efficiency, delivery, and safety. Ethical concerns regarding the clinical manipulation of RNA modifications must also be considered, necessitating robust regulatory frameworks and guidelines for the responsible application of these emerging technologies.

9 Conclusion and Future Directions

The field of epitranscriptomics has advanced rapidly since the 2011 discovery that m6A is a reversible RNA modification. Innovations in detection methods, such as long-read nanopore sequencing, have enabled deeper mechanistic insights into RNA modifications. This has fueled the development of small-molecule inhibitors targeting the RNA modification machinery, highlighting their therapeutic potential, particularly in cancer treatment. While initial studies focused on m6A, research has expanded to explore other RNA modifications in various biological contexts, including human development, homeostasis, and disease. Advanced mapping techniques have revealed complex landscapes of RNA modifications, leading to better understanding of gene expression and its impact on disease. This new knowledge has the potential to revolutionize cancer diagnosis and treatment by providing precision medicine tools based on RNA modification biomarkers. As research continues, the ability to engineer and manipulate RNA modifications could lead to new therapeutic strategies and more effective interventions. This expanding toolkit is crucial in uncovering the roles of modifications like m6A, m5C, and Ψ in regulating gene expression and disease progression. By leveraging these insights, scientists aim to create tailored treatments that can improve cancer care and patient outcomes. The convergence of advanced technologies and RNA modification research signals a new era in understanding and combating a wide range of diseases.

Acknowledgments We sincerely thank all the authors whose work we reviewed for their insightful feedback and suggestions, which greatly enhanced our manuscript. The authors confirm that there are no conflicts of interest related to this review, and we have taken every precaution to ensure the research's objectivity and integrity. Special thanks to Neb Burke Zell for editing, revising the manuscript, and adjusting the grammar.

Author Contributions O.S. and S.F. were responsible for the conceptualization and design of this review, carried out the literature search, and wrote the initial draft of the manuscript. M.A., V.T., and A.A. made substantial contributions by rigorously reviewing and editing the manuscript. O.S., Y.L., E-S.C., and S.F. gave valuable feedback and revised the manuscript. All authors have read and approved the final version for publication.

Institutional Review Board Statement Not applicable.

Informed Consent Statement Not applicable.

Funding The research endeavors of S.F. were made possible through the generous backing of the Metro Health Medical Center's startup fund, the American Cancer Society Research Scholar Grant (RSG-18-238-01-CSM), and the National Cancer Institute Research Grant (R01CA248304).

References

Alemu E, He C, Klungland A (2016) ALKBHs-facilitated RNA modifications and de-modifications. DNA Repair 44:87–91. https://doi.org/10.1016/j.dnarep.2016.05.026

Barbieri I, Kouzarides T (2020) Role of RNA modifications in cancer. Nat Rev Cancer 20(6): 303–322. https://doi.org/10.1038/s41568-020-0253-2

Bautista-Sánchez D, Arriaga-Canon C, Pedroza-Torres A, De La Rosa-Velázquez IA, González-Barrios R, Contreras-Espinosa L, Montiel-Manríquez R, Castro-Hernández C, Fragoso-Ontiveros V, Álvarez-Gómez RM, Herrera LA (2020) The promising role of miR-21 as a cancer biomarker and its importance in RNA-based therapeutics. Mol Ther Nucleic Acids 20: 409–420. https://doi.org/10.1016/j.omtn.2020.03.003

Boo SH, Kim YK (2020) The emerging role of RNA modifications in the regulation of mRNA stability. Exp Mol Med 52(3):400–408. https://doi.org/10.1038/s12276-020-0407-z

Booth BJ, Nourreddine S, Katrekar D, Savva Y, Bose D, Long TJ et al (2023) RNA editing: expanding the potential of RNA therapeutics. Mol Ther 31(6):1533–1549. https://doi.org/10.1016/j.ymthe.2023.01.005

Cayir A (2022) RNA modifications as emerging therapeutic targets. Wiley Interdisc Rev RNA 13(4):e1702. https://doi.org/10.1002/wrna.1702

Chiavetta RF, Titoli S, Barra V, Cancemi P, Melfi R, Di Leonardo A (2023) Site-specific RNA editing of stop mutations in the CFTR mRNA of human bronchial cultured cells. Int J Mol Sci 24(13):10940. https://doi.org/10.3390/ijms241310940

Deng X, Su R, Weng H, Huang H, Li Z, Chen J (2018) RNA N6-methyladenosine modification in cancers: current status and perspectives. Cell Res 28(5):507–517. https://doi.org/10.1038/s41422-018-0034-6

Deng X, Qing Y, Horne D, Huang H, Chen J (2023) The roles and implications of RNA m6A modification in cancer. Nat Rev Clin Oncol 20(8):507–526. https://doi.org/10.1038/s41571-023-00774-x

Dominissini D, Moshitch-Moshkovitz S, Amariglio N, Rechavi G (2011) Adenosine-to-inosine RNA editing meets cancer. Carcinogenesis 32(11):1569–1577. https://doi.org/10.1093/carcin/bgr124

El Dirani-Diab R, Sarih-Cottin L, Delord B, Dumon B, Moreau S, Toulme JJ, Fleury H, Litvak S (1997) Phosphorothioate oligonucleotides derived from human immunodeficiency virus type 1 (HIV-1) primer tRNA(Lys3) are strong inhibitors of HIV-1 reverse transcriptase and arrest viral replication in infected cells. Antimicrob Agents Chemother 41(10):2141–2148. https://doi.org/10.1128/AAC.41.10.2141

Elliott BA, Holley CL (2021) Assessing 2′-O-methylation of mRNA using quantitative PCR. Methods Mol Biol 2298:171–184. https://doi.org/10.1007/978-1-0716-1374-0_11

Elliott EK, Haupt LM, Griffiths LR (2021) Mini review: genome and transcriptome editing using CRISPR-Cas systems for hematological malignancy gene therapy. Transgenic Res 30(2):129–141. https://doi.org/10.1007/s11248-020-00232-9

Elsharawy KA, Mohammed OJ, Aleskandarany MA, Hyder A, El-Gammal HL, Abou-Dobara MI, Green AR, Dalton LW, Rakha EA (2020) The nucleolar-related protein dyskerin pseudouridine synthase 1 (DKC1) predicts poor prognosis in breast cancer. Br J Cancer 123(10):1543–1552. https://doi.org/10.1038/s41416-020-01045-7

Fritzell K, Xu LD, Lagergren J, Öhman M (2018) ADARs and editing: the role of A-to-I RNA modification in cancer progression. Semin Cell Dev Biol 79:123–130. https://doi.org/10.1016/j.semcdb.2017.11.018

Gatsiou A, Vlachogiannis N, Lunella FF, Sachse M, Stellos K (2018) Adenosine-to-inosine RNA editing in health and disease. Antioxid Redox Signal 29(9):846–863. https://doi.org/10.1089/ars.2017.7295

Gregorova P, Sipari NH, Sarin LP (2021) Broad-range RNA modification analysis of complex biological samples using rapid C18-UPLC-MS. RNA Biol 18(10):1382–1389. https://doi.org/10.1080/15476286.2020.1853385

Gupta D, Bhattacharjee O, Mandal D, Sen MK, Dey D, Dasgupta A et al (2019) CRISPR-Cas9 system: a new-fangled dawn in gene editing. Life Sci 232:116636. https://doi.org/10.1016/j.lfs.2019.116636

Han J, Wang JZ, Yang X, Yu H, Zhou R, Lu HC, Yuan WB, Lu JC, Zhou ZJ, Lu Q, Wei JF, Yang H (2019) METTL3 promotes tumor proliferation of bladder cancer by accelerating pri-miR221/222 maturation in an m6A-dependent manner. Mol Cancer 18(1):110. https://doi.org/10.1186/s12943-019-1036-9

Han F, Hu M, Zhang L, Fan X, Wang J, Lou Z et al (2022) A-to-I RNA editing of BLCAP promotes cell proliferation by losing the inhibitory effect on Rb1 in colorectal cancer. Exp Cell Res 417(2):113209. https://doi.org/10.1016/j.yexcr.2022.113209

He R, Qiao J, Wang X, Chen W, Yin T (2022) A new quantitative method for pseudouridine and uridine in human serum and its clinical application in acute myeloid leukemia. J Pharm Biomed Anal 219:114934. https://doi.org/10.1016/j.jpba.2022.114934

Hu C, Ke A (2022) Reconstitution and biochemical characterization of the RNA-guided helicase-nuclease protein Cas3 from type I-A CRISPR-Cas system. Methods Enzymol 673:405–424. https://doi.org/10.1016/bs.mie.2022.03.059

Hu Z, Sun A, Yang J, Naz G, Sun G, Li Z, Gogo Liu JJ, Zhang S, Zhang X (2023) Regulation of the CRISPR-Cas12a system by methylation and demethylation of guide RNA. Chem Sci 14(22):5945–5955. https://doi.org/10.1039/d3sc00629h

Huang H, Weng H, Chen J (2020) m6A modification in coding and non-coding RNAs: roles and therapeutic implications in cancer. Cancer Cell 37(3):270–288. https://doi.org/10.1016/j.ccell.2020.02.004

Huang Z, Pan J, Wang H, Du X, Xu Y, Wang Z, Chen D (2021) Prognostic significance and tumor immune microenvironment heterogenicity of m5C RNA methylation regulators in triple-negative breast cancer. Front Cell Dev Biol 9:657547. https://doi.org/10.3389/fcell.2021.657547

Huang M, Ming L, Jiang H, Jiang P, Jiang X, Yin H, Hong H (2023) Diagnostic value of aberrant decreased 5-Methylcytosine RNA modification in leukocytes for non-small cell lung cancer. J Cancer 14(12):2198–2208. https://doi.org/10.7150/jca.85681

Hwang W, Calza S, Silvestri M, Pawitan Y, Lee Y (2019) CREDO: highly confident disease-relevant A-to-I RNA-editing discovery in breast cancer. Sci Rep 9(1):5064. https://doi.org/10.1038/s41598-019-41294-y

Jin Z, MacPherson K, Liu Z, Vu LP (2023) RNA modifications in hematological malignancies. Int J Hematol 117(6):807–820. https://doi.org/10.1007/s12185-023-03576-0

Kara G, Calin GA, Ozpolat B (2022) RNAi-based therapeutics and tumor targeted delivery in cancer. Adv Drug Deliv Rev 182:114113. https://doi.org/10.1016/j.addr.2022.114113

Kasowitz SD, Ma J, Anderson SJ, Leu NA, Xu Y, Gregory BD, Schultz RM, Wang PJ (2018) Nuclear m6A reader YTHDC1 regulates alternative polyadenylation and splicing during mouse oocyte development. PLoS Genet 14(5):e1007412. https://doi.org/10.1371/journal.pgen.1007412

Khan P, Siddiqui JA, Lakshmanan I, Ganti AK, Salgia R, Jain M, Batra SK, Nasser MW (2021) RNA-based therapies: a cog in the wheel of lung cancer defense. Mol Cancer 20(1):54. https://doi.org/10.1186/s12943-021-01338-2

Körtel N, Rücklé C, Zhou Y, Busch A, Hoch-Kraft P, Sutandy FXR, Haase J, Pradhan M, Musheev M, Ostareck D, Ostareck-Lederer A, Dieterich C, Hüttelmaier S, Niehrs C, Rausch O, Dominissini D, König J, Zarnack K (2021) Deep and accurate detection of m6A RNA modifications using miCLIP2 and m6Aboost machine learning. Nucleic Acids Res 49(16):e92. https://doi.org/10.1093/nar/gkab485

Lee SH, Kim HP, Kang JK, Song SH, Han SW, Kim TY (2017) Identification of diverse adenosine-to-inosine RNA editing subtypes in colorectal cancer. Cancer Res Treat 49(4):1077–1087. https://doi.org/10.4143/crt.2016.301

Lennox KA, Behlke MA (2020) Chemical modifications in RNA interference and CRISPR/Cas genome editing reagents. Methods Mol Biol 2115:23–55. https://doi.org/10.1007/978-1-0716-0290-4_2

Li W, Zhang X, Lu X, You L, Song Y, Luo Z, Zhang J, Nie J, Zheng W, Xu D, Wang Y, Dong Y, Yu S, Hong J, Shi J, Hao H, Luo F, Hua L, Wang P, Qian X, Yuan F, Wei L, Cui M, Zhang T, Liao Q, Dai M, Liu Z, Chen G, Meckel K, Adhikari S, Jia G, Bissonnette M, Zhang X, Zhao Y, Zhang W, He C, Liu J (2017) 5-Hydroxymethylcytosine signatures in circulating cell-free DNA as diagnostic biomarkers for human cancers. Cell Res 27(10):1243–1257. https://doi.org/10.1038/cr.2017.121

Li Z, Peng Y, Li J, Chen Z, Chen F, Tu J, Lin S, Wang H (2020) N6-methyladenosine regulates glycolysis of cancer cells through PDK4. Nat Commun 11(1):2578. https://doi.org/10.1038/s41467-020-16306-5

Li X, Ma S, Deng Y, Yi P, Yu J (2022a) Targeting the RNA m6A modification for cancer immunotherapy. Mol Cancer 21(1):76. https://doi.org/10.1186/s12943-022-01558-0

Li B, Zhao R, Qiu W, Pan Z, Zhao S, Qi Y, Qiu J, Zhang S, Guo Q, Fan Y, Xu H, Li M, Li G, Xue H (2022b) The N6-methyladenosine-mediated lncRNA WEE2-AS1 promotes glioblastoma progression by stabilizing RPN2. Theranostics 12(14):6363–6379. https://doi.org/10.7150/thno.74600

Li T, Chen Z, Wang Z, Lu J, Chen D (2023a) Combined signature of N7-methylguanosine regulators with their related genes and the tumor microenvironment: a prognostic and therapeutic biomarker for breast cancer. Front Immunol 14:1260195. https://doi.org/10.3389/fimmu.2023.1260195

Li B, Xi W, Bai Y, Liu X, Zhang Y, Li L et al (2023b) FTO-dependent m6A modification of Plpp3 in circSCMH1-regulated vascular repair and functional recovery following stroke. Nat Commun 14(1):489. https://doi.org/10.1038/s41467-023-36008-y

Liu F, Su X (2021) Effects of m6A modifications on signaling pathways in human cancer (review). Oncol Rep 45(4):36. https://doi.org/10.3892/or.2021.7987

Liu Z, Wang T, She Y, Wu K, Gu S, Li L, Dong C, Chen C, Zhou Y (2021a) N6-methyladenosine-modified circIGF2BP3 inhibits CD8+ T-cell responses to facilitate tumor immune evasion by promoting the deubiquitination of PD-L1 in non-small cell lung cancer. Mol Cancer 20(1):105. https://doi.org/10.1186/s12943-021-01398-4

Liu X, Xiao M, Zhang L, Li L, Zhu G, Shen E, Lv M, Lu X, Sun Z (2021b) The m6A methyltransferase METTL14 inhibits the proliferation, migration, and invasion of gastric cancer by regulating the PI3K/AKT/mTOR signaling pathway. J Clin Lab Anal 35(3):e23655. https://doi.org/10.1002/jcla.23655

Liu X, He H, Zhang F, Hu X, Bi F, Li K, Yu H, Zhao Y, Teng X, Li J, Wang L, Zhang Y, Wu Q (2022) m6A methylated EphA2 and VEGFA through IGF2BP2/3 regulation promote vasculogenic mimicry in colorectal cancer via PI3K/AKT and ERK1/2 signaling. Cell Death Dis 13(5):483. https://doi.org/10.1038/s41419-022-04950-2

Majd N, Yap TA, Yung WKA, De Groot J (2020) The promise of poly(ADP-ribose) polymerase (PARP) inhibitors in gliomas. J Immunother Precis Oncol 3(4):157–164. https://doi.org/10.36401/JIPO-20-20

Marsh S, Hanson B, Wood MJA, Varela MA, Roberts TC (2020) Application of CRISPR-Cas9-mediated genome editing for the treatment of myotonic dystrophy type 1. Mol Ther 28(12): 2527–2539. https://doi.org/10.1016/j.ymthe.2020.10.005

Mathis S, Le Masson G (2018) RNA-targeted therapies and amyotrophic lateral sclerosis. Biomedicines 6(1):9. https://doi.org/10.3390/biomedicines6010009

Medina-Munoz HC, Kofman E, Jagannatha P, Boyle EA, Yu T, Jones KL et al (2023) Expanded palette of RNA base editors for comprehensive RBP-RNA interactome studies. Preprint. https://doi.org/10.1101/2023.09.25.558915

Meng Y, Yang W, Li J, Chai W (2023) KIAA1429 facilitates progression of hepatocellular carcinoma by modulating m6A levels in HPN. Heliyon 9(11):e22084. https://doi.org/10.1016/j.heliyon.2023.e22084

Orsolic I, Carrier A, Esteller M (2023) Genetic and epigenetic defects of the RNA modification machinery in cancer. Trends Genet 39(1):74–88. https://doi.org/10.1016/j.tig.2022.10.004

Peng Y, Meng H, Ge R, Liu S, Chen M, He C, Hu L (2022) Detection of m6A RNA modifications at single-nucleotide resolution using m6A-selective allyl chemical labeling and sequencing. STAR Protoc 3(4):101677. https://doi.org/10.1016/j.xpro.2022.101677

Pfaller CK, George CX, Samuel CE (2021) Adenosine deaminases acting on RNA (ADARs) and viral infections. Annu Rev Virol 8(1):239–264. https://doi.org/10.1146/annurev-virology-091919-065320

Platt RJ, Chen S, Zhou Y, Yim MJ, Swiech L, Kempton HR et al (2014) CRISPR-Cas9 knockin mice for genome editing and cancer modeling. Cell 159(2):440–455. https://doi.org/10.1016/j.cell.2014.09.014

Qiu L, Jing Q, Li Y, Han J (2023) RNA modification: mechanisms and therapeutic targets. Mol Biomed 4(1):25. https://doi.org/10.1186/s43556-023-00139-x

Qu L, Yi Z, Zhu S, Wang C, Cao Z, Zhou Z et al (2019) Programmable RNA editing by recruiting endogenous ADAR using engineered RNAs. Nat Biotechnol 37(9):1059–1069. https://doi.org/10.1038/s41587-019-0178-z

Raghava Kurup R, Oakes EK, Manning AC, Mukherjee P, Vadlamani P, Hundley HA (2022) RNA binding by ADAR3 inhibits adenosine-to-inosine editing and promotes expression of immune response protein MAVS. J Biol Chem 298(9):102267. https://doi.org/10.1016/j.jbc.2022.102267

Schlegel MK, Janas MM, Jiang Y, Barry JD, Davis W, Agarwal S et al (2022) From bench to bedside: improving the clinical safety of GalNAc-siRNA conjugates using seed-pairing destabilization. Nucleic Acids Res 50(12):6656–6670. https://doi.org/10.1093/nar/gkac539

Somasekharan SP, Saxena N, Zhang F, Beraldi E, Huang JN, Gentle C, Fazli L, Thi M, Sorensen PH, Gleave ME (2022) Regulation of AR mRNA translation in response to acute AR pathway inhibition. Nucleic Acids Res 50(2):1069–1091. https://doi.org/10.1093/nar/gkab1247

Stockert JA, Gupta A, Herzog B, Yadav SS, Tewari AK, Yadav KK (2019) Predictive value of pseudouridine in prostate cancer. Am J Clin Exp Urol 7(4):262–272. PMC

Stockert JA, Weil R, Yadav KK, Kyprianou N, Tewari AK (2021) Pseudouridine as a novel biomarker in prostate cancer. Urol Oncol 39(1):63–71. https://doi.org/10.1016/j.urolonc.2020.06.026

Sun T, Wu R, Ming L (2019) The role of m6A RNA methylation in cancer. Biomed Pharmacother 112:108613. https://doi.org/10.1016/j.biopha.2019.108613

Teng PC, Liang Y, Yarmishyn AA, Hsiao YJ, Lin TY, Lin TW, Teng YC, Yang YP, Wang ML, Chien CS, Luo YH, Chen YM, Hsu PK, Chiou SH, Chien Y (2021) RNA modifications and epigenetics in modulation of lung cancer and pulmonary diseases. Int J Mol Sci 22(19):10592. https://doi.org/10.3390/ijms221910592

Tusup M, Kundig T, Pascolo S (2018) Epitranscriptomics of cancer. World J Clin Oncol 9(3): 42–55. https://doi.org/10.5306/wjco.v9.i3.42

Wang YN, Yu CY, Jin HZ (2020) RNA N6-Methyladenosine modifications and the immune response. J Immunol Res 2020:6327614. https://doi.org/10.1155/2020/6327614

Wang Y, Mao Y, Wang C, Jiang X, Tang Q, Wang L, Zhu J, Zhao M (2023) RNA methylation-related genes of m6A, m5C, and m1A predict prognosis and immunotherapy response in cervical cancer. Ann Med 55(1):2190618. https://doi.org/10.1080/07853890.2023.2190618

Wei H, Xie H, Qu J, Xie A, Xie S, Huang H, Li J, Fang C, Shi F, Qiu H, Qi Y, Tian X, Yang Q, Huang J (2021) TLR7 modulating B-cell immune responses in the spleen of C57BL/6 mice infected with Schistosoma japonicum. PLoS Negl Trop Dis 15(11):e0009943. https://doi.org/10.1371/journal.pntd.0009943

Wen J, Rusch M, Brady SW, Shao Y, Edmonson MN, Shaw TI et al (2021) The landscape of coding RNA editing events in pediatric cancer. BMC Cancer 21(1):1233. https://doi.org/10.1186/s12885-021-08956-5

Wu Z, Ren J, Liu GH (2023) Deciphering RNA m6A regulation in aging: perspectives on current advances and future directions. Aging Cell 22(10):e13972. https://doi.org/10.1111/acel.13972

Xiang Y, Laurent B, Hsu CH, Nachtergaele S, Lu Z, Sheng W, Xu C, Chen H, Ouyang J, Wang S, Ling D, Hsu PH, Zou L, Jambhekar A, He C, Shi Y (2017) RNA m6A methylation regulates the ultraviolet-induced DNA damage response. Nature 543(7646):573–576. https://doi.org/10.1038/nature21671

Xu W, Lai Y, Pan Y, Tan M, Ma Y, Sheng H, Wang J (2022) m6A RNA methylation-mediated NDUFA4 promotes cell proliferation and metabolism in gastric cancer. Cell Death Dis 13(8): 715. https://doi.org/10.1038/s41419-022-05132-w

Yang C, Panwar N, Wang Y, Zhang B, Liu M, Toh H, Yoon HS, Tjin SC, Chong PH, Law WC, Chen CK, Yong KT (2016) Biodegradable charged polyester-based vectors (BCPVs) as an efficient non-viral transfection nanoagent for gene knockdown of the BCR-ABL hybrid oncogene in a human chronic myeloid leukemia cell line. Nanoscale 8(17):9405–9416. https://doi.org/10.1039/c6nr00996d

Yang Z, Wang T, Wu D, Min Z, Tan J, Yu B (2020) RNA N6-methyladenosine reader IGF2BP3 regulates cell cycle and angiogenesis in colon cancer. J Exp Clin Cancer Res 39(1):203. https://doi.org/10.1186/s13046-020-01714-8

Yang B, Wang JQ, Tan Y, Yuan R, Chen ZS, Zou C (2021) RNA methylation and cancer treatment. Pharmacol Res 174:105937. https://doi.org/10.1016/j.phrs.2021.105937

Yang C, Yu T, Li Q, Xie F, Lin Q (2022) A signature based on m6A pattern and tumor microenvironment infiltration in clear cell renal cell carcinoma. Am J Transl Res 14(7): 4931–4947. PMC

Yang YH, Ma CY, Gao D, Liu XW, Yuan SS, Ding H (2023) i2OM: toward a better prediction of 2′-O-methylation in human RNA. Int J Biol Macromol 239:124247. https://doi.org/10.1016/j.ijbiomac.2023.124247

Yu D, Pan M, Li Y, Lu T, Wang Z, Liu C, Hu G (2022) RNA N6-methyladenosine reader IGF2BP2 promotes lymphatic metastasis and epithelial-mesenchymal transition of head and neck squamous carcinoma cells via stabilizing slug mRNA in an m6A-dependent manner. J Exp Clin Cancer Res 41(1):6. https://doi.org/10.1186/s13046-021-02212-1

Zhang C, Zhang B (2023) RNA therapeutics: updates and future potential. Sci China Life Sci 66(1): 12–30. https://doi.org/10.1007/s11427-022-2171-2

Zhang Q, Liu F, Chen W, Miao H, Liang H, Liao Z, Zhang Z, Zhang B (2021) The role of RNA m5C modification in cancer metastasis. Int J Biol Sci 17(13):3369–3380. https://doi.org/10.7150/ijbs.61439

Zhao J, Han H, Wang R, Wang Y, Zhang Y, Li N, Wang B, Chu Z, Zhang Y, Zhang H (2023) Identification of N1-methyladenosine-related biomarker predicting overall survival outcomes and experimental verification in ovarian cancer. J Obstet Gynaecol Res 49(10):2457–2467. https://doi.org/10.1111/jog.15745

Zhu S, Rooney S, Michlewski G (2020) RNA-targeted therapies and high-throughput screening methods. Int J Mol Sci 21(8):2996. https://doi.org/10.3390/ijms21082996

The Different Aspects of Telomerase Inhibitors in Cancer Treatment

Anahita Radmehr and Amir Reza Safdarian

Abstract

Telomeres are the sticky ends of chromosomes that, after time and with age increasing, get shorter, and this shortening is directly related to aging and disease. Telomeres, which shield the ends of chromosomes in mammals, are nucleoprotein complexes. Telomere length varies between species. Telomerase is a reverse ribonucleic transcriptase enzyme that elongates telomeres by postponing their shortening. In some diseases like cancer, telomerase gets overexpressed, and a mass of immortal cells will be made. These cells, with unlimited replication, will migrate to other parts of the body and metastasize. In the later steps, angiogenesis occurs, and the cancer cells supply the needed blood. Angiogenesis is one of the most common causes of cancer, and if it can be controlled, it can help with cancer care. Some chemical signals control the process of angiogenesis, and many strategies have been suggested to defeat these signals. Since telomerase is overexpressed in 85–95% of cancerous tumors, telomerase inhibitors may be used to combat cancer. These inhibitors can be natural, synthetic, or modified oligonucleotides. Some telomerase inhibitors can simultaneously target telomerase and the Wnt signaling pathway, essential in angiogenesis.

Keywords

Angiogenesis · Cancer · Natural products · Telomerase · Telomerase inhibitors · Telomeres · Wnt signaling pathway

A. Radmehr
Islamic Azad University, Parand Branch, Tehran, Iran
e-mail: annaradmehr@gmail.com

A. R. Safdarian (✉)
Immunology Board for Transplantation and Cell-Based Therapeutics (immuno_TACT), Universal Scientific Education and Research Network (USERN), Tehran, Iran
e-mail: Safdarian.amir.r@ut.ac.ir; amirrezasafdarian@gmail.com

Interdisciplinary Cancer Research, https://doi.org/10.1007/16833_2024_480
Published online: 01 December 2024

1 Introduction

Telomerase is a ribonucleoprotein made of telomerase RNA component (TERC) noncoding RNA used as a frame for the protein compounds telomerase reverse transcriptase (TERT), telomerase cajal body protein 1 (TCAB1), dyskerin, NOP10, and NHP2. Dyskerin and attributed proteins are the main reasons for the formation and firmness of TERC, while TCAB assists in transporting telomerase-to-telomere. TERT is a catalytic subunit, and TERC encodes the reverse transcription pattern (Grill and Nandakumar 2021). Telomerase is a reverse ribonucleic transcriptase enzyme that extends telomere DNA sequences, TTAGGG, to the end of 3′ chromosomes by using a full RNA factor as a model. Most tumors in humans and cell lines derived from them express significant concentrations of telomerase. As a consequence, they may be linked to the development of cancer cells. Regular somatic cells often lack telomerase activity except in germ and stem cells. This form of expression has been used to develop unique and effective cancer therapies. Apoptosis occurs when cancer cells lose their intact telomeres, while cell cycle arrest occurs when normal cells lose their telomeres (Seimiya 2020). However, 5–15% of neoplasms, mostly sarcomas and gliomas, lack telomerase and must rely on a telomerase-independent pathway called alternative telomere lengthening (ALT) to preserve telomere length. Telomerase is constantly used by proliferating cells to handle the problem of terminal replication. Cancer cells maintain telomere length for unlimited growing by reactivating telomerase or using a recombination-based pathway (Zhang and Zou 2020). Telomerase regulates gene expression, cell proliferation, apoptosis, Wnt/β-catenin signaling, NF-κB signaling, MYC-derived carcinogenesis, cell adhesion, cell migration, and epithelial-mesenchymal transmission (EMT), among other roles (Yuan and Xu 2019). Mammalian telomeres are nucleoprotein complexes that protect the ends of chromosomes. Telomeres include guanine-rich nucleotide replicates performing as binding sites for a protein complex called shelterin, which is a six subunit–protein complex consisting of TRF1, TRF2, RAP1, TIN2, POT1, and TPP1 supporting chromosome ends and controlling telomerase performances. As a cell divides, telomeres progressively get shorter, resulting in aging or apoptosis (de Lange 2018). Via its interplay with the TPP1 localization protein, telomerase recruits single-stranded telomere DNA (Xu et al. 2019). Several telomere proteins indicate specific binding activity for telomere DNA series. TRF1 and TRF2 bind to the DNA of the double-stranded telomere, while POT1 binds to the end of the free telomere single-strand. In connection with other signaling proteins, these proteins protect the end of the chromosome and control its length (Srinivas et al. 2020). TRF2 and POT1 are basic proteins for end protection against ataxia-telangiectasia mutated (ATM)- and ataxia-telangiectasia and Rad3-related (ATR)-dependent DNA damage response (DDR), followed by DNA repair ways: nonhomologous end joining and homologous recombination, respectively. TPP1-POT1 has a positive and negative influence on telomerase function. POT1 binds to single-stranded telomeres and restricts telomerase from reaching G-overhangs, while TPP1 interacts with telomerase to improve its motion (Frescas and de Lange 2014). In insufficient telomerase levels, telomere DNA repeats decrease with each cell division, and the telomere cap eventually loses its protective function. Telomerase is needed to increase the proliferative ability of tumors and immortal cells. DNA damage can regulate telomerase activity; consequently, additional pieces of telomere DNA are added directly to non-telomere fractures (Jafri et al. 2016). ATM and ATR are two major DNA damage response proteins in telomerase assembly and recruitment (Blackford and Jackson 2017). Telomerase is the favorite target for drug design in cancer treatment because it guarantees the progression of unspecified cells throughout malignancy, which is a characteristic of cancer (Guterres and Villanueva 2020). In 1989, researchers investigated the telomerase enzyme in the HeLa cervical cancer cells (Ganesan and Xu 2017). Telomerase utilizes the RNA pattern to bind nucleotide copies to telomeres, sustaining the karyotype and offsetting DNA failure (Wu et al. 2017). Telomeres are unencrypted DNA regions at the end of every chromosome that indicate life expectancy and general well-being. In structure and function, telomeres are distinct from other chromosomal sequences. They are essential components that stabilize the eukaryotic chromosome ends and prevent genetic material from being lost (Procházková Schrumpfová et al. 2019). Telomeres usually secure chromosomes from DNA damage and degradation of terminal nucleotides and avoid irrelevant recombination and chromosome-to-chromosome fusion. The length of telomeres differs between species. The proliferative potential of healthy somatic cells is controlled and regulated by telomeres. In human tumors, telomere length is kept by mechanisms other than telomerase activity (Verma et al. 2022). Telomerase activity is pretty limited in natural stem cells (Lupatov and Yarygin 2022). Without telomerase action, chromatin regeneration and methylation of catalytic proteins, hTERT and hTR, occur in ALT (Ganesan and Xu 2017). In tumor tissue, telomere length is highly variable regarding catalytic activity and recombination effects. In cancer, unregulated cell multiplication happens, according to telomere preservation (Bordeira Gaspar et al. 2018). Telomerase has the potential to be a reliable marker and a possible treatment for several serious malignancies (Judasz et al. 2022). The majority of telomere-related anticancer methods rely on telomerase to preserve telomere length (Martínez and Blasco 2017). At the end of the chromosome, the t-loop structure creates a cap that protects against degradation, recombination, and end-to-end fusion (Aksenova and Mirkin 2019). Tumor behavior, including cell differentiation and metastasis, can be predicted based on telomerase enzyme levels (Noureen et al. 2021). Telomerase expression is connected to hTERT mRNA expression in most cancer cells (Yuan et al. 2019). Malignant tumors have specific biological features, including growth signal autonomy, evasion of inhibitory growth signals, evasion of apoptosis, unlimited replicative potential, angiogenesis, invasion, and metastasis (Sameri et al. 2021). Adult hTR requires DKC1 for proper assembly and stability, essential for telomerase activity (MacNeil et al. 2019). Short telomeres and decreased telomerase function define dyskeratosis congenita (DC) and Hoyeraal-Hreidarsson (HHS) disorders, suggesting that the hDKC1 protein plays a fundamental role in telomere preservation (Olivieri et al. 2017). Almost all advanced malignancies need the presence of a telomere retention mechanism during DNA replication (Sugarman et al. 2019). The most prevalent noncoding mutation in cancer is telomerase promoter mutations (Lorbeer and Hockemeyer 2020). The telomeres' length and the cell's age seem proportional to the number of mutations (Aviv et al. 2017). Shorter telomeres have been linked to increased genomic alterations and may explain the regular occurrence of hTERT promoter mutations during periods of reduced telomere length (Rachakonda et al. 2018). EMT is defined by epithelial cells losing cell-to-cell connection and their capability to move, resulting in invasion and metastasis, a critical hallmark of different tumors. The Wnt/b-catenin pathway is activated, the transcription factors Slug and Twist are stabilized, and metastasis and invasion are boosted (Leggett et al. 2021). Telomerase activity is positively related to age (Denham and Sellami 2021). Over the last few years, the study of telomerase's function in carcinogenesis has made excellent strides, and enough data has been collected to suggest that telomerase and telomere preservation are acceptable options for designing personalized cancer treatments (Saretzki 2023). Utilizing electron microscope scans, a 3D model of human telomerase has assisted researchers in better comprehending the structure of telomerase (Ghanim et al. 2021).

2 The Telomerase Inhibition Manners

Technological advancements and biological visions have opened up new medical research prospects, and attempts to find new telomerase inhibitors have accelerated. Experimental research revealed that telomerase inhibitors are secure and well tolerated (Dratwa et al. 2020). Numerous natural products, small molecules, immunotherapeutics, and oligonucleotides are in progressive clinical trials to treat various cancers (Wang et al. 2023). The discovery of innovative diagnostic tools and potent prospective antitumor therapeutics has resulted from more excellent knowledge of telomere biology and telomerase activity (Trybek et al. 2020). Still, due to the considerable delay between supplying and therapeutic effects, the FDA has yet to approve any telomerase-based cancer drugs for clinical usage in the United States. Extra-telomeric activities may sidestep these postponed therapeutic qualities by focusing on telomerase-associated proteins, resulting in a comprehensive anticancer impact (Ataker and Simsek 2020). Dyskerin has been investigated as a possible cancer target, which has cleared the path for developing new inhibitors. Because of their higher expression in malignant cells than normal cells, both hTERT and dyskerin are intriguing targets (Chen et al. 2020). Expanding gene therapy and utilizing the hTERT promoter's cancer-fighting abilities as an effective viral vector are promising directions for future research (Hacker et al. 2020). Moreover, immunotherapies that target hTERT antigens showed promising outcomes and can revolutionize cancer treatment in the coming years (Carrozza et al. 2018). Telomerase inhibitors based on small molecules have had little success but may soon contribute to clinical factors (Neidle 2020).

The idea of creating rational structure-based telomerase inhibitors is to increase selectivity, bioavailability, and inhibitory effectiveness, and compared to the present arsenal of small-molecule inhibitors, they might give more significant results (Baginski and Serbakowska 2020). G4 stabilizers have a big future as anticancer drugs due to their propensity to trigger telomere structural disruption. TRF2 and POT1 are telomerase-binding proteins with a significant threshold in the in vivo experiments (Fernandes et al. 2020). As a result, targeting telomere and telomerase activities might be clinically advantageous in expanding practical and powerful anticancer medications with cancer cell-specific toxicity (Guterres and Villanueva 2020). The initiation of senescence, suppression of cell growth, and end-to-end chromosomal fusion can all be induced by small ligands stabilizing telomeres into G-4 structures (Bryan 2020). The stability of G-4 inside c-myc and c-kit can inhibit gene transcription and downregulate the production of these proteins (Monsen et al. 2022). Cancer risk rises with age, and genetic problems, habits, smoking, and surroundings are all major contributors to cancer development (Lewandowska et al. 2018). The ability to utilize the differences in telomerase activity in normal and malignant cells to expand new anticancer drugs is critical (Vishwakarma et al. 2023). Inhibiting telomerase activity can be accomplished in various ways, including targeting the catalytic activity of TERT, targeting TERC interactions, straightly targeting TERC, and targeting DKC1 in RNP biogenesis (Eitsuka et al. 2018). Synthetic oligonucleotides (e.g., imetelstat), nucleoside analogs (e.g., zidovudine), small molecules (e.g., BIBR1532), natural compounds (rhodocyanine, curcumin, and genistein), G-4 stabilizers (telomestatin), and vaccines are all examples of inhibitors (Saraswati et al. 2019).

2.1 The Natural-Based Inhibitors

Inactivation of telomerase and telomere instability by natural products provides an opportunity to achieve new goals in cancer therapy (Mustafa 2024). Many telomerase inhibitors exist, and they target the enzyme's catalytic components or RNA to prevent it from catalyzing. Natural and synthetic materials, as well as modified oligonucleotides, are widely used as telomerase inhibitors (Bajaj et al. 2020). G-quadruplex (G4) ligands, which attach to telomeres, may be implicated in telomerase-positive and ALT cells. For the ALT pathway, there are no specific inhibitors yet (Yang et al. 2021). Most cancer cells have telomerase, which is required for cancer cell development. Telomerase inactivation and telomere destabilization by natural/synthetic products provide many opportunities for achieving new goals in cancer therapy. Several chemical compounds are now available for commercial use in cancer treatment. However, many of these chemicals cause or exacerbate adverse effects in cancer patients (Ali and Walter 2023). Consequently, natural products such as herbs must be studied to determine their beneficial effects on cancer cells and combat cancer with them. Also, natural products commonly consumed as part of a traditional medicine diet are eatable, safe to digest, and generally well accepted by individuals (Lee et al. 2018). Different natural compounds suppress telomerase activity in cancer cells, and there is a link between this activity and decreased cell viability. Natural ingredients limit telomerase function when used to treat different malignancies via downregulating hTERT mRNA synthesis, inducing apoptosis, and inducing senescence through DNA damage response. Additionally, these natural ingredients promote the production of p53, which limits cell cycle, migration, and metastasis (Yan et al. 2022).

Secondary metabolites are prevalent telomerase inhibitors produced from natural plant components like polyphenols (curcumin, quercetin, resveratrol, and tannic acid), alkaloids (boldine and berberine), triterpenoid (pristimerin and oleanane), xanthones (gambogic acid and gambogenic acid), and sesquiterpene (Parekh et al. 2023). Plant metabolites include medicinal compounds, and a large portion of their research focuses on the inhibition of telomerase, including hTERT and hTR, telomerase substrates, and related proteins (Savelyev et al. 2018). Plant secondary metabolites are critical in decreasing telomerase activity and inducing apoptosis in an anti-telomerase screening investigation. Studies show that secondary metabolites in vivo and in vitro can inhibit telomerase and prevent proliferation (Wani et al. 2023).

2.2 Synthetic Sources of Telomerase Inhibitors

By exploiting the Protein Data Bank (PDB) and the hTERT-BIBR1532 complex, researchers studied the small molecules as inhibitors of the hTERT catalytic subunit. Telomeres can form secondary structures called G4s due to their G-rich and repetitive character (Tan and Lan 2020). By pairing four guanines with Hoogsteen base pairing, G4s form stacks of G-quartets (Lerner and Sale 2019). G4 stabilization at telomeres causes telomere dysfunction, disrupting recombination, replication, and association, manifesting as incomplete replication, DNA fragmentation, telomere cap loss, or shortening of telomeres. As telomeres get defective, DDR components, including 53BP1, γ-H2AX, and the MRN complex, are employed to create telomere dysfunction-induced foci (TIFs) (Liu et al. 2019). Apoptosis and genetic instability can arise from incorrect telomere repair. G4s at telomere ends may also obstruct telomerase detection and prevent telomere extension, resulting in telomere shortening (Berardinelli et al. 2017). Thus, applying G4 ligands, which maintain the G4 structure, stops the cloning fork and damages the DNA in the telomere. G4 fixation in telomeres is thought to be a viable strategy to eliminate quickly proliferating cells in anticancer therapy (Pavlova et al. 2021).

G-Quadruplex Stabilizers

For different G4 topologies, the fluorescence resonance energy transfer (FRET) approach is used to measure the stability and selection of quaternary ligands (Umar et al. 2019). Specific prospective G4 stabilizers have been created to understand the interaction between G4 stabilizers and their impact on numerous biological processes.

3 Vaccine-Based Strategies to Telomerase Inhibition

Immune defense systems have a significant role in treating cancer. The active site of telomerase in cancer cells is a target for making vaccines (Kailashiya et al. 2017). The human leukocyte antigen (HLA) class-1 pathway expresses telomerase fragments on the surface of tumor cells as antigens as a result of telomerase breakdown via proteasomes (Bauer et al. 2019). Telomerase antigen epitopes will be known by cytotoxic T lymphocytes (CTLs), and then they begin to attack cancer cells (Dosset et al. 2020). There are two main techniques for immunotherapy based on telomerase: first, direct in vivo immune system activation, and second, immune system activation and proliferation in an ex vivo setting. The two most studied vaccination approaches are GRNVAC1 and GV1001 (Negrini et al. 2020).

3.1 In Vivo Induction of the Immune Cells Directly

GV1001 directly stimulates the immune system with 16 amino acids (p611-EARPALLTSRLRFIPK-p626) and a restricted peptide generated from TERT (Chen et al. 2018). Due to its recognition by primary MHC class I and class II molecules, this vaccine triggers CD4+ and CD8+ T cell responses (Kyte et al. 2019). Pancreatic cancer, hepatocellular carcinoma, malignant melanoma, and non-small cell lung cancer are among the malignancies for which GV1001 is currently being tested (Shou et al. 2024). Presently, GV1001 therapy has not been associated with any adverse effects (Kim et al. 2019). According to recent research, GV1001 permeates the cell membrane and lowers the amounts of the heat shock proteins (HSPs) HSP70 and HSP90 on the surface and within cells. In cancer cells exposed to hypoxia, GV1001 dramatically lowers the levels of VEGF and HIF-1α (Mizukoshi and Kaneko 2019). Through inhibiting free radicals and modulation of life and death signals, it also demonstrates antioxidant capabilities and protection of nerves in neural stem cells (Shaban et al. 2017).

3.2 Ex Vivo Immune Cell Activation and Proliferation

As part of the GRNVAC1 treatment, patients get intradermal injections of mature autologous dendritic cells extracted from them and transfected ex vivo with mRNA that encodes hTERT and LAMP1 (Al-Khafaf et al. 2021). This unique strategy elicits CD4+ and CD8+ responses that are specific to TERT. Patients with acute myelogenous leukemia (AML) participated in a phase II research of GRNVAC1. The patients who took GNVAC1 showed high levels of tolerance and safety, according to the findings (Witkowska 2021). Since DNA vaccine allows for the flexible incorporation of numerous genes, it is a successful developing strategy in cancer immunotherapy (Pandya et al. 2023). INVAC-1, an enhanced DNA plasmid that encodes the inactive version of hTERT, stimulates cellular defense against malignancies. In several mice models, an intradermal injection of INVAC-1, accompanied by electro-gene-transfer (EGT), induced an immune cell response particular to hTERT characterized by increased numbers of CD8+ memory T cells and CD4 + Th1 effector. Furthermore, INVAC-1 is a potential vaccination volunteer to treat cancer since it reduced tumor development and raised the survival rate of mice with tumors by 50% when administered to a spontaneous and invasive HLA-A2 sarcoma mouse model (Teixeira et al. 2020).

4 Control of Telomerase and Tumor Angiogenesis Through Wnt Signaling

Proteins that deliver signals to cells through cell surface receptors are the starting point of a class of signal transduction pathways called Wnt signaling pathways. Wnt signaling pathways may employ same-cell (autocrine) or nearby cell-cell (paracrine) communication (Gajos-Michniewicz and Czyz 2020). The pathology and average growth of many diseases, including cancer, are significantly influenced by the signaling pathways of Wnts, which are crucial components of angiogenesis. Cell survival, differentiation, migration, apoptosis, and proliferation are all impacted by Wnt pathways. These pathways significantly influence angiogenesis and vessel regeneration (Olsen et al. 2017). Secreted glycoproteins called Wnt ligands bind to frizzled receptors (FZDs) and prompt LRP5/6 to form a larger complex on the cell surface with it. The inactive canonical pathway: no signal is transduced through Dvl without Wnt ligand activation via the FZD-LRP5/6 receptor complex. As a result, the destruction complex of Axin, APC, GSK3, and CK1 stabilizes, phosphorylating β-catenin and causing its eventual disintegration. Active canonical Wnt signaling: the activation of FZD receptor and LRP5/6 co-receptors is triggered by Wnt ligand stimulation; the destabilization of the destruction complex results from a signal transduced through Dvl. Wnt target gene transcription is initiated by non-phosphorylated (active) β-catenin, which migrates to the cell nucleus and interacts with TCF/LEF transcription factors (Hayat et al. 2022). Recent research demonstrated that Wnt signaling pathways, whether active or inactive, contribute to angiogenesis in a variety of organs in both normal and pathological conditions (Muccioli et al. 2021). Many biological processes contribute to inducing tumor vascularization, which develops concurrently inside the same malignancy. A variety of secreted compounds and signaling pathways control these processes (Lugano et al. 2020). Many cancer types can now be treated with anti-angiogenic drugs that use antibodies or tyrosine kinase inhibitors (TKIs). However, the effects of the therapy have been marginal thus far, and some patients refuse to improve (Liu et al. 2023). Keeping cancers from reaching the bloodstream is a complex undertaking. When analyzing diverse cancer subtypes, tumor vascular function and gene expression can vary greatly, and vascular phenotype inside the same tumor can likewise differ (Roda et al. 2021). Angiogenesis-related signaling pathway suppression may prevent the growth of fresh veins and trigger cancer dormancy (Li et al. 2022).

5 Discussion

It is clear that telomeres and telomerase play a key role in health and longevity. Telomerase is an enzyme that can add repetitive noncoding DNA sequences to the ends of chromosomes, called telomeres, using its RNA template, and delay their shortening following cell divisions. Since more than 85% of cancers have overexpressed telomerase, telomerase inhibitor drugs have been developed as promising targets for the treatment of various malignancies. Today, there are countless drugs whose function is to inhibit telomerase, from natural products to synthetic and modified oligonucleotides. Among these drugs, natural products have greater efficacy and acceptability, and there is more scope for research and clinical trials with synthetic drugs. Telomeres, which are rich in guanine, form structures called G-quadruplexes (G4s) that protect the vulnerable ends of telomeres and help maintain genome integrity. By using G4 ligands to stabilize G4s, the DNA replication fork is stalled, and telomeres are damaged. Hence, the stabilization of G4s provides a hopeful outlook for the development of anticancer drugs that target highly proliferative cells. Wnts are potent angiogenic factors, and their signaling pathways have a major part in the pathogenesis of numerous cancers. Some telomerase inhibitors have the ability to inhibit telomerase and the Wnt signaling pathway simultaneously. Recently, a telomerase inhibitor, imetelstat (Rytelst), has been approved by the FDA. Given that telomerase is implicated in the majority of malignancies, telomerase inhibitors represent an impressive potential for future research and development as well as a viable treatment for a wide range of tumors. Utilizing artificial intelligence and machine learning, we have innumerable opportunities to design and manufacture such drugs, which puts a positive perspective in front of us.

References

Aksenova AY, Mirkin SM (2019) At the beginning of the end and in the middle of the beginning: structure and maintenance of telomeric DNA repeats and interstitial telomeric sequences. Genes 10(2):118

Ali JH, Walter M (2023) Combining old and new concepts in targeting telomerase for cancer therapy: transient, immediate, complete and combinatory attack (TICCA). Cancer Cell Int 23(1):197

Al-Khafaf MN, Abubaker SR, Ahmed A (2021) A significance correlation between malignant tumors and telomerase. Annals Roman Soc Cell Biol:3822–3842

Ataker Y, Simsek R (2020) Telomere, telomerase and telomerase inhibitors. Bioorganic Med Chem Report 3(1):1

Aviv A, Anderson JJ, Shay JW (2017) Mutations, cancer and the telomere length paradox. Trends Cancer 3(4):253–258

Baginski M, Serbakowska K (2020) In silico design of telomerase inhibitors. Drug Discov Today 25(7):1213–1222

Bajaj S, Kumar MS, Peters G, Mayur Y (2020) Targeting telomerase for its advent in cancer therapeutics. Med Res Rev 40(5):1871–1919

Bauer J, Nelde A, Bilich T, Walz JS (2019) Antigen targets for the development of immunotherapies in leukemia. Int J Mol Sci 20(6):1397

Berardinelli F, Coluzzi E, Sgura A, Antoccia A (2017) Targeting telomerase and telomeres to enhance ionizing radiation effects in in vitro and in vivo cancer models. Mutat Res Rev Mutat Res 773:204–219

Blackford AN, Jackson SP (2017) ATM, ATR, and DNA-PK: the trinity at the heart of the DNA damage response. Mol Cell 66(6):801–817

Bordeira Gaspar T, Sá A, Lopes JM, Sobrinho-Simões M, Soares P, Vinagre J (2018) Telomere maintenance mechanisms in cancer. Genes 9(5):241

Bryan TM (2020) G-quadruplexes at telomeres: friend or foe? Molecules 25(16):3686

Carrozza F, Santoni M, Piva F, Cheng L, Lopez-Beltran A, Scarpelli M, Montironi R, Battelli N, Tamberi S (2018) Emerging immunotherapeutic strategies targeting telomerases in genitourinary tumors. Crit Rev Oncol Hematol 131:1–6

Chen W, Shin KH, Kim S, Shon WJ, Kim RH, Park NH, Kang MK (2018) hTERT peptide fragment GV1001 demonstrates radioprotective and antifibrotic effects through suppression of TGF-β signaling. Int J Mol Med 41(6):3211–3220

Chen X, Tang WJ, Shi JB, Liu MM, Liu XH (2020) Therapeutic strategies for targeting telomerase in cancer. Med Res Rev 40(2):532–585

de Lange T (2018) Shelterin-mediated telomere protection. Annu Rev Genet 52:223–247

Denham J, Sellami M (2021) Exercise training increases telomerase reverse transcriptase gene expression and telomerase activity: a systematic review and meta-analysis. Ageing Res Rev 70: 101411

Dosset M, Castro A, Carter H, Zanetti M (2020) Telomerase and CD4 T cell immunity in cancer. Cancers 12(6):1687

Dratwa M, Wysoczańska B, Łacina P, Kubik T, Bogunia-Kubik K (2020) TERT—regulation and roles in cancer formation. Front Immunol 11:589929

Eitsuka T, Nakagawa K, Kato S, Ito J, Otoki Y, Takasu S, Shimizu N, Takahashi T, Miyazawa T (2018) Modulation of telomerase activity in cancer cells by dietary compounds: a review. Int J Mol Sci 19(2):478

Fernandes SG, Dsouza R, Pandya G, Kirtonia A, Tergaonkar V, Lee SY, Garg M, Khattar E (2020) Role of telomeres and telomeric proteins in human malignancies and their therapeutic potential. Cancers 12(7):1901

Frescas D, de Lange T (2014) TRF2-tethered TIN2 can mediate telomere protection by TPP1/POT1. Mol Cell Biol 34(7):1349–1362

Gajos-Michniewicz A, Czyz M (2020) WNT signaling in melanoma. Int J Mol Sci 21(14):4852

Ganesan K, Xu B (2017) Telomerase inhibitors from natural products and their anticancer potential. Int J Mol Sci 19(1):13

Ghanim GE, Fountain AJ, Van Roon A-MM, Rangan R, Das R, Collins K, Nguyen THD (2021) Structure of human telomerase holoenzyme with bound telomeric DNA. Nature 593(7859): 449–453

Grill S, Nandakumar J (2021) Molecular mechanisms of telomere biology disorders. J Biol Chem 296:100064

Guterres AN, Villanueva J (2020) Targeting telomerase for cancer therapy. Oncogene 39(36): 5811–5824

Hacker UT, Bentler M, Kaniowska D, Morgan M, Büning H (2020) Towards clinical implementation of adeno-associated virus (AAV) vectors for cancer gene therapy: current status and future perspectives. Cancers 12(7):1889

Hayat R, Manzoor M, Hussain A (2022) Wnt signaling pathway: a comprehensive review. Cell Biol Int 46(6):863–877

Jafri MA, Ansari SA, Alqahtani MH, Shay JW (2016) Roles of telomeres and telomerase in cancer, and advances in telomerase-targeted therapies. Genome Med 8:1–18

Judasz E, Lisiak N, Kopczyński P, Taube M, Rubiś B (2022) The role of telomerase in breast cancer's response to therapy. Int J Mol Sci 23(21):12844

Kailashiya C, Sharma HB, Kailashiya J (2017) Telomerase based anticancer immunotherapy and vaccines approaches. Vaccine 35(43):5768–5775

Kim JW, Yadav DK, Kim SJ, Lee M-Y, Park J-M, Kim BS, Kim M-h, Park H-g, Kang KW (2019) Anti-cancer effect of GV1001 for prostate cancer: function as a ligand of GnRHR. Endocr Relat Cancer 26(2):147–162

Kyte JA, Fåne A, Pule M, Gaudernack G (2019) Transient redirection of T cells for adoptive cell therapy with telomerase-specific T helper cell receptors isolated from long term survivors after cancer vaccination. Onco Targets Ther 8(4):e1565236

Lee KW, Ching SM, Hoo FK, Ramachandran V, Swamy MK (2018) Traditional medicinal plants and their therapeutic potential against major cancer types. Antican Plants Nat Prod Biotechnol Implement 2:383–410

Leggett SE, Hruska AM, Guo M, Wong IY (2021) The epithelial-mesenchymal transition and the cytoskeleton in bioengineered systems. Cell Commun Signal 19(1):32

Lerner LK, Sale JE (2019) Replication of G quadruplex DNA. Genes 10(2):95

Lewandowska AM, Rudzki M, Rudzki S, Lewandowski T, Laskowska B (2018) Environmental risk factors for cancer-review paper. Ann Agric Environ Med 26(1):1–7

Li Y, Lin M, Wang S, Cao B, Li C, Li G (2022) Novel angiogenic regulators and anti-angiogenesis drugs targeting angiogenesis signaling pathways: perspectives for targeting angiogenesis in lung cancer. Front Oncol 12:842960

Liu R, Liu J, Wang S, Wang Y, Zhang T, Liu Y, Geng X, Wang F (2019) Combined treatment with emodin and a telomerase inhibitor induces significant telomere damage/dysfunction and cell death. Cell Death Dis 10(7):527

Liu Z-L, Chen H-H, Zheng L-L, Sun L-P, Shi L (2023) Angiogenic signaling pathways and anti-angiogenic therapy for cancer. Signal Transduct Target Ther 8(1):198

Lorbeer FK, Hockemeyer D (2020) TERT promoter mutations and telomeres during tumorigenesis. Curr Opin Genet Dev 60:56–62

Lugano R, Ramachandran M, Dimberg A (2020) Tumor angiogenesis: causes, consequences, challenges and opportunities. Cell Mol Life Sci 77:1745–1770

Lupatov AY, Yarygin KN (2022) Telomeres and telomerase in the control of stem cells. Biomedicines 10(10):2335

MacNeil DE, Lambert-Lanteigne P, Autexier C (2019) N-terminal residues of human dyskerin are required for interactions with telomerase RNA that prevent RNA degradation. Nucleic Acids Res 47(10):5368–5380

Martínez P, Blasco MA (2017) Telomere-driven diseases and telomere-targeting therapies. J Cell Biol 216(4):875

Mizukoshi E, Kaneko S (2019) Telomerase-targeted cancer immunotherapy. Int J Mol Sci 20(8): 1823

Monsen RC, DeLeeuw LW, Dean WL, Gray RD, Chakravarthy S, Hopkins JB, Chaires JB, Trent JO (2022) Long promoter sequences form higher-order G-quadruplexes: an integrative structural biology study of c-Myc, k-Ras and c-kit promoter sequences. Nucleic Acids Res 50(7): 4127–4147

Muccioli S, Brillo V, Chieregato L, Leanza L, Checchetto V, Costa R (2021) From channels to canonical Wnt signaling: a pathological perspective. Int J Mol Sci 22(9):4613

Mustafa YF (2024) Nutraceutical-based telomerase inhibitors: renewed hope for cancer therapy. Phytomedicine Plus:100537

Negrini S, De Palma R, Filaci G (2020) Anti-cancer immunotherapies targeting telomerase. Cancers 12(8):2260

Neidle S (2020) Challenges in developing small-molecule quadruplex therapeutics. Ann Rep Med Chem Elsevier 54:517–546

Noureen N, Wu S, Lv Y, Yang J, Alfred Yung W, Gelfond J, Wang X, Koul D, Ludlow A, Zheng S (2021) Integrated analysis of telomerase enzymatic activity unravels an association with cancer stemness and proliferation. Nat Commun 12(1):139

Olivieri C, Mondino A, Chinello M, Risso A, Finale E, Lanciotti M, Guala A (2017) Clinical heterogeneity in a family with DKC1 mutation, dyskeratosis congenita and Hoyeraal-Hreidarsson syndrome in first cousins. Pediatric Reports 9(3):7301

Olsen JJ, Pohl SÖ-G, Deshmukh A, Visweswaran M, Ward NC, Arfuso F, Agostino M, Dharmarajan A (2017) The role of Wnt signalling in angiogenesis. Clin Biochem Rev 38(3):131

Pandya A, Shah Y, Kothari N, Postwala H, Shah A, Parekh P, Chorawala MR (2023) The future of cancer immunotherapy: DNA vaccines leading the way. Med Oncol 40(7):200

Parekh N, Garg A, Choudhary R, Gupta M, Kaur G, Ramniwas S, Shahwan M, Tuli HS, Sethi G (2023) The role of natural flavonoids as telomerase inhibitors in suppressing cancer growth. Pharmaceuticals 16(4):605

Pavlova AV, Kubareva EA, Monakhova MV, Zvereva MI, Dolinnaya NG (2021) Impact of G-quadruplexes on the regulation of genome integrity, DNA damage and repair. Biomol Ther 11(9):1284

Procházková Schrumpfová P, Fojtová M, Fajkus J (2019) Telomeres in plants and humans: not so different, not so similar. Cells 8(1):58

Rachakonda S, Kong H, Srinivas N, Garcia-Casado Z, Requena C, Fallah M, Heidenreich B, Planelles D, Traves V, Schadendorf D (2018) Telomere length, telomerase reverse transcriptase promoter mutations, and melanoma risk. Genes Chromosom Cancer 57(11):564–572

Roda N, Blandano G, Pelicci PG (2021) Blood vessels and peripheral nerves as key players in cancer progression and therapy resistance. Cancers 13(17):4471

Sameri S, Mohammadi C, Mehrabani M, Najafi R (2021) Targeting the hallmarks of cancer: the effects of silibinin on proliferation, cell death, angiogenesis, and migration in colorectal cancer. BMC Complement Med Therap 21(1):160

Saraswati AP, Relitti N, Brindisi M, Gemma S, Zisterer D, Butini S, Campiani G (2019) Raising the bar in anticancer therapy: recent advances in, and perspectives on, telomerase inhibitors. Drug Discov Today 24(7):1370–1388

Saretzki G (2023) Role of telomeres and telomerase in cancer and aging. MDPI 24:9932

Savelyev N, Baykuzina P, Dokudovskaya S, Lavrik O, Rubtsova M, Dontsova O (2018) Comprehensive analysis of telomerase inhibition by gallotannin. Oncotarget 9(27):18712

Seimiya H (2020) Crossroads of telomere biology and anticancer drug discovery. Cancer Sci 111(9):3089–3099

Shaban S, El-Husseny MWA, Abushouk AI, Salem AMA, Mamdouh M, Abdel-Daim MM (2017) Effects of antioxidant supplements on the survival and differentiation of stem cells. Oxidative Med Cell Longev 2017(1):5032102

Shou S, Li Y, Chen J, Zhang X, Zhang C, Jiang X, Liu F, Yi L, Zhang X, Geer E (2024) Understanding, diagnosing, and treating pancreatic cancer from the perspective of telomeres and telomerase. Cancer Gene Ther 31:1–14

Srinivas N, Rachakonda S, Kumar R (2020) Telomeres and telomere length: a general overview. Cancers 12(3):558

Sugarman ET, Zhang G, Shay JW (2019) In perspective: an update on telomere targeting in cancer. Mol Carcinog 58(9):1581–1588

Tan J, Lan L (2020) The DNA secondary structures at telomeres and genome instability. Cell Biosci 10(1):47

Teixeira L, Medioni J, Garibal J, Adotevi O, Doucet L, Durey M-AD, Ghrieb Z, Kiladjian J-J, Brizard M, Laheurte C (2020) A first-in-human phase I study of INVAC-1, an optimized human telomerase DNA vaccine in patients with advanced solid tumors. Clin Cancer Res 26(3): 588–597

Trybek T, Kowalik A, Góźdź S, Kowalska A (2020) Telomeres and telomerase in oncogenesis. Oncol Lett 20(2):1015–1027

Umar MI, Ji D, Chan C-Y, Kwok CK (2019) G-quadruplex-based fluorescent turn-on ligands and aptamers: from development to applications. Molecules 24(13):2416

Verma AK, Singh P, Al-Saeed FA, Ahmed AE, Kumar S, Kumar A, Dev K, Dohare R (2022) Unravelling the role of telomere shortening with ageing and their potential association with diabetes, cancer, and related lifestyle factors. Tissue Cell 79:101925

Vishwakarma K, Dey R, Bhatt H (2023) Telomerase: a prominent oncological target for development of chemotherapeutic agents. Eur J Med Chem 249:115121

Wang F, Fu K, Wang Y, Pan C, Wang X, Liu Z, Yang C, Zheng Y, Li X, Lu Y (2023) Small-molecule agents for cancer immunotherapy, vol 14, Acta Pharmaceutica Sinica B, p 905

Wani AK, Akhtar N, Sharma A, El-Zahaby SA (2023) Fighting carcinogenesis with plant metabolites by weakening proliferative signaling and disabling replicative immortality networks of rapidly dividing and invading cancerous cells. Curr Drug Deliv 20(4):371–386

Witkowska M (2021) Biologically active compounds based on the carbazole scaffold-synthetic and mechanistic aspects

Wu RA, Upton HE, Vogan JM, Collins K (2017) Telomerase mechanism of telomere synthesis. Annu Rev Biochem 86:439–460

Xu M, Kiselar J, Whited TL, Hernandez-Sanchez W, Taylor DJ (2019) POT1-TPP1 differentially regulates telomerase via POT1 His266 and as a function of single-stranded telomere DNA length. Proc Natl Acad Sci 116(47):23527–23533

Yan S, Lin S, Chen K, Yin S, Peng H, Cai N, Ma W, Songyang Z, Huang Y (2022) Natural product library screens identify sanguinarine chloride as a potent inhibitor of telomerase expression and activity. Cells 11(9):1485

Yang SY, Chang EY, Lim J, Kwan HH, Monchaud D, Yip S, Stirling PC, Wong JM (2021) G-quadruplexes mark alternative lengthening of telomeres. NAR Cancer 3(3):zcab031

Yuan X, Xu D (2019) Telomerase reverse transcriptase (TERT) in action: cross-talking with epigenetics. Int J Mol Sci 20(13):3338

Yuan X, Larsson C, Xu D (2019) Mechanisms underlying the activation of TERT transcription and telomerase activity in human cancer: old actors and new players. Oncogene 38(34):6172–6183

Zhang J-M, Zou L (2020) Alternative lengthening of telomeres: from molecular mechanisms to therapeutic outlooks. Cell Biosci 10(1):30

Intricate Relationship Between Radiation-Induced Trismus and Inflammation

Efsun Somay, Erkan Topkan, Duriye Ozturk, and Ugur Selek

Abstract

Radiation therapy is an essential component of multimodality cancer treatment, as it can potentially eliminate tumors and improve patient outcomes. However, radiation therapy may induce severe side effects, such as highly debilitating radiation-induced trismus. Radiation-induced trismus, characterized by restricted jaw movement and muscular rigidity, represents a severe challenge in cancer treatment and may threaten an affected patient's life in certain conditions like emergencies. The medical literature has researched and documented the mechanisms that cause radiation-induced trismus, a hyperinflammatory disease, by inducing and maintaining inflammation after head and neck irradiation. Significant labor has been undertaken to elucidate the series of events that play crucial roles in the development and progression of this unfortunate condition, with particular emphasis on critical factors such as oxidative stress, cytokine dysregulation, damage to salivary glands and soft tissues, and the triggers of a hyper-inflammatory state. However, too many unknowns remain about the exact relationship between radiation-induced trismus and hyperinflammation caused by head and neck irradiation. Hence, this chapter aims to provide an evidence-based

E. Somay (✉)
Department of Oral and Maxillofacial Surgery, Faculty of Dentistry, Baskent University, Ankara, Turkey
e-mail: efsuner@gmail.com; esomay@baskent.edu.tr

E. Topkan
Department of Radiation Oncology, Faculty of Medicine, Baskent University, Adana, Turkey

D. Ozturk
Department of Radiation Oncology, Faculty of Medicine, Afyonkarahisar Health Sciences University, Afyonkarahisar, Turkey

U. Selek
Department of Radiation Oncology, Faculty of Medicine, Koc University, Istanbul, Turkey

Interdisciplinary Cancer Research, https://doi.org/10.1007/16833_2023_198
Published online: 17 November 2023

review of the intricate and multifaceted interactions between radiation-induced hyperinflammation and the development of radiation-induced trismus in head and neck cancer patients treated with radiation or chemoradiotherapy.

Keywords

Cytokines · Inflammation · Radiation therapy · Radiation-induced trismus

1 Introduction

Radiation therapy (RT), a crucial tool in combating cancer, is an indispensable component of treatment for patients presenting with head and neck cancers (HNC), which may be used in adjuvant, definitive, or palliative settings with or without systemic therapies. Patients undergoing RT for head and neck cancer (HNC) may experience radiation-induced trismus (RIT), a well-known and challenging side effect (Louise Kent et al. 2008). RIT is a highly detrimental complication of RT or chemo-RT (CRT), which can harm various aspects of daily life, such as oral hygiene, eating, speaking, chewing, and swallowing. Furthermore, RIT has the potential to significantly impact multiple aspects of patients' quality of life (QoL), including social interactions, psychological health, and economic well-being (Raj et al. 2020; Johnson et al. 2015). Nutritional problems associated with RIT can contribute to the development or progression of cancer cachexia, which can worsen the prognosis for patients (van de Worp et al. 2020). Additionally, RIT poses a potential threat to the lives of patients with respiratory issues during emergencies, as it can be challenging to ensure an open airway (Graham et al. 2006).

While RT is intended to target cancer cells and treat the disease, it can also result in unwarranted severe adverse effects beyond the intended treatment area (Baskar et al. 2012). High doses of RT or CRT may gradually damage nearby healthy tissues by triggering a cascade of pathologic processes that can lead to trismus, a condition characterized by limited mouth opening due to muscle stiffness and fibrosis in the jaw and temporomandibular joint region, namely the masticatory apparatus (Fig. 1) (Brook 2020). Inflammation plays a crucial physiologic role in the body's defense, healing, and restoration of injured tissues (Nepon et al. 2021; Straub et al. 2015; Somay et al, 2022a, b). However, when the delicate balance of this response is disrupted, inflammation may have adverse effects apart from its positive impacts on the body's defense. This disruption can occur in irradiated tissues, where cellular stress and DNA damage provide a favorable environment for subsequent events like RIT (Kim et al. 2019).

Inflammation is widely considered to have a substantial role in the development of RIT via many mechanisms (Nepon et al. 2021). According to previous research, the primary cellular stress response involves the synthesis of proinflammatory cytokines and chemokines, which function as signaling molecules to attract immune cells to the site of injury (Zhang et al. 2021a). Moreover, immune cells, including neutrophils and macrophages, infiltrate irradiated tissues and secrete supplementary inflammatory mediators, perpetuating the inflammatory cascade (Su et al. 2020).

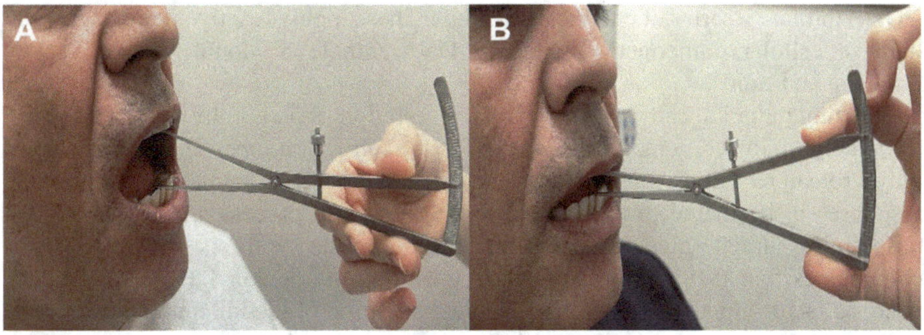

Fig. 1 Representative assessment of maximum mouth opening before and after treatment in a 48-year-old male patient treated with concurrent chemoradiotherapy for locally advanced nasopharyngeal cancer: (**a**) He had a maximum mouth opening of 46 mm before the commencement of the chemoradiotherapy. (**b**) It was proved that he had radiation-induced trismus with a maximum mouth opening of only 19 mm at the post-chemoradiotherapy 5-month evaluations

Despite the fact that the precise mechanisms of RIT development and progression remain largely unresolved, it exemplifies the intricate connection between the inflammatory cascade occurring in the oral and maxillofacial areas and exposure to high-dose radiation. Because radiation-induced inflammation and RIT development are firmly interrelated conditions, this chapter aims to illuminate the complex landscape of inflammation's contribution to RIT development and comprehend the pathways regulating this dynamic interaction, which may guide the future evolution of novel preventive and treatment strategies in HNC patients.

2 Cellular Response to Radiation

The ionizing radiation exhibits an array of mechanisms to interact with biological tissues by depositing energy. The consequential effects of these interactions are contingent on the dose and the intended purpose of the radiation exposure, which can vary from beneficial to harmful. The following are the primary mechanisms of ionizing radiation tissue interactions.

Direct ionization is a significant radiation effect, accounting for approximately one-third of all such occurrences. It takes place when high-energy photons or particles, such as X-rays, gamma rays, alpha particles, and beta particles, collide with atoms in the tissue, resulting in the ejection of electrons from the atoms. This interaction generates an ion pair, consisting of a positively charged ion and a free electron within the tissue. The resulting ions and free electrons can cause further damage by interacting with other nearby atoms and molecules, thereby exacerbating the destruction wrought by direct ionization. However, most ionization events are indirect, corresponding to two-thirds of all. In this process, the ionizing radiation interacts with water molecules (which make up 60–70% of biological tissues) and generates free radicals such as hydroxyl radicals (•OH) and superoxide radicals

(•O2–) through a series of chemical reactions. These highly reactive free radicals can damage cellular components including DNA (single or double-strand breaks), proteins, and lipids.

Ionizing radiation can induce chemokine secretion as part of the cellular response to radiation-induced damage irrespective of the ionization type. These chemokines play a role in recruiting immune cells and modulating the inflammatory and immune responses in irradiated tissues. In brief, the ionization process and the associated tissue injury initiate a cascade of events leading to the synthesis of cytokines and chemokines that facilitate inflammation, including interleukin-1 (IL-1) and tumor necrosis factor-alpha (TNF-α), marking the beginning of the inflammatory process. Moreover, after ionizing radiation, inflammatory chemokines such as interleukin-8 (IL-8 or CXCL8) are secreted in response to radiation-induced tissue damage, which recruits neutrophils and other immune cells to the injury site. Radiation-induced chemokines can attract immune cells like T cells, B cells, and dendritic cells to areas of radiation injury and further worsen the ongoing inflammatory process. As this process progresses, symptoms of acute inflammation manifest, such as increased vascular permeability, localized edema, endothelial cell apoptosis, and vascular thrombosis (Baskar et al. 2012; Brook 2020; Nepon et al. 2021). In non-tumorous tissues, these deleterious modifications culminate in a diminished capacity for tissue regeneration, primarily attributable to tissue hypoxia and inadequate nutrient supply. This phenomenon can elicit apoptotic cascades or necrosis, leading to the formation of fibrotic tissue during the subsequent reparative phase. Therefore, RT may lead to RIT formation by inducing tissue injury, hypoxia, hyperinflammation, and inappropriate tissue repair via fibrosis in the masticatory apparatus components.

3 Inflammatory Mediators and Immune Cell Infiltration

Inflammation is a multifaceted biological reaction that plays a crucial role in various physiological processes, such as immune response, tissue regeneration, and defense against infections (Chen et al. 2017). Inflammatory cytokines are attractant proteins that have the ability to recruit immune cells to the area injured by ionizing radiation, such as neutrophils and macrophages (Kim et al. 2019). Upon arrival at the site of injury, these immune cells secrete supplementary inflammatory mediators, sustaining the progression of the inflammatory cascade. Macrophages, specifically, have dual functionality in tissue repair and fibrosis processes, as they release pro-inflammatory and anti-inflammatory substances (Chen et al. 2017; Wynn and Vannella 2016). Following radiation exposure, neutrophils exhibit rapid migration toward the damaged region and often demonstrate prompt arrival at the injury site (Nguyen et al. 2017). Despite their effectiveness in fighting microbial infections, polymorphonuclear leukocytes can potentially exacerbate tissue damage due to releasing proteases and reactive oxygen species (ROS). Neutrophils have a crucial role in regulating the inflammatory milieu, facilitating immunological responses, and promoting tissue healing (Mittal et al. 2014).

RT can also induce the secretion of a wide range of cytokines and other mediators by cells, such as endothelial cells of tumor stroma and infiltrating immune cells, including the dendritic cells surrounding the tumor. These cytokines can be either immune-stimulating, pro-inflammatory, such as interleukin (IL)-6, tumor necrosis factor (TNF)-α, or IL-1, or immune suppressive, anti-inflammatory (e.g., IL-10) (Sologuren et al. 2014). Many cell types of the immune system produce cytokines and chemokines, including macrophages, lymphocytes, and granulocytes. Nevertheless, other cells, not necessarily from the immune system, such as endothelial cells and fibroblasts, may also produce a vast array of cytokines and chemokines (Sologuren et al. 2014).

4 Fibroblast Activation and Collagen Deposition

Fibroblasts are the primary source of inflammatory cytokines and chemokines in inflammatory disorders due to their ability to generate larger quantities of inflammatory factors compared to leukocytes (Nygaard and Firestein 2020; Nguyen et al. 2017). Persistent inflammation creates an unfavorable microenvironment that stimulates fibroblasts to become hyperactive (Schuster et al. 2021). Although fibroblasts play a crucial role in tissue repair through collagen synthesis, excessive collagen production can lead to fibrosis, causing tissue stiffness and impaired muscular function, as evidenced in cases of RIT (Shih et al. 2019). Kumar et al. demonstrated in an in vitro experiment that fibroblasts exposed to radiation had a fibrotic phenotype characterized by elevated collagen deposition of TGF-β, enhanced cell proliferation, migration, and invasion (Raj et al. 2020). Initial inflammation triggered by radiation causes fibroblasts to proliferate, migrate, and transdifferentiate into myofibroblasts. In response to TGF-β, myofibroblasts produce excess collagen, fibronectin, and proteoglycans responsible for the increased stiffness and thickening of the tissue and are in abundance in the fibrotic region (Kumar et al. 2018; Wynn 2007). In addition, TGF-β exacerbates the excessive deposition of extracellular matrix by promoting reduced activity of matrix metalloproteinases (MMPs), namely MMP-2 and MMP-9, and increased activity of tissue inhibitors of metalloproteinases (TIMPs) (Pardo 2006). Myofibroblasts have a crucial role in promoting angiogenesis and the development of endothelial cells via the secretion of essential fibroblast growth factors.

Fibroblasts may also secrete large amounts of IL-6 and IL-11, which are key drivers of hyperinflammatory and hyperfibrotic diseases, respectively (Choy et al. 2020; Cook and Schafer 2020). Leukocyte-recruiting chemokines such as CCL2 and CXCL12 are another class of fibroblast-derived factors critical for tissue inflammation (Szekanecz and Koch 2016; Haringman et al. 2006). However, regardless of the underlying pathological mechanisms and the specific inflammatory and fibrogenic pathways triggered, the outcome consistently involves an augmented synthesis and buildup of collagen inside the afflicted region. An excessive buildup of collagen indicates an elevated collagen production and results in a reduction in the blood supply to the tissues and a state of low oxygen levels, namely hypoxia (Toussaint et al. 2002). If the affected area is the masticatory apparatus, then RIT is unfortunately unavoidable in HNC patients undergoing RT or CRT.

5 Signaling Pathways

The activation of signaling pathways such as TGF-β and nuclear factor-kappa B (NF-κB) has been shown in the context of radiation-induced inflammation and fibrosis. The activation of fibroblasts and the subsequent synthesis of extracellular matrix proteins play a crucial role in initiating the fibrotic process (Zhang et al. 2021b). When living cells are exposed to high doses of ionizing radiation, they experience detrimental effects that lead to the production of specific molecules called damage-associated molecular pattern molecules (DAMPs). These chemicals function as signaling agents, attracting diverse immune cells, including neutrophils, macrophages, leukocytes, and lymphocytes, to the location of tissue injury. Research findings have shown that many cytokines, including interleukin 3 (IL-3), IL-6, interferon-γ (IFN-γ), TGF-β, and TNF-α, are detected inside the irradiated tissue and have a significant impact on aiding the process of immune cell transmigration. The initiation of an inflammatory response, which ultimately results in the formation of chronic fibrosis, is mediated by many signaling pathways (Barker et al. 2015). Moreover, hypoxia-inducible factors (HIFs) are of utmost importance in the response of immune cells to hypoxic conditions since they facilitate their migration (Moeller et al. 2004). Hence, as we delve deeper into the RIT mechanisms, we realize the significant impact of inflammatory biomarkers, which are crucial in initiating the fibrotic process and creating a hypoxic background on the way to mature RIT formation (Fig. 2).

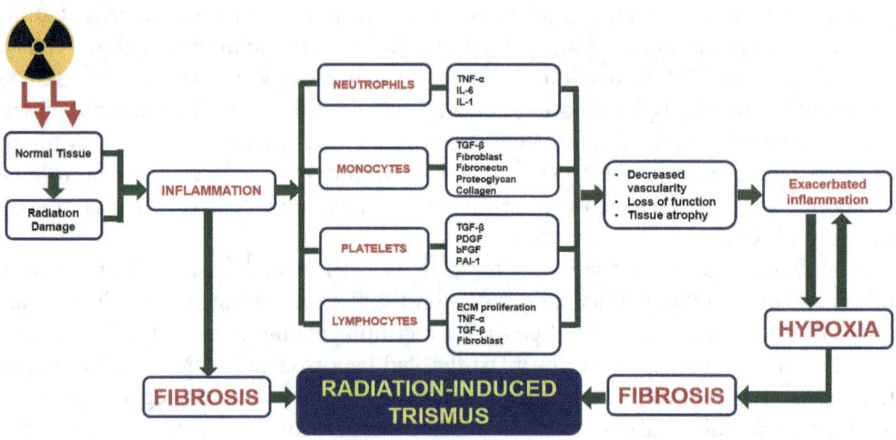

Fig. 2 Possible pathophysiological mechanisms underlying radiation-induced trismus. **Abbreviations**: *IL-1* Interleukin-1, *IL-6* Interleukin-6, *TNF-α* Tumor necrosis factor-alpha, *TGF-β* Transforming growth factor beta, *PDGF* Platelet-derived growth factor, *bFGF*, basic fibroblast growth factor, *PAI-1* Plasminogen activator inhibitor type, *ECM* extracellular matrix

6 The Role of Chronic Inflammation on Radiation-Induced Trismus Pathogenesis

Inflammation is a critical physiological response of the immune system against tissue injury or infection. The acute inflammation serves as a defensive mechanism that facilitates the body's healing process. However, the persistence of inflammation over an extended period, known as chronic inflammation, may lead to tissue damage and the emergence of several health issues.

The precise mechanism behind RIT remains unknown, but it is thought to originate from inflammatory processes, hypoxia, and fibrosis associated with inflammation. Theoretically, it is hypothesized that fibrotic activation may take place in several anatomical structures, including the synovial fluid, temporomandibular joint, temporomandibular joint ligaments, and other components of the masticatory apparatus after exposure to high RT doses. This fibrotic activation is believed to be one of the key contributors to the development of RIT (Mack 2018; van der Geer et al. 2019). Numerous preclinical investigations have shown that low-dose RT has an inflammation-modulating or anti-inflammatory impact through various pathways, while high-dose RT induces the release of pro-inflammatory cytokines, signaling molecules responsible for regulating immunological responses. After RT, there is a surge in cytokines such as interleukin-1 (IL-1), interleukin-6 (IL-6), and tumor necrosis factor-alpha (TNF-α) levels, which promote inflammation and may contribute to tissue damage in the irradiated area (Carvalho and Villar 2018). RT can also harm blood vessels in the treated area, leading to impaired circulation and decreased oxygen delivery to the masticatory muscles caused by the injury to the vascular endothelium, reduced formation of new blood vessels (angiogenesis), and ultimately insufficient oxygen supply (hypoxia). Additionally, it is widely recognized that hypoxia manifests in both synovial and muscle tissues via the activation of hypoxia-inducible factors (HIF). Hypoxia, particularly when experienced over a prolonged period (chronic hypoxia), exacerbates cellular injury, inflammation, and fibrogenesis. The initiation, acceleration, and exacerbation of tissue fibrosis may be attributed to the intrusion of fibrotic inflammatory mediators into the hyperinflammatory tissue state, such as vascular endothelial growth factor (VEGF). This process ultimately results in the advancement of fibrosis and the eventual development of RIT (Gilkes et al. 2014; Moon et al. 2022). The presence of persistent inflammation inside the irradiated region has the potential to induce the synthesis of collagen, a fibrous protein responsible for the formation of scar tissue. Collagen buildup has been seen to manifest in the masticatory muscles after RT within the context of RIT, resulting in restricted mobility and the development of stiffness (Ramia et al. 2022). It should also be noted that the aforementioned inflammatory processes have the potential to elicit the recruitment of immune cells toward irradiated tissues, hence prolonging the cycle of inflammation and subsequent tissue damage and further accumulation of collagen in the irradiated area (Lumniczky et al. 2021). Therefore, the self-perpetuating process of exacerbated inflammation and collagen synthesis (fibrosis) will unavoidably and ultimately manifest as RIT in the long term (Table 1 and Fig. 2).

Table 1 Functions of cytokines in radiation-induced trismus development

Cytokines	Functions in radiation-induced trismus
IL-1	Starts the inflammatory process (increased vascular permeability, localized edema, endothelial cell death, and vascular thrombosis occurred)
	Triggers tissue fibrosis
	Has synergistic effects on the expression of profibrotic and inflammatory mediators in fibroblasts
IL-6	Promotes the transformation of fibroblasts into myofibroblasts through the JAK/STAT3 signaling pathway
	Stimulates the proliferation of fibroblasts and triggers tissue fibrosis
IL-10	Limits host immune response to pathogens
	Activates inflammation
	Has no direct effect, but it regulates TGF-beta and MCP-1 differently in the modulation of ECM proteins and indirectly causes fibrosis.
IL-11	Has fibrotic effects
	Stimulation of IL-11 upregulates expression of collagen type 1
	Has a key regulator role in tissue fibrosis such as the proliferation of fibroblasts, deposition of collagen
CCL2	The effect of CCL2 on fibrosis is not straightforward and can vary depending on the specific disease or tissue context
	Attracts monocytes and macrophages to sites of inflammation
	Leads to the production of pro-fibrotic factors, such as TGF-β
	Activates fibroblasts
CXCL12	Has a key role in the recruitment of fibroblasts
	Stimulates fibroblasts and produces ECM proteins
	Activates TGF-β and increases fibroblast activation and collagen deposition
	Attracts monocytes and macrophages
TNF-α	Exerts inflammation, proliferation, and apoptosis
	Starts the inflammatory process (increased vascular permeability, localized edema, endothelial cell death, and vascular thrombosis occurred)
	Increases collagen synthesis
IFN-γ	Inhibits angiogenesis
	Induces MHC-I expression
TGF-β	In response to TGF-β, myofibroblasts produce excess collagen, fibronectin, and proteoglycans which are responsible for the increased stiffness and thickening of the tissue and are in abundance in the fibrotic region
	Worsens the already excessive extracellular matrix deposition by encouraging decreased matrix metalloproteinase (MMP) activity (particularly MMP-2 and MMP-9) and increased activity of tissue inhibitors of metalloproteinases
	Increases activity of tissue inhibitors of metalloproteinases stimulates angiogenesis and endothelial cell development by secreting basic fibroblast growth factors, and the excessive amount of collagen lowers vascularity
NF-κB	Contributes to the activation of fibroblasts and the synthesis of extracellular matrix proteins, driving the fibrotic process
	Mediates transactivation of pro-fibrotic genes in fibroblastic cells

(continued)

Table 1 (continued)

Cytokines	Functions in radiation-induced trismus
HIF	Aggravates cell damage, inflammation, and fibrogenesis
	Stimulates excessive amount of ECM, vascular remodeling, and futile angiogenesis with further exacerbation of chronic hypoxia and deteriorated pathofibrogenesis
VGEF	Has profibrotic effects on fibroblasts
	Promotes fibrogenesis
	With the triggering effect of chronic hypoxia, VGEF-induced vascular remodeling leads to progressive luminal narrowing and occlusion and may exacerbate local hypoxia.

Abbreviations: *IL-1* Interleukin-1, *IL-6* Interleukin-6, *IL-10* Interleukin-10, *IL-11* Interleukin-11, *CCL2* C-C Motif chemokine ligand-2, *CXCL12* C-C Motif chemokine ligand-12, *TNF-α* Tumor necrosis factor-alpha, *IFN-γ* interferon gamma, *TGF- β* Transforming growth factor beta, *NF-κB* Nuclear factor-kappa B, *HIF* Hypoxia-inducible factor, *VGEF* Vascular endothelial growth factor

7 Discussion

The primary treatment modality for most individuals diagnosed with head and neck cancer (HNC) involves external beam RT. The observed decrease in mandibular function and range of motion resulting from RT seems to be associated with injury and fibrosis in the masticatory muscles (Wang et al. 2005). The RT has a notable impact on the masticatory apparatus, either entirely or partially, due to its inclusion inside the radiation field. A hypothesis suggests that specific components of the masticatory system, namely the masseter muscles and the pterygoids, have a more significant role in RIT development than other anatomical structures (Teguh et al. 2008; van Der Molen et al. 2013). The research done by Okineff et al. (2004) showed that RT might give rise to fibrotic consequences, which are characterized by the appearance of edema and discomfort. These issues subsequently lead to trismus and muscular weakness in the masticatory system. According to the authors, the potential reason behind this occurrence was the damage caused by high doses of radiation on the fibrovascular system, which may have been facilitated by increased levels of proinflammatory TNF-α and fibrosis-inducing fibroblast growth factor 2 (FGF2) in irradiated tissues. These findings emphasize the significance of muscular and vascular injury and the crucial roles that inflammatory and fibrogenic factors play in RIT's initiation and progression steps.

The temporomandibular joint (TMJ) is a crucial non-muscular component of the jaw that, when injured, can cause acute or progressive trismus. Research conducted by Wu et al. (2017) indicates that radiation-induced TMJ injury may lead to RIT, a prevalent complication that often arises after radical head and neck RT or CRT in patients with nasopharyngeal carcinoma (NPC). The researchers administered an average total dosage of 41.4 Gy to the temporomandibular joint (TMJ) group of patients and compared the results with those of unirradiated controls. They observed via ultrasound assessments conducted after radiotherapy that the TMJ disc thickness in the patient group was considerably reduced compared to the control group. According to the authors, the thinning of the disc might be attributed to the depletion of collagen fibers caused by radiation-induced damage to TMJ cartilage, where collagen fibers and proteoglycans are abundantly present. The investigators of this study have pointed out that the fiber system of the disc plays a crucial role in distributing stress and maintaining joint movement, and they have implied that the loosening or injury of fibers inside the disc can lead to RIT. This is because the fiber system inside the disc acts as a stress dispersal function, and the relaxation of these fibers can impact the joint's mobility, leading to RIT. Furthermore, during the same research investigation, it was observed that patients who had RT exhibited mandibular condyle erosion, sclerosis, and disc thinning. The patients also displayed abnormalities on the surface of the mandibular condyle. These pathological findings have been linked to the inflammatory process created by radiation, which results in the degradation of proteoglycans and collagen fibers. These results collectively indicate that the development of RIT may be influenced not only by the diminished functions of the muscular components of the masticatory apparatus but also by the damage caused to the vascular structures and TMJ.

RIT represents a significant but sometimes overlooked complication within the spectrum of RT-associated toxicities. Despite the recognized impact of inflammation on the progression of RIT, there is a dearth of research investigating this relationship. The hemoglobin-to-platelet ratio (HPR) was studied to see if it could be used to accurately predict the occurrence of RIT in 198 patients with locally advanced NPC (LA-NPC) (Somay et al. 2022b), primarily based on previous research results that showed how inflammatory response and fibrosis cause trismus after C-CRT (Darby and Hewitson 2016; Haubner et al. 2012). This study diagnosed 43 patients (21.7%) with RIT during the follow-up period, and the rate of RIT was significantly higher in the group with HPR ≤ 0.54 compared to the group with HPR >0.54 (34.1% vs. 12.9%; HR: 2.86; $p < 0.001$). This result can be explained by considering that hemoglobin and platelets, components of the HPR formula, play crucial roles in tissue oxygenation, vascular patency, and immune and inflammatory responses (Mo et al. 2020). Radiation-induced thrombosis and ischemia, caused by vascular occlusion and/or low hemoglobin levels, can exacerbate damage to the masticatory apparatus, leading to increased production of inflammatory cytokines and chemokines and the recruitment of inflammatory cells to the affected area (Raj et al. 2020). Consequently, attracted monocytes may undergo a process of differentiation into M2 cells. These M2 cells are responsible for releasing TGF-ß, which is a critical element in the development of radiation-induced fibrosis. This process of differentiation is set off by localized inflammation and may be sped up by the production and release of proinflammatory cytokines like TNF-α, IL-1, and IL-6 in the area of interest, which in the case of RIT is the masticatory apparatus (Toussaint et al. 2002). Hence, although the precise mechanism may possess more intricacy, the existing body of research indicates that a confluence of tissue hypoxia and fibrosis, instigated by heightened systemic and/or local inflammation, may engender an elevated susceptibility to RIT in HNC patients treated with radical RT or CRT.

The investigation pertaining to the potential impact of tissue hypoxia on RIT development has entailed the scrutiny of hemoglobin, which is widely recognized as a pivotal marker of hypoxia. Somay et al. (2023) have published compelling research results highlighting the crucial role of inflammatory and hypoxic conditions before RT in the development of RIT. They used receiver operating characteristic (ROC) curve analysis to stratify patients into two groups with significantly distinct RIT, revealing a hemoglobin cutoff of 12.05 g/dL [area under the curve (AUC): 82.7%; sensitivity: 72.9%; and specificity: 71.3%]. The findings of this insightful research underscore the significance of pretreatment hemoglobin levels in identifying high-risk patients for RIT after treatment. The incidence of RIT was found to be significantly higher in the Hb $\leq$ 12 g/dL group compared to the Hb $>$ 12 g/dL group (41.9% vs. 7.3%; $p < 0.001$), indicating a strong association between lower hemoglobin levels and a higher risk of RIT. According to the study results, the authors hpothesized that the condition might have caused a prolonged hypoxic state in the affected masticatory apparatus, which may have been further exacerbated by the use of RT, which prevented or delayed healthy tissue repair and triggered the fibrosis cascade, as previously explained by Lo and colleagues (Lo et al. 2008). In support of the hypothesis put forth by Somay and colleagues, Sharma and Radhakrishnan examined trismus in individuals with oral submucosal fibrosis and discovered that fibrosis occurs in the muscles due to ischemia caused by hypoxia in the region (Sharma and Radhakrishnan 2017). While it is important to acknowledge that more work is necessary before drawing definitive conclusions, these study results play a crucial role in enhancing our understanding of the underlying mechanisms of RIT. Consequently, they are poised to make significant contributions to the progress of medical knowledge and the development of preventative measures and treatment strategies for this particular ailment.

An increasing body of evidence has been accumulating in recent years, which enables us to confidently suggest that an overly active inflammatory response plays a significant role in the onset and advancement of RIT. To investigate this relationship further, recently, Somay et al. conducted a study on 51 patients with parotid gland cancer to see how their pre-treatment neutrophil-to-platelet ratio (NLR) levels affected their risk of RIT (Somay et al. 2022a). According to the comparative analysis, the incidence of RIT was significantly higher among patients with NLR >2.7 as compared to those with NLR ≤ 2.7 (35.2% vs. 5.8%; rs:0.79; $p < 0.001$), which indicates that an increased NLR level, an established inflammatory marker, could have contributed to the development of RIT. Although similar studies are limited, Kawashita et al. (2021). have investigated the role of NLR in predicting radiation-related toxicities and their severity. The authors noted that high NLR values before RT were associated with significantly higher rates of grade 3 mucositis than low NLR levels ($p = 0.045$) in hypopharyngeal and laryngeal cancer patients. Together, these research results suggest that pre-RT high NLR values may play significant roles in developing radiation-induced toxicities, including oral mucositis and RIT.

Based on the existing, albeit limited, robust evidence, it can be deduced that a mutually reinforcing connection exists between radiation-induced hypoxia and inflammation. This interplay gives rise to a detrimental cycle of hypoxia and inflammation, which subsequently upregulates the expression of hypoxia-related genes, triggers the synthesis of profibrotic molecules, and ultimately culminates in the development of tissue fibrosis, the ultimate fate in the pathogenesis of RIT development. Hence, it is imperative to conduct future research encompassing multidisciplinary, large-scale prospective studies, specifically emphasizing inhibiting the underlying mechanisms involved in the genesis of RIT. Such studies should aim to develop interventions that can effectively prevent or mitigate the development of RIT, thereby minimizing its adverse impact on various aspects of the QoL measures among patients with HNC undergoing RT or CRT (Table 2).

Table 2 Studies on radiation-induced trismus

Author	Year	Aim	Findings	Conclusion
Somay et al. (2022a)	2022	To investigate the link between pretreatment NLR and RIT in parotid gland cancer patients after postoperative RT	The incidence of RIT was found to be statistically higher in the NLR >2.7 than its counterpart (35.2% vs.5.8%; $p < 0.001$)	High pre-RT NLR levels were a robust and independent predictor of significantly elevated rates of RIT.
Somay et al. (2022b)	2022	The significance of HPR in predicting the occurrence of RIT in LA-NPC patients who received C-CRT.	RIT incidence was found to be significantly higher in the HPR ≤0.54 group than its HPR >0.54 counterpart ($p < 0.001$)	The risk of post-C-CRT RIT may be significantly increased when pre-treatment HPR levels are low.
Topkan et al. (2023)	2023	To assess the H-Index's (calculated using neutrophils, monocytes, lymphocytes, hemoglobin, and albumin) predictive significance for RIT in patients with LA-NPC receiving C-CRT.	The patients in the H-index >5.5 group had significantly higher rates of either RIT (31.8% vs. 5.9%; $p < 0.001$) than their H-index ≤5.5 counterparts.	Pre-C-CRT H-index >5.5 is associated with significantly increased RIT rates in LA-NPC patients receiving C-CRT.
Somay et al. (2023)	2023	To investigate the predictive significance of Hb values in the incidence of RIT in LA-NPC patients who received C-CRT.	RIT was significantly more prevalent in the Hb ≤ 12 g/dL group than in its counterpart (41.9% vs. 7.3%; $p < 0.001$)	Low pre-C-CRT Hb and anemia status are novel biological markers that independently predict higher RIT rates in LA-NPC undergoing C-CRT.

Abbreviations: *NLR* neutrophil-to-lymphocyte ratio, *RIT* radiation-induced trismus, *RT* radiotherapy, *HPR* pre-hemoglobin-to-platelet ratio, *LA-NPC* locally advanced nasopharyngeal carcinoma, *Hb* hemoglobin, *C-CRT* concurrent chemoradiotherapy

8 Emerging Trends and Future Directions

In recent years, research has been increasing on the association between RIT development and exacerbated inflammation. The ultimate goal of such research has been to identify new therapeutic targets and interventions for preventing or managing RIT in HNC patients. In the future, there could be potential developments that might be summarized as follows:

1. *Targeted therapies*: Conducting investigations into specific biological pathways and developing targeted therapeutic interventions that impede the processes of fibrosis and inflammation could provide more effective treatment options characterized by a reduced occurrence of undesirable side effects, including the hard-to-manage RIT.
2. *Personalized diagnoses and therapies*: Optimization of outcomes, management of side effects, and reduction of the risk of RIT may be achieved by customizing treatment plans to accommodate the individual features of patients and their respective radiation protocols.
3. *Telehealth and Rehabilitation*: The use of telehealth technology in the context of physical therapy and rehabilitation has the potential to enhance healthcare accessibility, particularly for individuals residing in rural regions.
4. *Implementation of multidisciplinary patient care*: Every patient with HNC must have an assessment conducted by a proficient multidisciplinary team to predict the risk of RIT after RT or CRT and promptly initiate appropriate preventative measures. The composition of this team should include a range of professionals, such as radiation oncologists, medical oncologists, head and neck surgeons, dental oncologists, physical therapists, psychiatrists, and supportive care teams, among others.

9 Conclusion

In conclusion, RIT is a demanding and apprehensive adverse effect of RT or CRT experienced by patients with HNC. Although the precise processes responsible for its development are still being investigated, recent research indicates a significant association between inflammation and the pathophysiology of this particular malady. Comprehending the intricate relationship among radiation-induced inflammation, fibrosis, chronic hypoxia, and immune responses is paramount to advancing efficacious preventive and therapeutic strategies for RIT in individuals with HNC. Future research endeavors are expected to persistently investigate the complex molecular and cellular mechanisms involved, which may reveal valuable insights into the RIT pathogenesis and the resultant demarcation of innovative targeted preventive and/or therapeutic interventions that will ultimately enhance the well-being of patients receiving RT or CRT.

Acknowledgments None.

Funding This research received no external funding.

Conflict of Interests The authors declared that they had no conflict of interest.

References

Barker HE, Paget JT, Khan AA et al (2015) The tumour microenvironment after radiotherapy: mechanisms of resistance and recurrence. Nat Rev Cancer 15:409–425. https://doi.org/10.1038/nrc3958

Baskar R, Lee KA, Yeo R et al (2012) Cancer and radiation therapy: current advances and future directions. Int J Med Sci 9:193–199

Brook I (2020) Late side effects of radiation treatment for head and neck cancer. Radiat Oncol J 38: 84–92

Carvalho HA, Villar RC (2018) Radiotherapy and immune response: the systemic effects of a local treatment. Clinics (Sao Paulo) 73:e557s. https://doi.org/10.6061/clinics/2018/e557s

Chen L, Deng H, Cui H et al (2017) Inflammatory responses and inflammation-associated diseases in organs. Oncotarget 9:7204–7218. https://doi.org/10.18632/oncotarget.23208

Choy EH, De Benedetti F, Takeuchi T et al (2020) Translating IL-6 biology into effective treatments. Nat Rev Rheumatol 16:335–345

Cook SA, Schafer S (2020) Hiding in plain sight: interleukin-11 emerges as a master regulator of fibrosis, tissue integrity, and stromal inflammation. Annu Rev Med 71:263–276. https://doi.org/10.1146/annurev-med-041818-011649

Darby IA, Hewitson TD (2016) Hypoxia in tissue repair and fibrosis. Cell Tissue Res 365:553–562. https://doi.org/10.1007/s00441-016-2461-3

Gilkes DM, Semenza GL, Wirtz D (2014) Hypoxia and the extracellular matrix: drivers of tumour metastasis. Nat Rev Cancer 14:430–439. https://doi.org/10.1038/nrc3726

Graham CA, Yu AH, Chan SS et al (2006) Primary emergency surgical airway for trismus caused by electrical burn. Burns 32:1062–1063

Haringman JJ, Gerlag DM, Smeets TJ (2006) A randomized controlled trial with an anti-CCL2 (anti-monocyte chemotactic protein 1) monoclonal antibody in patients with rheumatoid arthritis. Arthritis Rheum 54:2387–2392. https://doi.org/10.1002/art.21975

Haubner F, Ohmann E, Pohl F et al (2012) Wound healing after radiation therapy: review of the literature. Radiat Oncol 7:162

Johnson J, Johansson M, Rydén A et al (2015) Impact of trismus on health-related quality of life and mental health. Head Neck 37:1672–1679

Kawashita Y, Kitamura M, Soutome S et al (2021) Association of neutrophil-to-lymphocyte ratio with severe radiation-induced mucositis in pharyngeal or laryngeal cancer patients: a retrospective study. BMC Cancer 21:1064. https://doi.org/10.1186/s12885-021-08793-6

Kim W, Lee S, Seo D et al (2019) Cellular stress responses in radiotherapy. Cell 8:1105. https://doi.org/10.3390/cells8091105

Kumar D, Yalamanchali S, New J, Parsel S et al (2018) Development and characterization of an in vitro model for radiation-induced fibrosis. Radiat Res 189:326–336. https://doi.org/10.1667/RR14926.1

Lo LJ, Lin CL, Chen YR (2008) A device for temporomandibular joint exercise and trismus correction: design and clinical application. J Plast Reconstr Aesthet Surg 61:297–301. https://doi.org/10.1016/j.bjps.2007.05.009

Louise Kent M, Brennan MT, Noll JL et al (2008) Radiation-induced trismus in head and neck cancer patients. Support Care Cancer 16:305–309

Lumniczky K, Impens N, Armengol G et al (2021) Low dose ionizing radiation effects on the immune system. Environ Int 149:106212. https://doi.org/10.1016/j.envint.2020.106212

Mack M (2018) Inflammation and fibrosis. Matrix Biol 68:106–121. https://doi.org/10.1016/j.matbio.2017.11.010

Mittal M, Siddiqui MR, Tran K et al (2014) Reactive oxygen species in inflammation and tissue injury. Antioxid Redox Signal 20:1126–1167. https://doi.org/10.1089/ars.2012.5149

Mo CJ, Hu ZJ, Qin SZ et al (2020) Diagnostic value of platelet-lymphocyte ratio and hemoglobin-platelet ratio in patients with rectal cancer. J Clin Lab Anal 34:e23153. https://doi.org/10.1002/jcla.23153

Moeller BJ, Cao Y, Li CY et al (2004) Radiation activates HIF-1 to regulate vascular radiosensitivity in tumors: role of Reoxygenation, free radicals, and stress granules. Cancer Cell 5:429–441. https://doi.org/10.1016/S1535-6108(04)00115-1

Moon EJ, Petersson K, Olcina MM (2022) The importance of hypoxia in radiotherapy for the immune response, metastatic potential and FLASH-RT. Int J Radiat Biol 98:439–451. https://doi.org/10.1080/09553002.2021.1988178

Nepon H, Safran T, Reece EM et al (2021) Radiation-induced tissue damage: clinical consequences and current treatment options. Semin Plast Surg 35:181–188

Nguyen HN, Noss EH, Mizoguchi F et al (2017) Autocrine loop involving IL-6 family member LIF, LIF receptor, and STAT4 drives sustained fibroblast production of inflammatory mediators. Immunity 46:220–232. https://doi.org/10.1016/j.immuni.2017.01.004

Nygaard G, Firestein GS (2020) Restoring synovial homeostasis in rheumatoid arthritis by targeting fibroblast-like synoviocytes. Nat Rev Rheumatol 16:316–333. https://doi.org/10.1038/s41584-020-0413-5

Okunieff P, Augustine E, Hicks JE et al (2004) Pentoxifylline in the treatment of radiation-induced fibrosis. J Clin Oncol 22:2207–2213. https://doi.org/10.1200/JCO.2004.09.101

Pardo A (2006) Matrix metalloproteases in aberrant fibrotic tissue remodeling. Proc Am Thorac Soc 3:383–388

Raj R, Thankappan K, Janakiram C, Iyer S et al (2020) Etiopathogenesis of trismus in patients with head and neck cancer: An exploratory literature review. Craniomaxillofac Trauma Reconstr 13:219–225

Ramia P, Bodgi L, Mahmoud D (2022) Radiation-induced fibrosis in patients with head and neck cancer: a review of pathogenesis and clinical outcomes. Clin Med Insights Oncol 16:11795549211036898. https://doi.org/10.1177/11795549211036898

Schuster R, Rockel JS, Kapoor M et al (2021) The inflammatory speech of fibroblasts. Immunol Rev 302:126–146

Sharma M, Radhakrishnan R (2017) Limited mouth opening in oral submucous fibrosis: reasons, ramifications, and remedies. J Oral Pathol Med 46:424–430. https://doi.org/10.1111/jop.12513

Shih YH, Wang TH, Shieh TM et al (2019) Oral submucous fibrosis: a review on etiopathogenesis, diagnosis, and therapy. Int J Mol Sci 20:2940. https://doi.org/10.3390/ijms20122940

Sologuren I, Rodríguez-Gallego C, Lara PC (2014) Immune effects of high dose radiation treatment: implications of ionizing radiation on the development of bystander and abscopal effects. Transl Cancer Res 3:18–31

Somay E, Yilmaz B, Topkan E et al (2022a) Initial neutrophil-to-lymphocyte ratio predicts radiation-induced trismus in parotid gland cancer. Oral Dis 29:2772

Somay E, Yilmaz B, Topkan E et al (2022b) Hemoglobin-to-platelet ratio in predicting the incidence of trismus after concurrent chemoradiotherapy. Oral Dis 29:2962. https://doi.org/10.1111/odi.14363

Somay E, Yilmaz B, Topkan E et al (2023) Low hemoglobin levels predict increased radiation-induced trismus rates in nasopharyngeal cancer. Oral Dis. https://doi.org/10.1111/odi.14605

Straub JM, New J, Hamilton CD et al (2015) Radiation-induced fibrosis: mechanisms and implications for therapy. J Cancer Res Clin Oncol 141:1985–1994

Su Y, Gao J, Kaur P et al (2020) Neutrophils and macrophages as targets for development of nanotherapeutics in inflammatory diseases. Pharmaceutics 12:1222. https://doi.org/10.3390/pharmaceutics12121222

Szekanecz Z, Koch AE (2016) Successes and failures of chemokine-pathway targeting in rheumatoid arthritis. Nat Rev Rheumatol 12(1):5–13. https://doi.org/10.1038/nrrheum.2015.157

Teguh DN, Levendag PC, Voet P et al (2008) Trismus in patients with oropharyngeal cancer: relationship with dose in structures of mastication apparatus. Head Neck 30:622–630

Topkan E, Somay E, Yilmaz B et al (2023) Valero's host index is useful in predicting radiation-induced trismus and osteoradionecrosis of the jaw risks in locally advanced nasopharyngeal carcinoma patients. BMC Cancer 23:651. https://doi.org/10.1186/s12885-023-11155-z

Toussaint O, Remacle J, Dierick JF et al (2002) Approach of evolutionary theories of ageing, stress, senescence-like phenotypes, calorie restriction, and hormesis from the viewpoint of far-from-equilibrium thermodynamics. Mech Ageing Dev 123:937–946

van de Worp WRPH, Schols AMWJ, Theys J et al (2020) Nutritional interventions in cancer cachexia: evidence and perspectives from experimental models. Front Nutr 7:601329

van der Geer SJ, van Rijn PV, Kamstra JI et al (2019) Prevalence and prediction of trismus in patients with head and neck cancer: a cross-sectional study. Head Neck 41:64–71. https://doi.org/10.1002/hed.25369

van Der Molen L, Heemsbergen WD, de Jong R et al (2013) Dysphagia and trismus after concomitant chemo-intensity-modulated radiation therapy (chemo-IMRT) in advanced head and neck cancer dose–effect relationships for swallowing and mastication structures. Radiother Oncol 106:364–369

Wang CJ, Huang EY, Hsu HC et al (2005) The degree and time-course assessment of radiation-induced trismus occurring after radiotherapy for nasopharyngeal cancer. Laryngoscope 115:1458–1460

Wu VW, Ying MT, Kwong DL (2017) A study on the post-radiotherapy changes of temporomandibular joint in nasopharyngeal carcinoma patients. Br J Radiol 90:20170375. https://doi.org/10.1259/bjr.20170375

Wynn TA (2007) Common and unique mechanisms regulate fibrosis in various fibroproliferative diseases. J Clin Investig 117:524–529

Wynn TA, Vannella KM (2016) Macrophages in tissue repair, regeneration, and fibrosis. Immunity 44:450–462. https://doi.org/10.1016/j.immuni.2016.02.015

Zhang C, Liang Z, Ma S et al (2021a) Radiotherapy and cytokine storm: risk and mechanism. Front Oncol 11:670464. https://doi.org/10.3389/fonc.2021.670464

Zhang Z, Zhou J, Verma V et al (2021b) Crossed pathways for radiation-induced and immunotherapy-related lung injury. Front Immunol 12:774807. https://doi.org/10.3389/fimmu.2021.774807

Current Overview of the Biological Effects of GRID, Microbeam, and FLASH Radiotherapy

Meryem Cansu Sahin and Selami Eken

Abstract

External beam radiation has long been a linchpin in cancer treatment, demanding not just efficacy in tumor control but also precision to minimize damage to healthy tissues. To achieve this, several methods have been developed, such as particle therapy, stereotactic body radiation therapy, and intensity-modulated radiation therapy.

Recent studies in technology and research into radiobiology have focused on three distinct modalities: GRID radiotherapy, microbeam radiotherapy, and ultra-high dose rate radiotherapy. These new methods are also called spatial fractionation. A type of external beam radiation therapy known as GRID radiotherapy uses sieve-like collimators and non-uniform dose distribution. By delivering high-dose and dose rate beams that are micron-sized, the application of spatially fractionated beams, also referred to as Microbeam radiation therapy, has the potential to raise the therapeutic ratio. FLASH radiotherapy uses ultra-high dose rate radiation on the target to reduce radiation-induced toxicity.

These methods, each of which has unique physical and biological bases, collectively offer a comprehensive approach to achieving effective tumor control while protecting healthy tissues. The most crucial topic in all these studies is normal tissue toxicity. Because of this, research is being done on biological response mechanisms in addition to ultra-high dose rate. The critical relationship between clinical results and physical parameters in the tumor and normal tissue

M. C. Sahin (✉)
Usak University, Department of Medical Services and Techniques, Vocational School of Health Services, Usak, Turkey
e-mail: meryem.sahin@usak.edu.tr

S. Eken
Department of Radiation Oncology, Faculty of Medicine, Kahramanmaras Sutcu Imam University, Kahramanmaras, Turkey

Interdisciplinary Cancer Research, https://doi.org/10.1007/16833_2024_299
Published online: 02 July 2024

response is the subject of ongoing study. The research involves the biological basis and modeling the dose-effect to better understand these relationships.

These innovative methods, based on technology and biological research, could be acknowledged as a significant development in the history of radiation treatment and could have great potential going forward.

Keywords

FLASH · GRID · Microbeam · Radiobiology · Radiotherapy

1 Introduction

One of the most significant treatment techniques for cancer is external beam radiation. Increasing the precision and accuracy with which consistent radiation doses are delivered to target tumor volumes has been the main focus of radiotherapy technology development. There are two approaches to achieving this: different biological radiation response within healthy tissue and the tumor and precise deposition of ionizing radiation energy limited to the tumor site and sparing no harm to the surrounding healthy tissue. For this reason, several methods have been developed, such as Intensity-Modulated Radiation Therapy, Stereotactic Body Radiation Therapy, and Particle Therapy. However, the impact of external beam radiation is often limited by normal tissue toxicity in organs at risk. For decades, the field of radiation oncology has aimed to maximize the death of tumor cells while minimizing adverse effects on healthy tissues.

Advances in today's technology and a better understanding of radiobiology play an essential role in radiation therapy's future, and studies on new technologies are ongoing for this purpose. Recently, various treatment modalities have been explored with modern-day technology. These approaches focus on delivering high doses quickly (high dose rate) and using different fraction schemes. One of these approaches is GRID radiotherapy, which involves using multiple smaller fields. The other is microbeam radiotherapy (MRT). It has different spatial fractionation and uses the micro-beams. The last method in this chapter is FLASH radiotherapy, which uses ultra-high dose rates.

1.1 Spatially Fractionated Conventional Radiotherapy (GRID)

Spatially fractionated irradiation (GRID) is a therapeutic approach that involves administering a concentrated radiation dosage by partitioning a sizable treatment region into multiple smaller fields. The GRID technique aims to mitigate the overall toxicity associated with the treatment (Penagaricano et al. 2010; Laissue et al. 2012). The GRID technique has demonstrated efficacy in managing voluminous and deeply located neoplasms. The integration of GRID therapy with conventional dose/time fractionated radiation therapy, as well as its utilization in conjunction with other treatment modalities like chemotherapy, has demonstrated enhanced management of large tumors while minimizing the extension of the treatment duration. The initial documented instance of employing spatially fractionated or GRID therapy may be traced back to 1909, as recorded by Alban Kohler (Laissue et al. 2012). Kohler utilized an attenuating grid positioned directly on the skin to mitigate tissue harm while treating tumors at significant depths. During the period characterized by kilovoltage, a novel strategy was implemented to mitigate the adverse effects on healthy tissues (Marks 1952). However, as megavoltage linear accelerator-generated beams emerged, researchers led by Mohiuddin and his team conducted a series of sophisticated investigations to investigate the effectiveness of this technique further (Mohiuddin et al. 1999; Meigooni et al. 2002; Sathishkumar et al. 2002; Zwicker et al. 2004; Neuner et al. 2012). During the 1950s, GRID was commonly employed in addition to orthovoltage radiation therapy to treat deeply located cancers while minimizing adverse effects on the skin and subcutaneous tissues (Marks 1952). Nevertheless, utilizing megavoltage radiation has facilitated the attainment of improved depth dose distribution and minimized skin toxicity. This approach has been implemented in a GRID configuration to enhance the efficacy of treating voluminous and advanced malignancies (Becker and Kuttig 1965). The GRID technique entails the administration of elevated levels of radiation using a specifically designed GRID or a multileaf collimator. This approach ensures that the radiation dose is not uniformly distributed across the target area. In contrast, solely the specific target located right beneath the exposed regions is subjected to irradiation. Several additional centers have also collaborated to enhance antitumor control for patients while maintaining appropriate levels of normal tissue responses. This is exemplified by Penagaricano et al. in a limited sample of individuals (Penagaricano et al. 2010). The methodology was initially executed in three-dimensional blueprints featuring one or two fields generated through the utilization of MLC shaping, cerrobend, or customized blocks that are capable of being positioned within the linear accelerator head (Trapp et al. 2004; Neuner et al. 2012). The utilization of MLC or cerrobend-based GRID facilitates the deployment process in a straightforward manner.

GRID use in underdeveloped countries is potentially advantageous, particularly when financial limitations restrict the adoption of advanced GRID methodologies. A recent study showed that the GRID technique can be effectively utilized for the treatment of deep-seated and irregular geometries by leveraging the additional functionalities offered by a tomotherapy system (Zhang et al. 2016).

The current clinical findings of GRID have yielded auspicious outcomes. Significantly, integrating GRID therapy inside a radiation oncology clinic does not necessitate allocating supplementary clinical personnel. The existing clinical personnel is deemed adequate for implementing a GRID therapy program (Asur et al. 2015). Regarding therapeutic outcomes, Mohiuddin et al. (Mohiuddin et al. 1990, 1999) developed a specialized GRID collimator comprising 7 cm lead material with 250 evenly spaced apertures. A total of 71 individuals diagnosed with advanced bulky tumors had treatment with a radiation dose of 15 Gy, administered using 6 MV photons and given by GRID technique. The treatment was administered to several anatomical areas, including the lung, head and neck, gastrointestinal region, sarcomas, gynecologic area, genitourinary system, and skin. The patients received treatment with GRID as a standalone therapy, GRID followed by fractionated radiation therapy, or GRID followed by fractionated radiation therapy in combination with surgery. After the trial, a response rate of 75.7% was recorded overall. Specifically, a response rate of 78% was observed for palliative treatment, while a response rate of 72.5% was observed for mass effect. A uniform response rate of 16% was recorded across all treatment groups. In a subsequent trial, a cohort of 27 individuals diagnosed with advanced head and neck cancer underwent treatment with GRID in combination with radiation therapy. The participants were divided into two groups: Group 1 received GRID alongside radiation therapy, while Group 2 received GRID followed by radiation therapy and a scheduled neck dissection. This study was referenced by (Huhn et al. 2006). Group 1 had an overall neck control rate of 93% and a disease-specific survival rate of 50%. Notably, the observed morbidity was confined to modest soft tissue injury. Group 2 had an 85% rate of pathologic complete response and a 92% rate of neck control. Additionally, the group demonstrated an 85% rate of disease-specific survival, whereas surgical morbidity was confined to issues related to wound healing. In a separate investigation, a cohort of 79 individuals afflicted with sizable tumors underwent treatment with spatially fractionated radiation (Neuner et al. 2012). The comparative analysis revealed that the efficacy of pain and tumor mass control was similar between the groups treated with GRID utilizing a cerrobend block and a multi-leaf collimator.

Although it is valuable to utilize a commercially manufactured cerrobend block that has the necessary opening-to-opening distance (on/off ratio) and opening diameter for administering GRID therapy, it is important to note that the use of such a block is not obligatory. This is because the method may be efficiently conducted by utilizing the pre-existing multi-leaf collimators often present on most linear accelerators, adopting a step-and-shoot technique. Subsequently, the utilization of a multileaf collimator was employed in GRID research to manipulate the beams and administer dosage patterns that are spatially fractionated. In their study, Penagaricano et al. (Penagaricano et al. 2010) employed a GRID design with a multileaf collimator, which was constructed using a cerrobend alloy with a thickness of 7 cm. A total of 14 individuals diagnosed with advanced head and neck malignancies underwent evaluation. The patients in this study were administered GRID treatment using 6 MV photons, followed by chemo-radiotherapy. The GRID treatment demonstrated an overall control rate of 93% for the tumor volume, while the combined control rate for the neck and primary tumor was 86%. The study saw an overall survival rate of 64%, with disease-specific survival rates of 79%. Additionally, 57% of patients demonstrated disease-free survival. Neuner et al. (Neuner et al. 2012) reported more positive outcomes from a clinical study examining several collimation methods.

While the dose distribution of this technique is known to be non-uniform, clinical observations have shown that the reduction of tumor mass undergoing GRID treatment is uniform (Huhn et al. 2006; Penagaricano et al. 2010). One potential rationale could be the heightened reoxygenation of the tumor after GRID, as the tumor underwent conventional chemoradiation treatment after the administration of the GRID dose. The findings of a recent study utilizing spatially fractionated microbeam therapy showed significant enhancements in tumor oxygenation throughout the initial 2-week period after exposure (Griffin et al. 2012). This observation implies that applying spatial fractionation on a larger scale could potentially enhance tumor physiology. However, further investigation is necessary as the impacts of high-dose microbeams, both in direct and bystander effects, are expected to differ significantly from those of GRID doses.

Patients who have undergone GRID treatment have shown an increase in the production of tumor necrosis factor α and ceramide, as well as a decrease in the expression of transforming growth factor β1 (Sathishkumar et al. 2002, 2005). Furthermore, it has been observed that GRID treatment induces heightened cytokine production, leading to extensive systemic effects (Penagaricano et al. 2010). The potential involvement of bystander effects in destroying neighboring non-irradiated or partially irradiated cells cannot be ruled out. Research investigations that center on the intercellular communication occurring between adjacent cells in the open and closed regions of GRID have the potential to yield significant insights into the underlying mechanisms responsible for the encouraging therapeutic outcomes reported.

1.2 Microbeam (MRT)

Utilizing ionizing radiation in radiotherapy has proven to be an effective method for treating cancer. MRT has seen considerable improvements as a result of the increased understanding of its effects, which advancements in epidemiology and radiobiology have facilitated (Dauer et al. 2018). The interest in employing micro-irradiation techniques for radiobiological studies stems from the ongoing progression of technology and the emergence of novel radiobiology difficulties. The use of microbeams in studies has provided researchers with distinctive investigation techniques owing to their minimal beam size and precise targeting capabilities within cellular environments (Ghita et al. 2018). The correct administration of dosage has been of utmost importance in examining nontargeted effects, wherein the cellular response to ionizing radiation is triggered in cells that were not directly exposed to such radiation (Ghita et al. 2018). In recent times, technological advancements have played a significant role in identifying crucial and time-sensitive interaction mechanisms between ionizing radiation and cells and tissues (Ghita et al. 2017; Walsh et al. 2017). Several technical elements are essential to ensure that microbeams possess the adaptability and high specificity required for contemporary radiobiological studies. The parameters encompassed in this set are the precision of targeting, the efficiency of particle counting, the rate of dose delivery, and the speed at which cellular targets can be recognized and exposed to radiation. A diverse array of facilities has been established globally to provide charged particles (such as protons and helium ions), X-rays, and electrons for various particular purposes in vitro and in vivo. Contemporary microbeams are categorized into different types depending on the beam's source, including cyclotron or accelerator-based microbeams for particle applications, compact X-ray source-based microbeams for soft X-ray applications, and synchrotron-based facilities.

MRT is a novel preclinical radiotherapy approach that utilizes synchrotron X-rays with spatial fractionation. Previous studies by Serduc et al. (2008a, b) and Bouchet et al. (2016) have demonstrated the ability of MRT to protect radiosensitive organs, such as mammalian brains effectively. In MRT, the tumor is exposed to arrays of planar beams with micrometer-wide dimensions. These beams deliver very high doses, reaching up to a few hundred Gy, and are interspersed with low-dose zones of several hundred micrometers in width (Brauer-Krisch et al. 2005). One of the primary advantages of MRT compared to traditional radiotherapy methods is its ability to exploit the dose-volume effect. This effect arises from using a micrometer-scale treatment beam width, which results in a greater tolerance of normal tissue to radiation compared to tumor tissue (Serduc et al. 2008a, b; Bouchet et al. 2010; Schultke et al. 2017). The rat skin has demonstrated a high tolerance for doses ranging from 835 to 1335 Gy in MRT, significantly exceeding the doses utilized in preclinical investigations (350 Gy) (Zhong et al. 2003). Additionally, the immediate impacts on the skin caused by high doses of MRT were shown to be comparable to the effects of moderate doses of wide beam radiation, as observed in a study conducted by Priyadarshika et al. (2011). Hence, the capacity of the organ, specifically the healthy brain, to withstand radiation could potentially enable the possibility of re-irradiating the tumor. Magnetic resonance-guided radiation (MRT) in small animal models has demonstrated therapeutic ratios that surpass those attained using conformal preclinical radiotherapy with uniform dose distributions in several types of cancers (Grotzer et al. 2015).

At present, the generation of clinical microbeams is limited to prominent synchrotron establishments such as the European Synchrotron (ESRF) in Grenoble and the Imaging and Medical Beamline (IMBL) at the Australian Synchrotron, primarily due to the demanding criteria for beam flux and quality. Nevertheless, researchers have also investigated the feasibility of utilizing a traditional X-ray tube or carbon nanotubes (Wang et al. 2011) for generating microbeams in preclinical trials. In this study, Bartzsch et al. employed an X-ray tube featuring a diminutive focal point and a meticulously crafted collimator to generate microbeams for preclinical investigation (Bartzsch et al. 2016). The increasing fascination with vibrant monochromatic and adjustable X-ray sources for application in imaging and radiation therapy has prompted the convergence of research institutes and partners in the ThomX project. This collaborative effort aims to construct a compact Compton Backscattering Source (CBS) in France (Variola et al. 2014). The aim of this project is to develop a functional hard X-ray Compton Backscattering (CBS) system that can be upgraded at a relatively low cost (Alagoz et al. 2016). A recent study conducted by Bartzsch and Oelfke introduces a new technical approach for line focus X-ray tubes, with the primary objective of facilitating the clinical implementation of microbeam radiotherapy (MRT) (Bartzsch and Oelfke 2017). In the long run, this advancement has the potential to facilitate the creation of clinical microbeams without relying on a synchrotron facility.

1.3 Ultra-High Dose Rate Radiotherapy (FLASH RT)

Clinical radiotherapy technology is being developed to prevent damage to normal tissue by changing the types of irradiation and maximizing the precision of radiation applied to malignant tissue. Ultra-high dose rate (HDR) radiation, or FLASH radiotherapy (FLASH-RT), has developed as a novel technique in recent years—the first studies on FLASH effect date back to 1958.

Kirby-Smith and Dolphin conducted a comparison of the dose rates of 1×10^6 rads per second and 4×10^8 rads per second on the two-hit. The recent advancements in dosimetric techniques and the availability of radiation sources with high intensity have enabled the extension of the spectrum of aberrations in this study on chromosomal breakage to exceptionally high dose rates. This study can be accepted as the first step of FLASH-RT (Kirby-Smith and Dolphin 1958). Also in 1966, Horsney et al. investigated the survival of mice under 500 Gy/min (Hornsey and Alper 1966). Such works were published until 1970. It is thought that it has been put on the back burner due to insufficient clinical practice. In particular, it is believed that technological insufficiency is the reason for this (Hornsey and Alper 1966; Berry 1973). However, the potential of FLASH-RT for clinical radiotherapy has once again been acknowledged because of advancements in radiobiology research, in-depth advancements in radiation source research, and improved technology in radiotherapy equipment.

FLASH RT uses a dose rate of >50 Gy/s. and a dose greater than 8 Gy (<1 s) can be applied (Kurup et al. 2019). Recently, FLASH radiation, or FLASH-RT, has received significant attention for much interest as a potentially effective method for maintaining healthy tissues and achieving tumor control that is comparable to conventional radiotherapy (Bourhis et al. 2019a, b).

Dr. Vozenin's group and Favaudon et al. published some new studies examining FLASH-RT in 2014. According to these in vivo studies, FLASH has an average tissue-sparing capacity while maintaining tumor cytotoxicity compared to conventional radiation (Favaudon et al. 2014; Montay-Gruel et al. 2017; Bourhis et al. 2019a, b; Vozenin et al. 2019a, b). The effects of FLASH on normal tissues have been the subject of several research, which Yinghao Lv et al. have summarized (Lv et al. 2022). Although the precise mechanism underlying the reaction is yet unknown, it is believed to be caused by radiochemical oxygen depletion at highly high dose rates, which influences the radioresistance given to irradiated normal tissue more so than malignant tissues (Spitz et al. 2019; Adrian et al. 2020; Griffin et al. 2020a, b; Petersson et al. 2020).

More comprehensive studies were continuing to be carried out on this issue. A mechanistic radiobiological model expansion was presented by Liew et al., "UNified and VERSatile Bio Response Engine" (UNIVERSE), which reproduces the dose, dose rate, and oxygen tension-dependent influence on cell killing in order to explore the radiobiological aspect of FLASH and evaluate its clinical relevance (Liew et al. 2021). Rothwell et al. additionally created a model incorporating parameters related to radiochemical oxygen dynamics, dose transfer, oxygen consumption, and tissue-specific biological properties (Rothwell et al. 2021). With the help of such studies dating back to 1958, the responses of normal and cancerous tissue can be better understood. The first mechanism involves inhibiting cytokine activation, which includes the production of transforming growth factor-beta. In a normal lung, this process does not begin after FLASH irradiation. An additional and more plausible mechanism pertains to the function of oxygen. In comparison to standard dosage rates, it released a large number of electrons and consumed all available oxygen, leading to a large number of ionizations. This increases the changes in the deterioration of the oxidation process between malignancies and healthy tissue. This mechanism makes FLASH RT, which also has the benefit of protecting healthy tissue, more successful than conventional dose-rate radiation therapy in eliminating hypoxic malignant cells (Vozenin et al. 2019a, b). These studies helped to highlight the possible advantages of FLASH-RT and gave rise to more research on the treatment's effects in clinics. It is known that various national and international associations (AAPM, ESTRO, etc.) conduct studies to evaluate treatment plans and clinical results.

The FLASH effect is thought to exist in electron-wire radiotherapy, X-ray, and proton beam radiotherapy. A summary of the many techniques for producing X-rays has been provided by Montay-Gruel et al. (Montay-Gruel et al. 2022). Depending on the apparatus, 10 MeV electron beam is generated for FLASH RT. Beyreuther et al. used the conventional dose rate proton beam and a proton FLASH beam with 100 Gy/s dose rate (Beyreuther et al. 2019). They observed that there was no difference between toxicity. The preclinical results of different types of radiation have been studied in a large number of studies. However, the agreement for the normalization and standardization of radiation types is still unclear. This situation leads to uncertainty in clinic FLASH-RT use dose rates a thousand times higher than those used in conventional dose rate (e.g. 50 Gy/s vs 0.01 Gy/s). The dosage time is very short (<200 milliseconds). Standard LINACs are insufficient to provide these values. This is one of the critical reasons why FLASH RT cannot be used in clinical applications. Achieving precise and accurate dosimetry at the increased dose rates required for FLASH is one of the additional problems.

Dosimetry devices for UHDR have not yet been produced, so it is difficult for us to quantify the precise dosage. Studies are still ongoing on this issue (Konradsson et al. 2020; McManus et al. 2020; Kranzer et al. 2021). It is necessary to determine the measuring equipment and calibration protocols, such as conventional radiotherapy protocols, which should be prepared separately for photons, electrons, protons, and heavy ions (Almond et al. 1999, International Atomic Energy Agency 2001, McEwen et al. 2014). FLASH irradiation is the most important recent development in radiation treatment history, and it has excellent potential for the future.

1.4 Biological Response Mechanisms

1.4.1 Bystander Effects

The investigation of bystander responses, wherein cells react to the irradiation of their neighboring cells, has been a significant focus in the field of radiation biology (Prise et al. 2009). The bystander effect has been identified as one of the biological phenomena linked to reactions to spatial fractionation—the initial studies on bystander effects primarily involved in vitro experimentation and predominantly utilized modest dosage levels (Mothersill and Seymour 1998; Seymour and Mothersill 2000; Mothersill and Seymour 2001; Brenner and Sachs 2002). The whole understanding of the possible clinical implications of the bystander effect has yet to be fully clarified. Nevertheless, several groups have shown evidence of bystander effects, such as cell death, resulting from the administration of high-dose spatial fractionation in laboratory settings (in vitro) and living organisms (in vivo) (Asur et al. 2012, 2015; Autsavapromporn et al. 2013). Moreover, there have been observations of adaptive and bystander-like reactions inside and between modulated fields, which hold significant implications for implementing GRID therapeutic techniques.

Research conducted using microbeams has provided evidence to support the significant involvement of gap-junction communications in the bystander effect observed between cancer cells and normal cells (Zhang et al. 2022). The experiment involved subjecting confluent cells to various microbeams, such as X-ray, carbon ion, neon ion, or argon ion. The results indicated that a higher proportion of cells developed micronuclei than what would be anticipated solely based on the fraction of cells directly exposed to primary radiation. This observation suggests the existence of a bystander effect. In the cell culture experiment, the application of 18-α-glycyrrhetinic acid (AGA), an inhibitor of gap junctional intercellular communication (GJIC), resulted in the suppression of micronuclei induction at high mean absorbed doses of heavy-ion radiotherapy. However, no significant difference was observed in the case of X-ray radiotherapy. These findings suggest that GJIC specifically involves the bystander effect induced by high-linear energy transfer (LET) irradiation. The bystander effect resulting from low LET irradiation can be influenced by factors secreted by the irradiated cells. This is evident from observations where non-irradiated surrounding cells, when exposed to the growth medium obtained from irradiated cells, displayed the bystander effect characterized by increased micronucleus formation (Autsavapromporn et al. 2013). The application of proton microbeams on confluent A549 cells resulted in the suppression of cytotoxic effects, including the formation of colonies, micronuclei, and chromosome aberrations in bystander A549 cells. This suppression was observed when the inhibition of gap junction was implemented, indicating the potential involvement of gap junctional intercellular communication (GJIC) (Autsavapromporn et al. 2019). The involvement of gap-junction communication in a secondary bystander impact is also possible. A radiation-induced secondary bystander effect occurs when main bystander cells emit secondary bystander signals to adjacent cells, leading to modified biological outcomes. Following the generation of primary bystander cells using human lung cancer cells A549, either a single dosage or fractionated doses of a proton were administered. Subsequently, the bystander cancer cells were placed on the upper surface of the insert together with secondary bystander WI-38 cells. The study revealed that administering fractionated doses resulted in a 20% reduction in micronucleus development in the secondary bystander WI-38 cells compared to applying a single irradiation dose. Nevertheless, including AGA in the co-culture system may effectively mitigate the secondary bystander effect (Autsavapromporn et al. 2019).

1.4.2 Vascular and Angiogenic Effects

The utilization of stereotactic radiosurgery, high-dose radiation has highlighted the possible implications of vascular injury as a critical factor in elucidating the phenomenon of tumor control at cumulative doses that do not align with mathematical predictions for complete cell eradication (Song et al. 2015, 2019; Griffin et al. 2020a, b).

High-dose-per-fraction irradiation has been found to elicit antitumor immune responses by the induction of immunologic cell death, which occurs by directly destroying the DNA of tumor cells and by producing vascular injury (Song et al. 2023). The release of tumor-specific antigens and "danger signs" from tumor cells undergoing immunologic cell death initiates and facilitates a cascade of immune responses. These responses include the release of cytokines, activation of antigen-presenting cells, stimulation of cytotoxic T cells, migration of immune cells toward tumor targets, and, ultimately, the immune-mediated destruction of tumor cells (Song et al. 2021, 2022). Nevertheless, it is essential to acknowledge that the occurrence of radiation-induced vascular injury and subsequent increase in hypoxic inducible factors following high-dose irradiation triggers a wide range of transcriptional processes, increasing immune suppressive pathways, such as the upregulation of immune checkpoints within tumors (Song et al. 2021, 2022). This suggests that the enhanced antitumor immune response caused by radiation may be offset by the potent immune suppressive effect observed in tumors subjected to high-dose-per-fraction irradiation. Hence, the precise magnitude of the antitumor immune response's involvement in tumor management through SABR, SFRT, and FLASH-RT remains uncertain.

The evidence suggests that vascular damage is a crucial factor in both conventional X-ray spatial fractionation and extreme high-dose, spatially fractionated microbeam applications (Serduc et al. 2008a, b; Lemasson et al. 2010). Several studies have been published that examine the vascular disturbances, damage, and inflammation caused by spatial fractionation. Furthermore, it has been seen in various preclinical investigations that there is a vascular response to stress or injury, which resembles the wound-healing process. This angiogenic response has significant implications for tumor control in the context of spatially fractionated radiation (Fontanella et al. 2015).

1.4.3 Immune and Abscopal Effect of Local/Spatial Exposures

The immune response strongly correlates with vascular damage and is pivotal in the reactions to high and ultra-high-dose rate exposures. The response may exhibit significant variations in amplitude and results as a result of regional fractionation. The extent of the abscopal impact in whole tumor exposures may be influenced by the occurrence of significant vascular injury and inflammation throughout the tumor volume (Demaria and Formenti 2020). In contrast, it is worth noting that both GRID and microbeam treatment modalities have the potential to elicit a more preserved physiological response to radiation fields. It can be inferred that the potential for improving the occurrence of an abscopal response against tumors located at a distance could be heightened due to the irradiated tumor's capacity to effectively attract immune cells or facilitate antigen-immune system interactions, thereby augmenting a systemic response. This is primarily because these techniques enable the retention of live vasculature and immune cells inside the low-dose volumes. Several studies have supported this idea, demonstrating that spatial fractionation elicits a more advantageous immune response than alternative methods.

The potential involvement of inflammatory and immunological responses has been proposed as underlying mechanisms contributing to the FLASH effect. The role of transforming growth factor beta (TGF-β), a significant proinflammatory cytokine, has been specifically associated with modifying the impacts of FLASH in contrast to conventional dose-rate irradiation. A prior study has revealed a decrease in TGF-β signaling in mice exposed to FLASH irradiation compared to those exposed to standard dose rates (Favaudon et al. 2014). A study was conducted to examine the effects of whole brain irradiation on C57BL/6 J mice, focusing on the transition from a proinflammatory to an anti-inflammatory phenotype (Simmons et al. 2019). The results demonstrated that FLASH irradiation led to a decrease in pro-inflammatory cytokine levels in the hippocampus, as compared to standard dose-rate irradiation. According to the paper, a statistically significant increase in five out of ten measured cytokines was observed at 10 weeks post-irradiation when standard dose rates were used. In contrast, the use of FLASH increased just three cytokines.

The involvement of TGF-β and its related signaling cascade in the anti-tumor immune response after conventional radiation is widely recognized. However, the specific consequences remain a topic of ongoing discussion (Vanpouille-Box et al. 2015). According to a particular study, the role of TGF-β in conferring radio-resistance to tumor-infiltrating T cells has been highlighted, but other studies propose that TGF-β signaling exerts immunosuppressive effects and facilitates the progression of cancer, hence emphasizing the necessity of employing TGF-β pathway inhibitors (Holmgaard et al. 2018). Therefore, it is imperative to thoroughly evaluate the changes in TGF-β signaling and immune system activation resulting from FLASH irradiation to effectively implement FLASH in clinical settings, particularly when paired with immunotherapy in radiotherapy treatments. There has been a suggestion that using FLASH radiotherapy may potentially enhance the immune response by minimizing the irradiation of circulating immune cells, owing to its rapid exposure time. However, it is worth noting that this effect might be diminished when employing fractionated FLASH radiotherapy (Durante et al. 2018).

1.4.4 Oxygen Availability and Radiochemistry Considerations

The complete understanding of the biochemical mechanisms underlying the FLASH effect remains a subject of ongoing research. However, the prevailing idea gaining significant support suggests that oxygen plays a crucial role as a molecule in the biological response to FLASH irradiation (Wilson et al. 2019). Typically, in the context of ionizing radiation, indirect DNA damage arises from the radiolysis of water, which leads to the creation of reactive oxygen species (ROS), including hydroxyl radicals (Morgan and Sowa 2005). These ROS then proceed to initiate an attack on the DNA. According to estimates, a significant proportion of DNA damage caused by low LET radiation, specifically photons and electrons, is attributed to producing reactive oxygen species (ROS), accounting for around 60–70% of the damage. The remaining 30–40% of DNA damage is directly caused by the interaction between the radiation and DNA (Santivasi and Xia 2014; Spitz et al. 2019). According to the oxygen fixation hypothesis, when indirect DNA damage occurs due to free radical reaction, the presence of molecular oxygen leads to the fixation of the damage by facilitating the development of a more harmful peroxyl radical (Grimes and Partridge 2015). This factor significantly contributes to the higher radioresistance observed in hypoxic tumors compared to well-oxygenated tumors, which exhibit an oxygen enhancement ratio of approximately 2–3 (Bristow and Hill 2008; Antonovic et al. 2014). The oxygen depletion concept posits that within the context of FLASH (ultra-high dose rate), the modulation of immediate radiochemical reactions in irradiated tissue occurs. During a brief period of exposure, the rate at which local oxygen is used exceeds the rate at which reoxygenation occurs (Bourhis et al. 2019a, b). As a result, a temporary condition of radiation-induced hypoxia arises, resulting in the development of radioresistance and safeguarding normal tissues from FLASH irradiation (Pratx and Kapp 2019).

The correlation between escalating dose rates and the oxygen depletion concept was observed in initial investigations on bacteria. This research demonstrated that exposure to extremely high radiation levels resulted in a survival curve resembling that of organisms irradiated in an oxygen-deprived (hypoxic) setting (Phillips and Worsnop 1969). Nevertheless, there has been a dearth of in vitro evidence utilizing mammalian cell lines to investigate the occurrence of the FLASH effect, and the findings have been inconclusive about the presence or absence of this phenomenon (Buonanno et al. 2019; Adrian et al. 2020). The discrepancy can be partially attributed to the utilization of cells cultivated in atmospheric oxygen concentrations (~20%) in FLASH research, whereas the in vivo observation of normal tissue sparing often occurs within physiological oxygen tensions ranging from 3% to 7% (McKeown 2014; Petersson et al. 2020). This implies that the FLASH dosages employed in the in vitro experiments were inadequate to substantially reduce oxygen tension. Following this assertion, a recent investigation conducted on prostate cancer cells subjected to irradiation at a dose rate 600 Gy/s and 10 MeV electrons demonstrated notable improvements in cell survival compared with conventional dose-rate irradiation administered at 14 Gy/min. These findings were observed under oxygen concentrations of 1.6%, 2.7%, and 4.4%. However, no statistically significant disparity was observed at higher oxygen concentrations of 8.3% and 20% (Adrian et al. 2020).

The concept of oxygen depletion raises a significant concern regarding the clinical translatability of FLASH. The reason behind this phenomenon is that in tumors with a heterogeneous cell population exhibiting varying levels of oxygen concentrations, the FLASH effect could potentially harm therapy by promoting an increase in tumor radioresistance. Hence, it is imperative to conduct further experimental investigations in order to delve into the relationship between oxygen tension and its influence on FLASH radiotherapy. A comprehensive comprehension of the dose-response relationship and the distribution of radiation exposure to physiological changes inside targeted tissues would significantly enhance the advancement of these strategies as feasible clinical treatment options for specific types of tumors.

1.5 Future Developments and Clinical Utility

The utilization of SFRT and FLASH-RT in everyday clinical practice necessitates thoroughly examining their new biological mechanisms through meticulously prepared controlled clinical trials. The radiation therapy techniques being discussed bear a resemblance to the biological hypotheses examined in extensive trials involving time-dose-fractionation over the past 25 years across various tumor locations. Similarly, they align with combined modality trials involving chemo-radiation therapy and radiation-immune-oncology combinations, compared to radiation therapy in isolation, which have yielded successful outcomes. After establishing the clinical target volume, a conventional radiation therapy regimen can be characterized by a limited number of parameters, including the radiation modality, total dose, fraction dose, treatment time, and an indicator of dose homogeneity within the target volume. On the other hand, SFRT encompasses a greater number of degrees of freedom, such as the contrast between the peak and valley doses, the spatial frequency at which these peaks and valleys occur, and the three-dimensional arrangement of dose peaks administered. The relative biological significance of these metrics and their potential interactions with dose-fractionation in the temporal domain and other anticancer methods have yet to be determined. One salient matter requiring elucidation is the potential nullification of the impact by a spatial displacement of the dose-lattice between successive fractions. In the preclinical context, it is common practice to administer FLASH-RT as a single fraction. This would render the 4Rs of radiation (repair, reoxygenation, regeneration, and redistribution) inconsequential.

Nevertheless, when considering the matter from a clinical standpoint, it might be argued that the appropriate point of comparison would be a fractionated schedule, potentially hypofractionated, administered at a typical acute dose rate. The extent to which the "FLASH" impact diminishes as the ultra-high dosage rate decreases remains uncertain. The inclusion of various delivery systems necessitates the implementation of meticulously designed and executed preclinical in vivo investigations. These experiments are essential to establish a logical framework for the transition from preclinical to clinical translation.

The need for precise dose delivery and accurate dosimetry has always been prioritized in clinical safety and practice. However, it is crucial not to impede the progress of these emerging modalities by solely focusing on associated concerns. The necessity for ongoing change persists as a recurring subject, as it is crucial for the continuous progress of emerging technologies in the healthcare field, to enhance its quality.

2 Conclusion

Radiotherapy techniques such as GRID, microbeam, and FLASH are all fascinating approaches that try to maximize the therapeutic index of radiation treatment. The use of charged particles has the potential to generate additional benefits, such as more conformal dose distributions and radiobiological advantages; however, these have not yet been proved in their entirety.

Compliance with Ethical Standards

Funding None.

Disclosure of Interests All authors declare they have no conflict of interest.

Ethical Approval This article does not contain any studies with human participants and animals performed by any of the authors.

References

Adrian G, Konradsson E, Lempart M, Back S, Ceberg C, Petersson K (2020) The FLASH effect depends on oxygen concentration. Br J Radiol 93:20190702

Alagoz E, Brauer-Krisch E, Bravin A, Cornelius I, Fournier P, Hansen TE, Kok A, Lerch M, Monakhov E, Morse J, Pacifico N, Petasecca M, Povoli M, Requard H, Rozenfeld AD, Salome M, Sandaker H, Stugu B (2016) Multi-strip silicon sensors for beam array monitoring in micro-beam radiation therapy. Phys Med 32:1795–1800

Almond PR, Biggs PJ, Coursey BM, Hanson WF, Huq MS, Nath R, Rogers DW (1999) AAPM's TG-51 protocol for clinical reference dosimetry of high-energy photon and electron beams. Med Phys 26:1847–1870

Antonovic L, Lindblom E, Dasu A, Bassler N, Furusawa Y, Toma-Dasu I (2014) Clinical oxygen enhancement ratio of tumors in carbon ion radiotherapy: the influence of local oxygenation changes. J Radiat Res 55:902–911

Asur RS, Sharma S, Chang CW, Penagaricano J, Kommuru IM, Moros EG, Corry PM, Griffin RJ (2012) Spatially fractionated radiation induces cytotoxicity and changes in gene expression in bystander and radiation adjacent murine carcinoma cells. Radiat Res 177:751–765

Asur R, Butterworth KT, Penagaricano JA, Prise KM, Griffin RJ (2015) High dose bystander effects in spatially fractionated radiation therapy. Cancer Lett 356:52–57

Autsavapromporn N, Suzuki M, Funayama T, Usami N, Plante I, Yokota Y, Mutou Y, Ikeda H, Kobayashi K, Kobayashi Y, Uchihori Y, Hei TK, Azzam EI, Murakami T (2013) Gap junction communication and the propagation of bystander effects induced by microbeam irradiation in human fibroblast cultures: the impact of radiation quality. Radiat Res 180:367–375

Autsavapromporn N, Liu C, Kobayashi A, Ahmad TAFT, Oikawa M, Dukaew N, Wang J, Wongnoppavichb A, Konishic T (2019) Emerging role of secondary bystander effects induced by fractionated proton microbeam radiation. Radiat Res 191:211–216

Bartzsch S, Oelfke U (2017) Line focus x-ray tubes-a new concept to produce high brilliance x-rays. Phys Med Biol 62:8600–8615

Bartzsch S, Cummings C, Eismann S, Oelfke U (2016) A preclinical microbeam facility with a conventional x-ray tube. Med Phys 43:6301

Becker J, Kuttig H (1965) The use of the grid in Supervoltage therapy. Prog Radiat Ther 3:50–67

Berry RJ (1973) Effects of radiation dose-rate from protracted, continuous irradiation to ultra-high dose-rates from pulsed accelerators. Br Med Bull 29:44–47

Beyreuther E, Brand M, Hans S, Hideghety K, Karsch L, Lessmann E, Schurer M, Szabo ER, Pawelke J (2019) Feasibility of proton FLASH effect tested by zebrafish embryo irradiation. Radiother Oncol 139:46–50

Bouchet A, Lemasson B, Le Duc G, Maisin C, Brauer-Krisch E, Siegbahn EA, Renaud L, Khalil E, Remy C, Poillot C, Bravin A, Laissue JA, Barbier EL, Serduc R (2010) Preferential effect of synchrotron microbeam radiation therapy on intracerebral 9L gliosarcoma vascular networks. Int J Radiat Oncol Biol Phys 78:1503–1512

Bouchet A, Brauer-Krisch E, Prezado Y, El Atifi M, Rogalev L, Le Clec'h C, Laissue JA, Pelletier L, Le Duc G (2016) Better efficacy of synchrotron spatially microfractionated radiation therapy than uniform radiation therapy on glioma. Int J Radiat Oncol Biol Phys 95:1485–1494

Bourhis J, Montay-Gruel P, Gonçalves Jorge P, Bailat C, Petit B, Ollivier J, Jeanneret-Sozzi W, Ozsahin M, Bochud F, Moeckli R, Germond J-F, Vozenin M-C (2019a) Clinical translation of FLASH radiotherapy: why and how? Radiother Oncol 139:11–17

Bourhis J, Sozzi WJ, Jorge PG, Gaide O, Bailat C, Duclos F, Patin D, Ozsahin M, Bochud F, Germond JF, Moeckli R, Vozenin MC (2019b) Treatment of a first patient with FLASH-radiotherapy. Radiother Oncol 139:18–22

Brauer-Krisch E, Requardt H, Regnard P, Corde S, Siegbahn E, LeDuc G, Brochard T, Blattmann H, Laissue J, Bravin A (2005) New irradiation geometry for microbeam radiation therapy. Phys Med Biol 50:3103–3111

Brenner DJ, Sachs RK (2002) Do low dose-rate bystander effects influence domestic radon risks? Int J Radiat Biol 78:593–604

Bristow RG, Hill RP (2008) Hypoxia and metabolism. Hypoxia, DNA repair and genetic instability. Nat Rev Cancer 8:180–192

Buonanno M, Grilj V, Brenner DJ (2019) Biological effects in normal cells exposed to FLASH dose rate protons. Radiother Oncol 139:51–55

Dauer LT, Yorke E, Williamson M, Gao Y, Dauer ZL, Miller DL, Vano E (2018) Radiotherapeutic implications of the updated ICRP thresholds for tissue reactions related to cataracts and circulatory diseases. Ann ICRP 47:196–213

Demaria S, Formenti SC (2020) The abscopal effect 67 years later: from a side story to center stage. Br J Radiol 93:20200042

Durante M, Bräuer-Krisch E, Hill MJT (2018) Faster and safer? FLASH ultra-high dose rate in radiotherapy. Br J Radiol 91:20170628

Favaudon V, Caplier L, Monceau V, Pouzoulet F, Sayarath M, Fouillade C, Poupon MF, Brito I, Hupe P, Bourhis J, Hall J, Fontaine JJ, Vozenin MC (2014) Ultrahigh dose-rate FLASH irradiation increases the differential response between normal and tumor tissue in mice. Sci Transl Med 6:245ra293

Fontanella AN, Boss MK, Hadsell M, Zhang J, Schroeder T, Berman KG, Dewhirst MW, Chang S, Palmer GM (2015) Effects of high-dose microbeam irradiation on tumor microvascular function and angiogenesis. Radiat Res 183:147–158

Ghita M, McMahon SJ, Taggart LE, Butterworth KT, Schettino G, Prise KM (2017) A mechanistic study of gold nanoparticle radiosensitisation using targeted microbeam irradiation. Sci Rep 7: 44752

Ghita M, Fernandez-Palomo C, Fukunaga H, Fredericia PM, Schettino G, Brauer-Krisch E, Butterworth KT, McMahon SJ, Prise KM (2018) Microbeam evolution: from single cell irradiation to pre-clinical studies. Int J Radiat Biol 94:708–718

Griffin RJ, Koonce NA, Dings RP, Siegel E, Moros EG, Brauer-Krisch E, Corry PM (2012) Microbeam radiation therapy alters vascular architecture and tumor oxygenation and is enhanced by a galectin-1 targeted anti-angiogenic peptide. Radiat Res 177:804–812

Griffin RJ, Ahmed MM, Amendola B, Belyakov O, Bentzen SM, Butterworth KT, Chang S, Coleman CN, Djonov V, Formenti SC, Glatstein E, Guha C, Kalnicki S, Le QT, Loo BW Jr, Mahadevan A, Massaccesi M, Maxim PG, Mohiuddin M, Mohiuddin M, Mayr NA,

Obcemea C, Petersson K, Regine W, Roach M, Romanelli P, Simone CB 2nd, Snider JW, Spitz DR, Vikram B, Vozenin MC, Abdel-Wahab M, Welsh J, Wu X, Limoli CL (2020a) Understanding high-dose, ultra-high dose rate, and spatially fractionated radiation therapy. Int J Radiat Oncol Biol Phys 107:766–778

Griffin RJ, Prise KM, McMahon SJ, Zhang X, Penagaricano J, Butterworth KT (2020b) History and current perspectives on the biological effects of high-dose spatial fractionation and high dose-rate approaches: GRID, microbeam & FLASH radiotherapy. Br J Radiol 93:20200217

Grimes DR, Partridge M (2015) A mechanistic investigation of the oxygen fixation hypothesis and oxygen enhancement ratio. Biomed Phys Eng Expr 1:045209

Grotzer MA, Schultke E, Brauer-Krisch E, Laissue JA (2015) Microbeam radiation therapy: clinical perspectives. Phys Med 31:564–567

Holmgaard RB, Schaer DA, Li Y, Castaneda SP, Murphy MY, Xu X, Inigo I, Dobkin J, Manro JR, Iversen PW (2018) Targeting the TGFβ pathway with galunisertib, a TGFβRI small molecule inhibitor, promotes anti-tumor immunity leading to durable, complete responses, as monotherapy and in combination with checkpoint blockade. 6:1–15

Hornsey S, Alper T (1966) Unexpected dose-rate effect in the killing of mice by radiation. Nature 210:212–213

Huhn JL, Regine WF, Valentino JP, Meigooni AS, Kudrimoti M, Mohiuddin M (2006) Spatially fractionated GRID radiation treatment of advanced neck disease associated with head and neck cancer. Technol Cancer Res Treat 5:607–612

International Atomic Energy Agency (2001) Absorbed dose determination in external beam radiotherapy. International Atomic Energy Agency, Vienna

Kirby-Smith JS, Dolphin GW (1958) Chromosome breakage at high radiation dose-rates. Nature 182:270–271

Konradsson E, Ceberg C, Lempart M, Blad B, Back S, Knoos T, Petersson K (2020) Correction for ion recombination in a built-in monitor chamber of a clinical linear accelerator at ultra-high dose rates. Radiat Res 194:580–586

Kranzer R, Poppinga D, Weidner J, Schuller A, Hackel T, Looe HK, Poppe B (2021) Ion collection efficiency of ionization chambers in ultra-high dose-per-pulse electron beams. Med Phys 48: 819–830

Kurup A, Pasternak J, Taylor R, Murgatroyd L, Ettlinger O, Shields W, Nevay L, Gruber S, Pozimski J, Lau HT, Long K, Blackmore V, Barber G, Najmudin Z, Yarnold J (2019) Simulation of a radiobiology facility for the Centre for the Clinical Application of particles. Phys Med 65:21–28

Laissue JA, Blattmann H, Slatkin DN (2012) Alban Kohler (1874-1947): inventor of grid therapy. Z Med Phys 22:90–99

Lemasson B, Serduc R, Maisin C, Bouchet A, Coquery N, Robert P, Le Duc G, Tropres I, Remy C, Barbier EL (2010) Monitoring blood-brain barrier status in a rat model of glioma receiving therapy: dual injection of low-molecular-weight and macromolecular MR contrast media. Radiology 257:342–352

Liew H, Mein S, Dokic I, Haberer T, Debus J, Abdollahi A, Mairani A (2021) Deciphering time-dependent DNA damage complexity, repair, and oxygen tension: a mechanistic model for FLASH-dose-rate radiation therapy. Int J Radiat Oncol Biol Phys 110:574–586

Lv Y, Lv Y, Wang Z, Lan T, Feng X, Chen H, Zhu J, Ma X, Du J, Hou G, Liao W, Yuan K, Wu H (2022) FLASH radiotherapy: a promising new method for radiotherapy. Oncol Lett 24:419

Marks H (1952) Clinical experience with irradiation through a grid. Radiology 58:338–342

McEwen M, DeWerd L, Ibbott G, Followill D, Rogers DW, Seltzer S, Seuntjens J (2014) Addendum to the AAPM's TG-51 protocol for clinical reference dosimetry of high-energy photon beams. Med Phys 41:041501

McKeown SR (2014) Defining normoxia, physoxia and hypoxia in tumours-implications for treatment response. Br J Radiol 87:20130676

McManus M, Romano F, Lee ND, Farabolini W, Gilardi A, Royle G, Palmans H, Subiel A (2020) The challenge of ionisation chamber dosimetry in ultra-short pulsed high dose-rate very high energy electron beams. Sci Rep 10:9089

Meigooni AS, Parker SA, Zheng J, Kalbaugh KJ, Regine WF, Mohiuddin M (2002) Dosimetric characteristics with spatial fractionation using electron grid therapy. Med Dosim 27:37–42

Mohiuddin M, Curtis DL, Grizos WT, Komarnicky L (1990) Palliative treatment of advanced cancer using multiple nonconfluent pencil beam radiation. A pilot study Cancer 66:114–118

Mohiuddin M, Fujita M, Regine WF, Megooni AS, Ibbott GS, Ahmed MM (1999) High-dose spatially-fractionated radiation (GRID): a new paradigm in the management of advanced cancers. Int J Radiat Oncol Biol Phys 45:721–727

Montay-Gruel P, Petersson K, Jaccard M, Boivin G, Germond JF, Petit B, Doenlen R, Favaudon V, Bochud F, Bailat C, Bourhis J, Vozenin MC (2017) Irradiation in a flash: unique sparing of memory in mice after whole brain irradiation with dose rates above 100Gy/s. Radiother Oncol 124:365–369

Montay-Gruel P, Corde S, Laissue JA, Bazalova-Carter M (2022) FLASH radiotherapy with photon beams. Med Phys 49:2055–2067

Morgan WF, Sowa MB (2005) Effects of ionizing radiation in nonirradiated cells. Proc Natl Acad Sci USA 102:14127–14128

Mothersill C, Seymour CB (1998) Cell-cell contact during gamma irradiation is not required to induce a bystander effect in Normal human keratinocytes: evidence for release during irradiation of a signal controlling survival into the medium. Radiat Res 149:256–262

Mothersill C, Seymour C (2001) Radiation-induced bystander effects: past history and future directions. Radiat Res 155:759–767

Neuner G, Mohiuddin MM, Vander Walde N, Goloubeva O, Ha J, Yu CX, Regine WF (2012) High-dose spatially fractionated GRID radiation therapy (SFGRT): a comparison of treatment outcomes with Cerrobend vs. MLC SFGRT. Int J Radiat Oncol Biol Phys 82:1642–1649

Penagaricano JA, Moros EG, Ratanatharathorn V, Yan Y, Corry P (2010) Evaluation of spatially fractionated radiotherapy (GRID) and definitive chemoradiotherapy with curative intent for locally advanced squamous cell carcinoma of the head and neck: initial response rates and toxicity. Int J Radiat Oncol Biol Phys 76:1369–1375

Petersson K, Adrian G, Butterworth K, McMahon SJ (2020) A quantitative analysis of the role of oxygen tension in FLASH radiation therapy. Int J Radiat Oncol Biol Phys 107:539–547

Phillips TL, Worsnop BR (1969) Ultra-high dose-rate effects in radiosensitive bacteria. Int J Radiat Biol Relat Stud Phys Chem Med 14:573–575

Pratx G, Kapp DS (2019) A computational model of radiolytic oxygen depletion during FLASH irradiation and its effect on the oxygen enhancement ratio. Phys Med Biol 64:185005

Prise KM, Schettino G, Vojnovic B, Belyakov O, Shao C (2009) Microbeam studies of the bystander response. J Radiat Res 50(Suppl A):A1-6

Priyadarshika RC, Crosbie JC, Kumar B, Rogers PA (2011) Biodosimetric quantification of short-term synchrotron microbeam versus broad-beam radiation damage to mouse skin using a dermatopathological scoring system. Br J Radiol 84:833–842

Rothwell BC, Kirkby NF, Merchant MJ, Chadwick AL, Lowe M, Mackay RI, Hendry JH, Kirkby KJ (2021) Determining the parameter space for effective oxygen depletion for FLASH radiation therapy. Phys Med Biol 66

Santivasi WL, Xia F (2014) Ionizing radiation-induced DNA damage, response, and repair. Antioxid Redox Signal 21:251–259

Sathishkumar S, Dey S, Meigooni AS, Regine WF, Kudrimoti MS, Ahmed MM, Mohiuddin M (2002) The impact of TNF-alpha induction on therapeutic efficacy following high dose spatially fractionated (GRID) radiation. Technol Cancer Res Treat 1:141–147

Sathishkumar S, Boyanovsky B, Karakashian AA, Rozenova K, Giltiay NV, Kudrimoti M, Mohiuddin M, Ahmed MM, Nikolova-Karakashian M (2005) Elevated sphingomyelinase activity and ceramide concentration in serum of patients undergoing high dose spatially fractionated radiation treatment: implications for endothelial apoptosis. Cancer Biol Ther 4: 979–986

Schultke E, Balosso J, Breslin T, Cavaletti G, Djonov V, Esteve F, Grotzer M, Hildebrandt G, Valdman A, Laissue J (2017) Microbeam radiation therapy – grid therapy and beyond: a clinical perspective. Br J Radiol 90:20170073

Serduc R, Christen T, Laissue J, Farion R, Bouchet A, Sanden B, Segebarth C, Brauer-Krisch E, Le Duc G, Bravin A, Remy C, Barbier EL (2008a) Brain tumor vessel response to synchrotron microbeam radiation therapy: a short-term in vivo study. Phys Med Biol 53:3609–3622

Serduc R, van de Looij Y, Francony G, Verdonck O, van der Sanden B, Laissue J, Farion R, Brauer-Krisch E, Siegbahn EA, Bravin A, Prezado Y, Segebarth C, Remy C, Lahrech H (2008b) Characterization and quantification of cerebral edema induced by synchrotron x-ray microbeam radiation therapy. Phys Med Biol 53:1153–1166

Seymour CB, Mothersill C (2000) Relative contribution of bystander and targeted cell killing to the low-dose region of the radiation dose–response curve. J Radiat Res 153:508–511

Simmons DA, Lartey FM, Schüler E, Rafat M, King G, Kim A, Ko R, Semaan S, Gonzalez S, Jenkins M (2019) Reduced cognitive deficits after FLASH irradiation of whole mouse brain are associated with less hippocampal dendritic spine loss and neuroinflammation. Radiother Oncol 139:4–10

Song CW, Lee YJ, Griffin RJ, Park I, Koonce NA, Hui S, Kim MS, Dusenbery KE, Sperduto PW, Cho LC (2015) Indirect tumor cell death after high-dose Hypofractionated irradiation: implications for stereotactic body radiation therapy and stereotactic radiation surgery. Int J Radiat Oncol Biol Phys 93:166–172

Song CW, Griffin RJ, Lee YJ, Cho H, Seo J, Park I, Kim HK, Kim DH, Kim MS, Dusenbery KE, Cho LC (2019) Reoxygenation and repopulation of tumor cells after ablative Hypofractionated radiotherapy (SBRT and SRS) in murine tumors. Radiat Res 192:159–168

Song CW, Glatstein E, Marks LB, Emami B, Grimm J, Sperduto PW, Kim M-S, Hui S, Dusenbery KE, Cho LC (2021) Biological principles of stereotactic body radiation therapy (SBRT) and stereotactic radiation surgery (SRS): indirect cell death. Int J Radiat Oncol Biol Phys 110:21–34

Song CW, Kim H, Cho H, Kim M-S, Paek S-H, Park H-J, Griffin RJ, Terezakis S, Cho LC (2022) HIF-1α inhibition improves anti-tumor immunity and promotes the efficacy of stereotactic ablative radiotherapy (SABR). Cancers 14:3273

Song CW, Terezakis S, Park WY, Paek SH, Kim MS, Cho LC, Griffin RJ (2023) Preferential tumor vascular damage is the common antitumor mechanism of high-dose Hypofractionated radiation therapy: SABR, spatially fractionated radiation therapy, and FLASH radiation therapy. Int J Radiat Oncol Biol Phys 117:701–704

Spitz DR, Buettner GR, Petronek MS, St-Aubin JJ, Flynn RT, Waldron TJ, Limoli CL (2019) An integrated physico-chemical approach for explaining the differential impact of FLASH versus conventional dose rate irradiation on cancer and normal tissue responses. Radiother Oncol 139: 23–27

Trapp JV, Warrington AP, Partridge M, Philps A, Glees J, Tait D, Ahmed R, Leach MO, Webb S (2004) Measurement of the three-dimensional distribution of radiation dose in grid therapy. Phys Med Biol 49:N317–N323

Vanpouille-Box C, Diamond JM, Pilones KA, Zavadil J, Babb JS, Formenti SC, Barcellos-Hoff MH, Demaria S (2015) TGFβ is a master regulator of radiation therapy-induced antitumor immunity. Cancer Res 75:2232–2242

Variola AAD, Blin A, Bonis J, Bouaziz S, Bruni C, Cassou K, Chaikovska I, Chance S, Chaumat V (2014) The ThomX project status. 5th international particle accelerator conference, IPAC 2014, Dresden, Germany

Vozenin MC, De Fornel P, Petersson K, Favaudon V, Jaccard M, Germond JF, Petit B, Burki M, Ferrand G, Patin D, Bouchaab H, Ozsahin M, Bochud F, Bailat C, Devauchelle P, Bourhis J (2019a) The advantage of FLASH radiotherapy confirmed in mini-pig and cat-cancer patients. Clin Cancer Res 25:35–42

Vozenin MC, Hendry JH, Limoli CL (2019b) Biological benefits of ultra-high dose rate FLASH radiotherapy: sleeping beauty awoken. Clin Oncol (R Coll Radiol) 31:407–415

Walsh DWM, Siebenwirth C, Greubel C, Ilicic K, Reindl J, Girst S, Muggiolu G, Simon M, Barberet P, Seznec H, Zischka H, Multhoff G, Schmid TE, Dollinger G (2017) Live cell imaging of mitochondria following targeted irradiation in situ reveals rapid and highly localized loss of membrane potential. Sci Rep 7:46684

Wang XF, Li JQ, Wang JZ, Zhang JX, Liu A, He ZJ, Zhang W, Zhang B, Shao CL, Shi LQ (2011) Current progress of the biological single-ion microbeam at FUDAN. Radiat Environ Biophys 50:353–364

Wilson JD, Hammond EM, Higgins GS, Petersson K (2019) Ultra-high dose rate (FLASH) radiotherapy: silver bullet or Fool's gold? Front Oncol 9:1563

Zhang X, Penagaricano J, Yan Y, Sharma S, Griffin RJ, Hardee M, Han EY, Ratanatharathom V (2016) Application of spatially fractionated radiation (GRID) to helical Tomotherapy using a novel TOMOGRID template. Technol Cancer Res Treat 15:91–100

Zhang Z, Li K, Hong M (2022) Radiation-induced bystander effect and cytoplasmic irradiation studies with microbeams. Biology 11:945

Zhong N, Morris GM, Bacarian T, Rosen EM, Dilmanian FA (2003) Response of rat skin to high-dose unidirectional x-ray microbeams: a histological study. Radiat Res 160:133–142

Zwicker RD, Meigooni A, Mohiuddin M (2004) Therapeutic advantage of grid irradiation for large single fractions. Int J Radiat Oncol Biol Phys 58:1309–1315

Bioimplants for the Reconstructive Surgery and Local Delivery of Chemo-Immunoagents

Natalia Yu. Anisimova, Natalia S. Martynenko, Olga V. Rybalchenko, Fedor S. Senatov, Boris B. Straumal, Nariman A. Enikeev, Keryam M. Novruzov, and Mikhail V. Kiselevskiy

Abstract

This chapter is devoted to the description of directions of bioimplants development in oncology, methods of their production, and materials used. The results of both own research in this field and achievements of other researchers are analyzed. Special attention is paid to the description of developments in the field of bioimplants and their scaffolds for the replacement of bone, cartilage, and trachea defects. Innovative solutions providing depot injection of bioactive components and drugs for therapy of cancer patients and preventing the

N. Y. Anisimova (✉) · M. V. Kiselevskiy
N.N. Blokhin National Medical Research Center of Oncology of the Ministry of Health of the Russian Federation (N.N. Blokhin NMRCO), Moscow, Russia

Center for Biomedical Engineering, National University of Science and Technology "MISIS", Moscow, Russia
e-mail: n.anisimova@misis.ru

N. S. Martynenko · O. V. Rybalchenko
A.A. Baikov Institute of Metallurgy and Materials Science of the Russian Academy of Sciences (IMET RAS), Moscow, Russia

F. S. Senatov
Center for Biomedical Engineering, National University of Science and Technology "MISIS", Moscow, Russia

B. B. Straumal
Osipyan Institute of Solid State Physics, Russian Academy of Sciences, Chernogolovka, Russia

N. A. Enikeev
Laboratory for Metals and Alloys under Extreme Impacts, Ufa University of Science and Technology, Ufa, Russia

K. M. Novruzov
N.N. Blokhin National Medical Research Center of Oncology of the Ministry of Health of the Russian Federation (N.N. Blokhin NMRCO), Moscow, Russia

Interdisciplinary Cancer Research, https://doi.org/10.1007/16833_2024_374
Published online: 20 September 2024

development of side effects are also described. The possibilities of using extracellular matrix implants, synthetic and natural polymers, titanium alloys, and biodegradable alloys based on Fe-Mn system and magnesium for the development of scaffolds were thoroughly discussed. The properties of compact and porous scaffolds based on titanium alloys were described in detail in separate sections. Recent advances in this field have been critically analyzed, including approaches to model design, testing of the resulting developments, the possibilities of machining and 3D printing to modify the structure and properties of scaffolds, and the problems of their biocorrosion, biocompatibility, and functionality. Special attention is paid to highlighting current problems in the industry and ways to solve them.

Keywords

Bioimplant · Bioresorbable alloy · Bone defect · Drug-device release system · Polymer · Porous structures · Reconstruction · Scaffold · Titanium alloys

1 Introduction

The development of implants for clinical medical practice is an urgent task of modern medicine. The purposes of application of such products are diverse. The important direction is the development of implants that can play the role of platforms for local injection or prolonged release of drugs used in the therapy of cancer patients. It is generally recognized that systemic chemotherapy is the most commonly used treatment for malignant neoplasms. However, only an insignificant part of cytostatic drug entering the bloodstream and producing a systemic toxic effect reaches tumor cells. Along with targeting therapy, other methods of targeted delivery of antitumor drugs to the tumor are being developed. One such approach is intratumoral administration of nonspecific cytotoxic agents. In clinical practice, there is a well-established method of brachytherapy, which consists in percutaneous injection of radioactive implants into the tumor node. Currently, the possibilities of targeted administration of cytostatic drugs used for systemic chemotherapy of malignant neoplasms are also being investigated. This is due to the fact that local administration, providing an effective dosage of the drug directly in the tumor area, causes minimal side effects (Hohenforst-Schmidt et al. 2015). Chemotherapy in many cases causes adverse effects when administered systemically, requiring discontinuation of treatment and additional costs to the health care system to treat side effects. Attempts to improve the efficacy of conventional chemotherapy by combining it with immunomodulators or anti-angiogenic or other targeted agents have not yielded the expected results (Boutsikou et al. 2013). The revolutionary trend in immuno-oncology—immune checkpoint inhibitors—has yet to prove itself as an effective treatment for various forms of malignant neoplasms, and the high cost of this type of therapy significantly limits the prospects of its use in clinical practice. These circumstances make us turn again to traditional cytostatics and solve the problem of their targeted delivery to the tumor (Hohenforst-Schmidt et al. 2013).

The accumulated experimental and clinical data testify to the effectiveness of intratumoral chemotherapy. In particular, in a recent clinical study, it was shown that intratumoral needle administration of 0.5–1% cisplatin solution to patients with non-small cell lung cancer caused regression or stabilization of the tumor, with no significant side effects. This simple and non-toxic method of treatment was superior to standard intravenous treatment regimens, not only improving the quality of life of patients, but also in terms of overall survival, and was significantly less costly in comparison with the so-called personalized tumor therapy with modern targeted agents. However, despite the simplicity and obviousness of intratumoral administration of chemopreparations, there are a number of unsolved problems. In particular, there are often difficulties in injecting the necessary volumes of cytostatic drug into tumor nodules, especially those with a pronounced stromal component or in bone or cartilage tumors. Fluid injection into the tumor can lead to increased interstitial pressure, pronounced hypoxia, which in combination with abnormal blood supply of the tumor causes uneven distribution of the drug and the formation of local necrosis with subsequent ulceration of the tumor. In addition, maintenance of effective drug concentration in the tumor requires repeated injections, i.e., constant traumatization of the tumor (Hohenforst-Schmidt 2011). In this regard, the task arises of both targeted delivery of a chemopreventive agent and its gradual release in the tumor site in order to maintain the effective concentration of cytostatic agent for a long time. Currently, approaches are being developed for targeted delivery of nanoparticles conjugated with antitumor drugs when a magnetic field is applied to the tumor site. However, it is difficult to control the concentration of cytostatics in the tumor, and the safety of using nanoparticles in clinical practice has not been confirmed. By analogy with brachytherapy it seems promising to create intratumoral implants saturated with cytotoxic agent, characterized by controlled biodegradation, providing a sufficient level of cytostatic concentration for a long time. Promising materials for this purpose are biodegradable alloys or other materials possessing a given level of biodegradation. Such structures saturated with cytostatic can be used in adjuvant chemotherapy of osteogenic sarcomas, aimed at reducing the volume of surgical interventions, which corresponds to the modern trends of performing salvage operations without amputation of the limb (He et al. 2017). Biodegradable materials saturated with cytostatic drugs can also be used to prevent local recurrences of osteogenic sarcoma, while simultaneously acting as anchoring elements or implants replacing bone tissue defects.

One of the difficult problems of clinical medicine is the task of compensating for tissue defects destroyed due to the progression of tumor process and removed after resection during surgical interventions. Osteochondroma accounts for 20–50% of benign bone tumors (Murphey et al. 2000) and 10–15% of all tumors in general. The second place in prevalence is occupied by enchondroma, which accounts for 13% and 3–10% (Hong et al. 2011), respectively. Osteoblastoma accounts for about 14% of benign bone tumors, which is approximately the same as the prevalence of giant cell tumors (Nandi et al. 2010; De Salvo et al. 2022). In addition, bone lesions in cancer patients may be a consequence of the development of metastases. In this case, along with the proximal part of the femur and humerus, the spine and pelvic bones are most often affected. The diagnosis is usually made when there is significant local spread of the tumor, which requires resection of significant areas of bone. This causes a high level of disability in patients after resection of bone tissue destroyed by a tumor, a significant decrease in motor activity, and a deterioration in the patient's quality of life. These patients require constant care, including the participation of medical workers of various qualifications. Therefore, this category of patients is in dire need of reconstructive surgeries to restore significant bone defects using implants, which is a complex and unresolved problem in the treatment of patients with malignant neoplasms. In some cases, the volume of tissue or organ to be reconstructed is very significant, which prevents not only the normal functioning of the organ, but also the viability of the organism as a whole. The optimal implant should keep biocompatibility, not cause inflammation, keep physical properties of the initial sample, and not possess carcinogenic properties; if the matrix is bioresorbable, the rate of resorption should coincide with the rate of tissue restoration. The limited availability of effective implants for bone defects replacement leads to a significant reduction in the quality of life of patients and significant economic losses due to the high cost of long-term treatment and rehabilitation measures, exclusion from the real sector of economy not only of patients themselves, but also of caregivers and social services. In the world practice several methods of reconstruction of tubular and flat bones are used, each of them has its own advantages and disadvantages. That is why no universal technique of bone defects compensation satisfying the requirements of modern medicine has been developed so far. The currently developed approaches to solve this problem provide for the use of implants based on synthetic and biological tissues.

2 Extracellular Matrix

Autologous bone is usually considered as the most optimal material because it has adequate mechanical properties and contains the main components for bone regeneration (viable osteogenic cells, osteoinductive growth factors), which provide a high probability of its integration. However, this approach is applicable only for the repair of adult bone defects not more than 5–6 cm in length (Nandi et al. 2010). This is explained by the possibility of removing a very limited amount of autogenous tissues from the body without functional damage, the danger of prolonging the time of surgery, increasing the likelihood of complications in the form of shock, pain, and infection with additional trauma to the patient (Habibovic and De Groot 2007). Consideration should also be given to the possibility of the presence of pathology of the donor tissue section not identified by the surgeon at the time of resection, as well as the need to give the removed material the required anatomical shape (Schwartz et al. 2009). The use of own tissue after specific treatment (liquid nitrogen treatment, irradiation of a bone fragment in osteosarcoma, bone freezing, bone boiling) has found its application in various years in medicine (Abdel Rahman et al. 2009; Böhm et al. 1998, 2003). This approach involved removing from the patient a portion of bone affected by a neoplastic or infectious process. After physical treatment, tumor cells and microorganisms were killed, the destructured part of tissue was removed in a minimal manner and the bone was transplanted back to the patient. In this way, the following main goals were sought to be achieved: tumor removal and preservation of framework properties. However, since to preserve the mechanical properties of the bone it was necessary to apply influencing factors in a mild mode, in a large percentage of cases the bone did not have time to be completely desellized and disinfected, which entailed frequent development of sepsis. At the same time, the possibility of using foreign tissues taken from cadavers or removed organs significantly expands the possibilities of plastic and reconstructive surgery. This approach is used to obtain material of allogenic or xenogenic origin. However, this approach poses new problems for researchers: reduction of immunogenicity while preserving mechanical characteristics peculiar to the original bone, combined with the need to develop methods of sterilization and preservation of tissues. Tissue incompatibility is the main cause of difficulties arising in allogeneic and xenogeneic tissue transplants, which requires long-term use of immunosuppressive therapy. It is necessary that the processing of tissues of biological origin by physical or chemical methods along with preserving the integrity and durability of the implant provides also its functionality. To reduce immunogenicity, it is necessary not only to kill donor cells, but also to remove their components from the structureless extracellular matrix as much as possible. Such an approach to the creation of naturally occurring implants is currently recognized as one of the most promising. There are reports on the promising application of decellularized tissues for the reconstruction of heart valves, trachea, muscles, tendons, and abdominal wall (Badylak et al. 2012; D'Onofrio et al. 2011; Macchiarini et al. 2008). However, the greatest interest is in the application of this approach for the replacement of bone and cartilage defects (Kim et al. 2003; Benders et al. 2013). There are many methods of cell removal, divided into three main categories: chemical, enzymatic, and physical (Gilbert 2012). To this date, such methods used in practice are able to provide plastic material with osteoconductive and osteoinductive properties of varying degrees of expression, but not having sufficient strength to independently provide the supporting function. They are used mainly in dentistry, so they are produced in the form of granules, crumbs, chips, small blocks, and plates, and, therefore, the final product does not have anatomical features peculiar to bone, is not able to fulfill the supporting function, and cannot be used for the replacement of significant area defects.

Previously we developed a method of obtaining deimmunized extracellular scaffold by chemical treatment of cadaver bone material (Anisimova et al. 2013). For this purpose, the bones were cleaned from soft tissues and bone marrow remnants. When the thickness of the bone wall was more than 5 mm, it was perforated. The bones were then treated with a solution based on a mixture of sodium chlorite and sodium perchlorate, which destroyed cells and promoted the removal of their remnants from the extracellular bone matrix. The bone was completely immersed in the prepared solution and incubated in the dark for 1 to 4 months depending on the size and thickness of the bone wall. Then the prepared matrix was repeatedly washed with sterile 0.9% sodium chloride solution. The tests

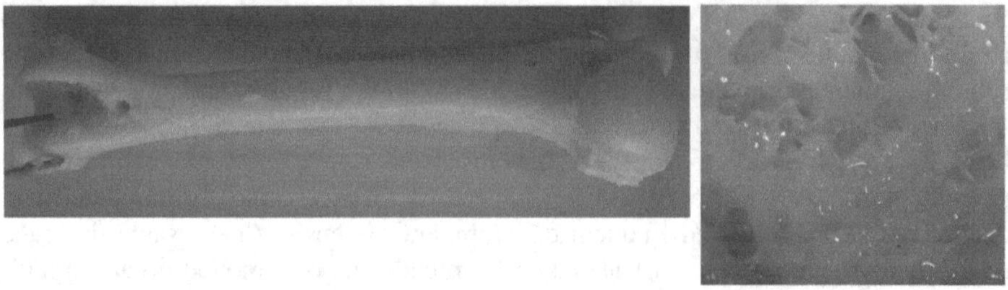

a b

Fig. 1 Morphology of the extracellular matrix with preservation of the configuration (**a**) and internal structure (**b**) of the original bone

performed by the researchers showed that the strength properties of the obtained material did not reliably ($p > 0.05$) differ from the characteristics of the original bone preserving the morphological features and the configuration (Fig. 1).

To evaluate the reduction of immunogenicity of the obtained bone matrix, it was implanted subcutaneously into laboratory mice for 3 months. The study of the morphology of the implant itself and the adjacent tissue showed that there were no signs of the development of local or systemic rejection or inflammation reactions. This approach leaves the possibility of creating a bank of scaffolds of different genesis, sizes, and configurations. The introduction of a cellular component into a bioconstruction for the replacement of tissue defects is, according to a number of specialists, one of the necessary factors (D'Onofrio et al. 2011; Macchiarini et al. 2008). It can contribute to the protection of the matrix surface from humoral and cellular biodegradation factors, as well as accelerate its adaptation in the recipient's body. Multipotent mesenchymal stromal cells (MMSC) are currently considered one of the most promising types of autologous material for cell therapy and tissue engineering (Ricchetti et al. 2012). Their use in bioimplants is intended to reduce the formation of granulations in the area of anastomoses and promote epithelialization and revascularization of the graft.

This approach was tested in organ-preserving surgeries for the treatment of dogs diagnosed with appendicular sarcoma (Kornyushenkov et al. 2023). It is known that osteosarcoma is the most common primary tumor of malignant bone tissue neoplasms in dogs, accounting for about 80-85%. Kornyushenkov E. et al. published the data of a study in which 25 dogs were treated with combined treatment of appendicular osteosarcoma, including chemotherapy with cisplatin (60-70 mg/m2, intravenous, dropwise, at intervals of 14–21 days, up to 4 cycles in total) and wide segmental resection of the affected bone with replacement of the defect with an allogeneic implant populated with cell culture of autologous bone marrow. The authors evaluated the efficacy of this technology by assessing overall survival, progression-free survival, and local recurrence rate in the group. The median overall survival in the group of animals with implants was 321 days, and the median progression-free survival was 222 days. In the course of the study 4 cases of local recurrences (16, 6%) were diagnosed, of which 2 diagnoses were confirmed by morphologic methods and 2 were established by clinical and radiologic data. At the same time, according to the literature data given by the authors, the average survival time of dogs with the diagnosis of appendicular osteosarcoma after amputation without specialized therapy, in the absence of radiologically detected metastases at the time of surgery, is 4 months. According to the results of the study, the authors concluded that the use of scaffold from extracellular allogeneic matrix populated with autologous MSCs contributed to the improvement of the quality of life of diseased animals and increased the median survival rate.

A similar approach was proposed to use for the development of an implant for the replacement of dilated segmental defects of the trachea and bronchi. It is known that in the development of tracheal stenosis caused by malignant neoplasms, infectious diseases, postoperative complications, or trauma, there is a need for resection of significant parts of the organ. In some cases it is impossible to form a primary anastomosis and it is necessary to replace the defect with a graft. To solve this problem, attempts have been made to replace tracheal defects with autologous tissues such as periosteum, small intestine, muscle, esophagus, bronchial, and aortic tissues. However, these methods were generally ineffective because they did not allow the formation of a complete tracheal skeleton. In addition, these grafts were further replaced by connective tissue blocking the air-conducting pathways (Grillo 2002). There have been attempts to use allografts containing epithelium and cartilage rings of the donor to replace tracheal defects (Sykes 2010). However, in this case, as well as in the majority of similar cases, rejection of the transplanted tissues was observed after discontinuation of immunosuppressive therapy, as the targets for the development of this process remained. To prevent allograft rejection, it is necessary to carry out long-term nonspecific immunosuppressive therapy causing a number of negative side effects. To obtain a non-immunogenic matrix, it was proposed to subject donor organs to chemical treatment. P. Macchiarini et al. incubated a trachea sample in distilled water for 72 h to reduce immunogenicity and remove molecules of the major histocompatibility complex MHC I and II classes, then performed desellitization by incubating the trachea in a mixture of 4% sodium deoxycholate solution and 2000 units of deoxyribonuclease in 1 mM/L sodium chloride, a total of 25 cycles for 6 weeks (Macchiarini et al. 2008). Subsequently, the obtained matrix was populated with autologous chondrocytes generated from bone marrow stem cells and epithelial cells of the mucous membrane of the recipient's airways. The main bronchus bioimplant was transplanted into the patient. However, attempts to routinely use this approach to fill large tracheal defects failed due to the development of implant matrix failure and adverse complications in the form of inflammation. We had experience in developing an extracellular tracheal matrix populated with patient cells (Kisilevskiĭ et al. 2012). After removal of fat and connective tissue, the trachea/bronchi sample was washed with distilled water, incubated for 10–14 days in 5–10% solution of chlorine oxidant, and finally washed with physiological solution. Stem mesenchymal CD271+ cells were isolated from the recipient's bone marrow by immunomagnetic separation and a culture of the recipient's mesenchymal cells was generated. The sterile tracheobronchial matrix was coated by the blood serum protein and the suspension of the recipient's epithelial and mesenchymal cells; the

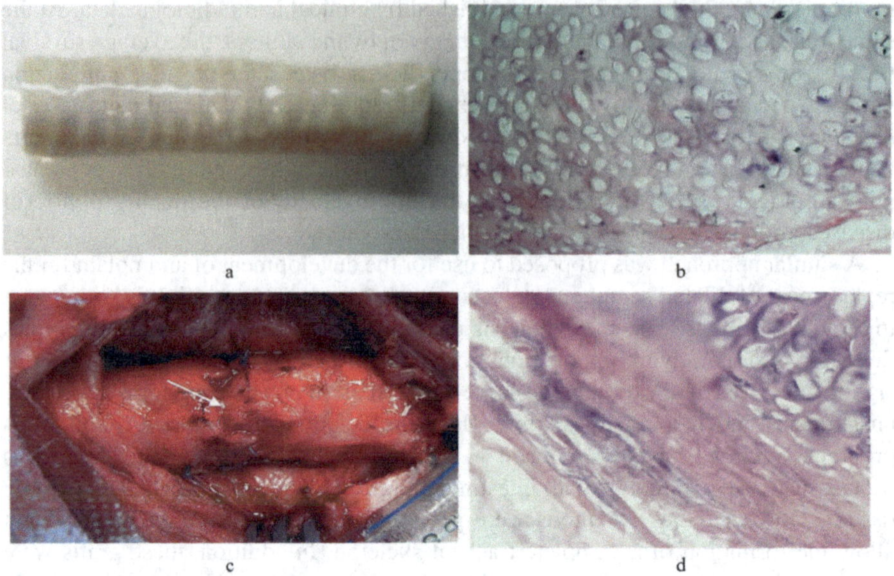

Fig. 2 Extracellular matrix of dog trachea (**a**) containing the cartilaginous half-rings without donor's cells before surgery (**b**) (Kisilevskiĭ et al. 2012) and after 3 weeks of implantation into the defect of a dog's trachea (the arrow shows the degraded matrix in the reconstructed area) (**c**) with the signs of degradation of the cartilage (**d**)

obtained product was incubated in growth medium until implantation. The scaffold thus obtained retained the mechanical properties, configuration, and morphology of the original organ. Unfortunately, implantation of such a cell-populated matrix into the defect of dog's trachea demonstrated fairly rapid (within 2–3 weeks) degradation of the cartilaginous half-rings, which led to partial loss of structure and reduction of the internal diameter and length of the implant, with the subsequent development of respiratory insufficiency (Fig. 2). Based on this obtained experience, in our opinion, the use of artificial scaffolds based on alloys or polymers seems more promising for the routine clinical practice.

3 Bioimplants Based on Synthetic and Natural Polymers

In case of damage of bones, cartilage, or soft tissues due to the development of cancer or tissue resection, the need arises for reconstruction of tissue and organ areas. In cases where the body's own regenerative abilities are insufficient or when reconstruction of extended tissue defects, there may be a need to install implants. Recently, bioimplants based on synthetic or natural polymers have become particularly important, which is associated with the high variability of their mechanical properties, which allow them to imitate the biomechanics of different native tissues (Zou et al. 2019), as well as with the presence of different functional properties and high manufacturability. The high manufacturability allows the use of different technologies for producing implants: molding, subtractive, and additive technologies.

Polymer implants for bone reconstruction. When reconstructing bones, important requirements for materials are: imitation of the architecture of bone tissue (cortical and spongy layer), individualization of shape, correspondence of mechanical properties to native tissues, the possibility of intraoperative modeling, induction of specific cellular reactions, osseointegration, and bioactivity. Polymer materials are used to replace defects in both tubular bones (e.g., limb bones) and flat bones (e.g., pelvis, calvarium, ribs).

Both bioinert and bioactive polymeric materials are used for bone tissue reconstruction. Bioinert materials based on synthetic polymers are usually used for the reconstruction of extended bone defects after resection (Maksimkin et al. 2017). In this case, bioinertness and bioresistance are necessary for long-term trouble-free functioning of the implant in the patient's body without changing the structure (microstructure and geometry) and properties (mechanical, physical-mechanical, biological, etc.) during the entire period of implantation. In orthopedics, ultra-high molecular weight polyethylene (UHMWPE), HDPE, and PTFE are used (Senatov et al. 2020). Polysulfone is used as fastening plates, pins, and bolts. A number of studies have noted the use of polyetheretherketone (PEEK) (Chubrik et al. 2020; Senatov et al. 2019), which has an increased modulus of elasticity, close to the modulus of elasticity of bone. In order to increase mechanical strength and wear resistance, reinforcement of the polymer matrix with dispersed fillers and fibers is used. This is especially important when forming implants of loaded bones (Luo et al. 2014).

Bioactive materials are often used for small (<3 cm^3) or non-loaded bone defects reconstruction. Among bioactive polymers the most used in clinical practice are synthetic polymers polylactide (PLA), polyhydroxybutyrate (PHB), polycaprolactone (PCL), polyglycolide (PG), and natural hydrogels based on collagen, sodium alginate, chitosan, etc. (Senatov et al. 2017a, b; Bitar and Zakhem 2014; Chen et al. 2015; Nijhuis et al. 2019) with different fillers. Bioactive polymers, as a rule, not only help induce specific cellular reactions and osseointegration, but are also bioresorbable. Bioresorption, which can develop due to the influence of enzymes, hydrolysis and be enhanced due to the development of microcracks under mechanical stress, makes it difficult to predict the resorption time, and therefore the stability of properties. The resorption time is also affected by changes in pH level during inflammatory processes, and the influence of bacterial and cellular destruction. All this complicates the predictability of the behavior of implants under load, and therefore limits the potential size of repairable tissue defects. The rate of resorption will be influenced by the hydrophilicity of the surface, hygroscopicity of the material, access to the body's environment, chemical composition, degree of crystallinity, the presence of a connected pore system, the presence of load, etc. However, due to this entire complex system of factors, it is also possible to adjust the rate of resorption for individual cases.

A separate potentially interesting direction is the creation of "self-aligning" implants based on polymer materials with shape memory, which can be installed minimally invasively with subsequent opening and filling of the cavity inside the body under the influence of body temperature, humidity, radiation, etc. However, the use of such materials is greatly limited by the difficulty of reducing activation temperature of the polymer shape memory to body temperature while maintaining biomechanical characteristics (Senatov et al. 2017a, b).

Polymer implants for reconstructive surgery of cartilage tissue. Cartilage tissue has significantly greater restrictions on regeneration compared to bone. In this regard, if there is significant damage to the cartilage or tissue resection, it may be necessary to install implants, including those combined with bone implants in the area of the epiphysis of the bone. The most important characteristics of the material for cartilage implants are the correspondence of the elastic modulus to native cartilage and wear resistance. In particular, physicomechanical and tribological characteristics are important in the case of hyaline cartilage reconstruction (Senatov et al. 2015). The elastic modulus and compressive strength of cartilage are 0.2–0.3 GPa and 0.01–3 MPa, while the Young's modulus and compressive strength of cortical bone are 15–20 GPa and 100–200 MPa, respectively (Tran et al. 2020). This must be taken into account when forming hybrid implants from dissimilar polymer materials.

Among bioinert polymeric materials, the most commonly used is ultra-high molecular weight polyethylene (UHMWPE). Its use is justified in the reconstruction of large areas of hyaline cartilage or in total joint replacement, since UHMWPE has increased impact strength (more than 80 kJ/m2 in the Charpy notch test), a low coefficient of friction (from 0.01 to 0.3) and good wear resistance in cross-linked state (Kurtz 2016). However, in the case of small cartilage defects, when a regenerative approach is still possible, the use of hydrogels in combination with a cellular component is promising.

Among natural polymer hydrogels, various articles describe the use of hyaluronic acid, gelatin, alginate, collagen, chitosan, silk fibroin, chondroitin sulfate, and dextran. Among the synthetic polymers, the most used are poly(ethylene glycol), poly(vinyl alcohol), poly(α-hydroxyether), poly(N-isopropylacrylamide), and polypeptide (Tran et al. 2020).

However, due to the low mechanical strength of hydrogels and their fluidity under load, only injecting hydrogels or hydrogels with cells is possible as a short-term therapeutic procedure. In the case of a long-term regenerative approach, ensuring a gradual release of drugs and uniform distribution of the cellular component, it is necessary to use polymer scaffolds in the pores of which the hydrogel and cellular components are distributed (Yang et al. 2020; Li et al. 2014, 2020). The most commonly used are polylactide and its copolymers. The requirements for such scaffolds in these cases are similar to bone implants. However, despite the above advantages of polymer scaffolds, it should be recognized that at present, mainly different alloys are used as the basis of products for orthopedics.

4 Stable Bioimplants Based on Compact Scaffolds Made of Titanium Alloys

Titanium alloys have played a crucial role in medical applications for over six decades. They have been extensively utilized in the fabrication of various medical devices, including artificial heart valves, blood vessel stents, endoprostheses for bones and joints (such as shoulder, knee, hip, and elbow), ear reconstruction, facial surgery, and dental implants. In the initial phase of development, first-generation materials like commercially pure titanium or Ti64 alloys predominantly consisted of the α-Ti phase or a combination of α and β phases. However, a drawback was identified as implants made from these materials required replacement within 10–15 years due to degradation and loss of contact with the bone. Addressing these concerns, second-generation materials, particularly β-titanium alloys, have emerged. These alloys mitigate the adverse effects caused by the release of aluminum and vanadium ions during gradual corrosion. Moreover, their elastic modulus closely aligns with that of living bone, distinguishing them from the earlier α and α + β alloys. The ongoing advancements in the field focus on enhancing the mechanical strength, fatigue resistance, corrosion resistance, and biocompatibility of β-titanium alloys. Innovative production methods and thermo-mechanical processing techniques, such as additive technologies and severe plastic deformation, are gaining prominence. A notable development is the substitution of expensive components like tantalum, zirconium, or niobium with more cost-effective alternatives such as chromium and manganese. This substitution trend is rapidly progressing, resulting in titanium implants exhibiting properties that increasingly resemble those of human bone, thereby extending their service life. In summary, the evolution from first-generation to second-generation titanium alloys, coupled with ongoing research and development, is steadily advancing the field of medical implants. The continuous refinement of alloy compositions and manufacturing techniques holds promise for further improving the performance, longevity, and biocompatibility of titanium implants in medical applications.

Advantages of Titanium Alloys In the current landscape of surgical implant development, metal alloys such as chromium-nickel stainless steels (like 316LSS), cobalt-chromium alloys, and various titanium alloys are commonly employed (Kolachev and Lyasotskaya 2003; Egorova et al. 2003; Fishgoit et al. 1990). Nevertheless, issues have arisen with implants made from stainless steel and cobalt-chromium alloys, as elements like nickel, cobalt, and chromium are gradually released due to corrosion in human body fluids, resulting in potential toxic effects (Okazaki and Gotoh 2005). Moreover, both chromium-nickel stainless steel and chromium-cobalt alloys exhibit a significantly higher modulus of elasticity compared to bone. This disparity leads to an inadequate transfer of mechanical stress from the prosthesis to the surrounding human or animal bones. Consequently, bone resorption and the detachment of the implant from skeletal bones may occur several years after the operation. Fatigue failure, particularly evident in prostheses like hip joint implants subjected to numerous load and unload cycles over many years, poses a significant challenge (Teoh 2000). Presently, titanium-based alloys are widely acknowledged as superior materials for prosthetics in clinical practice. This recognition is attributed to the exceptional combination of properties inherent to titanium and its alloys. These properties include high strength, low density (resulting in high specific strength), remarkable corrosion resistance, inertness to the biological environment (i.e., tissues surrounding the implant), enhanced biocompatibility, low elastic modulus, and a remarkable ability to integrate with bones and other tissues (Fishgoit et al. 1990; Sehitoglu et al. 2001). For instance, the modulus of elasticity of titanium alloys ranges from 110 to 55 GPa, a notable contrast to the 210 GPa exhibited by chromium-nickel stainless steels and the 240 GPa seen in chromium-cobalt alloys. This distinct property underscores the attractiveness of titanium alloys in the realm of surgical implants.

The initial exploration of titanium's utility in crafting bone prostheses dates back to the late 1930s. During this period, it was observed that titanium proved effective in replacing femur bones in cats, alongside alternative materials like stainless steel or vitallium—a cobalt, chromium, and molybdenum alloy. In contemporary applications, commercial-grade titanium and the Ti64 alloy (also known as Ti–6Al–4V ELI) are predominant choices for implant manufacturing. Despite Ti64's original development for aviation purposes, its elevated corrosion resistance and biocompatibility have secured a pivotal role in the biomedical industry. Beyond implant production, titanium alloys find extensive use in diverse medical products, including wheelchairs and removable limb prostheses. The breadth of applications for titanium alloys in medicine is truly remarkable. These alloys play crucial roles in dental implants, endoprostheses for facial surgery, as well as prosthetics for hip joints, knees, shoulder joints, spine, elbow joints, and wrists. Additionally, they contribute to osteosynthesis elements for bone fixation, such as pins, screws, and plates, and serve in the manufacturing of housings for pacemakers and artificial heart valves. Titanium alloys are also integral in producing surgical instruments and components of high-speed centrifuges for blood component separation (Maehara et al. 2002; Akahori et al. 2005). While commercially pure titanium and its alloys, like Ti64, have garnered acclaim for their high corrosion resistance and biocompatibility, concerns arise regarding the long-term use of implants and prostheses made from these materials due to the gradual release of aluminum and vanadium ions. Notably, research indicates that the release of aluminum and vanadium ions from the Ti64 alloy could lead to potential health issues, including the development of conditions such as Alzheimer's disease, neuropathy, and osteomalacia—a systemic disease linked to inadequate mineralization of bone tissue, resulting in bone softening (Nag et al. 2005). Furthermore, vanadium poses a significant toxicity risk in both its elemental state and as V_2O_5 oxide, a compound present on the surface of products fabricated from the Ti64 alloy (Eisenbarth et al. 2004). It is crucial to highlight that titanium exhibits low shear strength, rendering it less suitable for the manufacturing of screws, plates, and similar fixation components for osteosynthesis. Additionally, products made of titanium are prone to rapid wear when subjected to friction against each other or other metal parts.

The utilization of titanium alloys with a high coefficient of friction can lead to the generation of wear debris—small metal particles or filings. This, in turn, triggers an inflammatory reaction, causing pain and implant loosening due to osteolysis. The enumerated drawbacks of first-generation materials have constrained the service life of implants to a mere 10–15 years. This limitation prompted biomedical material developers to embark on creating novel alloys for prosthetics that closely mirror the properties of human bone. Consequently, low-modulus β-titanium alloys have been innovated, incorporating only alloying additives compatible with the human body and boasting an elastic modulus in close proximity to that of bone.

The phase composition of titanium alloys plays a pivotal role in determining their mechanical properties, wear resistance, and corrosion resistance. Titanium alloys offer significant appeal in this regard, as a diverse range of microstructures can be achieved by altering the alloy composition and engaging in thermo-mechanical processing. Titanium exhibits two allotropic modifications: α-titanium, characterized by a close-packed hexagonal structure, exists at low temperatures, while above 883 °C, β-titanium, with a body-centered cubic structure, is in equilibrium. The temperature at which the transformation from α to β occurs in titanium alloys varies depending on the alloying elements. Elements that stabilize α-titanium, such as aluminum, oxygen, and nitrogen, are referred to as alpha stabilizers. The inclusion of these elements raises the β-transus temperature, marking the transition from the α + β region to the β region in the phase diagram. Conversely, elements that stabilize the β-phase, such as vanadium, molybdenum, niobium, iron, and chromium, are termed β-stabilizers. Their addition to titanium lowers the β-transus temperature, allowing the β-phase to persist at room temperature in alloys with rapid cooling. Titanium alloys are categorized into three main classes based on their phase content: α, α + β, and β. Apart from the α and β phases, there is an additional high-pressure ω phase in titanium. This ω phase can manifest as a metastable phase even under small deformations in titanium alloys and endure as a metastable phase at atmospheric pressure and temperatures up to 550 °C, close to room temperature. The formation of the ω phase is particularly pronounced under conditions of substantial shear strains and high pressure (Kilmametov et al. 2018; Kriegel et al. 2019).

Transition from α and α + β to β Titanium Alloys The Ti64 alloy remains the predominant titanium biomedical alloy, commonly supplied in the α + β annealed state. Regrettably, the use of α + β titanium alloys with a high elastic modulus often results in bone resorption at the prosthesis interface, destabilizing the implant consolidation area and compromising its fixation to the bone. Hence, there is a notable interest in single-phase alloys characterized by a low elastic modulus and a β-microstructure, achievable through rapid cooling from elevated temperatures. Theoretical predictions suggest that neodymium, zirconium, molybdenum, and tantalum are optimal alloying elements, effectively reducing the elastic modulus of β-titanium without compromising the alloy's strength (Niinomi et al. 2012). Studies have further demonstrated that minor additions of these metals to titanium contribute to a decreased elastic modulus. However, an increase in the concentration of these alloying elements can elevate the elastic modulus due to the formation of the ω-phase and the release of α-phase particles during aging (Sakaguchi et al. 2005). Crucially, these alloying elements exhibit low toxicity, enhancing their appeal for implant manufacturing. In line with these considerations, material scientists have successfully developed a range of biomedical titanium alloys incorporating titanium, niobium, tantalum, and zirconium. Notable examples include thoroughly studied alloys like Ti–29Nb–13Ta–4.6Zr and Ti–35Nb–7Zr–5Ta (Tang et al. 2000).

Features of the Multicomponent β-Titanium Alloys Characteristics of recently developed multicomponent β-titanium alloys are noteworthy, with examples including Ti–Mo–6Zr–2Fe (TMZF), Ti–15Mo–5Zr–Al, Ti–15Mo–3Nb–3O, TIMETAL 21SRx, and Ti–13Nb–13Zr (Mishra et al. 1993). In the realm of biocompatible titanium alloys, the repertoire of alloying elements has expanded to encompass molybdenum, tin, and hafnium, in addition to the traditional niobium, tantalum, and zirconium (Morinaga et al. 1988). Notably, there has been a recent trend toward incorporating cost-effective alloying elements like chromium and manganese to mitigate the expenses associated with medical titanium alloys (Morinaga et al. 1988). Ongoing and robust research is actively exploring the realm of β-titanium alloys, investigating the intricate interplay of alloying elements, machining parameters, and heat treatment protocols on phase transformations, microstructure development, elastic modulus, and deformation behavior of the alloys. The selection of the optimal chemical composition for titanium alloys is not confined to experimental approaches but is also informed by theoretical methods such as the molecular orbital method or ab initio calculations (Morinaga et al. 1988). For instance, the Ti-29Nb-13Ta-4.6Zr alloy, commonly referred to as TNTZ, emerged through the application of the d-electron concentration alloy design method (Kuroda et al. 1998). A primary objective of these extensive studies is to formulate biomedical alloys possessing the requisite mechanical properties for sustained utilization as implants and bone prostheses over an extended duration.

Following this, β-titanium alloys characterized by a low and adjustable Young's modulus, such as Ti-12Cr and Ti-11Cr-0.2O (oxygen), have been introduced. These alloys find specific applications in the manufacturing of rods utilized for securing spinal elements (Liu et al. 2014). Additionally, β-titanium alloys featuring a low Young's modulus and elevated zirconium content, such as Ti-30Zr-7Mo, Ti-30Zr-5Cr, and Ti-30Zr-3Cr-3Mo, have been developed for the production of removable implants (Zhao et al. 2011a, b, c). Notably, titanium alloys with a zirconium content surpassing 25 wt. % hinder the formation of calcium phosphate on the surface. This implies a reduced adhesion of such alloys to bone, facilitating the removal of temporary titanium implants after achieving bone fusion and rendering them unnecessary (e.g., in fixing facial bone fragments). Various other titanium-zirconium alloys, including Ti-Zr-Nb, Ti-Zr-Nb-Ta, and Ti-Zr-Al-V, serve as temporary implants (Yang and Zhang 2005). The Young's moduli of β-titanium alloys like Ti-30Zr-7Mo, Ti-30Zr-3Cr-3Mo, and Ti-30Zr-3Cr-3Mo can be adjusted within broad ranges. These alloys were primarily developed for application as rods in spinal surgery.

The aforementioned low Young's modulus β-titanium alloys employed in the medical field (excluding titanium-chromium alloys) incorporate substantial quantities of costly alloying elements such as niobium, tantalum, molybdenum, and zirconium. Consequently, there arose a necessity to devise titanium alloys with a low Young's modulus that also integrate cost-effective alloying additives. In response to this demand, alloys such as Ti-Mn, Ti-Mn-Fe, Ti-Mn-Mo, and Ti-Mn-Al were developed. Additionally, budget-friendly alternatives encompass Ti-10Cr-Al, Ti-Cr-Al, Ti-Sn-Cr, Ti-Cr-Sn-Zr, and Ti-12Cr (Hieda et al. 2013; Santos et al. 2017; Nakai et al. 2011). These alloys feature elevated concentrations of economically viable components like manganese, chromium, and tin. A recent breakthrough involves the development of a method for fabricating gradient implants with varying chromium concentrations, allowing for the adjustment of mechanical properties. This groundbreaking technique utilizes additive technologies, specifically layer-by-layer laser fusion (Thomas et al. 2020).

Derived from multicomponent titanium alloys like Ti–Nb–Ta–Zr–Mo and Co–Cr–Mo alloys, high-entropy biocompatible alloys have been innovatively formulated (Nagase et al. 2020. High-entropy alloys, characterized by the absence of a primary component, exhibit comparable concentrations of various metals. These alloys effectively address the constraints of conventional metallic biomaterials by concurrently enhancing mechanical hardness and biocompatibility. In comparison to commercial-grade titanium, these compositions demonstrate superior biocompatibility, making them well-suited for applications as diverse orthopedic implants with a range of functionalities (Nagase et al. 2020).

Typically, β-titanium alloys undergo annealing in the β region to create a solid solution based on the β phase, followed by aging to decompose metastable phases and achieve heightened strength. Appropriate heat treatment can yield various structures in β-titanium alloys, with particular emphasis on the appealing properties of the equiaxed grain structure, as opposed to the lamellar structure, in titanium alloys. Research has revealed that the equiaxed structure exhibits the most favorable combination of mechanical properties in $\alpha + \beta$ alloys. It is noteworthy that thermo-mechanical processing of biomedical titanium alloys has not been a focal point for researchers for an extended period. The initial investigation into the impact of thermo-mechanical treatment on the formation of an equiaxial structure in the Ti–13Nb–13Zr alloy was conducted in 2001 (Geetha et al. 2001). In this study, the authors also explored the formation of an equiaxed grain structure in two other β-Ti-based alloys, namely Ti–13Nb–20Zr and Ti–20Nb–20Zr. By carefully selecting an appropriate "window" for the heat treatment of these alloys, specifically Ti–13Nb–20Zr and Ti–20Nb–20Zr, small equiaxed grains were achieved. Conversely, under identical conditions, the Ti–13Nb–13Zr alloy exhibited a mixture of large equiaxed and elongated grains. The inclusion of niobium in these alloys facilitated processing at low temperatures, resulting in the formation of a structure comprising small equiaxed grains (Geetha et al. 2001). It's crucial to note that the concentrations of alloying elements were capped at 20 wt. % to prevent the formation of the ω-phase, which could otherwise elevate the strength and elastic modulus of the alloy.

The elastic modulus of β-titanium alloys is contingent upon the quantity of β-phase within the microstructure. The aging process in β-titanium alloys results in heightened hardness and elastic modulus due to the release of small α-phase particles. However, the presence of these small α-phase grains does not consistently translate to an increase in strength and elastic modulus. These properties hinge on both the origin of the α-phase and other microstructural parameters. A notable example is observed in the aging of the Ti–34Nb–9Zr–8Ta (TNZT) alloy, where the aging process correlates with a reduction in both strength and elastic modulus. This phenomenon has been attributed to the dissolution of the ordered B2 phase (Nag et al. 2005). It is noteworthy that, following homogenization, the B2 phase exhibits higher hardness compared to its state after aging.

In contrast to the TNZT alloy, the Ti–29Nb–13Ta–4.6Zr alloy exhibits an augmentation in both strength and elastic modulus with aging. This enhancement results from the precipitation of small α-phase particles emerging from the ω-phase within the β-matrix. Notably, the Ti-15-Mo alloy presents an intriguing behavior whereby strength decreases while the elastic modulus increases (Nag et al. 2005). The reduction in strength in this alloy is attributed to the absence of nanometer-sized particles of ω-phase precipitates during aging, while the elevation in the elastic modulus is ascribed to the substantial volume fraction of small α-phase particles.

Biocompatibility In Vivo In vivo testing of a femoral head endoprosthesis crafted from the TNTZ alloy was conducted on Suffolk sheep (Hattori et al. 2009). The endoprosthesis was implanted by press-fitting it into the remaining femur of the experimental animal. Unfortunately, the animal succumbed to traumatic bleeding and intestinal obstruction three years after the implantation, leading to its demise. During the necropsy of the animal, the endoprosthesis was removed, subsequently dissected to examine its composition, and the concentration of metal elements in the bone surrounding the prosthesis was measured. Additionally, the concentrations of titanium alloy alloying elements in the liver, kidneys, and soft tissues of the animal were also assessed.

X-ray images of the prosthesis within the femur, as well as cross-sections of the femur around the midsection of the prosthesis, revealed congruence and secure fixation of the prosthesis in the bone, indicating the success of the endoprosthetic procedure. Metal element concentrations were measured in the liver, kidneys, acetabulum-forming bone tissue, and the distal femoral cortex. Except for titanium and zirconium, present in the experimental animal's food, no other foreign metal elements were detected in the sheep's liver or kidneys. Niobium and tantalum were identified in the inner cortical region of the femur. It is hypothesized that the release of metal ions primarily occurred in the interface between the bone of the experimental animal and the prosthesis. Consequently, prosthetics with the experimental product did not lead to the accumulation of its metal elements in the liver and kidneys, preserving the structural integrity of these organs. The results from these in vivo experiments affirm the biocompatibility of the rod made from the TNTZ alloy with a low Young's modulus. Furthermore, excellent compatibility was also demonstrated in experiments involving the implantation of intramedullary rods and plates for the fixation of bone fragments in a tibia fracture model in Japanese white rabbits (Niinomi and Nakai 2011).

Optimal Surface Roughness of Titanium Alloys In the study documented in reference (Straumal et al. 2022), the influence of surface roughness on the adhesion of mouse MC3T3-pre-osteoblasts cells on cold-wrought Ti6Al4V alloy was thoroughly examined. The substrate surface was intentionally modified by creating an array of linear grooves with varying depths, achieved using abrasive SiC papers and diamond pastes. These abrasives featured a gradient in grain size, spanning from 68 μm (for 200 grit paper) to a fine 1 μm for the most refined diamond paste. The intriguing aspect of this research lies in the non-linear relationship between the relative fraction of adhered mouse MC3T3-pre-osteoblasts cells and abrasive grain size. At a grain size of 1 μm, the adhesion fraction measured approximately 0.35. This fraction progressively increased to 0.95 at a grain size of 7 μm, followed by a gradual decline to 0.55 for an abrasive grain size of 68 μm. Surprisingly, the surface ground with a grinding medium aligned with a grain size of approximately 10 μm exhibited the highest cell adhesion. Notably, this grain size closely matched the dimensions of the studied MC3T3-pre-osteoblasts cells, typically measuring around ~14 μm. This investigation underscores the potential of manipulating surface roughness to precisely control and customize the fraction of adhered cells, catering to diverse requirements in medical techniques. Such nuanced control over surface properties could pave the way for tailored cellular adhesion strategies in various biomedical applications.

Hence, in the realm of medical applications, titanium alloys primarily grounded in β-Ti have become the preferred substitute for first-generation alloys based on α-Ti or a combination of α and β phases, including commercially pure titanium or Ti64 alloys. Implants fashioned from first-generation materials occasionally necessitate replacement after a decade or more of use, as they may release aluminum or vanadium ions into the body. β-Titanium alloys, characterized by a lower elastic modulus compared to α and α + β alloys, closely align with the elastic modulus of living bone. The development of novel β-titanium alloys facilitates the enhancement of mechanical strength, fatigue resistance, corrosion resistance, and biocompatibility in implants. Emerging techniques in the production and thermo-mechanical processing of titanium alloys, such as additive technologies and severe plastic deformation, are gaining prominence. The substitution of costly alloy components (like tantalum, zirconium, or niobium) with more economical alternatives (such as chromium and manganese) has proven highly successful. Consequently, the properties of titanium implants are progressively converging with those of human or animal bone, contributing to a prolonged service life. The quest to create titanium alloys mirroring the properties of living tissue stands out as one of the most compelling and coveted challenges in contemporary science and healthcare.

5 Porous Bioactive Ti-Based Scaffolds by Additive Manufacturing

The review above testifies that the functional performance of Ti and Ti-based alloys makes them appear to be among the best biocompatible materials to develop permanent orthopedic implants. However, their orthopedic application is still limited by the level of stiffness—the Young's modulus (E) comprises about 100–140 GPa for popular two-phase Ti alloys, which far exceeds that value typical for bone tissues (0.5–20 GPa) (Zysset et al. 1999; Olszta et al. 2007). Moreover, there is a considerable scattering in elastic and strength properties of different bone tissues—from cancellous to cortical ones. For the latter case $E \sim 15–20$ GPa, while for the former it ranges from 0.1 to 2 GPa (Olszta et al. 2007; Bose et al. 2012). Similar trend is observed for compressive strength, which comprises 100–200 MPa and 2–20 MPa for cortical and cancellous bones, respectively (Olszta et al. 2007; Bose et al. 2012). Such scattering in the mechanical performance of the remodeled bones complicates reliable application of Ti-based materials in bone tissue engineering.

Mismatch in elastic properties between an implant and bone can entail highly undesired stress-shielding effect (Savio and Bagno 2022) which can result in osteoporosis and resorption or poor osseointegration followed by the implant failure under long-term operation (Kim et al. 2020). Even with the very recent progress with developing low-E β-type Ti alloys, the stiffness can hardly be reduced below 40–50 GPa, with the lowest achievable values reported to be about $E = 14$ GPa demonstrated by specific Ti-Nb-Zr alloys (Ma et al. 2013). However, as denoted in the previous chapter, these materials are at the intensive research stage, often contain expensive elements, still cannot fit full range for values of bone elastic moduli, and can hardly be certified and brought into healthcare markets in the near future.

Another effective approach to adjust stiffness of metallic materials is related to purposeful engineering of porous structures. As denoted in Fougere et al. (1995), pores can dramatically reduce Young's modulus of various metals with power function relationship to the reference value of a fully dense material. Introducing percolated network of pores with a regulated elementary unit size and internal geometry into certified biocompatible materials, such as Ti-6Al-4V, allows reducing E down to several or even tenths of a GPa (Timercan et al. 2023; Koju et al. 2022). Another major advantage of porous materials relates to their capability to be loaded with antibiotic or antitumor compounds allowing targeted drug delivery to provide local antimicrobial or chemotherapy (Lv et al. 2021; du Plessis et al. 2022). Besides, porous architecture of an implant can facilitate enhanced cell proliferation and differentiation of mesenchymal stem cells (MSCs) as well as promote better vascularization and osteointegration (du Plessis et al. 2022; Murr 2019). Thus, introduction of porous structures into Ti-based materials opens promising prospects of engineering bioactive implants/scaffolds to be applied in orthopedic oncology (Kiselevskiy et al. 2023).

Development of new metallurgical technologies such as additive manufacturing (AM) substantially levels up the opportunities to design and produce porous metallic materials. Such techniques as Laser or Electron Beam Powder Bed Fusion

(L/EB-PBF) are capable of highly precise prototyping of metallic specimens with pre-designed shape and sophisticated internal cellular topology hardly reproducible though conventional methods (Koju et al. 2022; Lv et al. 2021; du Plessis et al. 2022; Murr 2019; Kiselevskiy et al. 2023). Research in this field represents a burning topic for modern multidisciplinary area combining CAD, simulation, AM, physics, mechanics, chemistry, life sciences, and biomedical approaches (Koju et al. 2022; Lv et al. 2021; du Plessis et al. 2022; Murr 2019; Kiselevskiy et al. 2023). Numerous studies testify that pore design can tailor the mechanical performance of Ti alloys in a wide range. As mentioned above, stiffness of Ti-6Al-4V alloy can be radically reduced down, while the strength can be maintained at the reasonable level compatible with the fracture strength of bone allowing for successful tissue engineering, confirmed also by in-vivo tests (Taniguchi et al. 2016). CAD-based design of pore topology can also manage adjustable interconnection of internal cavities to keep a proper level of permeability, which is needed to improve osseointegration (Zhianmanesh et al. 2019) and reserve a capacity for the injected bioactive substances (Murr 2019).

A strategy to achieve a new generation of high-performance bioactive implants based on porous structures is presented in Fig. 3. As outlined in Kiselevskiy et al. (2023), it should cover several key activities:

- Computer-aided pore architecture guided by a feedback from AM fabrication of the designed products.
- Optimization of porous structures via virtual experiments to reveal desired pore geometry providing the best combination of mechanical parameters validated through experimental tests.

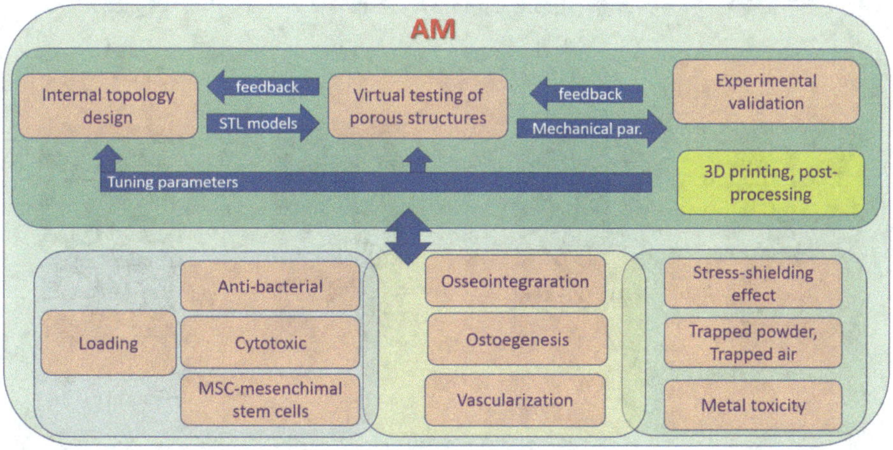

Fig. 3 A strategy of additive manufacturing (AM) for designing, manufacturing, and characterization of porous structures toward engineering advanced bioactive implants of a new generation

- Deliberate adjustment of AM procedure, printing, and post-processing parameters to ensure producing of high-quality defect-free fine structures matching the designed models.
- Careful examination of biomedical performance of the manufactured products to provide high levels of biocompatibility, cell proliferation, osseointegration, and vascularization as well as capacity for bearing bioactive compounds and their controllable release.

The CAD-assisted projecting of porous structures puts forward several different approaches, based on periodic structures consisting of elementary units composed by connected struts or triply periodic minimal surfaces (TPMS) calculated thanks to mathematical expressions as well as on bio-inspired stochastic or gradient pore distributions (du Plessis et al. 2022). Figure 4 represents different model examples of porous structures composing cylindrical specimens for compression tests as well as the corresponding L-PBF printed products.

Figure 4 indicates that AM enables coherent reproduction of variously designed porous structures different by pore geometry and pore dimensions numerously confirmed in the literature. However, even modern high-end AM equipment induces specific features into printed materials inherent to the L-PBF technology due to rapid melting and solidification processes of fine powders. AM products can be

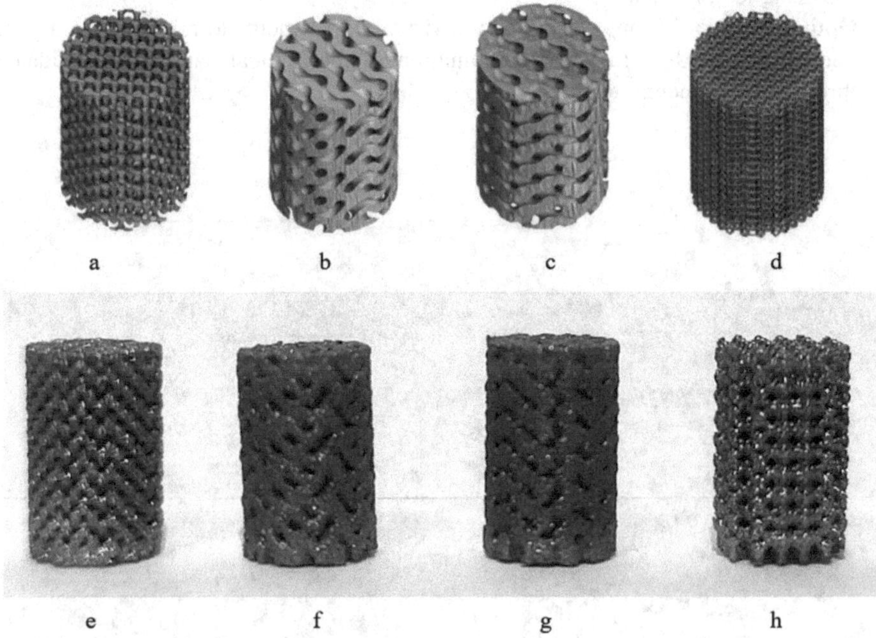

a b c d

e f g h

Fig. 4 Designed and printed specimens of Ti-6Al-4V alloy according to different designs (adopted from Kiselevskiy et al. 2023): TMPS-based Diamond (**a**, **e**), Gyroid Sheet (**b**, **f**) and Gyroid Skeletal (**c**, **g**) models; strut-based Octa model (**d**, **h**)

characterized by AM-induced voids, macro-stresses, unmelted particles, rough surfaces, and structural heterogeneity in different building directions. These features can result in a notable mismatch between the model and manufactures specimens; specific textures and defect configuration; internal imperfections such as voids and cracks. Additional difficulties arise in case of printing porous structures—AM resolution and powder size are often not enough to reproduce sophisticated internal topology with small unit wall dimensions; openwork configurations can exhibit critical heterogeneity accompanied with imperfections such as broken walls or sealed interconnectivity of cavities (du Plessis et al. 2022; Benedetti et al. 2021); a separate problem relates to residual powders trapped in the interiors of printed products (Khrapov et al. 2023). Despite the recent progress in the field, there is still a room to tune AM and post-processing procedures for reliable manufacturing porous Ti-based scaffolds.

The balance for the desired combination of properties often requires a reasonable trade-off between different properties. Increasing porosity allows significant reduction in elastic moduli of Ti alloys but being accompanied by a notable decrease in mechanical strength. Similar trend is observed in case of competing processes of cell colonization and vascularization (Barba et al. 2019). Despite tremendous activity in research carried out in this field, there are still many open questions on the way of implementing porous bioactive Ti scaffolds to the medical practice. Albeit optimization of mechanical behavior of porous materials is being successfully resolved through computer simulation (Timercan et al. 2023; Gryko et al. 2022), the biomedical performance of the developed structures is still not properly understood in terms of the optimal pore architecture.

Porous titanium L-PBF-produced mesh scaffolds provided a good survival and proliferation of osteoblasts in vitro and in vivo studies (Warnke et al. 2009). According to a number of dedicated studies, the minimal pore size is believed to be ranged from 50 to 100 μm to provide favorable bone ingrowth (Jones et al. 2009; Braem et al. 2014). However, some authors observed (Lee et al. 2016) better osteoinduction in PBF Ti implants with pore sizes exceeding 500 μm. At the same time, the other studies did not reveal a clear effect of a pore size ranging from 350 to 800 μm on osseointegration (Karageorgiou and Kaplan 2005; Wally et al. 2019).

Several studies report on better perfusion of body fluids and neoangiogenesis with changing pore dimensions from about 100 to 700 μm, while in vivo investigations of tissue ingrowth and neovascularization testify that a greater pore size facilitates the blood vessels growth (Barba et al. 2019). At the upper limit, an increase in porosity can entail abnormal growth of MSCs leading to undesired fibrosis instead of bone tissue neo-formation (Pilliar 1987). Up to now, the optimal geometric parameters of porous structures to ensure optimal biological performance of the AM scaffolds are still not identified. There are still many open questions on roughness of internal surfaces of porous AM structures and their interaction with bioactive coatings facilitating osteogenesis (Takemoto et al. 2005). The local drug delivery function of porous scaffolds can be highly demanded by orthopedic oncology (Kiselevskiy et al. 2023; Ma et al. 2021). The loaded compounds can feature cytostatic tumor inhibitors, growth stimulators for enhanced neoosteogenesis and vasculogenesis, immune and antimicrobial agents. This area is still needed in thorough systematic research including deliberate in-vivo studies. To sum up, the AM-driven development of bioactive porous Ti scaffolds appears to be an ambitious and challenging multidisciplinary task. Thoughtful solution of the facing problems with a special focus on biomedical performance of the new generation bioactive scaffolds would provide a sound pathway to their successful advancing to the clinic.

6 Scaffolds Based on Biodegradable Alloys

The development of biodegradable implants is relevant for osteosynthesis in orthopedics, as well as in oral and cranio-maxillo-facial surgery to eliminate the consequences of injuries, tumor processes, and hypoplasia for both adult patients and pediatric patients (Huang et al. 2024; Putra et al. 2020; Payr 1900; Lambotte 1932; Verbrugge 1934; McBride 1938; Virtanen 2011). Biodegradable implants are made from materials that dissolve and are absorbed by the body over time. This avoids the need to remove the worn-out implant in the future. Biodegradable implants are already actively used, for example, for bone reconstruction after fractures. They offer a number of benefits, including a reduced risk of infection, more natural healing processes of the injury, and reduced negative consequences for the patient. It is expected that in the coming years, the development of new technologies and materials will lead to a greater prevalence of biodegradable implants not only in orthopedics, but also in other areas. Such areas may include orthopedic oncology and creation of scaffolds for local delivery of chemo-immunological agents.

Currently, promising candidates for creating biodegradable implants are magnesium-, zinc-, and iron-based alloys, as well as polymers (Huang et al. 2024). Bioimplants based on these materials have good biocompatibility with the human body and are suitable for long-term stay in the patient's body. Ideally, these biomaterials should gradually decompose in vivo without harm to the human body. At the same time, metal biodegradable implants most often demonstrate higher mechanical characteristics compared to polymers (Putra et al. 2020). Thus, the latest advances in the design of Mg-, Fe-, and Zn-based biodegradable implants for orthopedic oncology and scaffolds for local delivery of chemo-immunological agents will be considered.

Historical background. One of the first research of the behavior of biodegradable metals was the study of magnesium as a medical material. It was performed in 1892 by the Austrian physician E. Payr, who conducted a comprehensive clinical trial of magnesium implants on rabbits and dogs (Payr 1900). A few years later, in 1906, Dr. A. Lambotte carried out the first clinical study on humans of fasteners for osteosynthesis developed by E. Payr (Lambotte 1932). Implantation of a magnesium plate resulted in the appearance of large subcutaneous gas cavities near the implants. This led to the need to remove the destroyed fragments of the plate on the eighth day. It was found that electrochemical interaction caused by the use of steel screws to fix the magnesium plate led to increased biodegradation of magnesium. Taking into account the obtained results, Magnesium Elektron Ltd. (British company) began the development of Mg-based alloys for orthopedic use in 1937. Clinical studies of pure magnesium, without steel screws, showed a more successful result (Verbrugge 1934). However, the high biodegradation rate still led to the accumulation of large amounts of hydrogen in the form of subcutaneous gas bubbles. This ultimately stopped research of magnesium as a material for biomedical purposes (McBride 1938). In addition, a new type of stainless steel was developed, which replaced magnesium alloys as materials for orthopedic implants. This led to the suspension of research in this area around the world for a long period.

At the turn of the twentieth and twenty-first centuries, scientists again became interested in bioresorbable alloys. The first work was carried out on magnesium alloys with aluminum and zinc (AZ series) and WE series alloys (in particular the WE43 alloy) due to their commercial availability (Virtanen 2011). Therefore, these alloys are currently among the most studied. In works carried out in the first decade of the 2000s, the effect of various alloying elements on the degradation rate and biocompatibility of magnesium alloys in vitro and in vivo was widely studied. It was shown that in addition to the AZ series alloys, magnesium alloys with rare earth metals, as well as alloys based on Mg-Ca, Mg-Zn-Ca, Mg-Zn-Mn, Mg-Ag, and Mg-Li are promising for medical application. However, despite the promising results, the question related to the rapid degradation of magnesium alloys and the accompanying hydrogen release process still remains open. That is why the views of many researchers have turned toward biodegradable materials that do not have this drawback.

At first, Fe-based alloys (in particular the Fe-Mn system) became such materials. Initially, Fe-based biomaterials were considered as materials for creating coronary stents (Hermawan et al. 2010a). In 2001 M. Peuster et al. conducted a study of corrodible iron stents ($> 99.8\%$ iron) by implanting them into the native descending aorta of New Zealand white rabbits. They concluded that these stents can be safely implanted without significant obstruction of the stented vessel (Peuster 2001). However, in vivo degradation rate of pure iron was too low (Kraus et al. 2014), and the mechanical properties of pure iron were not suitable for the manufacture of implants. Therefore, further research was aimed at studying the possibility of using Fe-based materials, including for osteoreconstructive medicine. One of these materials was Fe—Mn alloy, which had appropriate mechanical characteristics, good biocompatibility, and at the same time an increased degradation rate, although still insufficient and significantly lower in comparison with magnesium alloys (Hermawan et al. 2010c).

The "youngest" biodegradable materials are Zn and its alloys. The first mention of Zn-based alloys in the context of medical use was found in 2007 in an article written by Wang et al. (Wang et al. 2007). At the same time, Zn-based alloys were considered both as materials for creating coronary stents and as osteoreconstructive materials. Despite many in-depth and comprehensive studies conducted in recent decades, biodegradable metal materials are still being intensively researched. Currently, the subject of research includes both the development of new compositions and the determination of the effect of the manufacturing method and microstructure and surface modification of the alloys on its corrosion properties, especially under in vivo conditions. The promise of this area of research is confirmed by a large number of studies conducted by scientists from around the world.

Alloying is the main way to regulate the degradation rate of alloys. Additionally, the alloying elements should have a high level of biocompatibility. It is known that additives to pure magnesium such as Zn, Ca, Mn, Al, rare earth metals (REM), Ag, and others, which possess an acceptable level of biocompatibility, also significantly reduce its degradation rate (Tsakiris et al. 2021). Němec et al. showed that the addition of Zn to pure magnesium significantly improves not only its strength but also its corrosion resistance (Němec et al. 2017). Further study of the corrosion resistance of Mg-6%Zn and Mg-12%Zn alloys revealed the significantly high degradation rate of the latter due to the formation of a large amount of more corrosion-resistant $MgZn_2$ phase particles in the structure. The formation of a large amount of more (or less) resistant phase often leads to an increase in the degradation rate of magnesium alloys due to accelerated microgalvanic corrosion. In other studies, it has been shown that the optimal content of Ca in Mg-Ca alloys is in the range of 0.5–1.0 wt.%, while further increasing its content increases the biocorrosion rate of the alloy (Li et al. 2010). Investigation of the Mg-0.5%Ca-0.5%Zn alloy revealed an improvement in corrosion resistance compared to pure magnesium. However, an unevenness in the corrosion process due to the predominant location of Mg_2Ca and $Ca_2Mg_6Zn_3$ phase particles along the grain boundaries was observed (Školáková et al. 2020).

It is important to note that for iron-based alloys the corrosion process is, on the contrary, aimed at accelerating degradation. It is known that the addition of manganese to pure iron leads to its accelerated degradation (Hermawan et al. 2008; Hermawan et al. 2010b). Moreover, an increase in the manganese content in the alloy results in an increase in the degradation rate. It is also worth noting that Fe-Mn alloys with a manganese content higher than 25% (by weight) have non-magnetic properties, allowing for the potential use of MRI to observe the healing process of injuries (Youn et al. 2015). Additionally, Schinhammer et al. demonstrated that alloying 1% Pd into Fe-10%Mn alloys leads to the formation of dispersed intermetallics, which act as cathodic sites relative to the matrix, accelerating microgalvanic corrosion and further increasing the degradation rate (Schinhammer et al. 2010). It should be noted that these particles not only increase the rate of degradation, but also enhance the mechanical properties of the alloy. In a study (Caligari Conti et al. 2019), it was found that adding 2% and 5% of Ag to Fe-29%Mn and Fe-28%Mn alloys, and their subsequent pressing, respectively, can increase the corrosion current density by an average of 30%, indicating an increase in their degradation rate. In the case of the Fe-30%Mn-6%Si-1%Pd alloy, additions of silicon and palladium also lead to a decrease in the corrosion resistance of the alloy, manifested by a reduction in the corrosion potential (Feng et al. 2016). The subsequent deformation and thermomechanical processing, contributing to an increase in the density of defects in the crystalline structure and the precipitation of particles during aging, will further increase the rate of degradation. Therefore, in the case of iron-based alloys, one of the ways to increase the rate of degradation is to alloy them with elements that lead to the formation of more corrosion-resistant phases, the presence of which accelerates the degradation process (Kraus et al. 2014).

Another method of regulating corrosion rate is deformation processing. Properly selected deformation regimes allow both increasing and decreasing the degradation rate. In the case of magnesium alloys, it is promising to use deformation methods that allow obtaining an ultrafine-grained (UFG) structure in the alloy, for example, methods of severe plastic deformation (SPD). Among the most popular methods of severe plastic deformation (SPD), there are high-pressure torsion (HPT) (Zhilyaev and Langdon 2008) and equal channel angular pressing (ECAP) (Valiev and Langdon 2006). It has been previously shown that the application of HPT can lead to both an increase in the corrosion resistance of magnesium alloys (Gao et al. 2011) and a decrease in it (Lukyanova et al. 2017). The same situation has also been observed for the case of ECAP. Shahar et al. (2017) demonstrated in the example of the AZ31 alloy that ECAP and subsequent aging can lead not only to a decrease in degradation rate, but also to an increase. It was shown that an increase in temperature and aging time, which leads to particle coarsening and grain growth, deteriorates the corrosion resistance of the AZ31 alloy. Thus, by selecting appropriate deformation and/or subsequent aging conditions, it is possible to control the degradation rate to either accelerate or decelerate it depending on the goal of the developer. For iron-based biodegradable alloys, the goal is often to accelerate the corrosion process, whereas for magnesium-based alloys, both deceleration and acceleration may be desired. Increasing the degradation rate of magnesium alloys is necessary for consistently releasing a sufficient level of metal ions over an extended period or for maintaining a required concentration of a medicinal agent.

Biodegradable alloys for orthopedic oncology and for local delivery of chemo-immunoagents. There are several key characteristics that must meet materials for bioresorbable implants. Depending on the intended application the requirements for material properties may alter. In the case of bioresorbable orthopedic implants, the most important properties are biocompatibility, close to cortical bone mechanical characteristics and the ability to dissolve in physiological environments and to be absorbed by patient's body. In addition, implant materials should not suppress osteogenesis, but ideally promote it. In general, the requirements for orthopedic oncology implants are similar to those for orthopedic implants with one exception. The use of such implants is associated with partial bone resection for osteosarcoma or metastatic bone lesions in patients in advanced stages of cancer. In such cases, chemotherapy and radiation therapy can be prescribed immediately after diagnosis, but for severe metastatic bone lesions, reconstructive surgery is required in most cases. However, despite advances in cancer treatment and orthopedic surgery, patients who undergo reconstruction are still at risk of developing serious complications. This may include tumor recurrence or failed reconstruction. In such cases, postoperative radiation therapy or chemotherapy may be required after surgery. For more effective treatment, it is advisable to combine reconstructive surgery and therapy with antitumor drugs. Currently, a lot of research is aimed at creating implants that realize these two functions, ensuring the creation of a bone frame and the gradual supply of drugs to the implantation area. This can be achieved in different ways, for example, by doping the base metal with elements that exhibit cytotoxic activity toward tumor cells or by creating scaffolds containing an antitumor agent as part of the coating or directly in the implant body.

Local drug release systems based on bioresorbable metals have also attracted great interest in the last decade (Wu and Grainger 2006). Biodegradation of medical devices from bioresorbable metals provides a favorable environment that can allow drugs, bioactive materials, and therapeutic agents to be locally released at the implantation site. Compared with targeted drug delivery designs, the local drug-device release system allows to control the dose of the drug by regulating the degradation rate and reduce side effects on surrounding tissues not affected by the disease. The design of such systems varies from applying a special coating to the surface of the implant to loading porous frames made of biodegradable alloys uploaded by drugs. In most cases, drug release from bioresorbable metal implants occurs through drug diffusion within the coating or as a result of degradation of scaffold with gradual release of drug. Some studies have found that drugs are first released by diffusion within the carrier/coating and then continuously released due to degradation of the carrier/coating (Zhao et al. 2021). Based on numerous research studies dedicated to this topic, creating such products is a promising and potentially commercially viable task.

Currently, most research aimed at creating metal biodegradable implants that exhibit antitumor activity are focused on the study of magnesium alloys (Hsu et al. 2023). Qi et al. showed that a WE43 alloy implant coated with gelatin nanospheres uploaded by chitosan stimulated osteogenic activity (Qi et al. 2019). Peng et al. developed an implant based on a composite consisting of AZ31 magnesium alloy with a porous coating applied by plasma-electrolytic oxidation, that combines structural integrity and targeted drug release ability (Peng et al. 2017). Lee et al. created a medical device for local drug delivery with controlled corrosion rate based on pure magnesium, which effectively releases the drug within 21 days (Lee et al. 2016). These researches laid the foundation not only for the development of osteoreconstructive implants for orthopedic oncology, but also for products for local chemotherapy and the creation of an effective concentration of an antitumor agent directly in the tumor. Such products will make it possible to pre-treat unresectable and relatively chemo-resistant tumor nodes for subsequent surgical treatment, as well as to ensure the prevention of local relapse of cancer. In addition, studies conducted on magnesium alloys have made it possible to identify a number of metals with antitumor activity, for example, La, Y, Dy, Gd, Ag, Mn, etc. (Wu and Grainger 2006). It is interesting to note that extracts of Zn-containing Mg alloys inhibit cell proliferation by altering the cell cycle and inducing cell apoptosis via activation of the mitochondrial pathway (Wu et al. 2016). On the other hand, Elborolosy et al. showed that nanostructured biodegradable Fe-Mn-Cu, Fe-Mn-W, and Fe-Mn-Co alloys exhibited anticancer activity against the osteosarcoma MG-63 cell line (Elborolosy et al. 2023). The study noted a time-dependent selective cytotoxic effect on osteosarcoma cells rather than normal cell lines. This could be explained by the formation of Fe^{2+} and Fe^{3+} ions, as well as reactive oxygen species (ROS) and free radicals, which could have a cytotoxic effect on these cells. Thus, increased cell proliferation on normal cells and cytotoxic activity on tumor cells were shown. As a result, it can be concluded that these alloys are suitable for use in oncologic orthopedics for the reconstruction of bone defects after surgical removal of malignant tumors with a high recurrence rate. Thus, the above works suggest that the creation of scaffolds with antitumor activity based on Zn and Fe-Mn alloys is also a promising area of research.

Scaffolds based on Mg, Fe, and Zn alloys. Researchers from IMET RAS and N.N. Blokhin NMRCO are developing orthopedic implants with antitumor activity. By the end of 2023, the main studies were carried out on Mg-1%Zn-0.6%Ca, Mg-3.56%Y-2.20%Nd-0.47%Zr (Martynenko et al. 2020; Anisimova et al. 2020), Fe-Mn-C (Rybalchenko et al. 2022), Fe-Mn-Pd (Rybalchenko et al. 2023) alloys, and the alloys of the Zn-Mg system (Martynenko et al. 2023) (hereinafter, alloy compositions are presented in wt.%). It was shown that incubation of rotary swaged Mg-1%Zn-0.6%Ca alloy with the culture of K562 tumor cells led to a more noticeable increase in the level of dead and apoptotic cells in comparison with the effect obtained on MMSC, considered as a non-transformed cell model (Martynenko et al. 2020). At the same time, the alloy was as close as possible to the requirements for orthopedic implants in terms of strength (276 ± 6 MPa), ductility ($18.3 \pm 2.9\%$), and degradation rate (0.3–0.5 mm/year). It has also been shown that the contact with Mg-Y-Nd-Zr alloy reduces the viability of LNCaP human prostate carcinoma cells and MDA-MB-231 human breast adenocarcinoma cells (Anisimova et al. 2020). The choice of these cell lines is determined by the fact that these types of cancer often grow as metastases in bone. The cytotoxic effect of the Mg-Y-Nd-Zr alloy on tumor cells was accompanied by cell death associated with an increase in the apoptosis level (Fig. 5). The studies published in Anisimova et al. (2020) showed that incubation of tumor cells with an Mg-Y-Nd-Zr alloy was accompanied by a decrease in the release of oxygen radicals (ROS) by the cells. This may indicate that oxidative stress during incubation of tumor cells with the alloy was not the reason for the induction of apoptosis. In turn, it was found that incubation with the Mg-Y-Nd-Zr alloy led to a decrease in the Bcl-2 (+) cell concentration. That is, the probable reason for the increase in the level of apoptosis in tumor cells during incubation with the Mg-Y-Nd-Zr alloy is a decrease in the anti-apoptotic Bcl-2 protein expression (Fig. 6).

During research of the mechanical and functional properties of Fe-27Mn-C and Fe-36Mn-C alloys (Rybalchenko et al. 2022) in the coarse-grained and ultrafine-grained (UFG) states after ECAP, the proliferation of SKBR3 cells on the surface of these samples was additionally studied. The inhibition of the proliferative activity of SKBR3 cells on the surface of the Fe-36Mn-C alloy sample after ECAP was observed. The reason for this could be the high concentration of α-Mn on the surface of samples and its cytotoxic effect. UFG structure obtained by ECAP implies a high density of grain boundaries, and, accordingly, a more frequent appearance of them to the surface of the sample. As a result, it leads to a more active release of manganese into the medium.

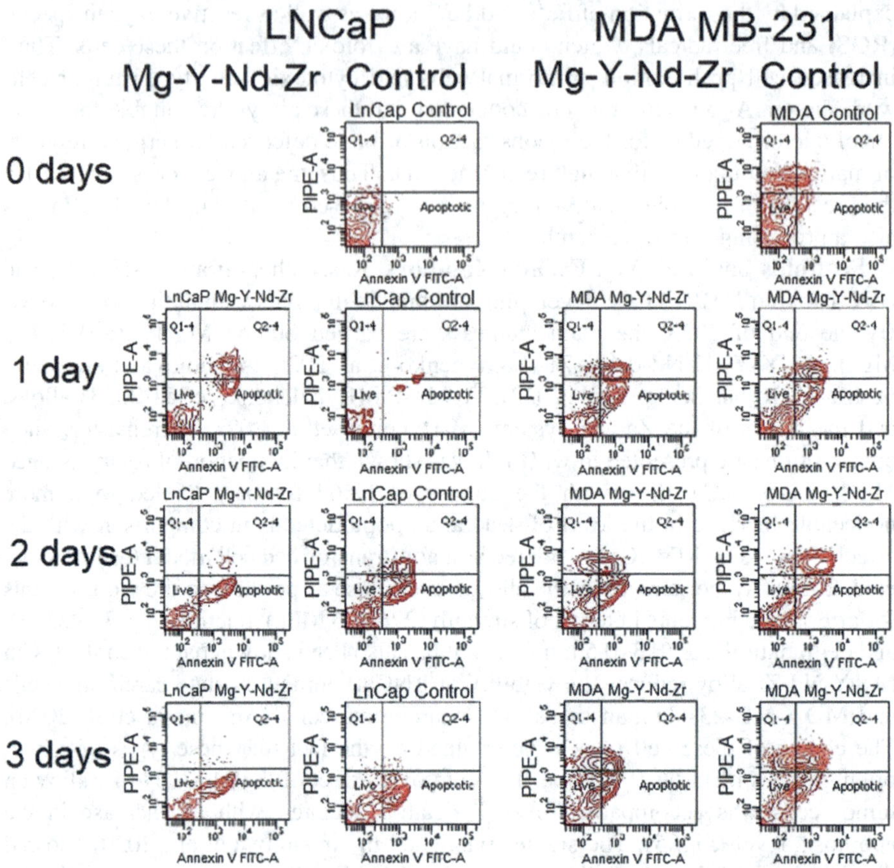

Fig. 5 Increase of Annexin V (+) tumor cells concentration after incubation with samples of Mg-3.56%Y-2.20%Nd-0.47%Zr alloy strengthened by equal-channel angular pressing (ECAP) compared to the control (intact cells)

It was shown that ECAP-strengthened Zn-1%Mg and Zn-1%Mg-0.1%Ca alloys inhibit the viability of SCOV3 human ovarian cancer cells after their joint incubation (Fig. 7) (Martynenko et al. 2023). This was confirmed by a significant decrease in the cell viability, based on the assessment of the metabolic activity of the cell culture after incubation on the surface of alloy samples in comparison with the control where cells were grown at the bottom of the plate wells. ECAP-treated Zn-Mg alloy inhibited cellular activity by an average of 49%, and ECAP-treated Zn-Mg-Ca alloy—by 59%. The study of the cells on the surface of alloys using fluorescence microscopy led to similar conclusions. At the same time, the samples of the Zn-Mg-Ca alloy had more pronounced signs of inhibition of cell viability.

In addition, as part of the joint work of researchers from IMET RAS and N.N. Blokhin NMRCO are conducting research on local delivery of chemo-immunoagents. For example, the work was carried out to create scaffolds based on

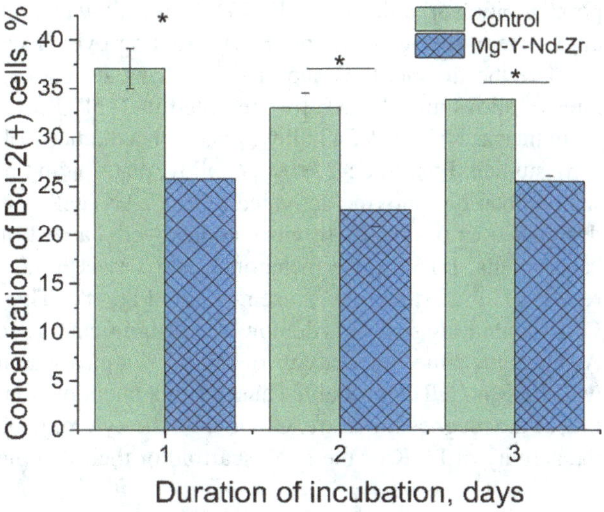

Fig. 6 The concentration of Bcl-2(+) LNCaP cells after coincubation with ECAP-treated Mg-Y-Nd-Zr alloy on comparison with the control (intact cells), $^*p < 0.05$

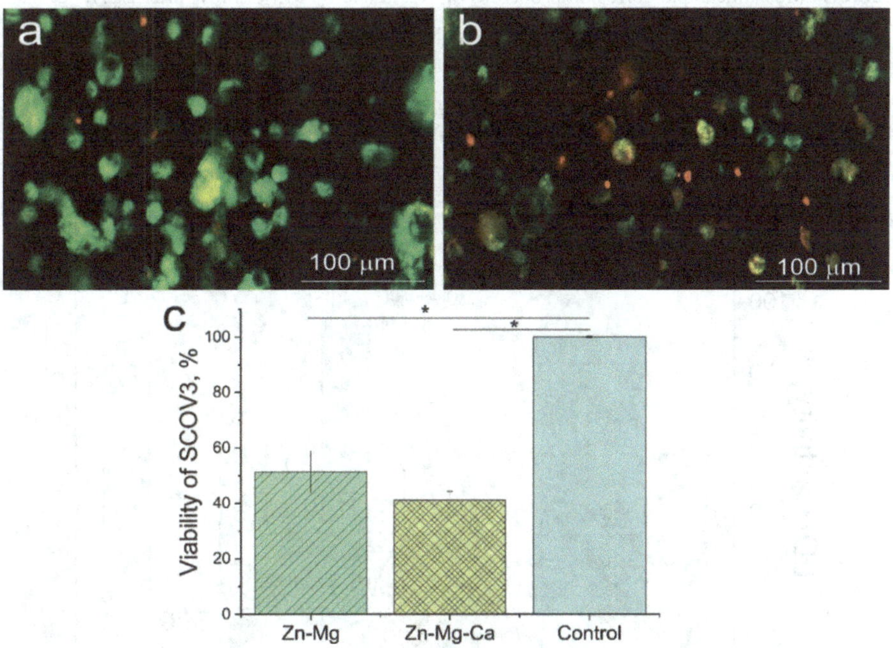

Fig. 7 SCOV3 cells on the surface of samples after 3 days of incubation: Zn-1%Mg (**a**) and Zn-1% Mg-0.1% Ca (**b**) alloys. Calcein AM and propidium iodide staining: *green* live cells; *red* dead cells. Viability of SCOV3 cells after coincubation with Zn-Mg and Zn-Mg-Ca alloys in comparison with the control where cells were grown at the bottom of the plate wells (**c**), $^*p < 0.05$

popular bioresorbable alloys: Fe-27%Mn-C alloy and magnesium WE43 alloy. Both alloys were strengthened by ECAP to improve their mechanical properties and regulate the degradation rate. The mechanical characteristics and the degradation rates of alloys after ECAP are presented in Table 1.

In the case of the WE43 alloy, pins with a diameter of 2 mm and a length of 5 mm were studied. For the Fe-27%Mn-C alloy, plates with transverse slits filled with a gel with human lymphokine-activated killer (LAK) cells were made. These samples are designated as Fe-Mn-C. In vitro studies were carried out on SKBR3 human breast cancer cells, B16 mouse melanoma, and Lewis lung carcinoma (LLC) cells. The result of the study is presented in Fig. 8. The studies showed that the LAK-containing scaffolds demonstrated significantly pronounced cytotoxic activity. At the same time, the activity of WE43 samples was more intense in comparison with Fe-Mn-C. The probable cause of this phenomenon was the higher degradation rate of the magnesium alloy. Obviously, the cytotoxic effect obtained may be due to the activity of LAK or the alloy scaffold or their complex effect. From this point of

Table 1 Mechanical and corrosion properties of WE43 and Fe-Mn-C alloys after ECAP

Alloy	Yield stress, MPa	Ultimate tensile strength, MPa	Elongation, %	Degradation rate, mm/y
WE43	260 ± 11	300 ± 5	13.2 ± 0.4	1.40 ± 0.11
Fe-27%Mn-C	1,327 ± 21	1,515 ± 20	12.5 ± 0.5	0.63 ± 0.10

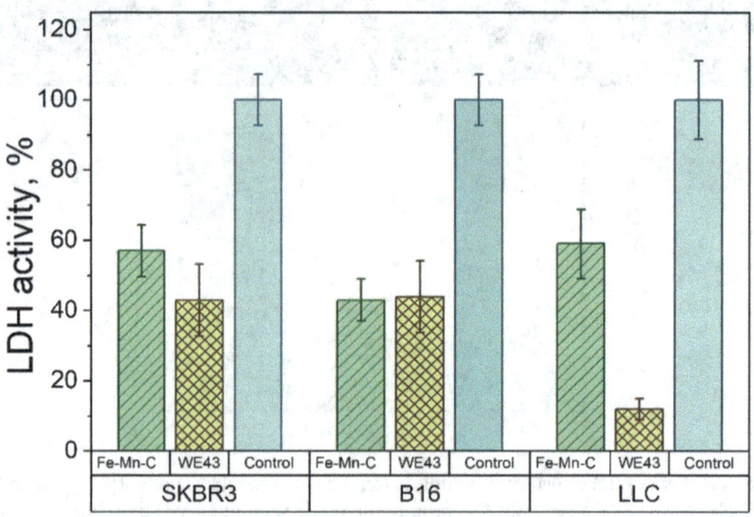

Fig. 8 Study of the antitumor cytotoxic bioactivity of scaffolds made from Fe-27%Mn-C and WE43 alloys loaded with lymphokine-activated killer (LAK) cells against SKBR3, B16, and Lewis lung carcinoma (LLC) cells. The samples based on Fe-27%Mn-C are designated as Fe-Mn-C. Tumor cell viability was determined in a test for assessing lactate dehydrogenase activity (LDH activity). Intact tumor cells were considered as control

view, it is interesting that the active cytotoxic effect of scaffolds loaded with human LAK was also recorded against B16 mouse melanoma cells. This led us to recognize that the alloy or its corrosion products are capable of suppressing the tumor cells viability and, therefore, is an important component of the bioconstruction, ensuring its activity in combination with immune cells.

Along with studies conducted under in vitro conditions, tests of these samples were carried out under in vivo ones. The studies of the antitumor properties of the bioresorbable cell-free scaffolds were first carried out on a mouse melanoma model. For this purpose, mice were subcutaneously inoculated with B16 melanoma, and then samples of the studied alloys were implanted into the formed tumor node (Fig. 9). At the end of the experiment, tumor nodes of mice with implanted alloys and a control group (without alloys samples) were examined using computed tomography (CT scan) to identify gas accumulations and comparatively assess the volume of melanoma mass. It was found that the structure of the melanoma node was homogeneous and did not contain gas bubbles only in the control group of animals. Single small-volume gas bubbles adjacent to the alloy samples were found in the tumor tissue of mice with implanted Fe-Mn-C scaffold. In the group of mice with implanted WE43 alloy samples, the gas content in the tumor node was significantly higher. The main volume of gas was concentrated around the scaffold.

The volumes of the tumor node and accumulated in this node gas were measured in each group of animals to calculate the volume of melanoma tumor tissue using special software. For this purpose, a three-dimensional model of the tumor node and the mouse body was built (Fig. 10a–c). This analysis showed that a significant part of the volume of tumor node was occupied by gas in the group of animals with implanted WE43 alloy scaffolds. This is accompanied by the scaffold destruction (Fig. 10d) and reduction in melanoma tissue volume (Fig. 10e). This made it possible to prove the fact of reliable inhibition of melanoma growth under the influence of the studied samples of bioresorbable alloys. The activity of WE43 alloy scaffold was higher than Fe-Mn-C and averaged 23% (Table 2).

The second stage of studying antitumor activity of LAK-loaded scaffolds was carried out on human adenocarcinoma transplanted into nude mice. The results of morphological analysis of tumor node tissue after paratumoral implantation of the

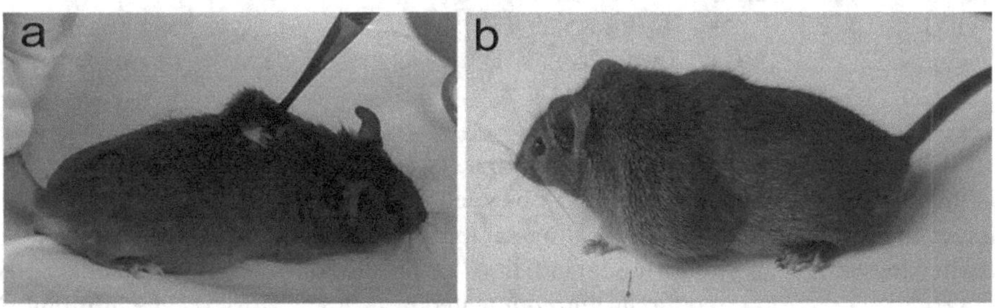

Fig. 9 The implantation of WE43 alloy scaffold near the melanoma node (**a**) and subcutaneous accumulation of gas 5 days after this procedure (**b**)

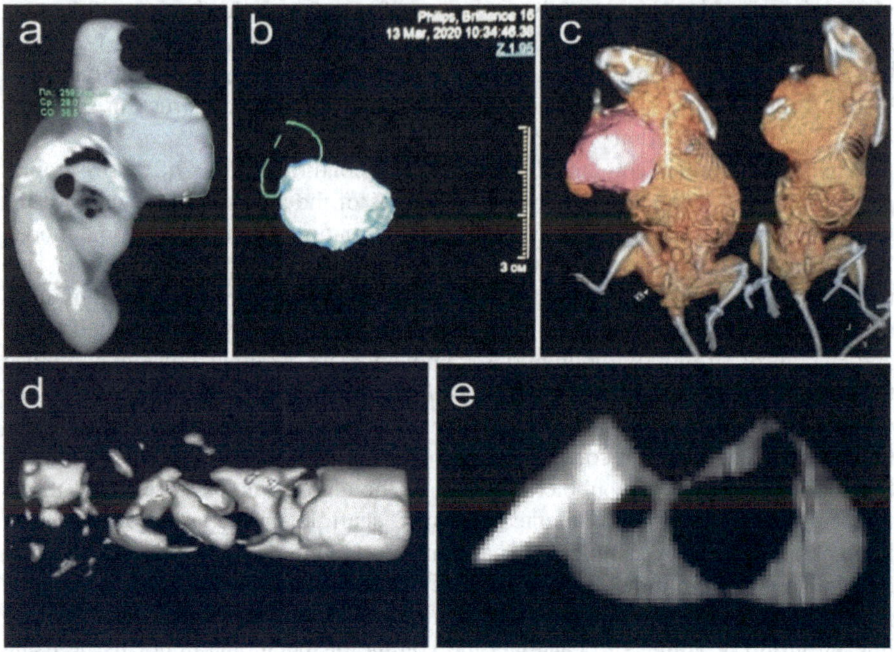

Fig. 10 The main stages of determining the homogeneity of B16 melanoma nodes: (**a**) highlighting the boundaries of the tumor node; (**b**) separation of a tumor node with included gas bubbles to determine the volume; (**c**) color localization of the tumor node in the mouse body. Micro CT of the WE43 alloy scaffolds injected paratumorally, after 10 days of implantation: destruction of the scaffold (**d**), gas accumulation within the tumor node (**e**)

Table 2 Calculation of tumor growth inhibition (TGI) and the volume of the melanoma tumor node of mice of different groups at the end of the experiment, measured by intravital measurements and by CT

Samples/groups	Intravital superficial tumor measurement			Measurement by CT		
	Volume, mm^3		TGI, %	Volume, mm^3		TGI, %
	M	SD		M	SD	
Fe-Mn-C	2,168	1732	84	5,247	693	5
WE43	2,623	1,628	80	4,266	564	23
Control	13,475	3,219	–	5,524	729	–

scaffolds are presented in Fig. 11. After 10 days it was demonstrated that the largest amount of necrotic tumor tissue was observed in the edge zone of the tumor node under the influence of the WE43 alloy samples. A marginal growth of connective tissue strands into the tumor node and signs of infiltration by lymphoid cells were observed in the group of animals with implanted Fe-Mn-C scaffolds. The infiltration by lymphoid cells can be explained both by the release of LAK from the scaffold cavity and by the homing of immunocompetent cells from the depot. In addition, it

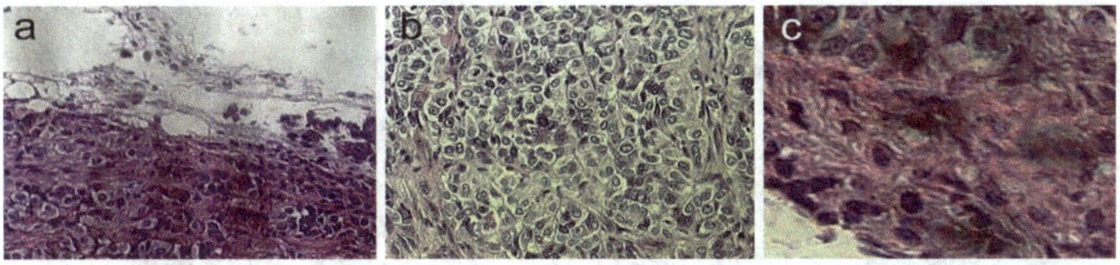

Fig. 11 Morphology of tumor tissue of mice after implantation of LAK-loaded scaffolds based on WE43 (**a**) and Fe-Mn-C (**b**) alloys in comparison with the control group of untreated animals (**c**)

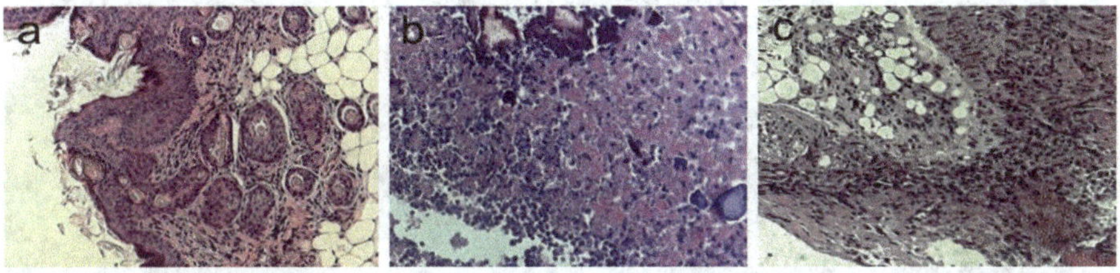

Fig. 12 Morphology of the capsule formed around samples of WE43 (**a**) and Fe-Mn-C (**b**) alloys in mice after implantation in comparison in comparison with the control group of untreated animals (**c**)

can be a reaction to the degradation of the Fe-Mn-C alloy. Only a fairly thin capsule of uniform thickness was observed surrounding the tumor mass with signs of intense peripheral cell division in the control group of untreated animals (Fig. 11).

The analysis of the capsule morphology covering the implants showed signs of intense vascularization of the area of WE43 alloy biodegradation and foci of accumulation of biocorrosion products of the alloy, surrounded by a large number of histiocytic cells (Fig. 12a). In the capsule surrounding the Fe-Mn-C scaffold, a large number of monocular lymphoid cells, as well as a number of foci of accumulation of alloy biodegradation products were also detected (Fig. 12b). The area of the formed subcutaneous pocket, where the absence of these signs can be seen, was shown for the control animal group for comparison (Fig. 12c).

The morphological studies were also carried out to evaluate the biocompatibility of bioresorbable alloys under in vivo conditions. The morphological analysis of the internal organs of mice of three groups did not reveal any significant signs of destruction of the main internal organs, indicating the development of organ failure in animals (Fig. 13). In particular, there were no signs of loss of airiness or swelling in the kidney tissue. The preservation of the morphology of the liver lobules without signs of bile stagnation or destruction of hepatocytes can be seen. There were no signs of destruction of the glomeruli and tubules, accumulation of amyloid, or other signs of disruption of their structure in the kidneys. The signs of increased red blood cell destruction or decreased lymphocyte counts were not also detected in the spleen. Thus, we found no signs of toxic effects after implantation of the developed biodegradable scaffolds loaded with cells.

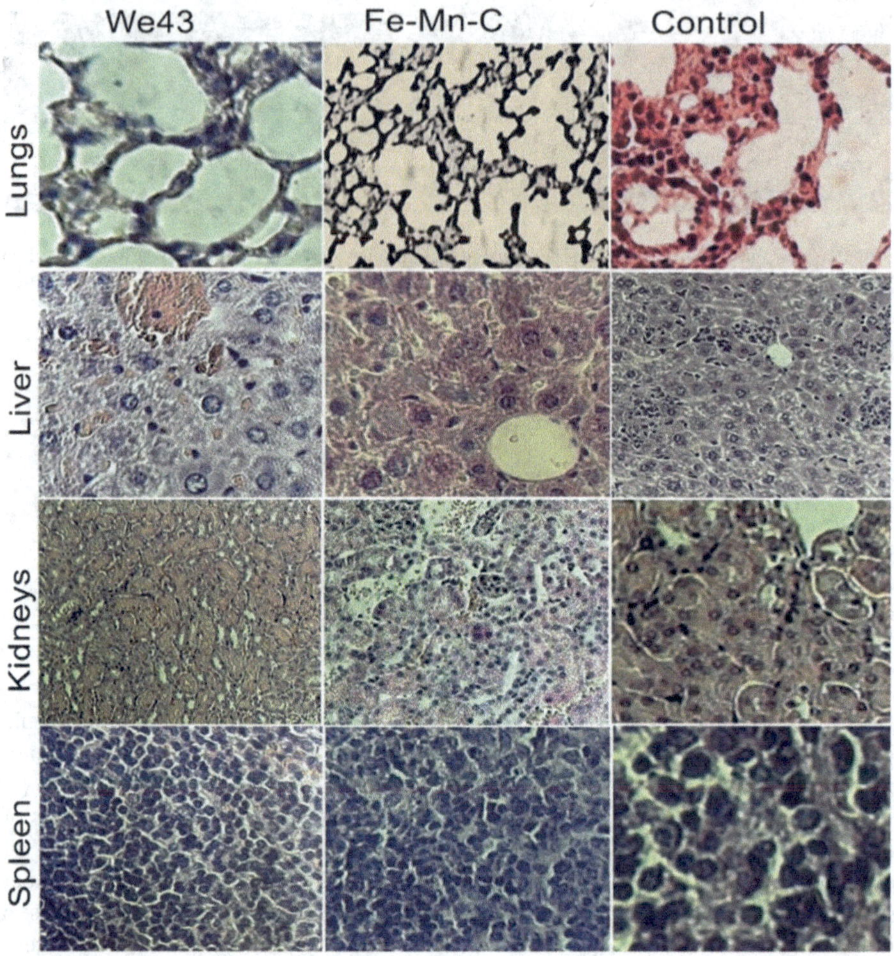

Fig. 13 Morphology of the internal organs of mice after implantation of the LAK-loaded scaffolds based on WE43 and Fe-Mn-C alloys in comparison with the control group of intact animals

To summarize the above biodegradable alloys based on Fe, Zn, and Mg are promising materials for creating a new generation of metal implants for various purposes. Currently, intensive research is being conducted aimed at regulating the corrosion resistance and mechanical characteristics of bioresorbable implants, as well as giving them additional functional properties, for example, antitumor activity. Promising methods for solving this issue are choosing the optimal alloying system, regulating the microstructure, and treating/coating the surface of materials. In addition, a competent choice of alloying and the creation of special designs allows to use the biodegradable alloys based on Fe, Zn, and Mg not only in orthopedics (including orthopedic oncology), but also for the creation of local chemo-immunological agents release systems. All these aspects are currently being methodically and deeply studied, including in joint work conducted by IMET RAS and N.N. Blokhin NMRCO. The results obtained on alloys based on Mg and Fe-Mn showed the promise of using typical biodegradable alloys (e.g., magnesium alloys WE43 and Mg-Zn-Ca or Fe-Mn-(C, Pd) alloys) developed for osteoreconstructive implants in the development scaffolds for the treatment of patients with cancer. Due to their good biocompatibility and bioresorption ability, these alloys allow to release gradually therapeutic agents aimed at treating tumor cells without harmful effects on healthy cells.

7 Conclusion

The above results achieved by various researchers demonstrate the prospects of using different modeling techniques, materials, and processing routes to develop bioimplants and their scaffolds for the treatment of cancer patients.

Approaches to obtain both stable and biodegradable implants for reconstructing parts of the skeleton and airways are described. For onco-orthopedics the described approach is of special interest, because it can provide not only replenishment of the destroyed tissues for restoration of the organ functions, but also prevention of local recurrences development after conditional radical resection of the affected bone area. It should be noted that the characterized scaffolds can serve for local administration of both pharmaceuticals and bioactive trace elements for chemotherapy or inhibition of tumor angiogenesis, and targeted immune drugs such as activated lymphocytes (cytokine-induced cellular killers, CIK) or genetically modified lymphocytes—CAR-T cells. At the same time, it has to be stated that there is still no method of creating ideal medical devices for reconstructive surgery and local drug delivery for therapy of cancer patients. In addition, there are a number of unresolved biomedical issues that hinder the active introduction of the new generation of bioactive implants into clinical practice.

The demonstrated advantages and disadvantages of the used approaches prove the relevance of continuing developments in this field and the necessity of using an interdisciplinary complete approach to achieve the set goals. The described approaches of creating advanced bioimplants look extremely promising not only for oncology, but also for other branches of medicine. Despite the positive results, there is still a lot of in-depth research to be done to create functional and safe products using modern technologies. Only a carefully thought-out solution to these challenges, with a special focus on the biomedical characteristics of the new generation of bioactive scaffolds, can provide a reliable path to their successful advancement into the clinic.

References

Abdel Rahman M, Bassiony A, Shalaby H (2009) Reimplantation of the resected tumour-bearing segment after recycling using liquid nitrogen for osteosarcoma. Int Orthop 33:1365–1370. https://doi.org/10.1007/s00264-009-0773-6

Akahori T, Niinomi M, Fukui H, Ogawa M, Toda H (2005) Improvement in fatigue characteristics of newly developed beta type titanium alloy for biomedical applications by thermo-mechanical treatments. Mater Sci Eng C 25(3):248–254. https://doi.org/10.1016/j.msec.2004.12.007

Anisimova NY, Kopylov AN, Kornyushenkov EA et al (2013) The sterile deimmunized matrix for the replacement of extended defects in bone. Bone and soft tissue sarcomas. In: Tumors of the Skin, vol 2, pp 49–54. (In Russ.)

Anisimova N, Kiselevskiy M, Martynenko N et al (2020) Cytotoxicity of biodegradable magnesium alloy WE43 to tumor cells in vitro: bioresorbable implants with antitumor activity? J Biomed Mater Res 108:167–173. https://doi.org/10.1002/jbm.b.34375

Badylak SF, Weiss DJ, Caplan A, Macchiarini P (2012) RETRACTED: engineered whole organs and complex tissues. Lancet 379:943–952. https://doi.org/10.1016/S0140-6736(12)60073-7

Barba D, Alabort E, Reed RC (2019) Synthetic bone: design by additive manufacturing. Acta Biomater 97:637–656. https://doi.org/10.1016/j.actbio.2019.07.049

Benders KEM, Weeren PRV, Badylak SF et al (2013) Extracellular matrix scaffolds for cartilage and bone regeneration. Trends Biotechnol 31:169–176. https://doi.org/10.1016/j.tibtech.2012.12.004

Benedetti M, Du Plessis A, Ritchie RO et al (2021) Architected cellular materials: a review on their mechanical properties towards fatigue-tolerant design and fabrication. Mater Sci Eng: R Rep 144:100606. https://doi.org/10.1016/j.mser.2021.100606

Bitar KN, Zakhem E (2014) Design strategies of biodegradable scaffolds for tissue regeneration. Biomed Eng Comput Biol 6:BECB.S10961. https://doi.org/10.4137/BECB.S10961

Böhm P, Springfeld R, Springer H (1998) Re-implantation of autoclaved bone segments in musculoskeletal tumor surgery. Arch Orthop Trauma Surg 118:57–65. https://doi.org/10.1007/s004020050312

Böhm P, Fritz J, Thiede S, Budach W (2003) Reimplantation of extracorporeal irradiated bone segments in musculoskeletal tumor surgery: clinical experience in eight patients and review of the literature. Langenbeck's Arch Surg 387:355–365. https://doi.org/10.1007/s00423-002-0332-8

Bose S, Roy M, Bandyopadhyay A (2012) Recent advances in bone tissue engineering scaffolds. Trends Biotechnol 30:546–554. https://doi.org/10.1016/j.tibtech.2012.07.005

Boutsikou E, Kontakiotis T, Zarogoulidis P (2013) Docetaxel-carboplatin in combination with erlotinib and/or bevacizumab in patients with non-small cell lung cancer. Onco Targets Ther 6: 125–134. https://doi.org/10.2147/OTT.S42245

Braem A, Chaudhari A, Vivan Cardoso M et al (2014) Peri- and intra-implant bone response to microporous Ti coatings with surface modification. Acta Biomater 10:986–995. https://doi.org/10.1016/j.actbio.2013.10.017

Caligari Conti M, Mallia B, Sinagra E et al (2019) The effect of alloying elements on the properties of pressed and non-pressed biodegradable Fe–Mn–Ag powder metallurgy alloys. Heliyon 5: e02522. https://doi.org/10.1016/j.heliyon.2019.e02522

Chen C-Y, Ke C-J, Yen K-C et al (2015) 3D porous calcium-alginate scaffolds cell culture system improved human osteoblast cell clusters for cell therapy. Theranostics 5:643–655. https://doi.org/10.7150/thno.11372

Chubrik A, Senatov F, Kolesnikov E et al (2020) Highly porous PEEK and PEEK/HA scaffolds with Escherichia coli-derived recombinant BMP-2 and erythropoietin for enhanced osteogenesis and angiogenesis. Polym Test 87:106518. https://doi.org/10.1016/j.polymertesting.2020.106518

D'Onofrio A, Cresce GD, Bolgan I et al (2011) Clinical and hemodynamic outcomes after aortic valve replacement with stented and stentless pericardial xenografts: a propensity-matched analysis. J Heart Valve Dis 20:319–325; discussion 326

De Salvo S, Pavone V, Coco S et al (2022) Benign bone tumors: an overview of what we know today. JCM 11:699. https://doi.org/10.3390/jcm11030699

Du Plessis A, Razavi N, Benedetti M et al (2022) Properties and applications of additively manufactured metallic cellular materials: a review. Prog Mater Sci 125:100918. https://doi.org/10.1016/j.pmatsci.2021.100918

Egorova YB, Il'in AA, Kolachev BA et al (2003) Effect of the structure on the cutability of titanium alloys. Met Sci Heat Treat 45:134–139. https://doi.org/10.1023/A:1024527807272

Eisenbarth E, Velten D, Müller M et al (2004) Biocompatibility of β-stabilizing elements of titanium alloys. Biomaterials 25:5705–5713. https://doi.org/10.1016/j.biomaterials.2004.01.021

Elborolosy SA, Hussein LA, Mahran H et al (2023) Evaluation of the biocompatibility, antibacterial and anticancer effects of a novel nano-structured Fe–Mn-based biodegradable alloys in-vitro study. Heliyon 9:e20932. https://doi.org/10.1016/j.heliyon.2023.e20932

Feng YP, Blanquer A, Fornell J et al (2016) Novel Fe–Mn–Si–Pd alloys: insights into mechanical, magnetic, corrosion resistance and biocompatibility performances. J Mater Chem B 4:6402–6412. https://doi.org/10.1039/C6TB01951J

Fishgoit AV, Maistrov VM, Il'in AA, Rozanov MA (1990) Interaction of short cracks with the structure of metals. Mater Sci 25:571–574. https://doi.org/10.1007/BF00727082

Fougere GE, Riester L, Ferber M et al (1995) Young's modulus of nanocrystalline Fe measured by nanoindentation. Mater Sci Eng A 204:1–6. https://doi.org/10.1016/0921-5093(95)09927-1

Gao JH, Guan SK, Ren ZW et al (2011) Homogeneous corrosion of high pressure torsion treated Mg–Zn–Ca alloy in simulated body fluid. Mater Lett 65:691–693. https://doi.org/10.1016/j.matlet.2010.11.015

Geetha M, Singh AK, Muraleedharan K et al (2001) Effect of thermomechanical processing on microstructure of a Ti–13Nb–13Zr alloy. J Alloys Compd 329:264–271. https://doi.org/10.1016/S0925-8388(01)01604-8

Gilbert TW (2012) Strategies for tissue and organ decellularization. J Cell Biochem 113:2217–2222. https://doi.org/10.1002/jcb.24130

Grillo HC (2002) Tracheal replacement: a critical review. Ann Thorac Surg 73:1995–2004. https://doi.org/10.1016/S0003-4975(02)03564-6

Gryko A, Prochor P, Sajewicz E (2022) Finite element analysis of the influence of porosity and pore geometry on mechanical properties of orthopaedic scaffolds. J Mech Behav Biomed Mater 132:105275. https://doi.org/10.1016/j.jmbbm.2022.105275

Habibovic P, De Groot K (2007) Osteoinductive biomaterials—properties and relevance in bone repair. J Tissue Eng Regen Med 1:25–32. https://doi.org/10.1002/term.5

Hattori T, Ito N, Morikawa K, Sato K, Akahori T, Niinomi M (2009) Animal study on biocompatibility of Ti-29Nb-13ta-4.6Zr titanium alloy. Bone tissue reaction and metal ion release in femoral head replacement of sheep. In: Proceedings 2nd European Conference On Biomaterials

He X, Gao Z, Xu H et al (2017) A meta-analysis of randomized control trials of surgical methods with osteosarcoma outcomes. J Orthop Surg Res 12:5. https://doi.org/10.1186/s13018-016-0500-0

Hermawan H, Alamdari H, Mantovani D, Dubé D (2008) Iron–manganese: new class of metallic degradable biomaterials prepared by powder metallurgy. Powder Metall 51:38–45. https://doi.org/10.1179/174329008X284868

Hermawan H, Dubé D, Mantovani D (2010a) Developments in metallic biodegradable stents. Acta Biomater 6:1693–1697. https://doi.org/10.1016/j.actbio.2009.10.006

Hermawan H, Dubé D, Mantovani D (2010b) Degradable metallic biomaterials: design and development of Fe–Mn alloys for stents. J Biomedical Materials Res 93A:1–11. https://doi.org/10.1002/jbm.a.32224

Hermawan H, Purnama A, Dube D et al (2010c) Fe–Mn alloys for metallic biodegradable stents: degradation and cell viability studies. Acta Biomater 6:1852–1860. https://doi.org/10.1016/j.actbio.2009.11.025

Hieda J, Niinomi M, Nakai M et al (2013) Improvement of adhesive strength of segmented polyurethane on Ti–29Nb–13Ta–4.6Zr alloy through H_2O_2 treatment for biomedical applications. J Biomed Mater Res 101B:776–783. https://doi.org/10.1002/jbm.b.32881

Hohenforst-Schmidt W (2011) Intratumoral chemotherapy (ITC) as adjunct therapy in NSCLC iiia–iv prolongs life; poster presented at: international conference and exhibition on cancer science and therapy, Las Vegas, NV

Hohenforst-Schmidt W, Zarogoulidis P, Darwiche K (2013) Intratumoral chemotherapy for lung cancer: re-challenge current targeted therapies. Drug Des Devel Ther 7:571–583. https://doi.org/10.2147/DDDT.S46393

Hohenforst-Schmidt W, Zarogoulidis P, Stopek J et al (2015) Enhancement of Intratumoral chemotherapy with cisplatin with or without microwave ablation and Lipiodol. Future concept for local treatment in lung cancer. J Cancer 6:218–226. https://doi.org/10.7150/jca.10970

Hong ED, Carrino JA, Weber KL, Fayad LM (2011) Prevalence of shoulder enchondromas on routine MR imaging. Clin Imaging 35:378–384. https://doi.org/10.1016/j.clinimag.2010.10.012

Hsu Y, Lu Y, Wang S et al (2023) Magnesium alloys in tumor treatment: current research status, challenges and future prospects. J Magnesium Alloys 11:3399–3426. https://doi.org/10.1016/j.jma.2023.08.008

Huang B, Yang M, Kou Y et al (2024) Absorbable implants in sport medicine and arthroscopic surgery: a narrative review of recent development. Bioact Mate 3:1272–1283

Jones AC, Arns CH, Hutmacher DW et al (2009) The correlation of pore morphology, interconnectivity and physical properties of 3D ceramic scaffolds with bone ingrowth. Biomaterials 30:1440–1451. https://doi.org/10.1016/j.biomaterials.2008.10.056

Karageorgiou V, Kaplan D (2005) Porosity of 3D biomaterial scaffolds and osteogenesis. Biomaterials 26:5474–5491. https://doi.org/10.1016/j.biomaterials.2005.02.002

Khrapov D, Paveleva A, Kozadayeva M et al (2023) Trapped powder removal from sheet-based porous structures based on triply periodic minimal surfaces fabricated by electron beam powder bed fusion. Mater Sci Eng A 862:144479. https://doi.org/10.1016/j.msea.2022.144479

Kilmametov AR, Ivanisenko Y, Mazilkin AA et al (2018) The $\alpha \to \omega$ and $\beta \to \omega$ phase transformations in Ti–Fe alloys under high-pressure torsion. Acta Mater 144:337–351. https://doi.org/10.1016/j.actamat.2017.10.051

Kim T-K, Sharma B, Williams CG et al (2003) Experimental model for cartilage tissue engineering to regenerate the zonal Organization of Articular Cartilage. Osteoarthr Cartil 11:653–664. https://doi.org/10.1016/S1063-4584(03)00120-1

Kim T, See CW, Li X, Zhu D (2020) Orthopedic implants and devices for bone fractures and defects: past, present and perspective. Eng Regener 1:6–18. https://doi.org/10.1016/j.engreg.2020.05.003

Kiselevskiy MV, Anisimova NY, Kapustin AV et al (2023) Development of bioactive scaffolds for orthopedic applications by designing additively manufactured titanium porous structures: a critical review. Biomimetics (Basel) 8:546. https://doi.org/10.3390/biomimetics8070546

Kisilevskiĭ MV, Anisimova NI, Lebedinskaia OV et al (2012) Heterotopic transplantation of non-immunogenic trachea populated with recipient bone marrow stromal cells. Morfologiia 141:66–70

Koju N, Niraula S, Fotovvati B (2022) Additively manufactured porous Ti6Al4V for bone implants: a review. Metals 12:687. https://doi.org/10.3390/met12040687

Kolachev BA, Lyasotskaya VS (2003) Correlation between diagrams of isothermal and anisothermal transformations and phase composition diagram of hardened titanium alloys. Met Sci Heat Treat 45:119–126. https://doi.org/10.1023/A:1024571622294

Kornyushenkov EA, Mitrushkin DE, Garanin DV et al (2023) Overall and relapse-free survival of dogs with appendicular osteosarcoma after limb-sparing bio-implantation treatment. Bone Soft

Tissue Sarcomas Tumors Skin 15(4):33–39. https://doi.org/10.17650/2219-4614-2023-15-4-33-39

Kraus T, Moszner F, Fischerauer S et al (2014) Biodegradable Fe-based alloys for use in osteosynthesis: outcome of an in vivo study after 52weeks. Acta Biomater 10:3346–3353. https://doi.org/10.1016/j.actbio.2014.04.007

Kriegel MJ, Kilmametov A, Klemm V et al (2019) Thermal stability of Athermal ω-Ti (Fe) produced upon quenching of β-Ti(Fe). Adv Eng Mater 21:1800158. https://doi.org/10.1002/adem.201800158

Kuroda D, Niinomi M, Morinaga M et al (1998) Design and mechanical properties of new β type titanium alloys for implant materials. Mater Sci Eng A 243:244–249. https://doi.org/10.1016/S0921-5093(97)00808-3

Kurtz SM (2016) UHMWPE biomaterials handbook: ultra-high molecular weight polyethylene in total joint replacement and medical devices, 3rd edn. Academic Press, Amsterdam Boston

Lambotte A (1932) L'utilisation du magnesium comme materiel perdu dans l'osteosynthese [the use of magnesium as material for osteosynthesis]. Bulletins et Mémoires de la Societe Nationale de Chirurgie 28:1325–1334

Lee WS, Park M, Kim MH et al (2016) Nanoparticle coating on the silane-modified surface of magnesium for local drug delivery and controlled corrosion. J Biomater Appl 30:651–661. https://doi.org/10.1177/0885328215582110

Li YC, Li MH, Hu WY et al (2010) Biodegradable mg-ca and mg-ca-Y alloys for regenerative medicine. MSF 654–656:2192–2195. https://doi.org/10.4028/www.scientific.net/MSF.654-656.2192

Li B, Li F, Ma L et al (2014) Poly(lactide- *co* -glycolide)/fibrin gel construct as a 3D model to evaluate gene therapy of cartilage in vivo. Mol Pharm 11:2062–2070. https://doi.org/10.1021/mp5000136

Li L, Zhang K, Wang T et al (2020) Biofabrication of a biomimetic supramolecular-polymer double network hydrogel for cartilage regeneration. Mater Des 189:108492. https://doi.org/10.1016/j.matdes.2020.108492

Liu H, Niinomi M, Nakai M et al (2014) Deformation-induced changeable Young's modulus with high strength in β-type Ti–Cr–O alloys for spinal fixture. J Mech Behav Biomed Mater 30:205–213. https://doi.org/10.1016/j.jmbbm.2013.11.001

Lukyanova EA, Martynenko NS, Serebryany VN et al (2017) Structure and mechanical and corrosion properties of a magnesium mg–Y–Nd–Zr alloy after high pressure torsion. Russ Metall 2017:912–921. https://doi.org/10.1134/S0036029517110088

Luo H, Xiong G, Yang Z et al (2014) Preparation of three-dimensional braided carbon fiber-reinforced PEEK composites for potential load-bearing bone fixations. Part I. Mechanical properties and cytocompatibility. J Mech Behav Biomed Mater 29:103–113. https://doi.org/10.1016/j.jmbbm.2013.09.003

Lv Y, Wang B, Liu G et al (2021) Metal material, properties and design methods of porous biomedical scaffolds for additive manufacturing: a review. Front Bioeng Biotechnol 9:641130. https://doi.org/10.3389/fbioe.2021.641130

Ma LW, Cheng HS, Chung CY (2013) Effect of thermo-mechanical treatment on superelastic behavior of Ti–19Nb–14Zr (at.%) shape memory alloy. Intermetallics 32:44–50. https://doi.org/10.1016/j.intermet.2012.07.024

Ma X, Gao Y, Zhao D et al (2021) Titanium implants and local drug delivery systems become mutual promoters in orthopedic clinics. Nano 12:47. https://doi.org/10.3390/nano12010047

Macchiarini P, Jungebluth P, Go T et al (2008) RETRACTED: clinical transplantation of a tissue-engineered airway. Lancet 372:2023–2030. https://doi.org/10.1016/S0140-6736(08)61598-6

Maehara K, Doi K, Matsushita T, Sasaki Y (2002) Application of vanadium-free titanium alloys to artificial hip joints. Mater Trans 43:2936–2942. https://doi.org/10.2320/matertrans.43.2936

Maksimkin AV, Senatov FS, Anisimova NY et al (2017) Multilayer porous UHMWPE scaffolds for bone defects replacement. Mater Sci Eng C 73:366–372. https://doi.org/10.1016/j.msec.2016.12.104

Martynenko N, Anisimova N, Kiselevskiy M et al (2020) Structure, mechanical characteristics, biodegradation, and in vitro cytotoxicity of magnesium alloy ZX11 processed by rotary swaging. J Magnesium Alloys 8:1038–1046. https://doi.org/10.1016/j.jma.2020.08.008

Martynenko NS, Anisimova NY, Rybalchenko OV et al (2023) Study of biocompatibility and antitumor cytotoxic activity *in vitro* of Zn—1 %mg and Zn—1 %mg—0.1 %ca alloys strengthened by equal angular pressing. Rossijskij bioterapevtičeskij žurnal 22:64–74. https://doi.org/10.17650/1726-9784-2023-22-3-64-74

McBride ED (1938) Absorbable metal in bone surgery: a further report on the use of magnesium alloys. JAMA 111:2464. https://doi.org/10.1001/jama.1938.02790530018007

Mishra AK, Davidson JA, Kovacs P, Poggie RA (1993) Beta titanium in the 1990s. Mineral, Metals and Materials Society, Warrendale, Pennsylvania, pp 61–66

Morinaga M, Yukawa N, Maya T, Sone K, Adachi H (1988) Theoretical design of titanium alloys. In: Proceedings Sixth World Conference on Titanium. Societe Francaise de Metallurgie, Paris, pp 1601–1606

Murphey MD, Choi JJ, Kransdorf MJ et al (2000) Imaging of Osteochondroma: variants and complications with radiologic-pathologic correlation. Radiographics 20:1407–1434. https://doi.org/10.1148/radiographics.20.5.g00se171407

Murr LE (2019) Strategies for creating living, additively manufactured, open-cellular metal and alloy implants by promoting osseointegration, osteoinduction and vascularization: an overview. J Mater Sci Technol 35:231–241. https://doi.org/10.1016/j.jmst.2018.09.003

Nag S, Banerjee R, Fraser HL (2005) Microstructural evolution and strengthening mechanisms in Ti–Nb–Zr–ta, Ti–Mo–Zr–Fe and Ti–15Mo biocompatible alloys. Mater Sci Eng C 25:357–362. https://doi.org/10.1016/j.msec.2004.12.013

Nagase T, Iijima Y, Matsugaki A et al (2020) Design and fabrication of Ti–Zr-Hf-Cr-Mo and Ti–Zr-Hf-co-Cr-Mo high-entropy alloys as metallic biomaterials. Mater Sci Eng C 107:110322. https://doi.org/10.1016/j.msec.2019.110322

Nakai M, Niinomi M, Zhao X, Zhao X (2011) Self-adjustment of Young's modulus in biomedical titanium alloys during orthopaedic operation. Mater Lett 65:688–690. https://doi.org/10.1016/j.matlet.2010.11.006

Nandi SK, Roy S, Mukherjee P et al (2010) Orthopaedic applications of bone graft & graft substitutes: a review. Indian J Med Res 132:15–30

Němec M, Jäger A, Tesař K, Gärtnerová V (2017) Influence of alloying element Zn on the microstructural, mechanical and corrosion properties of binary mg-Zn alloys after severe plastic deformation. Mater Charact 134:69–75. https://doi.org/10.1016/j.matchar.2017.10.017

Niinomi M, Nakai M (2011) Titanium-based biomaterials for preventing stress shielding between implant devices and bone. Int J Biomater 2011:1–10. https://doi.org/10.1155/2011/836587

Niinomi M, Nakai M, Hieda J (2012) Development of new metallic alloys for biomedical applications. Acta Biomater 8:3888–3903. https://doi.org/10.1016/j.actbio.2012.06.037

Nijhuis WH, Eastwood DM, Allgrove J et al (2019) Current concepts in osteogenesis imperfecta: bone structure, biomechanics and medical management. J Child Orthop 13:1–11. https://doi.org/10.1302/1863-2548.13.180190

Okazaki Y, Gotoh E (2005) Comparison of metal release from various metallic biomaterials in vitro. Biomaterials 26:11–21. https://doi.org/10.1016/j.biomaterials.2004.02.005

Olszta MJ, Cheng X, Jee SS et al (2007) Bone structure and formation: a new perspective. Mater Sci Eng: R: Rep 58:77–116. https://doi.org/10.1016/j.mser.2007.05.001

Payr E (1900) Beiträge zur Technik der Blutgefäss- und Nervennaht nebst Mittheilungen über die Verwendung eines resorbirbaren Metalles in der Chirurgie. Arch Klin Chir 62(S):67–93

Peng F, Wang D, Tian Y et al (2017) Sealing the pores of PEO coating with mg-Al layered double hydroxide: enhanced corrosion resistance, cytocompatibility and drug delivery ability. Sci Rep 7:8167. https://doi.org/10.1038/s41598-017-08238-w

Peuster M (2001) A novel approach to temporary stenting: degradable cardiovascular stents produced from corrodible metal—results 6–18 months after implantation into New Zealand white rabbits. Heart 86:563–569. https://doi.org/10.1136/heart.86.5.563

Pilliar RM (1987) Porous-surfaced metallic implants for orthopedic applications. J Biomed Mater Res 21:1–33

Putra NE, Mirzaali MJ, Apachitei I et al (2020) Multi-material additive manufacturing technologies for Ti-, Mg-, and Fe-based biomaterials for bone substitution. Acta Biomater 109:1–20. https://doi.org/10.1016/j.actbio.2020.03.037

Qi H, Heise S, Zhou J et al (2019) Electrophoretic deposition of bioadaptive drug delivery coatings on magnesium alloy for bone repair. ACS Appl Mater Interfaces 11:8625–8634. https://doi.org/10.1021/acsami.9b01227

Ricchetti ET, Aurora A, Iannotti JP, Derwin KA (2012) Scaffold devices for rotator cuff repair. J Shoulder Elb Surg 21:251–265. https://doi.org/10.1016/j.jse.2011.10.003

Rybalchenko OV, Anisimova NY, Kiselevsky MV et al (2022) Effect of equal-channel angular pressing on structure and properties of Fe-Mn-C alloys for biomedical applications. Mater Today Commun 30:103048. https://doi.org/10.1016/j.mtcomm.2021.103048

Rybalchenko O, Anisimova N, Martynenko N et al (2023) Structure optimization of a Fe–Mn–Pd alloy by equal-channel angular pressing for biomedical use. Materials (Basel) 16:45. https://doi.org/10.3390/ma16010045

Sakaguchi N, Niinomi M, Akahori T et al (2005) Relationships between tensile deformation behavior and microstructure in Ti–Nb–Ta–Zr system alloys. Mater Sci Eng C 25:363–369. https://doi.org/10.1016/j.msec.2004.12.014

Santos PF, Niinomi M, Cho K et al (2017) Effects of Mo addition on the mechanical properties and microstructures of Ti-Mn alloys fabricated by metal injection molding for biomedical applications. Mater Trans 58:271–279. https://doi.org/10.2320/matertrans.M2016286

Savio D, Bagno A (2022) When the Total hip replacement fails: a review on the stress-shielding effect. PRO 10:612. https://doi.org/10.3390/pr10030612

Schinhammer M, Hänzi AC, Löffler JF, Uggowitzer PJ (2010) Design strategy for biodegradable Fe-based alloys for medical applications☆. Acta Biomater 6:1705–1713. https://doi.org/10.1016/j.actbio.2009.07.039

Schwartz CE, Martha JF, Kowalski P et al (2009) Prospective evaluation of chronic pain associated with posterior autologous iliac crest bone graft harvest and its effect on postoperative outcome. Health Qual Life Outcomes 7:49. https://doi.org/10.1186/1477-7525-7-49

Sehitoglu H, Karaman I, Zhang X et al (2001) Deformation of NiTiCu shape memory single crystals in compression. Metall Mater Trans A 32:477–489. https://doi.org/10.1007/s11661-001-0064-3

Senatov FS, Kopylov AN, Anisimova NY et al (2015) UHMWPE-based nanocomposite as a material for damaged cartilage replacement. Mater Sci Eng C 48:566–571. https://doi.org/10.1016/j.msec.2014.12.050

Senatov F, Anisimova N, Kiselevskiy M et al (2017a) Polyhydroxybutyrate/hydroxyapatite highly porous scaffold for small bone defects replacement in the nonload-bearing parts. J Bionic Eng 14:648–658. https://doi.org/10.1016/S1672-6529(16)60431-6

Senatov FS, Zadorozhnyy MY, Niaza KV et al (2017b) Shape memory effect in 3D-printed scaffolds for self-fitting implants. Eur Polym J 93:222–231. https://doi.org/10.1016/j.eurpolymj.2017.06.011

Senatov FS, Chubrik AV, Maksimkin AV et al (2019) Comparative analysis of structure and mechanical properties of porous PEEK and UHMWPE biomimetic scaffolds. Mater Lett 239:63–66. https://doi.org/10.1016/j.matlet.2018.12.055

Senatov F, Amanbek G, Orlova P et al (2020) Biomimetic UHMWPE/HA scaffolds with rhBMP-2 and erythropoietin for reconstructive surgery. Mater Sci Eng C 111:110750. https://doi.org/10.1016/j.msec.2020.110750

Shahar IA, Hosaka T, Yoshihara S, MacDonald BJ (2017) Mechanical and corrosion properties of AZ31 mg alloy processed by Equal-Channel angular pressing and aging. Procedia Eng 184:423–431. https://doi.org/10.1016/j.proeng.2017.04.113

Školáková A, Lovaši T, Pinc J et al (2020) The effect of zinc and calcium addition on magnesium alloy. Manuf Technol 20:668–676. https://doi.org/10.21062/mft.2020.107

Straumal BB, Gornakova AS, Kiselevskiy MV et al (2022) Optimal surface roughness of Ti6Al4V alloy for the adhesion of cells with osteogenic potential. J Mater Res 37:2661–2674. https://doi.org/10.1557/s43578-022-00600-7

Sykes M (2010) Immune evasion by chimeric trachea. N Engl J Med 362:172–174. https://doi.org/10.1056/NEJMe0908366

Takemoto M, Fujibayashi S, Neo M et al (2005) Mechanical properties and osteoconductivity of porous bioactive titanium. Biomaterials 26:6014–6023. https://doi.org/10.1016/j.biomaterials.2005.03.019

Tang X, Ahmed T, Rack HJ (2000) Phase transformations in Ti–Nb–Ta and Ti–Nb–Ta–Zr alloys. J Mater Sci 35:1805–1811. https://doi.org/10.1023/A:1004792922155

Taniguchi N, Fujibayashi S, Takemoto M et al (2016) Effect of pore size on bone ingrowth into porous titanium implants fabricated by additive manufacturing: an in vivo experiment. Mater Sci Eng C 59:690–701. https://doi.org/10.1016/j.msec.2015.10.069

Teoh S (2000) Fatigue of biomaterials: a review. Int J Fatigue 22:825–837. https://doi.org/10.1016/S0142-1123(00)00052-9

Thomas J, Mogonye JE, Mantri SA et al (2020) Additive manufacturing of compositionally graded laser deposited titanium-chromium alloys. Addit Manuf 33:101132. https://doi.org/10.1016/j.addma.2020.101132

Timercan A, Terriault P, Brailovski V (2023) Axial tension/compression and torsional loading of diamond and gyroid lattice structures for biomedical implants: simulation and experiment. Mater Des 225:111585. https://doi.org/10.1016/j.matdes.2022.111585

Tran HDN, Park KD, Ching YC et al (2020) A comprehensive review on polymeric hydrogel and its composite: matrices of choice for bone and cartilage tissue engineering. J Ind Eng Chem 89:58–82. https://doi.org/10.1016/j.jiec.2020.06.017

Tsakiris V, Tardei C, Clicinschi FM (2021) Biodegradable mg alloys for orthopedic implants—a review. Journal of Magnesium and Alloys 9:1884–1905. https://doi.org/10.1016/j.jma.2021.06.024

Valiev RZ, Langdon TG (2006) Principles of equal-channel angular pressing as a processing tool for grain refinement. Prog Mater Sci 51:881–981. https://doi.org/10.1016/j.pmatsci.2006.02.003

Verbrugge J (1934) Le matériel métallique résorbable en chirurgie osseuse [Resorbable metallic material in bone surgery]. La Presse Medicale 23:460–465

Virtanen S (2011) Biodegradable mg and mg alloys: corrosion and biocompatibility. Mater Sci Eng B 176:1600–1608. https://doi.org/10.1016/j.mseb.2011.05.028

Wally ZJ, Haque AM, Feteira A et al (2019) Selective laser melting processed Ti6Al4V lattices with graded porosities for dental applications. J Mech Behav Biomed Mater 90:20–29. https://doi.org/10.1016/j.jmbbm.2018.08.047

Wang X, Lu H, Li X et al (2007) Effect of cooling rate and composition on microstructures and properties of Zn-Mg alloys. Trans Nonferrous Metals Soc China 17:122–125

Warnke PH, Douglas T, Wollny P et al (2009) Rapid prototyping: porous titanium alloy scaffolds produced by selective laser melting for bone tissue engineering. Tissue Eng Part C Methods 15:115–124. https://doi.org/10.1089/ten.tec.2008.0288

Wu P, Grainger DW (2006) Drug/device combinations for local drug therapies and infection prophylaxis. Biomaterials 27:2450–2467. https://doi.org/10.1016/j.biomaterials.2005.11.031

Wu Y, He G, Zhang Y et al (2016) Unique antitumor property of the Mg-Ca-Sr alloys with addition of Zn. Sci Rep 6:21736. https://doi.org/10.1038/srep21736

Yang G, Zhang T (2005) Phase transformation and mechanical properties of the Ti50Zr30Nb10Ta10 alloy with low modulus and biocompatible. J Alloys Compd 392:291–294

Yang R, Chen F, Guo J et al (2020) Recent advances in polymeric biomaterials-based gene delivery for cartilage repair. Bioactive Materials 5:990–1003. https://doi.org/10.1016/j.bioactmat.2020.06.004

Youn SW, Kim MJ, Yi S et al (2015) Effect of manganese content on the magnetic susceptibility of ferrous-manganese alloys: correlation between microstructure on X-ray diffraction and size of the low-intensity area on MRI. Investig Magn Reson Imaging 19:76. https://doi.org/10.13104/imri.2015.19.2.76

Zhao X, Niinomi M, Nakai M et al (2011a) Development of high Zr-containing Ti-based alloys with low Young's modulus for use in removable implants. Mater Sci Eng C 31:1436–1444. https://doi.org/10.1016/j.msec.2011.05.013

Zhao X, Niinomi M, Nakai M et al (2011b) Microstructures and mechanical properties of metastable Ti–30Zr–(Cr, Mo) alloys with changeable Young's modulus for spinal fixation applications. Acta Biomater 7:3230–3236. https://doi.org/10.1016/j.actbio.2011.04.019

Zhao X, Niinomi M, Nakai M (2011c) Relationship between various deformation-induced products and mechanical properties in metastable Ti–30Zr–Mo alloys for biomedical applications. J Mech Behav Biomed Mater 4:2009–2016. https://doi.org/10.1016/j.jmbbm.2011.06.020

Zhao Y, Yu S, Wu X et al (2021) Construction of macroporous magnesium phosphate-based bone cement with sustained drug release. Mater Des 200:109466. https://doi.org/10.1016/j.matdes.2021.109466

Zhianmanesh M, Varmazyar M, Montazerian H (2019) Fluid permeability of graded porosity scaffolds architectured with minimal surfaces. ACS Biomater Sci Eng 5:1228–1237. https://doi.org/10.1021/acsbiomaterials.8b01400

Zhilyaev AP, Langdon TG (2008) Using high-pressure torsion for metal processing: fundamentals and applications. Prog Mater Sci 53:893–979. https://doi.org/10.1016/j.pmatsci.2008.03.002

Zou L, Zhang Y, Liu X et al (2019) Biomimetic mineralization on natural and synthetic polymers to prepare hybrid scaffolds for bone tissue engineering. Colloids Surf B: Biointerfaces 178:222–229. https://doi.org/10.1016/j.colsurfb.2019.03.004

The Interplay of Ferroptosis and Cuproptosis in Cancer: Mechanisms and Therapeutic Implications

Jinjiang Wang, Loucia Kit Ying Chan, Tao Zhang, Jiaxi Li, Jiao Liu, Tat San Lau, and Chi Chiu Wang

Abstract

Ferroptosis and cuproptosis, two recently identified forms of non-apoptotic cell death, have significant relevance in cancer biology due to their higher demand for metal ions. Iron (Fe) and copper (Cu), as transition metals, are critical in cell proliferation, mitochondrial respiration, distant metastases, oxidative stress, and antioxidant defense, all contributing to the onset and advancement of cancer. Given the intertwined relationship of copper and iron in cancer biology, initially studied as independent phenomena, recent evidence suggests a linkage between ferroptosis and cuproptosis. Studies have shown a connection between copper accumulation in mitochondria and the process of ferroptosis. Co-targeting ferroptosis and cuproptosis can be a novel strategy to address refractory cancers by aiming at the vulnerabilities of cancer stem cells and drug-tolerant cells. A potential strategy involves the combination of sorafenib and elesclomol-Cu to target ferroptosis and cuproptosis at the same time. The combined application of iron chelators and copper-lowering agents with chemotherapeutic agents, immunotherapies, radiotherapies, and neoadjuvant therapies holds promise in enhancing antitumor effects across various malignancies. In this chapter, we explore the interconnection between ferroptosis and cuproptosis, elucidate their underlying mechanisms, and discuss their potential as druggable targets in both cancer research and clinical settings.

J. Wang · L. K. Y. Chan · T. Zhang · J. Liu · T. S. Lau · C. C. Wang (✉)
Department of Obstetrics & Gynaecology, The Chinese University of Hong Kong, Hong Kong, China
e-mail: ccwang@cuhk.edu.hk

J. Li
Department of Surgery, Li Ka Shing Faculty of Medicine, The University of Hong Kong, Pokfulam, Hong Kong, China

Interdisciplinary Cancer Research, https://doi.org/10.1007/16833_2024_233
Published online: 20 June 2024

Keywords

Cancer · Copper · Cuproptosis · Drug resistance · Ferroptosis · Iron

1 Introduction

In cancer biology, the regulation of cell death mechanisms has been a topic of great interest and study. In the study of regulated cell death (RCD), various mechanisms with unique characteristics and physiological importance have been discovered. Two notable forms of RCD, ferroptosis and cuproptosis, have emerged in cancer research. Both of these mechanisms rely on metal ions, iron and copper, respectively. Ferroptosis was discovered in 2012 along with selective inhibition of small molecules inducing non-apoptotic RCD which was iron dependent. It was introduced to be different from forms of RCD in terms of morphology, biochemistry, and genetics. Very recently, cuproptosis was described by Tsvetkov et al. in 2021 (Dixon et al. 2012; Tsvetkov et al. 2022). Understanding these pathways is crucial as it opens up possibilities for combined therapies and clinical trials. The ability to manipulate ferroptosis and cuproptosis in cancer treatment represents an exciting frontier that could revolutionize therapeutic approaches and improve patient outcomes (Tong et al. 2022; Xie et al. 2023). Nevertheless, the exploitability of iron- and copper-induced cell death for cancer patients can also pose serious risks and complications for normal cells and adjacent T cells and macrophages (Wang et al. 2020a; Murdoch and Skaar 2022). This chapter provides an in-depth review of the underlying mechanisms that drive ferroptosis and cuproptosis, their interplay, and the practical implications of harnessing these pathways for cancer treatment. By integrating molecular insights, case studies, state of the art, and future perspectives, this chapter underscores the importance of ferroptosis and cuproptosis in cancer research and therapeutic approaches.

2 Mechanisms of Ferroptosis and Cuproptosis

2.1 Comprehensive Overview of Ferroptosis

Ferroptosis is a unique form of iron-dependent regulated cell death, distinct from apoptosis, necrosis, and autophagy. Ferroptosis plays a role in neurodegeneration, ischemia-reperfusion injury, and cancer (Belaidi and Bush 2016; Ma et al. 2016; Li et al. 2019). The core machinery of ferroptosis includes lipid peroxidation, glutathione (GSH), glutathione peroxidase 4 (GPX4), iron metabolism, amino acid, and polyunsaturated fatty acid (PUFA) metabolism. These mechanisms and pathways collectively summarize the complex biological process of ferroptosis.

2.1.1 Lipid Peroxidation and Reactive Oxygen Species

Lipid peroxidation, driven by reactive oxygen species (ROS), acts as a key event in ferroptosis (Yang and Stockwell 2016). ROS, especially iron-derived ROS, can oxidize PUFA in phospholipids, resulting in the generation of lipid hydroperoxides (Latunde-Dada 2017). If these lipid hydroperoxides are not efficiently balanced, they can damage cellular membranes, causing ferroptosis (Li et al. 2020). The balance between production and removal of lipid ROS is crucial. GPX4 uses GSH to reduce lipid hydroperoxides, preventing lipid peroxidation. The Xc–antiporter system regulates cystine uptake for GSH synthesis (Wang et al. 2020b). Therapeutic investigations are underway to explore molecules targeting enzymes and transporters involved in regulating ferroptosis in cancer. Inhibitors of system Xc– (e.g., erastin, sorafenib, sulfasalazine) and direct GPX4 inhibitors (e.g., ML162, ML210) exhibit promise in modulating ferroptosis. Recent studies highlight the therapeutic potential of targeting these components in cancer. Repression of SLC7A11, a component of system Xc–, renders hepatocellular carcinoma (HCC) cells susceptible to GPX4 inhibition (Kim et al. 2020). The system Xc–/GSH/GPX4 axis has been identified as an important antioxidant system in ferroptosis, especially in drug-resistant solid tumors (Li et al. 2022a). Inhibitors of system Xc– or GPX4 disrupt antioxidants or elevate lipid hydroperoxides, selectively eliminating cancer cells while preserving healthy ones. Targeting cancer cell metabolism through this strategy presents a potential for more effective and less toxic treatments.

2.1.2 GSH and GPX4

GPX4 is a key enzyme in ferroptosis. It converts lipid hydroperoxides to lipid alcohols, preventing the formation of toxic lipid ROS that depends on iron. Inhibiting GPX4 induces lipid peroxidation and triggers ferroptosis (Forcina and Dixon 2019). Targeting GPX4 exhibits therapeutic potential in cancer cells. Activation of the Wnt/β-catenin pathway mitigates lipid ROS and impedes ferroptosis in gastric cancer cells. The β-catenin/TCF4 complex directly binds to the GPX4 promoter, inducing its expression (Wang et al. 2022b). Additionally, dihydroorotate dehydrogenase (DHODH) modulates ferroptosis induced by GPX4 inhibition. Modulating DHODH activity can either augment or mitigate the consequences of GPX4 inhibition in cellular contexts. The interplay between DHODH and GPX4 pathways adds complexity to the regulatory mechanisms influencing ferroptosis (Mao et al. 2021). Moreover, p53 also exerts a complex and bidirectional role in ferroptosis by regulating GSH and GPX4 (Liu and Gu 2022; Xu et al. 2023b). Chemotherapy-resistant cancer cells, characterized by heightened iron dependency, exhibit vulnerability to ferroptosis upon GPX4 inhibition. This strategy enhances iron-catalyzed lipid ROS production, providing a promising therapeutic avenue for combating cancer effectively (Hassannia et al. 2019; Seibt et al. 2019).

2.1.3 Iron Metabolism

Iron metabolism plays a crucial role in ferroptosis. Cells employ transferrin receptors (TfR1) for iron acquisition, directing it toward storage in ferritin or iron-containing proteins. Disruptions in this equilibrium elevate cellular iron levels, heightening susceptibility to ferroptosis (Chen et al. 2020). The labile iron pool (LIP) contains a fraction of cellular iron. This iron reservoir can engage in Fenton reactions, producing ROS that oxidizes polyunsaturated fatty acids in phospholipids, initiating lipid peroxidation (Masaldan et al. 2019). To maintain iron homeostasis, cells export excess iron through ferroportin and utilize iron regulatory proteins (IRPs) to modulate the expression of genes involved in iron metabolism (Fan et al. 2022). Moreover, strategies targeting iron metabolism, such as using iron chelators or modifiers of iron-associated proteins, hold promise despite inhibiting ferroptosis (Wang et al. 2020b; Chen et al. 2020). The significance of iron in cancer and how its metabolic modulation can offer therapeutic benefits has been widely investigated (Morales and Xue 2021). Advancements in nanotherapeutics hold a versatile platform for regulating iron metabolism in cancer biology (Lin et al. 2022). The intersection of iron metabolism with ferroptosis has also emphasized the role of iron in cancer pathogenesis and treatment (Luo et al. 2021).

2.1.4 PUFA Metabolism

As PUFAs, arachidonic acid and adrenic acid are highly susceptible to lipid peroxidation. The enzymes acyl-CoA synthetase long chain family member 4 (ACSL4) and lysophosphatidylcholine acyltransferase 3 (LPCAT3) are key drivers of this process, with ACSL4 enriching cellular membranes, particularly those containing arachidonic acid and adrenic acid, making them primary targets for lipid peroxidation (Yang et al. 2022a). Once these PUFAs are incorporated into phospholipids like phosphatidylethanolamine (PE) and phosphatidylcholine (PC), they become predisposed to oxidation. The equilibrium between PUFA incorporation, their subsequent oxidation, and the neutralization of these oxidized products is a determining factor in cell sensitivity to ferroptosis (Zhang et al. 2022b).

2.2 Comprehensive Overview of Cuproptosis

Cuproptosis is triggered by excessive intracellular copper in cancer cells (Tsvetkov et al. 2022). While an essential cofactor for many enzymes and proteins, excess copper can be toxic to cells. Copper-ion balance is vital for cellular health, as imbalances can lead to cell death or carcinogenesis. This section explores cuproptosis, focusing on intracellular copper accumulation and its impact on copper dynamics, mitochondrial metabolism, lipoylated proteins in the tricarboxylic acid (TCA) cycle, iron-sulfur cluster proteins, and oxidative phosphorylation.

2.2.1 Intracellular Copper Accumulation

Excess extracellular and consequently intracellular copper triggers cuproptosis, initiated by copper binding and transport to cell compartments, mainly facilitated by elesclomol, an investigational small molecule anticancer drug (Soma et al. 2018; Tsvetkov et al. 2022). In the extracellular environment, elesclomol, as a Cu ionophore, binds to copper and transports it to the intracellular compartment, causing copper accumulation within cells (Gohil 2021; Zulkifli et al. 2023).

Metallochaperones control intracellular copper levels by transporting copper ions and serving as buffers to regulate the transcriptional responsiveness and efficiency of copper efflux mechanisms (Pang et al. 2013). The regulation of copper trafficking and accumulation within cells is controlled by copper transporter 1 (Ctr1), ATP7A, and ATP7B. Ctr1 is a membrane copper transporter belonging to the SLC31 family of solute carriers (Bertinato and L'Abbe 2004). It serves as the primary channel for copper transportation into cells (La Fontaine and Mercer 2007). ATP7A and ATP7B are copper-exporting P-type ATPase pumps. Being primarily located in the trans-Golgi network, ATP7A and ATP7B, upon copper accumulation, these transporters relocate to vesicles, which eventually fuse with the cell membranes. They coordinate copper movement by adjusting its uptake, internal distribution, and export, being key in regulating and sustaining mammalian copper balance (La Fontaine and Mercer 2007). However, the expressions, distributions, and functions of ATP7A and ATP7B are not identical (Linz and Lutsenko 2007). Specifically, while ATP7A is vital for cuproenzyme creation and needed in enterocytes for copper export to portal blood, ATP7B mediates the secretion of excess copper into the bile in addition to the incorporation of copper into proteins (Lutsenko et al. 2007). ATP7A and ATP7B overexpression in cancers is associated with platinum drug resistance and impacts prognosis and treatment outcomes (Li et al. 2018).

2.2.2 Aggregation of Lipoylated Proteins

Aggregation of mitochondrial lipoylated proteins is a hallmark of cuproptosis (Li et al. 2022b; Tang et al. 2022). Lipoylation, a posttranslational modification involving the attachment of lipoic acid to mitochondrial proteins, is essential for their function. In cuproptosis, ferredoxin 1 (FDX1) mediates the reduction of copper ions from Cu2+ to Cu+, facilitating this modification. FDX1 serves as a protein target of elesclomol (Wu et al. 2023b). Lipoylation primarily targets enzymes involved in the TCA cycle, with dihydrolipoamide S-acetyltransferase (DLAT) being a key target. The interaction between copper ions and these enzymes, particularly DLAT, leads to the formation of lipoylated protein clusters through disulfide bonds. This process induces proteotoxic stress mainly within the mitochondria (Tsvetkov et al. 2022). Protein aggregation stresses mitochondria, impairing the TCA cycle and contributing to cuproptosis (Tsvetkov et al. 2022). FDX1 aids in toxic lipoylated DLAT buildup, contributing to cuproptotic cell death (Tang et al. 2022). Exploring the involvement of FDX1 in lipoylation and its link to copper-induced proteotoxic stress reveals insights into cuproptosis, suggesting possible therapeutic strategies (Wu et al. 2023b).

2.2.3 Destabilization of Iron-Sulfur Cluster Proteins

Copper has been found to directly bind to lipoylated TCA cycle proteins. This binding leads to a disulfide-bond-dependent aggregation of these proteins, causing the degradation of iron-sulfur (Fe-S) cluster proteins (Xiong et al. 2023). Copper also indirectly affects mitochondrial function regarding mitochondrial iron uptake, as it acts as a cofactor for ferroxidases (Xu et al. 2013). The transport of iron is crucial for the assembly of iron-sulfur (Fe-S) clusters, which are essential for various mitochondrial functions including heme biosynthesis (Lill and Freibert 2020). The primary characteristic of cuproptosis is the aggregation of copper-bound, lipoylated mitochondrial proteins and the loss of Fe-S cluster proteins. At a proteomic level, this loss includes proteins such as POLD1, NUBP2, CISD1, ISCU, GLRX3, SDHB, and PPAT, which verifies the occurrence of cuproptosis (Yang et al. 2022b). The degradation and loss of Fe-S cluster proteins disrupt various mitochondrial functions as Fe-S clusters are crucial cofactors for many mitochondrial enzymes.

2.2.4 Oxidative Phosphorylation Disruption

Cuproptosis disrupts oxidative phosphorylation, causing mitochondrial dysfunction and cell death by targeting and aggregating lipoylated proteins in the TCA cycle, impacting Fe-S clusters (Chen et al. 2022b; Tang et al. 2022). This occurs mainly in cells relying on oxidative phosphorylation for energy. The aggregation of lipoylated proteins and reduced Fe-S clusters disrupts the mitochondrial electron transport chain (mtETC) and the TCA cycle (Yang et al. 2023a). It has been noted that inhibitors of oxidative phosphorylation might inhibit cuproptosis by suppressing the protein stress response (Wang et al. 2023a). Genes like LIPT1, LIAS, DLD, DLAT, PDHA1, and PDHB are important in the lipoic acid pathway and lipoylation of proteins. The direct interaction between copper and lipoylated proteins in the TCA cycle results in disulfide-bond-driven aggregation and the collapse of Fe-S cluster proteins (Xiong et al. 2023). Researchers have developed cuproptosis-related signatures with cuproptosis-related genes (CRGs) to explore the link between cuproptosis and cancer. This sheds light on the genetic basis of cuproptosis and its association with the disruption of oxidative phosphorylation (Xie et al. 2023) (Fig. 1).

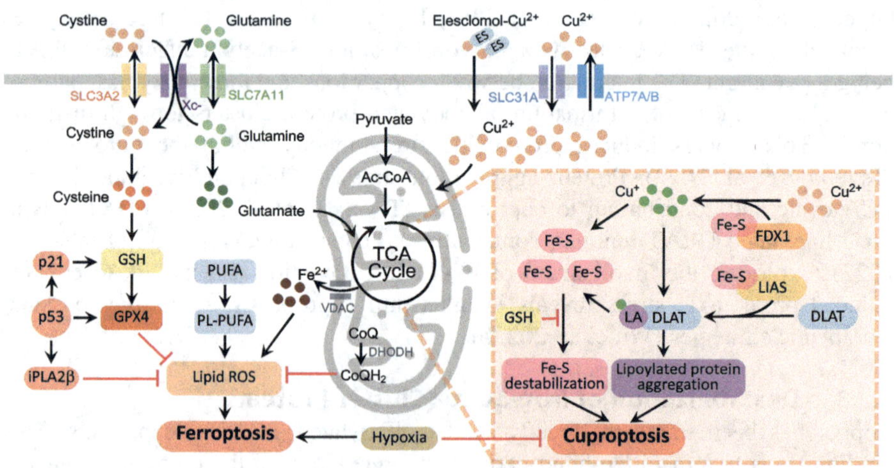

Fig. 1 Mechanisms of ferroptosis and cuproptosis. Ferroptosis is characterized by iron-dependent lipid peroxidation. Cystine uptake from the extracellular environment is facilitated by Xc−, composed of SLC3A2 and SLC7A11. GPX4 utilizes GSH synthesized from cystine to neutralize lipid peroxides. P53 regulates ferroptosis in canonical and non-canonical ways. VDAC regulates

3 Interplay Between Ferroptosis and Cuproptosis in Cancer

3.1 Crosstalk Between Ferroptosis and Cuproptosis

Distinct molecular signatures characterize ferroptosis and cuproptosis. Ferroptosis inducers can potentially amplify cuproptosis in liver cancer cells by promoting the aggregation of copper-dependent lipoylated proteins. Moreover, ferroptosis inducers enhance cellular copper by inhibiting cystine import for glutathione synthesis as an alternative intracellular copper chelator (Wang et al. 2023b). Combining ferroptosis inducers and cuproptosis-inducing agents significantly reduced liver cancer growth in vivo by enhancing cuproptosis. Copper plays a crucial role as a vital cofactor for metalloenzymes like cytochrome c oxidase (COX). Copper depletion also limited GPX4 expression, the sole enzyme, and the core molecule preventing lipid peroxidation. These links suggest synergistic therapeutic effects when co-targeting metal-induced cell deaths.

3.2 The Role of Cellular Metabolism and Microenvironment

The interplay between ferroptosis and cuproptosis might be crucial in the tumor microenvironment (TME) (Shen et al. 2022). A recent study identified three distinct clusters named CuFeclusters, representing three distinct gene subsets based on cuproptosis and ferroptosis regulation. These clusters align with three immune phenotypes of tumors (Shen et al. 2022). TME and cellular metabolism significantly influence ferroptosis and cuproptosis. The interplay between ferroptosis and the immune system in the TME affects tumor progression and antitumor immunity (Mbah and Lyssiotis 2022). Key metabolic pathways such as glycolysis, pentose phosphate pathway, and TCA cycle are involved in the regulation of ferroptosis markers including reduced nicotinamide adenine dinucleotide phosphate (NADPH), glutathione, and ROS (Yao et al. 2021). Other metabolic pathways including selenol/thiol metabolism, fatty acid metabolism, iron, mevalonate pathway, and mitochondrial respiration also impact ferroptosis and cell sensitivity to lipid peroxidation (Zheng and Conrad 2020). In an inflammatory milieu, ferroptosis modulation can be orchestrated by metabolic flux or the secretion and exchange of bioactive substances

Fig. 1 (continued) mitochondrial metabolism and iron homeostasis. When bound to copper, elesclomol generates ROS which can trigger cuproptosis. ATP7A and ATP7B serve as copper-transporter ATPases and maintain copper homeostasis. Mutations in these transporters can lead to copper overload, eventually leading to Fe-S cluster destabilization. Copper can enhance the lipoylation of proteins, leading to their aggregation. FDX1, LIAS, and DLAT are associated with mitochondrial function and iron-sulfur cluster synthesis. Copper-induced aggregation of lipoylated DLAT, mediated by FDX1, is known to contribute to the mechanism of cuproptosis. Alterations in TCA cycle enzymes or metabolites in addition to copper and iron dysregulation might affect the redox status of the cell, influencing susceptibility to ferroptosis or cuproptosis

between microorganisms and host cells, or intercellularly among host cells (Dou et al. 2022). Cuproptosis correlates with distinct TME patterns, influencing prognosis, tumor subtypes, immune response, and therapeutic outcomes. (Xiang et al. 2021; Zhu et al. 2022b; Nie et al. 2023).

3.3 Mitochondria as a Bridge Between Ferroptosis and Cuproptosis

Mitochondria connect ferroptosis and cuproptosis. Ferroptosis induces mitochondrial changes, shifting energy metabolism and causing oxidative stress. Cuproptosis, driven by intracellular copper overload, initiates FDX1-mediated mitochondrial proteotoxic stress, impairing functionality. Investigating mitochondrial mechanisms may reveal targeted oncology therapeutic strategies.

3.3.1 Mitochondria and Ferroptosis

Mitochondria and ferroptosis strongly impact each other by regulating iron metabolism and lipid peroxidation. This process triggers a shift in energy metabolism, reducing glycolysis and altering oxidative phosphorylation, highlighting mitochondria's role as primary ATP producers (Zhang et al. 2022b). Excessive stress causes irreversible damage to mitochondria, compromising their structure and function. As the main source of ROS, mitochondria play a central role in both the production and management of ROS during ferroptosis (Masaldan et al. 2019). During ferroptosis, mitochondria experience morphological alterations (Li et al. 2023). These changes include damage to mitochondrial cristae and a more condensed mitochondrial membrane density (Li et al. 2020; Yang et al. 2023b). The mitochondria also appear smaller in volume compared to their normal state, and there is a noticeable reduction or even disappearance of the mitochondrial cristae and outer membrane (Otasevic et al. 2021). The modulation of ferroptosis includes diverse cellular metabolic and signaling cascades, wherein processes such as mitochondrial fusion, fission, and mitophagy are crucial constituents of this modulation (Liu et al. 2023b). Mitochondrial dysfunction, triggered by factors such as reperfusion-induced ROS production, frequently surpasses the capabilities of cellular antioxidant defenses, thus highlighting the intricate connection between mitochondrial function and the modulation of ferroptosis (She et al. 2023). Certain mitochondrial lipids, notably cardiolipin, are direct substrates for lipid peroxidation, linking mitochondrial vitality to ferroptotic cell death. Peroxidation of cardiolipin damages and permeabilizes the mitochondrial membrane, impairing its structure and function (Rochette et al. 2022).

3.3.2 Mitochondria and Cuproptosis

Cuproptosis is initiated by the accumulation of copper within cytoplasm and organelles, leading to the aggregation of mitochondrial lipoylated modules and the destabilization of Fe-S cluster proteins, which are crucial for normal mitochondrial function (Chen et al. 2022b; Tang et al. 2022). Unlike ferroptosis, cuproptosis relies on galactose-mediated mitochondrial respiration, impacting cells using the TCA cycle more than those dependent on glucose-induced glycolysis (Lee et al. 2020; Song et al. 2021). Cuproptosis closely links to mitochondrial respiration, and its sensitivity is influenced by the mitochondrial respiratory state. Unlike ferroptosis, cuproptosis sensitivity decreases under hypoxia, which directs to glycolysis rather than oxidative phosphorylation, emphasizing the importance of mitochondrial respiration and oxygen involvement in the cuproptosis process (Tang et al. 2022; Yuan et al. 2022). Two mitochondrial proteotoxic stress pathways mediate cuproptosis. Copper overload increases mitochondrial protein lipoylation, causing disulfide-bond-dependent aggregation of lipoylated DLAT. This FDX1-mediated accumulation of toxic lipoylated DLAT, coupled with the degradation of Fe-S cluster proteins, underscores the unique cellular demise mechanism in cuproptosis (Tang et al. 2022).

3.3.3 Mitochondrial Crosstalk Between Ferroptosis and Cuproptosis

Mitochondria act as potential metal pools and mitochondrial respiratory chains work as oxygen sensors under hypoxia conditions. Due to their unique mechanisms related to mitochondrial metabolisms, ferroptosis and cuproptosis show distinct vulnerabilities when exposed to hypoxia (Oh et al. 2022; Tang et al. 2022). In cuproptosis, excess intracellular copper triggers lipoylated DLAT aggregation, causing proteotoxic stress. Mitochondrial dysfunction–associated ROS can induce various regulated cell deaths, including ferroptosis. Degradation of the copper-exporter ATP7A in colorectal cancer cells, in addition to inducing cuproptosis, increases ROS, inducing antitumor activity via ferroptosis (Chen et al. 2022b; Shen et al. 2022). A scoring scheme named CuFescore was established to predict the response to immunotherapy and chemotherapeutic drugs based on the regulators of cuproptosis and ferroptosis (Shen et al. 2022). While lipoylation proteins within the TCA cycle serve as a determinant in cuproptosis, ferroptosis inducers sorafenib or erastin could modulate protein lipoylation through FDX1 (Wang et al. 2023b). Mitochondria rely on iron, copper, and calcium for efficient ATP production. The mitochondrial electron transport chain and other mitochondrial functions are modulated by these metal ions, impacting both ferroptosis and cuproptosis (Prasad Panda and Kesharwani 2023). This also suggests a novel strategy to co-target cuproptosis and ferroptosis by aiming at mitochondria in cancer treatment.

4 Iron/Copper Addiction in Cancer

Iron, indispensable for DNA synthesis and cellular respiration, is essential for cancer progression. The metabolism of iron often exhibits dysregulation within cancer cells, leading to tumor initiation, proliferation, and metastasis (Torti and Torti 2020). On the other hand, excessive intracellular copper accumulation shares similar biological functions with iron overload, which makes the targeting of copper metabolism a promising therapeutic avenue for oncological intervention (Kong and Sun 2023).

4.1 Iron Addiction of Cancer Cells

The phenomenon of "iron addiction" in cancer cells refers to the heightened dependency on iron over benign cells (Torti and Torti 2020). Cancers such as gliomas (Han et al. 2018), breast cancer (Torti and Torti 2013), and prostate cancer (Tesfay et al. 2015) exhibit dysregulated iron homeostasis, necessitating excess iron for their metabolism and growth. In these cells, there is an increased pool of labile iron which catalyzes reactions generating ROS, potentially driving further malignancy (Salnikow 2021). Iron addiction in cancer cells has a strong interconnection with ferroptosis. The dependence on iron is not just for growth, but it also highlights various cell death pathways, including ferroptosis (Torti et al. 2018). Moreover, iron dependency is a vulnerability that can be therapeutically targeted either through the administration of iron-dependent anticancer agents or by manipulating iron concentrations within the neoplastic cells (Jiang et al. 2022).

4.2 Copper Addiction of Cancer Cells

Cancer cells exhibit a high dependency on copper, akin to their iron addiction. A study revealed the crucial role of mitochondrial copper in maintaining a mesenchymal state in cancer cells. Metformin was identified as a direct inhibitor of the epithelial-to-mesenchymal transition by targeting copper (Muller et al. 2018). Copper is a key nutrient limiting cancer cell growth. Oral copper chelators, when taken with food, show anti-neoplastic and anti-metastatic benefits in both animal and human studies (Shanbhag et al. 2021). Copper, a key cofactor for metalloenzymes, influences malignant progression. Depleting copper with agents like tetrathiomolybdate (TM) modulates mitochondrial oxidative phosphorylation in breast cancer cells, affecting cell metabolism (Ramchandani et al. 2021). Copper is a key component for enzymes controlling the tumor microenvironment and appears to play a role in cancer cell migration. Copper depletion has been shown to decrease breast cancer cell and prostate cancer cell proliferation (McCarty 2003; Lopez et al. 2019).

4.3 Iron and Copper Labile Pool

4.3.1 LIP in Cancer Cells

Labile iron pool (LIP) is identified as a determinant of the sensitivity of cancer cells to particular therapies such as intravenous ascorbate therapy (McCarty and Contreras 2014). LIP in cancer cells can transit certain compounds from nontoxic to toxic, and increased LIP levels in tumor cells can enable chemodynamic therapy of cancer (Lin et al. 2020). The labile iron pool in cancer cells is usually increased with the increasing amount of ROS, which can cause DNA mutations, damage proteins, and lipids, and lead to either cell death or transformation (Salnikow 2021). Iron, obtained through specific transporters, constitutes the metabolically active cytoplasmic LIP. Malignant tumors exhibit aberrant regulation of iron metabolism-related proteins, highlighting the increased need for iron in cancer cell proliferation (Wang et al. 2018). In these cells, the labile iron pool represents no more than 5% of the total iron content, and due to imbalanced iron metabolism, cancer cells exhibit an increased dependence on iron compared with normal cells (Salnikow 2021).

4.3.2 Labile Copper Pool in Cancer Cells

Changes to the labile copper pool can be analyzed using fluorescent small-molecule indicators, emphasizing the growing importance of copper in cancer as a regulator of tumor cell proliferation (Ackerman and Chang 2018). Bioluminescent probes have also been utilized to measure the labile copper concentration in cells, as discussed in a study on mitochondrial copper depletion suppressing triple-negative breast cancer (TNBC) (Cui et al. 2021). Cellular copper ions are found in either a static pool or a labile pool where it is weakly bound to cellular ligands and is mobile. Mismanagement of cellular copper pools can result in oxidative stress and the formation of ROS (Priessner et al. 2021).

4.3.3 Clinical Implications

One of the strategies targeting LIP to enhance the chemodynamic therapy and in situ Near-Infrared-II (NIR-II) photothermal therapy is through the development of a novel nanomedicine (CuHCF) based on a mixed-metal (Cu2+/ Fe3+) Prussian blue analog. It has provided a promising approach for precise medicine in cancer (Chen et al. 2023). Another strategy has been presented that employs the intracellular LIP as the endogenous source of Fenton-reactive metals to trigger free radical generation. Hydroperoxides have been identified as an optimal agent for LIP-mediated chemodynamic therapy against cancer cells (Lin et al. 2020). Various promising approaches are being explored in cancer therapeutics to modulate iron metabolism (Morales and Xue 2021). A potential strategy involves the enhancement of intracellular LIP that subsequently drives the ferroptotic death of cancer cells. Strategies like copper chelation therapy and nanotechnology for targeted delivery of copper-targeting agents are also being explored (Kong and Sun 2023). Copper ionophores, as metal-binding compounds, have shown potential for cancer treatment. However, copper ionophores are still in the early stages of development, with the lack of selectivity being one of the major challenges in this area (Oliveri 2022).

5 Targeting Cancer Stem Cells (CSCs) and Drug Resistance Through Ferroptosis/Cuproptosis

CSCs possess unique features rendering them sensitive to certain cell death mechanisms, which can be exploited to overcome drug resistance and eradicate tumors (Elgendy et al. 2020). Ferroptosis has shown promise in targeting drug-resistant cancer cells (Ozkan and Bakar-Ates 2022). It is believed that complete tumor eradication could be achieved by targeting CSCs which could be through the induction of ferroptosis in these cells (Elgendy et al. 2020). Researchers are investigating the link between ferroptosis and drug resistance in tumors (Nie et al. 2022). High mitochondrial respiratory status in breast cancer cells causes resistance to antitumor drugs like proteasome inhibitors. Yet, these drug-resistant cancer cells show sensitivity toward copper ionophore and cuproptosis inducer, elesclomol, suggesting a novel therapeutic role of cuproptosis for overcoming drug resistance (Tsvetkov et al. 2019).

5.1 Drug Resistance and Ferroptosis

Iron metabolism is expected to be disrupted in cancer cells, which often causes multidrug resistance in cancer. Manipulate pathophysiology related to iron holds the promise to overcome drug resistance in cancer (Brown et al. 2020; Roemhild et al. 2021). Unbalanced ferroptosis inevitably leads to chemotherapy resistance and tumor recurrence, largely due to aberrant iron metabolism and lipid peroxidation (Friedmann Angeli et al. 2019; Nie et al. 2022; Zhang et al. 2022a). High hydrogen peroxide levels in cancer cells can induce ferroptosis by interacting with iron ions. Modulating ferroptosis may reverse cancer resistance to standard treatments, offering a promising approach to overcome drug resistance by targeting redox homeostasis (Nie et al. 2022). Carcinoma cells show maximum drug resistance when their epithelial-to-mesenchymal transition (EMT) program is activated to an intermediate level. Targeting specific stages of EMT could help overcome drug resistance. Mesenchymal cancer cells are more prone to ferroptosis, suggesting a potential therapeutic strategy for targeting and inducing ferroptosis in mesenchymal rather than epithelial cells (Shibue and Weinberg 2017; Ren et al. 2023).

5.2 Drug Resistance and Cuproptosis

Copper exerts its role as a tumor promoter primarily by modulating cellular proliferation and promoting the development of drug resistance. Cuproptosis has been suggested to potentially impact tumor drug resistance behavior (Zhang et al. 2023a). In particular, nano-drug-based cuproptosis targeting approaches are expected to be combined with conventional treatments to improve the efficiency of anticancer therapeutics (Lu et al. 2022). Some studies have constructed prediction models of different types of cuproptosis to address these approaches (Qi et al. 2022). Drug-resistant tumors often exhibit heightened mitochondrial metabolism. Treatment of tumor cells with specific antitumor drugs, like proteasome inhibitors, increases mitochondrial metabolism. This suggests a crucial link between cuproptosis and cancer progression (Xie et al. 2023). The discovery of cuproptosis opens up possibilities for clinical applications, including the use of copper ion ionophores to induce cuproptosis in combination with small molecule drugs for targeted therapy (Wang et al. 2024).

5.3 Persister Cells

Cancer persister cells are a subpopulation of cancer cells that can survive despite anticancer treatments, contributing to treatment resistance and cancer recurrence. These cells exhibit a unique metabolic state compared to the bulk tumor cells, which includes an addiction to metal ions (Rodriguez et al. 2022). Targeting iron metabolism could potentially induce ferroptosis in persister cells, offering a strategy to challenge drug-resistant cancer cells (Rodriguez et al. 2022). The crosstalk between lipid metabolism reprogramming and ferroptosis is deemed significant, with ongoing research exploring its potential in antitumor immunity and cancer therapy, by potentially exploiting the metabolic vulnerabilities of persister cells to enhance treatment outcomes (Tousignant et al. 2020; You et al. 2021; Rodriguez et al. 2022; Lee et al. 2023a).

5.4 Cancer Stem Cells

CSCs are found in tumors or hematological cancers that have characteristics akin to normal stem cells. CSCs contribute to conventional therapy–acquired resistance and are partially responsible for tumor heterogeneity (Kusoglu and Biray Avci 2019; Elgendy et al. 2020). Furthermore, targeting ferroptosis has shown promising results in eradicating CSCs (Xu et al. 2023a). Given potential alterations in lipid metabolism, CSCs might exhibit heightened susceptibility to lipid peroxidation, and eventually, ferroptosis. Leveraging this weakness of CSCs and developing strategies to exploit the sensitivity of CSCs to ferroptosis could potentially unveil a new horizon in cancer therapeutics (Elgendy et al. 2020). Excessive intracellular copper ions can be toxic to cells, and this toxicity could be harnessed to target CSCs, given their potential unique sensitivities to oxidative stress (Wang et al. 2023d).

6 Clinical Trials Targeting Ferroptosis and Cuproptosis

6.1 Ongoing Clinical Trials Targeting Ferroptosis and Iron Metabolism

Recently, ferroptosis-associated long noncoding RNAs (lncRNA) have been studied in different cancer types such as laryngeal squamous carcinoma (Dong et al. 2023), renal cell carcinoma (Zong et al. 2023; Ju et al. 2022), hepatocellular carcinoma (Lian et al. 2022), and lung adenocarcinoma (Gao et al. 2022) have been studied in clinical trials as prognostic and predictive models. Among them, multiple significant lncRNAs have been identified.

Clinical trials targeting iron metabolism are summarized in Table 1.

Table 1 Clinical trials targeting iron metabolism

Cancer type	Target	Substance	Phase	Outcome	Patients enrolled	Status	Reason for termination	References
Hematological malignancy, cancer-related anemia	Iron	Shengxuening tablet/ferrous succinate	Phase 3	Promoting hematopoietic function and potentially addressing anemia in hematological tumor patients	168	Recruiting	–	NCT05784870
Multiple types (e.g., colorectal, pancreatic, breast, gastric, cervical, lung, head and neck, prostate)	Iron metabolism	CNSI-Fe(II)	Phase I	CNSI-Fe (II) shows promise as an innovative tumor therapeutic agent due to its unique properties of ferroptosis (not yet finished)	24	Recruiting	–	NCT06048367
Gastrointestinal stromal tumor (GIST)	Iron deficiency anemia (IDA)	Ferric carboxymaltose	Phase 2	Not specified (the goal of this clinical research study is to compare Injectafer® (ferric carboxymaltose) with an iron supplement to learn which may be more effective in improving red blood cell counts in patients who have iron-deficiency anemia)	3	Terminated with results	Terminated per PI's request	NCT02949947

Gynecologic cancer, anemia, iron-deficiency	Iron-deficiency anemia	Ferric derisomaltose	Phase 3	The study aims to assess the effectiveness of preoperative ferric derisomaltose/iron isomaltoside compared to placebo in correcting preoperative hemoglobin in patients undergoing surgery for gynecologic malignancy	82	Not yet recruiting	–	NCT05407987
Colorectal cancer	Iron-deficiency	Iron (III) isomaltoside	Phase 2	Investigate the effects of intravenously administered iron on physical capacity and immune function prior to surgery	134	Not yet recruiting	–	NCT05220800
Ovarian, pancreatic, colorectal, head and neck, lung neoplasms	Hepcidin /IL-6	Siltuximab (CNTO 328)	Phase 1/2	Improves cancer patient anemia	84	Completed	–	NCT00841191
Myelodysplastic syndromes	Iron overload	Iron chelation therapy	Phase 3	MDS event-free survival (EFS)	225	Completed	–	NCT00940602

(continued)

Table 1 (continued)

Cancer type	Target	Substance	Phase	Outcome	Patients enrolled	Status	Reason for termination	References
Solid tumors	Liposomal drug functionalized with transferrin	SGT-94 (*RB94* gene in a liposome targeted to tumor cells)	Phase 1	Evaluate safety & MTD of SGT-94, seek evidence of RB94 expression in tumor tissue	13	Completed	–	NCT01517464
Anemia of chronic disease	Hepcidin/ Ferroportin (FPN)	Spiegelmer NOX-H94 (Lexaptepid Pegol)	Phase 1	This study aims to determine the safety, tolerability, and efficacy of NOX-H94 in patients with anemia of chronic disease (ACD). The treatment with NOX-H94 is expected to inhibit the patho-mechanism by binding and inactivating hepcidin	12	Completed	–	NCT01691040
Anemia of chronic disease	Hepcidin/FPN	Spiegelmer NOX-H94 (Lexaptepid Pegol)	Phase 2	This study aims to determine the safety, tolerability, and efficacy of NOX-H94 in patients with anemia of chronic disease (ACD). The treatment with	64	Completed	–	NCT01372137

				NOX-H94 is expected to inhibit the patho-mechanism by binding and inactivating hepcidin				
Triple-negative inflammatory breast cancer	TfR	Transferrin receptor–targeted liposomal p53 cDNA (SGT-53)	Phase 1	Feasibility and preliminary activity of SGT-53 with carboplatin and pembrolizumab in metastatic triple-negative inflammatory breast cancer	0	Withdrawn	Funding issues and pharmacy preparation for the drug	NCT05093387
Chronic myeloproliferative disorders, leukemia, lymphoma, multiple myeloma, and plasma cell neoplasm	Antitransferrin receptor	Monoclonal antibodies E2.3 and A27.15	Phase 1	Determine the toxicities associated with a 4-h infusion of antitransferrin receptor antibodies. Determine the pharmacokinetics of monoclonal antibodies E2.3 and A27.15	27	Completed	–	NCT00003082

(continued)

Table 1 (continued)

Cancer type	Target	Substance	Phase	Outcome	Patients enrolled	Status	Reason for termination	References
Iron overload, accelerated phase chronic myelogenous leukemia, adult acute lymphoblastic leukemia in remission, adult acute myeloid leukemia in remission, and others	Iron overload	Deferasirox	Phase 2	Determine labile plasma iron (LPI) levels in iron-overloaded patients after allogeneic hematopoietic stem cell transplantation (HSCT). Determine the safety and tolerability of low-dose deferasirox in the post-allogeneic HSCT setting	1	Terminated with results	Low enrollment	NCT01159067
Hemochromatosis, myelodysplastic syndromes	Iron overload	Deferasirox	Not specified (observational study)	The study terminated due to challenges in recruiting patients with hemochromatosis	1	Terminated	Failure to recruit patients with hemochromatosis to the deferasirox arm	NCT01892644
Anemia, colorectal neoplasm	Iron overload	Ferric carboxymaltose, ferrous sulfate	Phase 4	The study aimed to investigate the efficacy of intravenous iron in treating preoperative anemia in colorectal patients	116	Completed	–	NCT01701310

Iron deficiency anemia secondary to IBD or gastric bypass	Iron overload	Injectafer, ferrous sulfate tablets	Phase 4	Evaluate the treatment response of Injectafer vs. oral iron in patients with varying hepcidin levels correlating the treatment response/hepcidin levels to more common laboratory parameters such as ferritin and C-reactive protein (CRP) levels	198	Completed with results	–	NCT02086968
Anemia of chronic disease in patients with cancer	Iron overload	NOX-H94	Phase 2	Determine the safety, tolerability, and efficacy of NOX-H94 in patients with anemia of chronic disease (ACD)	116	Completed	–	NCT01701310
Refractory advanced solid tumors	Iron chelation	VLX600	Phase 1	Evaluate the safety and tolerability of VLX600 in patients with refractory advanced solid tumors	19	Terminated	Slow recruitment and lack of efficacy despite the completion of several dose steps	NCT02222363

(continued)

Table 1 (continued)

Cancer type	Target	Substance	Phase	Outcome	Patients enrolled	Status	Reason for termination	References
Advanced solid tumors	Iron chelation	DpC	Phase 1	Evaluate the safety, tolerability, and evidence of antitumor activity of DpC in patients with advanced solid tumors	14	Completed	–	NCT02688101
Myelodysplastic syndromes	Iron overload	Deferasirox	Phase 4	Assess the safety and tolerability of oral deferasirox in adult transfusion-dependent myelodysplastic syndrome (MDS) patients with iron overload	24	Completed	–	NCT00117507
MDS	Iron	Deferiprone	Phase 2	Change in serum ferritin levels	19	Completed	–	NCT02477631
High-risk MDS or AML	Iron overload	Exjade (deferasirox)	Early phase 1	Examine the hematologic response rate of Exjade in patients with AML and high-risk MDS with chronic iron overload from blood transfusions	25	Completed	–	NCT02233504

6.2 Ongoing Clinical Trials Targeting Cuproptosis and Copper Metabolism

Clinical trials targeting cuproptosis and copper metabolism are less common than those focusing on iron metabolism.

Like ferroptosis, most clinical trials assessing cuproptosis are focused on recognizing the prognostic value of cuproptosis-associated lncRNAs. Cuproptosis-associated lncRNAs have been identified as prognostic markers of clinical outcomes and immunotherapeutic responses in cervical cancer (Kong et al. 2023), pancreatic adenocarcinoma (Cui et al. 2023), prostate carcinoma (Cheng et al. 2023), bladder cancer (Jiang et al. 2023), and breast cancer (Pan et al. 2023).

Clinical trials targeting copper metabolism are summarized in Table 2.

6.3 Iron and Copper Toxicity as a Challenge in Clinical Applications

The prooxidant activity of iron can cause oxidative DNA damage, posing high risks for developing cancerous cells. Individuals with conditions like hemochromatosis or iron overload have an increased risk of developing liver cancer due to iron toxicity (Fonseca-Nunes et al. 2014). Iron overload is related to hypoxia, autoxidation, and production of pro-inflammatory cytokines; thus, it is considered as a high-risk factor for tumorigenesis, e.g., colorectal cancer, liver cancer, and kidney cancer (Huang 2003). Iron is fundamental to cancer cell proliferation, metabolism, and metastasis. Its excess can be toxic, leading to malignant transformation, cancer progression, drug resistance, and immune evasion (Brown et al. 2020). While the ferroptosis-related gene, iron exporter Ferroportin (FPN) has low baseline expression levels (Gao et al. 2021), its inhibitor, hepcidin, is being more actively transcribed (Vela and Vela-Gaxha 2018). In cancer cells, the iron importer protein TFR1 is elevated, associated with a worse prognosis. Additionally, STEAPs and DMT1, two other proteins involved in iron transport and metabolism, are also increased in several cancers including colon cancer (Torti et al. 2018). Even though iron-induced ferroptosis can be exploited as a novel strategy for cancer treatment, high iron levels can also cause tissue damage and organ failure. Iron overload also disrupts the immune system, increasing susceptibility to infections and worsening tissue damage (Puliyel et al. 2015; Haschka et al. 2021). Copper's redox properties also make it both beneficial and toxic to cells. Tumor growth and metastasis have a heightened requirement for copper, making it a critical element in cancer biology. As a result, copper chelation therapy has shown promise as a cancer treatment by targeting the heightened copper demand in tumor cells, impacting cellular metabolism, and synergizing with other cancer therapies (Ge et al. 2022; Tang et al. 2023). On the other hand, copper ionophores, as another approach, offer promising potential as potent anticancer agents. Copper ionophores take advantage of the therapeutic window between normal and cancerous cells when increasing intracellular copper levels. They show superior efficacy compared to platinum-based drugs with reduced

Table 2 Clinical trials targeting copper metabolism

Cancer type	Target	Substance	Phase	Outcome	Patients enrolled	Status	Reason for termination	Reference
Head and neck tumors	Not specified	Copper isotope	Not specified	Determine if the distribution of 65Cu/63Cu is modified in tumoral tissues compared to healthy tissues	7	Unknown	–	NCT02864836
Glioblastoma multiforme	Radiation therapy	Disulfiram/copper with temozolomide	Phase 1/2	Determine drug uptake in tumor samples during surgery	35	Active, not recruiting	–	NCT02715609
Cervical cancer	64Cu-ATSM PET/CT	64Cu-ATSM PET/CT	Phase 2	Predict disease progression in patients undergoing standard-of-care treatment with cisplatin and radiation therapy	73	Terminated	Transfer of funding	NCT00794339
Melanoma	BRAF V600 mutation	Vemurafenib and trientine	Phase 1	Evaluate the safety of combination therapy with vemurafenib and trientine in patients with BRAF-mutated metastatic melanoma	0	Withdrawn	–	NCT02068079

Relapsed multiple myeloma	Not specified	Copper 64Cu-DOTA-daratumumab	Phase 1	Evaluate the extent of multiple myeloma in patients prior to the initiation of treatment and monitor disease status/response during and posttreatment	21	Active, not recruiting	–	NCT03311828
Breast carcinoma	Breast calcifications	64 cu-DOTA-alendronate PET imaging	Early phase 1	Evaluate the uptake of 64Cu-DOTA-alendronate in female patients with biopsy-proven malignant breast calcifications	1	Active, not recruiting	–	NCT03542695
Cancer cachexia	Not specified	Not specified	Not specified	Quality of life in cancer cachexia	80	Not yet recruiting	–	NCT05262192
Brain and central nervous system tumors	Not specified	Penicillamine, low copper diet	Phase 2	Effect of penicillamine and copper reduction on survival and time to progression	40	Completed	–	NCT00003751
Prostate cancer	Not specified	ATN-224	Phase 2	Determine the proportion of patients who do not have PSA progression for 24 weeks	50	Unknown status	–	NCT00405574

(continued)

Table 2 (continued)

Cancer type	Target	Substance	Phase	Outcome	Patients enrolled	Status	Reason for termination	Reference
Fallopian tube cancer, ovarian neoplasms malignant, peritoneal carcinoma	Not specified	Trientine, pegylated liposomal doxorubicin, carboplatin	Phase 1/phase 2	Determine the dose-limited toxicities and maximal toxicity dosage and explore the combination's applicability	18	Completed with results	–	NCT03480750
Esophageal carcinoma	Not specified	Tetrathiomolybdate (TM)	Phase 2	Evaluate the safety of combination therapy with chemotherapy, radiation, and tetrathiomolybdate (TM)	69	Completed with results	–	NCT00176800
Melanoma	Not specified	ATN-224 and temozolomide	Phase 2	Evaluate the safety and efficacy of oral ATN-224 plus temozolomide in patients with advanced melanoma	60	Unknown status	–	NCT00383851
Breast cancer	Not specified	Exemestane with or without ATN-224	Phase 2	Evaluate the safety and efficacy of exemestane given together with or without ATN-224 in treating postmenopausal	111	Terminated	Withdrawn as the clinical development of ATN-224 was terminated by the drug company that	NCT00674557

				women with recurrent or advanced breast cancer			was providing ATN-224 for the study	
Colorectal carcinoma	Not specified	Irinotecan, 5-fluorouracil, leucovorin	Phase 2	Evaluate the safety and tolerability of the combination of these drugs in the treatment of metastatic colorectal cancer	24	Completed		NCT00176774
Carcinoma, hepatocellular	Not specified	Tetrathiomolybdate	Phase 2	Evaluate the safety and efficacy of tetrathiomolybdate (TM) in treating hepatocellular carcinoma. The primary outcome is to prevent tumor progression	Not specified	Completed		NCT00006332

toxicity toward normal cells and the ability to overcome chemoresistance associated with recurrent platinum treatment (Denoyer et al. 2015; Ge et al. 2022).

7 Combined Therapeutic Strategy

Combining ferroptosis and cuproptosis with conventional cancer treatments, chemotherapy, immunotherapy, radiotherapy, and nanotherapeutics is an emerging strategy in the field of oncology. This combination therapy approach seeks to enhance the effectiveness of cancer treatment by exploiting the unique vulnerabilities of cancer cells.

7.1 Combining Ferroptosis with Chemotherapy

Conventional chemotherapeutic drugs like cisplatin could trigger mitochondrial damage and induce ferroptosis in ovarian cells (Zhang et al. 2023b). The mechanism of combining ferroptosis inducers with conventional anticancer drugs to treat prostate cancer and halting its progression is largely driven by lipid peroxidation that triggers ferroptosis, thereby inhibiting key cellular pathways that support cancer growth and drug resistance (Zaffaroni and Beretta 2022). Further studies suggest that the strategic incorporation of ferroptosis inducers with chemotherapy drugs could provide a more effective treatment approach for hepatocellular carcinoma (Huang et al. 2023). Ferroptosis induction has been shown as a potential strategy to address chemotherapy resistance (Wang et al. 2023c).

7.2 Combining Ferroptosis with Immunotherapy

Inducing ferroptosis through radiotherapy and targeted therapy can enhance immunotherapies like anti-PD-1/PD-L1 treatments (Sun et al. 2021). Induction of ferroptosis strengthens immune cell activity such as T cells or macrophages, which is associated with the signal of damage-associated molecular patterns (DAMPs) and IFNγ secretion (Gong et al. 2022). Ferroptosis serves as a double-edged sword in immunotherapies; while the combination of ferroptosis-inducers and immune-checkpoint inhibitors can efficiently kill cancer cells, T cells could get exhausted and damaged by the production of ROS and over-activation of ferroptosis. GPX4 (the master regulator of ferroptosis) inhibition-driven death in liver tumors is triggered through a tumor-suppressive immune response with CD8+ T cell infiltration. Blocking PD-1 or HMGB1 activates T cells and improves survival in GPX4-deficient liver tumor mice. A combination therapy involving a ferroptosis inducer (withaferin A), a CXCR2 inhibitor (SB225002), and an anti-PD-1 antibody significantly improved the survival rate of mice with liver tumors. This combination therapy displayed a differential effect based on the tumor location and growth phase, indicating a need for further exploration of the underlying mechanisms and potential applications in human cancer therapy (Conche et al. 2023). PRMT5 activation in TNBC (triple-negative breast cancer) drives resistance to ferroptosis inducers and immunotherapy. Targeting PRMT5 could enhance the effectiveness of combined ferroptosis induction and immunotherapy in TNBC (Wang et al. 2023e).

7.3 The Combination of Ferroptosis with Radiotherapy

Recent studies have found the induction of ferroptosis radiation. Meanwhile, ferroptosis inducers show promise as radiosensitizers, enhancing the antitumor effects of radiation in lung adenocarcinoma and glioma. By inhibiting system Xc– or GPX4 activity, certain small molecules can activate ferroptosis, which amplifies the efficacy of radiation in murine xenograft and human patient-derived tumors (Ye et al. 2020). However, activation of the ferroptosis defensive system induced by radiation confines the synergistic effect of radiotherapy and ferroptosis. This indicates the need for a combination strategy potentially improving the overall efficacy of radiotherapy (Zeng et al. 2023). In an animal study of glioma, the combination of iron ion therapy with radiotherapy strengthened the antitumor effects, while the administration of iron chelator together with radiotherapy reduced the cancer-killing effects largely due to its inhibition of ferroptosis (Ivanov et al. 2015).

7.4 The Combination of Ferroptosis with Nanotherapy

Ferroptosis-based nanotherapeutics can be exploited to eliminate highly aggressive and drug-resistant tumors. These nanotherapeutics induce the accumulation of ROS and lipid peroxidation products within the TME. The induction of ferroptosis in cancer cells relies on the Fenton reaction, inhibition of GPX4, and exogenous regulation of lipid peroxidation (Zhu et al. 2022a). Nanoparticles possess distinctive characteristics that make them highly suitable for loading anticancer drugs by enhancing tumor-targeting efficiency. This enables more accurate and precise delivery of therapeutics to cancer cells, potentially leading to a reduction in adverse effects when compared to conventional treatments (Zaffaroni and Beretta 2021). Fundamental insights are needed for the design of nanomaterials with the capability to either induce or alleviate ferroptosis (Zheng et al. 2021).

7.5 Combining Cuproptosis with Chemotherapy

Copper intricately contributes to cancer chemoresistance. Copper-based treatments disrupt cellular processes, induce oxidative stress, and interfere with signaling pathways inhibiting tumor growth. This strategy shows promise for addressing chemotherapy-insensitive tumors, offering a unique avenue for targeted cancer therapy by modulating copper dynamics to overcome resistance challenges

(Kuo et al. 2007; Wang et al. 2024). A combination strategy termed "cuproptosis-inducible chemotherapeutic/cascade catalytic reactor system" has been developed for breast cancer treatment. A hydrogel system, utilizing glucose oxidase, cupric sulfate, and berberine hydrochloride, offers a targeted cancer therapy with combined effects of starvation, chemodynamic therapy, and cuproptosis. Its slow biodegradation reduces the dosing frequency and extends retention time for the effective treatment of breast cancer tumors (Lee et al. 2023b).

7.6 Combining Cuproptosis with Immunotherapy

A recent study developed cuproptosis subtypes and a cuproptosis-related risk signature based on the expression of cuproptosis regulators. The risk signature associated with cuproptosis could help to assess each risk score for each patient, paving the way for more individualized and effective immunotherapy (Wang et al. 2022a). A study explored the correlation between cuproptosis-related genes and the prognosis of melanoma, highlighting the potential of targeting cuproptosis for immunotherapy (Lv et al. 2022). Zhao et al. reported cuproptosis-related genes (CRGs), along with ferroptosis-related genes (FRGs), being able to predict the prognosis and immune profile of HCC patients (Zhao et al. 2022). Another recent study showed cuproptosis score as a prognostic and predictive marker with immune checkpoint inhibitor therapy in patients with lung adenocarcinoma (Wu et al. 2023a). A study developed a nanoparticle platform through which cuproptosis was induced using ROS-responsive polymer co-encapsulating elesclomol and copper. The combination treatment with anti-PD-L1 antibody for enhanced cancer immunotherapy demonstrated a novel approach to integrating cuproptosis with immunotherapy (Guo et al. 2023).

7.7 Combining Cuproptosis with Radiotherapy

Understanding radiotherapy-related cell fate decisions can potentially improve the efficiency of radiotherapy for cancer treatment (Chen et al. 2022a). A study proposed a model to independently predict the prognosis of non-small cell lung cancer (NSCLC) patients post-radiotherapy. This model explored the role of cuproptosis-related lncRNAs in NSCLC post-radiotherapy and provided a clinical strategy for combining radiotherapy with cuproptosis in NSCLC patients (Xu et al. 2022). Another study generated a cuproptosis-related lncRNA signature to not only predict the survival and immunotherapy responses in patients with cervical cancer but also predict the prognosis in patients treated with radiotherapy (Liu et al. 2023a).

7.8 Combining Cuproptosis with Nanotherapy

Nanotechnology can potentially mediate cell death via the cuproptosis pathway. A recent study developed the use of a DNAzyme-mediated cascade nanoreactor for promoting cuproptosis in pancreatic cancer (Yu et al. 2023). Nanotherapeutics could potentially address the short blood half-lives of existing copper ionophores like elesclomol and ensure more effective delivery of copper ions to cancer cells (Guo et al. 2023). Cancers that rely on oxidative phosphorylation for energy production can be ideal targets for inducing cuproptosis. Applying copper ionophores to such cancers through nanotherapeutic platforms could provide a new treatment paradigm (Xu et al. 2023a).

8 Conclusion and Perspectives

The crosstalk between ferroptosis and cuproptosis regulators has demonstrated molecular correlations at a multiomic level, which may significantly influence the tumor microenvironment and the prediction of prognosis and therapies. Researchers are working toward understanding the association between cuproptosis and cancer, exploring the therapeutic potential of employing copper ion ionophores with cuproptosis-inducing functions in combination with small molecule drugs for targeted therapy (Xie et al. 2023). This also indicates a move toward more personalized cancer treatment strategies (Ma et al. 2023). The unique vulnerabilities of cancer cells related to iron and copper addiction open up opportunities for more tumor-targeted therapies with less toxicity toward normal cells. As the mechanisms of oxidative stress and mitochondrial respiratory dysfunction have been further illustrated, new strategies targeting key molecular elements in ferroptosis and cuproptosis are expected to target cancer cell vulnerabilities, with the potential to limit or reverse malignancy. This results in improved clinical outcomes when synergistically combined with other strategies. Despite the progress, these metal-induced types of cell death remain not fully understood. An interdisciplinary approach that connects genomics, transcriptomics, proteomics, and metabolomics is required for innovative oncological therapeutics designed for precision medicine, potentially overcoming the challenge of pharmacoresistance in oncological practice.

Acknowledgment None

Disclosure of Potential Conflicts of Interest The authors declare no conflict of interest.

References

Ackerman CM, Chang CJ (2018) Copper signaling in the brain and beyond. J Biol Chem 293(13): 4628–4635

Belaidi AA, Bush AI (2016) Iron neurochemistry in Alzheimer's disease and Parkinson's disease: targets for therapeutics. J Neurochem 139(Suppl 1):179–197

Bertinato J, L'Abbe MR (2004) Maintaining copper homeostasis: regulation of copper-trafficking proteins in response to copper deficiency or overload. J Nutr Biochem 15(6):316–322

Brown RAM, Richardson KL, Kabir TD, Trinder D, Ganss R, Leedman PJ (2020) Altered iron metabolism and impact in cancer biology, metastasis, and immunology. Front Oncol 10:476

Chen X, Yu C, Kang R, Tang D (2020) Iron metabolism in ferroptosis. Front Cell Dev Biol 8: 590226

Chen H, Han Z, Luo Q, Wang Y, Li Q, Zhou L, Zuo H (2022a) Radiotherapy modulates tumor cell fate decisions: a review. Radiat Oncol 17(1):196

Chen L, Min J, Wang F (2022b) Copper homeostasis and cuproptosis in health and disease. Signal Transduct Target Ther 7(1):378

Chen J, Xue F, Du W, Deng X, Wu Y, Chen H (2023) Endogenous Fe2+—activated nanomedicine to amplify ROS generation and in-situ response NIR-II photothermal therapy of tumor. Chem Eng J 471:144358

Cheng X, Zeng Z, Yang H, Chen Y, Liu Y, Zhou X, Zhang C, Wang G (2023) Novel cuproptosis-related long non-coding RNA signature to predict prognosis in prostate carcinoma. BMC Cancer 23(1):105

Conche C, Finkelmeier F, Pesic M, Nicolas AM, Bottger TW, Kennel KB, Denk D, Ceteci F, Mohs K, Engel E, Canli O, Dabiri Y, Peiffer KH, Zeuzem S, Salinas G, Longerich T, Yang H, Greten FR (2023) Combining ferroptosis induction with MDSC blockade renders primary tumours and metastases in liver sensitive to immune checkpoint blockade. Gut 72(9): 1774–1782

Cui L, Gouw AM, LaGory EL, Guo S, Attarwala N, Tang Y, Qi J, Chen YS, Gao Z, Casey KM, Bazhin AA, Chen M, Hu L, Xie J, Fang M, Zhang C, Zhu Q, Wang Z, Giaccia AJ et al (2021) Mitochondrial copper depletion suppresses triple-negative breast cancer in mice. Nat Biotechnol 39(3):357–367

Cui W, Wang Y, Guo J, Zhang Z (2023) Construction of a cuproptosis-associated long non-coding RNA risk prediction model for pancreatic adenocarcinoma based on the TCGA database. Medicine (Baltimore) 102(5):e32808

Denoyer D, Masaldan S, La Fontaine S, Cater MA (2015) Targeting copper in cancer therapy: 'copper that cancer'. Metallomics 7(11):1459–1476

Dixon SJ, Lemberg KM, Lamprecht MR, Skouta R, Zaitsev EM, Gleason CE, Patel DN, Bauer AJ, Cantley AM, Yang WS, Morrison B 3rd, Stockwell BR (2012) Ferroptosis: an iron-dependent form of nonapoptotic cell death. Cell 149(5):1060–1072

Dong Y, Zhao K, Qiu Q, Zheng S, Zhang X, Liu J, Xu H, Pan X, Liu M (2023) Ferroptosis-associated lncRNA prognostic signature predicts prognosis and immune response in laryngeal squamous carcinoma. Cell Mol Biol (Noisy-le-Grand) 69(12):223–231

Dou J, Liu X, Yang L, Huang D, Tan X (2022) Ferroptosis interaction with inflammatory microenvironments: mechanism, biology, and treatment. Biomed Pharmacother 155:113711

Elgendy SM, Alyammahi SK, Alhamad DW, Abdin SM, Omar HA (2020) Ferroptosis: an emerging approach for targeting cancer stem cells and drug resistance. Crit Rev Oncol Hematol 155:103095

Fan X, Li A, Yan Z, Geng X, Lian L, Lv H, Gao D, Zhang J (2022) From iron metabolism to ferroptosis: pathologic changes in coronary heart disease. Oxidative Med Cell Longev 2022: 6291889

Fonseca-Nunes A, Jakszyn P, Agudo A (2014) Iron and cancer risk--a systematic review and meta-analysis of the epidemiological evidence. Cancer epidemio Biomarkers Prev 23(1):12–31

Forcina GC, Dixon SJ (2019) GPX4 at the crossroads of lipid homeostasis and ferroptosis. Proteomics 19(18):e1800311

Friedmann Angeli JP, Krysko DV, Conrad M (2019) Ferroptosis at the crossroads of cancer-acquired drug resistance and immune evasion. Nat Rev Cancer 19(7):405–414

Gao J, Luo T, Wang J (2021) Gene interfered-ferroptosis therapy for cancers. Nat Commun 12(1): 5311

Gao C, Kong N, Zhang F, Tang T, Li J, Ding H, Sun Z, Wu L, Xu M (2022) Risk stratification of lung adenocarcinoma using a nomogram combined with ferroptosis-related LncRNAs and subgroup analysis with immune and N6-methyladenosine modification. BMC Med Genet 15(1):15

Ge EJ, Bush AI, Casini A, Cobine PA, Cross JR, DeNicola GM, Dou QP, Franz KJ, Gohil VM, Gupta S, Kaler SG, Lutsenko S, Mittal V, Petris MJ, Polishchuk R, Ralle M, Schilsky ML, Tonks NK, Vahdat LT, Van Aelst L, Xi D, Yuan P, Brady DC, Chang CJ (2022) Connecting copper and cancer: from transition metal signalling to metalloplasia. Nat Rev Cancer 22(2): 102–113

Gohil VM (2021) Repurposing elesclomol, an investigational drug for the treatment of copper metabolism disorders. Expert Opin Investig Drugs 30(1):1–4

Gong D, Chen M, Wang Y, Shi J, Hou Y (2022) Role of ferroptosis on tumor progression and immunotherapy. Cell Death Discov 8(1):427

Guo B, Yang F, Zhang L, Zhao Q, Wang W, Yin L, Chen D, Wang M, Han S, Xiao H, Xing N (2023) Cuproptosis induced by ROS responsive nanoparticles with elesclomol and copper combined with alphaPD-L1 for enhanced cancer immunotherapy. Adv Mater 35(22):e2212267

Han M, Xu R, Wang S, Yang N, Ni S, Zhang Q, Xu Y, Zhang X, Zhang C, Wei Y, Ji J, Huang B, Zhang D, Chen A, Li W, Bjerkvig R, Li X, Wang J (2018) Six-transmembrane epithelial antigen of prostate 3 predicts poor prognosis and promotes glioblastoma growth and invasion. Neoplasia 20(6):543–554

Haschka D, Hoffmann A, Weiss G (2021) Iron in immune cell function and host defense. Semin Cell Dev Biol 115:27–36

Hassannia B, Vandenabeele P, Vanden Berghe T (2019) Targeting ferroptosis to iron out cancer. Cancer Cell 35(6):830–849

Huang X (2003) Iron overload and its association with cancer risk in humans: evidence for iron as a carcinogenic metal. Mutat Res 533(1–2):153–171

Huang Z, Xia H, Cui Y, Yam JWP, Xu Y (2023) Ferroptosis: from basic research to clinical therapeutics in hepatocellular carcinoma. J Clin Transl Hepatol 11(1):207–218

Ivanov SD, Semenov AL, Kovan'ko EG, Yamshanov VA (2015) Effects of iron ions and iron chelation on the efficiency of experimental radiotherapy of animals with gliomas. Bull Exp Biol Med 158(6):800–803

Jiang H, Muir RK, Gonciarz RL, Olshen AB, Yeh I, Hann BC, Zhao N, Wang YH, Behr SC, Korkola JE et al (2022) Ferrous iron-activatable drug conjugate achieves potent MAPK blockade in KRAS-driven tumors. J Exp Med *219*(4):e20210739

Jiang S, Zhang J, Fan Q, Li Z, Dou R, Lin Z, Chen Z, Xu Y, Huang Z, Lan J, Lin W, Xu S, Gao X, Li M (2023) A prognostic cuproptosis-related lncRNA predictive signature for bladder cancer patients. Hum Cell 36(2):798–811

Ju L, Shi Y, Liu G (2022) Identification and validation of a ferroptosis-related lncRNA signature to robustly predict the prognosis, immune microenvironment, and immunotherapy efficiency in patients with clear cell renal cell carcinoma. PeerJ 10:e14506

Kim DH, Kim WD, Kim SK, Moon DH, Lee SJ (2020) TGF-beta1-mediated repression of SLC7A11 drives vulnerability to GPX4 inhibition in hepatocellular carcinoma cells. Cell Death Dis 11(5):406

Kong R, Sun G (2023) Targeting copper metabolism: a promising strategy for cancer treatment. Front Pharmacol 14:1203447

Kong X, Xiong Y, Xue M, He J, Lu Q, Chen M, Li L (2023) Identification of cuproptosis-related lncRNA for predicting prognosis and immunotherapeutic response in cervical cancer. Sci Rep 13(1):10697

Kuo MT, Chen HH, Song IS, Savaraj N, Ishikawa T (2007) The roles of copper transporters in cisplatin resistance. Cancer Metastasis Rev 26(1):71–83

Kusoglu A, Biray Avci C (2019) Cancer stem cells: a brief review of the current status. Gene 681: 80–85

La Fontaine S, Mercer JF (2007) Trafficking of the copper-ATPases, ATP7A and ATP7B: role in copper homeostasis. Arch Biochem Biophys 463(2):149–167

Latunde-Dada GO (2017) Ferroptosis: role of lipid peroxidation, iron and ferritinophagy. Biochim Biophys Acta Gen Subj 1861(8):1893–1900

Lee H, Zandkarimi F, Zhang Y, Meena JK, Kim J, Zhuang L, Tyagi S, Ma L, Westbrook TF, Steinberg GR, Nakada D, Stockwell BR, Gan B (2020) Energy-stress-mediated AMPK activation inhibits ferroptosis. Nat Cell Biol 22(2):225–234

Lee J, Shin D, Roh JL (2023a) Lipid metabolism alterations and ferroptosis in cancer: paving the way for solving cancer resistance. Eur J Pharmacol 941:175497

Lee SY, Seo JH, Kim S, Hwang C, Jeong DI, Park J, Yang M, Huh JW, Cho HJ (2023b) Cuproptosis-inducible chemotherapeutic/cascade catalytic reactor system for combating with breast cancer. Small 19(35):e2301402

Li YQ, Yin JY, Liu ZQ, Li XP (2018) Copper efflux transporters ATP7A and ATP7B: novel biomarkers for platinum drug resistance and targets for therapy. IUBMB Life 70(3):183–191

Li Y, Feng D, Wang Z, Zhao Y, Sun R, Tian D, Liu D, Zhang F, Ning S, Yao J, Tian X (2019) Ischemia-induced ACSL4 activation contributes to ferroptosis-mediated tissue injury in intestinal ischemia/reperfusion. Cell Death Differ 26(11):2284–2299

Li J, Cao F, Yin HL, Huang ZJ, Lin ZT, Mao N, Sun B, Wang G (2020) Ferroptosis: past, present and future. Cell Death Dis 11(2):88

Li FJ, Long HZ, Zhou ZW, Luo HY, Xu SG, Gao LC (2022a) System X(c) (−)/GSH/GPX4 axis: an important antioxidant system for the ferroptosis in drug-resistant solid tumor therapy. Front Pharmacol 13:910292

Li SR, Bu LL, Cai L (2022b) Cuproptosis: lipoylated TCA cycle proteins-mediated novel cell death pathway. Signal Transduct Target Ther 7(1):158

Li J, Jia YC, Ding YX, Bai J, Cao F, Li F (2023) The crosstalk between ferroptosis and mitochondrial dynamic regulatory networks. Int J Biol Sci 19(9):2756–2771

Lian J, Zhang C, Lu H (2022) A Ferroptosis-related LncRNA signature associated with prognosis, tumor immune environment, and genome instability in hepatocellular carcinoma. Comput Math Methods Med 2022:6284540

Lill R, Freibert SA (2020) Mechanisms of mitochondrial iron-sulfur protein biogenesis. Annu Rev Biochem 89:471–499

Lin L, Wang S, Deng H, Yang W, Rao L, Tian R, Liu Y, Yu G, Zhou Z, Song J, Yang HH, Chen ZY, Chen X (2020) Endogenous labile iron pool-mediated free radical generation for cancer chemodynamic therapy. J Am Chem Soc 142(36):15320–15330

Lin L, Chen H, Zhao R, Zhu M, Nie G (2022) Nanomedicine targets iron metabolism for cancer therapy. Cancer Sci 113(3):828–837

Linz R, Lutsenko S (2007) Copper-transporting ATPases ATP7A and ATP7B: cousins, not twins. J Bioenerg Biomembr 39(5–6):403–407

Liu Y, Gu W (2022) p53 in ferroptosis regulation: the new weapon for the old guardian. Cell Death Differ 29(5):895–910

Liu L, Zheng J, Xia H, Wu Q, Cai X, Ji L, Sun Y (2023a) Construction and comprehensive analysis of a curoptosis-related lncRNA signature for predicting prognosis and immune response in cervical cancer. Front Genet 14:1023613

Liu Y, Lu S, Wu LL, Yang L, Yang L, Wang J (2023b) The diversified role of mitochondria in ferroptosis in cancer. Cell Death Dis 14(8):519

Lopez J, Ramchandani D, Vahdat L (2019) Copper depletion as a therapeutic strategy in cancer. Met Ions Life Sci 19:327–338

Lu Y, Pan Q, Gao W, Pu Y, He B (2022) Reversal of cisplatin chemotherapy resistance by glutathione-resistant copper-based nanomedicine via cuproptosis. J Mater Chem B 10(33): 6296–6306

Luo L, Wang H, Tian W, Zeng J, Huang Y, Luo H (2021) Targeting ferroptosis for cancer therapy: iron metabolism and anticancer immunity. Am J Cancer Res 11(11):5508–5525

Lutsenko S, Barnes NL, Bartee MY, Dmitriev OY (2007) Function and regulation of human copper-transporting ATPases. Physiol Rev 87(3):1011–1046

Lv H, Liu X, Zeng X, Liu Y, Zhang C, Zhang Q, Xu J (2022) Comprehensive analysis of Cuproptosis-related genes in immune infiltration and prognosis in melanoma. Front Pharmacol 13:930041

Ma S, Henson ES, Chen Y, Gibson SB (2016) Ferroptosis is induced following siramesine and lapatinib treatment of breast cancer cells. Cell Death Dis 7(7):e2307

Ma Q, Hui Y, Huang BR, Yang BF, Li JX, Fan TT, Gao XC, Ma DY, Chen WF, Pei ZX (2023) Ferroptosis and cuproptosis prognostic signature for prediction of prognosis, immunotherapy and drug sensitivity in hepatocellular carcinoma: development and validation based on TCGA and ICGC databases. Transl Cancer Res 12(1):46–64

Mao C, Liu X, Zhang Y, Lei G, Yan Y, Lee H, Koppula P, Wu S, Zhuang L, Fang B, Poyurovsky MV, Olszewski K, Gan B (2021) DHODH-mediated ferroptosis defence is a targetable vulnerability in cancer. Nature 593(7860):586–590

Masaldan S, Bush AI, Devos D, Rolland AS, Moreau C (2019) Striking while the iron is hot: iron metabolism and ferroptosis in neurodegeneration. Free Radic Biol Med 133:221–233

Mbah NE, Lyssiotis CA (2022) Metabolic regulation of ferroptosis in the tumor microenvironment. J Biol Chem 298(3):101617

McCarty MF (2003) A wholly nutritional 'multifocal angiostatic therapy' for control of disseminated cancer. Med Hypotheses 61(1):1–15

McCarty MF, Contreras F (2014) Increasing superoxide production and the labile iron pool in tumor cells may sensitize them to extracellular ascorbate. Front Oncol 4:249

Morales M, Xue X (2021) Targeting iron metabolism in cancer therapy. Theranostics 11(17): 8412–8429

Muller S, Versini A, Sindikubwabo F, Belthier G, Niyomchon S, Pannequin J, Grimaud L, Caneque T, Rodriguez R (2018) Metformin reveals a mitochondrial copper addiction of mesenchymal cancer cells. PLoS One 13(11):e0206764

Murdoch CC, Skaar EP (2022) Nutritional immunity: the battle for nutrient metals at the host-pathogen interface. Nat Rev Microbiol 20(11):657–670

Nie Z, Chen M, Gao Y, Huang D, Cao H, Peng Y, Guo N, Wang F, Zhang S (2022) Ferroptosis and tumor drug resistance: current status and major challenges. Front Pharmacol 13:879317

Nie H, Wang H, Zhang M, Ning Y, Chen X, Zhang Z, Hu X, Zhao Q, Chen P, Fang J, Wang F (2023) Comprehensive analysis of cuproptosis-related genes in prognosis, tumor microenvironment infiltration, and immunotherapy response in gastric cancer. J Cancer Res Clin Oncol 149(8):5453–5468

Oh SJ, Ikeda M, Ide T, Hur KY, Lee MS (2022) Mitochondrial event as an ultimate step in ferroptosis. Cell Death Discov 8(1):414

Oliveri V (2022) Selective targeting of cancer cells by copper Ionophores: an overview. Front Mol Biosci 9:841814

Otasevic V, Vucetic M, Grigorov I, Martinovic V, Stancic A (2021) Ferroptosis in different pathological contexts seen through the eyes of mitochondria. Oxidative Med Cell Longev 2021:5537330

Ozkan E, Bakar-Ates F (2022) Ferroptosis: a trusted ally in combating drug resistance in cancer. Curr Med Chem 29(1):41–55

Pan Y, Zhang Q, Zhang H, Kong F (2023) Prognostic and immune microenvironment analysis of cuproptosis-related LncRNAs in breast cancer. Funct Integr Genomics 23(1):38

Pang WL, Kaur A, Ratushny AV, Cvetkovic A, Kumar S, Pan M, Arkin AP, Aitchison JD, Adams MW, Baliga NS (2013) Metallochaperones regulate intracellular copper levels. PLoS Comput Biol 9(1):e1002880

Prasad Panda S, Kesharwani A (2023) Micronutrients/miRs/ATP networking in mitochondria: clinical intervention with ferroptosis, cuproptosis, and calcium burden. Mitochondrion 71:1–16

Priessner M, Summers PA, Lewis BW, Sastre M, Ying L, Kuimova MK, Vilar R (2021) Selective detection of cu(+) ions in live cells via fluorescence lifetime imaging microscopy. Angew Chem Int Ed Engl 60(43):23148–23153

Puliyel M, Mainous AG 3rd, Berdoukas V, Coates TD (2015) Iron toxicity and its possible association with treatment of cancer: lessons from hemoglobinopathies and rare, transfusion-dependent anemias. Free Radic Biol Med 79:343–351

Qi X, Wang J, Che X, Li Q, Li X, Wang Q, Wu G (2022) The potential value of cuprotosis (copper-induced cell death) in the therapy of clear cell renal cell carcinoma. Am J Cancer Res 12(8): 3947–3966

Ramchandani D, Berisa M, Tavarez DA, Li Z, Miele M, Bai Y, Lee SB, Ban Y, Dephoure N, Hendrickson RC, Cloonan SM, Gao D, Cross JR, Vahdat LT, Mittal V (2021) Copper depletion modulates mitochondrial oxidative phosphorylation to impair triple negative breast cancer metastasis. Nat Commun 12(1):7311

Ren Y, Mao X, Xu H, Dang Q, Weng S, Zhang Y, Chen S, Liu S, Ba Y, Zhou Z, Han X, Liu Z, Zhang G (2023) Ferroptosis and EMT: key targets for combating cancer progression and therapy resistance. Cell Mol Life Sci 80(9):263

Rochette L, Dogon G, Rigal E, Zeller M, Cottin Y, Vergely C (2022) Lipid peroxidation and iron metabolism: two corner stones in the homeostasis control of Ferroptosis. Int J Mol Sci 24(1):1–12

Rodriguez R, Schreiber SL, Conrad M (2022) Persister cancer cells: iron addiction and vulnerability to ferroptosis. Mol Cell 82(4):728–740

Roemhild K, von Maltzahn F, Weiskirchen R, Knuchel R, von Stillfried S, Lammers T (2021) Iron metabolism: pathophysiology and pharmacology. Trends Pharmacol Sci 42(8):640–656

Salnikow K (2021) Role of iron in cancer. Semin Cancer Biol 76:189–194

Seibt TM, Proneth B, Conrad M (2019) Role of GPX4 in ferroptosis and its pharmacological implication. Free Radic Biol Med 133:144–152

Shanbhag VC, Gudekar N, Jasmer K, Papageorgiou C, Singh K, Petris MJ (2021) Copper metabolism as a unique vulnerability in cancer. Biochim Biophys Acta, Mol Cell Res 1868(2):118893

She R, Liu D, Liao J, Wang G, Ge J, Mei Z (2023) Mitochondrial dysfunctions induce PANoptosis and ferroptosis in cerebral ischemia/reperfusion injury: from pathology to therapeutic potential. Front Cell Neurosci 17:1191629

Shen Y, Li D, Liang Q, Yang M, Pan Y, Li H (2022) Cross-talk between cuproptosis and ferroptosis regulators defines the tumor microenvironment for the prediction of prognosis and therapies in lung adenocarcinoma. Front Immunol 13:1029092

Shibue T, Weinberg RA (2017) EMT, CSCs, and drug resistance: the mechanistic link and clinical implications. Nat Rev Clin Oncol 14(10):611–629

Soma S, Latimer AJ, Chun H, Vicary AC, Timbalia SA, Boulet A, Rahn JJ, Chan SSL, Leary SC, Kim BE, Gitlin JD, Gohil VM (2018) Elesclomol restores mitochondrial function in genetic models of copper deficiency. Proc Natl Acad Sci USA 115(32):8161–8166

Song X, Liu J, Kuang F, Chen X, Zeh HJ 3rd, Kang R, Kroemer G, Xie Y, Tang D (2021) PDK4 dictates metabolic resistance to ferroptosis by suppressing pyruvate oxidation and fatty acid synthesis. Cell Rep 34(8):108767

Sun LL, Linghu DL, Hung MC (2021) Ferroptosis: a promising target for cancer immunotherapy. Am J Cancer Res 11(12):5856–5863

Tang D, Chen X, Kroemer G (2022) Cuproptosis: a copper-triggered modality of mitochondrial cell death. Cell Res 32(5):417–418

Tang X, Yan Z, Miao Y, Ha W, Li Z, Yang L, Mi D (2023) Copper in cancer: from limiting nutrient to therapeutic target. Front Oncol 13:1209156

Tesfay L, Clausen KA, Kim JW, Hegde P, Wang X, Miller LD, Deng Z, Blanchette N, Arvedson T, Miranti CK, Babitt JL, Lin HY, Peehl DM, Torti FM, Torti SV (2015) Hepcidin regulation in prostate and its disruption in prostate cancer. Cancer Res 75(11):2254–2263

Tong X, Tang R, Xiao M, Xu J, Wang W, Zhang B, Liu J, Yu X, Shi S (2022) Targeting cell death pathways for cancer therapy: recent developments in necroptosis, pyroptosis, ferroptosis, and cuproptosis research. J Hematol Oncol 15(1):174

Torti SV, Torti FM (2013) Cellular iron metabolism in prognosis and therapy of breast cancer. Crit Rev Oncog 18(5):435–448

Torti SV, Torti FM (2020) Iron and cancer: 2020 vision. Cancer Res 80(24):5435–5448

Torti SV, Manz DH, Paul BT, Blanchette-Farra N, Torti FM (2018) Iron and cancer. Annu Rev Nutr 38:97–125

Tousignant K, Rockstroh A, Poad B, Talebi A, Young R, Taherian Fard A, Gupta R, Zang T, Wang C, Lehman M, Swinnen J, Blanksby S, Nelson C, Sadowski MJC (2020) Therapy-induced lipid uptake and remodeling underpin ferroptosis hypersensitivity in prostate cancer. Cancer Metab 8:11

Tsvetkov P, Detappe A, Cai K, Keys HR, Brune Z, Ying W, Thiru P, Reidy M, Kugener G, Rossen J, Kocak M, Kory N, Tsherniak A, Santagata S, Whitesell L, Ghobrial IM, Markley JL, Lindquist S, Golub TR (2019) Mitochondrial metabolism promotes adaptation to proteotoxic stress. Nat Chem Biol 15(7):681–689

Tsvetkov P, Coy S, Petrova B, Dreishpoon M, Verma A, Abdusamad M, Rossen J, Joesch-Cohen L, Humeidi R, Spangler RD, Eaton JK, Frenkel E, Kocak M, Corsello SM, Lutsenko S, Kanarek N, Santagata S, Golub TR (2022) Copper induces cell death by targeting lipoylated TCA cycle proteins. Science 375(6586):1254–1261

Vela D, Vela-Gaxha Z (2018) Differential regulation of hepcidin in cancer and non-cancer tissues and its clinical implications. Exp Mol Med 50(2):e436

Wang Y, Yu L, Ding J, Chen Y (2018) Iron metabolism in cancer. Int J Mol Sci 20(1):95–105

Wang C, Zhang R, Wei X, Lv M, Jiang Z (2020a) Metalloimmunology: the metal ion-controlled immunity. Adv Immunol 145:187–241

Wang Y, Wei Z, Pan K, Li J, Chen Q (2020b) The function and mechanism of ferroptosis in cancer. Apoptosis 25(11–12):786–798

Wang G, Xiao R, Zhao S, Sun L, Guo J, Li W, Zhang Y, Bian X, Qiu W, Wang S (2022a) Cuproptosis regulator-mediated patterns associated with immune infiltration features and construction of cuproptosis-related signatures to guide immunotherapy. Front Immunol 13:945516

Wang Y, Zheng L, Shang W, Yang Z, Li T, Liu F, Shao W, Lv L, Chai L, Qu L, Xu Q, Du J, Liang X, Zeng J, Jia J (2022b) Wnt/beta-catenin signaling confers ferroptosis resistance by targeting GPX4 in gastric cancer. Cell Death Differ 29(11):2190–2202

Wang D, Tian Z, Zhang P, Zhen L, Meng Q, Sun B, Xu X, Jia T, Li S (2023a) The molecular mechanisms of cuproptosis and its relevance to cardiovascular disease. Biomed Pharmacother 163:114830

Wang W, Lu K, Jiang X, Wei Q, Zhu L, Wang X, Jin H, Feng L (2023b) Ferroptosis inducers enhanced cuproptosis induced by copper ionophores in primary liver cancer. J Exp Clin Cancer Res 42(1):142

Wang Y, Wu X, Ren Z, Li Y, Zou W, Chen J, Wang H (2023c) Overcoming cancer chemotherapy resistance by the induction of ferroptosis. Drug Resist Updat 66:100916

Wang Z, Jin D, Zhou S, Dong N, Ji Y, An P, Wang J, Luo Y, Luo J (2023d) Regulatory roles of copper metabolism and cuproptosis in human cancers. Front Oncol 13:1123420

Wang Z, Li R, Hou N, Zhang J, Wang T, Fan P, Ji C, Zhang B, Liu L, Wang Y, Kong J, Yao Q, Duan J, Zhao G, Ling R, Zhang J (2023e) PRMT5 reduces immunotherapy efficacy in triple-negative breast cancer by methylating KEAP1 and inhibiting ferroptosis. J Immunother Cancer 11(6):e006890

Wang Y, Chen Y, Zhang J, Yang Y, Fleishman JS, Wang Y, Wang J, Chen J, Li Y, Wang H (2024) Cuproptosis: a novel therapeutic target for overcoming cancer drug resistance. Drug Resist Updat 72:101018

Wu G, Hu Q, Chen H, He M, Ma H, Zhou L, Xu K, Ren H, Qi J (2023a) Cuproptosis-related signature predicts prognosis, immunotherapy efficacy, and chemotherapy sensitivity in lung adenocarcinoma. Front Oncol 13:1127768

Wu Z, Li W, Zhu H, Li X, Zhou Y, Chen Q, Huang H, Zhang W, Jiang X, Ren C (2023b) Identification of cuproptosis-related subtypes and the development of a prognostic model in glioma. Front Genet 14:1124439

Xiang R, Ge Y, Song W, Ren J, Kong C, Fu T (2021) Pyroptosis patterns characterized by distinct tumor microenvironment infiltration landscapes in gastric cancer. Genes (Basel) 12(10):1471–1482

Xie J, Yang Y, Gao Y, He J (2023) Cuproptosis: mechanisms and links with cancers. Mol Cancer 22(1):46

Xiong C, Ling H, Hao Q, Zhou X (2023) Cuproptosis: p53-regulated metabolic cell death? Cell Death Differ 30(4):876–884

Xu W, Barrientos T, Andrews NC (2013) Iron and copper in mitochondrial diseases. Cell Metab 17(3):319–328

Xu Q, Liu T, Wang J (2022) Radiosensitization-related cuproptosis LncRNA signature in non-small cell lung cancer. Genes (Basel) 13(11):1904–1915

Xu L, Liu K, Wang F, Su Y (2023a) Cuproptosis and its application in different cancers: an overview. Mol Cell Biochem 478:2683

Xu R, Wang W, Zhang W (2023b) Ferroptosis and the bidirectional regulatory factor p53. Cell Death Discov 9(1):197

Yang WS, Stockwell BR (2016) Ferroptosis: death by lipid peroxidation. Trends Cell Biol 26(3): 165–176

Yang J, Dai X, Xu H, Tang Q, Bi F (2022a) Regulation of ferroptosis by amino acid metabolism in cancer. Int J Biol Sci 18(4):1695–1705

Yang Y, Liang S, Geng H, Xiong M, Li M, Su Q, Jia F, Zhao Y, Wang K, Jiang J, Qin S, Li X (2022b) Proteomics revealed the crosstalk between copper stress and cuproptosis, and explored the feasibility of curcumin as anticancer copper ionophore. Free Radic Biol Med 193(Pt 2): 638–647

Yang L, Yang P, Lip GYH, Ren J (2023a) Copper homeostasis and cuproptosis in cardiovascular disease therapeutics. Trends Pharmacol Sci 44(9):573–585

Yang P, Li J, Zhang T, Ren Y, Zhang Q, Liu R, Li H, Hua J, Wang WA, Wang J, Zhou H (2023b) Ionizing radiation-induced mitophagy promotes ferroptosis by increasing intracellular free fatty acids. Cell Death Differ 30:2432

Yao X, Li W, Fang D, Xiao C, Wu X, Li M, Luo Z (2021) Emerging roles of energy metabolism in ferroptosis regulation of tumor cells. Adv Sci (Weinh) 8(22):e2100997

Ye LF, Chaudhary KR, Zandkarimi F, Harken AD, Kinslow CJ, Upadhyayula PS, Dovas A, Higgins DM, Tan H, Zhang Y, Buonanno M, Wang TJC, Hei TK, Bruce JN, Canoll PD, Cheng SK, Stockwell BR (2020) Radiation-induced lipid peroxidation triggers ferroptosis and synergizes with ferroptosis inducers. ACS Chem Biol 15(2):469–484

You JH, Lee J, Roh JL (2021) PGRMC1-dependent lipophagy promotes ferroptosis in paclitaxel-tolerant persister cancer cells. J Exp Clin Cancer Res 40(1):350

Yu Q, Zhou J, Liu Y, Li XQ, Li S, Zhou H, Kang B, Chen HY, Xu JJ (2023) DNAzyme-mediated cascade nanoreactor for cuproptosis-promoted pancreatic cancer synergistic therapy. Adv Healthc Mater 12:e2301429

Yuan HJ, Xue YT, Liu Y (2022) Cuproptosis, the novel therapeutic mechanism for heart failure: a narrative review. Cardiovasc Diagn Ther 12(5):681–692

Zaffaroni N, Beretta GL (2021) Nanoparticles for ferroptosis therapy in cancer. Pharmaceutics 13(11):1785–1795

Zaffaroni N, Beretta GL (2022) Ferroptosis inducers for prostate cancer therapy. Curr Med Chem 29(24):4185–4201

Zeng L, Ding S, Cao Y, Li C, Zhao B, Ma Z, Zhou J, Hu Y, Zhang X, Yang Y, Duan G, Bian XW, Tian G (2023) A MOF-based potent ferroptosis inducer for enhanced radiotherapy of triple negative breast cancer. ACS Nano 17(14):13195–13210

Zhang C, Liu X, Jin S, Chen Y, Guo R (2022a) Ferroptosis in cancer therapy: a novel approach to reversing drug resistance. Mol Cancer 21(1):47

Zhang Y, Xin L, Xiang M, Shang C, Wang Y, Wang Y, Cui X, Lu Y (2022b) The molecular mechanisms of ferroptosis and its role in cardiovascular disease. Biomed Pharmacother 145: 112423

Zhang P, Zhao JH, Yuan LX, Ju LL, Wang HX, Wang F, Chen L, Cai WH (2023a) DLAT is a promising prognostic marker and therapeutic target for hepatocellular carcinoma: a comprehensive study based on public databases. Sci Rep 13(1):17295

Zhang S, Liu Q, Chang M, Pan Y, Yahaya BH, Liu Y, Lin J (2023b) Chemotherapy impairs ovarian function through excessive ROS-induced ferroptosis. Cell Death Dis 14(5):340

Zhao C, Zhang Z, Jing T (2022) A novel signature of combing cuproptosis- with ferroptosis-related genes for prediction of prognosis, immunologic therapy responses and drug sensitivity in hepatocellular carcinoma. Front Oncol 12:1000993

Zheng J, Conrad M (2020) The metabolic underpinnings of ferroptosis. Cell Metab 32(6):920–937

Zheng H, Jiang J, Xu S, Liu W, Xie Q, Cai X, Zhang J, Liu S, Li R (2021) Nanoparticle-induced ferroptosis: detection methods, mechanisms and applications. Nanoscale 13(4):2266–2285

Zhu L, Meng D, Wang X, Chen X (2022a) Ferroptosis-driven nanotherapeutics to reverse drug resistance in tumor microenvironment. ACS Appl Bio Mater 5(6):2481–2506

Zhu Z, Zhao Q, Song W, Weng J, Li S, Guo T, Zhu C, Xu Y (2022b) A novel cuproptosis-related molecular pattern and its tumor microenvironment characterization in colorectal cancer. Front Immunol 13:940774

Zong H, Li A, Huang Y, Che X, Zhang Y, Ma G, Zhou Z (2023) Analysis of lncRNAs profiles associated with ferroptosis can predict prognosis and immune landscape and drug sensitivity in patients with clear cell renal cell carcinoma. J Biochem Mol Toxicol 37(11):e23464

Zulkifli M, Spelbring AN, Zhang Y, Soma S, Chen S, Li L, Le T, Shanbhag V, Petris MJ, Chen TY, Ralle M, Barondeau DP, Gohil VM (2023) FDX1-dependent and independent mechanisms of elesclomol-mediated intracellular copper delivery. Proc Natl Acad Sci USA 120(10): e2216722120

Biologically Active Metallic Cu(II) Complexes in Cancer: Past, Present, and Future

Adriana Corina Hangan, Luminița Simona Oprean, Bogdan Sevastre, Lucia Maria Procopciuc, Lucia Dican, and Roxana Liana Lucaciu

Abstract

More than 200 types of cancer are known today. Cancer represents the second cause of death in Europe. Statistical studies indicate that by 2035, the number of cancers in Europe could double and thus cancer would represent the first cause of death, before cardiovascular diseases. The use of metal complexes in therapy is increasing and this fact puts hope in the discovery of a new copper-based anticancer drug. The current chapter provides an overview of the types of DNA-metal complex interactions, of the antitumor mechanisms of action for the copper complexes, and presents the copper compounds in clinical study and targeted drug delivery systems based on copper in cancer treatment. PubMed, Scopus, and Web of Science databases were used to find suitable articles for this topic. The following keywords were used: cancer, Cu(II) complexes, DNA-Cu(II) complex interactions, mechanisms of action, clinical studies, and targeted drug delivery systems concerning anticancer Cu(II) complexes. Although the copper complexes have the expected antitumor activity, the problem of their toxicity is

A. C. Hangan (✉) · L. S. Oprean
Department of Inorganic Chemistry, Faculty of Pharmacy, "Iuliu-Hațieganu" University of Medicine and Pharmacy, Cluj-Napoca, Romania
e-mail: adriana.hangan@umfcluj.ro

B. Sevastre
Department of Pathophysiology, Faculty of Veterinary Medicine, University of Agricultural Science and Veterinary Medicine, Cluj-Napoca, Romania

L. M. Procopciuc · L. Dican
Department of Medical Biochemistry, Faculty of Medicine, "Iuliu-Hațieganu" University of Medicine and Pharmacy, Cluj-Napoca, Romania

R. L. Lucaciu
Department of Pharmaceutical Biochemistry and Clinical Laboratory, Faculty of Pharmacy, "Iuliu-Hațieganu" University of Medicine and Pharmacy, Cluj-Napoca, Romania

Interdisciplinary Cancer Research, https://doi.org/10.1007/16833_2024_405
Published online: 18 October 2024

raised. Classical chemotherapy doesn't present selectivity only for the tumor cells; therefore, the discovery of a Cu(II) complex with selectivity only for tumor cells is desirable. With the help of molecular analysis, immunotherapy, and personalized therapy, remarkable progress has been made in the treatment of cancer, but the fight against this merciless disease continues.

Keywords

Cancer · Clinical studies · Cu(II) complexes · DNA interactions · Mechanisms of action · Targeted drug delivery systems

1 Introduction

More than 200 types of cancer are known today. Cancer represents the second cause of death in Europe. Statistical studies indicate that by 2035, the number of cancers in Europe could double and thus cancer would represent the first cause of death, before cardiovascular diseases (Hangan et al. 2023). Fortunately, thanks to the innovative therapies discovered in the last decades, the life expectancy of cancer patients has increased considerably and also their quality of life (Siegel et al. 2019).

Metal complexes present a multitude of optimal properties for the synthesis of compounds with antitumor activity. For example, they are characterized by different modes of coordination and reactivity toward an organic compound and they have different redox proprieties. They must selectively act at the tumor level and arrest or diminish the tumor cell proliferation and be free of toxicity for healthy cells. Nowadays, Cisplatin is widely used as an anticancer agent, but unfortunately the treatment is limited by the presence of adverse effects and by the resistance of tumor cells to therapy. These disadvantages are only partially eliminated with the use of new anticancer drugs derived from platinum. Thus, it is desirable to obtain a new anticancer drug with the best effectiveness and minimal adverse effects (Dilruba and Kalayda 2016).

Copper is a necessary and indispensable element for the human body. Regarding its antitumor activity it is involved in the death of tumor cells through different mechanisms (Fig. 1). The apoptosis of tumor cells can be consecutive to DNA damage, cell cycle arrest, and activation of stress pathways (oxidative stress and endoplasmic reticulum stress). The participation of copper ion in Haber–Weiss reaction explains the involvement of copper in oxidative stress. Intracellular protein homeostasis is disrupted by endoplasmic reticulum stress. Also, endoplasmic reticulum stress influences regulatory signals in apoptosis, determining in this way the apoptosis of tumor cells (Tsvetkov et al. 2022).

At the tumor level, there is a lack of oxygen due to the presence of a low number of vessels. This determines multiplication of tumor cells, the formation of metastasis, and a metabolic change due to hypoxia, a process named "Warburg effect" (Schwartz et al. 2017). Tumor hypoxia presents the advantage to allow the discovery of antitumor prodrugs which become active in the reducing medium of the tumor

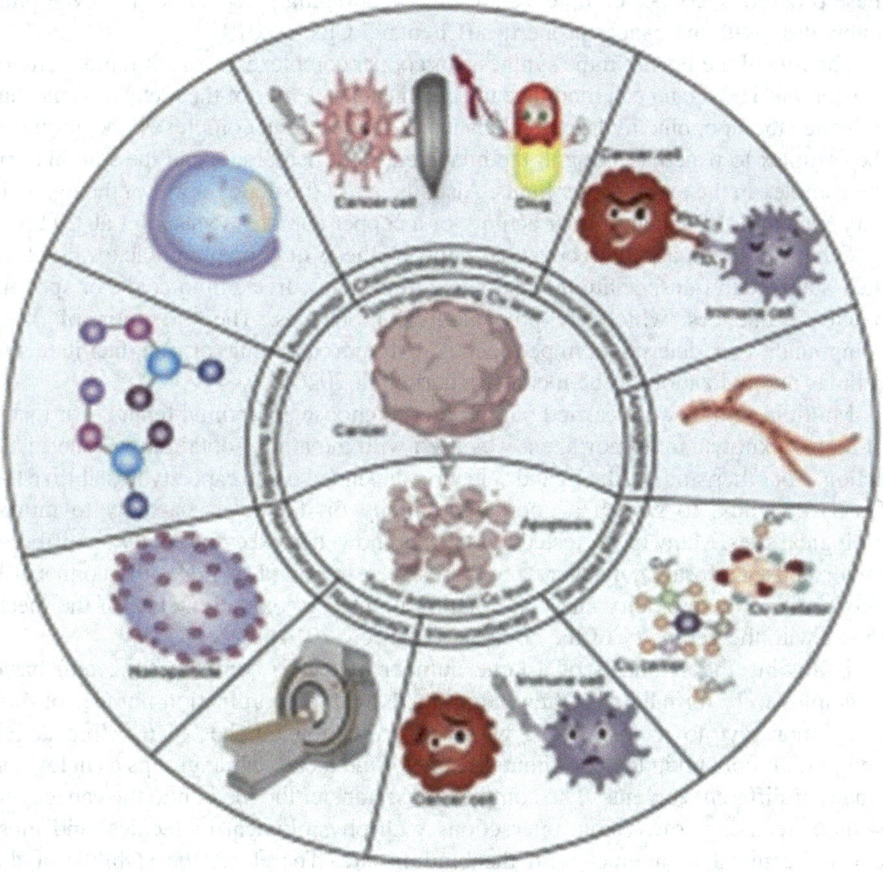

Fig. 1 Role of copper compounds in cancer therapy. (Guan et al. 2023)

cells. To this end, copper ion can be used because it exists under different oxidation states in tumor cells. When Cu(II) arrives in the hypoxic medium of the tumor cells it is reduced to Cu(I). The reduction of Cu(II) does not occur in healthy cells and thus the chance of targeted therapy is offered (Graf and Lippard 2012).

Cu(I) is involved in the formation of ROS and RNS and therefore in the production of pro-apoptotic oxidative stress. The affinity of copper for ligands is modulated by its redox state. Cu(I) presents a high affinity for sulfur ligands due to the fact that Cu(I) is a softer Lewis acid compared to Cu(II). Cu(II), in general, prefers the coordination with nitrogen and oxygen from proteins and DNA (Tabti et al. 2017). Copper complexes are known as "artificial nucleases". They present in vitro cytotoxicity on different tumor cell lines and in vivo good antitumor activity. Their cytotoxicity is manifested only on tumor cells, not affecting healthy cells. Some of the Cu complexes proved their activity against tumor cell lines resistant to Cisplatin and platinum analogs, being less toxic than them. Taking into account these properties, copper complexes present encouraging perspectives in developing a new drug with anticancer properties (Chen and Chang 2019).

The role of the ligand in the synthesis of copper complexes with antitumor activity is essential. The ligand can modulate the chemical properties of the metal ion, and can influence the lipophilic/hydrophilic balance of the resulting complexes, the ability of the complex to penetrate through the bilayered lipid membrane, and the solubility of the complex in the extracellular fluids. Also, the set of the donor atoms of the ligand is very important for the antitumor activity of a copper complex (Masuri et al. 2022).

Other important aspect to consider in the synthesis of copper complexes involves their stability to transchelation reactions with proteins, free amino acids, or specific peptide sequences, which are physiological molecules. The formation of these compounds can determine impediments in tumor targeting or can facilitate the cellular internalization of the metal (Baldari et al. 2020).

Multiple studies were carried out in order to choose an optimal ligand. For many of them, a known antitumor agent was used with the aim of obtaining a synergistic action. For other studies, the ligand selection depended on its capacity to stabilize the Cu(II) complex, to give it a good lipophilicity or due to its capacity to mimic biological sites. Many of the tested complexes showed good cytotoxicity on different tumor cells. Unfortunately, very few cases were reported to make the connection between their cytotoxicity and coordination number or oxidation state of the metal ion or with the geometry of the complex (Renfrew 2014).

Following the synthesis of a large number of Cu(II) complexes, several basic principles were formulated. Often, compounds with a coordination number of 4 or 5 are more cytotoxic than those with a coordination number of 6. More active compounds contain in the coordination zone of the metal, labile groups as halogens, water, or different solvents. The complex must transfer the metal into the cancer cell without realizing irreversible interactions with physiological molecules, and must allow the metal to interact with the binding site. Therefore, the stability of the complex must be optimal. In some cases, the cytotoxicity of the complexes was decreased by the presence of voluminous ligands. No link between the antiproliferative activity of the complex and the oxidation state of the metal was demonstrated. However, a high cytotoxicity was found for the copper(I) complexes which contain ligands as heterocyclic phosphine or carbene (Balsa et al. 2023).

The current cancer therapies cause a series of unwanted adverse reactions and this is the reason why more advanced treatments must be found. Nowadays, many copper complexes were synthetized and was demonstrated that some of them induce the death of tumor cells, while normal cells remain unaffected. In this context, the potential of copper complexes in cancer treatment gives us hope for treating cancer in the future.

The current chapter presents past, present, and future aspects concerning biologically active metallic Cu(II) complexes in cancer therapy, and addresses the types of DNA-metal complex interactions, the antitumor mechanisms of action for copper complexes, copper compounds in clinical study, and targeted drug delivery systems based on copper in cancer treatment. PubMed, Scopus, and Web of Science databases were used to find suitable articles for this topic. The following keywords were used: cancer, Cu(II) complexes, DNA-Cu(II) complex interactions, mechanisms of action, clinical studies, and targeted drug delivery systems concerning anticancer Cu(II) complexes.

2 Types of DNA-Metal Complex Interactions

DNA is the genetic information carrier in living organisms. In the normal flow of biological information, upon DNA replication, the information coded in DNA is copied in messenger-RNA (transcription). RNA information is then interpreted and translated into a sequence of amino acids; proteins are thus synthesized using the information in the messenger-RNA as template (translation). The genetic information is carried by genes, which are DNA sequences. Other DNA sequences participate in regulating the use of genetic information or have a structural role (Sugimoto 2023).

DNA structure has a large number of potential binding sites for endogenous compounds and also for xenobiotics. Therefore, xenobiotics take advantage of the binding sites along the nucleic acid molecule in order to modify its structure, its genetic message, and, implicitly, its functions. Copper complexes bind to specific sites on DNA having as goal reversibly or irreversible DNA damage.

Currently, there are several mechanisms known to be involved in DNA binding. They are covalent and non-covalent interactions. The covalent interaction or metal base coordination is an irreversible binding and it is represented by an intra–/inter-strand cross-link. The non-covalent interaction is generally a reversible binding and it is represented by intercalation between DNA base pairs, insertion, major and/or minor groove-binding, and electrostatic interactions with the sugar-phosphate DNA backbone.

Some anticancer drugs act by covalently binding to DNA. Through intra- or inter-chain alkylation, cross-linking adducts are formed. The irreversible covalent binding determines the DNA destruction and cells death. For the metal complexes, the covalent binding to the nucleic acid is kinetically controlled. The rate and site where the metal binds can be modulated by an initial reversible noncovalent binding. If the metal complex is positively charged, an electrostatic interaction takes place between the metal complex and DNA (DNA is known as a polyanion) (Barone et al. 2013).

In general, the non-covalent binding is less cytotoxic and for this reason is preferred over covalent adduct formation. It determines abnormalities in DNA structure and interferes with DNA functions, namely with DNA replication and with protein interactions. The forces that hold together such complexes are π-stacking interactions, hydrophobic bonds, van der Waals bonds, hydrogen bonds, and/or charge transfer forces (Nelson et al. 2007).

Around 1980 Sigman et al. synthesized the $[Cu(1,10\text{- phenanthroline})_2]^{2+}$ complex and demonstrated that it binds to DNA in a non-covalent manner. A partial intercalation and a minor groove binding are characteristics of this complex (Sigman et al. 1996).

2.1 Intercalators and Insertors

Intercalators are extended planar aromatic structures that stack between adjacent base pairs and are located perpendicularly to the DNA backbone. They don't form covalent bonds between the DNA bases and they don't break the hydrogen bonds located between the DNA bases. Van der Waals interactions made between the heterocyclic rings of the nucleobases and the π-electron systems of the intercalator stabilize the DNA-intercalator complex. The stability of the DNA-intercalator complex is reinforced by the presence of charge-transfer interactions, of hydrogen bonding, and hydrophobic and electrostatic forces (Nakamoto et al. 2008).

Metallo-intercalators are metal complexes which contain minimum one intercalating ligand. 1,10-phenantroline, 9,10-phenanthrenequinone diimine, dipyrido(3,2-a:2′,3′-c)phenazine, etc. can be intercalating ligand(s). They are orientated parallel to the base pairs, can π-stack in the DNA helix, and act as a new base pair. To keep the complex in the proximity of the DNA, at binding, the ligands act as an anchor for the metal complex. Metallo-intercalators usually enter into the double helix through the major groove. Their intercalation through the minor groove is also possible. Intercalation requires a minimum distortion of the DNA's structure, for example, an opening of the phosphate angles, without perturbation of the nucleobases or of the sugar residues. No nucleobase is removed from the helix. Following the process takes place a modification of axial distance between base pairs and a broadening at the binding site of the groove (Shobha Devi et al. 2018).

Although the most common way of binding small molecules to DNA is represented by intercalation, each structure may have its own preference for the binding site. Some structures prefer the intercalation between a 5′-pyrimidine-purine-3′base step while others prefer the intercalation between a 5′-purine-pyrimidine-3′base step. There are structures which prefer certain base-pair sequences and they have no preference for order (Biver et al. 2008).

At the level of a DNA double-strand, insertion determines a separation and a displacement of a base pair.

As metallo-intercalators, metallo-insertors contain a ligand with a planar aromatic structure which enters the base-stack when it binds to DNA. Metallo-intercalators produce relaxation of DNA helix and then insert their planar-ligand between two intact base pairs. Metallo-insertors remove the bases which correspond to a single base pair. The planar ligand of the insertor acts as a π-stacking replacement of a nitrogenous base in the DNA base stack (Zeglis et al. 2007).

Metallo-insertors are able to recognize the mismatched sites in DNA structure and to bind selectively at this level. As examples of mismatched sites in DNA structure are adenine-cytosine or cytosine-cytosine pairs which are formed as a result of errors during replication or upon exposure to genotoxic agents. They can accumulate if the cells' defense mechanism is disabled. In this case, a specific type of site is recognized by the metal complex, rather than a certain base sequence. The recognition site is a thermodynamically destabilized area in the DNA double helix realized by the imperfect hydrogen bonding between the mismatched nucleobases. The complex removes the mismatched base pair and makes a slighter DNA distortion compared to a metallo-intercalator. This way, selective mismatch detection agents can be used for diagnostic of mismatch repair deficiency and cancer (Modrich 2006).

2.2 Major and Minor Groove Binders

The minor and the major DNA grooves have different widths and depths, and represent important binding domains on nucleic acids. They also present structural features that may be used for molecular recognition of base sequences. Groove binders contain in their structure electron-donating and electron-accepting groups capable to form hydrogen bonds with the nucleic acid. Their structure contains aromatic rings, as for example benzene or furan, which present bonds with torsional freedom. Compared to the intercalators, groove binders have flexible structures, which allow them to lodge along the three-dimensional shape of the DNA grooves (Khan et al. 2012).

Several bonds are involved in the DNA groove-binding. These are the hydrogen, hydrophobic, van der Waals bonds, and electrostatic forces. Factors such as groove hydration and steric differences also characterize the interaction of a small compound with the DNA groove (Morris 2014).

In the minor and major grooves some atoms participate as hydrogen acceptors during the hydrogen bond formation, while others participate as hydrogen donors. As hydrogen acceptor participate O2 atom from pyrimidine ring and N3 atom from purine ring and as hydrogen donor participate the amino group of the guanine ring. Minor grooves have few binding sites and they have the advantage to bind small molecules.

In the case of the major groove, the N7 atom from purine ring, O6 atom from guanine, or O4 atom from thymine serve as potential hydrogen acceptor in hydrogen bonds formation. The amino groups from adenine and cytosine structure participate as hydrogen donors in hydrogen bond formation. Major grooves have a large number of binding sites and because of their larger size, they can accommodate bulky molecules (Pages et al. 2015).

Sequences rich in adenine-thymine are preferred by the groove-binding agents. This affinity is explained by the fact that these regions contain electronegative pockets and van der Waals bonds made between the groove wall and the ligand. Adenine-thymine regions are narrower than guanine-citosine ones and the steric hindrance is absent in the latter. The amino group in the C2 position of guanidine determines a steric hindrance (Khan et al. 2012).

Generally, the binding of a Cu(II) heterocyclic complex to the minor groove requires for its structure to have a shape that complements the convex surface of the groove (Erxleben 2018).

The way of binding the Cu(II) complex to the base pairs in the DNA structure is important. Firstly, the Cu(II) complex binds to the minor groove of the DNA. The binding takes place by the coordination of the phosphate's oxygen atom to the metal center and is stabilized by CH···π interactions with the backbone. Then, the Watson–Crick pairing takes place, when the ligands of the Cu(II) complex push an adenine-thymine base pair, until eventually it's broken. The action of the Cu

(II) complex continues at the level of the double helix by directing both nucleobases to the major groove and then by its insertion in the newly formed cavity. The possibility that the Cu(II) complex to be retained at the level of this cavity is due to the stacking interactions and electron depletion of the planar ligand because of charge transfer (Galindo-Murillo et al. 2020). For [Cu(4,4-dimethyl-2,2′-bipyridine)(acetylacetonate)(H_2O)]$^+$, [Cu(1,10-phenanthroline)(acetylacetonate)(H_2O)]$^+$, [Cu(5-methyl-1,10-phenanthroline)-(acetylacetonate)(H_2O)]$^+$ and [Cu(4,7-diphenyl-1,10-phenanthroline)(acetylacetonate)(H2O)]$^+$ complexes was found this type of interaction. These Cu(II) complexes contain acetylacetonate as the secondary ligand (Galindo-Murillo et al. 2015).

2.3 Electrostatic Interactions with the Sugar-Phosphate DNA Backbone

External binding, of electrostatic nature, between the negatively charged sugar-phosphate backbone of the nucleic acid represents non-specific interactions that usually enhance the stability of a DNA-small molecule complex formed through intercalation and/or groove binding, but is not considered to be the main binding mode. The electrostatic interactions are essential in the case of positively charged ligands or metal complexes. There are, however, very few examples of compounds which interact with DNA exclusively through electrostatic forces (von Hippel and Marcus 2019).

Although extensive research was done concerning drug-DNA binders, the studies concerning the interaction between the Cu(II) coordination compounds and DNA are still considered to be useful. In most cases, experimental techniques and analysis used for routine DNA studies can be extrapolated to coordination complexes. This statement is also valid for the Computational Chemistry tools, specifying that it must be taken into account that transition metals are difficult to simulate due to their multiple oxidation states and resulting geometry changes. To apply a Quantum Mechanical method to such a compound special care must be taken (Sponer et al. 2006).

For many years the main objective in cancer treatment was centered on arresting the reproductive cycle. Nowadays, when new antitumor compounds are studied, researchers must take into account that nucleic acids must be one of the main targets. Cu(II) complexes are excellent choices in the field of antineoplastic drug development taking into account the fact that Cu(II) are dynamic in geometry, electron affinity, and reactivity (Garcia-Ramos et al. 2013).

3 Copper(II) Complexes and Their Mechanisms of Action

The antitumor activity of Cu(II) complexes is due to several mechanisms of action: oxidative or hydrolytic degradation of DNA, apoptosis or autophagy in tumor cells, or topoisomerase/proteasome inhibition. The oxidative degradation of DNA requires the formation of ROS (reactive oxygen species) obtained as a result of some redox reactions. The obtained ROS are involved in the degradation of the helical structure of DNA. The hydrolytic degradation of DNA is an oxygen-independent process, a non-oxidative one. Activation of stress pathways, arrest of cell cycle, inhibition of angiogenesis, cuproptosis, and paraptosis can induce apoptosis or autophagy in tumor cells through different mechanisms of action (Brissos et al. 2015).

3.1 The Oxidative Cleavage Mechanism

Numerous toxic substances, besides being capable of transforming into free radicals during metabolization, can participate in redox cycles, generating superoxide anion radicals, which can in turn determine the formation of other reactive oxygen species (ROS), involved in numerous cytotoxic processes. ROS, as for example superoxide ion radical O2. -, hydroxyl radical OH., oxygen peroxide H2O2, is formed during some normal and pathologic metabolic processes that include the activity of oxidase and of electron transporter systems. ROS can also be produced due to external factors: exposure to radiation, polluting agents, and drugs. The organism has mechanisms which allow it to protect itself from the aggression of reactive oxygen species. These can be enzymatic or non-enzymatic mechanisms (Nakamura and Takada 2021). Following the changes in the ratio between oxidants and antioxidants that occur in the body, markers of oxidative stress are formed. These markers may indicate the presence of cancer (Cheung and Vousden 2022).

It is important to know that DNA-cleaving oxidants produce fragments that, unlike those produced by natural hydrolases, cannot be enzymatically repaired. Through electron spin resonance (RES) it was demonstrated that the formation of hydroxyl radicals mainly occurs in the process of reducing the Cu(II) ion to Cu(I) in the presence of reducing agents (e.g., H_2O_2) (Sies et al. 2022). The copper ions are involved in the Haber–Weiss reaction, which determines the ROS formation (Szewczyk et al. 2022). The presence of an excessive amount of copper/copper complexes in the cells will determine the formation of a large number of ROS which will produce cytotoxicity and finally apoptosis. So, probably by increasing the concentration of copper in the cells, a new anticancer drug can be obtained (Hangan et al. 2015).

The first Cu(II) complex recognized as "chemical nuclease" is Cu(1,10-phenantroline)$_2$. This complex destroys the DNA molecule through a mechanism which requires a reducing agent and O_2 (Scheme 1). During this process, Cu(II) is reduced to Cu(I) by a molecule which contains a thiol moiety. The resulting compound, (phen)$_2$Cu$^+$, which enters the DNA's double helix, joins it and then reacts with H_2O_2 (the reducing agent), forming hydroxyl radicals ($^{\bullet}OH^{\cdot}$). Studies performed on the activity of this complex show that the catalase and some other compounds that have an affinity for hydroxyl radicals (DMSO, tert-butanol) inhibit DNA degradation. This confirms the involvement of ROS in DNA destruction (Sigman et al. 1996).

Scheme 1 The nuclease activity of the Cu(1,10-phen)$_2$ complex, explained its mechanism of action. (Sigman et al. 1996)

$$(phen)_2Cu^{++} \overset{1e^-}{\leftrightarrow} (phen)_2Cu^+$$

$$(phen)_2Cu^+ + ADN \leftrightarrow (phen)_2Cu^+\text{- } ADN$$

$$(phen)_2Cu^+\text{- } ADN + H_2O_2 \rightarrow (phen)_2Cu^{++}\, OH - ADN + HO^\bullet$$

$$2\,(phen)_2Cu^+ + O_2 + 2H^+ \rightarrow 2\,(phen)_2Cu^{++} + H_2O_2$$

H_2O_2 can be added as reducing agent or can be produced in situ.

Scheme 2 Degradation mechanism: (**a**) Fenton and (**b**) Haber-Weiss. (Hangan et al. 2016)

(a) $Cu(II)(L) + e^- \rightarrow Cu(I)(L)$
$Cu(I)(L) + H_2O_2 \rightarrow Cu(II)(L) + HO^- + HO^\bullet$

(b) $Cu(I)(L) + O_2 \leftrightarrow Cu(II)\,(L) + O_2^{\cdot -}$
$O_2^{\cdot -} + H_2O_2 \rightarrow O_2 + HO^- + HO^\bullet$

The reaction products obtained after the degradation of DNA are free bases, 5′- and 3′-phosphorilated rests, which are compounds resulting from the oxidation of ribose or even of 5-methylfuran (Pitie et al. 2003).

Other oxidative degradation mechanisms of DNA proposed for Cu(II) complexes, which contain sulfonamide and phenanthroline ligands with nuclease activity, imply Fenton reactions (Scheme 2a) or Haber-Weiss reactions (Scheme 2b; Szewczyk et al. 2022).

These reaction mechanisms imply the reduction of Cu(II) to Cu(I) and elimination of a sulfonamide or phenantroline molecule which will interpose themselves between the nucleotides from the DNA molecule following certain "π-stacking" interactions or the formation of hydrogen bonds. The reduced copper ion, the Cu(I) ion, will react with reducing agent H_2O_2, generating ions, hydroxyl radicals, or superoxide anion radicals which will break the DNA helix, obtaining first its circular form, then its linear form (Fig. 2) (Srivatsan et al. 2003).

Due to its ability to oscillate between oxidized and reduced states in the biological environment, copper acts as a co-factor for enzymes involved in energy metabolism (C oxidase), ROS destruction (superoxide dismutase 1), melanin synthesis (tyrosinase), dopamine synthesis (dopamine-β-hydroxylase), etc. However, an excess of copper can be toxic to normal cells due to the generation of reactive oxygen or nitrogen species (RNS) (Oe et al. 2016).

Unlike normal cells, tumor cells show a reduced vascularity that results in a low level of oxygen, a fact that explains invasion, metastasis, and a metabolic shift toward an anaerobic process known as the Warburg effect. As a result, tumor hypoxia can be exploited to develop new prodrugs that become active in the reducing environment of cancer cells. In this sense, copper as a metal becomes very attractive because it can exist in two different oxidation states in cells. The presence of hypoxia in cancer cells promotes the reduction of Cu(II) to Cu(I), which is not possible in normal cells, and thus provides a therapeutic opportunity for copper

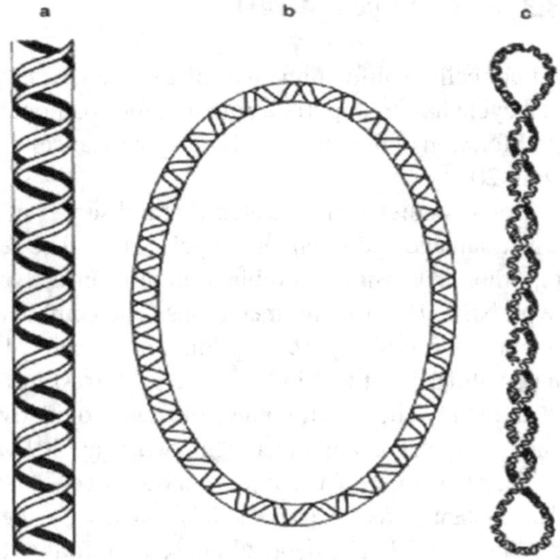

Fig. 2 DNA helicoidal (**a**), circular (**b**), linear (**c**) structures. (National Research Council 1995)

compounds to act targeted at tumors (Wu et al. 2021). The Cu(I) ion, once formed, can catalyze the formation of ROS and RNS, to induce a pro-apoptotic oxidative stress. Wei and Fang (2021) demonstrated that the permeability of the endoplasmic reticulum increases in the presence of copper. Consecutive, protein misfolding inhibits the correction ability of the endoplasmic reticulum, the regulatory signals pass into pro-apoptotic, the damaged cells are removed and the number of ROS species will increase.

3.2 The Hydrolytic Cleavage Mechanism

The hydrolytic cleavage mechanism of the DNA molecule was observed in the case of metallic complexes where metallic ions were connected through hydroxyl bridges $[Cu_2(\mu\text{-}OH)_2^{2+}]$. These complexes have a high nucleasic activity even in the presence of inhibitors like DMSO or sodium azide. This proves that in this case the cleavage of DNA is done independently of oxygen, through a process different from oxidative degradation. Literature shows the participation of the Cu(II) complexes (where Cu(II) ions are connected through hydroxyl bridges) in the hydrolysis of phospho-diesteric bonds (Thomas et al. 2004). The Cu(II) ion forms covalent bonds with the phosphate moiety from the nucleotides of the DNA structure, leading to the cleavage of the phospho-diesteric bonds and finally destroying the nucleic acid molecule.

Following the discovery of the reaction mechanism, the mono- or di-nuclear Cu (II) complexes which contain labile bonds can be used as accelerators of the hydrolysis of the phospho-diesteric groups and can finally lead to the destruction of DNA.

3.3 Cell Cycle Arrest

Tumor cells proliferation takes place when the cell cycle is no longer controlled. The cell cycle has an important role in tumor pathogenesis. For this reason, to inhibit the proliferation of the tumor cells many anticancer drugs aim to arrest the cell cycle (Liu et al. 2022a, b).

Some studies demonstrated that a disorder in copper metabolism can determine DNA damage and finally cell cycle arrest. The researchers tried to induce the death of tumor cells using a combination of an effective cancer cell cycle growth inhibitor (e.g., NSC319726) with metal ions. The combination with copper ions presented an important inhibitory activity on tumor cells due to the production of ROS at intracellular level that induces the cell arrest in G phase and apoptosis. The results of the study show that copper-mediated oxidative stress determines DNA damage and finally cell cycle arrest (Shimada et al. 2018).

The Disulfiram Cu complex induces cell death via instant and delayed phases. The instant phase may be solely caused by the Disulfiram Cu complex reaction generated ROS. The delayed phase may follow the rule of conventional anticancer drugs, which may interfere with the vital molecular pathways within the cancer cells and induce apoptosis. The cell cycle was arrested in G2/M phase. Protein blotting showed that Disulfiram Cu complex activates exogenous and intrinsic apoptotic pathways by cleavage of cystatin-8 and by disrupting the mitochondrial membrane of the myeloma cells. This complex demonstrated a good in vitro and in vivo anti-myeloma activity, which may be recommended as a treatment in the future (Xu et al. 2020).

3.4 Inhibition of Topoisomerase I or II

Topoisomerases are a group of enzymes responsible for maintaining the compact informational integrity of cellular DNA. They have the ability to break or repair one or both strands of DNA to keep genetic information compact during replication, transcription, or recombination. Since their discovery in 1971, DNA topoisomerases represent molecular targets for anticancer drugs discovery (Wang 1971).

Topoisomerases I have the ability to cleave and rejoin one of the two DNA strands. Topoisomerases II can pass one of the two helical segments, through a portion at the level of the two segments, in a reaction ATP dependent, breaking the interchromosomal bonds. Strand transfer through the breaking of a single strand in a reversible manner is catalyzed by type I topoisomerase and strand transfer through the double-strand port of DNA is catalyzed by type II topoisomerase (Ceramella et al. 2020).

During many profound physiological processes, type I topoisomerase is needed for DNA relaxation. Type I topoisomerase scaffolds are involved in a transitory cleavage reaction via a reversible *trans*-esterification reaction that produces an intermediate covalent compound with the tyrosine from the enzyme's structure, enzyme attached to the 3′-terminal of the DNA strand. The formed compound is unstable and persists only until the newly synthesized strand passes through the cut before type I topoisomerase reseals the cleavage (Thomas and Pommier 2019). Without ATP presence, the type I topoisomerase improves DNA supercoiling by cutting the DNA and allows the broken strands to rotate around the type I topoisomerase-bound DNA strand. In this way, topoisomerase I achieves the positive or negative relaxation of DNA. The inhibition of type I topoisomerases prevents the conversion of relaxed DNA into supercoiled DNA. The fact that type I topoisomerase is a cell cycle-independent enzyme is desired to be exploited to develop a new anticancer drug (Liang et al. 2019).

Type II topoisomerase is a ATP-dependent enzyme which catalyze different ATP-dependent DNA topoisomerization processes, like positively and negatively supercoiled DNA relaxing, ligation or religation, and raveling or unraveling via a double-strand-passing mechanism. Type II topoisomerases cut some complete DNA strands at the level of a single duplex segment. Then, a DNA double-strand is left by the protein, and one of the strands is cut off and re-enter in the main DNA section (Calderwood 2016). Only in the presence of ATP and divalent ions, type II topoisomerases produce the relaxation or decatenation of supercoiled DNA. From viruses to humans, type II topoisomerases are structurally and transitionally linked. Type II topoisomerases of human origin, are presented under the form of two isoforms: alpha hTOPIIα (known as α) and hTOPIIβ (known as β). They both act as type IIA topoisomerase (Konkolova et al. 2018). In vitro, these isoforms showed analogous properties, but they differ in their formation during the cell cycle. In interphase, both isoforms worked in the same way. In mitoses, α isoform was chromosome syndicated to a key part. At the chromosome level, type II topoisomerases had an equal distribution and were completely mobile. Although they are encoded by different genes, both α and β isoforms have a similarity of 70% in terms of amino acid sequence. They can be differentiated by their protomer molecular weights, 170 kDa for α type and 180 kDa for β type (Burden and Sullivan 1994).

It seems that type IIα topoisomerase is involved in the anticancer activity of type II topoisomerase inhibitors (Skok et al. 2020). Concerning type II β topoisomerase, besides the fact that it is expressed independently from the cell cycle, it plays important roles in transcriptional revival caused by heat shock and nuclear receptor activation (Hu et al. 2018).

The drugs that act by inhibiting topoisomerase, act by stabilizing the topoisomerase DNA complexes, causing lethal DNA damage during replication. The lack of ATP and divalent ions determines the relaxation of positive and negative supercoils of DNA, similar to the relaxation found in the case of the supercoiled plasmid pBR322 (Khadka and Cho 2013) (Molinaro et al. 2022).

For Cu(II) complexes with salicylaldoxime and resorcilaldoxime a similar cytotoxicity to that of Adriamycin was evident. Cytotoxicity consists in arresting the cell cycle and inducing apoptosis (Elo 2004). Both complexes act as topoisomerase II inhibitors, by preventing the formation of the enzyme dimer and by preventing its interaction with DNA. Therefore, Cu(II) complexes stabilize the cleavage complex from the topoisomerase II level and inhibit proper DNA replication (Jayaraju and Kondapi 2001).

Copper complexes with aminothioureas are good inhibitors of topoisomerase IIα. The movement of topoisomerase IIα is weaker if the metal ligands are absent (Qi et al. 2022).

The copper complexes which act as topoisomerase I, topoisomerase II, or topoisomerase I and II inhibitors are in general mononuclear Cu(II) complexes with different ligands. At present, the different properties of the ligands are exploited with the aim of synthesizing topoisomerase inhibitors (Hu et al. 2018).

Ceramella et al. (2020) demonstrated that the copper complexes which inhibit both topoisomerase I and topoisomerase II mainly aim to target DNA by cleavage or intercalation, a direct mode of interaction. The copper complexes' antiproliferative activity is potentiated by ROS production and other antitumor molecular mechanisms.

3.5 Proteasome Inhibition

Structurally, the proteasome is a multiprotein complex. It is located in the cytoplasm and in the nucleus. Its role is to selectively degrade and recycle intracellular proteins. It is involved in a special mechanism by which at the cellular level the concentration and stability of particular proteins is regulated and at the same time useless proteins are broken down. In tumor cell proliferation, apoptosis, angiogenesis, and metastasis formation, in a word in carcinogenesis, the ubiquitin-dependent proteasome degradation system is essential. It was demonstrated that cancer cells are more sensitive to proteasome inhibition than normal cells. Well known is the fact that copper is a cofactor for tumor angiogenesis processes. With all these, many Cu(II) binary complexes act as proteasome inhibitors, causing apoptosis in different types of human cancer cells. In these kinds of complexes, the metal is coordinated to ligands such as 8-hydroxyquinolinate, pyrrolidine dithiocarbamate, phenanthroline, or (pyridin-2-yl-methylamino) phenolate (Zhang and Burke 2023). The formation of the complex is required to facilitate the transport across the cell membrane, because free ligands are not active inhibitors (Shagufta and Ishrad 2020). Proteasome inhibitory activity mediated by copper ion complexes is superior when using the appropriate bidentate ligands and is blocked in the presence of polydentate ligands such as EDTA. Because the metal can't react with the cellular substrates at the molecular level, inert copper complexes cannot function as proteasome inhibitors. It was demonstrated that the purified 20S proteasome protein is implicated in the reduction of Cu(II) to Cu(I), a fact which suggests that Cu(I) ion reacts with the proteasome (Verani 2012).

Dithiocarbamates were used as a potential class of agents that target the ubiquitin-proteasome pathway in cancer treatment. They are a class of metal-chelating compounds which interact with metal ions and form metal complexes. Pyrrolidine dithiocarbamate binds to cooper and proved its efficacy in human breast and prostate cancers through inhibition of cancer-specific proteasome and inducing cellular apoptosis (Daniel et al. 2005; Chen et al. 2005).

The relation structure activity was studied for a number of pyrrolidine dithiocarbamate analogs with different substitutions at the pyrrolidine ring level. It was observed that the polarity and the size of the pyrrolidine ring from pyrrolidine dithiocarbamate structure affect the Cu complexes activity once they are formed. The inhibitory effect of the formed Cu complexes on proteasome activity was decreased when the substituents at the level of the pyrrolidine ring were large and polar groups. In human breast cancer cells, some novel Cu(II) complexes of pyrrolidine dithiocarbamate analogs inhibited the CT-like activity of the proteasome and showed a lower capacity to inhibit aldehyde dehydrogenase (Wang et al. 2011).

The proteasome CT-like activity was inhibited by diethyldithiocarbamate-Cu(II) (Pang et al. 2007) and diethyldithiocarbamate-Cu (Han et al. 2013) complexes. The complexes also induced apoptosis in prostate, breast, and pancreatic tumor cell lines. The expression of AR protein in prostate cancer cells and estrogen receptor proteins in breast cancer cells were successfully inhibited by the diethyldithiocarbamate-Cu (II) complex.

The proteasome inhibition activity of [Cu(pyrrolidine-dithiocarbamate)$_2$] and [Cu (diethyl-dithiocarbamate)$_2$] complexes on human cancer cells was investigated. They confirmed their proteasome inhibition activity (Frezza et al. 2010).

Schiff base Cu complexes were investigated for their action over the ubiquitin-proteasome pathway. In the structure of the Schiff base, there is a double bond between carbon and nitrogen. This bond can be formed following a condensation reaction between an amine (aliphatic or aromatic) and a compound containing a carbonyl group. The anticancer activity was attributed to the entire complex. A series of Cu complexes containing Schiff bases of quinoline-2-carboxaldehyde were synthesized and their cytotoxicity against PC-3 and LNCaP prostate cancer cell lines was studied. The complexes showed good antiproliferative activity. The type of side chains linked at C2 influences the biological activity of these complexes. The greatest cytotoxicity was obtained when a thiocarbonyl group was linked at the C2 position in the quinoline moiety upon Cu complexation. In LNCaP prostate cancer cells, Schiff base Cu complexes caused apoptosis by inhibiting the activity of CT-like proteasome. Instead, they didn't induce apoptosis through oxidative stress pathways (Adsule et al. 2006).

A compound that works as a metal chelator is represented by 1,10-phenanthroline. A copper complex with strong inhibitory activity over proteasome is represented by [Cu(taurine salicylic Schiff-base)(1,10-phenanthroline)(H_2O). It was also demonstrated that this complex causes apoptosis in human breast cancer cells (MDA-MB-231) and in leukemia cells (Jurkat T) (Zhang et al. 2008).

Cytotoxicity and antiproliferative studies on breast and prostate cancer cells (MDA-MB-231, MCF-7, PC-3) were performed using some amino acid Schiff base Cu complexes, namely: Cu(L-methionine-o-vanillin Schiff base)(2,2′--bipyridine), Cu(valine-2-hydroxy-1-naphthaldehyde Schiff base)(2,2′-bipyridine), Cu(L-methionine-o-vanillin Schiff base)(1,10-phenanthroline), and Cu(valine-2-hydroxy-1-naphthaldehyde Schiff base)(1,10-phenanthroline). 1,10-phenanthroline and 2,2′-bipyridine represent the second ligand for each complex. Following the studies, different activities were found for the complexes. Cu(L-methionine-o-vanillin Schiff base)(1,10-phenanthroline) and Cu(valine-2-hydroxy-1-naphthaldehyde Schiff base)1,10-phenanthroline) complexes had the ability to inhibit proteasome activity and cell growth and to determine cell death. The other two complexes do not have these properties. Thus, it was concluded that 1,10-phenanthroline is responsible for the cytotoxicity of the complex. Docking studies showed that Cu(L-methionine-o-vanillin Schiff base)(1,10-phenanthroline) makes significant intermolecular interactions at the level of the enzyme pocket and that it fits perfectly to the CT-like binding pocket. These interactions lead to a reversible inhibitory activity. Such interactions weren't evident for Cu(L-methionine-o-vanillin Schiff base)(2,2′-bipyridine) complex (Zuo et al. 2013).

It was also found that the participation of 1,10-phenanthroline as a ligand alongside two molecules of 3-acetic acid or 3-propionic acid favored the ability of the Cu(II) complex to inhibit proteasome activity and determine apoptosis in human cancer cells (Chen et al. 2021).

For [Cu(2,4-diiodo-6-((pyridine-2-ylmethylamino)methyl)phenol))Cl], [Cu(2,4-diiodo-6-((pyridine-2-ylmethylamino)methyl)phenol))OAc], and [Cu(H2,4-diiodo-6-((pyridine-2-ylmethylamino)methyl) phenol))(2,4-diiodo-6-((pyridine-2-ylmethylamino)methyl) phenol))]Oac complexes, a good cytotoxicity was demonstrated on human prostate cancer cells and leukemia cells. The 1:1 metal-to-ligand complexes were more effective than the 1:2 metal-to-ligand complexes. Due to the different stoichiometry, the three compounds show different cytotoxicity. Taking into account that the ligand works as a carrier, the Cu(II) ion must interact with the ligand to be able to cross the cell membrane and to reach the proteasome of the tumor cell. Once the metal center of the complex reaches the proteasome, it coordinates with different amino acids and this interaction enables Cu-N, Cu-S, or Cu-O bonds to form and finally determine proteasome inhibition (Hindo et al. 2009).

cis-[Cu(4-amino-1,4-dihidro-3-(2-pyridyl)-5-thioxo-1,2,4-triazole)Cl_2]Cl complex presented a better cytotoxicity than Cisplatin (Tardito et al. 2009). Its cytotoxicity is due to the ubiquitinated proteins accumulation and to the inhibition of the ubiquitin-proteasome pathway in human cancer cells (Gandin et al. 2012).

3.6 Anti-angiogenesis

Many new blood vessels are formed in the case of tumor development and growth. The role of these blood vessels is to ensure the transport of nutrients and water, needed for the tumor growth and to carry tumor cells at the distance, forming in this way metastases. It can be stated that the initial process of tumor cell proliferation and metastases is represented by angiogenesis. Copper complexes have an important role in the neovascularization of the cells because they have a unique proteasome inhibition capacity. These characteristics provide a possibility to discover a new antitumor treatment (Hariprabu et al. 2021; Fig. 3).

The usefulness of copper complexes in anti-angiogenesis therapy is related to the vascular endothelial growth factor (VEGF) (Tardito and Marchiò 2009). Zimbone et al. evaluated the ionophoretic activity of the pro-apoptotic bifunctional peptide, which can both chelate the Cu(II) ions and inhibit HUVEC viability. The results showed a correlation between the lipophilic character of the ligands and an increase in the cytotoxic activity of the corresponding copper complexes. The supplementation of copper amplified the artificial membrane damage VEGF73-101 (a fragment of vascular endothelial growth factor (VEGF165) induced, and intensified the cell viability reduction and the pro-apoptotic effect. The VEGF73-101 behaves as a copper ionophore and could be used as an anti-angiogenesis drug in antitumor treatment (Zimbone et al. 2020).

3.7 Cuproptosis and Paraptosis

Cuproptosis is a way of regulating cell death. It depends on the presence of copper and of the mitochondria respiration. At the level of Krebs cycle pathway, copper ions bind to lipid-acylated components, determining an abnormal aggregation of lipid-acylated proteins and the loss of iron–sulfur cluster proteins. In this way results a proteotoxic stress response which causes cuproptosis (Yang et al. 2023).

The role of copper in the process of paraptosis in tumor cells is due to the fact that it causes endoplasmic reticulum stress, unfolded protein responses, and massive

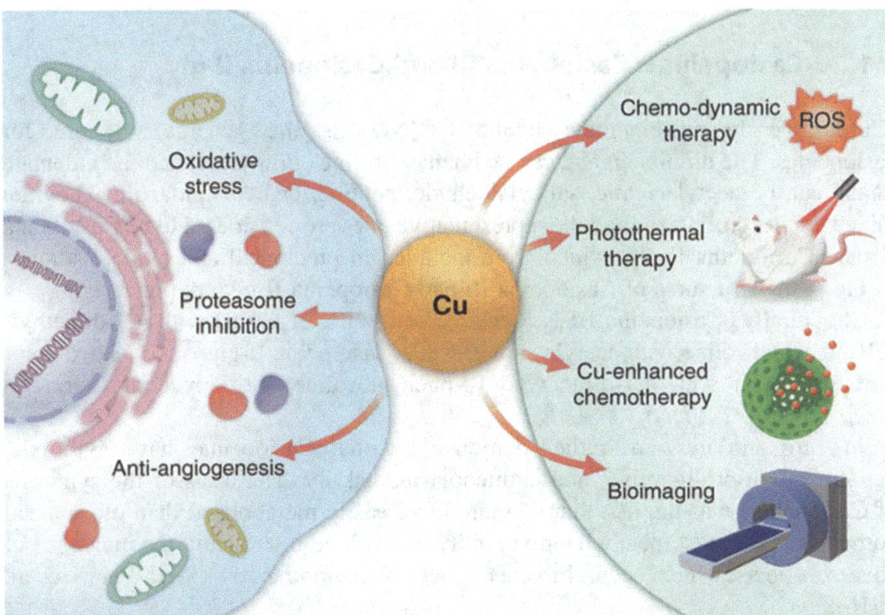

Fig. 3 Copper-induced tumor cell death mechanisms. (Jiang et al. 2022)

vacuolization in the cytoplasm (Hanson et al. 2023). Paraptosis is known as type III programmed cell death and consists of non-apoptotic programmed cell death. In vitro studies demonstrated that some copper complexes determine paraptosis by inhibiting the proteasome activity in tumor cells and also act as inhibitory in the accumulation of misfolded proteins, while being able to induce endoplasmic reticulum homeostasis to play the same function (Gandin et al. 2012). On human fibrosarcoma cells (HT1080), a copper complex with 4-amino-1,4-dihydro-3-(2-pyridyl)-5-thioxo-1,2,4-triazole ligand presented an important vacuolization and a change in the morphology of endoplasmic reticulum, which leads to tumor cells paraptosis. The activity of the complex was comparable to that obtained after the administration of Cisplatin (Tardito and Marchiò 2009). To develop a new anticancer drug which contains copper, the induction of paraptosis in tumor cells may be a possibility.

4 Copper Compounds in Clinical Study

The copper compounds showed a good selectivity for the tumor cells. Some of them showed cytotoxicity on tumor cell lines resistant to Cisplatin or other platinum derivatives and lower toxicity (Denoyer et al. 2018). Due to the good results obtained after their in vitro and in vivo testing and despite their toxicity, some of the compounds entered in preclinical and clinical studies. Preclinical and clinical studies provide encouraging results and for this reason the prospects of obtaining a new copper compound with anticancer activity are promising (Anthony et al. 2020).

4.1 Casiopeinas: Casiopeina III and Casiopeina II-gly

[Cu(diimine ligand)(bidentate ligand)H_2O]NO_3 is the general structure for casiopeinas. The diimine ligand can be phenanthroline or dipyridyl and the bidentate ligand can be acetylacetone, salicylaldehyde, peptide, or benzimidazole. They are mixed copper complexes and the representative ones are considered to be Casiopeina III and Casiopeina II-gly, which were included in preclinical and clinical studies. In Fig. 4 the structures of Casiopeina III and Casiopeina II-gly are presented.

Structurally, Casiopeina III is a chelated complex of Cu(II) with 4,7-dimethyl-1,10-phenanthroline with acetylacetone, while Casiopeina II-gly is a chelated complex of Cu(II) with 4,7-dimethyl-1,10-phenanthroline with glycocol (Serment-Guerrero et al. 2017).

In vitro and in vivo studies demonstrated that Casiopeinas have cytotoxic, genotoxic, antiproliferative, and antineoplastic activity. The basis of the synthesis of Casiopeinas was the fact that they are more easily metabolized than other metal complexes. This fast metabolization ability is involved in reducing the incidence of adverse effects which occur in other types of chemotherapy (Silva-Platas et al. 2016).

The activation of pro-apoptotic pathways in malignant cells represents the main way of acting as cytotoxic for Casiopeins. Casiopeins intercalate into the DNA

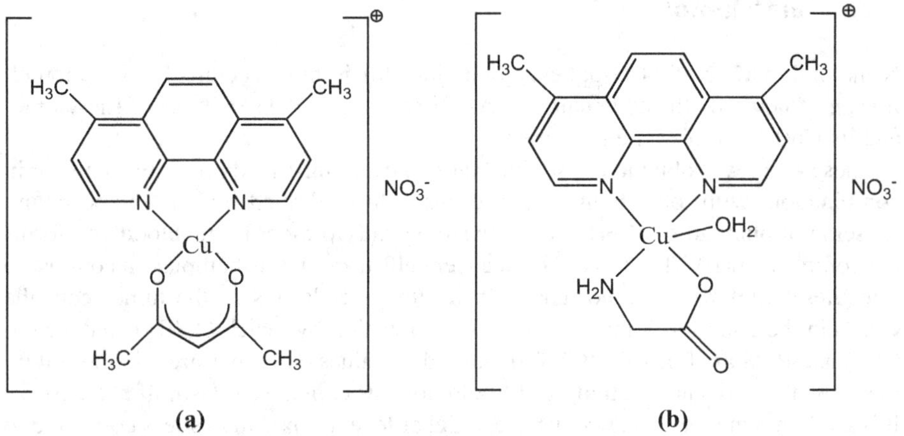

Fig. 4 The structures of Casiopeinas: (**a**) Casiopeina III; (**b**) Casiopeina II-gly

structure, prevent its correct replication, and act on the biochemical mechanisms involved in apoptosis. Because Casiopeinas contain copper, the Cu(II) ion is involved in a redox mechanism, which generates and increases the ROS level near DNA. ROS will react with DNA, damaging its structure, most often attacking deoxyribose residues. Cell apoptosis occurs by oxidation of –SH residues of the proteins located in the mitochondria due to the increased level of mitochondrial ROS. Another mechanisms of action were later discovered and consist in DNA fragmentation and apoptosis through caspase-dependent pathways or of the inhibition of energetic metabolism or could be due to mitochondrial toxicity (Aguilar-Jimenez et al. 2023). The antitumor activity of Casiopeina II-gly consists also in inhibiting the cell cycle, reducing the migration of tumor cells, and regulating the transformation processes in fibroblasts (Vértiz et al. 2014).

Due to the fact that for Casiopeina II-gly the researchers demonstrated that it blocks the migration and the proliferation of HeLa cells, it was included in clinical trials with the aim of treating cervical cancer (de Anda-Jáuregui et al. 2019). In turn, Casiopeina III was included in a phase I clinical trial to test its efficacy against acute myeloid leukemia and colon cancer (Chavez-Gonzalez et al. 2017).

Concerning toxicity studies on humans, Casiopeina II-gly was included in phase I clinical trials. The studies proved that Casiopeina II-gly inhibits energy metabolism and causes high cardiotoxicity. For these reasons, the studies were stopped (Guerrero et al. 2017).

After performing the clinical trials on Casiopeinas comparative to other anticancer drugs, it was found that its administration raises the patient's immunity and also realizes liver protection by regenerating damaged cells (Campero-Peredo et al. 2016).

4.2 Elesclomol

N-malonil-bis(N-methyl-N-tiobenzoyl hydrazide) is the structure for Elesclomol. It is also known by the code name STA-4783. In Fig. 5 the structures of Elesclomol and its Cu(II) complex are presented.

Elesclomol was obtained as sodium salt to be administrated injectable alone or in combination with other anticancer drugs. Once arrived in the bloodstream, Elesclomol binds to the Cu(II) ions physiologically present in the blood and forms the complex Cu(II)-Elesclomol. The cancer cells take up this complex in contrast to free Elesclomol which is not taken up by tumor cells. Inside the tumor cell, the Cu(II) in the complex is involved in a redox reaction by which Cu(II) is reduced to Cu(I) and ROS are formed. ROS formation determines oxidative stress in the cell. In this way, the anticancer activity of Elesclomol was explained (Hasinoff et al. 2015). It is well known that cancer cells have a higher level of oxidative stress compared to normal cells. After administration of Elesclomol, the level of ROS exceeds a critical threshold in cancer cells. The excessive presence of ROS increases the sensitivity of tumor cells to common anticancer agents and causes tumor cell death. Normal cells remain unaffected (Monk et al. 2018).

The anticancer activity of Elesclomol is also explained by disturbing the metabolism of mitochondria. This activity requires the presence of O_2 that results in energetic metabolism being driven primarily through oxidative phosphorylation at the mitochondria level. Elesclomol activity is diminished under hypoxic conditions, usually associated with elevated levels of lactate dehydrogenase. In a phase III study carried out on patients with metastatic melanoma, Elesclomol activity was highlighted only for subjects with normal baseline lactate dehydrogenase levels. Elesclomol and Cu(II)-Elesclomol present an in vitro good cytotoxicity on many types of tumor cells, in nanomolar concentrations. In human tumor xenograft models, Elesclomol potentiated the antitumor action of other chemotherapeutic drugs, for example, Paclitaxel (Kirshner et al. 2008). In preclinical studies, Elesclomol was found to be a good antitumor activity when was administrated alone or when was administrated in association with Paclitaxel or Docetaxel.

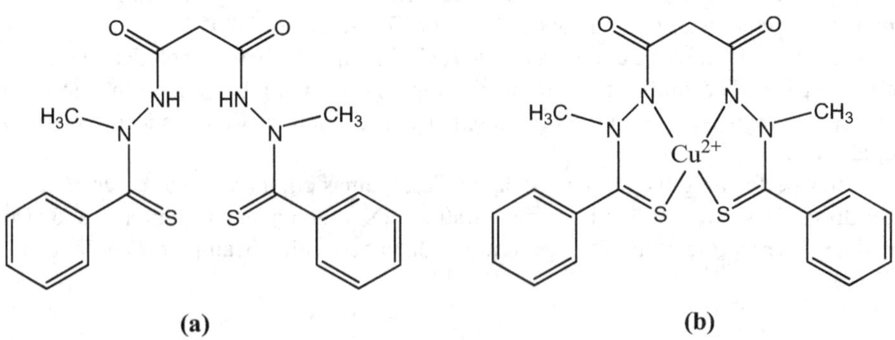

Fig. 5 The structures of: (**a**) Elesclomol; (**b**) Complex Cu(II)-Elesclomol

Moreover, following the association with Paclitaxel or Docetaxel, a synergistic activity was found (O'Day et al. 2013).

A number of patients with refractory solid tumors were included into a phase I clinical trial and a combination of Paclitaxel with Elesclomol was administrated. The combination was well tolerated, and the side effects were comparable to those that appeared following the administration of Paclitaxel as monotherapy (Berkenblit et al. 2007).

Eighty-one patients diagnosed with metastatic melanoma (stage IV) were included in a phase II clinical trial, a double-blinded, randomized study. A combination of Paclitaxel with Elesclomol was administrated. It was demonstrated that the administration of the combination Paclitaxel with Elesclomol doubled the median progression-free survival compared to the administration of Paclitaxel as monotherapy. Melanoma is a form of skin cancer with a starting point from melanocytes. Although it presents a high degree of malignancy, if it is diagnosed while it is still located in the superficial layer of the skin and can be surgically removed with a margin of safety, it can be curable. Unfortunately, for the patients with metastatic melanoma the evolution is unfavorable with a median survival of approximately 6–9 months (Korn et al. 2008). It was demonstrated that in hypoxic medium which is associated with lactate dehydrogenase increased levels the antitumor activity of Elesclomol is decreased. This is the reason why only for patients with normal lactate dehydrogenase values the antitumor effect of the combination of Paclitaxel with Elesclomol proved its efficacy. The trials carried out in order to improve disease prognosis in patients with elevated lactate dehydrogenase values did not give good results (Hasinoff et al. 2015).

For women with refractory ovarian cancer, a combination of Paclitaxel with Elesclomol was administrated. The patients were included in a phase I study and the obtained results were promising showing antitumor efficacy and a good tolerance concerning the adverse effects. In another phase II study, women with peritoneal, ovarian, or fallopian cancer were included. The women were diagnosed with recurrent cancer or cancer resistant to Cisplatin treatment and must have physiological levels of lactate dehydrogenase. Elesclomol combined with Paclitaxel was administrated. Good results were obtained from the point of view of therapeutic efficacy and also for drug tolerance (Monk et al. 2018). A phase I study was planned for patients with metastatic prostate cancer for which the administration of the combination of Docetaxel, Elesclomol, and Prednisone was desired. No results were reported (Rae and Mairs 2017).

5 Targeted Drug Delivery Systems

In parallel with the considerable efforts invested in the discovery of new molecules with anticancer efficacy, the attention of researchers is channeled toward the discovery of different kinds of delivery systems of antitumor compounds which deliver the drug directly into the tumor. From the patient's point of view, the use of targeted antitumor drug delivery systems presents a series of advantages, namely: administration of a smaller amount of antitumor drug, the presence of a larger amount of antitumor agent at the level of the tumor cells, the increase of treatment effectiveness, and decrease of the frequency of adverse effects. Therefore, the use of such targeted drug delivery systems would increase the treatment compliance and would improve the patient's quality of life. From the drug formulation point of view, the targeted delivery of the therapeutic compound through different mechanisms aims to protect the antitumor drug from degradation/inactivation and insurance a selective absorption at the level of tumor cells. In this way, the bioavailability and the bioactivity of the antitumor drug is assured (Dzhardimalieva et al. 2019).

With the help of nanomedicine, using photodynamic, photothermal, or chemodynamic therapy the possibility to treat advanced cancers or cancers resistant to classical chemotherapy appears (Fig. 3). It was also demonstrated that these modern therapies have reduced toxicity (Pan et al. 2021).

5.1 Photodynamic Therapy

In the last century, photodynamic therapy was discovered based on the therapeutic properties of light. Cancer photodynamic therapy requires selective localization of the photosensitizing drug in the tumor followed by drug activation in the presence of visible radiation. It results in a photocytotoxic effect on tumor cells, without affecting healthy cells (Monro et al. 2019). Using photodynamic therapy many types of tumors may be treated and in particular the tumors resistant to classical chemotherapy (Poblocki et al. 2021). It is a noninvasive therapy which requires the following conditions:

- Using a photosensitizer with photodamage selectivity for the tumor cells, without selectivity for the normal cells.
- Knowing the optimal period that must be waited after injecting the photosensitizer so that to act only on tumor cells.
- Formation of ROS species involved in the cell death. In this aim the tumor cells are irradiated with visible light (using a high wavelength) (Abdel-Kader 2016).

Regarding the photosensitizer, it must show DNA cleavage only under irradiation. The photosensitizer must not undergo DNA degradation through hydrolytic or chemical pathways in the presence of an external agent. A high-performance photosensitizer in photodynamic therapy must fulfill the following properties:

- Considering the fact that the penetration into the skin increases with the increase of the wavelength, the absorption must be carried out at a wavelength greater than 650 nm. Thus, a strong absorption takes place in the red part of the visible spectrum.
- The quantum yield of triplet formation must be high. The triplet energy >94 kJ M-1.
- The singlet oxygen quantum yield must be high.
- To present low toxicity in the dark.

- To show selectivity for the tumor tissue.
- Must have a pharmacokinetic profile which ensures its quick excretion from the body.
- To be synthesized with available starting materials.
- To have a long validity and to be formulated as simply as possible to be further transformed, with the aim to improve the requirements listed above (Dang et al. 2017).

Initially, the photosensitizer is found in a fundamental singlet form. Upon light absorption, it is excited to a higher energy level and finally reaches a short-lived first excited singlet state. The photosensitizer can return to the initial state by internal conversion or by emitting the absorbed energy as fluorescence. By intersystem crossing, the short-lived first excited singlet state can be converted to the first excited triplet state. The photosensitizer in its first excited triplet state can form energy by following the phosphorescence pathway or return to the initial state through a nonradiative path. The generation of reactive and cytotoxic singlet oxygen ($^1O_2$) takes place after the energy transfer from the triplet state of the photosensitizer to O_2. O_2 can be also reduced to $O_2^{\bullet -}$ which after dismutation generates H_2O_2. In the presence of copper and light, H_2O_2 is reduced to •OH. Electron transfer from the base to the photocleaver in the excited state also distorts the DNA structure (McFarland et al. 2020).

Since 1990, the usefulness of copper complexes in photodynamic therapy has been reported (Dolmans et al. 2003). To treat a deep tumor located inside the skin, Cu(II) complexes might be of interest, because the complex possesses d-d bands in the red region of Vis electromagnetic spectrum, which could lead to the use of Cu(II) complexes as photodynamic therapy. Once the Cu(II) complexes arrive inside the skin, they are easily activated due to the absorption of red light, which has the power of deep penetration into the tissues (DeRosa and Crutchley 2002).

[Cu(Ferrocene conjugated reduced Schiff base)(B)](NO3) with 1,10-phenanthroline derivatives presents a significant chemical nuclease activity in the presence of both oxidizing (H_2O_2) and reducing (GSH) agents. The complexes bind to DNA through different groove binding modes, being involved in the redox-active Fe(II) and Cu(II) centers with the observed redox couples of Cu(II)-Cu(I) and F_c^+-Fc 0.0 and 0.05 in DMF. PUC19 DNA photocleavage was observed at 454, 568, and 647 nm by $^{\bullet}$OH, which was formed during the photoredox pathways (Goswami et al. 2012). The formation of $^{\bullet}$OH by excited ferrocene-conjugated Cu-terpyridine complexes was also explained (Maity et al. 2010). Under photoexcitation, redox-active ferrocene moiety is oxidized and redox-active Cu(II) center is reduced to Cu(I), which determine the formation of $^{\bullet}$OH from O_2. Cu(I) center donates electrons to O_2 and in this way superoxide radical are formed. This finally generates $^{\bullet}$OH. Due to ferrocenyl moieties, the DNA cleavage activity at 454 nm was recorded. Using photoirradiation with Vis light (400–700 nm), photocytotoxicity of the complexes was demonstrated. The results obtained showed that the cytotoxicity of HeLa cells in Vis light increased approximately two to fourfold compared to dark toxicity (Goswami et al. 2012).

Under exposure of a ternary copper complex with antraquinone to Vis light (400–700 nm, 10Jcm^{-2}), using diphenylisobenzofuran, oxygen singlet was generated. Values between 0.157 and 0.629 were found for quantum yield.

The cytotoxicity of the complex on human breast adenocarcinoma (MCF-7) and human keratinocyte (HaCaT) cell lines conducted in Vis (400–700 nm, 10Jcm^{-2}) and dark light proved a very good efficacy in Vis (400–700 nm, 10Jcm^{-2}) light. This can be explained due to the presence of anthraquinone and S-coordination, which both present a photosensitizing capacity (Devi et al. 2020).

DNA binding capacity for some Cu(II) complexes containing Schiff base of salicylaldehyde and tryptophan and different kinds of phenanthroline bases was demonstrated by UV-visible absorption titration method. The cytotoxicity of the complexes on human cervical adenocarcinoma (HeLa) cell lines using MTT-method was determined in Vis(400–700 nm). The cytotoxicity of the complexes on HeLa cell lines was demonstrated also in dark light. This fact is due to the reduction of Cu (II) by cellular thiols which determine the ROS formation by using the Fenton reaction. However, when the cytotoxicity study was carried out under Vis light (400–700 nm) a 1–1.8 times higher cytotoxicity was found. DCFDA assay confirmed the ROS formation and the use of Annexin-V confirmed the apoptosis (Banaspati et al. 2019).

Several Cu(II) complexes with different ligands present good photocytotoxicity in visible light. So, the current results give hope to the researchers.

5.2 Photothermal Therapy

Photothermal therapy consists in the thermal damage of the tissues following irradiation with electromagnetic radiation (Chen et al. 2018). Photothermal agents (PTAs) irradiated by specific light wavelengths can induce local hyperthermia by absorbing photon energy and converting the increased kinetic energy into thermal energy. This process, known as photothermal therapy (PTT), is a highly effective and non-invasive treatment method that can induce cancer cell or pathogenic bacterial death. Moreover, PTT can facilitate other therapies by improving tissue perfusion and enhancing cell membrane permeability. Various synergistic therapies have been developed by combining PTT with other modalities, such as chemotherapy, chemodynamic therapy (CDT), and photodynamic therapy (PDT) (Ma et al. 2022).

Compared with other noble metal nanoparticles, copper nanoparticles have gained significant attention due to their high natural content and cost-effectiveness. Copper-incorporated nanomaterials (CINMs) have an intense and tunable localized surface plasmon resonance in the near-infrared biological window, which brings excellent photothermal conversion efficiency for PTT. CINMs have good catalytic properties and mediate Fenton-like reactions more efficiently than iron-based nanomaterials under a wide range of pH conditions (Doughty et al. 2019). Given these properties, the significance of CINMs has been investigated in various biomedical applications, such as tumor imaging and treatment, and tissue regeneration (Hu et al. 2021).

Au@MSNCu/PEG/DSF is a nano-platform whose antitumor action is triggered photothermally. In situ, it was shown that the release of DSF determines its chelation with Cu(II) and the generation of bis(diethyl-dithiocarbamate)-Cu, a cytotoxic compound which determines apoptosis and also the formation of Cu(I) species which are involved in the aggregation of toxic mitochondrial proteins which leads to cuproptosis at the cellular level. A new type of programmed cell death is represented by cuproptosis. This aims targeting the tumor cells and avoiding the action on healthy cells. In vivo studies also demonstrated the Au@MSNCu/PEG/DSF ability to kill tumor cells and to inhibit tumor growth (Xu et al. 2022).

5.3 Chemo-Dynamic Therapy

Chemo-dynamic therapy (CDT) represents a new kind of antitumor treatment. It is based on the Fenton reaction, namely on the decomposition of H_2O_2 with $^{\bullet}OH$ generation, which is implicated in DNA and protein damage from cancer cells (Dong et al. 2019). Fenton reaction takes place quickly only in acid medium. The tumor cells are known for their acid medium, so this therapy may be selective on tumor cells and avoid the destruction of normal cells. Other advantages of chemo-dynamic therapy are: an easy generation of $^{\bullet}OH$, capacity for deep tissue penetration, the method does not require other exogenous stimuli, and drug resistance is difficult to establish (Jana and Zhao 2022). Several in vivo studies demonstrated that Cu(I) ion-mediated Fenton-like reactions present kinetic and thermodynamic advantages in the acid medium of the tumor cells. Unfortunately, the method presents a disadvantage, namely, a low quantity of H_2O_2 was found and this determined a weak catalytic capacity which limits the development of chemo-dynamic therapy (Hwang and Jung 2020).

Glucose oxidase/CuFe-layered double hydroxides is a multifunctional nano-system obtained by loading glucose oxidase onto CuFe-LDH nanosheets, which is involved in a synchronous acid-enhanced/responsive chemo-dynamic/photothermal synergistic treatment. Layered double hydroxides are some two-dimensional nanomaterials, known under the formula [bivalent cation$_{1-x}$trivalen cation$_x$(OH)$_2$] (exchangeable interlaminar anion $^{n-}$)$_{x/n}$·mH_2O. The exchangeable interlaminar anion can balance the charge of the host layer. Due to their good biocompatibility, the layered double hydroxides were studied as inorganic biological composite nanomaterials (Mei et al. 2018). CuFe-layered double hydroxides determined the decomposition of H_2O_2 into $^{\bullet}OH$, being involved in the Fenton reaction. Using high-resolution transmission electron microscopy and atomic force microscopy for CuFe-LDHs a thickness of ~ 1.3 nm and a lateral size about ~ 65 nm were found. At the level of tumor cells, where the environment is acidic, glucose oxidase is involved in the decomposition of glucose with H_2O_2 formation. In this way, the problem of the low amount of H_2O_2 is solved. Moreover, glucose oxidase/CuFe-layered double hydroxides own an acid-enhanced near infrared photothermal treatment effect based on the defect-induced increase of photogenerated electron–hole pairs. The efficacy of the photothermal conversion was great and the heat released after the photothermal treatment stimulates the Fenton reaction, obtaining in this way a good chemo-dynamic treatment. Studying the cytotoxicity and the antitumor activity of glucose oxidase/CuFe-layered double hydroxides in vitro and in vivo, it was demonstrated that the nanosystem produced significant apoptosis and inhibition of tumor growth. Through this nanosystem, the possibility to associate the photothermal therapy with the chemo-dynamic therapy within the same nanoplatform, having as a goal to increase the efficacy of antitumor therapy, was demonstrated (Hu et al. 2021).

5.4 Nanoparticles

The use of nanoparticles in the formulation of anticancer drugs is studied by many researchers nowadays. Copper-based nanoparticles have inspired great interest in the area of antitumor therapy in recent decades, and their unique physicochemical features and remarkable biocompatibility make them suitable for biomedical applications, particularly tumor imaging and antitumor treatment (Zhang et al. 2019).

BSA-CuNPs were synthesized by a simple 2-step process that included the stable complex formation of Cu(II) with BSA and, subsequently, the reduction of the Cu (II) in ambient conditions. The CuNPs possessed superior photothermal activity over the Cu(II) and BSA/Cu(II) complex. The CuNPs, by themselves, showed significant cytotoxicity on the tested cancer cell lines; however, even higher anticancer effects were achieved with laser treatment. It was found that the photothermal activity could be retained for 5 days in storage conditions. Finally, the preliminary animal study results revealed that it is potentially safe to administer the BSA-CuNPs and these nanoparticles possess a relatively long plasma half-life. In these conditions, BSA-CuNPs could potentially serve as an effective PTT agent for cancer therapy.

Multifunctional copper-based nanomaterials have made significant progress in developing antitumor therapy during the previous decade. Compared with conventional copper complex, copper-based nanoplatforms provided efficient $^1O_2$ quantum yield and promising energy absorption in NIR, which could enable better cancer selectivity and lowered cytotoxicity, thus showing outstanding imaging and antitumor agent to diagnose and prevent cancer recurrence. The obtained results showed that copper was involved in multi-cell death pathways causing devastating injury to cancer cells, including mitochondrial dysfunction, indicating that copper-based nanomaterials theragnostics was a prospective antitumor approach when combined with drug delivery systems such as tumor-targeted drugs with genetic modification (McMahon et al. 2020).

Although the copper complexes have the expected antitumor activity, their biocompatibility and toxicity have not been enough studied. Considering the fact that classical chemotherapy also attacks normal cells, the discovery of a new anticancer compound with targeted action on tumor cells is very important. Synthesis of multifunctional copper nano-formulations will improve the availability of copper ions by targeted therapy, will decrease the toxicity of the compound, and finally will improve the anticancer treatment.

6 Conclusion

Considering that the number of people with cancer is increasing worldwide, the discovery of a new anticancer drug is imperative. Due to different mechanisms of action of the complexes, researchers synthetized and characterized different multi-functional copper complexes which induce tumor cell death and therefore have an antitumor effect. Many Cu(II) compounds possess promising physical and catalytic properties and their mechanism of action does not involve a single molecular target. In order to develop this kind of new drugs, the complexity of their mechanism of action must be understood and these mechanisms of action must be exploited in the new formulation. A large number of researchers were involved in studying the anticancer activity of copper complexes and many preclinical and clinical studies proved their anticancer activity. For this reason in the future it is desired to obtain copper compounds with better in vivo anticancer activity.

References

Abdel-Kader MH (2016) The journey of PDT throughout history: PDT from Pharos to present. In: Photodynamic medicine: from bench to clinic. Royal Society of Chemistry, Washington, DC, pp 1–21

Adsule S, Barve V, Chen D, Ahmed F, Dou QP, Padhye S, Sarkar FH (2006) Novel Schiff base copper complexes of quinoline-2 carboxyaldehyde as proteasome inhibitors in human prostate cancer cells. J Med Chem 49(24):7242–7246. https://doi.org/10.1021/jm060712l

Aguilar-Jimenez Z, Espinoza-Guillen A, Resendiz-Acevedo K, Fuentes-Noriega I, Mejia C, Ruiz-Azuara L (2023) The importance of being casiopeina as polypharmacologycal profile (Mixed chelate-copper (II) complexes and their *in vitro* and *in vivo* activities). Inorganics 11(10):394. https://doi.org/10.3390/inorganics11100394

Anthony EJ, Bolitho EM, Bridgewater HE, Carter OWL, Donnelly JM, Imberti C, Lant EC, Lermyte F, Needham RJ, Palau M, Sadler PJ, Shi H, Wang FX, Zhang WY, Zhang Z (2020) Metallodrugs are unique: opportunities and challenges of discovery and development. Chem Sci 11:12888–12017. https://doi.org/10.1039/d0sc04082g

Baldari S, Di Rocco G, Toietta G (2020) Current biomedical use of copper chelation therapy. Int J Mol Sci 21(3):1069. https://doi.org/10.3390/ijms21031069

Balsa LM, Baran EJ, Leon IE (2023) Copper complexes as antitumor agents: *In vitro* and *In vivo* evidence. Curr Med Chem 30(5):510–557. https://doi.org/10.2174/0929867328666211117094550

Banaspati A, Das D, Choudhury CJ, Bhattacharyya A, Goswami TK (2019) Photocytotoxic copper (II) complexes of N-salicylyl-l-tryptophan and phenanthroline bases. J Inorg Biochem 191:60–68. https://doi.org/10.1016/j.jinorgbio.2018.11.005

Barone G, Terenzi A, Lauria A, Almerico AM, Leal JM, Busto N, Garcia B (2013) DNA-binding of nickel(II), copper(II) and zinc(II) complexes: structure–affinity relationships. Coord Chem Rev 257(19–20):2848–2862. https://doi.org/10.1016/j.ccr.2013.02.023

Berkenblit A, Eder JP Jr, Ryan DP, Seiden MV, Tatsuta N, Sherman ML, Dahl TA, Dezube BJ, Supko JG (2007) Phase I clinical trial of STA-4783 in combination with paclitaxel in patients with refractory solid tumors. Clin Cancer Res 13(2 Pt1):584–590. https://doi.org/10.1158/1078-0432.CCR-06-0964

Biver T, Secco F, Venturini M (2008) Mechanistic aspects of the interaction of intercalating metal complexes with nucleic acids. Coord Chem Rev 252(10–11):1163–1177. https://doi.org/10.1016/j.ccr.2007.10.008

Brissos RF, Caubet A, Gamez P (2015) Possible DNA-interacting pathways for metal-based compounds exemplified with copper coordination compounds. Eur J Inorg Chem 16:2633–2645. https://doi.org/10.1002/ejic.201500175

Burden DA, Sullivan DM (1994) Phosphorylation of the alpha and beta isoforms of DNA topoisomerase II is qualitatively different in interphase and mitosis in Chinese hamster ovary cells. Biochemistry 33:14651–14655. https://doi.org/10.1021/bi00253a001

Calderwood SK (2016) A critical role for topoisomerase IIb and DNA double strand breaks in transcription. Transcription 7(3):75–83. https://doi.org/10.1080/21541264.2016.1181142

Campero-Peredo C, Bravo-Gómez ME, Hernández-Ojeda SL, Olguin-Reyes SR, Espinosa-Aguirre JJ, Ruiz-Azuara L (2016) Effect of [Cu(4,7-dimethyl-1,10-phenanthroline)(acetylacetonato)](NO_3), Casiopeína III-Ea, on the activity of cytochrome P450. Toxicol Vitro 33:16–22. https://doi.org/10.1016/j.tiv.2016.02.008

Ceramella J, Mariconda A, Iacopetta D, Saturnino C, Barbarossa A, Caruso A, Rosano C, Sinicropi MS, Longo P (2020) From coins to cancer therapy: gold, silver and copper complexes targeting human topoisomerases. Bioorg Med Chem Lett 30(3):126905. https://doi.org/10.1016/j.bmcl.2019.126905

Chavez-Gonzalez A, Centeno-Llanos S, Moreno-Lorenzana D, Sandoval-Esquivel MA, Aviles-Vazquez S, Bravo-Gomez ME, Ruiz-Azuara L, Ayala-Sanchez M, Torres-Martinez H, Mayani H (2017) Casiopeina III-Ea, a copper-containing small molecule, inhibits the *in vitro* growth of primitive hematopoietic cells from chronic myeloid leukemia. Leuk Res 52:8–19. https://doi.org/10.1016/j.leukres.2016.11.001

Chen SH, Chang JY (2019) New insights into mechanisms of cisplatin resistance: from tumor cell to microenvironment. Int J Mol Sci 20(17):4136. https://doi.org/10.3390/ijms20174136

Chen D, Peng FY, Cui QC, Daniel KG, Orlu S, Liu JG, Dou QP (2005) Inhibition of prostate cancer cellular proteasome activity by a pyrrolidine dithiocarbamate-copper complex is associated with suppression of proliferation and induction of apoptosis. Front Biosci 10:2932–2939. https://doi.org/10.2741/1749

Chen W, Yang W, Chen P, Huang Y, Li F (2018) Disulfiram copper nanoparticles prepared with a stabilized metal ion ligand complex method for treating drug-resistant prostate cancers. ACS Appl Mater Interfaces 10(48):41118–41128. https://doi.org/10.1021/acsami.8b14940

Chen X, Dou QP, Liu J, Tang D (2021) Targeting ubiquitin–proteasome system with copper complexes for cancer therapy. Front Mol Biosci 8:article 649154. https://doi.org/10.3389/fmolb.2021.649151

Cheung EC, Vousden KH (2022) The role of ROS in tumour development and progression. Nat Rev Cancer 22(5):280–297. https://doi.org/10.1038/s41568-021-00435-0

Dang J, He H, Chen D, Yin L (2017) Manipulating tumor hypoxia toward enhanced photodynamic therapy (PDT). Biomater Sci 5(8):1500–1511. https://doi.org/10.1039/c7bm00392g

Daniel KG, Chen D, Orlu S, Cui QC, Miller FR, Dou QP (2005) Clioquinol and pyrrolidine dithiocarbamate complex with copper to form proteasome inhibitors and apoptosis inducers in human breast cancer cells. Breast Cancer Res 7:R897–R908. https://doi.org/10.1186/bcr1322

de Anda-Jáuregui G, Espinal-Enríquez J, Hur J, Alcalá-Corona SA, Ruiz-Azuara L, Hernández-Lemus E (2019) Identification of Casiopeina II-gly secondary targets through a systems pharmacology approach. Comput Biol Chem 78:127–132. https://doi.org/10.1016/j.compbiolchem.2018.11.021

Denoyer D, Clatworthy SAS, Cater MA (2018) Copper complexes in cancer therapy. Met Ions Life Sci 18:469–506. https://doi.org/10.1515/9783110470734-022

DeRosa MC, Crutchley RJ (2002) Photosensitized singlet oxygen abd its applications. Coord Chem Rev 233–234:351–371. https://doi.org/10.1016/S0010-8545(02)00034-6

Devi LR, Raza MK, Musib D, Ramu V, Devi J, Roy M (2020) Novel targeting-based copper (II) complexes as the potent PDT agents: synthesis, photo-physical and theoretical evaluation. Inorg Chim Acta 500:119208. https://doi.org/10.1016/j.ica.2019.119208

Dilruba S, Kalayda GV (2016) Platinum-based drugs: past, present and future. Cancer Chemother Pharm 77(6):1103–1124. https://doi.org/10.1007/s00280-016-2976-z

Dolmans DE, Fukumura D, Jain RK (2003) Photodynamc therapy for cancer. Nat Rev Cancer 3(5): 380–387. https://doi.org/10.1038/nrc1071

Dong S, Xu J, Jia T, Xu M, Zhong C, Yang G, Li J, Yang D, He F, Gai S, Yang P, Lin J (2019) Upconversion-mediated $ZnFe_2O_4$ nanoplatform for NIR-enhanced chemodynamic and photodynamic therapy. Chem Sci 10:4259–4271. https://doi.org/10.1039/C9SC00387H

Doughty ACV, Hoover AR, Layton E, Murray CK, Howard EW, Chen WR (2019) Nanomaterial applications in photothermal therapy for cancer. Materials 12(5):779. https://doi.org/10.3390/ma12050779

Dzhardimalieva GI, Rabinskiy LN, Kydralieva KA, Uflyand IE (2019) Recent advances in metallopolymer-based drug delivery systems. RSC Adv 9(63):37009–37051. https://doi.org/10.1039/C9RA06678K

Elo H (2004) The antiproliferative agents trans-bis(resorcylaldoximato)copper(II) and trans-bis (2,3,4- trihydroxybenzaldoximato)copper(II) and cytopathic effects of HIV. Zeitschrift f¨ur Naturforschung 59(7–8):609–611. https://doi.org/10.1515/znc-2004-7-828

Erxleben A (2018) Interactions of copper complexes with nucleic acids. Coord Chem Rev 360:92–121. https://doi.org/10.1016/j.ccr.2018.01.008

Frezza M, Hindo S, Chen D, Davenport A, Schmitt S, Tomco D, Dou QP (2010) Novel metals and metal complexes as platforms for cancer therapy. Curr Pharm Des 16(16):1813–1825. https://doi.org/10.2174/138161210791209009

Galindo-Murillo R, Garcia-Ramos JC, Ruiz-Azuara L, Cheatham TE, Cortes-Guzman F (2015) Intercalation processes of copper complexes in DNA. Nucleic Acids Res 43:5364–5376. https://doi.org/10.1093/nar/gkv467

Galindo-Murillo R, Winkler L, Garcia-Ramos JC, Ruiz-Azuara L, Cortes-Guzman F, Cheatham TE (2020) Ancillary ligand on thernary Cu(II) complexes guides binding selectivity toward minor-grove DNA. J Phys Chem B 124:11648–11658. https://doi.org/10.1021/acs.jpcb.0c09296

Gandin V, Pellei M, Tisato F, Porchia M, Santini C, Marzano C (2012) A novel copper complex induces paraptosis in colon cancer cells via the activation of ER stress signalling. J Cell Mol Med 16(1):142–151. https://doi.org/10.1111/j.1582-4934.2011.01292.x

Garcia-Ramos JC, Galindo-Murillo R, Cortes-Guzman F, Ruiz-Azuara L (2013) Metal-based drug-DNA interactions. J Mex Chem Soc 57(3):245–259

Goswami TK, Gadadhar S, Roy M, Nethaji M, Karande AA, Chakravarty AR (2012) Ferrocene-conjugated copper(II) complexes of l-methionine and phenanthroline bases: synthesis, structure, and photocytotoxic activity. Organometallics 31:3010–3021. https://doi.org/10.1021/om201102k

Graf N, Lippard SJ (2012) Redox activation of metal-based prodrugs as a strategy for drug delivery. Adv Drug Deliv Rev 64:993–1004. https://doi.org/10.1016/j.addr.2012.01.007

Guan D, Zhao L, Shi X, Ma X, Chen Z (2023) Copper in cancer: from pathogenesis to therapy. Biomed Pharmacother 163:114791. https://doi.org/10.1016/j.biopha.2023.114791

Han J, Li L, Yue X, Chang J, Shi W, Hua Y (2013) A binuclear complex constituted by diethyldithiocarbamate and copper(I) functions as a proteasome activity inhibitor in pancreatic cancer cultures and xenografts. Toxicol Appl Pharmacol 273(3):477–483. https://doi.org/10.1016/j.taap.2013.09.009

Hangan AC, Turza A, Stan RL, Ştefan R, Oprean LS (2015) Synthesis, crystal structure, properties and nuclease activity of a new Cu(II) complex $[Cu(L)_2(py)_2(H_2O)]$. (HL=N-(5-(4-methylphenyl)-[1,3,4]–thiadiazole–2-yl)-toluenesulfonamide). Russ J Coord Chem 41(6):395–404. http://link.springer.com/journal/11173/41/6/page/1

Hangan AC, Turza A, Stan RL, Sevastre B, Páll E, Cetean S, Oprean LS (2016) Synthesis, crystal structure and characterization of new biologically active Cu(II) complexes with ligand derived from N-substituted sulfonamide. J Chem Sci 128(5):815–824. http://link.springer.com/article/10.1007/s12039-016-1077-1

Hangan AC, Lucaciu RL, Turza A, Dican L, Sevastre B, Páll E, Oprean LS, Borodi G (2023) New copper complexes with antibacterial and cytotoxic activity. Int J Mol Sci 24:13819. https://doi.org/10.3390/ijms241813819

Hanson S, Dharan A, Jinsha PV, Pal S, Nair BG, Kar R, Mishra N (2023) Paraptosis: a unique cell death mode for targeting cancer. Front Pharmacol 14:1159409. https://doi.org/10.3389/fphar.2023.1159409

Hariprabu KNG, Sathya M, Vimalraj S (2021) CRISPR/Cas9 in cancer therapy: a review with a special focus on tumor angiogenesis. Int J Biol Macromol 192:913–930. https://doi.org/10.1016/j.ijbiomac.2021.10.029

Hasinoff BB, Wu X, Yadav AA, Patel D, Zhang H, Wang DS, Chen ZS, Yalowich JC (2015) Cellular mechanisms of the cytotoxicity of the anticancer drug elesclomol and its complex with Cu(II). Biochem Pharmacol 93(3):266–276. https://doi.org/10.1016/j.bcp.2014.12.008

Hindo SS, Frezza M, Tomco D, Heeg MJ, Hryhorczuk L, McGarvey BR, Dou QP, Verani CN (2009) Metals in anticancer therapy: copper(II) complexes as inhibitors of the 20S proteasome. Eur J Med Chem 44:4353–4361. https://doi.org/10.1016/j.ejmech.2009.05.019

Hu W, Huang XS, Wu JF, Yang L, Zheng YT, Shen YM, Li ZY, Li X (2018) Discovery of novel topoisomerase II inhibitors by medicinal chemistry approaches. J Med Chem 61(20): 8947–8980. https://doi.org/10.1021/acs.jmedchem.7b01202

Hu T, Yan L, Wang Z, Shen W, Liang R, Yan D, Wei M (2021) A pH-responsive ultrathin Cu-based nanoplatform for specific photothermal and chemodynamic synergistic therapy. Chem Sci 12:2594–2603. https://doi.org/10.1039/d0sc06742c

Hwang E, Jung HS (2020) Metal-organic complex-based chemodynamic therapy agents for cancer therapy. Chem Commun 56:8332–8341. https://doi.org/10.1039/D0CC03012K

Jana D, Zhao Y (2022) Strategies for enhancing cancer chemodynamic therapy performance. Exploration 2:20210238. https://doi.org/10.1002/EXP.20210238

Jayaraju D, Kondapi AK (2001) Anti-cancer copper salicylaldoxime complex inhibits topoisomerase II catalytic activity. Curr Sci 81(7):787–792

Jiang Y, Huo Z, Qi X, Zuo T, Wu Z (2022) Copper-induced tumor cell death mechanisms and antitumor theragnostic applications of copper complexes. Nanomedicine (Lond) 7(5):303–324. https://doi.org/10.2217/nnm-2021-0374

Khadka DB, Cho WJ (2013) Topoisomerase inhibitors as anticancer agents: a patent update. Expert Opin Ther Pat 23:1033–1056. https://doi.org/10.1517/13543776.2013.790958

Khan GS, Shah A, Zia-ur-Rehman BD (2012) Chemistry of DNA minor groove binding agents. J Photochem Photobiol B 115:105–118. https://doi.org/10.1016/j.jphotobiol.2012.07.003

Kirshner JR, He S, Balasubramanyam V, Kepros J, Yang CY, Zhang M, Du Z, Barsoum J, Bertin J (2008) Elesclomol induces cancer cell apoptosis through oxidative stress. Mol Cancer Ther 7(8): 2319–2327. https://doi.org/10.1158/1535-7163.MCT-08-0298

Konkolova E, Janockova J, Perjesi P, Vaskova J, Kozurkova M (2018) Selected ferrocenyl chalcones as DNA/BSA-interacting agents and inhibitors of DNA topoisomerase I and II activity. J Organomet Chem 861:1–9. https://doi.org/10.1016/j.jorganchem.2018.01.031

Korn EL, Liu PY, Lee SJ, Chapman JAW, Niedzwiecki D, Suman VJ, Moon J, Sondak VK, Atkins MB, Eisenhauer EA, Parulekar W, Markovic SN, Saxman S, Kirkwood JM (2008) Meta-analysis of phase II cooperative group trials in metastatic stage IV melanoma to determine progression-free and overall survival benchmarks for future phase II trials. J Clin Oncol 26(4): 527–534. https://doi.org/10.1200/JCO.2007.12.7837

Liang X, Wu Q, Luan S, Yin Z, He C, Yin L, Zou Y, Yuan Z, Li L, Song X, He M, Lv C, Zhang W (2019) A comprehensive review of topoisomerase inhibitors as anticancer agents in the past decade. Eur J Med Chem 171:129–168. https://doi.org/10.1016/j.ejmech.2019.03.034

Liu H, Jiang R, Lu Y, Shan B, Wen Y, Li M (2022a) Biodegradable amorphous copper iron tellurite promoting the utilization of Fenton-like ions for efficient synergistic cancer theranostics. ACS Appl Mater Interfaces 14(25):28537–28547. https://doi.org/10.1021/acsami.2c03975

Liu J, Peng Y, Wei W (2022b) Cell cycle on the crossroad of tumorigenesis and cancer therapy. Trends Cell Biol 32(1):30–44. https://doi.org/10.1016/j.tcb.2021.07.001

Ma G, Liu Z, Zhu C, Chen H, Kwok RTK, Zhang P, Tang BZ, Cai L, Gong P (2022) H_2O_2 -Responsive NIR-II AIE nanobomb for carbon monoxide boosting low-temperature photothermal therapy. Angew Chem 61:e202207213. https://doi.org/10.1002/anie.202207213

Maity B, Roy M, Banik B, Majumdar R, Dighe RR, Chakravarty AR (2010) Ferrocene-promoted photoactivated DNA cleavage and anticancer activity of terpyridyl copper(II) phenanthroline complexes. Organometallics 29(16):3632–3641. http://pubs.acs.org/doi/abs/10.1021/om100524x

Masuri S, Vanhara P, Cabiddu MG, Moran L, Havel J, Cadoni E, Pivetta T (2022) Copper (II) phenantroline-based complexes as potential anticancer drugs: a walkthrough on the mechanisms of action. Molecules 27(1):49. https://doi.org/10.3390/molecules27010049

McFarland SA, Mandel A, Dumoulin-White R, Gasser G (2020) Metal-based photosensitizers for photodynamic therapy: the future of multimodal oncology? Curr Opin Chem Biol 56:23–27. https://doi.org/10.1016/j.cbpa.2019.10.004

McMahon A, Chen W, Li F (2020) Old wine in new bottles: advanced drug delivery systems for disulfiram-based cancer therapy. J Control Release 319:352–359. https://doi.org/10.1016/j.jconrel.2020.01.001

Mei X, Ma J, Bai X, Zhang X, Zhang S, Liang R, Wei M, Evans DG, Duan X (2018) A bottom-up synthesis of rare-earth-hydrotalcite monolayer nanosheets toward multimode imaging and synergetic therapy. Chem Sci 9:5630–5639. https://doi.org/10.1039/c8sc01288a

Modrich P (2006) Mechanisms in eukaryotic mismatch repair. J Biol Chem 281(41):30305–30309. https://doi.org/10.1074/jbc.R600022200

Molinaro C, Wambang N, Bousquet T, Vercoutter-Edouart AS, Pélinski L, Cailliau K, Martoriati AA (2022) Novel Copper(II) indenoisoquinoline complex inhibits topoisomerase I, induces G2 phase arrest, and autophagy in three adenocarcinomas. Front Oncol 12:837373. https://doi.org/10.3389/fonc.2022.837373

Monk BJ, Kauderer JT, Moxley KM, Bonebrake AJ, Dewdney SB, Secord AA, Ueland FR, Johnston CM, Aghajanian C (2018) A phase II evaluation of elesclomol sodium and weekly paclitaxel in the treatment of recurrent or persistent platinum resistant ovarian, fallopian tube or primary peritoneal cancer: an NRG oncology/gynecologic oncology group study. Gynecol Oncol 151(3):422–427. https://doi.org/10.1016/j.ygyno.2018.10.001

Monro S, Colon KL, Yin H, Roque J III, Konda P, Gujar S, Thummel RP, Lilge L, Cameron CG, McFarland SA (2019) Transition metal complexes and photodynamic therapy from tumor-centered ppproach: challenges, opportunities, and highlights from the development of TLD1433. Chem Rev 119(2):797–828. https://doi.org/10.1021/acs.chemrev.8b00211

Morris DL (2014) DNA-bound metal ions: recent developments. Biomol Concepts 5(5):397–407. https://doi.org/10.1515/bmc-2014-0021

Nakamoto K, Tsuboi M, Strahan GD (2008) Drug-DNA interactions. structures and spectra. Wiley, New York

Nakamura H, Takada K (2021) Reactive oxygen species in cancer: current findings and future directions. Cancer Sci 112(10):3945–3952. https://doi.org/10.1111/cas.15068

National Research Council (1995) Calculating the secrets of life: contributions of the mathematical sciences to molecular biology. The National Academies Press, Washington, DC

Nelson SM, Ferguson LR, Denny WA (2007) Non-covalent ligand/DNA interactions: minor groove binding agents. Mutat Res 623(1–2):24–40. https://doi.org/10.1016/j.mrfmmm.2007.03.012

O'Day SJ, Eggermont AM, Chiarion-Sileni V, Kefford R, Grob JJ, Mortier L, Robert C, Schachter J, Testori A, Mackiewicz J, Friedlander P, Garbe C, Ugurel S, Collichio F, Guo W, Lufkin J, Bahcall S, Vukovic V, Hauschild A (2013) Final results of phase III SYMMETRY study: randomized, double-blind trial of elesclomol plus paclitaxel versus paclitaxel alone as treatment for chemotherapy-naive patients with advanced melanoma. J Clin Oncol 31(9): 1211–1218. https://doi.org/10.1200/JCO.2012.44.5585

Oe S, Miyagawa K, Honma Y, Harada M (2016) Copper induces hepatocyte injury due to the endoplasmic reticulum stress in cultured cells and patients with Wilson disease. Exp Cell Res 347(1):192–200. https://doi.org/10.1016/j.yexcr.2016.08.003

Pages BJ, Ang DL, Wright EP, Aldrich-Wright JR (2015) Metal complex interactions with DNA. Dalton Trans 44(8):3505–3526. https://doi.org/10.1039/c4dt02700k

Pan P, Svirskis D, Rees SWP, Barker D, Waterhouse GIN, Wu Z (2021) Photosensitive drug delivery systems for cancer therapy: mechanisms and applications. J Control Release 338:446–461. https://doi.org/10.1016/j.jconrel.2021.08.053

Pang H, Chen D, Cui QC, Dou QP (2007) Sodium diethyldithiocarbamate, an AIDS progression inhibitor and a copper-binding compound, has proteasome-inhibitory and apoptosis-inducing activities in cancer cells. Int J Mol Med 19(5):809–816. https://doi.org/10.3892/ijmm.19.5.809

Pitie M, Boldron C, Gornitzka H, Hemmert C, Donnadieu B, Meunier B (2003) DNA cleavage by copper complexes of 2- and 3-clip-phen derivatives. Eur J Inorg Chem 3:528–540. https://doi.org/10.1002/ejic.200390075

Poblocki K, Drzezdzon J, Kostrzewa T, Jacewicz D (2021) Coordination complexes as a new generation photosensitizer for photodynamic anticancer therapy. Int J Mol Sci 22:8052. https://doi.org/10.3390/ijms22158052

Qi J, Zheng Y, Li B, Ai Y, Chen M, Zheng X (2022) Pyridoxal hydrochloride thiosemicarbazones with copper ions inhibit cell division via Topo-I and Topo-IIα. J Inorg Biochem 232:111816. https://doi.org/10.1016/j.jinorgbio.2022.111816

Rae C, Mairs RJ (2017) Evaluation of the radiosensitizing potency of chemotherapeutic agents in prostate cancer cells. Int J Radiat Biol 93(2):194–203. https://doi.org/10.1080/09553002.2017.1231946

Renfrew AK (2014) Transition metal complexes with bioactive ligands: mechanisms for selective ligand release and applications for drug delivery. Metallomics 6(8):1324–1335. https://doi.org/10.1039/c4mt00069b

Schwartz L, Supuran CT, Alfarouk KO (2017) The Warburg effect and the hallmarks of cancer. Anti Cancer Agents Med Chem 17(2):164–170. https://doi.org/10.2174/1871520616666161031143301

Serment-Guerrero J, Bravo-Gomez ME, Lara-Rivera E, Ruiz-Azuara L (2017) Genotoxic assessment of the copper chelated compounds Casiopeinas: clues about their mechanisms of action. J Inorg Biochem 166:68–75. https://doi.org/10.1016/j.jinorgbio.2016.11.007

Shagufta W, Ishrad A (2020) Transition metal complexes as proteasome inhibitors for cancer treatment. Inorg Chim Acta 506:119521. https://doi.org/10.1016/j.ica.2020.119521

Shimada K, Reznik E, Stokes ME, Krishnamoorthy L, Bos PH, Song Y, Quartararo CE, Pagano NC, Carpizo DR, deCarvalho AC, Lo DC, Stockwell BR (2018) Copper-binding small molecule induces oxidative stress and cell-cycle arrest in glioblastoma-patient-derived cells. Cell Chem Biol 25:585–594.e587. https://doi.org/10.1016/j.chembiol.2018.02.010

Shobha Devi C, Thulasiram B, Aerva RR, Nagababu P (2018) Recent advances in copper intercalators as anticancer agents. J Fluoresc 28(5):1195–1205. https://doi.org/10.1007/s10895-018-2283-7

Siegel RL, Miller KD, Jemal A (2019) Cancer Statistics CA Cancer J Clin 69:7–34. https://doi.org/10.3322/caac.21442

Sies H, Belousov VV, Chandel NS, Davies MJ, Jones DP, Mann GE, Murphy MP, Yamamoto M, Winterbourn C (2022) Defining roles of specific reactive oxygen species (ROS) in cell biology and physiology. Nat Rev Mol Cell Biol 23(7):499–515. https://doi.org/10.1038/s41580-022-00456-z

Sigman DS, Landgraf R, Perrin DM, Perason L (1996) Nucleic acid chemistry of the cuprous complexes of 1,10-phenanthroline and derivatives. Met Ions Biol Syst 33:485–513

Silva-Platas C, Guerrero-Beltrán CE, Carrancá M, Castillo EC, Bernal-Ramírez J, Oropeza-Almazán Y, González LN, Rojo R, Martínez LE, Valiente-Banuet J, Ruiz-Azuara L, Bravo-Gomez ME, Garcia N, Carvajal K, Garcia-Rivas G (2016) Antineoplastic copper coordinated complexes (Casiopeinas) uncouple oxidative phosphorylation and induce mitochondrial permeability transition in cardiac mitochondria and cardiomyocytes. J Bioenerg Biomembr 48(1): 43–54. https://doi.org/10.1007/s10863-015-9640-x

Skok Z, Zidar N, Kikelj D, Ilas J (2020) Dual Inhibitors of human DNA topoisomerase II and other cancer-related targets. J Med Chem 63:884–904. https://doi.org/10.1021/acs.jmedchem.9b00726

Sponer J, Burda JV, Leszczynski J (2006) Interactions of metal cations with nucleic acids and their building units. In: Šponer J, Lankaš F Computational Studies of RNA and DNA. Springer, pp 389–409

Srivatsan SG, Parvez M, Verma S (2003) Adenine-copper coordination polymer as an oxidative nucleozyme: implications for simple prebiotic catalytic units. J Inorg Biochem 97(4):340–344. https://doi.org/10.1016/S0162-0134(03)00285-X

Sugimoto N (2023) Handbook of chemical biology of nucleic acids. Springer, Singapore

Szewczyk OK, Roszczenko P, Czarnomysy R, Bielawska A, Bielawski K (2022) An overview of the importance of transition-metal nanoparticles in cancer research. Int J Mol Sci 23(12):6688. https://doi.org/10.3390/ijms23126688

Tabti R, Tounsi N, Gaiddon C, Bentouhami E, Desaubry L (2017) Progress in copper complexes as anticancer agents. Med Chem 7:5. https://doi.org/10.4172/2161-0444.1000445

Tardito S, Marchiò L (2009) Copper compounds in anticancer strategies. Curr Med Chem 16(11): 1325–1348. https://doi.org/10.2174/092986709787846532

Tardito S, Isella C, Medico E, Marchiò L, Bevilacqua E, Hatzoglou M, Bussolati O, Franchi-Gazzola R (2009) The thioxotriazole copper(II) complex A_0 induces endoplasmic reticulum stress and paraptotic death in human cancer cells. J Biol Chem 284(36):24306–24319. https://doi.org/10.1074/jbc.M109.026583

Thomas A, Pommier Y (2019) Targeting topoisomerase I in the era of precision medicine. Clin Cancer Res 25(22):6581–6589. https://doi.org/10.1158/1078-0432.CCR-19-1089

Thomas AM, Nethaji M, Chakravarty AR (2004) Different modes of DNA cleavage activity of dihydroxo-bridged dicopper(II) complexes having phenanthroline bases. J Inorg Biochem 98(6):1087–1094. https://doi.org/10.1016/j.jinorgbio.2004.02.029

Tsvetkov P, Coy S, Petrova B, Dreishpoon M, Verma A, Abdusamad M, Rossen J, Joesch-Cohen L, Humeidi R, Spangler RD, Eaton JK, Frenkel E, Kocak M, Corsello SM, Lutsenko S, Kanarek N, Santagata S, Golub TR (2022) Copper induces cell death by targeting lipoylated TCA cycle proteins. Science 375(6586):1254–1261. https://doi.org/10.1126/science.abf0529

Verani CN (2012) Metal complexes as inhibitors of the 26 proteasome in tumor cells. J Inorg Biochem 106(1):59–67. https://doi.org/10.1016/j.jinorgbio.2011.09.003

Vértiz G, García-Ortuño LE, Bernal JP, Bravo-Gómez ME, Lounejeva E, Huerta A, Ruiz-Azuara L (2014) Pharmacokinetics and hematotoxicity of a novel copper-based anticancer agent: Casiopeina III-Ea, after a single intravenous dose in rats. Fundam Clin Pharmacol 28:78–87. https://doi.org/10.1111/j.1472-8206.2012.01075.x

von Hippel PH, Marcus AH (2019) The many roles of binding cooperativity in the control of DNA replication. Biophys J 117(11):2143–2146. https://doi.org/10.1016/j.bpj.2019.10.029

Wang JC (1971) Interaction between DNA and an Escherichia coli protein omega. J Mol Biol 55(3): 523–533. https://doi.org/10.1016/0022-2836(71)90334-2

Wang F, Zhai S, Liu X, Li L, Wu S, Dou QP, Yan B (2011) A novel dithiocarbamate analogue with potentially decreased ALDH inhibition has copper-dependent proteasome-inhibitory and apoptosis-inducing activity in human breast cancer cells. Cancer Lett 300(1):87–95. https://doi.org/10.1016/j.canlet.2010.09.010

Wei J, Fang D (2021) Endoplasmic reticulum stress signaling and the pathogenesis of hepatocarcinoma. Int J Mol Sci 22(4):1799. https://doi.org/10.3390/ijms22041799

Wu J, Qiao S, Xiang Y, Cui M, Yao X, Lin R, Zhang X (2021) Endoplasmic reticulum stress: multiple regulatory roles in hepatocellular carcinoma. Biomed Pharmacother 142:112005. https://doi.org/10.1016/j.biopha.2021.112005

Xu Y, Zhou Q, Feng X, Dai Y, Jiang Y, Jiang W, Liu X, Xing X, Wang Y, Ni Y, Zheng C (2020) Disulfiram/copper markedly induced myeloma cell apoptosis through activation of JNK and intrinsic and extrinsic apoptosis pathways. Biomed Pharmacother 126:110048. https://doi.org/10.1016/j.biopha.2020.110048

Xu Y, Liu SY, Zeng L, Ma H, Zhang Y, Yang H, Liu Y, Fang S, Zhao J, Xu Y (2022) An enzyme-engineered nonporous copper(I) coordination polymer nanoplatform for cuproptosis-based synergistic cancer therapy. Adv Mater 34:e2204733. https://doi.org/10.1002/adma.202204733

Yang Y, Li M, Chen G, Liu S, Guo H, Dong X, Wang K, Geng H, Jiang J, Li X (2023) Dissecting copper biology and cancer treatment: "Activating cuproptosis or suppressing cuproplasia". Coord Chem Rev 495:215395. https://doi.org/10.1016/j.ccr.2023.215395

Zeglis BM, Pierre VC, Barton JK (2007) Metallo-intercalators and metallo-insertors. Chem Commun (Camb) 44:4565–4579. https://doi.org/10.1039/b710949k

Zhang B, Burke R (2023) Copper homeostasis and the ubiquitin proteasome system. Metallomics 15(3):mfad010. https://doi.org/10.1093/mtomcs/mfad010

Zhang X, Bi CF, Fan Y, Cui Q, Chen D, Xiao Y, Dou QP (2008) Induction of tumor cell apoptosis by taurine Schiff base copper complex is associated with the inhibition of proteasomal activity. Int J Mol Med 22:677–682. https://doi.org/10.3892/ijmm_00000072

Zhang D, Zhang C, Liu J, Chen Q, Zhu X, Liang C (2019) Carbon-encapsulated metal/metal carbide/metal oxide core–shell nanostructures generated by laser ablation of metals in organic solvents. ACS Appl Nano Mater 2(1):28–39. https://doi.org/10.1021/acsanm.8b01541

Zimbone S, Santoro AM, La Mendola D, Giacomelli C, Trincavelli ML, Tomasello MF, Milardi D, García-Viñuales S, Sciacca MFM, Martini C, Grasso G (2020) The ionophoric activity of a pro-apoptotic VEGF165 fragment on HUVEC cells. Int J Mol Sci 21(8):2866. https://doi.org/10.3390/ijms21082866

Zuo J, Bi C, Fan Y, Buac D, Nardon C, Daniel KG, Dou QP (2013) Cellular and computational studies of proteasome inhibition and apoptosis induction in human cancer cells by amino acid Schiff base-copper complexes. J Inorg Biochem 118:83–93. https://doi.org/10.1016/j.jinorgbio.2012.10.006

Liquid Biopsy and Cancer

Robert H. Eibl and Markus Schneemann

Abstract

Liquid biopsy is a minimally invasive diagnostic tool for cancer that analyzes easily accessible fluids such as blood, urine, and cerebrospinal fluid for cancer-specific biomarkers. It provides real-time information on tumor progression and treatment response and has several advantages over tissue biopsy. Technological improvements and standardization are expected to make it widely available at affordable prices, potentially reducing cancer mortality and contributing to achieving Sustainable Development Goal 3 (SDG 3). While further advancements are needed to make it affordable, liquid biopsy has the potential to revolutionize the diagnosis and treatment of cancer globally, benefitting both high- and lower-income populations. Its immense potential can reduce the burden of cancer and improve health outcomes for all.

Keywords

Cancer · Diagnostic tool · Liquid biopsy · Real time

R. H. Eibl (✉)
c/o M. Schneemann, Department of Internal Medicine, Hospitals of Schaffhausen, Schaffhausen, Switzerland
e-mail: robert.eibl@alumni.dkfz.de

M. Schneemann
Department of Internal Medicine, Hospitals of Schaffhausen, Schaffhausen, Switzerland
e-mail: markus.schneemann@spitaeler-sh.ch

Interdisciplinary Cancer Research, https://doi.org/10.1007/16833_2024_288
Published online: 29 June 2024

1 Introduction

Cancer remains a global health challenge, as it is, after cardiovascular diseases, the second most common cause of death worldwide, accounting for ten million deaths in 2020 alone (Sung et al. 2021). Despite significant advances in surgery, radiation, and chemotherapy over the last century, as well as the recent addition of immunotherapy, there is a continuing need for improvement. This includes the necessary smaller steps of translational research for clinical applications (low-risk research), as well as the funding of basic research for more fundamental innovations in the long run (high-risk research). Prevention and early diagnosis, as well as close monitoring of individual tumor development and treatment response, remain key to improving overall survival (OS) and progression-free survival (PFS). However, there are also significant inequalities in cancer incidence, diagnosis, and treatment between social groups and countries, highlighting the urgent need for accessible and affordable diagnostic tools, disease monitoring, and treatment. In recent years, liquid biopsy has emerged as a promising diagnostic and monitoring tool for cancer. Unlike normal biopsy, the gold standard to obtain tumor tissue for microscopic evaluation, liquid biopsy involves the less invasive analysis of easily accessible body fluids such as blood, cerebrospinal fluid (CSF), or urine to detect cancer-specific biomarkers such as circulating tumor DNA (ctDNA), circulating tumor cells (CTCs), and extracellular vesicles (EVs) distant from the tumor (Fig. 1). This noninvasive technique can offer several advantages over tissue biopsy, including real-time information on tumor progression or treatment response, including resistance. After a slow start

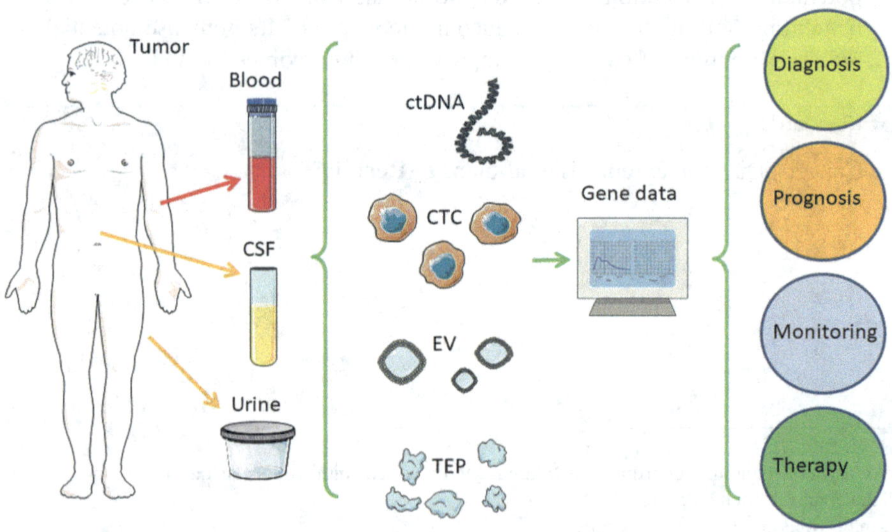

Fig. 1 Principles of liquid biopsy. Body fluids distant from the primary tumor can be easily obtained at low risk and analyzed for tumor-derived information. (Adapted from (Eibl and Schneemann 2021, 2022a), with modified images from Servier Med. Art. (https://smart.servier.com; CC BY 3.0))

two decades ago, a rapidly increasing number of publications over the last 5 years reflect this revolutionary development in medicine. Further improvement and standardization of technology allow the expectation of widespread applications with competitive pricing. The Sustainable Development Goals (SDGs) were adopted by the United Nations in 2015 to promote sustainable and equitable development worldwide (United Nations Department of Economic and Social Affairs 2016a). Among the 17 goals, SDG 3 aims to ensure healthy lives and well-being for all, including the prevention and treatment of cancer (United Nations Department of Economic and Social Affairs 2016b, p. 3). This goal comprises 13 specific targets and 27 goal indicators, including Target 3.4, which seeks to reduce premature mortality from noncommunicable diseases, such as cancer, by a third by 2030. Goal indicator 3.4.1 specifically measures mortality rates attributed to cardiovascular disease, cancer, diabetes, or chronic respiratory disease. Reducing cancer mortality can be achieved through prevention before the onset of the disease or an improved treatment after its development. To measure and compare this indicator across different regions and countries, mortality rates must be standardized, although prevention and treatment efforts can still be improved without complete data. For example, cigarette smoking and alcohol abuse are well-known risk factors for cancer and do not require further data from every country. However, improving early cancer detection and treatment approaches offers additional opportunities to reduce cancer mortality. While modern medicine has brought major advancements, such as computed tomography (CT) and magnetic resonance tomography (MRT) technologies, it also comes with significant additional costs. Health management expenses can quickly escalate, often resulting in increased disparities between high- and low-income countries. However, considering the dramatic reduction of costs for sequencing the human genome from the year 2000 until today (billions vs. a few hundred US dollars per genome sequencing), liquid biopsy may soon become an affordable diagnostic tool in personalized medicine, accompanied by an increasing number of targetable mutations and corresponding treatment options. Since liquid biopsy has the potential to facilitate not only the diagnosis and monitoring of cancer patients in countries with the highest medical standards but also in lower- and middle-income countries, it has the clear potential to bridge a major gap for better management of cancer patients in different parts of the world. Future directions may include establishing liquid biopsy in countries and regions even before patients can get easy and affordable access to otherwise established, but still hardly affordable methods of medical imaging such as magnetic resonance imaging (MRI) or tumor histopathology. Liquid biopsy has the potential to become a gamechanger in achieving at least some of the SDG 3 goals related to cancer prevention, early detection, and treatment. This chapter aims to summarize recent advances in liquid biopsy, including the analysis of ctDNA and CTCs, and their application in different types of cancer. The potential of liquid biopsy will be discussed to improve cancer outcomes and reduce health inequalities by making cancer diagnosis and monitoring more accessible and affordable in many countries.

2 Liquid Biopsy

The common principles of liquid biopsy are illustrated in Fig. 1.

In the past 20 years, liquid biopsy has encompassed a variety of techniques for detecting cancer-specific markers in biofluids such as blood, cerebrospinal fluid, or urine. Such probes are collected from locations far removed from the primary tumor and possible metastases, typically providing a simpler and safer means of access compared to more invasive tissue biopsy (Eibl and Schneemann 2021). As a result, liquid biopsy has evolved to encompass a much broader range of circulating biomarkers present in different body fluids (Alix-Panabières and Pantel 2021). The main targets of liquid biopsy are circulating tumor DNA (ctDNA), which is a subset of the entire cell-free DNA (cfDNA), and circulating tumor cells (CTC). Additional instances involve examining extracellular vesicles (EVs) and RNA molecules like microRNA (miRNA), along with tumor-educated platelets (TEPs). The shared objectives of liquid biopsy include detecting cancer early, diagnosing it accurately, and monitoring how well treatments are working. The ultimate goal is to develop a fast, dependable, and easily repeatable test that can track tumor progression in real time. This test would also help monitor treatment response, detect resistance, relapse, and metastasis sooner, and guide clinical decisions accordingly. Moreover, identifying specific markers after successful cancer treatment can confirm minimal residual disease (MRD), prompting further treatment before the tumor becomes untreatable (Bardelli and Pantel 2017). The prevailing protocol for addressing the majority of solid cancers involves conducting a more intrusive fine-needle biopsy or surgically extracting at least substantial portions of the tumor, followed by a meticulous microscopic examination performed by a tumor pathologist. Additionally, the analysis may encompass genetic molecular profiling of the primary tumor tissue. Notably, the 2016 revision of the WHO classification for nervous system tumors incorporated molecular and genetic profiling as a routine procedure for scrutinizing certain brain tumors like medulloblastomas and glioblastomas (Louis et al. 2016). Repeated acquisition of tumor tissues can present challenges and may not be ideal for continuous monitoring of tumor evolution. Moreover, rare, transthoracic lung biopsies can lead to the unintended spread of cancer cells (Müller et al. 1986), and fine-needle aspirations have been linked to an increase in circulating tumor cells (CTCs) in patients with prostate cancer (Joosse et al. 2020). Minor, but metastatically progressing, subpopulations of tumor cells with different genetic mutations may not be adequately sampled in a solitary biopsy (Eslami-S et al. 2020). Therefore, liquid biopsy is emerging as a potential new standard for tracking cancer progression. Current research efforts are focused on various methods for detecting and analyzing CTCs, enhancing our understanding of tumor growth and spread. This is supported by numerous clinical studies focused on establishing new standards for monitoring various types of cancers (Alix-Panabières and Pantel 2013; Denève et al. 2013; Ramirez et al. 2014; Cayrefourcq et al. 2015, 2019; Kuske et al. 2016; Garrel et al. 2019; Koch et al. 2020; Mazard et al. 2021). At present, the examination of cfDNA seems to be nearing broader clinical adoption due to its greater accessibility and the absence of intricate methodologies needed to capture the exceptionally scarce CTCs.

3 Markers

CTCs and ctDNA presently have a more established status in liquid biopsy compared to EVs and TEPs.

3.1 CTC

In the past two decades, clinical applications for detecting and quantifying circulating tumor cells (CTCs) have emerged, along with efforts to analyze their genetic profiles for prognostic purposes and informed clinical decision-making (Fig. 1). The metastatic process allows at least one tumor cell to leave its original location, either the primary tumor or a metastatic tumor site, before it can enter the bloodstream or the lymphatic system. Such a cell needs to be mobile enough to also migrate through the layers of a blood vessel wall. Then it needs to survive the shear forces of the bloodstream, perhaps due to a certain elasticity or rigidity, and then stop at a distant site to migrate again through a vessel wall and enter another tissue. Some of these steps are supposed to be due to simple mechanics. A tumor cell is usually much bigger than the diameter of a capillary, 10–20 μm vs. 7 μm (Chambers et al. 2002), but since red blood cells are also bigger than their capillary bed (7.7 vs. 7 μm), it is plausible that at least some metastatic tumor cells can pass through the capillary bed and may use adhesion molecules and chemokine receptors in different ways for their later stop and growth at distant sites (Eibl 2013). While only a small percentage of CTCs seem to contribute to the development of metastases, they can serve as indicators for predicting tumor progression (Fidler 1975; Alix-Panabieres et al. 2021; Yamamoto et al. 2023). The detection of rare CTCs is challenging and depends on enrichment steps, which usually target physical differences between CTCs and normal cells in the blood, like size, density, elasticity, or electric charges (Pantel and Alix-Panabières 2019; Deng et al. 2022). Some of these strategies also aim for functional biological differences, such as the presence or the absence of specific receptors: epithelium-derived carcinoma cells can be selected for the expression of EpCAM (positive selection), whereas removal of leukocytes expressing CD45 also helps to increase the concentration of CTCs (negative selection). EpCAM enrichment has already been used in various studies on metastatic and nonmetastatic breast cancer (Cristofanilli et al. 2004; Budd et al. 2006; Pachmann et al. 2008; Lucci et al. 2012; Bidard et al. 2014; Smerage et al. 2014), non-small-cell lung cancer (NSCLC) (Punnoose et al. 2012), small-cell lung cancer (Hou et al. 2012), metastatic and nonmetastatic colorectal cancer (Cohen et al. 2008; Bork et al. 2015), hepatocellular carcinoma (Kelley et al. 2015), and prostate cancer (Okegawa et al. 2014), although with variable predictive value. After enrichment, antibody-based direct immunological methods help to identify and further separate individual CTCs from contaminating leukocytes (Alix-Panabières et al. 2017). The CellSearch platform is the only FDA-approved clinical application for CTC detection, which uses fluorescently labeled antibodies to epithelial cytokeratin and CD45 for exclusion of leukocytes (Swennenhuis et al. 2016). However, this technology has limitations as it mainly relies on the expression of EpCAM, which decreases during metastasis, and has a low sensitivity for CTC detection. The CellSearch system also offers low purity of captured cells, resulting in captured CTCs being usually contaminated by blood cells or normally circulating epithelial cells. Manually isolating circulating tumor cells (CTCs) is a time-consuming process. An alternative method, called DEPArray, uses dielectrophoresis to trap single CTCs. However, this method has some limitations, such as low sample volumes and varying dielectric features of cells (Pethig 2010; Alshareef et al. 2013; De Luca et al. 2016). Flow cytometry and cell sorting can also detect and analyze CTCs, but a pre-enrichment step is required to achieve high initial CTC concentrations (Bhagwat et al. 2018). Immunomagnetic enrichment and laser technology can sort cells based on their properties, but the use of expensive antibodies makes it expensive. Additionally, real-time analysis of CTCs may not be possible since the cells are fixed during the assay process (Magbanua and Park 2013). CTCs can also be detected by targeting the mRNA or DNA level using polymerase chain reaction (PCR) tests with specific primers. These tests can identify tissue, organ, or tumor-specific transcriptions, as well as tumor-specific mutations, translocations, or methylation patterns (Mastoraki et al. 2018). Reverse transcription PCR (RT-PCR) can detect low-abundance mRNA, but the CTC number can only be estimated due to variations in gene expression levels (Bustin et al. 2004). Digital droplet PCR (ddPCR) is a newer technique that allows for faster quantification of low-abundance targets and with a lower sample requirement than other digital PCR assays (Siravegna and Bardelli 2014; Zhang et al. 2015). This method uses water-oil emulsion droplet technology, which reduces costs and preserves valuable samples (Hindson et al. 2011). The epithelial ImmunoSPOT (EPISPOT) assay is a functional assay that has been used for CTC detection in blood and bone marrow samples for over two decades (Soler et al. 2017). This assay provides quantitative and qualitative information about the number and types of viable CTCs present in the sample based on the fluorescence detection of specific epithelial proteins secreted by these cells. The EPIDROP assay is a newer (Eyer et al. 2017), more rapid and sensitive version of EPISPOT that allows for the capture and detection of CTCs at the single cell level by immunostaining prior to encapsulation in fluid microdroplets. This allows for the assessment of EMT status and the distinction between viable and apoptotic CTCs. However, there can be problems with lower antigen levels or reduced binding efficiency (Millner et al. 2013), and EPISPOT requires 3 days for analysis (Ramirez et al. 2014), making it unsuitable for clinical use in isolating more heterogeneous cells (Monteiro-Riviere et al. 2009). Future development of this innovative assay will incorporate molecular characterization of the captured CTCs. Despite the significant advantages of circulating tumor cells (CTCs) in diagnostics, prognostics, monitoring, and guiding therapy choices and delivery schedules, widespread use appears to be a distant goal. At present, only a limited number of well-equipped laboratories, backed by substantial research funds, seem capable of collecting and analyzing CTCs. A universally accepted standard is yet to be established. The introduction of CellSearch marked a milestone when both the European Medicines Agency and the US Food and Drug Administration granted approval for the first liquid biopsy in 2004. CellSearch was first licensed to identify and quantify CTCs in blood to estimate clinical outcome solely for patients with metastatic mammary carcinoma. Later, it was extended to track patients also with colorectal and prostate cancer.

3.2 ctDNA and cfDNA

The collective quantity of noncellular DNA found in samples like blood is referred to as cfDNA, encompassing all tumor-derived DNA in varying amounts, known as ctDNA in the case of tumor patients. Healthy individuals have highly fragmented cfDNA in their blood, with a peak of 166 bp and numerous smaller peaks. The fragment size of tumor-derived ctDNA shifts to a lower peak at 146 bp, allowing for increased sensitivity through selection strategies. The majority of cfDNA is produced by leukocytes, with minor contributions from many other cell types (Neuberger et al. 2022). Physical activity triggers cfDNA release primarily from granulocytes. ctDNA can originate from the original tumor mass, metastases, and CTCs. ctDNA is typically a small fraction of cfDNA, particularly in the early stages and after successful therapies. Therefore, the main obstacle to widespread tumor screening and treatment monitoring continues to be the detection of low concentrations of ctDNA. The development and application of several critical technologies have made it possible to identify possible micro-metastases and local relapses prior to clinical and radiological manifestations (Kwapisz 2017).

3.2.1 Targeted Analysis

The goal of targeted analysis is to locate methylations or mutations unique to a given tumor. Techniques employed for this purpose encompass digital PCR (dPCR), safe-sequencing system (Safe-SeqS), BEAMing (beads, emulsions, amplification, magnetics), and tagged-amplicon deep sequencing (Tam-Seq), as well as cancer personalized profiling by deep sequencing (CAPP-Seq). To act as a stand-in for tumor burden, ctDNA can also be examined for its proportion to total cfDNA. This enables early monitoring of therapy response or treatment failure, as well as risk assessment and staging. Vigilant monitoring aids in clinical decision-making by identifying mutations as potential targets or escape mechanisms, informing the treatment approach for NSCLC with tyrosine kinase inhibitors (TKIs) when specific *EGFR* gene mutations are detected in ctDNA (U.S. Federal Drug Administration – Center for Drug Evaluation and Research 2018; Lo et al. 2021). Treatment for breast cancer is guided by activating mutations of phosphatidylinositol-3-kinase catalytic subunit alpha, or PIK3CA. Unfortunately, through the acquisition of new mutations and clonal selection, resistant cancer cells can evade treatment. For instance, during the treatment of *EGFR* mutations, *KRAS* nucleotide changes may occur, leading to the evolution of tumor cell clones that become resistant under selective pressure (Diaz Jr. et al. 2012; Misale et al. 2012). By introducing methyl groups to the DNA, methylation is an epigenetic mechanism that controls the expression of genes (André et al. 2019). Tumors exhibit a reversed hyper- and hypomethylation pattern compared to normal tissue, influencing tumor development, progression, and clinical management. Since two decades, ctDNA was identified with typical methylation patterns, highlighting *MGMT* as a crucial druggable target in glioblastomas (Preuss et al. 1995, 1996; Balaña et al. 2003). In liquid biopsy for hepatocellular, pancreatic, and lung carcinomas, hydroxymethylation profiling—which finds 5-hydroxymethylcytosine (5hmC), a lesser-known epigenetic marker—has been used more recently (Song et al. 2017). While hepatocellular and pancreatic carcinoma showed increased 5hmC patterns typically associated with their diagnosis and dignity, lung carcinomas were identified by a reduced level of hydroxymethylation.

3.2.2 Non-targeted Analysis

Non-targeted methods attempt to explore the entire genome in the absence of prior knowledge about particular mutations. Examples of such methods include the detection of copy number aberrations (CNA) as well as whole exome or genome sequencing (WES, WGS) (Heitzer et al. 2019). These techniques make it possible to identify subclones that develop during treatment or as a tumor naturally progresses. Nevertheless, the low levels of ctDNA in patients without metastasis or relapse limit the sensitivity and usefulness of these methods. Certain techniques possess the ability to identify point mutations that were not previously detected in the initial tumor, offering beneficial options for treatment and prognosis (Ignatiadis et al. 2021).

3.2.3 Fragmentomics

Tumor-derived cfDNA in plasma typically exhibits a shorter size compared to normal cfDNA (Jiang et al. 2015). Reduced levels of a secreted DNASE1-like nuclease, DNASE1L3, have been linked to these variations in DNA fragmentation in a variety of tumor types (Serpas et al. 2019; Jiang et al. 2020). To ensure clinical relevance in this field, upcoming research should further enhance the understanding of ctDNA and nucleases, taking into account factors such as fragment size, jagged ends, and end motifs (Lo et al. 2021).

3.3 MicroRNA

miRNAs are 20 to 24 nucleotides long, noncoding RNA strains that make less than 1% of the total genome; in both health and disease, they play a role in the control of mRNA translation and stability. The possible roles of miRNAs remain to be elucidated (Kitano et al. 2021). Prospective investigations might expand to encompass additional RNA molecules, such as larger and more stable circular RNAs (circRNAs). circRNAs can function as antagonistic sponges for miRNAs and participate in the gene regulation of tumor cells. Nevertheless, establishing common standards is crucial for validation, especially given that dysregulation of both miRNAs and circRNAs may also occur in inflammatory diseases.

3.4 Extracellular Vesicles

Both normal cells and tumors can release tiny EVs that are packed with common proteins and nucleic acids. The vesicle's membrane shields its contents from enzymes like nucleases. As a result, EVs can be examined to find a variety of possible markers. For the majority of solid tumors, the preferred technique is to separate EVs from blood. CSF analysis of EVs from brain tumors may provide better results than blood samples for tumors near the ventricles due to an increased relative amount of tumor-derived material (Chen et al. 2013).

3.5 Tumor-Educated Platelets

Platelets in the blood originate as anucleated cytoplasmic fragments derived from megakaryocytes. They can promote metastasis through various pathways. Platelets can shield tumor cells circulating in the bloodstream from leukocytes, also protecting against shear stress. They can also facilitate adhesion to the blood vessel wall or provide growth factors at metastatic sites. Remarkably, tumors can modify the RNA content of platelets, resulting in the term "tumor-educated platelets" (TEP) (Best et al. 2015). The precise pathways are far from being understood, but TEPs from patients with different cancers differ from those with inflammatory diseases (Calverley et al. 2010; Best et al. 2018) (Fig. 2).

4 Clinical Applications and Cancer Types

As of March 22, 2023, the US National Institutes of Health's (NIH) ClinicalTrials.gov registry contained information on over 1160 clinical trials associated with the search term "ctDNA." The majority (804) of these trials are presently underway. Most studies analyze ctDNA changes to rapidly identify the outcomes of a newly tested treatment, rather than relying on it as the primary measure of treatment success. This is especially useful when tissue biopsy data is not available. Early detection of MRD, often months before local relapse or metastasis, allows for earlier therapy decisions, potentially leading to cure. A parallel search for "liquid biopsy" and "cancer" reveals only 439 studies, suggesting that many studies from the previous search on "ctDNA" do not explicitly include the term "liquid biopsy." Once again, a majority of "liquid biopsy" studies are ongoing (293), strongly indicating the burgeoning nature of the liquid biopsy field. The substantial and

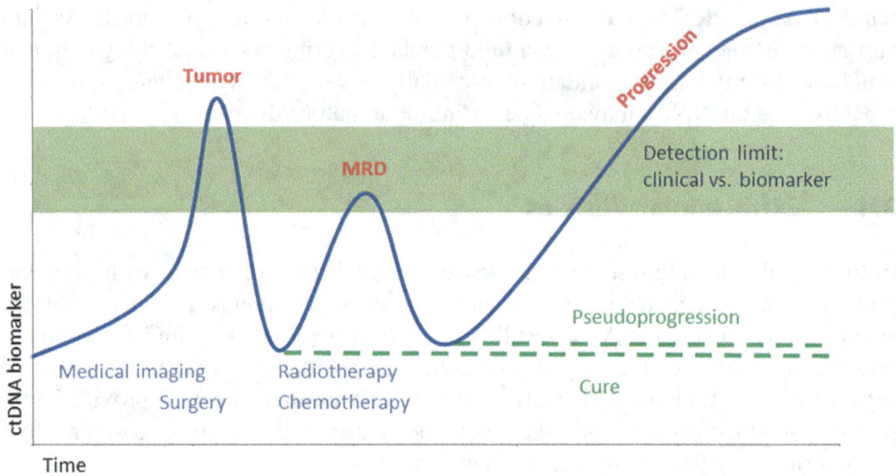

Fig. 2 Biomarker. A hypothetical biomarker released by the original tumor can be detected and monitored by liquid biopsy—just like the sun can be reflected on a mirror lake. The biomarker level typically drops after surgery, chemotherapy, or radiotherapy, but can increase again, somehow resembling the horizontal line of mountains. (Adapted from (Eibl and Schneemann 2022b), with permission)

rapidly increasing use of ctDNA detection in clinical studies suggests its potential to emerge as a new gold standard, especially as new therapy regimens gain approval, necessitating monitoring of ctDNA.

4.1 Lung Cancer

Lung cancer stands as the primary cause of cancer-related deaths, accounting for 18.4% of total cancer fatalities, and is the most prevalent cancer in both sexes combined, making up 11.6% of all cancer cases, with approximately 2.1 million new cases reported annually (Bray et al. 2018). A groundbreaking methodology in tumor evolution was employed to track genetic variations throughout tumor development and to discern early-stage predictors for non-small-cell lung cancer (NSCLC) in circulating tumor DNA (ctDNA) (Abbosh et al. 2017). In a separate study, a gene panel comprising 128 genes was employed in CAPSeq to evaluate relapse, demonstrating a lead time of about 5 months (Chaudhuri et al. 2017). The Cobas test was expanded in 2016 so that it could be used in tissue sections as well as serve as the initial liquid biopsy test for choosing appropriate treatments, allowing patients with advanced non-small-cell lung cancer to have their cfDNA tested for certain *EGFR* mutations (U.S. Federal Drug Administration – Center for Drug Evaluation and Research 2018). The ongoing SUMMIT study aims to enroll a large cohort of volunteers with an elevated risk of lung cancer in cigarette smokers.

The investigation focuses on validating GRAIL, LLC's blood test for early cancer detection using cell-free nucleic acids (cfNAs) and administering low-dose CT (LDCT) screening for lung cancer. The liquid biopsy evaluates the test quality and the efficacy, while LDCT screening effectiveness will be compared to established risk prediction measures. The study emphasizes maintaining ultralow radiation (University College, London 2021).

4.2 Colorectal Cancer

Colorectal cancer ranks as the second most common cancer in women and the third in men, with an annual incidence of almost two million new cases (Bray et al. 2018). In a 2016 prospective cohort study, individuals who had surgery for stage II colon cancer were investigated (Tie et al. 2016). The study employed advanced sequencing to find patient-specific mutations in their tumors, leading to the development of personalized assays for measuring circulating tumor DNA (ctDNA). In cases without adjuvant chemotherapy, ctDNA was found in almost 8% of cases and significantly linked with relapse within a median follow-up of slightly over 2 years, affecting about four quarters of all participants. Even among patients who received chemotherapy, ctDNA detection was associated with poor outcomes. Thus, ctDNA proves valuable for MRD and relapse. In a 2017 study, a patient primary-tumor-specific (PPS) assay was created to identify ctDNA in blood by monitoring patient-specific mutations present in tumor tissue (Ng et al. 2017). The investigation unveiled a robust association between ctDNA and clinical treatment outcomes, observable before surgery but not immediately post-surgery. Furthermore, ctDNA was identifiable before the clinical onset of recurrence, underscoring its potential for earlier detection of metastasis in comparison to existing imaging techniques and other markers such as carcinoembryonic antigen (CEA). In a 2017 study, the utility of ctDNA in monitoring colorectal cancer patients was further demonstrated (Schøler et al. 2017). Post-surgery, the detection of ctDNA indicated the presence of minimal residual disease (MRD), aiding in the identification of patients at a high risk of relapse. Monitoring ctDNA during a three-year follow-up, with a lead time of over 9 months in contrast to conventional medical imaging, facilitated early detection of relapse and tracking of treatment responses. Preoperative ctDNA detection rates proved to be more accurate in correlating with the disease stage than levels of CEA. The ongoing multicenter, prospective, randomized, controlled interventional trial known as CIRCULATing tumor DNA-based decision for adjuvant stage II Evaluation (CIRCULATE) aims to evaluate adjuvant therapy effectiveness in patients diagnosed with stage II colon cancer (Technische Universität Dresden 2020). This phase III study's primary goal is to compare disease-free survival (DFS) rates among patients testing positive for ctDNA with those who do not, particularly when treated with the drug capecitabine. The integration of ctDNA in clinical settings is demonstrated by the use of individual mutations that were previously determined from tumor blocks as eligibility criteria (Technische Universität Dresden 2020).

4.3 Breast Cancer

Breast cancer stands as the most prevalent cancer in women and is the leading cause of cancer-related deaths. Early detection and treatment offer the possibility of a cure for most patients. Additional treatments, such as chemotherapy, radiotherapy, and hormone therapy, can further diminish the risk of metastatic relapse post-surgical removal. However, avoiding overtreatment of cancer-free patients is crucial to mitigate unnecessary side effects. Therefore, personalized therapies tailored to individual patients are imperative, aiming for as many necessary treatments and as few as possible. The challenge for clinicians to identify residual disease (MRD) by measuring ctDNA has been addressed. In a preliminary study conducted in 2015, followed by a more extensive investigation in 2019, researchers monitored early breast cancer patients post-initial therapy by identifying ctDNA, which was associated with a high risk of relapse in all breast cancer subtypes (Garcia-Murillas et al. 2015; Coombes et al. 2019). This approach, linked to an elevated relapse risk across all breast cancer subtypes, involved pinpointing patient-specific somatic mutations. These mutations were initially identified through DNA sequencing of primary tumors and were subsequently tracked in blood samples using digital PCR (dPCR). The lead time for detecting these mutations was 10.7 months, providing substantial advance notice before any clinical signs of relapse. Notably, metastatic breast cancer is generally incurable once symptoms have become apparent. Recent research has shown promising results in the early detection of metastasis through ctDNA analysis. In a 2015 retrospective study, whole-genome sequencing of primary tumors was coupled with personalized dPCR from plasma ctDNA to quantify tumor-specific chromosomal rearrangements (Olsson et al. 2015). This method is capable of identifying as low as 0.01% of tumor DNA content, equivalent to detecting one rearranged sequence among 10,000 wild-type sequences. Metastatic recurrence was detected almost 1 year before its clinical presentation. No ctDNA was found in cancer-free long-term survivors, underscoring the need for additional tests to track early metastasis development, adjust therapy, and prevent unnecessary treatment. Tumor suppressor protein p53 (*TP53*) mutations are frequently found in a variety of malignant tumors, including mammary carcinoma (Ohgaki et al. 1991; Zhukova et al. 2013). A study investigated the high prevalence of TP53 mutations in a subset of mammary carcinoma, allowing for the monitoring of these mutations in ctDNA. Patient-specific *TP53* mutations were identified in nonmetastatic triple-negative breast cancer (TNBC) tumor tissue using massively parallel sequencing (MPS) (Riva et al. 2017). Ten milliliters of plasma were collected at four different times points to monitor these patient-specific *TP53* mutations before and after chemo- and surgical therapies. A sensitivity of 75% at baseline was attained with ctDNA dPCR. Tumor proliferation rate and tumor burden were both correlated with ctDNA levels. All patients experienced a decrease in ctDNA levels during Neutron capture therapy (NCT) treatment. After surgery, no minimal residual disease (MRD) was detected. However, a slow decrease in ctDNA during NCT was linked to shorter survival times. Another study further confirmed that ctDNA and CTC enumeration were independent factors associated with worse outcomes, including distant disease-free survival (DDFS), disease-free survival (DFS), and overall survival (OS) (Radovich et al. 2020).

4.4 Prostate Cancer

Prostate cancer ranks second globally among non-cutaneous cancers in men, causing over 350,000 deaths and an estimated 1.3 million new cases annually. It is identified in 7.1% of individuals diagnosed with cancer and represents 3.8% of fatalities associated with cancer (Bray et al. 2018). A phase III clinical study focusing on chemotherapies for metastatic castration-resistant prostate cancer (mCRPC) explored cfDNA levels (Mehra et al. 2018). It was found that the baseline concentration of cfDNA, partly derived from the tumor, independently served as a prognostic factor in both treatment settings, correlating with shorter radiological progression-free survival (rPFS) and overall survival. Elevated cfDNA levels prior to chemotherapy were associated with tumors displaying increased aggressiveness, while a decline in cfDNA levels at the onset of chemotherapy indicated a favorable response to treatment. While cfDNA can constitute 15%–20% of ctDNA, its efficacy in detecting or monitoring early-stage or less aggressive localized prostate cancers, which may have elevated prostate-specific antigen (PSA) levels, is currently limited (Hennigan et al. 2019). In a study involving cfDNA from metastatic castration-resistant prostate cancer (mCRPC) patients before novel androgen receptor (AR) therapy, whole-exome sequencing (WES) was employed to capture coding regions of 72 genes. It was found that mutations in *BRCA2*, *ATM*, and *TP53* were predictive of poorer outcomes with novel AR targeting. This implies the potential usefulness of liquid biopsy in guiding routine practice for AR-targeted therapy (Annala et al. 2018).

4.5 Brain Tumors

Only 1.6% of all cancers are brain or nervous system cancers, but they account for 2.5% of all cancer-associated fatalities. Despite their relatively low prevalence, the challenges presented by the location of these tumors within the brain, coupled with limited progress in treating aggressive cancers like glioblastoma, persist significantly. A recent review by Eibl and Schneemann (2021) explored the potential application of liquid biopsy in primary brain tumors. Detecting low-level circulating tumor DNA (ctDNA) in the blood faces challenges due to the blood-brain barrier (BBB) (Eibl and Schneemann 2021). However, cerebrospinal fluid (CSF) emerges as a more promising source due to the usual lack of leukocytes, significantly reducing background noise for cfDNA. Previous studies successfully identified specific mutations in serum (Balaña et al. 2003; Lavon et al. 2010; Majchrzak-Celińska et al. 2013; Bettegowda et al. 2014), plasma (Weaver et al. 2006; Boisselier et al. 2012; Schwaederle et al. 2017), or both (Bettegowda et al. 2014). In 1991, Eibl discovered the first *TP53* mutations in medulloblastoma samples, supporting his earlier rat tumor model where tumors induced by SV40 large T-antigen are histologically indistinguishable from primitive neuroectodermal tumors (PNET) (Ohgaki et al. 1991). While *TP53* mutations in medulloblastomas are now established as valuable prognostic and diagnostic markers, Eibl's early success underscored the complexity of this genetic landscape. Various oncogenic pathways in human brain tumors have been revealed and validated using similar models (von Deimling et al. 1992; Wiestler et al. 1992a, b; Ohgaki et al. 1993; Eibl et al. 1994).

5 Clinical Studies

An increasing number of clinical studies are utilizing liquid biopsy techniques to either assess their efficacy or monitor treatment outcomes (Table 1).

Table 1 Examples of using ctDNA in clinical studies

Year	Author	Tumor	Method	Findings
2016	Donaldson and Park (2018)	Advanced NSCL	ctDNA, cobas	Treatment selection for *EGFR* mutation
2017	Phallen et al. (2017)	Colon, mammary, lung, ovarian carcinoma	cfDNA, TEC-seq	Early-stage tumors detected
2017	Abbosh et al. (2017)	Early-stage NSCLC	ctDNA, multiplex-PCR, NGS	Detection of relapse
2017	Ng et al. (2017)	CRC	ctDNA, multiplex-PCR	Postoperative monitoring
2017	Schøler et al. (2017)	CRC	ctDNA, individual mutations	Detection of MRD, early recurrence after surgery; measuring therapy response
2017	Chaudhuri et al. (2017)	NSCLC stage I, II, III	ctDNA, CAPPseq, gene panel	Five months lead time prior relapse
2018	Mehra et al. (2018)	mCRPC, Prostate cancer	cfDNA	Prognosis for rPFS and OS after chemotherapy
2018	Annala et al. (2018)	mPRPC	ctDNA	Inferior prognosis on AR targeting
2019	Garcia-Murillas et al. (2019)	Early-stage breast cancer	cfDNA, dPCR mutation tracking	Prediction of relapse
2022	Pagès et al. (2022)	CNS tumors	ctDNA, ULP-WGS	CSF superior to blood, helpful for tumors of high grade
2022	Gale et al. (2022)	Early-stage NSCL	Monitoring individual mutations	MRD, treatment selection

Modified from (Eibl and Schneemann 2022a, 2023)

6 Ethical and Legal Considerations

As liquid biopsy becomes more widespread and integrated into clinical routine, there are important ethical and legal considerations that need to be addressed. Similar to other medical procedures, patients undergoing liquid biopsy testing should be fully informed about the procedure, the potential risks and benefits, and how the information will be used. It is important to obtain informed consent from patients before conducting any liquid biopsy testing. As liquid biopsy generates a large amount of medical data, there is a need to address issues related to data sharing and ownership. This may involve developing guidelines for data sharing and implementing secure systems for storing and sharing data. In addition, an unprecedented amount of data which contains sensitive patient information needs to be protected throughout the testing and storage. Data security measures and obtaining informed consent from patients need to be implemented. Meta-analysis of these data may also increase our knowledge of cancer epidemiology, prevention, and treatment and should meet the Findable, Accessible, Interoperable, and Reusable (FAIR) standards (Gonzalez-Beltran et al. 2020). Liquid biopsy is still a new and rapidly developing technology with ongoing debates about how it should be regulated. There is a major need for standardized testing procedures, quality control measures, and guidelines for interpreting test results. Continuing improvements in technology will increase the sensitivity and specificity of liquid biopsy, but a major hope includes a dramatic reduction of costs for at least some applications due to upscaling, standardization, and automation.

7 Public Health Implications

Apart from the direct effects of cancer on a patient's health and well-being, there are additional societal losses incurred when people leave their work due to cancer, as well as the tremendous costs of treatment. These costs are often paid, at least in part, by society through insurance programs and the infrastructure of hospitals or comprehensive cancer centers, as well as through the patient's savings. Furthermore, cancer research also requires significant funding. A current estimate projects the cost of cancer treatment to be 25.2 trillion international dollars over the next three decades, with half of this cost attributable to just five types of cancer: lung, colorectal, breast, liver, and leukemia (Chen et al. 2023). Over the past century, numerous environmental factors that contribute to cancer have been identified, including mutagenic chemical compounds, irradiation (UV and radioactivity), and certain infections. To prevent cancer, direct measures involve protecting people against cancer-causing agents, promoting safe work environments, creating smoke-free environments, and encouraging sun protection from a young age, as well as reducing alcohol consumption. Vaccination against some cancer-related viruses is also a recent development. Indirect measures include educating people about cancer-causing habits, such as smoking, alcohol consumption, and sun exposure. A simple ban on smoking or improved education in larger countries, for example, could have the greatest impact on reducing lung cancer. The sudden and devastating impact of a pandemic, such as COVID-19, can put cancer patients at a significant risk, especially those in advanced stages of the disease. Without regular vaccinations every 6 months following initial vaccination schemes and early treatment with antiviral drugs like nirmatrelvir/ritonavir or remdesivir, or with antibodies, many cancer patients succumb to the disease earlier than expected. Additionally, the pandemic has hindered early cancer diagnoses and reduced the likelihood of curative treatments, as patients have avoided seeking medical care to prevent infection. The potential for new pandemics or future waves of the current pandemic, with the SARS-CoV-2 virus continuing to mutate, poses a considerable threat to cancer patients who may be reluctant to seek medical care, especially when extensive medical imaging procedures like MRIs or multiple visits to specialized doctors are required. Although liquid biopsy methods cannot fully replace such examinations, some patients may benefit from simple blood screenings at their local doctor's office if they are unable to enter a hospital. The costs of diagnosing, monitoring, and treating illnesses are often significant and can add to the stress of patients. Inequalities in healthcare systems exist even within wealthier countries, but the challenges faced by low- and middle-income countries are far from being solved. Despite continued progress in medicine, the gap to implement new and often expensive applications in poor countries may not be closed anytime soon. For example, medical imaging with CT and MRI scans were once rare and expensive, but they are now considered a basic standard for many hospitals worldwide. However, these technologies may still be unaffordable in many regions, forcing patients to travel long distances to access them. In contrast, drawing blood and sending it to a central lab for analysis appears to be much easier to implement than providing the latest MRI technology in every poor region. In some parts of the world, accessing an MRI scan may still be impossible for many, while a simple blood test is readily available. Liquid biopsy has the potential to detect cancer at an earlier stage than other diagnostic methods. Depending on the tumor type, earlier and personalized treatment options, when available, can reduce mortality rates and improve overall health outcomes. Cost-effectiveness of liquid biopsy depends on the treatment options available. Screening for cancers without corresponding treatments with the intent to cure may not appear cost-effective. With limited resources, the focus should be on cancer types with significant treatment options. With new immunotherapies in parallel development, liquid biopsy has the potential to become a gamechanger, and in the middle or long run, it can be expected to be much cheaper than current medical standards. To achieve widespread implementation of liquid biopsy in clinical routines, common standards need to be developed, and healthcare professionals need to be trained to ensure that the results are interpreted correctly. However, covering the often-significant costs can be a challenge, especially in less wealthy countries, where cancer is a frequent disease, and different medical standards exist. Various concepts, such as solidarity sharing with society, have been proposed to address this issue. Despite these challenges, liquid biopsy has the potential to offer a tremendous impact on public health in any country. Potential solutions are as follows: The introduction and application of liquid biopsy for cancer detection and monitoring may vary depending on the available resources and the acceptance of health management practices in each country or region. High-income countries with good healthcare systems are likely to be the first to adopt this technology. Other countries may choose to start with the highest cost-benefit ratio. It is essential to note that implementing liquid biopsy should be accompanied by other measures to reduce cancer-related risks, such as a ban or regulation of cigarette smoking and alcohol consumption.

8 Challenges and Future Directions

The application of liquid biopsy in cancer management presents a promising opportunity to achieve some of the goals outlined in SDG 3 (Universal Good Health and Well-being). Over the past two decades, technological advances have enabled the development of liquid biopsy techniques to characterize the genomic and genetic features of tumors. These techniques have been used to detect and monitor disease progression, provide early detection of cancer recurrence, and assess treatment response in clinical settings. Liquid biopsy has also shown potential in improving patient outcomes by enabling personalized treatment strategies. However, despite these promising advances, there are still several challenges that need to be addressed before liquid biopsy can become a widely accessible and useful tool in cancer management. One major challenge is the lack of standardization and harmonization of liquid biopsy protocols, which can result in inconsistent results and hinder the comparability of data across studies. In addition, there is a need to develop less expensive and more accurate methods and technologies for liquid biopsy. Further development of methods, such as single-cell sequencing, may also help to expand the potential of liquid biopsy and provide rapid and low-cost analysis of genetic information from clinical samples. Standards may pose a challenge in the detection of brain tumor cells using the CellSearch system. As these cells originate from neural tissue, they do not possess the epithelial marker EpCAM that is typically used to isolate carcinoma cells. In order to improve the efficacy of the CellSearch system, it may be beneficial to incorporate an additional selection or enrichment marker. One potential option could be utilizing CD44v, splice variants of CD44 (Eibl et al. 1995). Recently, various nanotechnology methods have been discussed for the biophysical and functional characterization of circulating tumor cells (CTCs), including the use of atomic force microscopy (AFM) (Eibl and Benoit 2004; Eibl and Moy 2005; Pax et al. 2005; Eibl 2013, 2014; Di Santo et al. 2021; Li et al. 2021; Deliorman et al. 2022; Chowdhury et al. 2023). Ultimately, the continued development and implementation of liquid biopsy in cancer management has the potential to significantly improve patient outcomes and contribute to the achievement of SDG 3.

9 Conclusion

Liquid biopsy has the potential to revolutionize cancer diagnosis, monitoring, and treatment. Compared to tissue biopsy, it is less invasive, more easily accessible, and provides real-time information on tumor progression and drug resistance, enabling informed treatment decisions. However, sensitivity and specificity can vary. By leveraging technological advances, liquid biopsy offers a minimally invasive approach that helps us understand the unique genetic makeup of an individual's tumor, leading to personalized treatments and improved prognosis for cancer patients. In this way, liquid biopsy can contribute significantly to achieving Sustainable Development Goal 3 (SDG 3): Universal Good Health and Well-being, by reducing the burden of cancer and improving health outcomes worldwide. While the SDGs were proposed by the UN in 2015, it is too early to predict their future effects, especially in light of the COVID-19 pandemic and other potential political and environmental threats. However, with a longer perspective until 2050, liquid biopsy is likely to become a milestone in the global fight against cancer, benefiting not only high-income regions and populations but also many currently lower-income countries. Overall, the potential of liquid biopsy to revolutionize cancer diagnosis and treatment is immense. Providing a less invasive, more accessible, and more personalized approach to cancer care can help reduce the burden of cancer and improve health outcomes for all. Further development and accessibility of this technology should be pursued to maximize its potential for the benefit of individuals, families, and society as a whole.

Acknowledgments We gratefully acknowledge the introduction into the field of tumor research by Otmar D. Wiestler and the late Paul Kleihues, as well as discussions with Irving L. Weissman and Eugene C. Butcher on immune and tumor cell migration, metastasis, and stem cells, and Catherine Alix-Panabières on liquid biopsy.

Compliance with Ethical Standards The authors declare no conflict of interest. No external funding was received for writing this chapter.

References

Abbosh C, Birkbak NJ, Wilson GA et al (2017) Phylogenetic ctDNA analysis depicts early-stage lung cancer evolution. Nature 545:446–451. https://doi.org/10.1038/nature22364

Alix-Panabières C, Pantel K (2013) Circulating tumor cells: liquid biopsy of cancer. Clin Chem 59: 110–118. https://doi.org/10.1373/clinchem.2012.194258

Alix-Panabières C, Pantel K (2021) Liquid biopsy: from discovery to clinical application. Cancer Discov 11:858–873. https://doi.org/10.1158/2159-8290.CD-20-1311

Alix-Panabières C, Mader S, Pantel K (2017) Epithelial-mesenchymal plasticity in circulating tumor cells. J Mol Med 95:133–142. https://doi.org/10.1007/s00109-016-1500-6

Alix-Panabieres C, Magliocco A, Cortes-Hernandez LE et al (2021) Detection of cancer metastasis: past, present and future. Clin Exp Metastasis 39:21. https://doi.org/10.1007/s10585-021-10088-w

Alshareef M, Metrakos N, Perez EJ et al (2013) Separation of tumor cells with dielectrophoresis-based microfluidic chip. Biomicrofluidics 7:011803. https://doi.org/10.1063/1.4774312

André F, Ciruelos E, Rubovszky G et al (2019) Alpelisib for PIK3CA-mutated, hormone receptor–positive advanced breast cancer. N Engl J Med 380:1929–1940. https://doi.org/10.1056/NEJMoa1813904

Annala M, Vandekerkhove G, Khalaf D et al (2018) Circulating tumor DNA genomics correlate with resistance to abiraterone and enzalutamide in prostate cancer. Cancer Discov 8:444–457. https://doi.org/10.1158/2159-8290.CD-17-0937

Balaña C, Ramirez JL, Taron M et al (2003) O6-methyl-guanine-DNA methyltransferase methylation in serum and tumor DNA predicts response to 1,3-bis(2-chloroethyl)-1-nitrosourea but not to temozolamide plus cisplatin in glioblastoma multiforme. Clin Cancer Res Off J Am Assoc Cancer Res 9:1461–1468

Bardelli A, Pantel K (2017) Liquid biopsies, what we do not know (yet). Cancer Cell 31:172–179. https://doi.org/10.1016/j.ccell.2017.01.002

Best MG, Sol N, Kooi I et al (2015) RNA-seq of tumor-educated platelets enables blood-based pan-cancer, multiclass, and molecular pathway cancer diagnostics. Cancer Cell 28:666–676. https://doi.org/10.1016/j.ccell.2015.09.018

Best MG, Wesseling P, Wurdinger T (2018) Tumor-educated platelets as a noninvasive biomarker source for cancer detection and progression monitoring. Cancer Res 78:3407–3412. https://doi.org/10.1158/0008-5472.CAN-18-0887

Bettegowda C, Sausen M, Leary RJ et al (2014) Detection of circulating tumor DNA in early- and late-stage human malignancies. Sci Transl Med 6:224ra24. https://doi.org/10.1126/scitranslmed.3007094

Bhagwat N, Dulmage K, Pletcher CH et al (2018) An integrated flow cytometry-based platform for isolation and molecular characterization of circulating tumor single cells and clusters. Sci Rep 8:5035. https://doi.org/10.1038/s41598-018-23217-5

Bidard F-C, Peeters DJ, Fehm T et al (2014) Clinical validity of circulating tumour cells in patients with metastatic breast cancer: a pooled analysis of individual patient data. Lancet Oncol 15:406–414. https://doi.org/10.1016/S1470-2045(14)70069-5

Boisselier B, Gallego Perez-Larraya J, Rossetto M et al (2012) Detection of IDH1 mutation in the plasma of patients with glioma. Neurology 79:1693–1698. https://doi.org/10.1212/WNL.0b013e31826e9b0a

Bork U, Rahbari NN, Schölch S et al (2015) Circulating tumour cells and outcome in non-metastatic colorectal cancer: a prospective study. Br J Cancer 112:1306–1313. https://doi.org/10.1038/bjc.2015.88

Bray F, Ferlay J, Soerjomataram I et al (2018) Global cancer statistics 2018: GLOBOCAN estimates of incidence and mortality worldwide for 36 cancers in 185 countries. CA Cancer J Clin 68:394–424. https://doi.org/10.3322/caac.21492

Budd GT, Cristofanilli M, Ellis MJ et al (2006) Circulating tumor cells versus imaging—predicting overall survival in metastatic breast cancer. Clin Cancer Res 12:6403–6409. https://doi.org/10.1158/1078-0432.CCR-05-1769

Bustin SA, Siddiqi S, Ahmed S et al (2004) Quantification of cytokeratin 20, carcinoembryonic antigen and guanylyl cyclase C mRNA levels in lymph nodes may not predict treatment failure in colorectal cancer patients. Int J Cancer 108:412–417. https://doi.org/10.1002/ijc.11596

Calverley DC, Phang TL, Choudhury QG et al (2010) Significant downregulation of platelet gene expression in metastatic lung cancer. Clin Transl Sci 3:227–232. https://doi.org/10.1111/j.1752-8062.2010.00226.x

Cayrefourcq L, Mazard T, Joosse S et al (2015) Establishment and characterization of a cell line from human circulating colon cancer cells. Cancer Res 75:892–901. https://doi.org/10.1158/0008-5472.CAN-14-2613

Cayrefourcq L, De Roeck A, Garcia C et al (2019) S100-EPISPOT: a new tool to detect viable circulating melanoma cells. Cells 8:755. https://doi.org/10.3390/cells8070755

Chambers AF, Groom AC, MacDonald IC (2002) Dissemination and growth of cancer cells in metastatic sites. Nat Rev Cancer 2:563–572. https://doi.org/10.1038/nrc865

Chaudhuri AA, Chabon JJ, Lovejoy AF et al (2017) Early detection of molecular residual disease in localized lung cancer by circulating tumor DNA profiling. Cancer Discov 7:1394–1403. https://doi.org/10.1158/2159-8290.CD-17-0716

Chen WW, Balaj L, Liau LM et al (2013) BEAMing and droplet digital PCR analysis of mutant IDH1 mRNA in glioma patient serum and cerebrospinal fluid extracellular vesicles. Mol Ther Nucleic Acids 2:e109. https://doi.org/10.1038/mtna.2013.28

Chen S, Cao Z, Prettner K et al (2023) Estimates and projections of the global economic cost of 29 cancers in 204 countries and territories from 2020 to 2050. JAMA Oncol 9:465. https://doi.org/10.1001/jamaoncol.2022.7826

Chowdhury T, Cressiot B, Parisi C et al (2023) Circulating tumor cells in cancer diagnostics and prognostics by single-molecule and single-cell characterization. ACS Sens 8:406. https://doi.org/10.1021/acssensors.2c02308

Cohen SJ, Punt CJA, Iannotti N et al (2008) Relationship of circulating tumor cells to tumor response, progression-free survival, and overall survival in patients with metastatic colorectal cancer. J Clin Oncol Off J Am Soc Clin Oncol 26:3213–3221. https://doi.org/10.1200/JCO.2007.15.8923

Coombes RC, Page K, Salari R et al (2019) Personalized detection of circulating tumor DNA antedates breast cancer metastatic recurrence. Clin Cancer Res Off J Am Assoc Cancer Res 25:4255–4263. https://doi.org/10.1158/1078-0432.CCR-18-3663

Cristofanilli M, Budd GT, Ellis MJ et al (2004) Circulating tumor cells, disease progression, and survival in metastatic breast cancer. N Engl J Med 351:781–791. https://doi.org/10.1056/NEJMoa040766

De Luca F, Rotunno G, Salvianti F et al (2016) Mutational analysis of single circulating tumor cells by next generation sequencing in metastatic breast cancer. Oncotarget 7:26107–26119. https://doi.org/10.18632/oncotarget.8431

Deliorman M, Glia A, Qasaimeh MA (2022) Characterizing circulating tumor cells using affinity-based microfluidic capture and AFM-based biomechanics. STAR Protoc 3:101433. https://doi.org/10.1016/j.xpro.2022.101433

Denève E, Riethdorf S, Ramos J et al (2013) Capture of viable circulating tumor cells in the liver of colorectal cancer patients. Clin Chem 59:1384–1392. https://doi.org/10.1373/clinchem.2013.202846

Deng Z, Wu S, Wang Y, Shi D (2022) Circulating tumor cell isolation for cancer diagnosis and prognosis. EBioMedicine 83:104237. https://doi.org/10.1016/j.ebiom.2022.104237

Di Santo R, Romanò S, Mazzini A et al (2021) Recent advances in the label-free characterization of exosomes for cancer liquid biopsy: from scattering and spectroscopy to nanoindentation and nanodevices. Nano 11:1476. https://doi.org/10.3390/nano11061476

Diaz LA Jr, Williams RT, Wu J et al (2012) The molecular evolution of acquired resistance to targeted EGFR blockade in colorectal cancers. Nature 486:537–540. https://doi.org/10.1038/nature11219

Donaldson J, Park BH (2018) Circulating tumor DNA: measurement and clinical utility. Annu Rev Med 69:223–234. https://doi.org/10.1146/annurev-med-041316-085721

Eibl RH (2013) Single-molecule studies of integrins by AFM-based force spectroscopy on living cells. In: Bhushan B (ed) Scanning probe microscopy in nanoscience and nanotechnology 3. Springer, Berlin/Heidelberg, pp 137–169

Eibl RH (2014) Comment on "A method to measure cellular adhesion utilizing a polymer micro-cantilever" [Appl. Phys. Lett. 103, 123702 (2013)]. Appl Phys Lett 104:236103. https://doi.org/10.1063/1.4882182

Eibl RH, Benoit M (2004) Molecular resolution of cell adhesion forces. IEE Proc Nanobiotechnol 151:128–132. https://doi.org/10.1049/ip-nbt:20040707

Eibl RH, Moy VT (2005) Atomic force microscopy measurements of protein-ligand interactions on living cells. Methods Mol Biol (Clifton NJ) 305:439–450. https://doi.org/10.1385/1-59259-912-5:439

Eibl RH, Schneemann M (2021) Liquid biopsy and primary brain tumors. Cancers 13:5429. https://doi.org/10.3390/cancers13215429

Eibl RH, Schneemann M (2022a) Cell-free DNA as a biomarker in cancer. Extracell Vesicles Circ Nucleic Acids 3:178–198. https://doi.org/10.20517/evcna.2022.20

Eibl RH, Schneemann M (2022b) Liquid biopsy for monitoring medulloblastoma. Extracell Vesicles Circ Nucleic Acids 3:263–274. https://doi.org/10.20517/evcna.2022.36

Eibl RH, Schneemann M (2023) Medulloblastoma: from TP53 mutations to molecular classification and liquid biopsy. Biology 12:267. https://doi.org/10.3390/biology12020267

Eibl RH, Kleihues P, Jat PS, Wiestler OD (1994) A model for primitive neuroectodermal tumors in transgenic neural transplants harboring the SV40 large T antigen. Am J Pathol 144:556–564

Eibl RH, Pietsch T, Moll J et al (1995) Expression of variant CD44 epitopes in human astrocytic brain tumors. J Neuro-Oncol 26:165–170. https://doi.org/10.1007/BF01052619

Eslami-S Z, Cortés-Hernández LE, Cayrefourcq L, Alix-Panabières C (2020) The different facets of liquid biopsy: a kaleidoscopic view. Cold Spring Harb Perspect Med 10:a037333. https://doi.org/10.1101/cshperspect.a037333

Eyer K, Doineau RCL, Castrillon CE et al (2017) Single-cell deep phenotyping of IgG-secreting cells for high-resolution immune monitoring. Nat Biotechnol 35:977–982. https://doi.org/10.1038/nbt.3964

Fidler IJ (1975) Biological behavior of malignant melanoma cells correlated to their survival in vivo. Cancer Res 35:218–224

Gale D, Heider K, Ruiz-Valdepenas A et al (2022) Residual ctDNA after treatment predicts early relapse in patients with early-stage non-small cell lung cancer. Ann Oncol 33:500. https://doi.org/10.1016/j.annonc.2022.02.007

Garcia-Murillas I, Schiavon G, Weigelt B et al (2015) Mutation tracking in circulating tumor DNA predicts relapse in early breast cancer. Sci Transl Med 7:302ra133. https://doi.org/10.1126/scitranslmed.aab0021

Garcia-Murillas I, Chopra N, Comino-Méndez I et al (2019) Assessment of molecular relapse detection in early-stage breast cancer. JAMA Oncol 5:1473–1478. https://doi.org/10.1001/jamaoncol.2019.1838

Garrel R, Mazel M, Perriard F et al (2019) Circulating tumor cells as a prognostic factor in recurrent or metastatic head and neck squamous cell carcinoma: the CIRCUTEC prospective study. Clin Chem 65:1267–1275. https://doi.org/10.1373/clinchem.2019.305904

Gonzalez-Beltran AN, Masuzzo P, Ampe C et al (2020) Community standards for open cell migration data. GigaScience 9. https://doi.org/10.1093/gigascience/giaa041

Heitzer E, Haque IS, Roberts CES, Speicher MR (2019) Current and future perspectives of liquid biopsies in genomics-driven oncology. Nat Rev Genet 20:71–88. https://doi.org/10.1038/s41576-018-0071-5

Hennigan ST, Trostel SY, Terrigino NT et al (2019) Low abundance of circulating tumor DNA in localized prostate cancer. JCO Precis Oncol 1–13. https://doi.org/10.1200/PO.19.00176

Hindson BJ, Ness KD, Masquelier DA et al (2011) High-throughput droplet digital PCR system for absolute quantitation of DNA copy number. Anal Chem 83:8604–8610. https://doi.org/10.1021/ac202028g

Hou J-M, Krebs MG, Lancashire L et al (2012) Clinical significance and molecular characteristics of circulating tumor cells and circulating tumor microemboli in patients with small-cell lung cancer. J Clin Oncol 30:525–532. https://doi.org/10.1200/JCO.2010.33.3716

Ignatiadis M, Sledge GW, Jeffrey SS (2021) Liquid biopsy enters the clinic — implementation issues and future challenges. Nat Rev Clin Oncol 18:297–312. https://doi.org/10.1038/s41571-020-00457-x

Jiang P, Chan CWM, Chan KCA et al (2015) Lengthening and shortening of plasma DNA in hepatocellular carcinoma patients. Proc Natl Acad Sci USA 112:E1317–E1325. https://doi.org/10.1073/pnas.1500076112

Jiang P, Sun K, Peng W et al (2020) Plasma DNA end-motif profiling as a fragmentomic marker in cancer, pregnancy, and transplantation. Cancer Discov 10:664–673. https://doi.org/10.1158/2159-8290.CD-19-0622

Joosse SA, Beyer B, Gasch C et al (2020) Tumor-associated release of prostatic cells into the blood after transrectal ultrasound-guided biopsy in patients with histologically confirmed prostate cancer. Clin Chem 66:161–168. https://doi.org/10.1373/clinchem.2019.310912

Kelley RK, Magbanua MJM, Butler TM et al (2015) Circulating tumor cells in hepatocellular carcinoma: a pilot study of detection, enumeration, and next-generation sequencing in cases and controls. BMC Cancer 15:206. https://doi.org/10.1186/s12885-015-1195-z

Kitano Y, Aoki K, Ohka F et al (2021) Urinary microRNA-based diagnostic model for central nervous system tumors using nanowire scaffolds. ACS Appl Mater Interfaces 13:17316–17329. https://doi.org/10.1021/acsami.1c01754

Koch C, Kuske A, Joosse SA et al (2020) Characterization of circulating breast cancer cells with tumorigenic and metastatic capacity. EMBO Mol Med 12:e11908. https://doi.org/10.15252/emmm.201911908

Kuske A, Gorges TM, Tennstedt P et al (2016) Improved detection of circulating tumor cells in non-metastatic high-risk prostate cancer patients. Sci Rep 6:39736. https://doi.org/10.1038/srep39736

Kwapisz D (2017) The first liquid biopsy test approved. Is it a new era of mutation testing for non-small cell lung cancer? Ann Transl Med 5:10. https://doi.org/10.21037/atm.2017.01.32

Lavon I, Refael M, Zelikovitch B et al (2010) Serum DNA can define tumor-specific genetic and epigenetic markers in gliomas of various grades. Neuro-Oncology 12:173–180. https://doi.org/10.1093/neuonc/nop041

Li Y, Zhang T, Huang J et al (2021) Biostable double-strand circular aptamers conjugated onto dendrimers for specific capture and inhibition of circulating leukemia cells. Onco Targets Ther 13:13465–13477. https://doi.org/10.2147/OTT.S287720

Lo YMD, Han DSC, Jiang P, Chiu RWK (2021) Epigenetics, fragmentomics, and topology of cell-free DNA in liquid biopsies. Science 372:eaaw3616. https://doi.org/10.1126/science.aaw3616

Louis DN, Perry A, Reifenberger G et al (2016) The 2016 World Health Organization classification of tumors of the central nervous system: a summary. Acta Neuropathol (Berl) 131:803–820. https://doi.org/10.1007/s00401-016-1545-1

Lucci A, Hall CS, Lodhi AK et al (2012) Circulating tumour cells in non-metastatic breast cancer: a prospective study. Lancet Oncol 13:688–695. https://doi.org/10.1016/S1470-2045(12)70209-7

Magbanua MJM, Park JW (2013) Isolation of circulating tumor cells by immunomagnetic enrichment and fluorescence-activated cell sorting (IE/FACS) for molecular profiling. Methods 64:114–118. https://doi.org/10.1016/j.ymeth.2013.07.029

Majchrzak-Celińska A, Paluszczak J, Kleszcz R et al (2013) Detection of MGMT, RASSF1A, p15INK4B, and p14ARF promoter methylation in circulating tumor-derived DNA of central nervous system cancer patients. J Appl Genet 54:335–344. https://doi.org/10.1007/s13353-013-0149-x

Mastoraki S, Strati A, Tzanikou E et al (2018) *ESR1* methylation: a liquid biopsy–based epigenetic assay for the follow-up of patients with metastatic breast cancer receiving endocrine treatment. Clin Cancer Res 24:1500–1510. https://doi.org/10.1158/1078-0432.CCR-17-1181

Mazard T, Cayrefourcq L, Perriard F et al (2021) Clinical relevance of viable circulating tumor cells in patients with metastatic colorectal cancer: the COLOSPOT prospective study. Cancers 13:2966. https://doi.org/10.3390/cancers13122966

Mehra N, Dolling D, Sumanasuriya S et al (2018) Plasma cell-free DNA concentration and outcomes from taxane therapy in metastatic castration-resistant prostate cancer from two phase III trials (FIRSTANA and PROSELICA). Eur Urol 74:283–291. https://doi.org/10.1016/j.eururo.2018.02.013

Millner LM, Linder MW, Valdes R (2013) Circulating tumor cells: a review of present methods and the need to identify heterogeneous phenotypes. Ann Clin Lab Sci 43:295–304

Misale S, Yaeger R, Hobor S et al (2012) Emergence of KRAS mutations and acquired resistance to anti-EGFR therapy in colorectal cancer. Nature 486:532–536. https://doi.org/10.1038/nature11156

Monteiro-Riviere NA, Inman AO, Zhang LW (2009) Limitations and relative utility of screening assays to assess engineered nanoparticle toxicity in a human cell line. Toxicol Appl Pharmacol 234:222–235. https://doi.org/10.1016/j.taap.2008.09.030

Müller NL, Bergin CJ, Miller RR, Ostrow DN (1986) Seeding of malignant cells into the needle track after lung and pleural biopsy. Can Assoc Radiol J J Assoc Can Radiol 37:192–194

Neuberger EWI, Sontag S, Brahmer A et al (2022) Physical activity specifically evokes release of cell-free DNA from granulocytes thereby affecting liquid biopsy. Clin Epigenetics 14:29. https://doi.org/10.1186/s13148-022-01245-3

Ng SB, Chua C, Ng M et al (2017) Individualised multiplexed circulating tumour DNA assays for monitoring of tumour presence in patients after colorectal cancer surgery. Sci Rep 7:40737. https://doi.org/10.1038/srep40737

Ohgaki H, Eibl RH, Wiestler OD et al (1991) p53 mutations in nonastrocytic human brain tumors. Cancer Res 51:6202–6205

Ohgaki H, Eibl RH, Schwab M et al (1993) Mutations of the p53 tumor suppressor gene in neoplasms of the human nervous system. Mol Carcinog 8:74–80. https://doi.org/10.1002/mc.2940080203

Okegawa T, Itaya N, Hara H et al (2014) Circulating tumor cells as a biomarker predictive of sensitivity to docetaxel chemotherapy in patients with castration-resistant prostate cancer. Anticancer Res 34:6705–6710

Olsson E, Winter C, George A et al (2015) Serial monitoring of circulating tumor DNA in patients with primary breast cancer for detection of occult metastatic disease. EMBO Mol Med 7:1034–1047. https://doi.org/10.15252/emmm.201404913

Pachmann K, Camara O, Kavallaris A et al (2008) Monitoring the response of circulating epithelial tumor cells to adjuvant chemotherapy in breast cancer allows detection of patients at risk of early relapse. J Clin Oncol 26:1208–1215. https://doi.org/10.1200/JCO.2007.13.6523

Pagès M, Rotem D, Gydush G et al (2022) Liquid biopsy detection of genomic alterations in pediatric brain tumors from cell-free DNA in peripheral blood, CSF, and urine. Neuro-Oncology noab299. https://doi.org/10.1093/neuonc/noab299

Pantel K, Alix-Panabières C (2019) Liquid biopsy and minimal residual disease — latest advances and implications for cure. Nat Rev Clin Oncol 16:409–424. https://doi.org/10.1038/s41571-019-0187-3

Pax M, Rieger J, Eibl RH et al (2005) Measurements of fast fluctuations of viscoelastic properties with the quartz crystal microbalance. Analyst 130:1474–1477. https://doi.org/10.1039/b504302f

Pethig R (2010) Review article—dielectrophoresis: status of the theory, technology, and applications. Biomicrofluidics 4:022811. https://doi.org/10.1063/1.3456626

Phallen J, Sausen M, Adleff V et al (2017) Direct detection of early-stage cancers using circulating tumor DNA. Sci Transl Med 9:eaan2415. https://doi.org/10.1126/scitranslmed.aan2415

Preuss I, Eberhagen I, Haas S et al (1995) O6-methylguanine-DNA methyltransferase activity in breast and brain tumors. Int J Cancer 61:321–326. https://doi.org/10.1002/ijc.2910610308

Preuss I, Haas S, Eichhorn U et al (1996) Activity of the DNA repair protein O6-methylguanine-DNA methyltransferase in human tumor and corresponding normal tissue. Cancer Detect Prev 20:130–136

Punnoose EA, Atwal S, Liu W et al (2012) Evaluation of circulating tumor cells and circulating tumor DNA in non–small cell lung cancer: association with clinical endpoints in a phase II clinical trial of pertuzumab and erlotinib. Clin Cancer Res 18:2391–2401. https://doi.org/10.1158/1078-0432.CCR-11-3148

Radovich M, Jiang G, Hancock BA et al (2020) Association of circulating tumor DNA and circulating tumor cells after neoadjuvant chemotherapy with disease recurrence in patients with triple-negative breast cancer. JAMA Oncol 6:1–6. https://doi.org/10.1001/jamaoncol.2020.2295

Ramirez J-M, Fehm T, Orsini M et al (2014) Prognostic relevance of viable circulating tumor cells detected by EPISPOT in metastatic breast cancer patients. Clin Chem 60:214–221. https://doi.org/10.1373/clinchem.2013.215079

Riva F, Bidard F-C, Houy A et al (2017) Patient-specific circulating tumor DNA detection during neoadjuvant chemotherapy in triple-negative breast cancer. Clin Chem 63:691–699. https://doi.org/10.1373/clinchem.2016.262337

Schøler LV, Reinert T, Ørntoft M-BW et al (2017) Clinical implications of monitoring circulating tumor DNA in patients with colorectal cancer. Clin Cancer Res 23:5437–5445. https://doi.org/10.1158/1078-0432.CCR-17-0510

Schwaederle M, Chattopadhyay R, Kato S et al (2017) Genomic alterations in circulating tumor DNA from diverse cancer patients identified by next-generation sequencing. Cancer Res 77:5419–5427. https://doi.org/10.1158/0008-5472.CAN-17-0885

Serpas L, Chan RWY, Jiang P et al (2019) *Dnase1l3* deletion causes aberrations in length and end-motif frequencies in plasma DNA. Proc Natl Acad Sci 116:641–649. https://doi.org/10.1073/pnas.1815031116

Siravegna G, Bardelli A (2014) Minimal residual disease in breast cancer. Blood Veritas Clin Cancer Res 20:2505–2507. https://doi.org/10.1158/1078-0432.CCR-14-0370

Smerage JB, Barlow WE, Hortobagyi GN et al (2014) Circulating tumor cells and response to chemotherapy in metastatic breast cancer: SWOG S0500. J Clin Oncol 32:3483–3489. https://doi.org/10.1200/JCO.2014.56.2561

Soler A, Cayrefourcq L, Mazel M, Alix-Panabières C (2017) EpCAM-independent enrichment and detection of viable circulating tumor cells using the EPISPOT assay. In: Magbanua MJ M, Park J W (eds) Circulating tumor cells: methods and protocols. Springer, New York, NY, pp 263–276

Song C-X, Yin S, Ma L et al (2017) 5-hydroxymethylcytosine signatures in cell-free DNA provide information about tumor types and stages. Cell Res 27:1231–1242. https://doi.org/10.1038/cr.2017.106

Sung H, Ferlay J, Siegel RL et al (2021) Global cancer statistics 2020: GLOBOCAN estimates of incidence and mortality worldwide for 36 cancers in 185 countries. CA Cancer J Clin 71:209–249. https://doi.org/10.3322/caac.21660

Swennenhuis JF, van Dalum G, Zeune LL, Terstappen LWMM (2016) Improving the CellSearch® system. Expert Rev Mol Diagn 16:1291–1305. https://doi.org/10.1080/14737159.2016.1255144

Technische Universität Dresden (2020) Circulating tumour DNA based decision for adjuvant treatment in colon cancer stage II evaluation (CIRCULATE) AIO-KRK-0217. clinicaltrials.gov

Tie J, Wang Y, Tomasetti C et al (2016) Circulating tumor DNA analysis detects minimal residual disease and predicts recurrence in patients with stage II colon cancer. Sci Transl Med 8:346ra92. https://doi.org/10.1126/scitranslmed.aaf6219

U.S. Federal Drug Administration - Center for Drug Evaluation and Research (2018) cobas EGFR mutation test v2. [cited 2023 01 11]. https://www.fda.gov/drugs/resources-information-approved-drugs/cobas-egfr-mutation-test-v2. Accessed 3 Apr 2022

United Nations Department of Economic and Social Affairs (2016a) THE 17 GOALS. Transforming our world: the 2030 agenda for sustainable development. https://sdgs.un.org/goals. Accessed 5 Mar 2023

United Nations Department of Economic and Social Affairs (2016b) Goal 3. Ensure healthy lives and promote well-being for all at all ages. https://sdgs.un.org/goals/goal3. Accessed 5 Mar 2023

University College, London (2021) The SUMMIT study: cancer screening study with or without low dose lung CT to validate a multi-cancer early detection test. clinicaltrials.gov

von Deimling A, Eibl RH, Ohgaki H et al (1992) p53 mutations are associated with 17p allelic loss in grade II and grade III astrocytoma. Cancer Res 52:2987–2990

Weaver KD, Grossman SA, Herman JG (2006) Methylated tumor-specific DNA as a plasma biomarker in patients with glioma. Cancer Investig 24:35–40. https://doi.org/10.1080/07357900500449546

Wiestler OD, Aguzzi A, Schneemann M et al (1992a) Oncogene complementation in fetal brain transplants. Cancer Res 52:3760–3767

Wiestler OD, Brüstle O, Eibl RH et al (1992b) A new approach to the molecular basis of neoplastic transformation in the brain. Neuropathol Appl Neurobiol 18:443–453. https://doi.org/10.1111/j.1365-2990.1992.tb00810.x

Yamamoto A, Huang Y, Krajina BA et al (2023) Metastasis from the tumor interior and necrotic core formation are regulated by breast cancer-derived angiopoietin-like 7. Proc Natl Acad Sci 120:e2214888120. https://doi.org/10.1073/pnas.2214888120

Zhang B, Xu C-W, Shao Y et al (2015) Comparison of droplet digital PCR and conventional quantitative PCR for measuring EGFR gene mutation. Exp Ther Med 9:1383–1388. https://doi.org/10.3892/etm.2015.2221

Zhukova N, Ramaswamy V, Remke M et al (2013) Subgroup-specific prognostic implications of TP53 mutation in medulloblastoma. J Clin Oncol Off J Am Soc Clin Oncol 31:2927–2935. https://doi.org/10.1200/JCO.2012.48.5052

Mitochondrial Transplantation: A Breakthrough Approach for Cancer Treatment

Melika Mashhadi, Zahra Taheri, Taha Monadi, Niloofar Masoumi, Fatemeh Nosrati, Mohammadreza Heidari, and Jalal Pourahmad

Abstract

Mitochondria, essential organelles intricately involved in cellular processes, play a crucial role in cancer progression and the development of chemotherapeutic resistance. Mitochondrial transplantation, an innovative procedure to transfer healthy mitochondria to cells with dysfunctional counterparts, holds great potential in treating mitochondria-based diseases, including cancer. Various methods have been proposed for the isolation and transplantation of mitochondria, which differ depending on the type of study. Based on recent findings, four main mechanisms are involved in mitochondrial transplantation, which includes

M. Mashhadi · N. Masoumi
Network of Interdisciplinarity in Neonates and Infants (NINI), Universal Scientific Education and Research Network (USERN), Tehran, Iran

Student Research Committee, School of Pharmacy, Shahid Beheshti University of Medical Sciences, Tehran, Iran

Z. Taheri
Network of Interdisciplinarity in Neonates and Infants (NINI), Universal Scientific Education and Research Network (USERN), Tehran, Iran

Student Research Committee, Faculty of Pharmacy, Pharmaceutical Sciences Branch, Islamic Azad University (IAUPS), Tehran, Iran

T. Monadi
Network of Interdisciplinarity in Neonates and Infants (NINI), Universal Scientific Education and Research Network (USERN), Tehran, Iran

Student Research Committee, Faculty of Pharmacy, Mazandaran University of Medical Sciences, Sari, Iran

F. Nosrati
Network of Interdisciplinarity in Neonates and Infants (NINI), Universal Scientific Education and Research Network (USERN), Tehran, Iran

Faculty of Pharmacy, Tabriz University of Medical Sciences, Tabriz, Iran

Interdisciplinary Cancer Research, https://doi.org/10.1007/16833_2024_353
Published online: 02 October 2024

tunneling nanotubes (TNTs), extracellular vesicles, and cellular fusion. Preclinical studies have shown promising outcomes, including improvements in cell cycle regulation, cellular energy metabolism, and modulation of cancer progression. In this chapter, we aim to provide a comprehensive review of the pivotal role of mitochondria in cancer. We endeavor to investigate the impact of mitochondrial transplantation on targeted cells and cancer progression, explore diverse methods and mechanisms of mitochondrial transplantation, and discuss the challenges associated with implementing this approach.

Keywords

Cancer · Mitochondria · Mitochondrial transfer · Mitochondrial transplantation

1 Introduction

Cancer is a complex disease that arises from genetic and epigenetic alterations in cells. Despite the considerable progress made in comprehending its molecular mechanisms and developing novel therapeutic approaches, this devastating disease still claims the lives of millions every year (Tulsyan et al. 2022). Among the many mysteries surrounding cancer, the role of mitochondria has received much attention.

Mitochondria are crucial organelles involved in various cellular processes such as metabolism, energy generation, and cell death (Vakifahmetoglu-Norberg et al. 2017). It plays a vital role in the progression and chemotherapeutic resistance of cancer by regulating energy metabolism, calcium homeostasis, redox regulation, and apoptosis (Chang et al. 2019). In cancer cells, mitochondrial function is often compromised, which can actively promote tumor progression through several mechanisms (Celik et al. 2023). Hence, targeting mitochondria has become a hopeful approach for cancer treatment.

Mitochondrial transplantation is a procedure in which healthy mitochondria are transferred from a healthy cell to a damaged one to restore its normal function (Zampieri et al. 2021). This approach has gained significant interest in cancer research, particularly due to its potential in addressing cancer-specific mitochondrial abnormalities (Cruz-Gregorio et al. 2023). This technique has shown promising

M. Heidari
Network of Interdisciplinarity in Neonates and Infants (NINI), Universal Scientific Education and Research Network (USERN), Tehran, Iran

Student Research Committee, Alborz University of Medical Sciences, Karaj, Iran

J. Pourahmad (✉)
Network of Interdisciplinarity in Neonates and Infants (NINI), Universal Scientific Education and Research Network (USERN), Tehran, Iran

Department of Toxicology and Pharmacology, School of Pharmacy, Shahid Beheshti University of Medical Sciences, Tehran, Iran
e-mail: j.pourahmadjaktaji@alumni.utoronto.ca

results in preclinical studies, which have increased drug sensitivity and inhibited cancer cell growth (Zampieri et al. 2021). This technique, in addition to being considered a method for cancer treatment, also enhances the efficacy of conventional interventions like chemotherapy and radiotherapy. Moreover, it provides a new approach to overcome resistance to chemotherapy, which often impedes the success of cancer treatment (Tomita et al. 2021).

In this chapter, we discuss the latest studies on mitochondrial transplantation and its potential as a therapeutic strategy for cancer treatment. We will further discuss the underlying mechanisms, the results obtained in experimental models, and the challenges to be overcome for its clinical translation to develop more effective and targeted strategies to fight cancer.

2 Mitochondrial Dysfunction in Cancer

2.1 Role of Mitochondria in Cellular Energy Metabolism

Cellular metabolism consists of an elaborate network of biochemical reactions converting nutrients to metabolic precursors that promote the growth and survival of organisms. Mitochondria are considered a powerful primary energy source in various cell types, mainly found in significant numbers in major energy-consuming organs like myocardia, respiratory muscles, central nervous system (CNS), or liver. Mitochondria are in charge of diverse critical cellular mechanisms and metabolic processes. Predominantly, mitochondria are responsible for adenosine triphosphate (ATP) synthesis as a primary source of cellular energy through the oxidative phosphorylation known as “mitochondrial respiration.” Moreover, mitochondria play diverse roles in cellular processes, including inducing apoptosis, regulating temperature, generating reactive oxygen species (ROS), activating Ca^{2+} signaling pathways, and monitoring the presence of environmental growth factors (EGF) (Kuznetsov et al. 2022).

Three main steps are involved in mitochondrial ATP synthesis: nutrient entrance, mitochondrial tricarboxylic acid (TCA) cycle, and mitochondrial electron transport chain (ETC) (Spinelli and Haigis 2018).

Cells absorb various nutrients such as sugars, amino acids, and fatty acids to produce the energy required for cellular functions. These nutrients generate energy through ATP and guanosine triphosphate (GTP). Under normal oxygen availability and respiratory capacity, glucose can undergo glycolysis and generate pyruvate. At one end of the mitochondria, pyruvate can pass the inner mitochondrial membrane (IMM) with the aid of mitochondrial pyruvate carrier (MPC) and shuttle into the TCA cycle by the activity of pyruvate dehydrogenase complex (PDC) and pyruvate carboxylase (PC), which can catabolize pyruvate into acetyl CoA and oxaloacetate, respectively (Spinelli and Haigis 2018).

At the other end of the mitochondria, amino acids are catabolized by diverse mitochondrial enzymes to provide other precursors of TCA cycle intermediates. One such example is the catabolism of glutamine, the most abundant free amino acid in the body. Glutamine is broken down into glutamate and ammonia by the mitochondrial glutaminase (GLS). Afterward, glutamate is catabolized by glutamate dehydrogenase (GDH) to generate α-ketoglutarate, one of the critical mediators of the TCA cycle (DeBerardinis and Cheng 2010; Spinelli and Haigis 2018).

Since fatty acids are the other primary cellular sources of energy, the passage of fatty acids through the mitochondrial membrane indicates the metabolic adaptation to diverse cellular conditions. This process is mainly mediated by carnitine palmitoyl transferase 1 (CPT1), carnitine-acylcarnitine translocase (CACT), and CPT2. CPT1 can be found within the outer mitochondrial membrane (OMM) and converts fatty acyl CoA into acylcarnitine, facilitating the transport of long fatty acids through the IMM via the CACT. The fatty acid can later be liberated from entering acylcarnitine by the action of CPT2 and act as a substrate in the β-oxidation reaction (McGarry and Brown 1997; Spinelli and Haigis 2018).

Afterward, these catabolized sources will enter the anabolic mechanisms within the TCA cycle. Even though the TCA cycle does not directly produce a notable amount of ATP, it plays a significant role in gaining electrons from the substrates and transferring them to carriers such as NAD^+ and FAD. These carriers will further enter these electrons into the ETC and participate in the ATP production mechanism (Arnold and Finley 2023).

TCA cycles initiate with two molecular derivatives of pyruvate, oxaloacetate, and acetyl-CoA, which undergo oxidative reactions, convert to citrates, and later generate CO_2 and GTP or ATP molecule. In every cycle, three NADH and one $FADH_2$ are produced by transforming three hydride ions and two hydrogen atoms into these carriers, respectively. Ultimately, the round of each cycle terminates with the regeneration of oxaloacetate (Arnold and Finley 2023).

Later, these reduced carriers will enter the ETC in the IMM near the mitochondrial matrix. NADH will donate its electrons to complex I, regarded as NADH: ubiquinone oxidoreductase and FADH sub 2 will donate its electrons to complex II, called succinate dehydrogenase. The electron transfer within complex I leads to the pumping of the four H^+ ions to the intermembrane space. The same electron transfer process happens in complex II; however, no H^+ ion release occurs. Due to sequential oxidation and reduction mechanisms of the carrier coenzyme Q within complex I and II, electrons move to complex III, regarded as coenzyme Q: cytochrome c reductase, which pumps two H^+ ions in the intermembrane space. Furthermore, an electron shifts from complex III to IV, known as cytochrome c oxidase, which can pass eight protons through the IMM. Of these eight ions, four are used to reduce two oxygen molecules into two H_2O molecules. These secreted H^+ ions in the intermembrane space can cause an electrochemical gradient, known as the mitochondrial membrane potential (MMP). This potential can create a proton motive force resulting in the reentrance of H^+ ions to the matrix, the addition of phosphate to ADP, and ultimately, the synthesis of ATP by the complex V or ATP synthase through oxidative phosphorylation mechanism (Nolfi-Donegan et al. 2020).

These mechanisms exemplify the coordinated actions of these three steps in generating significant amounts of ATP (Fig. 1).

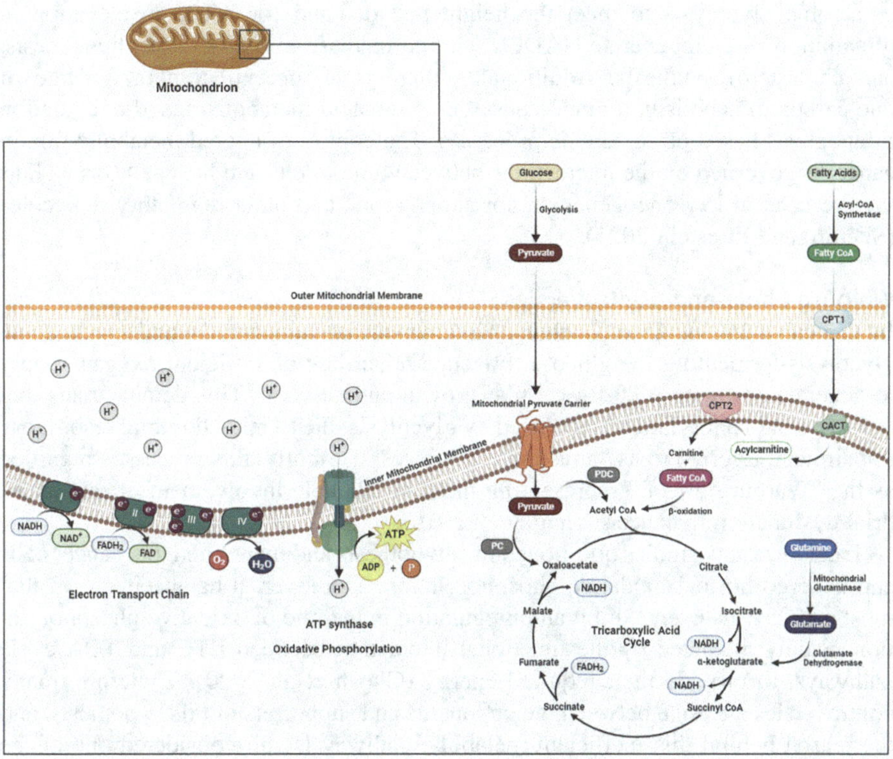

Fig. 1 Key steps in mitochondrial ATP synthesis, including nutrient entry, the tricarboxylic acid (TCA) cycle, and the electron transport chain (ETC), highlighting their roles in converting nutrients into ATP

2.2 Altered Mitochondrial Function in Tumor Growth and Progression

It has been widely accepted that alterations in mitochondria's bioenergetic, metabolic, and dynamic properties significantly promote tumorigenesis by providing cancer cells with ample ATP and essential building blocks. A broad range of human cancers have been found to exhibit mitochondrial dysfunction, which can be attributed to various factors such as defects in TCA cycle enzymes, genetic mutations, impaired ETC, oxidative stress, or abnormal signaling of oncogenes and tumor suppressor genes (Luo et al. 2020).

2.2.1 Metabolic Reprograming

Metabolic reprogramming denotes the capacity of tumorigenic cells to alter their metabolic processes to facilitate a pro-tumorigenic reaction while acquiring and sustaining malignant characteristics (DeBerardinis and Chandel 2016). These changes in metabolism encompass a transition from oxidative phosphorylation to aerobic glycolysis to meet the heightened demand for ATP, an elevation in glutaminolysis to regenerate NADPH, and an increase in lipid uptake, lipogenesis, and cholesterol synthesis. Additionally, there is an upregulation in the rate of one-carbon metabolism, a modification in amino acid metabolism, and a regulation of apoptosis based on metabolic processes. The control of altered metabolic flux in cancer is governed by the interactions between tumor cells and host cells, as well as the presence of key oncogenes, tumor suppressors, and other regulatory molecules (Schiliro and Firestein 2021).

Walburg Effect and Controversies

In the early 1920s, Otto Warburg discovered that tumor cells undergo aerobic glycolysis-fermenting the glucose to lactate regardless of sufficient oxygen supply to generate adequate ATP for cellular growth and survival. This demonstrates that oxidative phosphorylation is replaced by glycolysis due to mitochondrial respiratory impairment, referred to as "a respiratory injury." Currently, this process is regarded as the "Warburg effect," representing the first relatable involvement of mitochondrial dysfunction in cancer (Yang et al. 2016).

Later on, many studies questioned this hypothesis and mentioned that cancer cells can undergo normal oxidative phosphorylation. Moreover, it has been shown that most cancer cells even exhibit an upregulation in the rate of oxidative phosphorylation, mainly mediated by the functional interaction between ETC and TCA cycle pathways, to provide their required energy (Ghosh et al. 2020). Therefore, many controversies are gone between the opponents and supporters of this hypothesis, and the reason behind this inefficient metabolic pathway is still considered one of the current research interests of scientists.

The Warburg effect does not represent a compensatory increase of glycolysis following the persistent disruption of oxidative metabolism in tumor cells. Instead, it describes an aggressive phenotype with biosynthetic programs to maintain cell survival, proliferation, migration, invasion, metastasis, and immune suppression. The corresponding transcriptional response is mainly mediated by hypoxia-inducible factor (HIF), activated PI3K/Akt/mTOR and inactivated LKB1/AMPK pathways, and cMYC, as demonstrated in the last two decades (Vaupel et al. 2019).

Altered Metabolic Pathways

Cancer cells can modify the glycolysis pathway within the mitochondria to meet energy needs and ensure cell survival. Cancer cells have been demonstrated to alter glucose metabolism in mitochondria by redirecting glycolysis metabolites into pathways other than oxidation, such as pentose phosphate, serine anabolism, and lipid anabolism. For instance, some cancer cells reduce pyruvate consumption by upregulating pyruvate kinase (PKM) and downregulating MPC carriers. PKM is in charge of catalyzing the glycolysis reaction and producing pyruvate. The upregulation of PKM2 isoform results in the accumulation of glycolysis intermediates for anabolic pathways. Moreover, the reduced expression of MPC molecules activates mitochondrial metabolic reprogramming, which promotes the oxidation of other compounds, such as fatty acids and amino acids, through the TCA cycle (Vyas et al. 2016).

Under physiological circumstances, stimulation with growth factors leads to activation of phosphatidylinositol 3-kinase (PIK3) and AKT pathways. These pathways can trigger mammalian target of rapamycin (mTOR) and initiate anabolic mechanisms such as the activation of HIF-1 and sterol regulatory element-binding protein (SREBP) and further raise glycolysis and fatty acid formation. These signaling pathways are impressively upregulated in carcinoma cells, regardless of any stimulatory signals from growth factors (DeBerardinis and Chandel 2016).

MYC is responsible for the expression of anabolic-related enzymes, which contribute to glycolysis, glutaminolysis, fatty acid, and serin metabolism. Oncogenes such as KRAS can affect the MYC and PIK3 pathways and play a significant role in tumor development (DeBerardinis and Chandel 2016). Moreover, p53 is a novel identified tumor suppressor that affects the cellular metabolism and cycles by transcriptional stimulation of metabolic genes involved in reducing glycolysis (DeBerardinis and Chandel 2016; Vyas et al. 2016).

One-Carbon Metabolism

Mitochondria are also involved in tumorigenesis through the one-carbon metabolism, influencing the production of nucleotides. The mitochondrial one-carbon enzymes, serine hydroxymethyltransferase 2 (SHMT2), and methylenetetrahydrofolate dehydrogenase 2 (MTHFD2) are among the most prominently expressed in tumor cells. The primary source of the one-carbon pathway is serine; however, mitochondria can also activate this pathway using alternative donors, such as glycine and betaine. SHMT2 is activated in MYC-transformed cells due to hypoxia and ischemia, increasing the chance of cells' survival. Following SHMT2 activation, MTHFD2 is activated to fulfill three main functions: formylmethionine tRNA synthesis for mitochondrial transformation, NADPH synthesis by formyl-THF dehydrogenase (ALDH1L2), and release of formic acid. Recent studies have mentioned that ALDH1L2 contributes to mitochondrial redox homeostasis and metastasis (Zong et al. 2016).

Glutaminolysis in Cancer Cells

Along with glucose, malignant cells can activate glutaminolysis and consume a significant amount of glutamine. Glutaminolysis is vital to the extent that it has been observed that even though glutamine is not considered one of the essential amino acids in the body, the survival and growth of some cancer cells are entirely dependent on the presence of glutamine. As mentioned before, glutamine is involved as a substrate in the TCA cycle and aids the formation of NADPH. MYC oncogenes mediate glutamine-reprogrammed metabolism and promote the exhibition of glutamine addiction behavior in cancer cells (Yoshida 2015).

2.2.2 Cell Death and Apoptosis

Mitochondria are highly associated with the induction of cell death and apoptosis in tumor cells. The B cell lymphoma-2 (BCL-2) family consists of proteins that control the dynamic cellular decision-making processes between survival and mitochondrial apoptosis. The BCL-2-associated X protein (BAX) and BCL-2 antagonist killer 1 (BAK) are two proapoptotic members of this family, which are mainly located in the OMM and oligomerize to disturb OMM permeability by formatting pores within OMM and release cytochrome C to the cytoplasm to activate the apoptosis via caspases cascade. In healthy cells, this process is blocked by other members of the BCL-2 family, like BCL-extra-large (BCL-XL), which can bind to BAX and BAK and inhibit their actions. However, tumor cells can elevate their chance of survival by affecting apoptosis stimulatory and inhibitory mechanisms. Tumor cells can reduce the expression of the proapoptotic protein (BAX and BAK)-encoding genes while increasing the expression of the antiapoptotic protein (BCL-XL)-encoding gene, thus reducing the apoptosis rate, in favor of their survival (Lopez and Tait 2015).

Mitochondria are constantly changing, and their morphology depends upon the equilibrium of fission and fusion. However, this balance is disturbed by increased fission and reduced fusion rates in cancer cells, leading to a damaged mitochondrial network (Senft and Ronai 2016). The dynamin-like protein 1 (DRP1) maintains cell stability by playing a critical role in mitochondrial fission, fragmentation, and remodeling, which eases the release of cytochrome C in apoptosis. DRP1 and BAX represent a boosted interaction with each other during apoptosis. This interaction leads to the induction of mitochondrial remodeling and increased permeability, regardless of the existence of apoptosis stimulators. Therefore, DRP1 can promote apoptosis by inducing BAX activation and mitochondrial translocation (Jenner et al. 2022).

2.2.3 Reactive Oxygen Species (ROS)

ROS, highly reactive oxidant molecules mainly derived from impaired mitochondria, contribute to cancer progression. Although ROS can be produced by specific mechanisms such as electron transportation in ETC and NADH oxidases under physiological conditions, oncogenic pathways, mutational ETC, and hypoxic tumor microenvironment can also be regarded as contributors to excessive ROS production during the tumorigenesis phase. Excessive ROS in cancer cells can cause genomic instability and interact with receptors by oxidating cellular macromolecules like lipids, proteins, and DNA. In addition, ROS can impair vital processes in the progression of carcinoid tumors, including proliferation, apoptosis, and angiogenesis (Sullivan and Chandel 2014).

As mentioned earlier, in the process of mitochondrial respiration, almost all the oxygen consumed in that pathway is converted into water, and only a small portion is converted into ROS. However, this amount can rise significantly in cancer cells due to mitochondria or nucleus genome mutations. Moreover, any disruption in the TCA cycle or ETC may also block the proper oxidative phosphorylation mechanism and lead to the synthesis of superoxide (Yang et al. 2013; Yang et al. 2016).

Furthermore, increased mitochondrial ROS may also be correlated with oncogenic alteration. For instance, the hyperactivation of the *KRAS* gene can promote cancer progression by regulating the ERK/MAPK signaling pathway and, therefore, increase the production of complex III–derived ROS. Higher expressed ectopic

MYC may also be involved in DNA damage by elevating the production of ROS. Mitochondrial DNA (mtDNA) mutations like genes encoding NADH dehydrogenase 6 (ND6) can generate ROS through dysfunctional oxidative phosphorylation pathway (complex I) and promote cancer initiation and progression (Yang et al. 2016).

2.2.4 Mitochondrial DNA (mtDNA) Mutation

The presence of different mitochondrial genomes contributes to the unique biological complexity of this organelle. In mitochondria, 13 ETC subunits, mitochondrial ribosomes, and tRNA are encoded by multiple copies of a single circular DNA molecule. On that account, mutational alterations in mtDNA may contributed to the tumor formation and progression. Somatic mutations and decreased mtDNA copy numbers are common alterations associated with tumorigenesis. Differences in mtDNA copy numbers are involved in tumorigenesis, and both low and high numbers have been associated with different cancers. Additionally, there is a relationship between mitochondrial biogenesis and tumorigenesis. Even though the consequences underlying these mutations are poorly understood, as mentioned before, some modifications in the ETC subunit-encoding genes can result in dysfunctional oxidative phosphorylation and production of ROS, ultimately leading to the development of cancers. Mitochondria have multiple copies of mtDNA, and based on their conformations, cells can be divided into homoplastic or heteroplasmic. While the genome can transfer to other cells by fission and fusion, dominant genetic mutations are spread between different cells and reproduce a colony of mutated cells (van Gisbergen et al. 2015).

2.2.5 Elevated Heme Synthesis

According to recent studies, elevated levels of heme can also stimulate cancer cells' proliferation and tumorigenic potential. Heme is a cofactor in ETC's complex II, III, and IV, providing adequate oxygen for metabolic reactions. Moreover, heme has a crucial function in regulating the transportation of ADP and ATP between mitochondria and cytosol (Ghosh et al. 2020).

Regarding the involvement of heme in mitochondrial respiration and ADP/ATP exchange, heme anabolism and uptake are significantly elevated in non-small cell lung cancer (NSCLC) compared to nonneoplastic cells. This elevation was associated with the higher expression of the ALAS1 enzyme and SLC48A1 protein, which are in charge of the biosynthesis and uptake of heme and induce a higher rate of oxygen utilization and ATP generation in tumor cells (Sohoni et al. 2019).

3 Mitochondria-Targeted Strategies for Cancer Treatment

Experimental evidence highlights the critical significance of mitochondrial bioenergetics, dynamics, and signaling in initiating and progressing tumorigenesis (Ghosh et al. 2020). Recent research has presented compelling findings indicating that diverse cancer cells, including metastatic tumor cells, treatment-resistant tumor cells, and cancer stem cells, heavily rely on mitochondrial respiration. These cells notably amplify their oxidative phosphorylation (OXPHOS) activity to power the mechanisms underlying tumorigenesis. This heightened reliance on mitochondrial respiration and energy production is pivotal in supporting and advancing various types of cancer (Guerra et al. 2017; Dong and Neuzil 2019).

To counteract this dependence on mitochondrial function in cancer cells, multiple strategies have been developed for targeted cancer therapies. These strategies encompass a diverse array of agents and approaches aimed at disrupting specific facets of mitochondrial biology, including:

3.1 Electron Transport Chain (ETC) Inhibitors

The Electron transport chain (ETC) operates within mitochondria, generating ATP, the cell's energy currency. This chain comprises protein complexes situated in the inner mitochondrial membrane. Specifically, the respiratory chain consists of five complexes, three functioning as proton pumps and two as electron transporters (Grasso et al. 2020).

Its primary role involves transferring electrons from donors to oxygen, the ultimate electron acceptor. This electron movement creates a proton gradient across the inner mitochondrial membrane. In cancer cells, mitochondrial ETC alterations disrupt energy production and elevate reactive oxygen species (ROS) levels, potentially fueling cancer progression. By targeting particular ETC complexes or components, it is possible to interfere with cancer cell metabolism, prompting cell death (Grasso et al. 2020).

Compounds that interfere with the electron transport chain are a series of protein complexes critical for energy production in mitochondria. These inhibitors disrupt the generation of ATP and reduce the energy supply to cancer cells (Dong and Neuzil 2019).

3.2 Oxidative Phosphorylation (OXPHOS) Inhibitors

Substances are designed to inhibit OXPHOS, thereby hampering the production of ATP through mitochondrial respiration. This approach deprives cancer cells of the energy they require for proliferation and survival. The glycolysis metabolic pathway directly impacts mitochondrial function by supplying essential metabolic compounds, like pyruvate, necessary for mitochondrial processes. Additionally, the capacity of cancerous cells to efficiently switch between glycolysis and oxidative phosphorylation is a significant factor in various resistance mechanisms to treatments targeting cancerous mutations (Dong and Neuzil 2019).

3.3 Glycolysis Inhibition

Targeting the glycolytic pathway, another means cancer cells generate energy, can starve these cells of the glucose they need for their rapid growth. Targeting both glycolysis and oxidative phosphorylation (OXPHOS) in cancer treatment disrupts the cell's energy pathways crucial for cancer cell survival. By blocking glycolysis, cancer cells are deprived of their glucose-based energy, while inhibiting OXPHOS disrupts ATP production within mitochondria. Combining mitochondrial-targeted drugs (MTDs) with glycolytic inhibitors like 2-DG shows promise in starving cancer cells of energy, potentially boosting the effectiveness of chemotherapy. This dual approach aims to shut down multiple energy sources, hindering cancer growth and triggering cell death. However, fine-tuning doses and understanding potential side effects remain ongoing research areas for refining this combined therapy (Cheng et al. 2012; Dong and Neuzil 2019).

3.4 Tricarboxylic Acid (TCA) Cycle Disruption

Agents that interfere with the TCA cycle, a central metabolic pathway within mitochondria, can impair the generation of essential molecules required for cancer cell survival. The tricarboxylic acid (TCA) cycle is a vital part of cellular function, and manipulating its metabolism is being explored as a way to treat cancer. Mutations in Isocitrate Dehydrogenase 1 (*IDH1*) and Isocitrate Dehydrogenase 2 (*IDH2*) genes are found in cancers such as glioblastoma and acute myeloid leukemia (AML). Glutamine serves as a key fuel for cancer growth, and efforts to inhibit its breakdown, especially by targeting the enzyme GLS with drugs like CB-839 in clinical trials, show strong potential in fighting tumors. These strategies aim to disrupt cancer cell metabolism, offering promising avenues for cancer treatment (Ghosh et al. 2020).

3.5 Modulation of Apoptotic Pathways

Strategies that impact the regulation of apoptosis, the programmed cell death process. These approaches promote the death of cancer cells by influencing the balance of pro-survival and pro-death signals. Bcl-2, Bcl-xL, Bax, and Bak proteins regulate cell death through the intrinsic apoptotic pathway. Venetoclax and inhibitors like navitoclax, TW-37, GX15–070, and BM-1197 target these proteins, causing cancer cell death. Additionally, compounds such as gossypol, ABT-737, and others mimic parts of these proteins, prompting cancer cell death by activating specific signals. These approaches aim to induce apoptosis in cancer cells, offering potential treatments across various cancer types (Dong and Neuzil 2019).

3.6 Reactive Oxygen Species (ROS) Homeostasis

ROS are reactive molecules that can damage cellular structures, including mitochondria. Agents that modulate ROS levels in cancer cells can cause mitochondrial dysfunction and contribute to cell death. As mentioned, the electron transport chain is the primary source of reactive oxygen species (ROS). When the ECT complexes are disrupted, it leads to a high level of ROS release, causing cellular damage. Oxymatrine has been shown to efficiently eliminate human melanoma cells by substantially increasing ROS production. Capsaicin, casticin, and myricetin demonstrate anticancer effects by promoting ROS generation, which disrupts the mitochondrial transmembrane potential in cancer cells (Ramsay et al. 2011; Cui et al. 2017; Porporato et al. 2018; Dong and Neuzil 2019; Roth et al. 2020).

4 Mechanisms and Methods of Mitochondrial Transplantation in Cancer

4.1 Mitochondrial Isolation Techniques

The initial stage of mitochondrial transplantation involves the isolation of viable mitochondria from a cellular donor source. The isolation of mitochondria is an essential procedure in mitochondrial transplantation and other scientific endeavors involving mitochondria. This objective can be accomplished by utilizing diverse techniques (Kim et al. 2023). These multiple techniques have been devised to isolate mitochondria, each with distinct merits and drawbacks. The selection of a methodology is contingent upon the context in which it is to be applied and the accessibility of necessary resources. Density gradient ultracentrifugation, differential centrifugation, and fractionated mitochondrial magnetic separation are among the most used mitochondria isolation methods (Hubbard et al. 2019). Different isolation techniques were developed to protect intact and functional mitochondria and preserve their physical and biochemical characteristics (Hartwig et al. 2015).

4.1.1 Differential Centrifugation

Most mitochondrial isolation methods rely on differential centrifugation. This method uses a two-stage centrifuge at a speed of 1000 to 15,000 g. Initially, a low-speed centrifugation step is employed to eliminate intact cells and cellular debris consisting of cells, tissues, and nuclei, from the overall cellular debris. Subsequently, a high-speed centrifugation step is conducted to segregate mitochondria from other organelles. Although this method is inexpensive and fast, it may involve other cellular debris. The current challenge of this method is the inability to efficiently isolate mitochondrial pellets of high purity or specific mitochondrial subpopulations. As a result, more complex, expensive, and time-consuming processes are needed to isolate mitochondria (Liao et al. 2020).

4.1.2 Density Gradient High-Speed Ultracentrifugation

In this method, which is one of the most accurate and specific methods, a high-speed centrifuge is used. The isolation process in this method is time-consuming and expensive and requires high technical skill. The density of nonfunctional mitochondria, specifically those swollen, exhibits a drop after transferring. Consequently, using density-based approaches for isolating mitochondria may result in selecting intact mitochondria as nonfunctional and low-density mitochondria (Pour et al. 2021).

4.1.3 Fractionated Mitochondrial Magnetic Separation

In this method, the mitochondrial membrane is targeted by magnetically labeled antibodies such as anti-TOM 22. The mitochondria and the magnetically labeled antibody are incubated in this method for 30 min. Then, the contents pass through the magnetic field column, and the labeled mitochondria are attached to the column while other contents are separated. Although this method is more time-consuming than older methods, it produces a higher yield and purity of mitochondria. Accordingly, magnetic-activated cell sorting (MACS), one of the cell separation methods based on surface antigen, can also be used to isolate mitochondria (Hubbard et al. 2019).

4.1.4 Additional Approaches

Other techniques exist for isolating mitochondria, such as the fluorescence-based method, electrophoresis, field-flow fractionation-based method, and filter-based method (Bury et al. 2020; Bodenstein et al. 2023).

4.2 Mitochondrial Transplantation Methods

Transplantation of exogenous mitochondria to different cell types has succeeded in laboratory and animal models and clinical settings (Popov 2021). There are several methods for mitochondrial transplantation. Of them, the most commonly used are mentioned, and the summary of methods is provided in Table 1.

4.2.1 Direct Injection (Microinjection)

The procedure involves injecting isolated mitochondria into target cells or tissues through a fine needle or microinjection techniques. This method has been used in laboratory, animal, and human models, and the injection can be performed locally to specific tissue sites or systemically through the bloodstream. Local injection is employed in situations when there is localized and restricted tissue damage, whereas intravenous injection is utilized in the context of multi-organ mitochondrial disorders (Guariento et al. 2021).

4.2.2 Co-incubation

In this experimental procedure, extracted mitochondria and recipient cells are simultaneously subjected to incubation. Because mitochondria have a bacterial

Table 1 A comparison of mitochondrial transplantation methods

Mitochondrial transplantation Methods	Description	Advantages	Disadvantages	Ref.
Direct injection	Injecting isolated mitochondria into target cells or tissues using a fine needle or microinjection techniques	Used in preclinical and clinical studies Local or systemic injection Suitable for localized tissue damage or multi-organ mitochondrial disorders	Invasive procedure	Guariento et al. (2021)
Co-incubation	Simultaneous incubation of extracted mitochondria with recipient cells	Depends on physiological state of recipient cells Effective in controlled laboratory settings	High risk of mitochondria damage Limited applicability in animal models	Qin et al. (2021)
Centrifugation	Rapid procedure involving centrifugation of mitochondria and recipient cells	Convenient and rapid approach Preserves cell membrane integrity	Unsuitable for in vivo mitochondrial transfer	Kim et al. (2018)
Peptide-1 (pep-1)	Conjugation of mitochondria with peptide-1 to enhance permeability.	Increased uptake capacity rate of recipient cells Low manipulation	Potential immune reactions against the peptide Limited use in animal studies	Chang et al. (2013)
Biocompatible polymers	Use of dextran coating to enhance mitochondrial internalization	Protective effect on respiratory function Enhanced internalization	Not suitable for in vivo mitochondrial transfer	Wu et al. (2018)
Magnetomitotransfer	Magnetic-based approach for enhanced internalization of mitochondria	Rapid massively delivery	Potential transfer of dysfunctional mitochondria	Cowan et al. (2016)
Photothermal nanoblade	Mitochondrial transfer through a micropipette coated with titanium	High transfer Exceeds microinjection	Requires specialized equipment Not suitable for in vivo mitochondrial transfer	Wu et al. (2016)
FluidFM	Using special probes for minimally invasive access to cells	Mitochondria and cellular integrity preservation	Requires specialized equipment High cost	Gäbelein et al. (2022)

origin, the scenario resembles the physiological process by which eukaryotic cells acquire mitochondria. The standard protocol for this methodology is incubating a culture medium containing both mitochondria and the desired target cell. Subsequently, two rounds of centrifugation were performed with a force of 1,500 g for 15 min while maintaining a temperature of 4 °C. While co-incubation is a straightforward technique that can be effectively employed in controlled laboratory settings, its applicability in animal models is constrained (Qin et al. 2021).

4.2.3 Centrifugation

The delivery of mitochondria to target cells without co-incubation can be achieved using a straightforward and rapid procedure, including centrifugation of separated mitochondria and recipient cells in a microcentrifuge tube at 1500 g for 5 min at 4 °C. The aforementioned technique presents a highly convenient approach for transferring mitochondria to the desired cell while preserving membrane integrity without any detrimental effects. It is essential to acknowledge that this particular approach is unsuitable for transferring mitochondria in in vivo settings (Kim et al. 2018).

4.2.4 Peptide-1 (Pep-1)

This peptide is conjugated to mitochondria and enhances mitochondria permeability to the target cell. Small peptides and genetic content can enter the target cell using peptide conjugation without endocytosis. Various studies have shown that when peptide-1 is used, approximately 75% of mitochondria are successfully replaced, whereas the absorption rate is meager without using the peptide. The noteworthy point of this method is the immune reactions against the peptide, which limits its use in animal studies (Chang et al. 2013).

4.2.5 Biocompatible Polymers

Dextran, a naturally occurring polysaccharide, is employed in mitochondrial transplantation. Applying a dextran-triphenylphosphonium coating to mitochondria has been found to have a protective effect on their respiratory function and enhance their internalization, compared to mitochondria that are not coated. Nevertheless, this approach is unsuitable for in vivo mitochondrial transplantation (Wu et al. 2018).

4.2.6 Magnetomitotransfer

The present methodology employs a magnetic-based approach to facilitate the binding of TOM2244 to the protein located on the outer mitochondrial membrane. This approach has been observed to significantly enhance the internalization of mitochondria into recipient cells, resulting in a notable increase ranging from 78 to 92%. However, it should be noted that TOM22 is not exclusively found in target and healthy mitochondria but also in faulty mitochondria. This suggests that dysfunctional mitochondria have the potential to be transported to cells concurrently. Furthermore, it is essential to consider the potential magnetic toxicity connected with this particular approach. It should be noted that this specific approach is not appropriate for in vivo mitochondrial transfer (Macheiner et al. 2016).

4.2.7 Photothermal Nanoblade

The application of photothermal nanoblade entails the introduction of isolated mitochondria into cells using a micropipette coated with titanium. By rapidly heating the micropipette with a laser pulse, the cellular membrane is induced to open. This method exhibits a transfer efficiency of 2%, surpassing that of microinjection. However, it requires specialized equipment and is not suitable for in vivo mitochondrial transfer (Wu et al. 2016).

4.2.8 FliudFM

It is a new method for isolating, injecting, and transplanting mitochondria, which is highly efficient and does not cause damage to the membrane or the mitochondria. Specialized probes are utilized in this method to achieve minimally invasive access to cells and controlled fluid flow, facilitating the isolation and transplantation process. Unlike other strategies that require complex mitochondrial isolation processes, FluidFM enables mitochondria to remain outside the cell for a short time, so the transfer efficiency reaches 95%, much higher than microinjection or photothermal techniques. However, this method requires extensive equipment for successful implementation and is unsuitable for clinical studies (Gäbelein et al. 2022).

In brief, the administration of mitochondria in vivo can be achieved using direct injection methods, such as local injection and intravenous injection. Various techniques have been developed in laboratory settings to enhance mitochondrial internalization compared to co-incubation. These techniques include magneto-mitotransfer, cell-penetrating peptide, centrifugation, and biocompatible polymers. Invasive procedures, such as photothermal nanoblade, FluidFM, and microinjection, are less frequently employed in experimental settings due to their inherent limitations in terms of the number of transplanted cells and the potential harm inflicted upon recipient cells, as compared to the more commonly utilized approach of incubation (Zhang and Miao 2023).

4.3 Mitochondrial Internalization Mechanisms

Mitochondria can be transferred horizontally between different cells. The process of transfer described herein facilitates the incorporation of mitochondria into the cytoplasm of recipient cells, enhancing cellular functionality and energy production. Moreover, the intercellular transfer of mitochondria encompasses the horizontal transfer of genes within mitochondria (Torralba et al. 2016). According to most studies, mitochondrial uptake involves several mechanisms, including:

4.3.1 Tunneling Nanotube (TNTS) and Actin-Dependent Endocytosis

Tunneling nanotubes are tubular structures comprising cell membranes and actin that function as intercellular transport channels. The dimensions of these structures range from 100 to 800 nm in diameter and 100 μm in length. They can transfer RNA, proteins, or complete organelles such as mitochondria and lysosomes, lipid droplets, viruses, and calcium ions to the target cells. These structures have been observed in muscle cells, nerve cells, immune cells, and tumors, and they are known as one of the most critical mechanisms in mitochondrial transfer. These dynamic structures cause the fusion of two cells by forming cell membrane protrusions in response to cellular signals (Bittins and Wang 2017; Wang et al. 2022).

The formation of these structures occurs within a brief time frame, typically spanning a few minutes, and exhibits varying half-lives that can range from minutes to hours, depending on the cell types and the state of the target cell. Actin is one of the important subparts in the structure of nanotubes and enables the strength and structural stability of these nanotubes. On the other hand, these actins bind to the cellular skeleton and allow mitochondria to be transferred along the cellular skeleton structure (Drab et al. 2019). It should be noted that transfer in TNTs can occur unidirectionally or bidirectionally. The predominant transfer mode in unidirectional transfer is from viable cells to cells that have incurred harm. In the process of bidirectional mitochondrial transfer, a disparity exists in the quantity of mitochondria that is moved between the two distinct cell types. One of the aspects that has been investigated in various studies is the intercellular transfer of organelles under cellular stress conditions (Liu et al. 2022). The intracellular expression of p53 increases under oxidative stress conditions, and the signaling pathway (AKT-PI3K-mTOR) is activated, which leads to the formation of TNTs between cells under oxidative stress and healthy cells. Ultimately, several organelles, including the endoplasmic reticulum, Golgi, endosome, and mitochondria, are transferred to the target cell through the transcellular pathway and the formation of nanotubes. Mitochondrial transfer via TNTs between endothelium and cancer cells has been observed to confer resistance to chemotherapy in the cancer cells that receive the transferred mitochondria (Qin et al. 2021).

One distinctive feature of TNTs is that they only contain actin and do not include microtubules (Korenkova et al. 2020). Two studies were carried out to examine this unique characteristic of TNTs. In one experiment, the microtubule inhibitor paclitaxel was used, while in another experiment, the actin polymerization inhibitors cytochalasin B and D were used. The results of the experiments showed that cytochalasin prevents the formation of nanotubes; therefore, if mitochondria and other organelles are transferred through nanotubes, the use of cytochalasin prevents their transfer, and this mechanism called actin-dependent endocytosis (Bukoreshtliev et al. 2009; Kretschmer et al. 2019).

4.3.2 Extracellular Vehicles (EVs)

Circular phospholipid structures known as extracellular vesicles are actively secreted into the extracellular space by a wide range of cell types, regardless of whether the cellular environment is normal or diseased. These entities encompass diverse bioactive compounds, such as proteins, lipids, nucleic acids, metabolites, and mitochondria. Furthermore, it should be noted that EVs can maintain stability within the extracellular milieu and play a significant role as mediators in several cellular processes, such as intercellular communication, cell migration, angiogenesis, and proliferation of tumor cells. The categorization of these vesicles is determined by their size, contents, and mode of creation, resulting in the classification of exosomes, microvesicles, and apoptotic bodies. The first group is exosomes up to 150 nm in diameter, which have an endocytic origin through the budding of the endosomal membrane. The second group is microvesicles with a diameter of 150 to 1,000 nm, and the third group is apoptotic bodies, which are released from apoptotic cells and have a diameter greater than one micrometer. Due to the very small size of the exosomes, microvesicles may contain healthy and viable mitochondria and contribute to the intercellular transport of mitochondria. Mitochondria must be replaced or internalized after entering the target cell. Recent research has indicated that the transfer of mitochondria from one cell to another, specifically through extracellular vesicles, is a significant factor in mitochondrial transfer and uptake (Doyle and Wang 2019).

4.3.3 Gap Junctions

These junctions are tubular structures consisting of six proteins called connexin CX (cell surface protein) that provide a hydrophilic channel for intercellular transport. They allow the exchange of ions, especially calcium ions, and small molecules between two cells and facilitate chemical or electrical signal exchange between two cells. In clathrin-dependent endocytosis or Gap junctions, membrane vesicles enter the cell through the Gap junction and connexins. Subsequently, internalization of mitochondria occurs, and the cell includes small parts of the target cell. Although this mechanism is not fully known, clathrin and dynamin are factors involved in this process. Beta-cyclodextrins inhibit this internalization. These inhibitors do not affect mitochondrial transfer but limit internalization (Qin et al. 2021; Valenti et al. 2021).

4.3.4 Cellular Fusion

Cellular fusion is a biological process characterized by the fusion of the membranes of two distinct cells, merging intracellular organelles and cytoplasmic contents. Notably, the transfer of the nucleus does not occur during this event. Cellular fusion can generate cells with distinct karyotypes while maintaining comparable cytoplasmic composition. The precise mechanism behind cellular fusion remains elusive; nonetheless, it appears that surface proteins and the order and structure of the cellular skeleton are implicated in this phenomenon. One of the benefits associated with cell-to-cell fusion as a method for mitochondrial transfer is its ability to facilitate the transfer of mitochondria to preserve their health and functionality. Mitochondria, which can be moved through other routes such as exosomes or nanotubes, may have impairments or loss of functionality due to the pressures associated with the transportation process (Paliwal et al. 2018; Clemente-Suárez et al. 2023).

4.3.5 Mitochondria Transfer via Tunneling Nanotubes (TNTs) in Cancer

TNTs are critical for facilitating intercellular communication and promoting solid malignancies. The transportation of mitochondria by TNTs between endothelium and cancer cells has been associated with the development of resistance to chemotherapy in the cancer cells that receive the mitochondria. Several variables, including reduced ATP synthesis, inhibition of particular cellular mechanisms, and blockade of the mTOR pathway, can impede the creation of TNTs and hinder the transfer of organelles in cancer cells. However, hydrogen peroxide has been observed to facilitate TNT formation and induce intercellular mitochondrial transfer. Proteins like Miro1 and other accessory proteins contribute to mitochondrial movement through TNTs, and their absence reduces the mitochondrial transfer rate (Lou et al. 2017; Jash et al. 2018).

Chemoresistant ovarian cancer cells have been found to produce more TNT under hypoxic conditions. Pharmacologically blocking the mTOR pathway with medicines such as metformin or everolimus has demonstrated the ability to restrain the development of TNTs, indicating that TNTs can be specifically addressed as a potential approach for cancer treatment (Desir et al. 2016). Hypoxia can also play a role in the transportation of hypoxia-inducible factor-1α (HIF-1α) and vascular endothelial growth factor (VEGF) via TNTs, which may explain the transformation of healthy cells by cancer cells and their implications in invasion and metastasis (Lou et al. 2018). Additionally, TNTs participate in the transport of P-glycoprotein (P-gp) in certain cancers, indicating their potential as therapeutic targets for multidrug resistance (MDR) processes (Pasquier et al. 2012).

5 Preclinical Studies and Experimental Models

Many preclinical studies have demonstrated that mitochondrial transplantation may stimulate cell proliferation, reduce apoptosis, and raise the metabolic performance of cells (Liu et al. 2022). Other studies, on the other hand, have produced contradictory results suggesting that mitochondrial transfer may enhance the survival and proliferation of cancer cells. Based on these conflicting findings, it appears that the impact of mitochondrial transfer on cancer cells could differ by the particular cellular environment (Chang et al. 2019).

5.1 Impact of Transplanted Mitochondria on Cellular Energy Metabolism

As mentioned earlier, mitochondria are crucial in producing adenosine triphosphate (ATP) by oxidative phosphorylation processes. Impairment of energy production by dysfunctional mitochondria results in cellular dysfunction. Restoring energy production and supplying cells with the vitality required to carry out their functions efficiently can be achieved via the transplantation of healthy mitochondria (Liu et al. 2022). Metabolic rate, calcium balance, and signaling systems are additional cellular processes that require healthy mitochondria to function. Restoring cellular functions by replacing dysfunctional mitochondria with functional ones results in an overall enhancement of cellular health and function (Kim et al. 2023).

According to other in vitro research, this technique recovers the bioenergetics of impaired mammalian cells. Additionally, this study discussed that under oxygen-glucose deprivation (OGD) coculture conditions, mesenchymal stem cells (MSCs) transfer mitochondria directly into tunnel nanotubes (TNTs) or indirectly into motor neurons (Liu et al. 2022).

Therefore, through the restoration of bioenergetics, mitochondrial transplantation holds tremendous potential for preserving physiological homeostasis and can be used as a potential treatment for malignancies (Liu et al. 2022).

5.2 Impact of Transplanted Mitochondria on Redox Balance

Mitochondrial malfunction tends to raise amounts of reactive oxygen species (ROS), which subsequently causes oxidative stress. ROS can cause cell injury and contribute to the progression of disease. Mitochondrial transplantation can help reduce oxidative stress by providing healthy mitochondria that produce fewer ROS while restoring the balance of cellular redox status (Sinha et al. 2013; Chen et al. 2018).

In a study carried out by Elliott et al. (2012), mitochondrial dysfunction was assessed, and its effect on cancer cells was examined. Isolated mitochondria from normal breast epithelium MCF-12A were transferred into MCF-7, MDA-MB-231 breast cancer cells, and adriamycin-resistant NCI/ADR-Res ovarian cancer cells. They outlined the procedure of microinjecting mitochondria into the mouse embryo, showing the possibility for therapeutic application of mitochondrial transplant. Increased ROS production, decreased apoptosis, and drug resistance in cancer cells have been mentioned as several adverse effects of mitochondrial dysfunction (Elliott et al. 2012).

In another study by Liu et al. (2023), the researchers investigated the impact of transplanted mitochondria on cholangiocarcinoma (CCA). They extracted mitochondria from 143BρW cells and cultured them with the CCA cell line HuCCT1. The study evaluated various biological consequences of mitochondrial transplantation, including changes in the PTEN/PI3K/AKT signaling pathway, oxidative stress, cell proliferation, and apoptosis. The researchers observed that transferring healthy mitochondria into cancer cells enhanced apoptosis, suppressed cell growth, and reduced oxidative stress (Liu et al. 2023).

5.3 Impact of Transplanted Mitochondria on Metabolic Reprogramming

Mitochondrial transfer can potentially play a role in the metabolic reprogramming of cancer cells. Cancer cells can exploit the trafficking of mitochondria as they reconfigure their tumor microenvironment. An example of this can be seen in acute myeloid leukemia (AML), a malignant blood cancer known for its high dependence on oxidative phosphorylation. Interestingly, when exposed to inhibitors of oxidative phosphorylation, leukemia cells formed an increased number of tunneling nanotube (TNT) connections with mesenchymal stem cells (MSCs). In response, MSCs transferred their mitochondria to AML cells, aiding in the restoration of leukemic respiration and promoting cell proliferation. This demonstrates how mitochondrial transfer can support cancer cell metabolism and growth, particularly in cases like AML, where oxidative phosphorylation is a crucial component of their metabolic profile (Wang et al. 2021; Wang et al. 2022).

5.4 Impact of Transplanted Mitochondria on Cell Proliferation and Apoptosis

As mitochondria play a key role in the regulation of apoptosis, also known as programmed cell death, mitochondrial malfunction can lead to aberrant cell survival or death. Mitochondrial transplantation can restore normal apoptotic signaling pathways, inducing apoptosis in diseased cells and contributing to their elimination. For instance, it was discovered that mitochondrial transplantation inhibits the proliferation of MCF-7 breast cancer cells and promotes apoptosis (Wang and Youle 2009; Chang et al. 2019; Kim et al. 2023).

Zhou et al. (2022) conducted a study comparing the inhibiting effect of mitochondria isolated from male (M-Mito) and female (F-Mito) mice on hepatocellular cancer using male BABL/C mice. The activity was evaluated through analysis of succinate dehydrogenase (SDH), mitochondrial isocitrate dehydrogenase (Mito-ICDH), and mitochondrial membrane potential (MMP). The aforementioned measurements offer valuable insights into the respiration, oxidative phosphorylation (OXPHOS), and overall functionality of mitochondria. By monitoring shifts in tumor cell aerobic glycolysis, supply of energy, progression of the cell cycle, and apoptosis, the study evaluated the impact of the mitochondrial transplantation approach on tumor growth. The results show that healthy mitochondria can impede the growth of hepatocellular carcinoma cells in vitro and in vivo. This suppression is achieved by interrupting the cell cycle and triggering apoptosis (Zhou et al. 2022).

Mitochondrial transplantation has also been reported to impact the proliferation and survival of the host cells. Research in this field has produced varying results; in a study conducted by Elliot et al. (2012) (Elliott et al. 2012), isolated mitochondria from normal breast epithelium MCF-12A were introduced into MCF-7, MDA-MB-231 breast cancer cells, and adriamycin-resistant NCI/ADR-Res ovarian cancer cells. This transfer led to a decrease in the proliferation of MCF-7 and NCI/ADR Res cells and an increased sensitivity of MCF-7 cells to doxorubicin, paclitaxel, and carboplatin. The use of assisted mitochondrial transfer methods from healthy cells, facilitated by a Pep-1-mediated mechanism, further demonstrated impaired in vitro viability of MCF-7 breast cancer cells and a suppression of tumorigenicity in vivo. Interestingly, the viability of the nonmalignant MCF-12A human breast cell line remained unaffected following mitochondrial transfer (Elliott et al. 2012). Moreover, other studies have reported contradictory outcomes following mitochondrial transfer. For instance, in the work of Caicedo et al. (2015) (Caicedo et al. 2015), the transfer of mitochondria from mesenchymal stem cells (MSCs) to MDA-MB-231 cancer cells resulted in enhanced mitochondrial functions, such as increased oxidative phosphorylation (OXPHOS) and ATP production. This, in turn, led to heightened proliferation and invasive characteristics of the cancer cells. Similarly, Marlein et al. (2019) (Marlein et al. 2019) observed that mitochondrial transfer from bone marrow stromal cells (BMSCs) to primary myeloma cells led to increased ATP production and an increased proliferation rate, both in vitro and in vivo. Furthermore, Wang and Gerdes noted a reduction in apoptosis in UV-stressed PC12 pheochromocytoma cells after mitochondrial transfer when co-cultured with healthy cells, suggesting an increase in the survival of cancer cells. These findings indicate the complexity and context-dependent nature of the effects of mitochondrial transfer on various cell types (Wang and Gerdes 2015). Also, in a recent study conducted by Celik et al. (2023), which focused on the impact of human cardiac fibroblast (HCF) mitochondrial transplantation on chemotherapy in prostate and ovarian cancer DU145, PC3, and SKOV3 cells in both in vitro and in vivo settings, the findings indicated that the introduction of viable, respiration-competent mitochondria had no noticeable effect on cancer cell proliferation. However, it significantly reduced cell migration and alterations in cell cycle checkpoints (Zhou et al. 2022; Celik et al. 2023).

6 Mitochondrial Transplantation and Chemotherapy

6.1 Enhancing Chemotherapy and Radiotherapy Efficacy

Mitochondrial transplantation is intricately associated with cellular redox status, which paves the way for potential synergies with established anticancer treatments such as ionizing radiation, chemotherapy, and radiotherapy. The combination of mitochondrial transplantation with radiotherapy leads to the release of cytochrome C, an increase in cleaved-caspase nine levels, and the activation of the mitochondrial apoptotic pathway. As evidenced by the annexin V-FITC/PI assay, this collaboration can potentially intensify cell death induction by amplifying or mitigating oxidative stress. On the flip side, the natural process of mitochondrial transfer, involving the exchange of mitochondria among cells, may provoke heightened resistance to chemotherapy and an elevated invasive capacity in cancer cells that acquire mitochondria from neighboring cells within the tumor microenvironment (TME) (Cruz-Gregorio et al. 2023).

Additionally, there is a likelihood that mitochondrial transplantation may not be employed as an assertive treatment approach in the same manner as other established clinical methods. This is attributed to the fact that mitochondrial transplantation can return cancer cells to a more “inexperienced” state by equipping them with healthy mitochondria.

Consequently, it can alleviate the oxidative stress within cancer cells, thus reducing the side effects associated with chemotherapy and radiotherapy. Furthermore, mitochondrial transplantation can potentially improve the tumor microenvironment and hinder the progression of residual cancer cells toward more aggressive forms, thanks to this “inexperienced” cellular profile. These questions warrant further investigation to provide a more thorough understanding of the genuine impact of mitochondrial transplantation on the demise of cancer cells (Liu et al. 2022; Cruz-Gregorio et al. 2023).

6.2 Overcoming Chemoresistance After Mitochondrial Transfer

Overcoming resistance to chemotherapy in cancer is a vital challenge in cancer therapy. Mitochondrial transfer, a process where mitochondria are exchanged between cells, presents promise as a potential strategy to tackle this problem. Chemoresistance in cancer has two primary forms: intrinsic and acquired (Liu et al. 2022, Cruz-Gregorio et al. 2023).

6.2.1 Intrinsic Chemoresistance

This resistance is inherent to cancer cells due to preexisting factors in the tumor microenvironment, hampering chemotherapy's efficacy even before treatment. These preexisting factors can include genetic mutations, altered cellular signaling pathways, and protective mechanisms that enable cancer cells to evade the cytotoxic effects of chemotherapy drugs (Bahar et al. 2022).

6.2.2 Acquired Chemoresistance

This form develops over time as cancer cells adapt to chemotherapy, reducing effectiveness. Mitochondrial transfer primarily targets intrinsic chemoresistance by enhancing cellular energy production and apoptosis mechanisms. This makes cancer cells more responsive to chemotherapy, potentially overcoming inherent resistance and improving overall treatment effectiveness (Guerra et al. 2017; Genovese et al. 2021). On the contrary, acquired resistance, which emerges after administering treatment, typically stems from changes or mutations in the adaptive response mechanisms. These alterations involve an increase in the expression of therapeutic targets, deactivation of drugs, heightened expression of drug efflux transporters like MDR pumps, improvements in DNA damage repair, shifts in metabolic processes, and the activation of alternative pathways for cell survival (Bahar et al. 2022). Mitochondria occupy a pivotal position in connecting metabolism to the advancement of tumors, as they can determine the destiny of cells. Intriguingly, there has been an observation that cancer stem cells (CSCs) enhance the production of genes responsible for mitochondrial proteins, emphasizing the significant role of mitochondria in the survival, resistance, and dissemination of cancer cells. In recent years, there has been an increasing focus on mitochondria as potentially vital targets for cancer treatment. This is primarily due to mitochondria's ability to adjust to stressful conditions swiftly, enabling the survival of cells (Genovese et al. 2021; Bahar et al. 2022).

6.3 Challenges and Limitations in Clinical Implementation

Clinical implementation of mitochondrial transplantation presents several challenges and limitations. First, ensuring the safety and efficacy of this procedure is paramount. Mitochondrial transplantation is a relatively novel and complex technique, and thorough clinical trials are necessary to establish its safety profile and effectiveness in treating various diseases. Second, the availability of healthy donor mitochondria can be a significant limitation. Sourcing mitochondria for transplantation without introducing potential risks is a critical consideration. Another limitation is the potential for immunological responses. Mitochondrial antigens could trigger immune reactions, and strategies to minimize rejection and adverse immune responses need to be developed (Yamada et al. 2020). Furthermore, the cost and accessibility of mitochondrial transplantation as a therapeutic option may be limited. High costs and technical expertise required for the procedure may hinder its availability to a broader patient population (Clemente-Suárez et al. 2023).

7 Conclusion

Current evidence shows that mitochondrial transfer can positively impact malignancies' cellular energy metabolism, apoptosis, and cell proliferation. Furthermore, mitochondrial transplantation has the potential to synergize with established anticancer treatments by modulating cellular redox status, enhancing apoptotic pathways, mitigating oxidative stress, reducing side effects, and impeding the progression of aggressive cancer cells within the tumor microenvironment. However, the effectiveness of mitochondrial transfer in overcoming both intrinsic and acquired chemoresistance remains a subject of debate and requires further research. Various mechanisms for mitochondrial transfer in malignancies have been postulated, encompassing tunneling nanotubes (TNTs), extracellular vesicles, gap junctions, and cellular fusion. Within this array of mechanisms, TNTs have surfaced as a salient avenue facilitating intercellular communication and the exchange of vital mitochondrial constituents, including adenosine triphosphate (ATP), reactive oxygen species (ROS), and mitochondrial DNA (mtDNA). Moreover, TNTs are pivotal in transforming mitochondria, exhibiting noteworthy implications in chemotherapy resistance and holding promise as a prospective target for therapeutic intervention. Despite the promising outcomes, it is important to acknowledge the limitations of mitochondrial transplantation. These limitations include the need for optimized protocols, the potential risk of immune responses, the challenge of obtaining healthy donor mitochondria, and the high costs involved. Addressing these issues will be crucial for the successful clinical implementation of this therapy. Rigorous research and ongoing advancements are needed to overcome these hurdles and make mitochondrial transplantation a viable and effective medical intervention. Overall, mitochondrial transplantation represents a promising strategy for addressing mitochondrial dysfunction in cancer cells and offers new opportunities for innovative cancer therapies.

Acknowledgment We would like to thank Dr. Noosha Samieefar for her valuable comments on our chapter.

Conflict of Interest None to declare.

References

Arnold PK, Finley LWS (2023) Regulation and function of the mammalian tricarboxylic acid cycle. J Biol Chem 299:102838

Bahar E, Han S-Y, Kim J-Y, Yoon H (2022) Chemotherapy resistance: role of mitochondrial and autophagic components. Cancers 14:1462

Bittins M, Wang X (2017) TNT-induced phagocytosis: tunneling nanotubes mediate the transfer of pro-phagocytic signals from apoptotic to viable cells. J Cell Physiol 232:2271–2279

Bodenstein DF, Powlowski P, Zachos KA, El Soufi El Sabbagh D, Jeong H, Attisano L, Edgar L, Wallace DC, Andreazza AC (2023) Optimization of differential filtration-based mitochondrial isolation for mitochondrial transplant to cerebral organoids. Stem Cell Res Ther 14:202

Bukoreshtliev NV, Wang X, Hodneland E, Gurke S, Barroso JF, Gerdes H-H (2009) Selective block of tunneling nanotube (TNT) formation inhibits intercellular organelle transfer between PC12 cells. FEBS Lett 583:1481–1488

Bury AG, Vincent AE, Turnbull DM, Actis P, Hudson G (2020) Mitochondrial isolation: when size matters. Wellcome Open Res 5

Caicedo A, Fritz V, Brondello J-M, Ayala M, Dennemont I, Abdellaoui N, de Fraipont F, Moisan A, Prouteau CA, Boukhaddaoui H (2015) MitoCeption as a new tool to assess the effects of mesenchymal stem/stromal cell mitochondria on cancer cell metabolism and function. Sci Rep 5:9073

Celik A, Orfany A, Dearling J, del Nido PJ, McCully JD, Bakar-Ates F (2023) Mitochondrial transplantation: effects on chemotherapy in prostate and ovarian cancer cells in vitro and in vivo. Biomed Pharmacother 161:114524

Chang J-C, Liu K-H, Li Y-C, Kou S-J, Wei Y-H, Chuang C-S, Hsieh M, Liu C-S (2013) Functional recovery of human cells harbouring the mitochondrial DNA mutation MERRF A8344G via peptide-mediated mitochondrial delivery. Neurosignals 21:160–173

Chang J-C, Chang H-S, Wu Y-C, Cheng W-L, Lin T-T, Chang H-J, Kuo S-J, Chen S-T, Liu C-S (2019) Mitochondrial transplantation regulates antitumour activity, chemoresistance and mitochondrial dynamics in breast cancer. J Exp Clin Cancer Res 38:30

Chen Y, Zhou Z, Min WJ (2018) Mitochondria, oxidative stress and innate immunity. Front Physiol 9:1487

Cheng G, Zielonka J, Dranka BP, McAllister D, Mackinnon AC Jr, Joseph J, Kalyanaraman B (2012) Mitochondria-targeted drugs synergize with 2-deoxyglucose to trigger breast cancer cell death. Cancer Res 72:2634–2644

Clemente-Suárez VJ, Martín-Rodríguez A, Yáñez-Sepúlveda R, Tornero-Aguilera JF (2023) Mitochondrial transfer as a novel therapeutic approach in disease diagnosis and treatment. Int J Mol Sci 24:8848

Cowan DB, Yao R, Akurathi V, Snay ER, Thedsanamoorthy JK, Zurakowski D, Ericsson M, Friehs I, Wu Y, Levitsky SJ (2016) Intracoronary delivery of mitochondria to the ischemic heart for cardioprotection. PLoS One 11:e0160889

Cruz-Gregorio A, Aranda-Rivera AK, Amador-Martinez I, Maycotte P (2023) Mitochondrial transplantation strategies in multifaceted induction of cancer cell death. Life Sci 332:122098

Cui Q, Wen S, Huang P (2017) Targeting cancer cell mitochondria as a therapeutic approach: recent updates. Future Med Chem 9:929–949

DeBerardinis RJ, Chandel NS (2016) Fundamentals of cancer metabolism. Sci Adv 2:e1600200

DeBerardinis RJ, Cheng T (2010) Q's next: the diverse functions of glutamine in metabolism, cell biology and cancer. Oncogene 29:313–324

Desir S, Dickson EL, Vogel RI, Thayanithy V, Wong P, Teoh D, Geller MA, Steer CJ, Subramanian S, Lou EJ (2016) Tunneling nanotube formation is stimulated by hypoxia in ovarian cancer cells. Oncotarget 7:43150

Dong L, Neuzil J (2019) Targeting mitochondria as an anticancer strategy. Cancer Commun 39:1–3

Doyle LM, Wang MZ (2019) Overview of extracellular vesicles, their origin, composition, purpose, and methods for exosome isolation and analysis. Cells 8:727

Drab M, Stopar D, Kralj-Iglič V, Iglič A (2019) Inception mechanisms of tunneling nanotubes. Cells 8

Elliott R, Jiang X, Head J (2012) Mitochondria organelle transplantation: introduction of normal epithelial mitochondria into human cancer cells inhibits proliferation and increases drug sensitivity. Breast Cancer Res Treat 136:347–354

Gäbelein CG, Feng Q, Sarajlic E, Zambelli T, Guillaume-Gentil O, Kornmann B, Vorholt JA (2022) Mitochondria transplantation between living cells. PLoS Biol 20:e3001576

Genovese I, Carinci M, Modesti L, Aguiari G, Pinton P, Giorgi C (2021) Mitochondria: insights into crucial features to overcome cancer chemoresistance. Int J Mol Sci 22:4770

Ghosh P, Vidal C, Dey S, Zhang L (2020) Mitochondria targeting as an effective strategy for cancer therapy. Int J Mol Sci 21:3363

Grasso D, Zampieri LX, Capelôa T, Van de Velde JA, Sonveaux P (2020) Mitochondria in cancer Cell stress. Trends Cancer 4:114

Guariento A, Piekarski BL, Doulamis IP, Blitzer D, Ferraro AM, Harrild DM, Zurakowski D, Del Nido PJ, McCully JD, Emani SM (2021) Autologous mitochondrial transplantation for cardiogenic shock in pediatric patients following ischemia-reperfusion injury. J Thorac Cardiovasc Surg 162:992–1001

Guerra F, Arbini AA, Moro L (2017) Mitochondria and cancer chemoresistance. Biochimica et Biophysica Acta (BBA)-Bioenerg 1858:686–699

Hartwig S, Kotzka J, Lehr S (2015) Isolation and quality control of functional mitochondria. Methods Mol Biol 1264:9–23

Hubbard WB, Harwood CL, Prajapati P, Springer JE, Saatman KE, Sullivan PG (2019) Fractionated mitochondrial magnetic separation for isolation of synaptic mitochondria from brain tissue. Sci Rep 9:9656

Jash E, Prasad P, Kumar N, Sharma T, Goldman A, Sehrawat SJ (2018) Perspective on nanochannels as cellular mediators in different disease conditions. Cell Commun Signal 16:1–9

Jenner A, Peña-Blanco A, Salvador-Gallego R, Ugarte-Uribe B, Zollo C, Ganief T, Bierlmeier J, Mund M, Lee JE, Ries J, Schwarzer D, Macek B, Garcia-Saez AJ (2022) DRP1 interacts directly with BAX to induce its activation and apoptosis. EMBO J 41:e108587

Kim MJ, Hwang JW, Yun C-K, Lee Y, Choi Y-S (2018) Delivery of exogenous mitochondria via centrifugation enhances cellular metabolic function. Sci Rep 8:3330

Kim JS, Lee S, Kim W-K, Han B-S (2023) Mitochondrial transplantation: an overview of a promising therapeutic approach. BMB Rep 56:488

Korenkova O, Pepe A, Zurzolo C (2020) Fine intercellular connections in development: TNTs, cytonemes, or intercellular bridges? Cell Stress 4:30

Kretschmer A, Zhang F, Somasekharan SP, Tse C, Leachman L, Gleave A, Li B, Asmaro I, Huang T, Kotula L (2019) Stress-induced tunneling nanotubes support treatment adaptation in prostate cancer. Sci Rep 9:7826

Kuznetsov AV, Margreiter R, Ausserlechner MJ, Hagenbuchner J (2022) The complex interplay between mitochondria. ROS and Entire Cellular Metabolism, Antioxidants (Basel), p 11

Liao P-C, Bergamini C, Fato R, Pon LA, Pallotti F (2020) Isolation of mitochondria from cells and tissues. Methods Cell Biol 155:3–31

Liu Z, Sun Y, Qi Z, Cao L, Ding S (2022) Mitochondrial transfer/transplantation: an emerging therapeutic approach for multiple diseases. Cell Biosci 12:1–29

Liu X, Zhang Y, Yang X, Zhang Y, Liu Y, Wang L, Yi T, Yuan J, Wen W, Jian YJ, Cell (2023) Mitochondrial transplantation inhibits cholangiocarcinoma cells growth by balancing oxidative stress tolerance through PTEN/PI3K/AKT signaling pathway Tissue Cell 85:102243

Lopez J, Tait SW (2015) Mitochondrial apoptosis: killing cancer using the enemy within. Br J Cancer 112:957–962

Lou E, O'Hare P, Subramanian S, Steer CJ (2017) Lost in translation: applying 2D intercellular communication via tunneling nanotubes in cell culture to physiologically relevant 3D microenvironments. FEBS J 284:699–707

Lou E, Zhai E, Sarkari A, Desir S, Wong P, Iizuka Y, Yang J, Subramanian S, McCarthy J, Bazzaro M, Steer CJ (2018) Cellular and molecular networking within the ecosystem of cancer cell communication via tunneling nanotubes. Front Cell Dev Biol 6:95

Luo Y, Ma J, Lu W (2020) The significance of mitochondrial dysfunction in cancer. Int J Mol Sci 21

Macheiner T, Fengler VHI, Agreiter M, Eisenberg T, Madeo F, Kolb D, Huppertz B, Ackbar R, Sargsyan K (2016) Magnetomitotransfer: an efficient way for direct mitochondria transfer into cultured human cells. Sci Rep 6:35571

Marlein CR, Piddock RE, Mistry JJ, Zaitseva L, Hellmich C, Horton RH, Zhou Z, Auger MJ, Bowles KM, Rushworth SA (2019) CD38-driven mitochondrial trafficking promotes bioenergetic plasticity in multiple myeloma. Cancer Res 79:2285–2297

McGarry JD, Brown NF (1997) The mitochondrial carnitine palmitoyltransferase system. From concept to molecular analysis. Eur J Biochem 244:1–14

Nolfi-Donegan D, Braganza A, Shiva S (2020) Mitochondrial electron transport chain: oxidative phosphorylation, oxidant production, and methods of measurement. Redox Biol 37:101674

Paliwal S, Chaudhuri R, Agrawal A, Mohanty S (2018) Regenerative abilities of mesenchymal stem cells through mitochondrial transfer. J Biomed Sci 25:1–12

Pasquier J, Galas L, Boulangé-Lecomte C, Rioult D, Bultelle F, Magal P, Webb G, Le Foll F (2012) Different modalities of intercellular membrane exchanges mediate cell-to-cell p-glycoprotein transfers in MCF-7 breast cancer cells. J Biol Chem 287:7374–7387

Popov LD (2021) One step forward: extracellular mitochondria transplantation. Cell Tissue Res 384:607–612

Porporato PE, Filigheddu N, Pedro JMB-S, Kroemer G, Galluzzi L (2018) Mitochondrial metabolism and cancer. Cell Res 28:265–280

Pour PA, Hosseinian S, Kheradvar A (2021) Mitochondrial transplantation in cardiomyocytes: foundation, methods, and outcomes. Am J Physiol Cell Physiol 321(3):C489–C503

Qin Y, Jiang X, Yang Q, Zhao J, Zhou Q, Zhou Y (2021) The functions, methods, and mobility of mitochondrial transfer between cells. Front Oncol 11:672781

Ramsay EE, Hogg PJ, Dilda PJ (2011) Mitochondrial metabolism inhibitors for cancer therapy. Pharm Res 28:2731–2744

Roth KG, Mambetsariev I, Kulkarni P, Salgia R (2020) The mitochondrion as an emerging therapeutic target in cancer. Trends Mol Med 26:119–134

Schiliro C, Firestein BL (2021) Mechanisms of metabolic reprogramming in cancer cells supporting enhanced growth and proliferation. Cells 10

Senft D, Ronai ZA (2016) Regulators of mitochondrial dynamics in cancer. Curr Opin Cell Biol 39:43–52

Sinha K, Das J, Pal PB, Sil PC (2013) Oxidative stress: the mitochondria-dependent and mitochondria-independent pathways of apoptosis. Arch Toxicol 87:1157–1180

Sohoni S, Ghosh P, Wang T, Kalainayakan SP, Vidal C, Dey S, Konduri PC, Zhang L (2019) Elevated Heme synthesis and uptake underpin intensified oxidative metabolism and tumorigenic functions in non-small cell lung cancer cells. Cancer Res 79:2511–2525

Spinelli JB, Haigis MC (2018) The multifaceted contributions of mitochondria to cellular metabolism. Nat Cell Biol 20:745–754

Sullivan LB, Chandel NS (2014) Mitochondrial reactive oxygen species and cancer. Cancer Metab 2:17

Tomita K, Kuwahara Y, Igarashi K, Roudkenar MH, Roushandeh AM, Kurimasa A, Sato T (2021) Mitochondrial dysfunction in diseases, longevity, and treatment resistance: tuning mitochondria function as a therapeutic strategy. Genes 12:1348

Torralba D, Baixauli F, Sánchez-Madrid F (2016) Mitochondria know no boundaries: mechanisms and functions of intercellular mitochondrial transfer. Front Cell Dev Biol 4:107

Tulsyan S, Aftab M, Sisodiya S, Khan A, Chikara A, Tanwar P, Hussain S (2022) Molecular basis of epigenetic regulation in cancer diagnosis and treatment. Front Genet 13

Vakifahmetoglu-Norberg H, Ouchida AT, Norberg E (2017) The role of mitochondria in metabolism and cell death. Biochem Biophys Res Commun 482:426–431

Valenti D, Vacca RA, Moro L, Atlante A (2021) Mitochondria can cross cell boundaries: an overview of the biological relevance, pathophysiological implications and therapeutic perspectives of intercellular mitochondrial transfer. Int J Mol Sci 22:8312

van Gisbergen MW, Voets AM, Starmans MH, de Coo IF, Yadak R, Hoffmann RF, Boutros PC, Smeets HJ, Dubois L, Lambin P (2015) How do changes in the mtDNA and mitochondrial dysfunction influence cancer and cancer therapy? Challenges, opportunities and models. Mutat Res Rev Mutat Res 764:16–30

Vaupel P, Schmidberger H, Mayer A (2019) The Warburg effect: essential part of metabolic reprogramming and central contributor to cancer progression. Int J Radiat Biol 95:912–919

Vyas S, Zaganjor E, Haigis MC (2016) Mitochondria and cancer. Cell 166:555–566

Wang X, Gerdes H-H (2015) Transfer of mitochondria via tunneling nanotubes rescues apoptotic PC12 cells. Cell Death Diff 22:1181–1191

Wang C, Youle RJ (2009) The role of mitochondria in apoptosis. Annu Rev Genet 43:95–118

Wang Y-P, Sharda A, Xu S-N, Van Gastel N, Man CH, Choi U, Leong WZ, Li X, Scadden DT (2021) Malic enzyme 2 connects the Krebs cycle intermediate fumarate to mitochondrial biogenesis. Cell Metab 33(1027–1041):e1028

Wang Z-H, Chen L, Li W, Chen L, Wang Y-P (2022) Mitochondria transfer and transplantation in human health and diseases. Mitochondrion 65:80–87

Wu T-H, Sagullo E, Case D, Zheng X, Li Y, Hong JS, TeSlaa T, Patananan AN, McCaffery JM, Niazi K (2016) Mitochondrial transfer by photothermal nanoblade restores metabolite profile in mammalian cells. Cell Metab 23:921–929

Wu S, Zhang A, Li S, Chatterjee S, Qi R, Segura-Ibarra V, Ferrari M, Gupte A, Blanco E, Hamilton DJ (2018) Polymer functionalization of isolated mitochondria for cellular transplantation and metabolic phenotype alteration. Adv Sci 5:1700530

Yamada Y, Ito M, Arai M, Hibino M, Tsujioka T, Harashima H (2020) Challenges in promoting mitochondrial transplantation therapy. Int J Mol Sci 21:6365

Yang Y, Karakhanova S, Werner J, Bazhin AV (2013) Reactive oxygen species in cancer biology and anticancer therapy. Curr Med Chem 20:3677–3692

Yang Y, Karakhanova S, Hartwig W, D'Haese JG, Philippov PP, Werner J, Bazhin AV (2016) Mitochondria and mitochondrial ROS in cancer: novel targets for anticancer therapy. J Cell Physiol 231:2570–2581

Yoshida GJ (2015) Metabolic reprogramming: the emerging concept and associated therapeutic strategies. J Exp Clin Cancer Res 34:111

Zampieri LX, Silva-Almeida C, Rondeau JD, Sonveaux P (2021) Mitochondrial transfer in cancer: a comprehensive review. Int J Mol Sci 22:3245

Zhang T-g, Miao C-y (2023) Mitochondrial transplantation as a promising therapy for mitochondrial diseases. Acta Pharm Sin B 13:1028–1035

Zhou W, Zhao Z, Yu Z, Hou Y, Keerthiga R, Fu A (2022) Mitochondrial transplantation therapy inhibits the proliferation of malignant hepatocellular carcinoma and its mechanism. Mitochondrion 65:11–22

Zong WX, Rabinowitz JD, White E (2016) Mitochondria and cancer. Mol Cell 61:667–676

Steroids in Cancer: Mechanisms, Therapies, and Challenges in Hormone-Driven Malignancies

Michael Li and Jianneng Li

Abstract

Steroid hormones intricately shape the landscape of cancer in breast, prostate, ovarian, and endometrial tissues, playing a pivotal role in tumorigenesis and progression. The dynamic interplay between these hormones and cancer cells reveals a nuanced relationship where steroid hormones can both promote and inhibit cancer progression. Understanding the complex nature of this interaction is vital for unraveling the intricacies of tumor development in these hormone-driven malignancies. Dysregulation in steroid hormone signaling pathways is a key driver, contributing to the pathophysiology of hormone-driven cancers. The chapter delves into the multifaceted nature of steroid hormones and their dual impact on tumorigenesis. The therapeutic landscape for these cancers has been significantly influenced by insights into steroid hormone dynamics. Hormonal treatments, such as those tailored for breast and prostate cancers, exemplify strategies aimed at manipulating steroid hormone actions to impede cancer progression. However, the narrative is complex, with cancer cells being able to exploit steroid hormones, reminiscent of evasion mechanisms observed in the contexts of other cancers. This chapter comprehensively explores the intricate relationship between steroid hormones and cancers of the breast, prostate, ovarian, and endometrial tissues.

M. Li
Department of Biological Sciences, University of Notre Dame, Notre Dame, IN, USA

J. Li (✉)
Department of Biological Sciences, University of Notre Dame, Notre Dame, IN, USA

Harper Cancer Research Institute, University of Notre Dame, Notre Dame, IN, USA

Melvin and Bren Simon Comprehensive Cancer Center, Indiana University, Indianapolis, IN, USA
e-mail: jli33@nd.edu

Interdisciplinary Cancer Research, https://doi.org/10.1007/16833_2024_294
Published online: 10 July 2024

Keywords

Breast cancer · Endometrial cancer · Hormone-driven malignancies · Ovarian cancer · Prostate cancer · Steroid receptors · Steroidogenesis · Steroids

1 Introduction

Steroids are a class of small, lipophilic hormones that are involved in a wide range of human physiological processes, including reproductive functions, metabolic control, digestion, the body's stress responses, and many more (Adhya et al. 2018). Some examples of the most crucial steroid hormones include cortisol, which manages stress responses and regulates metabolism; aldosterone, responsible for controlling electrolyte balance and blood pressure; testosterone (T) and dihydrotestosterone (DHT), key hormones in the development of male secondary sexual characteristics and muscle mass; estrogen, governing female secondary sexual characteristics and reproductive function; progesterone, essential for regulating the menstrual cycle and supporting pregnancy. These hormones collectively play vital roles in the body's growth, development, immune function, metabolism, and sexual characteristics (Hiller-Sturmhöfel and Bartke 1998; Kinter et al. 2023; Csaba 2014).

Steroid hormones share a basic chemical structure called cyclopentanoperhydrophenanthrene or gonane, a compound with the formula $C_{17}H_{28}$. This structure features a set of fused rings, and different steroid hormone groups are classified based on the saturated ring structures of their base compounds (Fig. 1). Cholestanes, like cholesterol (5-cholesten-3β-ol), have 27 carbon atoms. Pregnanes, such as progesterone (4-pregnen-3-20-dione), have 21 carbon atoms. Androstanes, including testosterone (17β-hydroxy-4-androsten-3-one), contain 19 carbon atoms. Estranes, exemplified by estradiol (1,3,5-estratriene-3,17β-ol), have 18 carbon atoms. The backbone's nomenclature, however, doesn't always reflect biological activity, which depends on the specific nuclear transcription factors or classical steroid hormone receptors activated by these molecules. For example, cortisol and progesterone are both pregnanes but have different biological effects and interact with different receptors.

Steroid receptors (SRs), a subgroup of nuclear receptors, exhibit notable heterogeneity across their functional characteristics. A prominent feature distinguishing these receptors is their ligand specificity, with each receptor precisely binding to a particular steroid hormone (Eick et al. 2012). For instance, the estrogen receptor (ER) demonstrates a unique affinity for estrogen hormones, whereas the androgen receptor (AR) selectively engages with androgens, exemplified by T (Carson-Jurica et al. 1990). Additionally, SRs display distinctive patterns of tissue distribution—some receptors are predominantly localized within specific anatomical regions, while others are more ubiquitously expressed. This differential tissue distribution allows steroid hormones to exert their highly specialized effects on target tissues. Moreover, specific SRs exist in multiple isoforms, adding complexity to their functional diversity (Keightley 1998). The ER, for example, features two principal

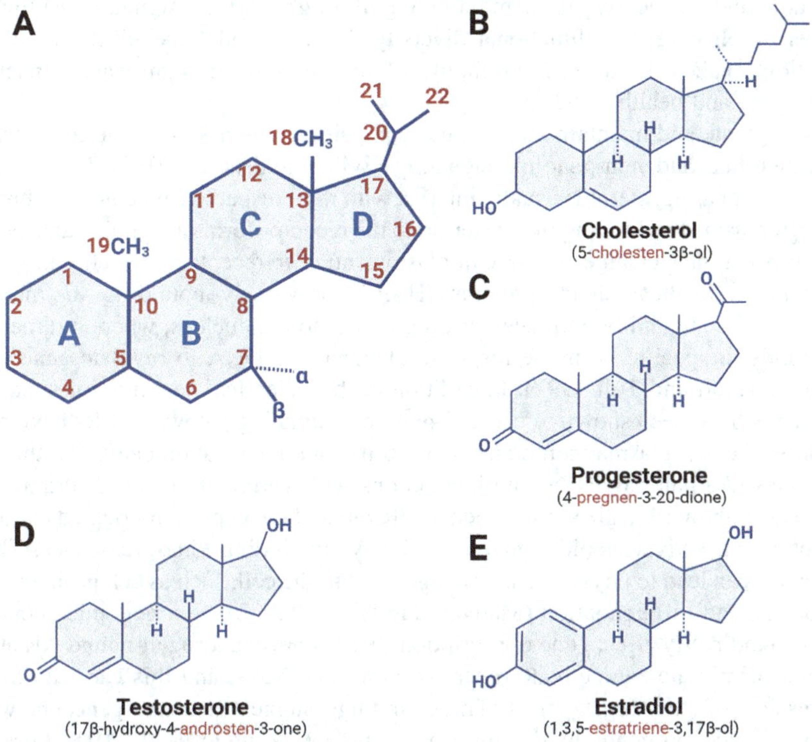

Fig. 1 The core of steroid hormones and examples. (**a**) Steroid hormone structure features a set of fused rings, each carbon atom numbered, and each ring marked by a capital letter. Substituents and hydrogens are shown projecting above (β solid line) or below (α, dashed line) the core plane. (**b, c, d,** and **e**) are the classic examples of steroids named (indicated in red) according to the saturated ring structures

subtypes, ERα and ERβ, each characterized by distinct tissue distribution patterns and functions. This array of subtypes potentially results in divergent responses to the same ligand in different tissues (Eyster 2016). Furthermore, the affinity of SRs for their ligands can differ, with consequences for target tissue sensitivity to the hormonal signal (Garabedian and Yamamoto 1992). Notably, these receptors exhibit disparate DNA-binding specificities, a trait that underpins their capacity to selectively regulate specific sets of genes in a tissue-specific manner (McKeown et al. 2014). Moreover, the recruitment of coactivators and corepressors by SRs can vary among tissues, exerting a pivotal role in modulating their transcriptional activities. The interplay between these co-regulatory proteins contributes to the receptor's functional versatility (Edwards 2000). SRs interact with other signaling pathways and receptors, resulting in crosstalk between distinct hormonal systems (Truong and Lange 2018). For instance, the ER has been shown to interface with the insulin-like growth factor receptor pathway, influencing cellular growth and proliferation (Martin and Stoica 2002). Beyond ligand-dependent activation, some SRs can also be activated independently of ligand binding through various signaling pathways, further amplifying their functional diversity (Treviño and Gorelick 2021). These variations make SRs a complex family of proteins with a significant impact on physiology and health.

To regulate and maintain many of these physiological processes, steroids rely on both genomic and non-genomic signaling (Wilkenfeld et al. 2018). In canonical genomic signaling, steroids usually interact with their respective receptors within the cell cytoplasm. The binding of the steroid to the receptor forms a complex and causes a conformational change in the cytoplasmic nuclear receptors, which causes the dissociation of heat shock proteins (HSPs), previously bound to the nuclear receptors. The ligand-bound receptor translocates to the nucleus, where it dimerizes and binds to specific hormone response elements on DNA to regulate gene transcription (Pratt and Toft 1997). In addition to their classical genomic roles, steroid hormones have been shown to use non-genomic signaling pathways. SRs have been found in the cell plasma membrane. This membrane localization can occur through processes like palmitoylation and interactions with various proteins (Pedram et al. 2007). Membrane-localized SRs, such as ERα36 and the G protein-coupled estrogen receptor, can activate rapid signaling pathways, including kinase cascades. These pathways can lead to physiological changes within the cell, such as cell proliferation, apoptosis, and differentiation (Mauvais-Jarvis et al. 2022). Non-genomic signaling can also indirectly affect gene transcription. For instance, androgen-bound AR at the plasma membrane can activate other signaling pathways, and this can lead to the expression of AR target genes. These findings suggest a convergence between genomic and non-genomic signaling pathways (Wilkenfeld et al. 2018; Foradori et al. 2008). Finally, many non-genomic signaling events can be initiated or augmented following the occurrence of classical genomic actions. For example, growth factor receptors like IGF-IR, EGFR, and VEGFR can be downstream targets of canonical genomic SR signaling, leading also to non-genomic effects (Fagan and Yee 2008; Filardo and Thomas 2005; Hernández-Hernández et al. 2012; Cookman and Belcher 2015). Genes encoding calcium channels or other proteins have also been shown to be transcriptional targets of SRs, which can further propagate non-genomic signals (Asuthkar et al. 2015; Zhang and Barritt 2004).

Steroid hormones are mainly synthesized in the adrenal cortex, placenta, and sexual organs (Hiller-Sturmhöfel and Bartke 1998; Ostróżka-Cieślik and Dolińska 2020). The production of steroids is the result of intricate negative regulatory mechanisms of the hypothalamus-pituitary-adrenal (HPA) and hypothalamus-pituitary-gonadal (HPG) axes (Fig. 2). In the HPA axis, the hypothalamus releases corticotropin-releasing hormone (CRH), which triggers the anterior pituitary to secrete trophic hormones. These trophic hormones, in turn, stimulate the adrenal cortex to synthesize and release steroid hormones like cortisol and aldosterone. Within the HPG axis, gonadotropin-releasing hormone (GnRH) from the hypothalamus stimulates the anterior pituitary to release additional trophic hormones, which similarly stimulate the gonads to release the sex steroid hormones (T, estrogen, progesterone, etc.) (Hiller-Sturmhöfel and Bartke 1998; Ostróżka-Cieślik and Dolińska 2020).

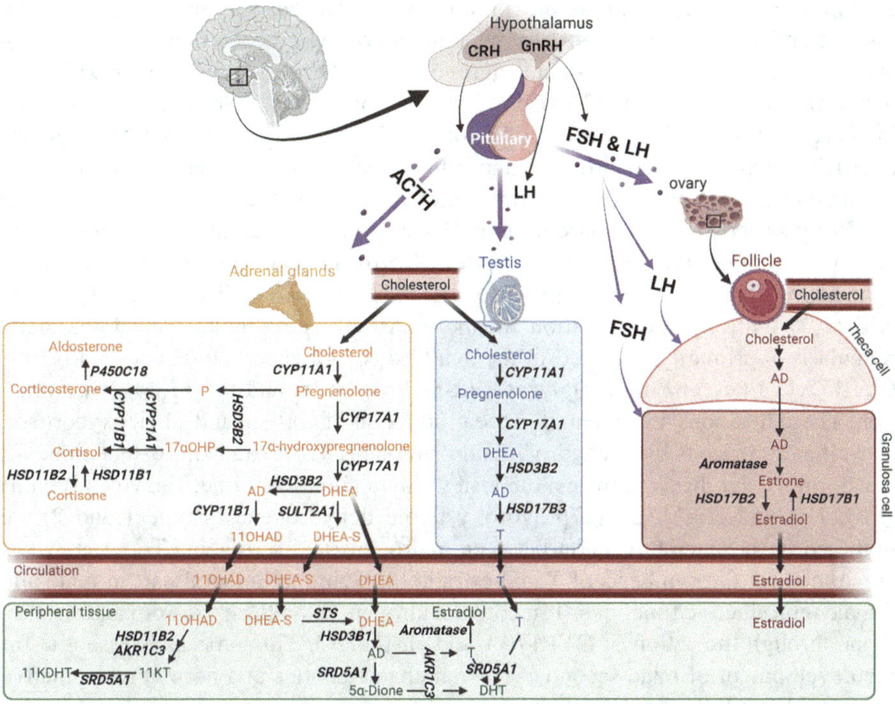

Fig. 2 Steroidogenesis pathways and their regulation by HPA and HPG axes. In the HPA axis, CRH released by the hypothalamus triggers the secretion of ACTH from the anterior pituitary to stimulate the adrenal cortex to synthesize and release steroid hormones utilizing cholesterol. It generates glucocorticoids and mineralocorticoids, as well as provides DHEA, DHEA-S, and 11OHAD for peripheral tissues to synthesize potent androgens. Within the HPG axis, GnRH from the hypothalamus instigates the anterior pituitary to release LH and FSH, which similarly stimulate the gonads (testes and ovaries) to release the well-known sex steroid hormones (T, estrogen, progesterone, etc.). Abbreviations of hormones: *CRH* corticotropin-releasing hormone, *GnRH* gonadotropin-releasing hormone, *ACTH* adrenocorticotropin, *LH* luteinizing hormone, *FSH* follicle-stimulating hormone, *P* progesterone, *DHEA* dehydroepiandrosterone, *DHEAS* dehydroepiandrosterone sulfate, *AD* androstenedione, *11OHAD* 11β-hydroxyandrostenedione, *11KT* 11-ketotestosterone, *11KDHT* 11-ketodihydrotestosterone, *5α-Dione* 5α-androstanedione, *DHT* 5α-dihydrotestosterone, *T* testosterone. Abbreviations of enzymes: *CYP* cytochrome P450, *HSD* hydroxysteroid dehydrogenase, *SULT* sulfotransferase, *STS* steroid sulfatase, *AKR* aldo-keto reductase, *SRD5A* 5α-reductase

All steroid hormones are synthesized through a series of closely interrelated enzymatic pathways that originate from cholesterol (Fig. 2; Payne and Hales 2004; Miller and Bose 2011; Hu et al. 2010). The synthesis starts from the conversion of cholesterol to pregnenolone catalyzed by CYP11A1, also known as P450scc or cholesterol side-chain cleavage enzyme, through a series of three oxygenation reactions involving hydroxylation at the C22 and C20 positions, followed by cleavage of the side chain, all of which requires molecular oxygen and electrons from NADPH, facilitated by redox partners. Then, pregnenolone serves as a pathway divergence point, heading to the production of various steroid hormones with distinct physiological functions. In the adrenal cortex, glucocorticoids like cortisol and mineralocorticoids such as aldosterone are synthesized, and 3β-hydroxysteroid dehydrogenase/isomerase (3β-HSD), mainly 3β-HSD2, plays a pivotal role in these pathways. It is responsible for the 3β-hydroxylation of intermediates, a crucial step in glucocorticoid and mineralocorticoid synthesis. In the zona glomerulosa of the adrenal cortex, aldosterone synthesis commences from 11-deoxycorticosterone. This compound is converted to aldosterone through the action of CYP11B1 (11β-hydroxylase). Cortisol, a major glucocorticoid, is synthesized from 17α-hydroxyprogesterone. The enzyme CYP21A1 catalyzes the critical 21-hydroxylation reaction in this pathway. The adrenal zona fasciculata/reticularis is primarily involved in the synthesis of glucocorticoids and androgens. CYP17A1, a key enzyme, catalyzes 17α-hydroxylation and the 17,20- lyase reaction. These reactions are essential in the production of cortisol and 11-deoxycortisol, as well as androgens like dehydroepiandrosterone (DHEA) and androstenedione. In sex hormone synthesis in males, the testes play a significant role. Enzymes such as HSD17B1 and HSD17B2 (17β-hydroxysteroid dehydrogenases type 1 and 2) are involved in the interconversion between androgens and estrogens. These enzymes are crucial for the synthesis of T and estradiol, playing an integral part in male and female reproductive functions. T, a potent androgen, is synthesized from androstenedione through the action of CYP17A1 and HSD17B3. This process is essential for the development of male secondary sexual characteristics and normal reproductive function. Estradiol, a major estrogen, is produced from estrone via CYP19A1, also known as aromatase. This enzyme is central to regulating the female reproductive system and the development of secondary sexual characteristics. Furthermore, enzymes such as HSD11B2 and HSD11B1 (111β-hydroxysteroid dehydrogenases type 1 and 2) are involved in the conversion of cortisol to cortisone and 11-deoxycortisol to cortisol, respectively, in specific tissues and are critical in regulating glucocorticoid levels. In addition, the enzyme SRD5A2 (5α-reductase type 2) is pivotal in the conversion of T to the more potent DHT, an androgen that significantly influences male sexual development and secondary sexual characteristics. These enzymes are crucial in their respective pathways, and their activity or regulation can significantly impact the production of specific steroid hormones. Many of the enzymatic conversions are rate-limiting steps that often determine the overall rate of hormone synthesis and thus are crucial for maintaining cellular homeostasis and physiological processes (Payne and Hales 2004; Miller and Bose 2011; Hu et al. 2010).

Steroid hormones are usually tightly regulated to maintain cellular homeostasis and normal physiological functions. Disruption of this tight control can significantly contribute to the development of cancer (Zubeldia-Brenner et al. 2016). This disruption of hormonal balance creates an environment where specific cancer risk factors can emerge and thrive, allowing conditions for uncontrolled cell proliferation and survival, hormone receptor aberrations (through genetic mutations, rearrangements, or overexpression), genetic and epigenetic alterations, and the overall progression of hormone-dependent cancers (Satpathi et al. 2023; Guerini-Rocco et al. 2021;

Takeshima and Ushijima 2019; Clusan et al. 2021; Jeong et al. 2014). Four cancer types, namely breast, prostate, ovarian, and endometrial cancers, present significant treatment challenges, each with unique hormonal underpinnings (Hormones and breast cancer 2004; Bosland 2000; Jeon et al. 2016; Thakur and Thakur 2023). Extensive research exploring the potential connections between most major steroids and their corresponding receptors in these cancers underscores that many major steroids contribute to their development. Understanding these hormonal intricacies holds promise for improving our approach to diagnosis and treatment in each of these cancer types. In the upcoming sections, we will delve into the critical factors and mechanisms, discussing the roles of different steroid hormones in the four cancer types.

2 Breast Cancer

Breast cancer (BC) is the predominant cancer affecting women and is a leading cause of cancer fatalities (Łukasiewicz et al. 2021). Women aged 50 and above, as well as those with a family history of breast or ovarian cancer, are at higher risk (Petrucelli et al. 1993). Additional risk factors encompass early onset of menstruation, never having given birth, having a first child after the age of 35, hormone therapies including estrogen (with or without progesterone), and late menopause (Feng et al. 2018). In postmenopausal women, adipose tissue becomes the primary source of estrogen, linking obesity in this demographic to elevated endogenous estrogen levels and an increased BC risk (Cleary and Grossmann 2009). A hormone-responsive malignancy, breast cancer constitutes roughly 25% of all female cancer cases (Sung et al. 2021; Kamińska et al. 2015). Although it is rare, only occurring in 1% of all BCs, male BC does occur. In the United States, about 2800 cases of male BC are diagnosed annually, most of which are late-stage and have high mortality. Similar to female BC, estrogen overexposure is one of the main causes of male BC (Fentiman 2009).

A multifaceted, heterogeneous disease, breast cancer can be divided into five main groups based on expression profiles: (I) luminal types A or B, characterized by the presence of estrogen receptor (ER), and/or progesterone receptor (PR), along with the absence of human epidermal growth factor receptor 2 (HER2); (II) basal-like, which lacks all three receptors, also referred to as triple-negative BC (TNBC); (III) HER2-enriched types; (IV) normal breast-like cancer, distinguished by diminished luminal epithelial gene expression and elevated basal epithelial and non-epithelial gene expression; and (V) claudin-low-expressed cancer, noted for its reduced expression of cell-cell junction proteins (Prat et al. 2015). Most recently, classifying BC based on the expression of steroid hormone receptors has been proven to be valuable for research (Valko-Rokytovská et al. 2021). ER, PR, and HER2 serve as vital biological markers to predict prognosis and survival. Leveraging these markers enables a more accurate categorization of BC into four distinct subtypes: ER+/PR+/HER2-, ER+/PR+/HER2+, ER-/PR-/HER2+, and ER-/PR-/HER2- (Johnson et al. 2020).

2.1 The Role of Estrogens in Breast Cancer

The prevailing standard paradigm regarding BC is that cumulative estrogen (and potentially progesterone) exposure leads to spontaneous mutations, triggering uncontrolled cell proliferation (Hevir et al. 2011). A range of biological and epidemiological evidence documents a key role of estrogen in BC etiology (Rice et al. 2016; Chen 2008; Suzuki et al. 2007; Miyoshi et al. 2001). Mechanistically, the increasing levels of circulating and intratumoral estrogens activate the ER, which produces a series of cascade effects (Ciucci et al. 2016). The molecular mechanisms involving the ERα, a transcription factor that is pivotal in regulating genes related to cell cycle, proliferation, and apoptosis, in BC are highly complex and involve both genomic and non-genomic pathways (Madhu Krishna et al. 2018). Estrogens are the principal ligands that activate ERα, changing the receptor's conformation to an active form, which then dimerizes, translocates to the nucleus, and interacts with transcriptional coactivators, leading to transcription of target genes (genomic pathways) (Fuentes and Silveyra 2019). Specifically, ERα interacts with estrogen-responsive elements (EREs) within the promoters of target genes, as well as other transcription factors, such as activator protein 1 and specific protein 1, via serum-responsive elements to regulate genes without EREs in their promoter region (Lin et al. 2004). Dysregulation of ERα expression, activity, or its coregulators and target genes is associated with the development of most BCs and is classified as ERα-positive or luminal cancer. ERα target genes in BC have oncogenic potential because they increase cell proliferation and DNA damage; they include MYC, cyclin D1, BCL2, IGF-1, and CXCL12 (Clusan et al. 2023). ERα also engages in non-genomic actions. In certain instances, ERα is anchored to the cell membrane, where it interacts with G proteins or growth factor receptors. This non-genomic activity of ERα initiates a cascade of molecular events that involve the production of second messengers like cyclic adenosine monophosphate and stimulates signaling pathways, including PI3K/AKT and Ras/MAPK, which have been shown in hormone receptor-positive cancers to increase cell proliferation and survival (Miricescu et al. 2020).

Two other estrogen receptors, ERβ and G protein-coupled estrogen receptor (GPER), are also activated by estrogens via non-genomic signaling. ERβ, a nuclear receptor similar to ERα, has been shown to influence cell proliferation and apoptosis, although its role isn't completely understood (Yujing Zhou and Liu 2020). GPER also plays a role in estrogen's rapid cellular effects. GPER activation has been shown to not only promote tumor growth but also potentially contribute to resistance to hormone therapy. Research has shown that selective estrogen receptor modulators, like tamoxifen, have been shown to exert agonistic effects on GPER, furthering the notion of GPER's involvement in BC development and providing a potential target for future therapeutics (Xu et al. 2019).

Evidence is growing that tumor tissues synthesize steroids locally (McNamara et al. 2013; Caceres et al. 2016). Enzymes like aromatase, which transforms androstenedione and testosterone into estrone and estradiol, respectively, steroid sulfatase which converts estrone sulfate into estrone, and HSD17B1 which converts estrone to estradiol, are responsible for producing biologically active estrogens in BC tumors (Takagi et al. 2010). It has also been found that androgen levels in BC tumors are notably elevated, as are those of androgen-synthesizing enzymes like HSD17B5, which converts androstenedione to testosterone, and 5α-reductase, which further processes testosterone into dihydrotestosterone, both of which are present in BC tumors (Suzuki et al. 2007). Chetrite and colleagues established that estradiol concentrations are substantially greater in tumors compared to normal breast tissue, further confirming that intratumoral steroid synthesis is another critical factor in BC progression and metastasis (Chetrite et al. 2000). All these preclinical findings indicate that the enzymes involved in steroid synthesis are likely potential therapeutic targets for BC.

2.2 The Role of Progesterone in Breast Cancer

Progesterone is central to biological processes, including the menstrual cycle, pregnancy, and embryonic development (Bulletti et al. 2022). Progesterone receptor (PR) serves as a critical prognostic marker in BC. Specifically, higher PR expression is more commonly observed in tumors with a more favorable prognosis (Purdie et al. 2014). PR, a conventional hormone-activated transcription factor, has two isoforms, PR-A and PR-B, which share the same gene but differ significantly in their transcriptional and biological activities. PR-B is the full-length receptor, whereas PR-A is a truncated form of PR-B with a 164 amino-acid deletion at the N-terminus (Jacobsen and Horwitz 2012). Interestingly, both isoforms are expressed in normal breast tissue, with a 1:1 ratio. However, in malignant transformation, a shift occurs toward a predominant expression of PR-A or PR-B, subsequently influencing the impact of progesterone on gene expression in reproductive tissue and cancer prognosis (Kariagina et al. 2008). Further evidence indicates that prolonged exposure to progesterone can elevate the risk of BC and lead to the development of both hormone receptor-negative and receptor-positive tumors (Li et al. 2022). Postmenopausal women with higher circulating progesterone levels are reported to have a 16% increased risk of BC (Trabert et al. 2020). In many breast target tissues, PR has been implicated as a direct estrogen-inducing gene and is capable of either synergizing with or antagonizing ER to affect downstream biological processes (Diep et al. 2016). Additionally, progesterone may not only interfere directly with ER transcription but also modulate Pol III-mediated transcription and downstream translation, impacting overall tumor growth (Li et al. 2022).

2.3 The Role of Androgens in Breast Cancer

The connection between circulating androgen levels and breast cancer risk remains ambiguous. However, given that AR is expressed in 60%–70% of BCs and may play a dual role in ER-positive cancers alongside estrogen receptors, it has garnered substantial attention (Iacopetta et al. 2012). AR-positive/ER-negative breast tumors exhibit apocrine characteristics and maintain an intact and active AR signaling pathway (Ni et al. 2011). Gene expression microarrays have revealed overexpression of steroid-response genes, such as AR and HER2, in approximately 50% of ER-negative BCs (Schettini et al. 2016). Androgens, such as DHT or R1881 (a synthetic androgen), cause nuclear accumulation of AR; the physical interaction between AR and β-catenin, mediating upregulation of HER3 and activation of HER2/HER3 signaling, along with downstream effectors like PI3K/AKT, ultimately contributes to increased cell growth (Ni et al. 2011). It has been demonstrated that loss of ER expression prompts cells to shift from ER-mediated transcription to an AR-mediated transcriptional priority, utilizing similar mechanisms and co-factors as ER, and thus promoting cell growth in ER-negative BC. When this shift occurs, cell growth becomes less responsive to traditional BC therapies like tamoxifen and aromatase inhibitors but potentially more susceptible to bicalutamide treatment (Cao et al. 2018; Iacopetta et al. 2012). Most recent clinical trials have shown promise in treating AR-positive BC with AR antagonists, which are already used for prostate cancer. First-generation AR antagonists like bicalutamide and second-generation antagonists like enzalutamide have demonstrated clinical benefits in AR-positive BC (Dai and Ellisen 2023). Selective AR modulators and CYP17A1 inhibitors like abiraterone acetate and seviteronel are also being investigated as potential therapies (Anestis et al. 2020). Most recent investigations also reveal that the presence of 3β-HSD1, one of the rate-limiting enzymes in androgen synthesis, in breast cancer is inversely related to patient outcomes, suggesting it to be a potential therapeutic target for AR-positive/ER-negative breast cancer (Chang et al. 2017; McManus et al. 2022). However, the need for predictive biomarkers to identify patients who would benefit most from AR-targeted therapies remains a research focus.

The prognosis is more favorable for women with AR expression in ER-positive tumors. Numerous immunohistochemistry studies correlate a decrease in AR expression with cancer progression, and androgens such as fluoxymesterone have been utilized as second-line hormonal therapy for advanced BC (Iacopetta et al. 2012). The tumor suppressor PTEN cell-signaling pathway, involved in cell proliferation, migration, and apoptosis, might be directly regulated by AR, which sheds light on the opposing effects of AR in the prostate and certain BCs (Iacopetta et al. 2012). In breast cancer, an AR-binding motif exists in the promoter region of PTEN and is positively associated with AR and PTEN transcription levels (Michmerhuizen et al. 2020). Furthermore, elevated expression of AR and PTEN is linked to more favorable clinical results (Wang et al. 2011). An important 2021 study supports the tumor suppressor role of AR in ER-positive BC because AR appears to alter the distribution of ER and vital co-activators (such as p300 and SRC-3) across the genome. This shift leads to the suppression of cell cycle genes regulated by ER, while simultaneously increasing the expression of genes targeted by AR, including tumor suppressors. In sum, these findings all indicate that AR agonism stands out as a very promising strategy for ER-positive BC (Hickey et al. 2021).

2.4 The Role of Glucocorticoids in Breast Cancer

Synthetic glucocorticoids like dexamethasone (DEX) and prednisone have been used for years to treat various diseases, including cancer, because of their anti-inflammatory properties. They are also used to mitigate the side effects of cytotoxic drugs. Glucocorticoids effectively reduce symptoms like vomiting, allergies, edema, and pain (Mitre-Aguilar et al. 2022). However, the role of glucocorticoids in certain cancers, including BC, is controversial. An evaluation of over 65,000 postmenopausal French women in the E3N cohort found that exposure to glucocorticoids was linked to a decreased risk of invasive breast cancer, specifically in ER-positive cases and in stage 1 or 2 tumors, but it was connected to an increased risk of in situ BC and stage 3 or 4 tumors, suggesting that the effect of glucocorticoids on BC varies, depending on the subtype (Cairat et al. 2021). In ER-positive BC, DEX has been shown to inhibit cell proliferation and alter cell cycle progression positively through repressing the ERα transcriptional program (Yang et al. 2017). In contrast, DEX has the opposite effect in ER-negative BC or TNBC, where DEX-bound GR induces the expression of pro-tumorigenic genes that drive chemotherapy resistance and TNBC progression (Noureddine et al. 2021). Additionally, GR activation can lead to increased heterogeneity and metastasis in TNBC, emphasizing the need for caution when administering glucocorticoids to patients receiving chemotherapy or advanced disease, and making GR a potential therapeutic target (Mitre-Aguilar et al. 2022). In conclusion, glucocorticoids and their receptors play complex roles in BC, with varying effects depending on the subtype. High GR expression can serve as a biomarker for prognosis, but the use of glucocorticoids in BC treatment is a topic of ongoing research and debate. These findings underscore the importance of tailoring treatments to the specific characteristics of each BC subtype.

2.5 The Role of the Mineralocorticoid Receptor in Breast Cancer

The mineralocorticoid receptor (MR) appears to be present in tumors in up to 90% of BC cases, making it a receptor of significant interest (Sasano et al. 1997). The direct interplay between ER and MR in BC models remains uninvestigated, yet one study reported that high MR and retinoic acid receptor (RAR) expression correlates with better survival outcomes specifically for ER-positive breast cancer (Doan et al. 2020). The authors suggested a potential interplay between MR and RAR signaling in normal breast tissue, a balance that was disrupted in BC. Subsequent expression profiling of MR-induced BC cells treated with aldosterone and retinoic acid demonstrated that MR and RAR signaling jointly regulate a unique set of genes, a regulation not significantly affected by either receptor individually. Interestingly, whereas the co-activation of MR and retinoic acid signaling inhibited BC proliferation, it promoted glycolysis and suppressed oxidative phosphorylation, a phenomenon contrary to observations in hepatocellular carcinoma (Nie et al. 2015). This unexpected result may be explained by the reverse Warburg effect model, where cancer-associated fibroblasts induce aerobic glycolysis in neighboring cells, leading to the observed metabolic profile in BC cells treated with aldosterone and retinoic acid. Furthermore, the study suggested that the metabolic phenotype observed in treated cells might be tumor-suppressive, possibly through the activation of HIF-1α and subsequent induction of autophagy. In addition to modulating metabolic responses, the tumor-suppressive effects of MR and RAR signaling in BC are likely mediated through other mechanisms, such as the regulation of apoptosis and angiogenesis. The combined treatment with mineralocorticoids and retinoic acid receptor-activating retinoids revealed a tumor-suppressing connection between these nuclear receptors, indicating a promising therapeutic route to explore for BC that is unresponsive to conventional ER-targeted treatments (Doan et al. 2020).

3 Prostate Cancer

Prostate cancer (PC) is the second most common cancer diagnosis in men and the fifth leading cause of death worldwide (Giona 2021). About 1 man out of 8 will be diagnosed with PC during his lifetime, and 1 in 41 will die from PC. Most PC cases remain within the prostate and surrounding areas, with these localized cases often having a favorable prognosis. Treatment options include surgery, radiation, or active surveillance. However, for the minority that develops metastatic disease, the condition is usually not curable, and bone metastasis is characteristic, leading to severe pain and complications (Rebello et al. 2021; Siegel et al. 2020).

3.1 The Role of Androgen in Prostate Cancer

Despite the significance of this cancer, its exact causes remain elusive. Androgens are believed to be critical in the development of PC (Dai et al. 2017). Yet, the specific ways in which they influence this process, as well as the potential role of other steroid hormones, are still not fully understood. Epidemiological research has consistently not supported the "androgen hypothesis," which suggests that elevated levels of androgens in the bloodstream heighten the risk of PC (Hsing et al. 2008). An examination of 10 epidemiological studies that measured blood androgen levels prior to PC diagnosis revealed no connection between the risk of developing PC and serum concentrations of naturally occurring sex hormones or their carrier protein, sex hormone-binding globulin (SHBG) (Eaton et al. 1999). Another study analyzed total androgens (including T, androstanediol glucuronide, androstenedione, DHEA sulfate), estradiol, and SHBG in plasma collected at baseline in a prospective cohort study of 17,049 men suggested that elevated T and adrenal androgen levels are linked with a decreased risk of aggressive PC, but they do not appear to affect the risk of developing nonaggressive disease (Severi et al. 2006).

Although neither androgen level nor activity has been conclusively linked to an increased risk for PC, the undoubted role of androgens in PC progression was established in 1941, when Huggins and Hodges demonstrated the central role of androgen signaling in PC, showing that gonadal depletion of androgens resulted in decreased progression of PC (Huggins and Hodges 1941). In humans, two primary androgens, T and the more potent DHT play vital roles (Banerjee et al. 2018). T is produced by the male gonad, although small quantities are also produced by the adrenal glands. After synthesis, T is released into the bloodstream, where it binds to SHBG and albumin, as well as passively diffused into peripheral tissues, where it exerts its effects (Handelsman 2000). T is converted to DHT in androgenic tissues with high 5α-reductase (SRD5A) expression, where androgen activates the androgen receptor (AR) (Sharifi 2012). Androgen binding to AR results in conformational changes that facilitate nuclear translocation and activation of AR target genes. AR signaling in PC is complex and dynamic. The classical genomic AR signaling model involves the recruitment of the AR to androgen-responsive elements to activate AR target genes (Dai et al. 2017). Chromosomal rearrangements, such as TMPRSS2-ERG fusions, can lead to the overexpression of oncogenic transcription factors and are common in PC (Sun et al. 2008). AR binding is context-dependent, with factors like FOXA1 and HOXB13 playing key roles in reprogramming the AR cistrome to resemble that of malignant tissue and assisting the AR in activating specific genes and maintaining cellular differentiation in PC (Shen et al. 2022). Furthermore, crosstalk between the AR pathway and other signaling pathways collectively promotes key processes in PC, including proliferation and invasion (Awad et al. 2018). As such, nearly all PCs are initially sensitive to androgen deprivation therapy (ADT) by way of medical or surgical castration (Harris et al. 2009). However, resistance to ADT eventually develops, and the disease progresses to castration-resistant PC (CRPC), which is lethal (Coutinho et al. 2016).

It has become overwhelmingly clear that AR signaling is also implicated in CRPC (Coutinho et al. 2016). Several mechanisms contribute to the restoration of functional AR signaling or sensitization of AR to lower androgen levels in CRPC. These mechanisms include the emergence of constitutively active AR splice variants, AR overexpression and amplification, gain-of-function mutations, dysregulated AR coactivators and corepressors, ligand-independent signaling, and crosstalk with downstream signaling pathways, like growth factor receptors and kinases (Ehsani et al. 2021). Furthermore, despite castration, significant levels of intratumoral androgens persist, which indicates the importance of upstream regulation of AR in fueling tumor growth (Dai et al. 2017).

Tumors can use various alternative pathways to produce these intratumoral androgens. One is the de novo pathway converts cholesterol into DHT via the "back door" route (Fiandalo et al. 2014). Backdoor androgen synthesis refers to an alternative pathway for producing T and DHT that bypasses the conventional or "front door" pathways (Fig. 2). In the backdoor pathway, androgen synthesis still begins with cholesterol, but different enzymes and intermediates are utilized to produce DHT directly without going through androstenedione or T as intermediates (Fig. 3). This pathway begins with the 5α-reduction of either progesterone or 17α-hydroxyprogesterone. This initial step produces 5α-C21 steroids, which are then processed by 3α-HSD enzymes (AKR1C2/4), creating precursors for P450c17 enzyme action. Androsterone, generated through the activity of P450c17, can subsequently be transformed into DHT by the enzyme HSD17B6. This pathway

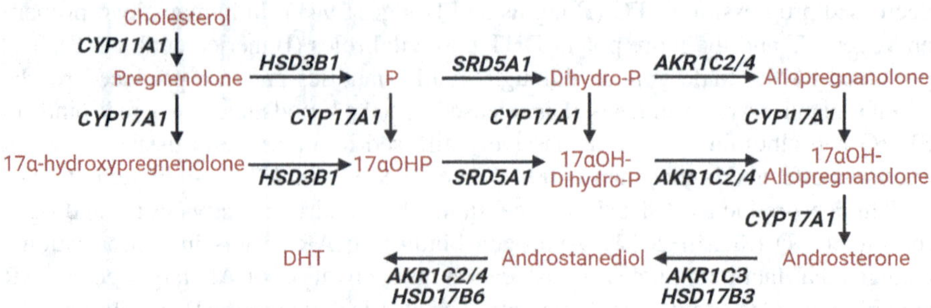

Fig. 3 The "backdoor" route for DHT synthesis. This pathway is significant for its involvement in the development of male traits and is also linked to various human health conditions, including androgen-secreting tumors (like prostate cancer) and specific types of congenital adrenal hyperplasia. Not the absence of androstenedione and T as intermediates. Abbreviations: *P* progesterone, *CYP* cytochrome P450, *HSD* hydroxysteroid dehydrogenase, *SRD5A* 5α-reductase, *AKR* aldo-keto reductase

is notable for its role in the development of male characteristics in some animals and can also be a factor in human disease states such as androgen-secreting tumors and certain forms of congenital adrenal hyperplasia (Wilson et al. 2003; Auchus 2004; Miller and Auchus 2019). Additionally, adrenal androgens, such as DHEA-S and DHEA, can be converted into DHT in prostate tumor tissues, which is supported by clinical findings that circulating adrenal androgen levels are linked to intratumoral androgen levels and poor prognosis (Mostaghel et al. 2021). Although the adrenal glands produce only a small amount of T directly, they secrete significant quantities of androstenedione (AD) and especially large levels of DHEA and its sulfate, DHEA-S, which are the second most and most abundant 19-carbon steroid, respectively. Consequently, if even just 10% of the circulating DHEA or 0.1% of circulating DHEA-S were converted into T or DHT within PC cells (Fig. 2), it would yield sufficient androgens to potentially nullify ADT. It's not unexpected, then, that PC cells, particularly CRPC cells, exhibit increased expression of the enzymes necessary for converting DHEA to T and DHT, compared to normal prostate cells (Lorence et al. 1990; Mitsiades et al. 2012). Moreover, studies have demonstrated that prostate tumor cells can also synthesize 11-ketotestosterone (an androgen that has a similar potency to T for activating AR) using adrenal-derived 11β-hydroxyandrostenedione, the third most abundant known steroid in adrenal, whose circulating concentrations generally exceed those of AD. This metabolic pathway begins with its oxidation by HSD11B2 to form 11β-ketoandrostenedione. Subsequently, the aldo-keto reductase 1C3 (AKR1C3), also known as HSD17B5, catalyzes the reduction of 11β-ketoandrostenedione to produce 11-ketotestosterone (Storbeck et al. 2013; du Toit et al. 2017). Notably, 11-ketotestosterone can also be metabolized via SRD5A1 to its more potent 5α-reduced metabolite (Turcu et al. 2016; Rege et al. 2018).

Intratumoral androgen synthesis requires various enzymes to complete the production of T or DHT or their 11-oxygenated forms from adrenal precursors. Among those enzymes, 3β-HSD1 has been widely studied in PC. A critical and indispensable step in the production of T or DHT from extragonadal precursor steroids—regardless of whether tumors employ de novo steroidogenesis, the adrenal 5-α-androstanedione route, or the traditional adrenal pathway involves the action of 3β-HSD. 3β-HSD performs two sequential reactions which collectively are essentially non-reversible. In the initial reaction, the 3β-hydroxyl group is oxidized to a 3-keto group, followed by isomerization from a Δ5 to a Δ4 bond (Lorence et al. 1990; Evaul et al. 2010). This enzymatic process is responsible for the conversion of DHEA to AD, Δ5-androstenediol to T, pregnenolone to progesterone, and 17-hydroxypregnenolone to 17-hydroxyprogesterone (Sharifi and Auchus 2012). Two human genes give rise to different isoenzymes of 3β-HSD. HSD3B2 is responsible for the isoenzyme found in the gonads and adrenal glands, while HSD3B1 encodes the isoenzyme predominantly expressed in peripheral tissues such as the prostate, skin, breast, and placenta (Simard et al. 2005). HSD3B1 features a widely occurring genetic variant that influences the metabolic pathway controlled by the enzyme 3β-HSD1. Specifically, the HSD3B1(1245A) variant is known as the "adrenal-restrictive" allele, producing an unstable protein that can be easily degraded via ubiquitination pathway, which limits the transformation of adrenal DHEA into AD, whereas the HSD3B1(1245C) variant is the "adrenal-permissive" allele, resulting in a stable enzyme that facilitates the enhanced production of AD from adrenal DHEA and subsequent steroid derivatives (Chang et al. 2013; Sabharwal and Sharifi 2019). Remarkably, multiple cohort investigations in the United States, Japan, and Spain (Hearn et al. 2016; Agarwal et al. 2017; Hearn et al. 2018; Shiota et al. 2019; Garcia Gil et al. 2018) revealed that inheriting the adrenal-permissive allele leads to swifter development of resistance to ADT and a reduced time to reach clinical milestones associated with CRPC in men with advanced disease. Most importantly, two back-to-back studies in the *Annals of Oncology* suggest that adrenal-permissive HSD3B1 allele is associated with poor response in some patients to enzalutamide and abiraterone (the main drugs for treating CRPC, which block AR and androgen synthesis, respectively) (Khalaf et al. 2020; Lu et al. 2020). Together, these findings offer genetic proof that androgens produced outside of the gonads contribute to the PC progression and suggest that HSD3B1 can serve as a potential biomarker for predicting disease course and may be a therapeutic vulnerability.

3.2 The Role of Estrogens and Their Receptors in Prostate Cancer

Estradiol, the most potent estrogen, also has been identified as a key player in PC development and progression based on extensive experimental data in animal models (Nelles et al. 2011). When low doses of T are chronically administered to noble rats, PC develops in about 35–40%, mainly in the form of high-grade prostatic intraepithelial neoplasia (HGPIN). However, when estradiol is given with low-dose testosterone, the incidence of PC significantly increases to nearly 100% (Bosland et al. 1995). This highlights the essential role of estrogens in eliciting a maximal carcinogenic response to androgens, at least in rat prostate. In a novel mouse model, chronic treatment with T and estradiol failed to induce HGPIN or PC when the ERα (estrogen receptor alpha) was knocked out, indicating that functional ERα is crucial to PC development in this model (Ricke et al. 2008). The conversion of T to estradiol is facilitated by aromatase, which is active in various tissues, including the prostate (Stocco 2012) where it has been implicated as a key regulator of the balance between androgen and estrogen levels. Studies in aromatase-knockout mice revealed a reduced incidence of PC, suggesting that in situ production of estradiol is vital for PC development (Ellem and Risbridger 2006).

In the context of human PC, ERα expression extends from basal to luminal cells during the malignant transformation of the prostatic epithelium (Bonkhoff 2018). This aberrant expression of ERα, along with ERα-regulated genes like TMPRSS2-ERG, indicates that functional ERα signaling pathways are involved in human PC progression (Zhou et al. 2019; Xu et al. 2018; Adamo and Ladomery 2016). ERα is not commonly expressed in low- to intermediate-grade PC but is detected in high-grade tumors, metastatic lesions, and CRPC. Furthermore, ERα-regulated genes like PR and TMPRSS2-ERG fusion are found in clinically aggressive tumors, suggesting the activation of ERα-signaling pathways during PC progression (St John et al. 2012; Bonkhoff 2018). Interestingly, ADT can rapidly induce the ERα gene, indicating high-grade PC cell plasticity and the ability to switch from AR to ERα signaling in response to ADT (Tian et al. 2022). ERβ also plays a role in PC biology. ERβ, which preferentially binds phytoestrogens, is thought to protect the prostate epithelium from malignant transformation. Phytoestrogens, such as genistein, indole-3-carbinol, and resveratrol, have been studied for their anticancer properties. ERβ-mediated preventive effects of phytoestrogens may depend on specific ERβ gene polymorphisms and ERβ status in patient tissues (Bonkhoff and Berges 2009; Christoforou et al. 2014).

In summary, while AR remains the primary target for PC treatment, estrogens and their receptors, ERα and ERβ, are implicated in PC development and progression. Estrogens have been shown to promote carcinogenesis in animal models, and functional ERα signaling pathways have been identified in human PC. The emergence of ERα and ERα-regulated genes in clinically aggressive tumors suggests a potential mechanism by which PC cells can bypass ADT. Moreover, ERβ, with its protective role, and the use of specific ERβ agonists, holds promise as potential therapeutic avenues. Further research is needed to fully understand the intricate role of estrogen receptors in PC and to explore targeted therapies based on these receptors.

3.3 The Role of Progesterone in Prostate Cancer

Progesterone's potential role in PC has been seldom considered due to its low endogenous levels in men (Oettel and Mukhopadhyay 2004). However, recent therapies using abiraterone treatment for PC have been shown to significantly increase the concentration of plasma progesterone, providing a unique scenario in which progesterone can exert a greater effect (Chen et al. 2015). Controversy remains over whether progesterone and PR serve an oncogenic role or a tumor-suppressor role, although more studies have shown PR to have oncogenic rather than tumor-suppressive effects (Liao et al. 2023). In patients treated with abiraterone, a progesterone-responsive mutant, ART878A, was identified, indicating a potential resistance mechanism related to abiraterone. Thus, patients expressing certain AR mutations might respond more favorably to abiraterone treatment than those expressing ART878A (Chen et al. 2015). The implication is that the response to abiraterone treatment may be influenced by the specific genetic mutations present in the androgen receptor along with patient progesterone levels. Furthermore, wild-type AR has been demonstrated to have a relatively weak affinity for progesterone, and increasing AR abundance enhances the oncogenic impact of progesterone, which corresponds with clinical observation increased AR expression following abiraterone treatment (Hou et al. 2022). Progesterone also uniquely regulates the expression of non-canonical AR target genes, which are crucial in cell cycle regulation and gene transcription (Thiebaut et al. 2021). Altogether, these findings suggest a complex interplay between progesterone, androgen receptor mutations, and the response to certain therapies in patients with PC.

Prolonged progesterone exposure may also result in irreversible genome or transcriptome changes in PC cells. For example, progesterone induces genes like MUC1, MDK, and HMGCS2, which are associated with the activated estrogen response pathway in PC cells (Hou et al. 2022). Those genes were found to promote advanced disease, including neuroendocrine PC (NEPC), progression and maintain PC stemness (Yasumizu et al. 2020; Nordin et al. 2013; Hagiwara et al. 2021; Broustas et al. 2019). Additionally, progesterone upregulates GATA2 expression, a gene that plays a role in activating the estrogen response pathway and has been linked to PC progression (Rodriguez-Bravo et al. 2017; Xiao et al. 2016). Inhibiting GATA2 with a chemical named K7174 reduced the cumulative effects of progesterone, offering a potential strategy for managing PC in the setting of abiraterone resistance (Hou et al. 2022). 3β-HSD1 is another promising target for counteracting the oncogenic effects of progesterone because it is essential in progesterone production. Although enzalutamide and K7174 only restrained transient and cumulative progesterone-driven oncogenic functions, respectively, inhibiting 3β-HSD1 to block the conversion of pregnenolone to progesterone appears to be a more promising strategy. Thus, targeting 3β-HSD1 offers a promising approach to enhance the clinical efficacy of abiraterone (Hou et al. 2022; Mei et al. 2022).

3.4 The Role of Glucocorticoids in Prostate Cancer

Glucocorticoids have been effectively used in PC treatment for years, not only to mitigate antiandrogen treatment side effects but also to suppress serum androgen levels. They are well-documented to reduce prostate-specific antigen levels and tumor volume, and preclinical studies indicate their direct inhibitory impact on PC cell proliferation and angiogenesis (Sakellakis and Flores 2022). Furthermore, GR is negatively regulated by active AR signaling (Guo et al. 2018; Xie et al. 2015), suggesting the competitive relationship between AR and GR pathways in PC. However, recent studies have also demonstrated that elevated GR expression and activity can rescue cancer cells from enzalutamide-induced death and confer resistance to chemotherapy and radiation therapy (Arora et al. 2013; Isikbay et al. 2014; Sakellakis and Flores 2022).

The metabolism of glucocorticoids themselves adds another layer of complexity to glucocorticoid signaling in PC. Our previous studies suggested that glucocorticoid metabolism is associated with enzalutamide resistance in CRPC (Li et al. 2017, 2021). Specifically, long-term enzalutamide exposure sustains tumor cortisol concentrations via downregulation of the 11β-HSD2 protein, the enzyme that metabolizes cortisol, as well as an increase in hexose-6-phosphate dehydrogenase (H6PD), the cofactor for 11β-HSD1, which is essential for cortisone activation (Bánhegyi et al. 2009). Further, the sustained tumor cortisol level stimulates upregulated GR to confer enzalutamide resistance. Our studies have also found that targeting 11β-HSD2 protein loss and/or inhibiting H6PD activity may be a way to reverse enzalutamide resistance safely and effectively (Li et al. 2017; Li et al. 2021). In summary, glucocorticoids, acting through GR, have diverse effects across different cell types (Sakellakis and Flores 2022). In PC, their role is intricate, and they can exert antitumor effects in the presence of active AR signaling, but under specific conditions, they contribute to resistance to antiandrogen therapies or become the primary driver of the disease.

4 Ovarian Cancers

The fifth most frequent cause of cancer death, ovarian cancer is the most lethal gynecologic cancer in women in the United States (Arora et al. 2023). Similar to breast and prostate, ovarian function in normal female reproductive health is highly dependent on sex hormones, specifically estrogen and progesterone, and dysfunction often leads to an imbalance and deregulation associated with cancer development and progression (McHann et al. 2021).

The ovary plays a major role in reproduction as well as the production of female sex hormones (Gibson and Mahdy 2023). As previously discussed, GnRH is synthesized and released by the hypothalamus. GnRH binds the anterior pituitary, and in response, the pituitary synthesizes and releases two essential gonadotropins: follicle-stimulating hormone (FSH) and luteinizing hormone (LH). FSH demonstrates a particular affinity for ovarian granulosa cells. FSH interaction stimulates the granulosa cells to support follicle growth and maturation. The granulosa cells provide the necessary microenvironment for the developing oocyte and actively participate in the production of various growth factors and hormones required for this process. On the other hand, LH influences the ovarian theca cells to synthesize and release androgens, which are precursors for the synthesis of estradiol (Fig. 2). Estradiol is the primary sex hormone in females and plays a central role in regulating the female reproductive system. Following ovulation, the ovarian follicle is transformed into the corpus luteum, a temporary structure, which, under the influence of LH, changes the structural and functional makeup of the granulosa and theca cells, leading to the production of progesterone, which prepares the endometrium for a fertilized egg (Marques et al. 2000).

The vast majority of ovarian carcinoma derives from the ovarian surface epithelium and its inclusion cysts and is classified as epithelial ovarian cancer (EOC). Over 80% of all new OC cases are identified as advanced EOC, which has spread to the lining of the abdomen (peritoneal metastases) or organs far from the original tumor site, as classified by stages III–IV of the International Federation of Gynecology and Obstetrics (FIGO) system. The FIGO staging system is the one most frequently applied in diagnosing EOC, which includes four stages based on the detection of carcinoma (Current FIGO Staging for Cancer of the Vagina, Fallopian Tube, Ovary, and Gestational Trophoblastic Neoplasia, 2009). Clinically, there are two serous subtypes of OC: low-grade serous carcinoma (LGSC) and high-grade serous carcinoma (HGSC). LGSC and HGSC are different types of cancers with unique origins and are not simply lower and higher severity forms of the same cancer. Both types are often diagnosed at stage III or IV. LGSC is often associated with mutations in the BRAF or KRAS genes, whereas HGSC, which is the more common type of OC, is usually linked to mutations in the p53 gene. HGSC originates from the epithelium of the distal fallopian tube, not the ovarian epithelial cells. In contrast to serous tumors, endometrial ovarian carcinoma (EC) and clear cell carcinoma (CCC) usually present earlier and often develop from endometriotic tissue. Ovarian mucinous carcinomas (MCs) are typically unilateral and are stage I tumors, developing gradually from pre-existing mucinous cystadenoma or mucinous borderline tumors. Furthermore, OCs are classified into type I and type II tumors based on disease aggressiveness. Type I tumors (LGSC, low-grade EC, CCC, and MC) are generally slow-growing and genetically more stable. They often develop in a stepwise progression from benign lesions to invasive tumors, involving mutations in genes like KRAS or BRAF. In contrast, type II tumors, including HGSC, high-grade EC, and undifferentiated carcinomas, are more aggressive, grow quickly, and have high genetic instability, frequently featuring p53 mutations (McCluggage 2011).

4.1 The Role of Estrogens in Ovarian Cancer

Robust epidemiological data indicate that estrogen activity heavily influences the development, underlying causes, and progression of OC. Additionally, the equilibrium between estrogen and progesterone plays a vital role in OC onset (Folkerd and Dowsett 2010). Hormone replacement therapy (HRT) has been identified as a risk factor for the development of OC. Postmenopausal women using estrogen-only HRT were observed to have an approximately 22% heightened risk of OC over 5 years (Lee et al. 2023). Even with the addition of progestin to the estrogen therapy, the risk remained significantly elevated, showing an approximate 10% increase (Zhou et al. 2008; Pearce et al. 2009). A comprehensive patient study conducted in England demonstrated that the likelihood of developing OC escalates with the extended use of HRT, particularly when the therapy extends beyond a decade. The relative risk was greater for EOC in contrast to MC, EC, or CCC (Beral et al. 2007). Recent research indicates that postmenopausal women taking unopposed oral estrogen therapy face a higher risk for HGSC, LGSC, and EC. The only decrease in risk was observed for MC. Similarly, an elevated risk for serous carcinoma and EC was noted among women who were on a combined HRT regimen of estrogen and progestin (Mørch et al. 2012). Together, all these clinical studies emphasize the etiological role of estrogen in OC.

Mechanistically, estrogen exerts its tumor-promoting effects either with the help of receptors or without them. In receptor-dependent mechanisms, estrogen binds ERα, which activates cell growth and development genes, including proto-oncogenes like c-fos, c-myc, and HER2/neu, as well as genes for cell cycle regulators like the cyclins and various growth factors (Chang and McDonnell 2012). Additionally, when estrogen binds to GPER, it sets off a chain of intracellular signals. GPER is responsible for the immediate, non-genetic effects of estrogens (Prossnitz et al. 2007). In receptor-independent mechanisms, estrogens can be metabolized by cytochrome P450 (CYP) enzymes, which can create harmful byproducts that can bind to DNA and cause mutations. These mutations can accumulate because the estrogen metabolism generates free radicals, leading to harmful changes in various genes in the cells of the fallopian tubes and ovaries, which can eventually cause transformation (Gajjar et al. 2012; Yager 2015; Cavalieri and Rogan 2011).

4.2 The Role of Progesterone in Ovarian Cancer

On the other hand, research has suggested progesterone protects against the development and progression of OC, specifically as a tumor suppressor (Han et al. 2013). Statistical data indicate that the occurrence of OC is significantly greater in industrialized nations, which may result from the fact that birth rates in industrialized countries are comparatively lower than those in developing nations. Substantial evidence supports the notion that multiple pregnancies offer a measure of defense against OC. The likelihood of OC is reduced by 10–16% with each subsequent pregnancy, and becoming pregnant at 35 years old provides double the protective benefit against OC compared to a pregnancy at 25 years old (Whiteman et al. 2003). Furthermore, OC incidence was reported to be correlated with progesterone deficiency, and increased progesterone was associated with a subsequent reduction in OC risk (Modan et al. 1998), suggesting a suppressive role of progesterone in OC incidence because progesterone levels increase hugely (six- to eight-fold) during pregnancy.

Studies have shown that progesterone can inhibit OC cell development and proliferation and increase apoptosis (Han et al. 2013). Interestingly, accumulated data show progesterone has a growth-promoting effect when given at low concentrations but a growth-inhibitory effect at higher concentrations (Ho 2003). Nevertheless, studies in SNU-840, OVCAR-3, and HOC7, OC cell lines show that high levels of progesterone treatment are associated with transient upregulation of p53 expression, and induction of apoptosis due to downregulation of the anti-apoptotic protein Bcl-2 and inhibition of cell proliferation (Formby and Wiley 1998; Yu et al. 2001; Ho 2003). Furthermore, reports have suggested that progesterone uses a unique extrinsic apoptosis-initiation pathway with caspase-8 activation that enhances Fas/FASL signaling, leading to apoptotic induction (McGlorthan et al. 2021). Progesterone was also shown to reduce plasma membrane fluid dynamics in OC cells. This is associated with the inhibition of exocytotic vesicle release by malignant cells and a decrease in cell invasiveness and colony formation in collagen matrices (McDonnel et al. 2003).

In conclusion, the effects of estrogen and progesterone in OC are complex. Estrogen, with its proliferative and pro-survival properties, has been implicated in promoting the development and growth of OC cells. On the flip side, progesterone appears to have antitumorigenic effects by reducing cell proliferation and increasing apoptosis in OC. The interplay between these hormones and their precise roles in OC progression is an area of active research, and the mechanisms involved are far from fully understood. Further investigations into the intricate hormone-dependent pathways in OC are essential for developing more targeted and effective therapeutic strategies.

4.3 The Role of Androgens in Ovarian Cancer

Although the clinical evidence regarding the association of androgen levels with ovarian tumorigenesis and cancer progression is inconsistent, *investigations* in animal models and observations in humans suggest that high androgen concentrations contribute to the initiation and development of OC (Mizushima and Miyamoto 2019). As such, numerous clinical trials have been carried out to evaluate the effectiveness of anti-androgens, alone or in combination with GnRH agonists. ADT employing anti-androgens like flutamide, bicalutamide, and enzalutamide, as well as GnRH agonists that ultimately reduce AR activity, has been extensively used in prostate cancer, generally without significant adverse effects (Miyamoto et al. 2004; Manning-Geist et al. 2022). Currently, many phase II trials of anti-androgen treatment for OC have been finished (Tumolo et al. 1994; Vassilomanolakis et al. 2000; Levine et al. 2007; Manning-Geist et al. 2022), and all these trials suggest that antiandrogen therapy only benefits a subset of OC patients. Therefore, additional research is needed to ascertain the true advantages of antiandrogen therapy, its most effective protocols, and methods to identify suitable patients. This could involve, for instance, evaluating AR expression, examining AR polymorphism/splice variants, and monitoring the activity of downstream targets of the AR pathway.

4.4 The Role of Glucocorticoids in Ovarian Cancer

Glucocorticoids are commonly used as an adjunct in OC treatment to reduce the unpleasant side effects of chemotherapy (Roila et al. 2016; Hesketh et al. 2020), increasing patient tolerance to higher doses and more frequent cycles of cytotoxic drugs. Nonetheless, many researchers suggest that glucocorticoids may protect tumor cells from cell death. This protective effect is thought to occur through mechanisms such as increased cell adhesion, stimulation of anti-inflammatory signals, and the suppression of apoptotic pathways. A link has been identified between GR expression and clinical outcomes in patients with OC, suggesting that GR activity may adversely impact tumor progression (Veneris et al. 2017). A study involving 481 patients with OC examined this relationship by assessing GR protein levels in tumor samples using immunohistochemistry and correlating these levels with progression-free survival and overall survival. Significantly, patients with higher GR protein expression experienced a notably shorter median progression-free survival (20.4 months) compared to those with lower GR expression, who had a median progression-free survival of 36 months. However, no significant link was found between GR expression levels and overall survival (Veneris et al. 2017). The effect of GR expression on patient outcomes appeared to vary depending on the OC histiotype. There was a marked association between GR expression and progression-free survival, particularly in low-grade and non-serous OC, but this was not the case in HGSC histology (Veneris et al. 2017). This connection between GR activity and poorer outcomes in OC may be partly due to glucocorticoids diminishing the effectiveness of chemotherapy. In clinical and preclinical studies, GR signaling has been demonstrated to interfere with the efficacy of chemotherapy by inhibiting the apoptotic pathways activated by cytotoxic agents (Zhang et al. 2006; Zhang et al. 2007). Additionally, several preclinical studies have reported that glucocorticoids may enhance tumor cell survival after radiotherapy and chemotherapy by creating an environment conducive to tumor cell adhesion, migration, and spread, by modifying the expression of cellular adhesion components (Chen et al. 2010; Herr and Pfitzenmaier 2006; Liotta and Kohn 2001). Given the critical role of GR signaling in conferring resistance to chemotherapy, targeting the GR has become a promising strategy to enhance the effectiveness of chemotherapy in patients with OC.

5 Endometrial Cancer

The endometrium, a dynamic and highly responsive tissue, undergoes cyclic changes in response to estrogen and hormonal fluctuations, including proliferation, differentiation, and shedding of the endometrial lining during the menstrual cycle (Cousins et al. 2021). Specifically, in response to steroid hormones, the endometrium has both proliferative and secretory phases. In premenopausal women, the ovaries actively synthesize and release estrogen during the menstrual cycle (Yu et al. 2022). Estrogen, in conjunction with progesterone, orchestrates the phases of the menstrual cycle, including the proliferation of the endometrial lining during the follicular phase. This proliferative phase is characterized by increased vascularity and glandular development (Yu et al. 2022). Estrogen's effect on the endometrium includes its ability to stimulate cell growth and angiogenesis, and to maintain a receptive environment for embryonic implantation (Yu et al. 2022). Finally, the cyclical fluctuations in estrogen levels, specifically the withdrawal of estrogen with the onset of menstruation, initiate the shedding of the endometrial lining, thereby renewing the cycle (Yu et al. 2022). Conversely, post-menopause is signaled by decreased levels of ovarian estrogen production. With declining estrogen levels, the endometrium undergoes profound atrophic changes, characterized by a decrease in glandular tissue, vascularization, and overall thickness. These structural modifications, collectively known as endometrial atrophy, occur due to the absence of estrogen's proliferative effects, as the postmenopausal endometrium becomes less responsive to hormonal cues (Wend et al. 2012).

Endometrial cancer (EC) is the most common gynecologic cancer in the United States (Schlumbrecht et al. 2023). This cancer is characterized by various histological subtypes and molecular profiles. Traditionally, EC has been classified as Type I or Type II. Type I EC, often linked to prolonged exposure to unopposed estrogen, typically features low-grade cells, is more prevalent, and generally has a better prognosis. On the other hand, Type II EC is not driven by estrogen, involves high-grade cells, is less common, and usually has a poorer prognosis (Oaknin et al. 2022). Type I EC mainly consists of grade I or II endometrioid adenocarcinomas, while Type II ECs encompass grade III endometrioid adenocarcinoma, along with serous, clear cell, undifferentiated carcinoma, and carcinosarcoma (Conlon et al. 2014; Makker et al. 2021). Although the precise causes of EC remain unclear, it is believed that factors such as obesity, infertility, hormone replacement therapy, and diabetes may contribute to its development. The risk of recurrence is higher in advanced stages of the disease, with established risk factors including obesity and prolonged exposure to high levels of estrogen (Merritt et al. 2021).

5.1 The Role of Estrogens in Endometrial Cancer

Consistent with the standard mechanistic paradigms that involve estrogen and sex hormones, it is widely held that many of the EC risk factors have some relation to excess estrogens or estrogen signaling (Rodriguez et al. 2019). These events are often accompanied by a reduction in progesterone, a balancing essential for normal physiological function (Cable and Grider 2023). Therefore, dysfunction of this balance in favor of estrogen leads to unopposed estrogen domination and the development of cancer. Due to the multiple similar phenotypic results of estrogen signaling in EC and breast cancer, many molecular details of EC are similar to those in breast cancer, suggesting the oncogenic role of the ER pathway in EC (Rodriguez et al. 2019).

ER genome binding exhibits a high degree of cell-type specificity. However, EC only shares 15–30% ER binding site similarity with breast cancer, even though ER has been shown to induce increased tumor cell proliferation in both cancers (Droog et al. 2016). In EC, the ER has been shown to interact with other steroid hormone receptors, and their expression levels can influence each other's actions (Sikora 2016). It is worth noting that high ER and PR expression is associated with better outcomes in EC (Vahrenkamp et al. 2018). In EC, however, ER can decrease PR activity, and even potentially alter PR-target genes (Prange-Kiel et al. 2001; Mohammed et al. 2015; Singhal et al. 2016). Furthermore, mutations in the ligand binding domain of the ER have been linked to hormone therapy resistance in both breast cancer and EC (Rodriguez et al. 2019). Studies have also suggested that these mutations can confer estrogen-independent activity to ER, leading to increased proliferation and altered gene expression, even without estrogen (Blanchard et al. 2019). Moreover, a higher incidence of advanced EC has been linked to the loss of estrogen and progesterone receptors (Di Donato et al. 2018).

In conclusion, the link between estrogen and EC arises from estrogen-driven cellular proliferation within the endometrial tissue, which can eventually result in the accumulation of genetic mutations and the alteration of gene expression patterns, thereby increasing the risk of malignant transformation (Makker et al. 2021). Conversely, progesterone functions as an antagonist by hindering cell division, reducing ER expression, and fostering cell differentiation (Kim et al. 2013). Understanding the intricate relationship among estrogen, progesterone, and EC is not only crucial for elucidating the disease's molecular mechanisms but also for identifying potential targets for therapeutic intervention.

5.2 The Role of Androgens in Endometrial Cancer

Evidence is emerging that AR expression in EC may influence its prognosis. Current research indicates that androgens play a role in various endometrial conditions, including endometriosis, EC, and endometrial dysfunction (Lv et al. 2022). Abnormal levels of androgens have been detected in EC cases, suggesting a close link between androgens and the onset and progression of EC (Wu et al. 2022). However, data regarding the specific role of androgens in the development of EC remain inconsistent and somewhat contradictory.

Some researchers have noted the highest AR expression in precursor lesions and well-differentiated primary EC tumors, with a subsequent decrease in expression as tumors become less differentiated (Tangen et al. 2016). This decline in AR expression suggests that androgens may play a role in tumor differentiation. Evidence, however, is conflicting. Hashmi et al. observed no correlation between AR expression and tumor differentiation (Hashmi et al. 2018). Furthermore, the loss of AR has been associated with reduced disease-specific survival in patients with EC, especially those with early-stage disease (Maček et al. 2023). AR expression is also reported to be more frequently associated with Type I EC and early tumor stages. It also correlates with the absence of lymphovascular invasion and reduced lymph node involvement, although some inconsistencies exist in these findings (Mahdi et al. 2017; Abu Shahin et al. 2021).

The metabolism and regulation of androgens are influenced by multiple elements. Obesity, often associated with elevated androgen levels, complicates the picture. Studies suggest that a particular visceral adiposity phenotype, irrespective of body mass index, is linked to lower SHBG levels. This, in turn, influences androgen delivery to target tissues (Pasquali and Oriolo 2019). Insulin resistance adds another layer of complexity. Insulin affects various hormone signaling pathways, such as increasing LH secretion and adrenal androgen production, potentially contributing to hyperandrogenism in women (Unluhizarci et al. 2021). Insulin resistance can impact tumor cell proliferation and promote cancer progression. Moreover, the conversion of androgens into estrogens within adipose tissue has implications for EC. Studies have demonstrated that the estrogenic pathway is more critical than the androgenic pathway in EC etiology (Michels et al. 2019). Androgens may contribute to EC by serving as precursors for estrogen synthesis, emphasizing the need to inhibit the aromatization of androgens. Additional work is required to decipher these intricate relationships.

5.3 The Role of Glucocorticoids in Endometrial Cancer

In the normal endometrium, ER and GR have opposing roles, with ER promoting growth and GR inhibiting it (Vahrenkamp et al. 2018). However, research reveals a more intricate scenario in EC, where GR expression is associated with adverse outcomes and higher-grade tumors. This association becomes prominent only when it coexists with high ER expression. These results seem contradictory to the anti-growth effects of corticosteroids, but they reveal a complex relationship between ER and GR (Vahrenkamp et al. 2018). One possible explanation for the contrasting effects of GR-induced growth lies in the distinct locations of ER and GR expression within the endometrium (Vahrenkamp et al. 2018). GR is primarily expressed in stromal cells, whereas ER is predominantly expressed in endometrial glands (Bamberger et al. 2001). In the normal uterus, GR signaling in stromal cells inhibits growth through autocrine or paracrine mechanisms. However, when GR and ER are co-expressed in hyperplastic or cancerous endometrial cells, GR's inhibitory effect on growth is no longer observed. This loss of inhibition may lead to the development of more aggressive tumors. Moreover, gene expression studies in which glucocorticoid and estrogen are co-administered have shown a decrease in the expression of genes associated with cell adhesion, which might encourage a more metastatic phenotype (Vahrenkamp et al. 2018). The interplay between ER and GR reflects a dominance of ER as the primary steroid hormone receptor, with its genomic binding remaining largely unaffected by GR activation. In contrast, over one-third of GR binding sites are altered by ER activation. This suggests that the recruitment of GR to ER-bound sites has functional consequences, possibly enhancing regulatory activity (Vahrenkamp et al. 2018). Further studies are essential to unravel the precise mechanisms underlying the dominance of ER or GR in different cancer settings and to explore their potential implications for treatment strategies.

6 Conclusion

In conclusion, steroid-driven cancers encompass a diverse spectrum of malignancies, each characterized by their intricate reliance on hormonal cues, specifically steroids. Recent advances have substantially increased our comprehension of their underlying mechanisms, culminating in the emergence of new targeted hormonal therapies. The strategic use of steroids and their antagonists in cancer management has already ushered in a transformative era, significantly improving patient prognosis, not only in survival rate but also in the prevention and control of these cancers. Nonetheless, formidable challenges, including the development of resistance to hormonal therapies and adverse side effects, underscore the ongoing necessity for research and the pursuit of truly innovative treatment modalities. With deepening insight into the intricate interplay of steroids in cancer etiology and the perpetual evolution of therapeutic strategies, even more efficacious and personalized interventions will be developed to treat steroid-driven malignancies.

References

Abu Shahin N, Aladily T, Abu Alhaj N, Al-Khader A, Alqaqa S, Aljaberi R et al (2021) Differential expression of androgen receptor in type I and type II endometrial carcinomas: a Clinicopathological analysis and correlation with outcome. Oman Med J 36(2):e245. https://doi.org/10.5001/omj.2021.53

Adamo P, Ladomery MR (2016) The oncogene ERG: a key factor in prostate cancer. Oncogene 35(4):403–414. https://doi.org/10.1038/onc.2015.109

Adhya D, Annuario E, Lancaster MA, Price J, Baron-Cohen S, Srivastava DP (2018) Understanding the role of steroids in typical and atypical brain development: advantages of using a "brain in a dish" approach. J Neuroendocrinol 30(2). https://doi.org/10.1111/jne.12547

Agarwal N, Hahn AW, Gill DM, Farnham JM, Poole AI, Cannon-Albright L (2017) Independent validation of effect of HSD3B1 genotype on response to androgen-deprivation therapy in prostate cancer. JAMA Oncol 3(6):856–857. https://doi.org/10.1001/jamaoncol.2017.0147

Anestis A, Zoi I, Papavassiliou AG, Karamouzis MV (2020) Androgen receptor in breast cancer-clinical and preclinical research insights. Molecules 25(2). https://doi.org/10.3390/molecules25020358

Arora VK, Schenkein E, Murali R, Subudhi SK, Wongvipat J, Balbas MD et al (2013) Glucocorticoid receptor confers resistance to antiandrogens by bypassing androgen receptor blockade. Cell 155(6):1309–1322. https://doi.org/10.1016/j.cell.2013.11.012

Arora T, Mullangi S, Lekkala MR (2023) Ovarian cancer. StatPearls Publishing, Treasure Island. Copyright © 2023, StatPearls Publishing LLC

Asuthkar S, Velpula KK, Elustondo PA, Demirkhanyan L, Zakharian E (2015) TRPM8 channel as a novel molecular target in androgen-regulated prostate cancer cells. Oncotarget 6(19): 17221–17236. https://doi.org/10.18632/oncotarget.3948

Auchus RJ (2004) The backdoor pathway to dihydrotestosterone. Trends Endocrinol Metab 15(9): 432–438. https://doi.org/10.1016/j.tem.2004.09.004

Awad D, Pulliam TL, Lin C, Wilkenfeld SR, Frigo DE (2018) Delineation of the androgen-regulated signaling pathways in prostate cancer facilitates the development of novel therapeutic approaches. Curr Opin Pharmacol 41:1–11. https://doi.org/10.1016/j.coph.2018.03.002

Bamberger AM, Milde-Langosch K, Löning T, Bamberger CM (2001) The glucocorticoid receptor is specifically expressed in the stromal compartment of the human endometrium. J Clin Endocrinol Metab 86(10):5071–5074. https://doi.org/10.1210/jcem.86.10.8101

Banerjee PP, Banerjee S, Brown TR, Zirkin BR (2018) Androgen action in prostate function and disease. Am J Clin Exp Urol 6(2):62–77

Bánhegyi G, Csala M, Benedetti A (2009) Hexose-6-phosphate dehydrogenase: linking endocrinology and metabolism in the endoplasmic reticulum. J Mol Endocrinol 42(4):283–289. https://doi.org/10.1677/jme-08-0156

Beral V, Bull D, Green J, Reeves G (2007) Ovarian cancer and hormone replacement therapy in the million women study. Lancet 369(9574):1703–1710. https://doi.org/10.1016/s0140-6736(07)60534-0

Blanchard Z, Vahrenkamp JM, Berrett KC, Arnesen S, Gertz J (2019) Estrogen-independent molecular actions of mutant estrogen receptor 1 in endometrial cancer. Genome Res 29(9):1429–1441. https://doi.org/10.1101/gr.244780.118

Bonkhoff H (2018) Estrogen receptor signaling in prostate cancer: implications for carcinogenesis and tumor progression. Prostate 78(1):2–10. https://doi.org/10.1002/pros.23446

Bonkhoff H, Berges R (2009) The evolving role of oestrogens and their receptors in the development and progression of prostate cancer. Eur Urol 55(3):533–542. https://doi.org/10.1016/j.eururo.2008.10.035

Bosland MC (2000) The role of steroid hormones in prostate carcinogenesis. J Natl Cancer Inst Monogr 27:39–66. https://doi.org/10.1093/oxfordjournals.jncimonographs.a024244

Bosland MC, Ford H, Horton L (1995) Induction at high incidence of ductal prostate adenocarcinomas in NBL/Cr and Sprague-Dawley Hsd:SD rats treated with a combination of testosterone and estradiol-17 beta or diethylstilbestrol. Carcinogenesis 16(6):1311–1317. https://doi.org/10.1093/carcin/16.6.1311

Broustas CG, Hopkins KM, Panigrahi SK, Wang L, Virk RK, Lieberman HB (2019) RAD9A promotes metastatic phenotypes through transcriptional regulation of anterior gradient 2 (AGR2). Carcinogenesis 40(1):164–172. https://doi.org/10.1093/carcin/bgy131

Bulletti C, Bulletti FM, Sciorio R, Guido M (2022) Progesterone: the Key factor of the beginning of life. Int J Mol Sci 23(22). https://doi.org/10.3390/ijms232214138

Cable JK, Grider MH (2023) Physiology, progesterone. StatPearls Publishing, Treasure Island. Copyright © 2023, StatPearls Publishing LLC

Biomed Res Int 2016:8909878. https://doi.org/10.1155/2016/8909878

Cairat M, Al Rahmoun M, Gunter MJ, Heudel PE, Severi G, Dossus L, Fournier A (2021) Use of systemic glucocorticoids and risk of breast cancer in a prospective cohort of postmenopausal women. BMC Med 19(1):186. https://doi.org/10.1186/s12916-021-02004-6

Cao L, Xu C, Xiang G, Liu F, Liu X, Li C et al (2018) AR-PDEF pathway promotes tumour proliferation and upregulates MYC-mediated gene transcription by promoting MAD1 degradation in ER-negative breast cancer. Mol Cancer 17(1):136. https://doi.org/10.1186/s12943-018-0883-0

Carson-Jurica MA, Schrader WT, O'Malley BW (1990) Steroid receptor family: structure and functions. Endocr Rev 11(2):201–220. https://doi.org/10.1210/edrv-11-2-201

Cavalieri EL, Rogan EG (2011) Unbalanced metabolism of endogenous estrogens in the etiology and prevention of human cancer. J Steroid Biochem Mol Biol 125(3–5):169–180. https://doi.org/10.1016/j.jsbmb.2011.03.008

Chang CY, McDonnell DP (2012) Molecular pathways: the metabolic regulator estrogen-related receptor α as a therapeutic target in cancer. Clin Cancer Res 18(22):6089–6095. https://doi.org/10.1158/1078-0432.Ccr-11-3221

Chang KH, Li R, Kuri B, Lotan Y, Roehrborn CG, Liu J et al (2013) A gain-of-function mutation in DHT synthesis in castration-resistant prostate cancer. Cell 154(5):1074–1084. https://doi.org/10.1016/j.cell.2013.07.029

Chang YC, Chen CK, Chen MJ, Lin JC, Lin CH, Huang WC et al (2017) Expression of 3-β-Hydroxysteroid dehydrogenase type 1 in breast cancer is associated with poor prognosis independent of estrogen receptor status. Ann Surg Oncol 24(13):4033–4041. https://doi.org/10.1245/s10434-017-6000-6

Chen WY (2008) Exogenous and endogenous hormones and breast cancer. Best Pract Res Clin Endocrinol Metab 22(4):573–585. https://doi.org/10.1016/j.beem.2008.08.001

Chen YX, Wang Y, Fu CC, Diao F, Song LN, Li ZB et al (2010) Dexamethasone enhances cell resistance to chemotherapy by increasing adhesion to extracellular matrix in human ovarian cancer cells. Endocr Relat Cancer 17(1):39–50. https://doi.org/10.1677/erc-08-0296

Chen EJ, Sowalsky AG, Gao S, Cai C, Voznesensky O, Schaefer R et al (2015) Abiraterone treatment in castration-resistant prostate cancer selects for progesterone responsive mutant androgen receptors. Clin Cancer Res 21(6):1273–1280. https://doi.org/10.1158/1078-0432.Ccr-14-1220

Chetrite GS, Cortes-Prieto J, Philippe JC, Wright F, Pasqualini JR (2000) Comparison of estrogen concentrations, estrone sulfatase and aromatase activities in normal, and in cancerous, human breast tissues. J Steroid Biochem Mol Biol 72(1–2):23–27. https://doi.org/10.1016/s0960-0760(00)00040-6

Christoforou P, Christopoulos PF, Koutsilieris M (2014) The role of estrogen receptor β in prostate cancer. Mol Med 20(1):427–434. https://doi.org/10.2119/molmed.2014.00105

Ciucci A, Zannoni GF, Buttarelli M, Lisi L, Travaglia D, Martinelli E et al (2016) Multiple direct and indirect mechanisms drive estrogen-induced tumor growth in high grade serous ovarian cancers. Oncotarget 7(7):8155–8171. https://doi.org/10.18632/oncotarget.6943

Cleary MP, Grossmann ME (2009) Minireview: obesity and breast cancer: the estrogen connection. Endocrinology 150(6):2537–2542. https://doi.org/10.1210/en.2009-0070

Clusan L, Le Goff P, Flouriot G, Pakdel F (2021) A closer look at estrogen receptor mutations in breast cancer and their implications for estrogen and antiestrogen responses. Int J Mol Sci 22(2). https://doi.org/10.3390/ijms22020756

Clusan L, Ferrière F, Flouriot G, Pakdel F (2023) A basic review on estrogen receptor signaling pathways in breast cancer. Int J Mol Sci 24(7). https://doi.org/10.3390/ijms24076834

Conlon N, Leitao MM Jr, Abu-Rustum NR, Soslow RA (2014) Grading uterine endometrioid carcinoma: a proposal that binary is best. Am J Surg Pathol 38(12):1583–1587. https://doi.org/10.1097/pas.0000000000000327

Cookman CJ, Belcher SM (2015) Estrogen receptor-β up-regulates IGF1R expression and activity to inhibit apoptosis and increase growth of Medulloblastoma. Endocrinology 156(7):2395–2408. https://doi.org/10.1210/en.2015-1141

Cousins FL, Pandoy R, Jin S, Gargett CE (2021) The elusive endometrial epithelial stem/progenitor cells. Front Cell Dev Biol 9:640319. https://doi.org/10.3389/fcell.2021.640319

Coutinho I, Day TK, Tilley WD, Selth LA (2016) Androgen receptor signaling in castration-resistant prostate cancer: a lesson in persistence. Endocr Relat Cancer 23(12):T179–t197. https://doi.org/10.1530/erc-16-0422

Csaba G (2014) Hormones in the immune system and their possible role. A critical review. Acta Microbiol Immunol Hung 61(3):241–260. https://doi.org/10.1556/AMicr.61.2014.3.1

Dai C, Ellisen LW (2023) Revisiting androgen receptor signaling in breast cancer. Oncologist 28(5):383–391. https://doi.org/10.1093/oncolo/oyad049

Dai C, Heemers H, Sharifi N (2017) Androgen signaling in prostate cancer. Cold Spring Harb Perspect Med 7(9). https://doi.org/10.1101/cshperspect.a030452

Di Donato V, Iacobelli V, Schiavi MC, Colagiovanni V, Pecorella I, Palaia I et al (2018) Impact of hormone receptor status and Ki-67 expression on disease-free survival in patients affected by high-risk endometrial cancer. Int J Gynecol Cancer 28(3):505–513. https://doi.org/10.1097/igc.0000000000001191

Diep CH, Ahrendt H, Lange CA (2016) Progesterone induces progesterone receptor gene (PGR) expression via rapid activation of protein kinase pathways required for cooperative estrogen receptor alpha (ER) and progesterone receptor (PR) genomic action at ER/PR target genes. Steroids 114:48–58. https://doi.org/10.1016/j.steroids.2016.09.004

Doan TB, Cheung V, Clyne CD, Hilton HN, Eriksson N, Young MJ et al (2020) A tumour suppressive relationship between mineralocorticoid and retinoic acid receptors activates a transcriptional program consistent with a reverse Warburg effect in breast cancer. Breast Cancer Res 22(1):122. https://doi.org/10.1186/s13058-020-01355-x

Droog M, Nevedomskaya E, Kim Y, Severson T, Flach KD, Opdam M et al (2016) Comparative Cistromics reveals genomic cross-talk between FOXA1 and ERα in tamoxifen-associated endometrial carcinomas. Cancer Res 76(13):3773–3784. https://doi.org/10.1158/0008-5472.Can-14-1813

du Toit T, Bloem LM, Quanson JL, Ehlers R, Serafin AM, Swart AC (2017) Profiling adrenal 11β-hydroxyandrostenedione metabolites in prostate cancer cells, tissue and plasma: UPC(2)-MS/MS quantification of 11β-hydroxytestosterone, 11keto-testosterone and 11keto-dihydrotestosterone. J Steroid Biochem Mol Biol 166:54–67. https://doi.org/10.1016/j.jsbmb.2016.06.009

Eaton NE, Reeves GK, Appleby PN, Key TJ (1999) Endogenous sex hormones and prostate cancer: a quantitative review of prospective studies. Br J Cancer 80(7):930–934. https://doi.org/10.1038/sj.bjc.6690445

Edwards DP (2000) The role of coactivators and corepressors in the biology and mechanism of action of steroid hormone receptors. J Mammary Gland Biol Neoplasia 5(3):307–324. https://doi.org/10.1023/a:1009503029176

Ehsani M, David FO, Baniahmad A (2021) Androgen receptor-dependent mechanisms mediating drug resistance in prostate cancer. Cancers (Basel) 13(7). https://doi.org/10.3390/cancers13071534

Eick GN, Colucci JK, Harms MJ, Ortlund EA, Thornton JW (2012) Evolution of minimal specificity and promiscuity in steroid hormone receptors. PLoS Genet 8(11):e1003072. https://doi.org/10.1371/journal.pgen.1003072

Ellem SJ, Risbridger GP (2006) Aromatase and prostate cancer. Minerva Endocrinol 31(1):1–12

Evaul K, Li R, Papari-Zareei M, Auchus RJ, Sharifi N (2010) 3beta-hydroxysteroid dehydrogenase is a possible pharmacological target in the treatment of castration-resistant prostate cancer. Endocrinology 151(8):3514–3520. https://doi.org/10.1210/en.2010-0138

Eyster K (2016) The estrogen receptors: an overview from different perspectives. (pp. 1-10). https://doi.org/10.1007/978-1-4939-3127-9_1

Fagan DH, Yee D (2008) Crosstalk between IGF1R and estrogen receptor signaling in breast cancer. J Mammary Gland Biol Neoplasia 13(4):423–429. https://doi.org/10.1007/s10911-008-9098-0

Feng Y, Spezia M, Huang S, Yuan C, Zeng Z, Zhang L et al (2018) Breast cancer development and progression: risk factors, cancer stem cells, signaling pathways, genomics, and molecular pathogenesis. Genes Dis 5(2):77–106. https://doi.org/10.1016/j.gendis.2018.05.001

Fentiman I (2009) Male breast cancer: a review. Ecancermedicalscience 3:140. https://doi.org/10.3332/ecancer.2009.140

Fiandalo MV, Wilton J, Mohler JL (2014) Roles for the backdoor pathway of androgen metabolism in prostate cancer response to castration and drug treatment. Int J Biol Sci 10(6):596–601. https://doi.org/10.7150/ijbs.8780

Filardo EJ, Thomas P (2005) GPR30: a seven-transmembrane-spanning estrogen receptor that triggers EGF release. Trends Endocrinol Metab 16(8):362–367. https://doi.org/10.1016/j.tem.2005.08.005

Folkerd EJ, Dowsett M (2010) Influence of sex hormones on cancer progression. J Clin Oncol 28(26):4038–4044. https://doi.org/10.1200/jco.2009.27.4290

Foradori CD, Weiser MJ, Handa RJ (2008) Non-genomic actions of androgens. Front Neuroendocrinol 29(2):169–181. https://doi.org/10.1016/j.yfrne.2007.10.005

Formby B, Wiley TS (1998) Progesterone inhibits growth and induces apoptosis in breast cancer cells: inverse effects on Bcl-2 and p53. Ann Clin Lab Sci 28(6):360–369

Fuentes N, Silveyra P (2019) Estrogen receptor signaling mechanisms. Adv Protein Chem Struct Biol 116:135–170. https://doi.org/10.1016/bs.apcsb.2019.01.001

Gajjar K, Ogden G, Mujahid MI, Razvi K (2012) Symptoms and risk factors of ovarian cancer: a survey in primary care. ISRN Obstet Gynecol 2012:754197. https://doi.org/10.5402/2012/754197

Garabedian MJ, Yamamoto KR (1992) Genetic dissection of the signaling domain of a mammalian steroid receptor in yeast. Mol Biol Cell 3(11):1245–1257. https://doi.org/10.1091/mbc.3.11.1245

Garcia Gil S, Ramos Rodriguez R, Plata Bello A, Nazco Casariego G, Garcia Marrero R, Cruz Jurado J et al (2018) Relationship between mutations in the HSD3B1 gene and response time to androgen deprivation therapy in the treatment of prostate cancer. Eur Soc Oncol Pharm:25–27

Gibson E, Mahdy H (2023) Anatomy, abdomen and pelvis, ovary. StatPearls Publishing, Treasure Island. Copyright © 2023, StatPearls Publishing LLC

Giona S (2021) The epidemiology of prostate cancer. In: Bott SRJ, Ng KL (eds) Prostate cancer. Exon Publications, Brisbane (AU). Copyright: The Authors. doi:10.36255/exonpublications.prostatecancer.epidemiology.2021

Guerini-Rocco E, Gray KP, Fumagalli C, Reforgiato MR, Leone I, Rafaniello Raviele P et al (2021) Genomic aberrations and late recurrence in postmenopausal women with hormone receptor-positive early breast cancer: results from the SOLE trial. Clin Cancer Res 27(2):504–512. https://doi.org/10.1158/1078-0432.Ccr-20-0126

Guo J, Ma K, Xia HM, Chen QK, Li L, Deng J et al (2018) Androgen receptor reverts dexamethasone-induced inhibition of prostate cancer cell proliferation and migration. Mol Med Rep 17(4):5887–5893. https://doi.org/10.3892/mmr.2018.8566

Hagiwara M, Yasumizu Y, Yamashita N, Rajabi H, Fushimi A, Long MD et al (2021) MUC1-C activates the BAF (mSWI/SNF) complex in prostate cancer stem cells. Cancer Res 81(4):1111–1122. https://doi.org/10.1158/0008-5472.Can-20-2588

Han KH, Kim MK, Kim HS, Chung HH, Song YS (2013) Protective effect of progesterone during pregnancy against ovarian cancer. J Cancer Prev 18(2):113–122. https://doi.org/10.15430/jcp.2013.18.2.113

Handelsman DJ (2000) Androgen physiology, pharmacology, use and misuse. In: Feingold KR, Anawalt B, Blackman MR, Boyce A, Chrousos G, Corpas E et al (eds) Endotext. MDText.com, Inc, South Dartmouth. Copyright © 2000–2023, MDText.com, Inc.

Harris WP, Mostaghel EA, Nelson PS, Montgomery B (2009) Androgen deprivation therapy: progress in understanding mechanisms of resistance and optimizing androgen depletion. Nat Clin Pract Urol 6(2):76–85. https://doi.org/10.1038/ncpuro1296

Hashmi AA, Hussain ZF, Qadri A, Irfan M, Ramzan S, Faridi N et al (2018) Androgen receptor expression in endometrial carcinoma and its correlation with clinicopathologic features. BMC Res Notes 11(1):289. https://doi.org/10.1186/s13104-018-3403-9

Hearn JWD, AbuAli G, Reichard CA, Reddy CA, Magi-Galluzzi C, Chang KH et al (2016) HSD3B1 and resistance to androgen-deprivation therapy in prostate cancer: a retrospective, multicohort study. Lancet Oncol 17(10):1435–1444. https://doi.org/10.1016/s1470-2045(16)30227-3

Hearn JWD, Xie W, Nakabayashi M, Almassi N, Reichard CA, Pomerantz M et al (2018) Association of HSD3B1 genotype with response to androgen-deprivation therapy for biochemical recurrence after radiotherapy for localized prostate cancer. JAMA Oncol 4(4):558–562. https://doi.org/10.1001/jamaoncol.2017.3164

Hernández-Hernández OT, González-García TK, Camacho-Arroyo I (2012) Progesterone receptor and SRC-1 participate in the regulation of VEGF, EGFR and cyclin D1 expression in human astrocytoma cell lines. J Steroid Biochem Mol Biol 132(1–2):127–134. https://doi.org/10.1016/j.jsbmb.2012.04.005

Herr I, Pfitzenmaier J (2006) Glucocorticoid use in prostate cancer and other solid tumours: implications for effectiveness of cytotoxic treatment and metastases. Lancet Oncol 7(5):425–430. https://doi.org/10.1016/s1470-2045(06)70694-5

Hesketh PJ, Kris MG, Basch E, Bohlke K, Barbour SY, Clark-Snow RA et al (2020) Antiemetics: ASCO guideline update. J Clin Oncol 38(24):2782–2797. https://doi.org/10.1200/jco.20.01296

Hevir N, Trošt N, Debeljak N, Rižner TL (2011) Expression of estrogen and progesterone receptors and estrogen metabolizing enzymes in different breast cancer cell lines. Chem Biol Interact 191(1–3):206–216. https://doi.org/10.1016/j.cbi.2010.12.013

Hickey TE, Selth LA, Chia KM, Laven-Law G, Milioli HH, Roden D et al (2021) The androgen receptor is a tumor suppressor in estrogen receptor–positive breast cancer. Nat Med 27(2): 310–320. https://doi.org/10.1038/s41591-020-01168-7

Hiller-Sturmhöfel S, Bartke A (1998) The endocrine system: an overview. Alcohol Health Res World 22(3):153–164

Ho SM (2003) Estrogen, progesterone and epithelial ovarian cancer. Reprod Biol Endocrinol 1:73. https://doi.org/10.1186/1477-7827-1-73

Hormones and Breast Cancer (2004) Hum. Reprod Update 10(4):281–293. https://doi.org/10.1093/humupd/dmh025

Hou Z, Huang S, Mei Z, Chen L, Guo J, Gao Y et al (2022) Inhibiting 3βHSD1 to eliminate the oncogenic effects of progesterone in prostate cancer. Cell Rep Med 3(3):100561. https://doi.org/10.1016/j.xcrm.2022.100561

Hsing AW, Chu LW, Stanczyk FZ (2008) Androgen and prostate cancer: is the hypothesis dead? Cancer Epidemiol Biomarkers Prev 17(10):2525–2530. https://doi.org/10.1158/1055-9965.Epi-08-0448

Hu J, Zhang Z, Shen WJ, Azhar S (2010) Cellular cholesterol delivery, intracellular processing and utilization for biosynthesis of steroid hormones. Nutr Metab (Lond) 7:47. https://doi.org/10.1186/1743-7075-7-47

Huggins C, Hodges CV (1941) Studies on prostatic cancer. I. The effect of castration, of estrogen and of androgen injection on serum phosphatases in metastatic carcinoma of the prostate*. Cancer Res 1(4):293–297

Iacopetta D, Rechoum Y, Fuqua SAW (2012) The role of androgen receptor in breast cancer. Drug Disc Today Dis Mech 9(1):e19–e27. https://doi.org/10.1016/j.ddmec.2012.11.003

Isikbay M, Otto K, Kregel S, Kach J, Cai Y, Vander Griend DJ et al (2014) Glucocorticoid receptor activity contributes to resistance to androgen-targeted therapy in prostate cancer. Horm Cancer 5(2):72–89. https://doi.org/10.1007/s12672-014-0173-2

Jacobsen BM, Horwitz KB (2012) Progesterone receptors, their isoforms and progesterone regulated transcription. Mol Cell Endocrinol 357(1–2):18–29. https://doi.org/10.1016/j.mce.2011.09.016

Jeon SY, Hwang KA, Choi KC (2016) Effect of steroid hormones, estrogen and progesterone, on epithelial mesenchymal transition in ovarian cancer development. J Steroid Biochem Mol Biol 158:1–8. https://doi.org/10.1016/j.jsbmb.2016.02.005

Jeong HM, Kwon MJ, Shin YK (2014) Overexpression of cancer-associated genes via epigenetic derepression mechanisms in gynecologic cancer. Front Oncol 4:12. https://doi.org/10.3389/fonc.2014.00012

Johnson KS, Conant EF, Soo MS (2020) Molecular subtypes of breast cancer: a review for breast radiologists. J Breast Imag 3(1):12–24. https://doi.org/10.1093/jbi/wbaa110

Kamińska M, Ciszewski T, Łopacka-Szatan K, Miotła P, Starosławska E (2015) Breast cancer risk factors. Prz Menopauzalny 14(3):196–202. https://doi.org/10.5114/pm.2015.54346

Kariagina A, Aupperlee MD, Haslam SZ (2008) Progesterone receptor isoform functions in normal breast development and breast cancer. Crit Rev Eukaryot Gene Expr 18(1):11–33. https://doi.org/10.1615/critreveukargeneexpr.v18.i1.20

Keightley M-C (1998) Steroid receptor isoforms: exception or rule? Mol Cell Endocrinol 137(1): 1–5. https://doi.org/10.1016/S0303-7207(97)00236-0

Khalaf DJ, Aragón IM, Annala M, Lozano R, Taavitsainen S, Lorente D et al (2020) HSD3B1 (1245A>C) germline variant and clinical outcomes in metastatic castration-resistant prostate cancer patients treated with abiraterone and enzalutamide: results from two prospective studies. Ann Oncol 31(9):1186–1197. https://doi.org/10.1016/j.annonc.2020.06.006

Kim JJ, Kurita T, Bulun SE (2013) Progesterone action in endometrial cancer, endometriosis, uterine fibroids, and breast cancer. Endocr Rev 34(1):130–162. https://doi.org/10.1210/er.2012-1043

Kinter KJ, Amraei R, Anekar AA (2023) Biochemistry, dihydrotestosterone. StatPearls Publishing, Treasure Island. Copyright © 2023, StatPearls Publishing LLC

Lee HJ, Lee B, Choi H, Kim T, Kim Y, Kim YB (2023) Impact of hormone replacement therapy on risk of ovarian cancer in postmenopausal women with De novo endometriosis or a history of endometriosis. Cancers (Basel) 15(6). https://doi.org/10.3390/cancers15061708

Levine D, Park K, Juretzka M, Esch J, Hensley M, Aghajanian C et al (2007) A phase II evaluation of goserelin and bicalutamide in patients with ovarian cancer in second or higher complete clinical disease remission. Cancer 110(11):2448–2456. https://doi.org/10.1002/cncr.23072

Li J, Alyamani M, Zhang A, Chang KH, Berk M, Li Z et al (2017) Aberrant corticosteroid metabolism in tumor cells enables GR takeover in enzalutamide resistant prostate cancer. elife 6. https://doi.org/10.7554/eLife.20183

Li H, Liu Y, Wang Y, Zhao X, Qi X (2021) Hormone therapy for ovarian cancer: emphasis on mechanisms and applications (review). Oncol Rep 46(4). https://doi.org/10.3892/or.2021.8174

Li Z, Wei H, Li S, Wu P, Mao X (2022) The role of progesterone receptors in breast cancer. Drug Des Devel Ther 16:305–314. https://doi.org/10.2147/dddt.S336643

Liao W, Sui X, Hou G, Yang M, Lin Y, Lu J, Yang Q (2023) Trends in estrogen and progesterone receptors in prostate cancer: a bibliometric analysis. Front Oncol 13:1111296. https://doi.org/10.3389/fonc.2023.1111296

Lin CY, Ström A, Vega VB, Kong SL, Yeo AL, Thomsen JS et al (2004) Discovery of estrogen receptor alpha target genes and response elements in breast tumor cells. Genome Biol 5(9):R66. https://doi.org/10.1186/gb-2004-5-9-r66

Liotta LA, Kohn EC (2001) The microenvironment of the tumour-host interface. Nature 411(6835): 375–379. https://doi.org/10.1038/35077241

Lorence MC, Murry BA, Trant JM, Mason JI (1990) Human 3 beta-hydroxysteroid dehydrogenase/delta 5----4isomerase from placenta: expression in nonsteroidogenic cells of a protein that catalyzes the dehydrogenation/isomerization of C21 and C19 steroids. Endocrinology 126(5): 2493–2498. https://doi.org/10.1210/endo-126-5-2493

Lu C, Terbuch A, Dolling D, Yu J, Wang H, Chen Y et al (2020) Treatment with abiraterone and enzalutamide does not overcome poor outcome from metastatic castration-resistant prostate cancer in men with the germline homozygous HSD3B1 c.1245C genotype. Ann Oncol 31(9): 1178–1185. https://doi.org/10.1016/j.annonc.2020.04.473

Łukasiewicz S, Czeczelewski M, Forma A, Baj J, Sitarz R, Stanisławek A (2021) Breast cancer-epidemiology, risk factors, classification, prognostic markers, and current treatment strategies-an updated review. Cancers (Basel) 13(17). https://doi.org/10.3390/cancers13174287

Lv C, Sun J, Ye Y, Lin Z, Li H, Liu Y et al (2022) Long noncoding RNA EIF1AX-AS1 promotes endometrial cancer cell apoptosis by affecting EIF1AX mRNA stabilization. Cancer Sci 113(4): 1277–1291. https://doi.org/10.1111/cas.15275

Maček P, Molinari N, Sobočan M, Knez J (2023) What role do androgens play in endometrial cancer? J Pers Med 13(2). https://doi.org/10.3390/jpm13020341

Madhu Krishna B, Chaudhary S, Mishra DR, Naik SK, Suklabaidya S, Adhya AK, Mishra SK (2018) Estrogen receptor α dependent regulation of estrogen related receptor β and its role in cell cycle in breast cancer. BMC Cancer 18(1):607. https://doi.org/10.1186/s12885-018-4528-x

Mahdi Z, Abdulfatah E, Pardeshi V, Hassan O, Schultz D, Morris R et al (2017) The impact of androgen receptor expression on endometrial carcinoma recurrence and survival. Int J Gynecol Pathol 36(5):405–411. https://doi.org/10.1097/pgp.0000000000000355

Makker V, MacKay H, Ray-Coquard I, Levine DA, Westin SN, Aoki D, Oaknin A (2021) Endometrial cancer. Nat Rev Dis Primers 7(1):88. https://doi.org/10.1038/s41572-021-00324-8

Manning-Geist BL, Gordhandas SB, Giri DD, Iasonos A, Zhou Q, Girshman J et al (2022) Phase II study of enzalutamide in androgen receptor positive, recurrent, high- and low-grade serous ovarian cancer. Gynecol Oncol 164(1):12–17. https://doi.org/10.1016/j.ygyno.2021.10.087

Marques P, Skorupskaite K, Rozario KS, Anderson RA, George JT (2000) Physiology of GnRH and gonadotropin secretion. In: Feingold KR, Anawalt B, Blackman MR, Boyce A, Chrousos G, Corpas E et al (eds) Endotext. MDText.com, Inc, South Dartmouth. Copyright © 2000–2023, MDText.com, Inc.

Martin MB, Stoica A (2002) Insulin-like growth factor-I and estrogen interactions in breast cancer. J Nutr 132(12):3799S–3801S. https://doi.org/10.1093/jn/132.12.3799S

Mauvais-Jarvis F, Lange CA, Levin ER (2022) Membrane-initiated estrogen, androgen, and progesterone receptor signaling in health and disease. Endocr Rev 43(4):720–742. https://doi.org/10.1210/endrev/bnab041

McCluggage WG (2011) Morphological subtypes of ovarian carcinoma: a review with emphasis on new developments and pathogenesis. Pathology 43(5):420–432. https://doi.org/10.1097/PAT.0b013e328348a6e7

McDonnel AC, Van Kirk EA, Isaak DD, Murdoch WJ (2003) Inhibitory effects of progesterone on plasma membrane fluidity and tumorigenic potential of ovarian epithelial cancer cells. Exp Biol Med (Maywood) 228(3):308–314. https://doi.org/10.1177/153537020322800310

McGlorthan L, Paucarmayta A, Casablanca Y, Maxwell GL, Syed V (2021) Progesterone induces apoptosis by activation of caspase-8 and calcitriol via activation of caspase-9 pathways in ovarian and endometrial cancer cells in vitro. Apoptosis 26(3–4):184–194. https://doi.org/10.1007/s10495-021-01657-1

McHann MC, Blanton HL, Guindon J (2021) Role of sex hormones in modulating breast and ovarian cancer associated pain. Mol Cell Endocrinol 533:111320. https://doi.org/10.1016/j.mce.2021.111320

McKeown AN, Bridgham JT, Anderson DW, Murphy MN, Ortlund EA, Thornton JW (2014) Evolution of DNA specificity in a transcription factor family produced a new gene regulatory module. Cell 159(1):58–68. https://doi.org/10.1016/j.cell.2014.09.003

McManus JM, Vargas R, Bazeley PS, Schumacher FR, Sharifi N (2022) Association between adrenal-restrictive HSD3B1 inheritance and hormone-independent subtypes of endometrial and breast cancer. JNCI Cancer Spectr 6(5). https://doi.org/10.1093/jncics/pkac061

McNamara KM, Yoda T, Takagi K, Miki Y, Suzuki T, Sasano H (2013) Androgen receptor in triple negative breast cancer. J Steroid Biochem Mol Biol 133:66–76. https://doi.org/10.1016/j.jsbmb.2012.08.007

Mei Z, Yang T, Liu Y, Gao Y, Hou Z, Zhuang Q et al (2022) Management of prostate cancer by targeting 3βHSD1 after enzalutamide and abiraterone treatment. Cell Rep Med 3(5):100608. https://doi.org/10.1016/j.xcrm.2022.100608

Merritt MA, Strickler HD, Hutson AD, Einstein MH, Rohan TE, Xue X et al (2021) Sex hormones, insulin, and insulin-like growth factors in recurrence of high-stage endometrial cancer. Cancer Epidemiol Biomarkers Prev 30(4):719–726. https://doi.org/10.1158/1055-9965.Epi-20-1613

Michels KA, Brinton LA, Wentzensen N, Pan K, Chen C, Anderson GL et al (2019) Postmenopausal androgen metabolism and endometrial cancer risk in the Women's Health Initiative observational study. JNCI Cancer Spectr 3(3):pkz029. https://doi.org/10.1093/jncics/pkz029

Michmerhuizen AR, Spratt DE, Pierce LJ, Speers CW (2020) ARe we there yet? Understanding androgen receptor signaling in breast cancer. NPJ Breast Cancer 6:47. https://doi.org/10.1038/s41523-020-00190-9

Miller WL, Auchus RJ (2019) The "backdoor pathway" of androgen synthesis in human male sexual development. PLoS Biol 17(4):e3000198. https://doi.org/10.1371/journal.pbio.3000198

Miller WL, Bose HS (2011) Early steps in steroidogenesis: intracellular cholesterol trafficking. J Lipid Res 52(12):2111–2135. https://doi.org/10.1194/jlr.R016675

Miricescu D, Totan A, Stanescu S II, Badoiu SC, Stefani C, Greabu M (2020) PI3K/AKT/mTOR signaling pathway in breast cancer: from molecular landscape to clinical aspects. Int J Mol Sci 22(1). https://doi.org/10.3390/ijms22010173

Mitre-Aguilar IB, Moreno-Mitre D, Melendez-Zajgla J, Maldonado V, Jacobo-Herrera NJ, Ramirez-Gonzalez V, Mendoza-Almanza G (2022) The role of glucocorticoids in breast cancer therapy. Curr Oncol 30(1):298–314. https://doi.org/10.3390/curroncol30010024

Mitsiades N, Sung CC, Schultz N, Danila DC, He B, Eedunuri VK et al (2012) Distinct patterns of dysregulated expression of enzymes involved in androgen synthesis and metabolism in metastatic prostate cancer tumors. Cancer Res 72(23):6142–6152. https://doi.org/10.1158/0008-5472.Can-12-1335

Miyamoto H, Messing EM, Chang C (2004) Androgen deprivation therapy for prostate cancer: current status and future prospects. Prostate 61(4):332–353. https://doi.org/10.1002/pros.20115

Miyoshi Y, Ando A, Shiba E, Taguchi T, Tamaki Y, Noguchi S (2001) Involvement of up-regulation of 17beta-hydroxysteroid dehydrogenase type 1 in maintenance of intratumoral high estradiol levels in postmenopausal breast cancers. Int J Cancer 94(5):685–689. https://doi.org/10.1002/ijc.1525

Mizushima T, Miyamoto H (2019) The role of androgen receptor signaling in ovarian cancer. Cells 8(2). https://doi.org/10.3390/cells8020176

Modan B, Ron E, Lerner-Geva L, Blumstein T, Menczer J, Rabinovici J et al (1998) Cancer incidence in a cohort of infertile women. Am J Epidemiol 147(11):1038–1042. https://doi.org/10.1093/oxfordjournals.aje.a009397

Mohammed H, Russell IA, Stark R, Rueda OM, Hickey TE, Tarulli GA et al (2015) Progesterone receptor modulates ERα action in breast cancer. Nature 523(7560):313–317. https://doi.org/10.1038/nature14583

Mørch LS, Løkkegaard E, Andreasen AH, Kjaer SK, Lidegaard O (2012) Hormone therapy and different ovarian cancers: a national cohort study. Am J Epidemiol 175(12):1234–1242. https://doi.org/10.1093/aje/kwr446

Mostaghel EA, Marck BT, Kolokythas O, Chew F, Yu EY, Schweizer MT et al (2021) Circulating and intratumoral adrenal androgens correlate with response to Abiraterone in men with castration-resistant prostate cancer. Clin Cancer Res 27(21):6001–6011. https://doi.org/10.1158/1078-0432.Ccr-21-1819

Nelles JL, Hu W-Y, Prins GS (2011) Estrogen action and prostate cancer. Exp Rev Endocrinol Metabol 6(3):437–451. https://doi.org/10.1586/eem.11.20

Ni M, Chen Y, Lim E, Wimberly H, Bailey ST, Imai Y et al (2011) Targeting androgen receptor in estrogen receptor-negative breast cancer. Cancer Cell 20(1):119–131. https://doi.org/10.1016/j.ccr.2011.05.026

Nie H, Li J, Yang XM, Cao QZ, Feng MX, Xue F et al (2015) Mineralocorticoid receptor suppresses cancer progression and the Warburg effect by modulating the miR-338-3p-PKLR axis in hepatocellular carcinoma. Hepatology 62(4):1145–1159. https://doi.org/10.1002/hep.27940

Nordin A, Wang W, Welén K, Damber JE (2013) Midkine is associated with neuroendocrine differentiation in castration-resistant prostate cancer. Prostate 73(6):657–667. https://doi.org/10.1002/pros.22607

Noureddine LM, Trédan O, Hussein N, Badran B, Le Romancer M, Poulard C (2021) Glucocorticoid receptor: a multifaceted actor in breast cancer. Int J Mol Sci 22(9). https://doi.org/10.3390/ijms22094446

Oaknin A, Bosse TJ, Creutzberg CL, Giornelli G, Harter P, Joly F et al (2022) Endometrial cancer: ESMO clinical practice guideline for diagnosis, treatment and follow-up. Ann Oncol 33(9): 860–877. https://doi.org/10.1016/j.annonc.2022.05.009

Oettel M, Mukhopadhyay AK (2004) Progesterone: the forgotten hormone in men? Aging Male 7(3):236–257. https://doi.org/10.1080/13685530400004199

Ostróżka-Cieślik A, Dolińska B (2020) The role of hormones and trophic factors as components of preservation solutions in protection of renal function before transplantation: a review of the literature. Molecules 25(9). https://doi.org/10.3390/molecules25092185

Pasquali R, Oriolo C (2019) Obesity and androgens in women. Front Horm Res 53:120–134. https://doi.org/10.1159/000494908

Payne AH, Hales DB (2004) Overview of steroidogenic enzymes in the pathway from cholesterol to active steroid hormones. Endocr Rev 25(6):947–970. https://doi.org/10.1210/er.2003-0030

Pearce CL, Chung K, Pike MC, Wu AH (2009) Increased ovarian cancer risk associated with menopausal estrogen therapy is reduced by adding a progestin. Cancer 115(3):531–539. https://doi.org/10.1002/cncr.23956

Pedram A, Razandi M, Sainson RCA, Kim JK, Hughes CC, Levin ER (2007) A conserved mechanism for steroid receptor translocation to the plasma membrane*. J Biol Chem 282(31): 22278–22288. https://doi.org/10.1074/jbc.M611877200

Petrucelli N, Daly MB, Pal T (1993) BRCA1- and BRCA2-associated hereditary breast and ovarian cancer. In: Adam MP, Feldman J, Mirzaa GM, Pagon RA, Wallace SE, Bean LJH et al (eds) GeneReviews(®). University of Washington, Seattle. Copyright © 1993–2023, University of Washington, Seattle. GeneReviews is a registered trademark of the University of Washington, Seattle. All rights reserved

Prange-Kiel J, Rune GM, Zwirner M, Wallwiener D, Kiesel L (2001) Regulation of estrogen receptor alpha and progesterone receptor (isoform A and B) expression in cultured human endometrial cells. Exp Clin Endocrinol Diabetes 109(4):231–237. https://doi.org/10.1055/s-2001-15111

Prat A, Pineda E, Adamo B, Galván P, Fernández A, Gaba L et al (2015) Clinical implications of the intrinsic molecular subtypes of breast cancer. Breast 24(Suppl 2):S26–S35. https://doi.org/10.1016/j.breast.2015.07.008

Pratt WB, Toft DO (1997) Steroid receptor interactions with heat shock protein and Immunophilin chaperones*. Endocr Rev 18(3):306–360. https://doi.org/10.1210/edrv.18.3.0303

Prossnitz ER, Arterburn JB, Sklar LA (2007) GPR30: a G protein-coupled receptor for estrogen. Mol Cell Endocrinol 265-266:138–142. https://doi.org/10.1016/j.mce.2006.12.010

Purdie CA, Quinlan P, Jordan LB, Ashfield A, Ogston S, Dewar JA, Thompson AM (2014) Progesterone receptor expression is an independent prognostic variable in early breast cancer: a population-based study. Br J Cancer 110(3):565–572. https://doi.org/10.1038/bjc.2013.756

Rebello RJ, Oing C, Knudsen KE, Loeb S, Johnson DC, Reiter RE et al (2021) Prostate cancer. Nat Rev Dis Primers 7(1):9. https://doi.org/10.1038/s41572-020-00243-0

Rege J, Turcu AF, Kasa-Vubu JZ, Lerario AM, Auchus GC, Auchus RJ et al (2018) 11-Ketotestosterone is the dominant circulating bioactive androgen during Normal and premature Adrenarche. J Clin Endocrinol Metab 103(12):4589–4598. https://doi.org/10.1210/jc.2018-00736

Rice MS, Eliassen AH, Hankinson SE, Lenart EB, Willett WC, Tamimi RM (2016) Breast cancer research in the nurses' health studies: exposures across the life course. Am J Public Health 106(9):1592–1598. https://doi.org/10.2105/ajph.2016.303325

Ricke WA, McPherson SJ, Bianco JJ, Cunha GR, Wang Y, Risbridger GP (2008) Prostatic hormonal carcinogenesis is mediated by in situ estrogen production and estrogen receptor alpha signaling. FASEB J 22(5):1512–1520. https://doi.org/10.1096/fj.07-9526com

Rodriguez AC, Blanchard Z, Maurer KA, Gertz J (2019) Estrogen signaling in endometrial cancer: a Key oncogenic pathway with several open questions. Horm Cancer 10(2–3):51–63. https://doi.org/10.1007/s12672-019-0358-9

Rodriguez-Bravo V, Carceles-Cordon M, Hoshida Y, Cordon-Cardo C, Galsky MD, Domingo-Domenech J (2017) The role of GATA2 in lethal prostate cancer aggressiveness. Nat Rev Urol 14(1):38–48. https://doi.org/10.1038/nrurol.2016.225

Roila F, Molassiotis A, Herrstedt J, Aapro M, Gralla RJ, Bruera E et al (2016) 2016 MASCC and ESMO guideline update for the prevention of chemotherapy- and radiotherapy-induced nausea and vomiting and of nausea and vomiting in advanced cancer patients. Ann Oncol 27(suppl 5):v119–v133. https://doi.org/10.1093/annonc/mdw270

Sabharwal N, Sharifi N (2019) HSD3B1 genotypes conferring adrenal-restrictive and adrenal-permissive phenotypes in prostate cancer and beyond. Endocrinology 160(9):2180–2188. https://doi.org/10.1210/en.2019-00366

Sakellakis M, Flores LJ (2022) Is the glucocorticoid receptor a key player in prostate cancer?: a literature review. Medicine (Baltimore) 101(29):e29716. https://doi.org/10.1097/md.0000000000029716

Sasano H, Frost AR, Saitoh R, Matsunaga G, Nagura H, Krozowski ZS, Silverberg SG (1997) Localization of mineralocorticoid receptor and 11 beta-hydroxysteroid dehydrogenase type II in human breast and its disorders. Anticancer Res 17(3c):2001–2007

Satpathi S, Gaurkar SS, Potdukhe A, Wanjari MB (2023) Unveiling the role of hormonal imbalance in breast cancer development: a comprehensive review. Cureus 15(7):e41737. https://doi.org/10.7759/cureus.41737

Schettini F, Buono G, Cardalesi C, Desideri I, De Placido S, Del Mastro L (2016) Hormone receptor/human epidermal growth factor receptor 2-positive breast cancer: where we are now and where we are going. Cancer Treat Rev 46:20–26. https://doi.org/10.1016/j.ctrv.2016.03.012

Schlumbrecht M, Wright K, George S (2023) Unique considerations in early detection, risk, and awareness of endometrial cancer in black women. Cancer Control 30:10732748231202952. https://doi.org/10.1177/10732748231202952

Severi G, Morris HA, MacInnis RJ, English DR, Tilley W, Hopper JL et al (2006) Circulating steroid hormones and the risk of prostate cancer. Cancer Epidemiol Biomarkers Prev 15(1): 86–91. https://doi.org/10.1158/1055-9965.Epi-05-0633

Sharifi N (2012) The 5α-androstanedione pathway to dihydrotestosterone in castration-resistant prostate cancer. J Investig Med 60(2):504–507. https://doi.org/10.2310/JIM.0b013e31823874a4

Sharifi N, Auchus RJ (2012) Steroid biosynthesis and prostate cancer. Steroids 77(7):719–726. https://doi.org/10.1016/j.steroids.2012.03.015

Shen M, Demers LK, Bailey SD, Labbé DP (2022) To bind or not to bind: Cistromic reprogramming in prostate cancer. Front Oncol 12:963007. https://doi.org/10.3389/fonc.2022.963007

Shiota M, Narita S, Akamatsu S, Fujimoto N, Sumiyoshi T, Fujiwara M et al (2019) Association of Missense Polymorphism in HSD3B1 with outcomes among men with prostate cancer treated with androgen-deprivation therapy or Abiraterone. JAMA Netw Open 2(2):e190115. https://doi.org/10.1001/jamanetworkopen.2019.0115

Siegel DA, O'Neil ME, Richards TB, Dowling NF, Weir HK (2020) Prostate cancer incidence and survival, by stage and race/ethnicity - United States, 2001-2017. MMWR Morb Mortal Wkly Rep 69(41):1473–1480. https://doi.org/10.15585/mmwr.mm6941a1

Sikora MJ (2016) Family matters: collaboration and conflict among the steroid receptors raises a need for group therapy. Endocrinology 157(12):4553–4560. https://doi.org/10.1210/en.2016-1778

Simard J, Ricketts ML, Gingras S, Soucy P, Feltus FA, Melner MH (2005) Molecular biology of the 3beta-hydroxysteroid dehydrogenase/delta5-delta4 isomerase gene family. Endocr Rev 26(4): 525–582. https://doi.org/10.1210/er.2002-0050

Singhal H, Greene ME, Tarulli G, Zarnke AL, Bourgo RJ, Laine M et al (2016) Genomic agonism and phenotypic antagonism between estrogen and progesterone receptors in breast cancer. Sci Adv 2(6):e1501924. https://doi.org/10.1126/sciadv.1501924

St John J, Powell K, Conley-Lacomb MK, Chinni SR (2012) TMPRSS2-ERG fusion gene expression in prostate tumor cells and its clinical and biological significance in prostate cancer progression. J Cancer Sci Ther 4(4):94–101. https://doi.org/10.4172/1948-5956.1000119

Stocco C (2012) Tissue physiology and pathology of aromatase. Steroids 77(1–2):27–35. https://doi.org/10.1016/j.steroids.2011.10.013

Storbeck K-H, Bloem LM, Africander D, Schloms L, Swart P, Swart AC (2013) 11-β-Hydroxydihydrotestosterone and 11-ketodihydrotestosterone, novel C19 steroids with androgenic activity: a putative role in castration resistant prostate cancer? Mol Cell Endocrinol 377(1):135–146. https://doi.org/10.1016/j.mce.2013.07.006

Sun C, Dobi A, Mohamed A, Li H, Thangapazham RL, Furusato B et al (2008) TMPRSS2-ERG fusion, a common genomic alteration in prostate cancer activates C-MYC and abrogates prostate epithelial differentiation. Oncogene 27(40):5348–5353. https://doi.org/10.1038/onc.2008.183

Sung H, Ferlay J, Siegel RL, Laversanne M, Soerjomataram I, Jemal A, Bray F (2021) Global cancer statistics 2020: GLOBOCAN estimates of incidence and mortality worldwide for 36 cancers in 185 countries. CA Cancer J Clin 71(3):209–249. https://doi.org/10.3322/caac.21660

Suzuki T, Miki Y, Moriya T, Akahira J, Hirakawa H, Ohuchi N, Sasano H (2007) In situ production of sex steroids in human breast carcinoma. Med Mol Morphol 40(3):121–127. https://doi.org/10.1007/s00795-007-0365-8

Takagi K, Miki Y, Nagasaki S, Hirakawa H, Onodera Y, Akahira J et al (2010) Increased intratumoral androgens in human breast carcinoma following aromatase inhibitor exemestane treatment. Endocr Relat Cancer 17(2):415–430. https://doi.org/10.1677/erc-09-0257

Takeshima H, Ushijima T (2019) Accumulation of genetic and epigenetic alterations in normal cells and cancer risk. *Npj precision*. Oncology 3(1):7. https://doi.org/10.1038/s41698-019-0079-0

Tangen IL, Onyango TB, Kopperud R, Berg A, Halle MK, Øyan AM et al (2016) Androgen receptor as potential therapeutic target in metastatic endometrial cancer. Oncotarget 7(31): 49289–49298. https://doi.org/10.18632/oncotarget.10334

Thakur L, Thakur S (2023) The interplay of sex steroid hormones and microRNAs in endometrial cancer: current understanding and future directions. Front Endocrinol (Lausanne) 14:1166948. https://doi.org/10.3389/fendo.2023.1166948

Thiebaut C, Vlaeminck-Guillem V, Trédan O, Poulard C, Le Romancer M (2021) Non-genomic signaling of steroid receptors in cancer. Mol Cell Endocrinol 538:111453. https://doi.org/10.1016/j.mce.2021.111453

Tian L, Peng Y, Yang K, Cao J, Du X, Liang Z et al (2022) The ERα-NRF2 signalling axis promotes bicalutamide resistance in prostate cancer. Cell Commun Signal 20(1):178. https://doi.org/10.1186/s12964-022-00979-0

Trabert B, Bauer DC, Buist DSM, Cauley JA, Falk RT, Geczik AM et al (2020) Association of circulating progesterone with breast cancer risk among postmenopausal women. JAMA Netw Open 3(4):e203645. https://doi.org/10.1001/jamanetworkopen.2020.3645

Treviño LS, Gorelick DA (2021) The Interface of nuclear and membrane steroid signaling. Endocrinology 162(8). https://doi.org/10.1210/endocr/bqab107

Truong TH, Lange CA (2018) Deciphering steroid receptor crosstalk in hormone-driven cancers. Endocrinology 159(12):3897–3907. https://doi.org/10.1210/en.2018-00831

Tumolo S, Rao BR, van der Burg ME, Guastalla JP, Renard J, Vermorken JB (1994) Phase II trial of flutamide in advanced ovarian cancer: an EORTC Gynaecological cancer cooperative group study. Eur J Cancer 30a(7):911–914. https://doi.org/10.1016/0959-8049(94)90112-0

Turcu AF, Nanba AT, Chomic R, Upadhyay SK, Giordano TJ, Shields JJ et al (2016) Adrenal-derived 11-oxygenated 19-carbon steroids are the dominant androgens in classic 21-hydroxylase deficiency. Eur J Endocrinol 174(5):601–609. https://doi.org/10.1530/eje-15-1181

Unluhizarci K, Karaca Z, Kelestimur F (2021) Role of insulin and insulin resistance in androgen excess disorders. World J Diabetes 12(5):616–629. https://doi.org/10.4239/wjd.v12.i5.616

Vahrenkamp JM, Yang CH, Rodriguez AC, Almomen A, Berrett KC, Trujillo AN et al (2018) Clinical and genomic crosstalk between glucocorticoid receptor and estrogen receptor α in endometrial cancer. Cell Rep 22(11):2995–3005. https://doi.org/10.1016/j.celrep.2018.02.076

Valko-Rokytovská M, Očenáš P, Salayová A, Kostecká Z (2021) Breast cancer: targeting of steroid hormones in Cancerogenesis and diagnostics. Int J Mol Sci 22(11). https://doi.org/10.3390/ijms22115878

Vassilomanolakis M, Koumakis G, Barbounis V, Demiri M, Pateras H, Efremidis AP (2000) Vinorelbine and cisplatin in metastatic breast cancer patients previously treated with anthracyclines. Ann Oncol 11(9):1155–1160. https://doi.org/10.1023/a:1008377724931

Veneris JT, Darcy KM, Mhawech-Fauceglia P, Tian C, Lengyel E, Lastra RR et al (2017) High glucocorticoid receptor expression predicts short progression-free survival in ovarian cancer. Gynecol Oncol 146(1):153–160. https://doi.org/10.1016/j.ygyno.2017.04.012

Wang Y, Romigh T, He X, Tan MH, Orloff MS, Silverman RH et al (2011) Differential regulation of PTEN expression by androgen receptor in prostate and breast cancers. Oncogene 30(42): 4327–4338. https://doi.org/10.1038/onc.2011.144

Wend K, Wend P, Krum SA (2012) Tissue-specific effects of loss of estrogen during menopause and aging. Front Endocrinol (Lausanne) 3:19. https://doi.org/10.3389/fendo.2012.00019

Whiteman DC, Siskind V, Purdie DM, Green AC (2003) Timing of pregnancy and the risk of epithelial ovarian cancer. Cancer Epidemiol Biomarkers Prev 12(1):42–46

Wilkenfeld SR, Lin C, Frigo DE (2018) Communication between genomic and non-genomic signaling events coordinate steroid hormone actions. Steroids 133:2–7. https://doi.org/10.1016/j.steroids.2017.11.005

Wilson JD, Auchus RJ, Leihy MW, Guryev OL, Estabrook RW, Osborn SM et al (2003) 5alpha-androstane-3alpha,17beta-diol is formed in tammar wallaby pouch young testes by a pathway involving 5alpha-pregnane-3alpha,17alpha-diol-20-one as a key intermediate. Endocrinology 144(2):575–580. https://doi.org/10.1210/en.2002-220721

Wu S, Yu K, Lian Z, Deng S (2022) Molecular regulation of androgen receptors in major female reproductive system cancers. Int J Mol Sci 23(14). https://doi.org/10.3390/ijms23147556

Xiao L, Feng Q, Zhang Z, Wang F, Lydon JP, Ittmann MM et al (2016) The essential role of GATA transcription factors in adult murine prostate. Oncotarget 7(30):47891–47903. https://doi.org/10.18632/oncotarget.10294

Xie N, Cheng H, Lin D, Liu L, Yang O, Jia L et al (2015) The expression of glucocorticoid receptor is negatively regulated by active androgen receptor signaling in prostate tumors. Int J Cancer 136(4):E27–E38. https://doi.org/10.1002/ijc.29147

Xu Z, Wang Y, Xiao ZG, Zou C, Zhang X, Wang Z et al (2018) Nuclear receptor ERRα and transcription factor ERG form a reciprocal loop in the regulation of TMPRSS2:ERG fusion gene in prostate cancer. Oncogene 37(48):6259–6274. https://doi.org/10.1038/s41388-018-0409-7

Xu S, Yu S, Dong D, Lee LTO (2019) G protein-coupled estrogen receptor: a potential therapeutic target in cancer. Front Endocrinol (Lausanne) 10:725. https://doi.org/10.3389/fendo.2019.00725

Yager, J. D. (2015). Mechanisms of estrogen carcinogenesis: The role of E2/E1-quinone metabolites suggests new approaches to preventive intervention--A review. Steroids, 99 (Pt A), 56–60. doi:https://doi.org/10.1016/j.steroids.2014.08.006

Yang F, Ma Q, Liu Z, Li W, Tan Y, Jin C et al (2017) Glucocorticoid receptor:MegaTrans switching mediates the repression of an ERα-regulated transcriptional program. Mol Cell 66(3):321–331.e6. https://doi.org/10.1016/j.molcel.2017.03.019

Yasumizu Y, Rajabi H, Jin C, Hata T, Pitroda S, Long MD et al (2020) MUC1-C regulates lineage plasticity driving progression to neuroendocrine prostate cancer. Nat Commun 11(1):338. https://doi.org/10.1038/s41467-019-14219-6

Yu S, Lee M, Shin S, Park J (2001) Apoptosis induced by progesterone in human ovarian cancer cell line SNU-840. J Cell Biochem 82(3):445–451. https://doi.org/10.1002/jcb.1171

Yu K, Huang ZY, Xu XL, Li J, Fu XW, Deng SL (2022) Estrogen receptor function: impact on the human endometrium. Front Endocrinol (Lausanne) 13:827724. https://doi.org/10.3389/fendo.2022.827724

Zhang L, Barritt GJ (2004) Evidence that TRPM8 is an androgen-dependent Ca2+ channel required for the survival of prostate cancer cells. Cancer Res 64(22):8365–8373. https://doi.org/10.1158/0008-5472.Can-04-2146

Zhang C, Marmé A, Wenger T, Gutwein P, Edler L, Rittgen W et al (2006) Glucocorticoid-mediated inhibition of chemotherapy in ovarian carcinomas. Int J Oncol 28(2):551–558

Zhang C, Wenger T, Mattern J, Ilea S, Frey C, Gutwein P et al (2007) Clinical and mechanistic aspects of glucocorticoid-induced chemotherapy resistance in the majority of solid tumors. Cancer Biol Ther 6(2):278–287. https://doi.org/10.4161/cbt.6.2.3652

Zhou Y, Liu X (2020) The role of estrogen receptor beta in breast cancer. Biomark Res 8(1):39. https://doi.org/10.1186/s40364-020-00223-2

Zhou B, Sun Q, Cong R, Gu H, Tang N, Yang L, Wang B (2008) Hormone replacement therapy and ovarian cancer risk: a meta-analysis. Gynecol Oncol 108(3):641–651. https://doi.org/10.1016/j.ygyno.2007.12.003

Zhou F, Gao S, Han D, Han W, Chen S, Patalano S et al (2019) TMPRSS2-ERG activates NO-cGMP signaling in prostate cancer cells. Oncogene 38(22):4397–4411. https://doi.org/10.1038/s41388-019-0730-9

Zubeldia-Brenner L, Roselli CE, Recabarren SE, Gonzalez Deniselle MC, Lara HE (2016) Developmental and functional effects of steroid hormones on the neuroendocrine axis and spinal cord. J Neuroendocrinol 28(7). https://doi.org/10.1111/jne.12401

Surgical Treatment and Innovations in Soft Tissue Sarcoma Care

Flemming Puscz, Marcus Lehnhardt, and Christoph Wallner

Abstract

The multimodal treatment of soft tissue sarcomas (STS) is subject to constant change and further development. The chapter "Surgical Treatment and Innovations in Soft Tissue Sarcoma Care" is intended to give the reader a basic insight into the various treatment algorithms for STS.

After a brief overview into the epidemiology, histology as well as pathophysiology of STS, the basic treatment algorithms are discussed. The various preoperative preparatory measures are presented followed by the actual surgical resection. Here, emphasis is placed on the importance of resection margins. In addition, new treatment measures such as preventive lymphovenous anastomosis and the possibilities of plastic-reconstructive surgery are presented. Finally, postoperative measures with a special focus on adjuvant therapy options are discussed. There is also an outlook on current research fields in adult STS as well as possible clinical implementation of experimental therapeutic approaches.

The treatment of STS remains an exciting and challenging field within the treatment of malignant diseases. After studying this chapter, the reader will have a comprehensive overview of the treatment of STS, with a specific focus on the role of resection margins.

Keywords

Plastic-reconstructive surgery · Resection margin · Sarcoma treatment · Soft tissue sarcoma

F. Puscz (✉) · M. Lehnhardt · C. Wallner
Department for Plastic and Hand Surgery, BG University Hospital Bergmannsheil Bochum, Ruhr-University Bochum, Bochum, Germany
e-mail: flemming.puscz@bergmannsheil.de

Interdisciplinary Cancer Research, https://doi.org/10.1007/16833_2024_208
Published online: 16 May 2024

1 Introduction

1.1 Overview of the Outline

Soft tissue sarcomas (STS) represent an extremely rare subgroup when measured against all adult tumor diseases. They are responsible for only 1% of all malignancies in adults, and up to 20% in children (Burningham et al. 2012). Due to their heterogeneity with more than 50 subtypes, the symptoms, diagnosis, and therapy of STS can also be heterogeneous. However, what all STS have in common is the fact that the only curative treatment approach is the complete surgical resection (Gronchi 2021). The purpose of this book chapter is to present an overview of the various treatment approaches of surgical STS therapy.

1.2 Evolution of the Concept and the Role of Resection Margins

As described above, complete surgical resection represents the basis in most cases in the treatment of STS (Gronchi et al. 2010). But how has this doctrine evolved over the decades, and how are these resection margins defined in the first place?

Enneking and colleagues postulated their approach of safe sarcoma resections in the 1980s (Enneking et al. 1981): They referred to the fact that a reactive tumor zone could be found outside the actual tumor, i.e., extracapsularly, which could still contain tumor cells and skip lesions. Resection in this reactive zone was thus understood as marginal resection. In contrast, wide resections included this reactive zone. According to these principles, skip lesions could still occur even with wide resections. Radical resections included the removal of the surrounding muscle compartments, leaving no surrounding tumor cells and no skip lesions. Yet, this was often equivalent to amputation in the extremities or great functional losses. For decades, there was a lack of robust data on which resection distances would provide better local control and/or survival benefit. This was also due to the fact that the terms marginal, wide, and radical resection were not used consistently (Harati and Lehnhardt 2017). In subsequent years, there was a trend toward non-ablative and function-preserving resection margins followed by adjuvant radiation. This approach was thus able to show advantages in local control but not in overall survival. However, against the background of limb and function preservation, this was an important step toward the improvement of surgical STS therapy (Rosenberg et al. 1982; Williard et al. 1992). At the beginning of the 2000s, the first retrospective data analyses were published to clarify the definition of resection distances. Initially, resection distances of >10 mm were declared as optimal for extremity STS resection (McKee et al. 2004). This meant that the paradigm of wide, radical resection distances was once again critically questioned. Studies by Harati and colleagues (Harati et al. 2017) as well as Ahmad and colleagues (Ahmad et al. 2016) were recently able to show that even resection margins <1 mm are sufficient and make no difference in terms of the local recurrence rate and the overall survival, "as long as the resected tumor has no ink on it" (Harati et al. 2017). Based on various, comprehensive cohort studies, a more accurate, precise, and quality-of-life-preserving therapy could be offered to many STS patients. Today we know that non-R0 resected tumors have a significantly increased risk of local recurrence, the formation of metastases, and a worse overall survival (Gronchi et al. 2010).

2 Basics of Soft Tissue Sarcomas

2.1 Pathology and Classification of Soft Tissue Sarcomas

As mentioned at the outset, STS are a very heterogeneous group of malignant tumors, but they all have in common that they are of mesenchymal origin, whereas cancer is of epithelial origin. The term sarcoma comes from the Greek word "sarx, sarkos" and means flesh. The suffix sarcoma indicates that it is a malignant tumor. For example, there is the malignant liposarcoma, whereas a lipoma is benign. The mesenchyme is a pluripotent filling and supporting tissue formed in the embryonic period. It essentially arises from the mesoderm. A variety of filling and supporting tissues arise from the mesenchyme, including musculature, tendons, fat, connective tissue, bone, cartilage, and blood. This explains on the one hand the enormous tumor heterogeneity within the group of STS, but also the ubiquity of their occurrence.

Since 1999, the World Health Organization (WHO) has periodically published reference books on the histological classification of soft tissue tumors, both benign and malign. The most recent edition is from 2020 and is indispensable for the histological classification of STS. Nevertheless, it should be noted that accurate identification of sarcoma grade always requires close interaction between the surgeon and an experienced sarcoma pathologist. Thus, due to the rarity of these tumors, well-established cooperation is necessary here to identify the correct tumor entity (Ray-Coquard et al. 2012). In the following, the different STS entities will be described using the 2020 WHO classification of soft tissue tumors (Sbaraglia et al. 2021). It should be noted that only tumors classified as malignant by the WHO, i.e., only "real" sarcomas, are discussed:

2.1.1 Malignant Adipocytic Tumors

This subgroup includes the following entities:

- Well-differentiated liposarcoma: lipoma-like, sclerosing, inflammatory
- Dedifferentiated liposarcoma
- Myxoid liposarcoma
- Pleomorphic liposarcoma
- Myxoid pleomorphic liposarcoma

Malignant adipocytic tumors make up about 10% of all STS, making them one of the largest subgroups. These tumors arise from fatty tissue, or its precursor cells. The listed five tumors are characterized by specific morphologies and gene expression patterns. At the genetic level, the first three tumors (well-differentiated liposarcoma:

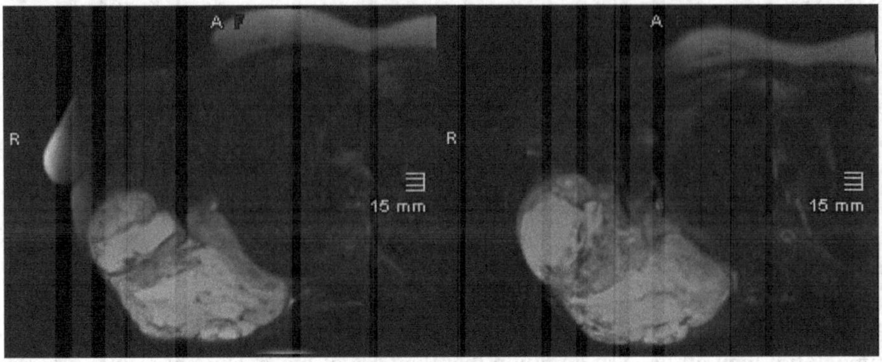

Fig. 1 Contrast-enhanced MRI images of a dedifferentiated liposarcoma on the trunk. Note the inhomogeneous contrast agent uptake of the tumor, a frequent indication of a high degree of aggressiveness, which in this case was confirmed by pathological grading G3

lipoma-like, sclerosing, inflammatory, dedifferentiated liposarcoma (cf. Fig. 1), myxoid liposarcoma) show *MDM2/CDK4* gene amplifications (Creytens 2020). Pleomorphic liposarcomas, on the other hand, are characterized by *FUS/EWSR1-DDIT3* gene fusions. The myxoid pleomorphic liposarcoma has been added as a new entity with the 2020 WHO classification. As the name describes, it represents a hybrid form of both myxoid and pleomorphic liposarcoma and accordingly presents portions of both types at the histologic level. Genetic aberrations for the identification of myxoid pleomorphic liposarcomas are not known so far. They represent a very rare entity that seems to occur mainly in young people, especially women (Alaggio et al. 2009).

2.1.2 Fibroblastic/Myofibroblastic Tumors

The following entities belong to fibroblastic and myofibroblastic STS:

- Solitary fibrous tumor, malignant
- Fibrosarcoma NOS
- Myxofibrosarcoma
- Low-grade fibromyxoid sarcoma
- Sclerosing epithelioid fibrosarcoma

These tumors arise from connective tissue cells and are characterized by immature proliferating fibroblasts or anaplastic spindle cells. Histologically fibrosarcomas appear as tumors composed of tightly packed spindle-shaped cells. These cells have increased nuclear density and may have atypia, indicating abnormal cellular structures. Fibrosarcomas are often surrounded by a collagenous stromal reaction emphasizing the connective tissue component. At the genetic level, we see chromosomal aberrations for the solitary fibrous tumor (*NAB2-STAT6*), the low-grade fibromyxoid sarcoma (*FUS-CREB3L2* and *EWSR1-CREB3L1*), and sclerosing epithelioid fibrosarcoma (*EWSR1-CREB3L1* and *EWSR1-CREB3L2*) (German Cancer Society, German Cancer Aid, AWMF 2022). It should be noted that there are some entities, such as the dermatofibrosarcoma protuberans, which has the suffix -sarcoma, but according to the WHO classification is categorized as an intermediate (locally aggressive) tumor. These are characterized by the fact that they rarely to never metastasize but can show aggressive and destructive growth locally.

2.1.3 So-Called Fibrohistiocytic Tumors

The malignant tenosynovial giant cell tumor is the only malignant tumor in the subgroup of the so-called fibrohistiocytic tumors. The giant cell tumors are a group of soft tissue tumors that can develop from joint, tendon, and bursa tissues (Salem et al. 2022). Accordingly, they often occur close to the joints. They are not to be confused with giant cell-rich tumors. Until 20 years ago, this group was among the largest subset of all sarcomas. The "malignant fibrous histiocytoma" accounted for approximately 50% of all sarcoma diagnoses until 2000 (Fletcher 1992; Dei Tos 2006; Sbaraglia et al. 2021). However, this entity was replaced in 2013 by the term undifferentiated pleomorphic sarcoma, which is now listed under "tumors of unclear differentiation".

2.1.4 Vascular Tumors

This subgroup includes:

- Epithelioid hemangioendothelioma
- Angiosarcoma

As the name implies, these tumors develop primarily from vascular tissues, therefore, their occurrence can be in almost any soft tissue. Epithelioid hemangioendothelioma represents an extremely rare tumor entity with an incidence of 0.1/100,000. At the genetic level, epithelioid hemangioendothelioma is known to have an aberration of the *WWTR1-CAMTA1* and *YAP1-TFE3* genes.

Angiosarcomas are accounting for 2% of all sarcomas. However, it should be noted that the incidence of angiosarcomas has increased significantly over the last 30 years (Young et al. 2010). This increase is demonstrably linked to the increase in the number of radiotherapies performed (Ronchi et al. 2020). A special problem is posed by radiation-associated angiosarcomas after therapy of breast carcinoma (Mergancová et al. 2022). These secondary angiosarcomas are significantly more common than the spontaneously occurring primary type (Arora et al. 2014). The risk of developing angiosarcoma for women with breast carcinoma and radiation is 26 times higher than for women with breast carcinoma without radiation. These tumors are always highly malignant and have a high rate of locoregional and distant metastases (cf. Fig. 2). Prospective study data are currently not available.

2.1.5 Pericytic/Perivascular Tumors

On the side of malignant neoplasms, this subgroup consists only of the malignant glomus tumor, which is an extremely rare condition as most glomus tumors are benign (Chen et al. 2020). They are characterized by a perivascular growth pattern. Glomus tumors originate from a glomus, which can be either vascular or nervous origin.

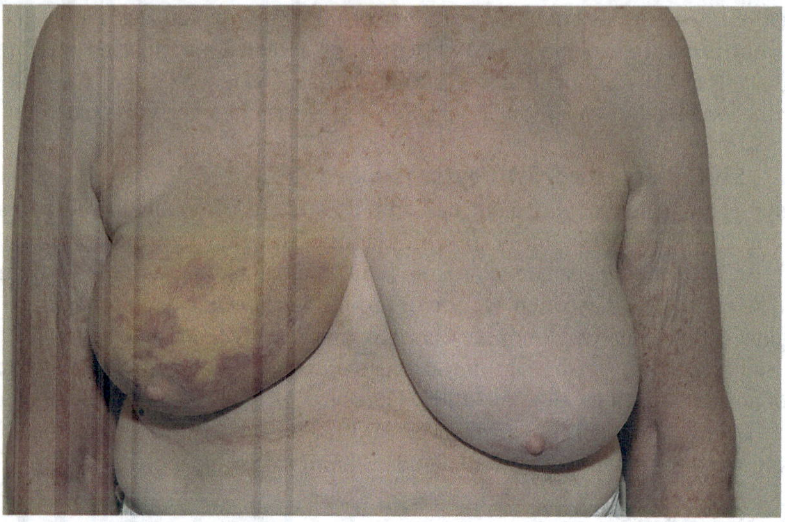

Fig. 2 Secondary angiosarcoma of the right breast after breast-conserving therapy including radiation for breast carcinoma

2.1.6 Smooth Muscle Tumors

On the malignant level, these include:

- Inflammatory leiomyosarcoma
- Leiomyosarcoma

Leiomyosarcomas arise from the smooth musculature. For this reason, the most common tumor locations are the uterus and the gastrointestinal tract (Serrano and George 2013). The inflammatory leiomyosarcoma is a rare subgroup of this entity that occurs primarily in the extremities, trunk, and retroperitoneum (Efstathopoulos et al. 2006). At the histological level, inflammatory leiomyosarcoma differs from "classic" leiomyosarcoma in lymphocyte infiltrates and reactivity for both smooth and skeletal muscle markers (Viljoen et al. 2021).

2.1.7 Skeletal Muscle Tumors

The best-known representative of this group is the rhabdomyosarcoma with its subtypes, as well as the very rare ectomesenchymoma:

- Embryonal rhabdomyosarcoma
- Alveolar rhabdomyosarcoma
- Pleomorphic rhabdomyosarcoma
- Spindle cell/sclerosing rhabdomyosarcoma
- Ectomesenchymoma

The tumors most commonly occur in the head and neck region and represent the most common entity of malignant soft tissue tumors in childhood. They are responsible for approx. only 1% of all adult STS. Histologically, all five malignant subtypes have in common the presence of portions of skeletal muscle differentiation (Kohashi et al. 2020). At the genetic level, a gene fusion to *PAX3-FOXO1* and *PAX7-FOXO1* in alveolar rhabdomyosarcoma is known to be specific for this entity.

2.1.8 Gastrointestinal Stromal Tumors (GIST)

This group includes only the GIST. As the name suggests, these tumors occur exclusively in the gastrointestinal tract. There they arise most frequently (50–70%) in the stomach, followed by the small intestine (20–30%). They are among the most common sarcomas in adults and are extremely rare in children. This entity originates from the intestinal cells of Cajal, which perform a mediating function between the smooth muscle and the autonomic nervous system. They are characterized by overexpression of the tyrosine kinase receptor KIT (Akahoshi et al. 2018).

2.1.9 Chondro-osseous Tumors

At the malignant level, this only includes extraskeletal osteosarcoma, which is an extremely rare form of STS. Due to its aggressive growth, it is often already metastasized at diagnosis. The recurrence rate is extremely high at 75% (Huvos 1986). At the histologic level, like skeletal osteosarcoma, it shows many portions of osteoid, cartilaginous, as well as fibrous tissue (Longhi et al. 2017). Overall, it accounts for just 1% of all STS in adulthood.

2.1.10 Peripheral Nerve Sheath Tumors

These include the following malignant entities:

- Malignant peripheral nerve sheath tumor
- Melanotic malignant nerve sheath tumor
- Granular cell tumor, malignant
- Perineurioma, malignant

The malignant peripheral nerve sheath tumor (MPNST) accounts for only 1% of all STS. The other three entities occur even less frequently. MPNSTs are frequently associated with the presence of a neurofibromatosis type 1 (Morbus Recklinghausen), which is why an additional genetic workup for the presence of neurofibromatosis should always be performed when peripheral nerve sheath tumors are diagnosed.

2.1.11 Tumors of Uncertain Differentiation

This group includes all tumors that cannot be assigned to the other groups based on their histology. Accordingly, it is large and heterogeneous:

- Phosphaturic mesenchymal tumor, malignant
- NTRK-rearranged spindle cell neoplasm (emerging)
- Synovial sarcoma

- Epithelioid sarcoma: proximal and classic variant
- Alveolar soft part sarcoma
- Clear cell sarcoma
- Extraskeletal myxoid chondrosarcoma
- Desmoplastic small round cell tumor
- Rhabdoid tumor
- Perivascular epithelioid tumor, malignant
- Intimal sarcoma
- Ossifying fibromyxoid tumor, malignant
- Myoepithelial carcinoma
- Undifferentiated sarcoma
- Spindle cell sarcoma, undifferentiated
- Pleomorphic sarcoma, undifferentiated
- Round cell sarcoma, undifferentiated

For reasons of clarity and comprehensibility, each individual entity will not be discussed in the following. However, the aforementioned work (Sbaraglia et al. 2021) provides a very good overview of the different tumors and their histological differences.

2.1.12 Ewing Sarcomas

Ewing sarcomas are solid malignant tumors that usually occur in the bone. Rarely, they also arise in soft tissues, i.e., connective tissue, fat tissue, muscle tissue, or peripheral nerves. The disease is named after James Ewing, an American cancer researcher who first described this tumor in 1921. Ewing sarcoma is classically described histologically as a small-blue-round-cell tumor. Most Ewing sarcomas grow and spread very rapidly. After osteosarcoma it is the second most common bone tumor in children and adolescents. The genetic aberrations for the "classic" Ewing sarcoma are *WSR1-ERG, EWSR1-ETV1, EWSR1-ETV4, EWSR1-FEV,* and *EWSR1-FLI1* gene fusions. However, other gene fusions also exist, which then allows the tumor to be assigned to the subgroup of Ewing-like sarcomas.

2.2 Epidemiology and Risk Factors

Regarding the overall epidemiology of STS, many different data and figures exist. Among others, population structure, geography but also the way of data acquisition depend on this. In the following, therefore, only a rough overview of the epidemiology can be given, noting that most of the sources refer to data from (Western-) Europe and Northern America.

Incidence rates for STS in adults usually range from 1.8 to 5.0 per 100.000 residents (Toro et al. 2006; Stiller et al. 2013). A study published in 2018 analyzed data on the presence of STS for the year 2013 in Germany (Ressing et al. 2018). It showed that GIST is the most common sarcoma entity with 22%. Besides GIST, fibrosarcomas (14%) and liposarcomas (12%) were most common in men, whereas non-uterine leiomyosarcomas (10%) and fibrosarcomas (9%) were among the most common entities in women. With the addition of further studies, a distinction can also be made between young adults, ranging from 15 to 39 years of age and adults over 39 years (Herzog 2005). This study showed that rhabdomyosarcomas and synovial sarcomas are most prevalent in the group of young adults. In older adults, however, undifferentiated sarcomas, leiomyosarcomas, liposarcomas, fibrosarcomas, and pleomorphic sarcomas are leading.

With regard to possible modifiable and non-modifiable risk factors, several studies have been published, which yet do not allow general statements to be made. Weskamp et al. carried out a meta-analysis for this purpose, in which over 6000 patients were included. In this analysis, they were able to demonstrate a general coincidence of risk factors that led to the development of STS. Yet, subgroup analysis of these risk factors did not meet statistical significances. But it revealed a greater magnitude with smoking, genetic predisposition, chronic inflammation, and toxins (Weskamp et al. 2022). In another study, an increased risk for the development of STS has been documented in patients with immunodeficiency (Selik et al. 1987; Bhatia et al. 2012). A review article from 2012 showed that leiomyosarcoma and angiosarcoma may occur disproportionately in immunodeficiency (Bhatia et al. 2012). Causes for this tumor development in immunodeficient patients are seen in viral infections with herpes viruses and the Epstein-Barr virus (EBV). For example, human herpesvirus 8 can be detected in 80% of all Kaposi sarcomas (Chang et al. 1994; Moore and Chang 1995), regardless of whether the affected individuals are HIV-positive or -negative. EBV has also been detected in various cases in immunosuppressed STS patients: approximately 85% of all leiomyomas and leiomyosarcomas contain the EBV (Bhatia et al. 2012), whereas it has not been detected in immunocompetent leiomyosarcomas (Stubbins et al. 2019). However, it is suggested that causal treatment of immunodeficiency may be associated with spontaneous remission of the sarcoma.

Another risk factor that has generated increasing attention in recent years is iatrogenic: radiotherapy. There are various case studies that have demonstrated an increased risk, especially for the occurrence of angiosarcomas after radiation in mamma carcinomas. Thus, the risk of angiosarcoma in the former radiation area is increased seven-fold for these patients (Rubino et al. 2005). These radiotherapy-associated angiosarcomas show a high recurrence rate with poor 5-year survival rates (D'Angelo et al. 2013). An association with chronic lymphedema has also been described previously and is called Stewart-Treves-Syndrome (Billings et al. 2004; Shavit et al. 2018). "Classic" predisposing factors such as tobacco and/or alcohol use or obesity have been studied in the past, but no sufficient associations between these factors and an increased incidence of sarcoma have been demonstrated.

2.3 Diagnosis and Staging of Sarcomas

Diagnosis of STS requires a standardized and focused approach, which should ideally be performed in a multidisciplinary setting at a center specialized in sarcoma care. Patients usually present with a swelling that has been present for a few weeks/

months and is often rapidly progressive in size. For a first rough assessment, the example of a golf ball is often used here: "If your lump is bigger than a golf ball and growing, think Sarcoma" (Nandra et al. 2015). Ideally, a contrast-enhanced MRI is obtained and the patient is referred to a sarcoma center. Another less preferable case here is the so-called "whoops" procedure (see next chapter). With regard to primary imaging for tumor visualization, the aforementioned contrast-enhanced MRI is the method of choice because it provides the best visualization of tumor margins and differentiation of fatty and cystic tumors but also necrotic and non-necrotic tumor components. After confirmation of the localization, specimen biopsy should be performed for definitive diagnosis and further histological and molecular pathological processing. Biopsy can be done either by (vacuum-assisted) punch biopsy or, e.g., in the case of complex anatomical conditions or inaccessibility of the tumor, by open biopsy. A fine-needle biopsy should no longer be performed, as this usually yields too little sample material. The advantages of vacuum-assisted punch biopsy in terms of a lower complication rate and faster performance have already been demonstrated (Simidjiiska-Belyaeva et al. 2019). The biopsy access should be selected in such a way that the biopsy channel can be resected during the definitive tumor removal *en bloc*. This is of importance, as tumor cell metastases can rarely be found in the biopsy channel after both punch biopsy and open biopsy (Barrientos-Ruiz et al. 2017). With regard to the number of samples, it has been shown that from a sample number of 3 (for bony tumors) and 4 (for soft tissue tumors) a plateau in diagnostic accuracy is reached (Wu et al. 2008). An excisional biopsy, i.e., the removal of the entire tumor and subsequent histological workup, can be performed for tumors <3 cm in diameter. However, the safe, R0 resection of the tumor must be ensured. After final confirmation of the diagnosis of STS by pathology, further staging should be based on the sarcoma entity and location. The procedure described here should always take place in a multidisciplinary setting and after discussing the relevant case in a tumor conference.

The specimens obtained in this way should be prepared, in the case of biopsies in 4% formalin, in the case of complete resections natively, and be taken directly to pathology. It is important that the specimen is clearly marked by the surgeon with regard to the resection boundaries. This can be done with thread markings or e.g. drawings on a corkboard (cf. Fig. 3). Further histopathological processing of the specimens or the entire tumor should be carried out by an experienced sarcoma pathologist. Due to the enormous complexity, the specific pathological procedure will not be examined in more detail here and can be reproduced in the relevant literature.

2.4 "Whoops" Procedures

So-called "whoops" procedures mean the accidental removal of a malignant tumor, often without prior imaging and further clarification in a specialized sarcoma unit. They are most often performed for superficial and small (<3 cm) STS under the suspected diagnosis of a benign lesion. In the event of unplanned resection of a soft

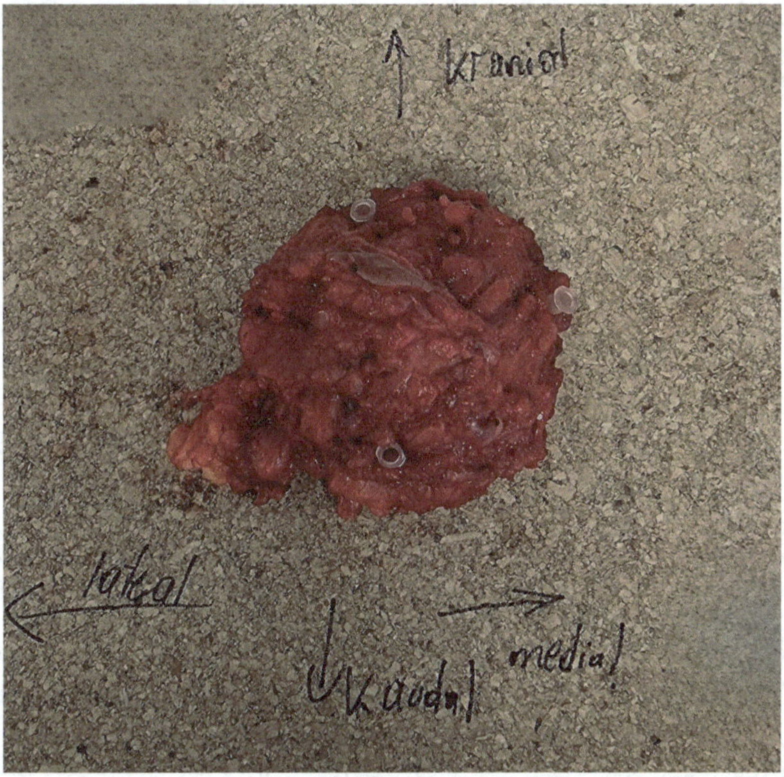

Fig. 3 Resected fibrosarcoma with excised skin that has been fixed to a cork plate to simplify orientation and providing anatomical relationship

tissue sarcoma, re-resection should be performed in order to achieve local tumor control. Several studies have shown that the local recurrence rate is significantly increased despite resection after primary unplanned resections compared to primary R0 resected tumors and that plastic reconstructions are required more often, but overall survival is not affected (Fiore et al. 2006; Cahlon et al. 2008).

3 Preoperative Preparation

3.1 Patient Selection and Assessment

Sarcomas can occur at any age in almost any location. Accordingly, the patient groups presenting for sarcoma treatment are also heterogeneous. Surgical therapy of STS should be performed when R0 resection is possible. In case of already occurred metastasis, surgical therapy should be critically evaluated.

After the diagnosis of a sarcoma has been confirmed, a genetic clarification regarding predisposing germline mutations should also be performed in certain patients. For this purpose, the Chompret criteria can be used, which are applied when the presence of a Li-Fraumeni syndrome (LFS) is suspected:

- A tumor of the LFS tumor spectrum (STS, osteosarcoma, brain tumor, choroid plexus tumor, premenopausal breast cancer, adrenocortical carcinoma, leukemia, bronchial carcinoma) before age 46 years and at least one first- or second-degree relative with an LFS tumor before age 56 years.
- Multiple tumors (other than breast cancer), two of which are on the LFS tumor spectrum and occurred before age 46.
- An adrenocortical tumor, choroid plexus tumor, or embryonal rhabdomyosarcoma regardless of family history.
- Breast cancer before the age of 31.

In addition, as mentioned above, genetic testing should be offered for rare STS entities (e.g., MPNST in neurofibromatosis type 1).

Regarding the preparations before surgical sarcoma treatment, the usual preoperative examinations should be performed. In this regard, patients with pre-existing conditions have a higher perioperative risk. Therefore, a precise anamnesis about previous diseases and previous operations must be taken before the operation. Of particular interest here are anticoagulants taken and previous thromboembolic events. Furthermore, an assessment of the bleeding risk should be made in consultation between the anesthesiologist and the surgeon in order to determine the blood group and, if necessary, prepare packed red blood cells.

In case of a retroperitoneal sarcoma and a (partial) nephrectomy might be possible in the context of the planned resection, it is essential to perform a detailed preoperative examination of the kidneys in order to ensure adequate renal function postoperatively. Furthermore, if the spleen is to be removed as well, vaccination against pneumococcus, haemophilus influenzae type B, and meningococcus should be performed.

4 Surgical Procedures and Resection Margins

4.1 Surgical Resection: Principles and Techniques for Achieving R0 Resections

The development of the concept of compartment resection by Enneking has already been discussed in the introduction. This treatment concept was initially developed for the surgical therapy of bone tumors and was thus not completely transferable to STS. Therefore, surgical resection distances have been repeatedly redefined and their advantages and disadvantages have been demonstrated on the basis of studies. As mentioned at the outset, surgical resection is the only curative therapeutic option in the treatment of adult STS, regardless of the tumor location (Gross et al. 2005). In this case, the tumor should be resected in one piece, i.e., *en bloc*, together with the above-mentioned biopsy access. The German guideline for the treatment of STS (German Cancer Society, German Cancer Aid, AWMF 2022) recommends the wide resection in this context. According to this, the tumor to be removed should at best not appear at all during the operation and should be completely surrounded by a layer of healthy tissue (e.g., muscle) (Kawaguchi et al. 2004). For successful R0 resection, knowledge of the exact anatomic location of the tumor is essential. Based on this, the experienced sarcoma surgeon must plan the procedure and can be prepared for any intraoperative problems. Preoperative planning based on the previously obtained MRI is therefore of great importance. Furthermore, this planning is important to inform the patient about possible postoperative functional limitations.

Accordingly, the actual operation already begins with the determination of the surgical position, which the surgeon has already determined in advance. After the skin incision has been drawn, further careful dissection is carried out in the direction of the tumor. In anatomically demanding regions, such as the distal forearm, this can be done under loupe magnification. In addition to the knowledge of precise anatomy, this requires a high level of expertise in the treatment of the various types of tissue in the resection area. Furthermore, a meticulous hemostasis should be performed in order to have a good overview in situ. In this context, bipolar diathermy is of particular importance. The tumor is then identified and exposed, considering its anatomical location. The actual tumor should not be revealed in the process. The surrounding capsule of the tumor should also be surrounded by a layer of healthy tissue (wide resection). Furthermore, the tumor itself should not be manipulated. This procedure is often described as a "no-touch technique". Once the tumor has been completely exposed, it is sent in its entirety as a specimen for histopathological examination. The tumor should be sent immediately and in native form. The pathologist must be informed of any anatomical peculiarities and the positional conditions. Suture marking, sketches, and drawing on a plate may help in this regard. After removal of the tumor, a change of all surgical instruments ("table change") and sterile gloves can be performed. Furthermore, the former tumor cavity is inspected. Here, it is still necessary to pay attention to a potential bleeding, which must be ligated. Under certain circumstances, the tumor cavity can be rinsed, e.g., with pure water, in order to achieve osmotic diffusion of the water into remaining tumor cells and thus cause them to burst. Various irrigations with different agents have also been attempted in connection with other tumors (Ganapathy et al. 2023), but these procedures have not yet progressed beyond the experimental stage and there is still a lack of real significance with regard to their efficacy.

The insertion of a wound drainage is not mandatory. However, for large tumor cavities, it should be done for hematoma and seroma prophylaxis. The drainage should be positioned close to the wound edge to enable resection of the drainage channel in the event of a necessary re-resection. The wound should then be closed in layers and without tension. The possibilities of defect reconstruction will be discussed later in chapter VI.

4.2 Significance of Resection Margins and Risks Associated with Positive Margins

It has already been explained that successful treatment of STS always involves R0 resection of the tumor. But what is the outcome in affected patients in the case of a marginal or even incomplete resection? A study on this was published in 2013 by Jebsen and colleagues (Jebsen et al. 2013). They carried out a retrospective analysis of a total of 462 STS patients and examined the rate of local recurrences with regard to the resection margins and the radiation dose administered postoperatively. They concluded that wide resections were more likely to ensure local recurrence-free survival than marginal resections. Furthermore, the authors concluded that marginal resections require higher adjuvant radiation doses. Another study examined tumor mortality of liposarcomas in 83 patients (Chang et al. 1990). Prognostic factors regarding favorable survival should be identified. According to their findings, five factors were significant for tumor mortality: tumor grade, histologic subtype, tumor size greater than or equal to 5 cm, type of surgery/margin, and invasion of vital structures. Adequate safety margins were associated with a lower local recurrence rate in contrast to marginal resection margins (Chang et al. 1990). In another large data analysis with 27.969 patients, the advantage of R0 resection over incomplete resections in terms of overall survival was also confirmed (Gingrich et al. 2017). Another factor for better overall survival was pre- and postoperative radiation. Interestingly, treatment in an academic facility was also mentioned as a prognostic factor for achieving R0 resection margins, which once again underlines the urgency of treatment at a specialized unit. A further retrospective analysis with 687 patients from 4 oncological centers also showed that not only pure R0 resection, but with a more generous safety margin of >2 mm had an additional benefit with regard to the occurrence of local recurrences (Willeumier et al. 2017). This once again reinforces the currently postulated approach of wide resection. What all given studies have in common is the fact that with an incomplete tumor resection, the likelihood of local recurrence is significantly higher. However, this also increases the risk of metastasis and ultimately leads to poorer long-term survival with higher mortality (Gronchi et al. 2010).

4.3 Lymph Nodes

The majority of all STS metastasize primarily hematogenously, which is why lymph node involvement is relatively rare and a preventive lymphadenectomy is therefore not recommended in current guidelines (German Cancer Society, German Cancer Aid, AWMF 2022). Nevertheless, various sarcoma entities, e.g., rhabdomyosarcoma, show an increased tendency to lymphogenic metastasis (Gandhi et al. 2017). In the data analysis of this study with 326 sarcoma patients, 19 (5.8%) showed lymph node involvement. Other entities that metastasized lymphogenically were synovial sarcoma, MPNST, and clear cell sarcoma (Gandhi et al. 2017). Other studies see similar incidences regarding lymph node involvement and the predestined entities (Daigeler et al. 2009). Since the lymph node metastases often metastasize further, a decision to undergo radical lymphadenectomy in the affected area must always be made against the background of operability and the overall metastasis status. Thus, even if lymph node involvement has been proven, no general statement can be made regarding radical lymphadenectomy. This decision should always be made in an interdisciplinary setting and regarding the individual patient situation.

4.4 Safeguarding Surrounding Critical Structures

Due to the relatively common location of STS in the extremities, these tumors are often located close to relevant functional structures (blood vessels, nerves, bones, etc.). These anatomic relationships must be known before the planned resection and possible consequences of a co-resection of the respective structure should be explained to the patient during the preoperative information. As mentioned above, R0 resection represents the most important goal of curative sarcoma surgery, and therefore the involvement of functional structures should not be an obstacle to the complete resection of the tumor.

In the case of affected blood vessels, reconstruction of the same, e.g., by vascular prostheses, should be considered to avoid amputation (German Cancer Society, German Cancer Aid, AWMF 2022). A vascular surgeon should always be involved in this decision-making process. It should be noted that vascular involvement of the STS alone does not predict a worse outcome of the disease (Poultsides et al. 2015), but is associated with higher perioperative mortality (Fujiki et al. 2020).

In the area of nerve involvement, Sweiti and colleagues have postulated the following classification of sciatic nerve affection by tumor (Sweiti et al. 2018):

- Type A: nerve encasement
- Type B: nerve contact
- Type C: no nerve involvement

The study examined a collective of 364 patients with STS of the lower extremity. Of these, 27 showed encasement or contact to the sciatic nerve. Of these 27 patients, 11.1% had local recurrence and 29.6% showed metastasis. Thus, overall, a worse outcome can be assumed in STS with nerve involvement, as this can usually be noticed from highly malignant STS with a high-grading status. Nevertheless, the authors concluded that nerve resection must always be critically evaluated, especially in view of the resulting loss of function. Furthermore, it must be pointed out that resection of the sciatic nerve does not yet imply a safe walking disability. Here, too, studies have demonstrated good to very good residual function after resection of the sciatic nerve (Bickels et al. 2002).

Anatomical proximity to the bone is reported with 5–6% in STS (German Cancer Society, German Cancer Aid, AWMF 2022). In this analysis, of 50 investigated STS with suspected bone infiltration, just 3 (6%) showed true bone involvement (Lin et al. 2007). Nevertheless, in these cases, co-resection of the adjacent periosteum is often necessary. Extensive bony resection is rarely indicated. Furthermore, in many cases, the muscle adjacent to the bone must also be resected to remove the tumor without affecting its capsule. In bony proximity, without true infiltration, neoadjuvant radiotherapy should be evaluated on an individual basis.

5 Prophylactic Lymphovenous Anastomosis

5.1 Concept of Prophylactic Lymphovenous Anastomosis

As one of the most current and innovative treatment concepts, prophylactic lymphovenous anastomosis (LVA) will be examined in this chapter. LVA describes a (micro-)surgical technique that creates a direct connection between the body's lymphatic system and venous system. This type of anastomosis was initially used to improve lymphatic drainage in the arm after lymphadenectomies, e.g., in the context of breast carcinoma (Scaglioni et al. 2020). During the procedure, which is carried out by an experienced microsurgeon using a microscope and microsurgical instruments, the surgeon connects a lymphatic vessel (usually a lymphatic vessel that leads to the damaged or swollen tissue) directly to a nearby venous vessel. This allows excess lymph fluid to be directed into the venous system, where it is more easily removed by the body. This connection allows swelling to decrease and the patient can benefit from improved lymphatic drainage (Jørgensen et al. 2018). In addition to LVA, it is also possible to perform a vascularized lymph node transfer. In this procedure, circumscribed lymph node packages (e.g., from the groin) are removed as part of a free flap and transplanted into the area affected by the lymphedema. This procedure is today mostly used after breast carcinomas (Liu et al. 2019).

5.2 Indications and Surgical Implementation

Patients should be screened for the presence of risk factors for the development of lymphedema before sarcoma resection. These risk factors include lymphadenectomy, radiotherapy, obesity, cardiac and renal diseases, thrombosis, chronic venous insufficiency, erysipelas, immobilization of the affected limb, trauma, and a family history of lymphedema. In patients who have already had trauma and/or surgery in the tumor area, imaging of lymphatic drainage, e.g., with indocyanine green (ICG), may be performed preoperatively. Thus, the lymphatic vessels can be specifically visualized with an infrared camera. Based on the classification of Yamamoto et al. (Yamamoto et al. 2020), possible lymphatic drainage disorders can be divided into different patterns and an LVA can be planned. Another method for visualizing the lymphatic vessels is MRI-supported lymphangiography. Here, the lymphatic pathways are visualized with the aid of a contrast agent in the MRI. However, this technique is relatively complex and the associated protocols are not yet widely used so far (Hsu and Itkin 2016). The lymphatic vessels are then redrawn prior to the actual LVA, whether as part of the tumor resection or as a single procedure. Intraoperatively, the lymphatic vessels can also

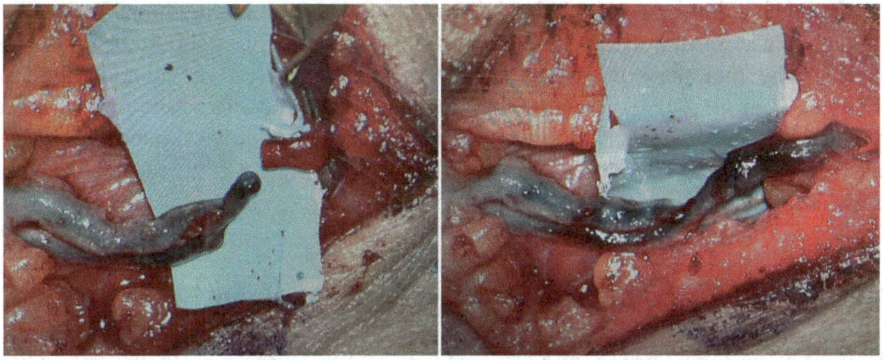

Fig. 4 Implementation of an LVA. The patent blue injected intracutaneously preoperatively reliably indicates the lymphatic vessel. A subcutaneously located vein can be used as a connecting vessel

be visualized by intracutaneous injection of patent blue. These superficially located lymphatic vessels are then precisely explored and anastomosed to a nearby vein using microsurgical techniques (cf. Fig. 4).

5.3 Evidence and Potential Benefits in Sarcoma Care

There are no reliable figures on the incidence of secondary lymphedema after sarcoma removal. However, it has already been explained that radical lymphadenectomy should not be performed as a standard procedure, which is why the proportion of affected patients with secondary lymphedema can be estimated as relatively low. That is why to date, LVAs are not performed as standard in the context of STS resections, although there might be a risk for STS patients to develop a secondary lymphedema postoperatively (Wan et al. 2023). However, recent studies have shown that LVAs can have a positive impact on the prevention of secondary lymphedema through prophylactic treatment, i.e., carried out at the same time as tumor resection (Wagner et al. 2022). However, the quantity and quality of the previous reports differ significantly, meaning that high-quality studies with large numbers of patients should be carried out in order to prove the presumed benefit of this procedure (Jørgensen et al. 2018).

6 Tissue Defect Reconstruction

6.1 Importance of Defect Coverage Following Extensive Resections

Due to the destructive growth of many sarcoma entities, resection of the same often results in a skin and soft tissue defect that necessitates plastic surgery. However, the frequently cited “reconstructive ladder” is not always meaningful and purposeful.

On the one hand, this is since with a primary wound closure no functional restoration can take place. Furthermore, the method of covering the defect should be chosen in such a way that the soft tissues can withstand postoperative radiation therapy (Lehnhardt et al. 2019). However, before planning a reconstructive measure, the probability of recurrence and the possible presence of a palliative situation should be taken into account. Therefore, even for small defects, defect coverage by means of free vascularized flaps must sometimes be considered.

6.2 Techniques for Tissue Defect and Functional Reconstruction

The entire armamentarium of plastic reconstructive surgery is then used in the reconstruction of these complex defects. As mentioned earlier, primary wound closure, while often the most obvious, is not the most useful method. Also, coverage with split skin grafts does not represent a sufficiently resistant wound bed for adjuvant radiotherapy. If primary wound closure and split skin grafts are not possible/reasonable, temporary closure is possible with the aid of a vacuum dressing. Thus, in the meantime, the resection status can be confirmed by pathology and the further reconstructive procedure can be determined. Local flaps are a good method for covering defects but are often not feasible due to a lack of mobilizable tissue surrounding the defect. This is often the case, especially on the distal arm and leg.

Therefore, free flaps play an increasingly important and indispensable role in defect reconstruction after STS resections. In particular, perforator-based flap surgery has experienced an upswing in the recent years, as it has allowed defects to be covered with thin yet resilient flaps. Here, the anterolateral thigh (ALT)- and the superficial circumflex iliac artery perforator (SCIP)-flap are of utter importance. However, classic myocutaneous flaps, such as the latissimus dorsi muscle flap, continue to be an excellent option for adequately restoring large, multi-layered defects (cf. Fig. 5). However, it should be noted here that myocutaneous flaps do not undergo adequate randomization of the supplying blood vessels. In contrast, most perforator flaps develop such randomization of the blood supply within 3 months, so that in case of recurrence, surgery can be performed through the flap without complications (German Cancer Society, German Cancer Aid, AWMF 2022).

However, in addition to the actual defect reconstruction, the restoration of function should also be considered. Here, too, various reconstruction methods can be used. Accordingly, the vascular reconstruction already mentioned above should not be mentioned here again. A co-resected nerve can, for example, be replaced by a nerve interposition of the sural nerve (Beris et al. 2019). With the use of synchronously performed tendon replacements, functional deficiencies can be minimized. It is yet to consider that many functions, due to the body's own compensation mechanisms, are self-restoring. An example is the thigh region, where the resection of several flexors or adductors without a recognizable functional deficit can be done. Some of the most frequently used motoric replacement plastics are, in the upper extremity, the relocation of the latissimus dorsi muscle to replace elbow flexion,

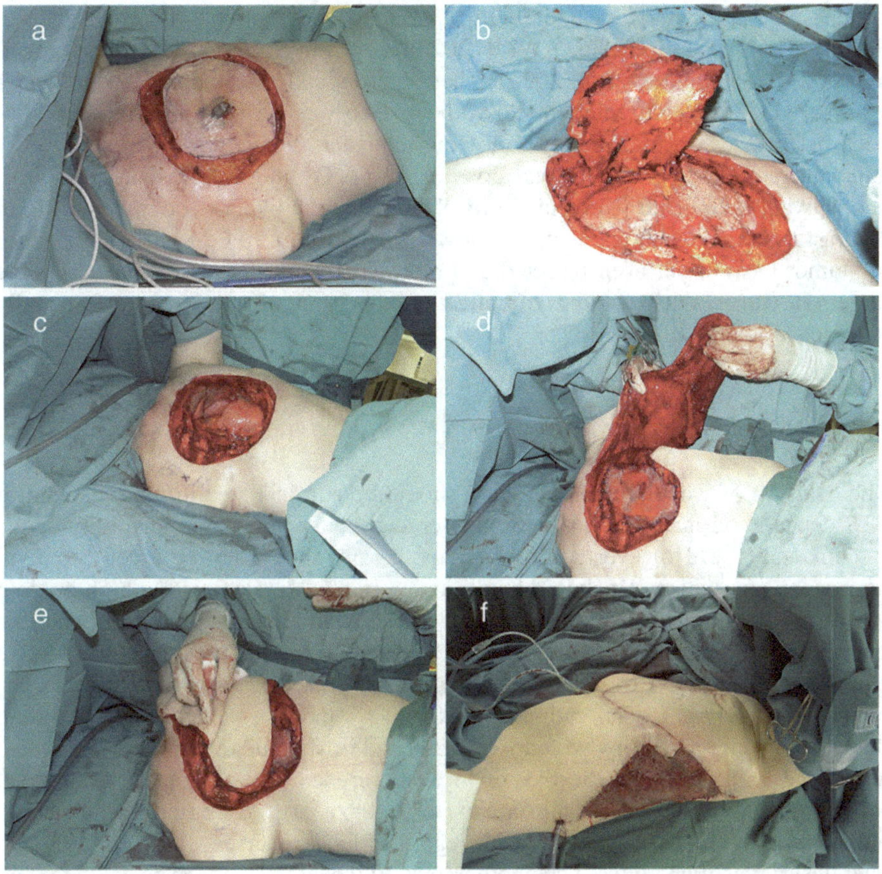

Fig. 5 Resection of an angiosarcoma with partial thoracic wall removal of the left breast with immediate defect coverage by pedicled latissimus dorsi flap. (**a**) Tumor resection with skin island, (**b**) Exposed parts of the lung after partial thoracic wall resection, (**c**) Tissue defect to be reconstructed, (**d**) Harvesting of the ipsilateral latissimus dorsi flap, (**e**) Fitting the flap into the defect, (**f**) Final defect reconstruction with split skin coverage of the donor area

flexor tendon transfer to reconstruct finger and hand extension and, in the lower extremity, transposition of the M. biceps femoris to restore knee joint extension.

7 Non-surgical Therapies

7.1 Role of Radiation Therapy

Adjuvant radiotherapy has been shown to significantly reduce local recurrence rates (Beane et al. 2014). Currently, its use is recommended in the German, ESMO (European Society for Medical Oncology) and NCCN (National Comprehensive

Cancer Network) guidelines for high-risk soft tissue sarcomas (German Cancer Society, German Cancer Aid, AWMF 2022; European Society for Medical Oncology 2021; von Mehren et al. 2022). These are defined as sarcomas ≥5 cm and a grade of G3. Adjuvant radiation should begin 3–6 weeks after tumor resection has been performed, or immediately following adjuvant chemotherapy. In addition to adjuvant radiotherapy with a total dose of 60–66 Gy, there is also the option of neoadjuvant radiotherapy, especially for STS that are unlikely to be resected R0. In contrast to the adjuvant application, a lower total dose of 50 Gy is used here, since the tumor has not yet been resected and represents a smaller and better accessible target. However, acute wound complications occur significantly more frequently with neoadjuvant radiotherapy.

7.2 Adjuvant Chemotherapy

The decision of whether chemotherapy should be administered in the treatment of STS depends on many factors, the most crucial being the chemosensitivity of the sarcoma subtype. However adjuvant chemotherapy should not be given for small tumors <5 cm, whereas it should be discussed in STS > 5 cm with a high grading (G3). The combination of doxorubicin and ifosfamide is reported as first-line therapy. Regarding the study situation, there is still a lack of large-scale prospective comparative studies. However, several meta-analyses have been performed (Sarcoma Meta-analysis Collaboration (SMAC) 2000), the last one in 2008 concluding that adjuvant chemotherapy with doxorubicin and ifosfamide represents a significant advantage with regard to the risk of local recurrence as well as overall survival (Pervaiz et al. 2008). These results are in contrast to a large-scale study, which could not show a significant advantage with regard to local recurrence-free survival and overall survival after adjuvant chemotherapy (Woll et al. 2012). The decision for and against adjuvant chemotherapy should therefore always be made on an individual patient basis and after interdisciplinary consultation.

7.3 Neoadjuvant Chemotherapy

Neoadjuvant chemotherapy is also generally used for high-risk sarcomas. Here too, the combination of an anthracycline with ifosfamide is most commonly used. The benefit of this combination was recently examined in a large-scale randomized trial (Gronchi et al. 2020): STS patients with an indication for neoadjuvant chemotherapy received either the combination of anthracycline + ifosfamide or a histotype-tailored chemotherapy. The results showed no significant differences in terms of disease-free survival and overall survival.

7.4 Novel Treatment Approaches

A possible non-invasive therapeutic approach is deep regional hyperthermia. In this procedure, electromagnetic waves heat defined body and tumor areas to temperatures of 40–43 °C for 60 min. This temperature increase is intended to activate the body's own immune cells. The temperature is measured by interventional radiological probes inserted into the tumor. Regional deep hyperthermia is usually combined with neoadjuvant chemotherapy. Unfortunately, there is only a limited number of studies available. These see significantly better overall survival rates with the addition of deep regional hyperthermia. Whole-body thermotherapy currently plays no role in the treatment of STS.

In isolated limb perfusion (ILP), a separate blood circulation is established in the affected limb. This is usually done by vascular surgery. The extremity affected by the tumor thus receives a separate circulation. This circuit is then heated slightly, to temperatures of up to 40 °C. Furthermore, recombinant tumor necrosis factor α (rTNFα) in combination with melphalan is injected into this separate circuit. With this procedure, the study situation is also not clear. However, several studies and reviews have demonstrated the potential benefit of ILP (Bhangu et al. 2013; Martin-Tellez et al. 2020). It seems to be particularly useful in cases of questionable amputation and in palliative therapy situations. However, ILP has not yet been integrated into standard therapy.

Unlike in other tumor entities, immunotherapy has not yet played a leading role in STS. This is due to the enormous heterogeneity of these tumors among themselves as well as the intratumoral heterogeneity, which is why it is complex to identify vulnerable immune mechanisms. The basic idea of immunotherapy in STS is to strengthen the patient's immune system to such an extent that it is able to recognize the tumor as "foreign" or "harmful" and fight it accordingly. Tumors try to prevent this by blocking certain immune mechanisms. To put it simply, "taking the brakes off" the immune system is therefore the starting point of many immunotherapies (Ayodele and Razak 2020). One receptor that is involved in this immune response and serves as a starting point for immunotherapy is programmed cell death protein-1 (PD-1). This receptor is primarily found on T and B cells and leads to apoptosis of the affected immune cell when the receptor is activated by the corresponding ligand (programmed cell death 1 ligand 1). Nivolumab, pembrolizumab, toripalimab, and other monoclonal antibodies occupy the PD-1 receptor in order to prevent inactivation of the body's own immune cells. This study by Ayodele and colleagues (Ayodele and Razak 2020) provides a good overview of the various approaches to immunotherapy for STS and the clinical trials currently being conducted. The implementation of biobanks is therefore an important step toward obtaining as much information as possible about the various tumor entities and their individual immune status and mechanisms.

8 Conclusion

In the present text, the different soft tissue sarcoma entities have been briefly explained and the different therapeutic algorithms with any special features have been presented. Due to the rarity of STS, it is even more important that patients with these tumors are treated in a multidisciplinary manner in specialized sarcoma centers. Furthermore, there is an everlasting urge to establish new studies on sarcoma therapy, on a clinical and on an experimental level. Only in this way, patients can be offered an increasingly successful therapy with a manageable side effect profile.

Compliance with Ethical Standards The authors declare that they have no competing interests. No fundings were received for the writing of this work.

References

Ahmad R, Jacobson A, Hornicek F et al (2016) The width of the surgical margin does not influence outcomes in extremity and truncal soft tissue sarcoma treated with radiotherapy. Oncologist 21: 1269–1276. https://doi.org/10.1634/theoncologist.2015-0534

Akahoshi K, Oya M, Koga T, Shiratsuchi Y (2018) Current clinical management of gastrointestinal stromal tumor. World J Gastroenterol 24:2806–2817. https://doi.org/10.3748/wjg.v24.i26.2806

Alaggio R, Coffin CM, Weiss SW et al (2009) Liposarcomas in young patients: a study of 82 cases occurring in patients younger than 22 years of age. Am J Surg Pathol 33:645–658. https://doi.org/10.1097/PAS.0b013e3181963c9c

Arora TK, Terracina KP, Soong J et al (2014) Primary and secondary angiosarcoma of the breast. Gland Surg 3:28–34. https://doi.org/10.3978/j.issn.2227-684X.2013.12.03

Ayodele O, Razak ARA (2020) Immunotherapy in soft-tissue sarcoma. Curr Oncol 27:17–23. https://doi.org/10.3747/co.27.5407

Barrientos-Ruiz I, Ortiz-Cruz EJ, Serrano-Montilla J et al (2017) Are biopsy tracts a concern for seeding and local recurrence in sarcomas? Clin Orthop Relat Res 475:511–518. https://doi.org/10.1007/s11999-016-5090-y

Beane JD, Yang JC, White D et al (2014) Efficacy of adjuvant radiation therapy in the treatment of soft tissue sarcoma of the extremity: 20-year follow-up of a randomized prospective trial. Ann Surg Oncol 21:2484–2489. https://doi.org/10.1245/s10434-014-3732-4

Beris A, Gkiatas I, Gelalis I et al (2019) Current concepts in peripheral nerve surgery. Eur J Orthop Surg Traumatol 29:263–269. https://doi.org/10.1007/s00590-018-2344-2

Bhangu A, Broom L, Nepogodiev D et al (2013) Outcomes of isolated limb perfusion in the treatment of extremity soft tissue sarcoma: a systematic review. Eur J Surg Oncol J Eur Soc Surg Oncol Br Assoc Surg Oncol 39:311–319. https://doi.org/10.1016/j.ejso.2012.12.018

Bhatia K, Shiels MS, Berg A, Engels EA (2012) Sarcomas other than Kaposi sarcoma occurring in immunodeficiency: interpretations from a systematic literature review. Curr Opin Oncol 24: 537–546. https://doi.org/10.1097/CCO.0b013e328355e115

Bickels J, Wittig JC, Kollender Y, Kellar-Graney K, Malawer MM, Meller I (2002) Sciatic nerve resection: is that truly an indication for amputation? Clin Orthop Relat Res 399:201–204. PMID: 12011710

Billings SD, McKenney JK, Folpe AL et al (2004) Cutaneous angiosarcoma following breast-conserving surgery and radiation: an analysis of 27 cases. Am J Surg Pathol 28:781–788. https://doi.org/10.1097/01.pas.0000126055.33916.0b

Burningham Z, Hashibe M, Spector L, Schiffman JD (2012) The epidemiology of sarcoma. Clin Sarcoma Res 2:14. https://doi.org/10.1186/2045-3329-2-14

Cahlon O, Spierer M, Brennan MF et al (2008) Long-term outcomes in extremity soft tissue sarcoma after a pathologically negative re-resection and without radiotherapy. Cancer 112: 2774–2779. https://doi.org/10.1002/cncr.23493

Chang HR, Gaynor J, Tan C et al (1990) Multifactorial analysis of survival in primary extremity liposarcoma. World J Surg 14:610–618. https://doi.org/10.1007/BF01658804

Chang Y, Cesarman E, Pessin MS et al (1994) Identification of herpesvirus-like DNA sequences in AIDS-associated Kaposi's sarcoma. Science 266:1865–1869. https://doi.org/10.1126/science.7997879

Chen J-H, Lin L, Liu K-L et al (2020) Malignant glomus tumor of the intestinal ileum with multiorgan metastases: a case report and review of literature. World J Gastroenterol 26:770–776. https://doi.org/10.3748/wjg.v26.i7.770

Creytens D (2020) What's new in adipocytic neoplasia? Virchows Arch 476:29–39. https://doi.org/10.1007/s00428-019-02652-3

D'Angelo SP, Antonescu CR, Kuk D et al (2013) High-risk features in radiation-associated breast angiosarcomas. Br J Cancer 109:2340–2346. https://doi.org/10.1038/bjc.2013.590

Daigeler A, Kuhnen C, Moritz R et al (2009) Lymph node metastases in soft tissue sarcomas: a single center analysis of 1,597 patients. Langenbeck's Arch Surg 394:321–329. https://doi.org/10.1007/s00423-008-0371-x

Dei Tos AP (2006) Classification of pleomorphic sarcomas: where are we now? Histopathology 48: 51–62. https://doi.org/10.1111/j.1365-2559.2005.02289.x

Efstathopoulos N, Lazarettos J, Nikolaou V, Chronopoulos E (2006) Inflammatory leiomyosarcoma of the ankle: a case report and review of the literature. J Foot Ankle Surg Off Publ Am Coll Foot Ankle Surg 45:127–130. https://doi.org/10.1053/j.jfas.2005.12.010

Enneking WF, Spanier SS, Malawer MM (1981) The effect of the anatomic setting on the results of surgical procedures for soft parts sarcoma of the thigh. Cancer 47:1005–1022. https://doi.org/10.1002/1097-0142(19810301)47:5<1005::aid-cncr2820470532>3.0.co;2-9

ESMO/European Sarcoma Network Working Group (2021) Soft tissue and visceral sarcomas: ESMO clinical practice guidelines for diagnosis, treatment and follow-up. Ann Oncol Off J Eur Soc Med Oncol 25(Suppl 3):iii102–12. https://doi.org/10.1093/annonc/mdu254

Fiore M, Casali PG, Miceli R et al (2006) Prognostic effect of re-excision in adult soft tissue sarcoma of the extremity. Ann Surg Oncol 13:110–117. https://doi.org/10.1245/ASO.2006.03.030

Fletcher CD (1992) Pleomorphic malignant fibrous histiocytoma: fact or fiction? A critical reappraisal based on 159 tumors diagnosed as pleomorphic sarcoma. Am J Surg Pathol 16:213–228

Fujiki M, Kimura T, Takushima A (2020) Limb-salvage surgery with vascular reconstruction after lower extremity sarcoma resection: a systematic review and meta-analysis. Microsurgery 40: 404–413. https://doi.org/10.1002/micr.30553

Ganapathy S, Venkataramana NK, Nagaraj A et al (2023) Post-resection cavity lavage of high grade glioma with a novel drug combination: a case report. Anticancer Res 43:3583–3588. https://doi.org/10.21873/anticanres.16537

Gandhi J, Mehta S, Patel T et al (2017) Metastasis of soft tissue sarcomas in lymph node: a cytomorphological study. Diagn Cytopathol 45:784–788. https://doi.org/10.1002/dc.23754

German Guideline Program in Oncology (German Cancer Society, German Cancer Aid, AWMF) (2022) Soft tissue sarcoma long version 1.1. AWMF Registration Number: 032/044OL. https://www.leitlinienprogrammonkologie.de/leitlinien/adulte-weichgewebesarkome/. Accessed 15 Nov 2023

Gingrich AA, Bateni SB, Monjazeb AM et al (2017) Neoadjuvant radiotherapy is associated with R0 resection and improved survival for patients with extremity soft tissue sarcoma undergoing surgery: a national cancer database analysis. Ann Surg Oncol 24:3252–3263. https://doi.org/10.1245/s10434-017-6019-8

Gronchi A (2021) Surgery in soft tissue sarcoma: the thin line between a surgical or more conservative approach. Future Oncol 17:3–6. https://doi.org/10.2217/fon-2021-0449

Gronchi A, Lo Vullo S, Colombo C et al (2010) Extremity soft tissue sarcoma in a series of patients treated at a single institution: local control directly impacts survival. Ann Surg 251:506–511. https://doi.org/10.1097/SLA.0b013e3181cf87fa

Gronchi A, Palmerini E, Quagliuolo V et al (2020) Neoadjuvant chemotherapy in high-risk soft tissue sarcomas: final results of a randomized trial from Italian (ISG), Spanish (GEIS), French (FSG), and polish (PSG) sarcoma groups. J Clin Oncol Off J Am Soc Clin Oncol 38:2178–2186. https://doi.org/10.1200/JCO.19.03289

Gross JL, Younes RN, Haddad FJ et al (2005) Soft-tissue sarcomas of the chest wall: prognostic factors. Chest 127:902–908. https://doi.org/10.1378/chest.127.3.902

Harati K, Lehnhardt M (2017) The changing paradigm of resection margins in sarcoma resection. Innov Surg Sci 2:165–170. https://doi.org/10.1515/iss-2017-0043

Harati K, Goertz O, Pieper A et al (2017) Soft tissue sarcomas of the extremities: surgical margins can be close as long as the resected tumor has no ink on it. Oncologist 22:1400–1410. https://doi.org/10.1634/theoncologist.2016-0498

Herzog CE (2005) Overview of sarcomas in the adolescent and young adult population. J Pediatr Hematol Oncol 27:215–218. https://doi.org/10.1097/01.mph.0000161762.53175.e4

Hsu MC, Itkin M (2016) Lymphatic anatomy. Tech Vasc Interv Radiol 19:247–254. https://doi.org/10.1053/j.tvir.2016.10.003

Huvos AG (1986) Osteogenic sarcoma of bones and soft tissues in older persons. A clinicopathologic analysis of 117 patients older than 60 years. Cancer 57:1442–1449. https://doi.org/10.1002/1097-0142(19860401)57:7<1442::aid-cncr2820570734>3.0.co;2-3

Jebsen NL, Engellau J, Engström K et al (2013) Patterns of local recurrence and dose fractionation of adjuvant radiation therapy in 462 patients with soft tissue sarcoma of extremity and trunk wall. Int J Radiat Oncol Biol Phys 86:949–955. https://doi.org/10.1016/j.ijrobp.2013.04.015

Jørgensen MG, Toyserkani NM, Sørensen JA (2018) The effect of prophylactic lymphovenous anastomosis and shunts for preventing cancer-related lymphedema: a systematic review and meta-analysis. Microsurgery 38:576–585. https://doi.org/10.1002/micr.30180

Kawaguchi N, Ahmed AR, Matsumoto S et al (2004) The concept of curative margin in surgery for bone and soft tissue sarcoma. Clin Orthop Relat Res 165–172:165. https://doi.org/10.1097/00003086-200402000-00027

Kohashi K, Kinoshita I, Oda Y (2020) Soft tissue special issue: skeletal muscle tumors: a clinicopathological review. Head Neck Pathol 14:12–20. https://doi.org/10.1007/s12105-019-01113-2

Lehnhardt M, Sogorski A, Wallner C et al (2019) Soft tissue sarcomas: limb salvage using reconstructive plastic surgery techniques. Chirurg 90:94–101. https://doi.org/10.1007/s00104-018-0769-0

Lin PP, Pino ED, Normand AN et al (2007) Periosteal margin in soft-tissue sarcoma. Cancer 109: 598–602. https://doi.org/10.1002/cncr.22429

Liu H-L, Pang S-Y, Lee C-C (2019) Donor limb assessment after vascularized groin lymph node transfer for the treatment of breast cancer-related lymphedema: clinical and lymphoscintigraphy findings. J Plast Reconstr Aesthet Surg 72:216–224. https://doi.org/10.1016/j.bjps.2018.10.013

Longhi A, Bielack SS, Grimer R et al (2017) Extraskeletal osteosarcoma: a European musculoskeletal oncology society study on 266 patients. Eur J Cancer 74:9–16. https://doi.org/10.1016/j.ejca.2016.12.016

Martin-Tellez KS, van Houdt WJ, van Coevorden F et al (2020) Isolated limb perfusion for soft tissue sarcoma: current practices and future directions. A survey of experts and a review of literature. Cancer Treat Rev 88:102058. https://doi.org/10.1016/j.ctrv.2020.102058

McKee MD, Liu DF, Brooks JJ et al (2004) The prognostic significance of margin width for extremity and trunk sarcoma. J Surg Oncol 85:68–76. https://doi.org/10.1002/jso.20009

Mergancová J, Lierová A, Coufal O et al (2022) Radiation-associated angiosarcoma of the breast: an international multicenter analysis. Surg Oncol 41:101726. https://doi.org/10.1016/j.suronc.2022.101726

Moore PS, Chang Y (1995) Detection of herpesvirus-like DNA sequences in Kaposi's sarcoma in patients with and those without HIV infection. N Engl J Med 332:1181–1185. https://doi.org/10.1056/NEJM199505043321801

Nandra R, Forsberg J, Grimer R (2015) If your lump is bigger than a golf ball and growing, think sarcoma. Eur J Surg Oncol J Eur Soc Surg Oncol Br Assoc Surg Oncol 41:1400–1405. https://doi.org/10.1016/j.ejso.2015.05.017

Pervaiz N, Colterjohn N, Farrokhyar F et al (2008) A systematic meta-analysis of randomized controlled trials of adjuvant chemotherapy for localized resectable soft-tissue sarcoma. Cancer 113:573–581. https://doi.org/10.1002/cncr.23592

Poultsides GA, Tran TB, Zambrano E et al (2015) Sarcoma resection with and without vascular reconstruction: a matched case-control study. Ann Surg 262:632–640. https://doi.org/10.1097/SLA.0000000000001455

Ray-Coquard I, Montesco MC, Coindre JM et al (2012) Sarcoma: concordance between initial diagnosis and centralized expert review in a population-based study within three European regions. Ann Oncol Off J Eur Soc Med Oncol 23:2442–2449. https://doi.org/10.1093/annonc/mdr610

Ressing M, Wardelmann E, Hohenberger P et al (2018) Strengthening health data on a rare and heterogeneous disease: sarcoma incidence and histological subtypes in Germany. BMC Public Health 18:235. https://doi.org/10.1186/s12889-018-5131-4

Ronchi A, Cozzolino I, Zito Marino F et al (2020) Primary and secondary cutaneous angiosarcoma: distinctive clinical, pathological and molecular features. Ann Diagn Pathol 48:151597. https://doi.org/10.1016/j.anndiagpath.2020.151597

Rosenberg SA, Tepper J, Glatstein E et al (1982) The treatment of soft-tissue sarcomas of the extremities: prospective randomized evaluations of (1) limb-sparing surgery plus radiation therapy compared with amputation and (2) the role of adjuvant chemotherapy. Ann Surg 196:305–315. https://doi.org/10.1097/00000658-198209000-00009

Rubino C, Shamsaldin A, Lê MG et al (2005) Radiation dose and risk of soft tissue and bone sarcoma after breast cancer treatment. Breast Cancer Res Treat 89:277–288. https://doi.org/10.1007/s10549-004-2472-8

Salem O, Kurdi K, Joudeh A et al (2022) Malignant diffuse-type tenosynovial giant cell tumor in the subcutaneous tissue of the midthigh: a report of a rare tumor in an unusual location. Case Rep Orthop 2022:6986741

Sarcoma Meta-Analysis Collaboration (SMAC) (2000) Adjuvant chemotherapy for localised resectable soft tissue sarcoma in adults. Cochrane Datab Syst Rev (4):CD001419. https://doi.org/10.1002/14651858.CD001419. PMID: 11034717

Sbaraglia M, Bellan E, Dei Tos AP (2021) The 2020 WHO classification of soft tissue tumours: news and perspectives. Pathologica 113:70–84. https://doi.org/10.32074/1591-951X-213

Scaglioni MF, Meroni M, Fritsche E (2020) Lymphaticovenous anastomosis (LVA) for breast cancer-related lymphedema treatment. Transl Cancer Res 9:3167–3171

Selik RM, Starcher ET, Curran JW (1987) Opportunistic diseases reported in AIDS patients: frequencies, associations, and trends. AIDS 1:175–182

Serrano C, George S (2013) Leiomyosarcoma. Hematol Oncol Clin North Am 27:957–974. https://doi.org/10.1016/j.hoc.2013.07.002

Shavit E, Alavi A, Limacher JJ, Sibbald RG (2018) Angiosarcoma complicating lower leg elephantiasis in a male patient: an unusual clinical complication, case report and literature review. SAGE Open Med Case Reports 6:2050313X18796343

Simidjiiska-Belyaeva M, Belyaev O, Lehnhardt M et al (2019) Use of a self-contained vacuum-assisted biopsy system in the assessment of soft tissue tumors. J Surg Oncol 120:740–745. https://doi.org/10.1002/jso.25609

Stiller CA, Trama A, Serraino D et al (2013) Descriptive epidemiology of sarcomas in Europe: report from the RARECARE project. Eur J Cancer 49:684–695. https://doi.org/10.1016/j.ejca.2012.09.011

Stubbins RJ, Alami Laroussi N, Peters AC et al (2019) Epstein-Barr virus associated smooth muscle tumors in solid organ transplant recipients: incidence over 31 years at a single institution and review of the literature. Transpl Infect Dis an Off J Transplant Soc 21:e13010. https://doi.org/10.1111/tid.13010

Sweiti H, Tamimi N, Bormann F et al (2018) Limb-salvage surgery of soft tissue sarcoma with sciatic nerve involvement. Sarcoma 2018:6483579. https://doi.org/10.1155/2018/6483579

Toro JR, Travis LB, Hongyu JW et al (2006) Incidence patterns of soft tissue sarcomas, regardless of primary site, in the surveillance, epidemiology and end results program, 1978–2001: an analysis of 26,758 cases. Int J Cancer 119:2922–2930. https://doi.org/10.1002/ijc.22239

Viljoen N, Viljoen G, Fagan JJ, Govender D (2021) Inflammatory leiomyosarcoma of the head and neck: case report. Int J Surg Case Rep 82:105907. https://doi.org/10.1016/j.ijscr.2021.105907

von Mehren M, Kane JM, Agulnik M et al (2022) Soft tissue sarcoma, version 2.2022, NCCN clinical practice guidelines in oncology. J Natl Compr Cancer Netw 20:815–833. https://doi.org/10.6004/jnccn.2022.0035

Wagner JM, Dadras M, Ufton D et al (2022) Prophylactic lymphaticovenous anastomoses for resection of soft tissue tumors of the thigh to prevent secondary lymphedema-a retrospective comparative cohort analysis. Microsurgery 42:239–245. https://doi.org/10.1002/micr.30850

Wan R, Hussain A, Kuruoglu D et al (2023) Prophylactic lymphaticovenous anastomosis (LVA) for preventing lymphedema after sarcoma resection in the lower limb: a report of three cases and literature review. Microsurgery 43:273–280

Weskamp P, Ufton D, Drysch M et al (2022) Risk factors for occurrence and relapse of soft tissue sarcoma. Cancers (Basel) 14. https://doi.org/10.3390/cancers14051273

Willeumier JJ, Rueten-Budde AJ, Jeys LM et al (2017) Individualised risk assessment for local recurrence and distant metastases in a retrospective transatlantic cohort of 687 patients with high-grade soft tissue sarcomas of the extremities: a multistate model. BMJ Open 7:e012930. https://doi.org/10.1136/bmjopen-2016-012930

Williard WC, Hajdu SI, Casper ES, Brennan MF (1992) Comparison of amputation with limb-sparing operations for adult soft tissue sarcoma of the extremity. Ann Surg 215:269–275. https://doi.org/10.1097/00000658-199203000-00012

Woll PJ, Reichardt P, Le Cesne A et al (2012) Adjuvant chemotherapy with doxorubicin, ifosfamide, and lenograstim for resected soft-tissue sarcoma (EORTC 62931): a multicentre randomised controlled trial. Lancet Oncol 13:1045–1054. https://doi.org/10.1016/S1470-2045(12)70346-7

Wu JS, Goldsmith JD, Horwich PJ et al (2008) Bone and soft-tissue lesions: what factors affect diagnostic yield of image-guided core-needle biopsy? Radiology 248:962–970. https://doi.org/10.1148/radiol.2483071742

Yamamoto T, Yamamoto N, Kageyama T et al (2020) Technical pearls in lymphatic supermicrosurgery. Glob Heal Med 2:29–32. https://doi.org/10.35772/ghm.2019.01010

Young RJ, Brown NJ, Reed MW et al (2010) Angiosarcoma. Lancet Oncol 11:983–991. https://doi.org/10.1016/S1470-2045(10)70023-1

The Importance of Drug Interactions During ALK Tyrosine Kinase Inhibitor Therapies

Francesco Ferrara, Roberto Langella, Roberta Pasquinucci, Mariavaleria Ziccardi, Gabriele Bagaglini, Giacomo Polito, Alessando Ottaiano, Maurizio Capuozzo, and Andrea Zovi

Abstract

The term "drug-drug interaction" (DDI) generally describes the occurrence when the therapeutic or harmful effects of a medication are changed by the simultaneous or prior administration of other pharmacologically active substances. These interactions can be generally categorized into two primary types: pharmacokinetic interactions (PKIs) and pharmacodynamic interactions (PDIs). Internationally, lung cancer remains among the most widespread and lethal malignancies,

F. Ferrara (✉) · R. Pasquinucci · M. Capuozzo
Pharmaceutical Department, Nola, Naples, Italy
e-mail: f.ferrara@aslnapoli3sud.it; r.pasquinucci@aslnapoli3sud.it; m.capuozzo@aslnapoli3sud.it

R. Langella
Italian Society of Hospital Pharmacy (SIFO), SIFO Secretariat of the Lombardy Region, Milan, Italy
e-mail: roberto.langella87@gmail.com

M. Ziccardi
Pharmaceutical Department, Bari BA, Italy
e-mail: mariavaleria.ziccardi@asl.bari.it

G. Bagaglini
ASL Latina, Pharmacy Unit, Latina, Italy
e-mail: dott.gabrielebagaglini@hotmail.it

G. Polito
Policlinico Umberto I Hospital, Pharmacy Unit, Rome, Italy
e-mail: gpolito1988@gmail.com

A. Ottaiano
Istituto Nazionale Tumori di Napoli, IRCCS "G. Pascale", Naples, Italy
e-mail: a.ottaiano@istitutotumore.na.it

A. Zovi
Ministry of Health, Rome, Italy
e-mail: zovi.andrea@gmail.com

Interdisciplinary Cancer Research, https://doi.org/10.1007/16833_2024_364
Published online: 12 September 2024

predominantly presenting as non-small cell lung cancer (NSCLC). Over the years, various anaplastic lymphoma kinase (ALK) tyrosine kinase inhibitors (ALK-TKIs) have been formulated and swiftly integrated into the field of oncology for treating NSCLC. Crucially, intestinal CYP-450 enzymes play a pivotal role in metabolizing a diverse array of orally administered drugs, including ALK-TKIs. Hence, it is imperative to avoid their concurrent use with potent CYP3A inhibitors or inducers. Pharmacokinetic drug-drug interactions can occur at various phases of the drug-body interaction, including absorption, distribution, metabolism, and excretion. Multiple factors, including food, acid-reducing agents (ARAs), transporter inhibitors/inducers, and cytochrome P450 (CYP) inhibitors/inducers, may contribute to the induction of DDIs upon the ingestion of ALK-TKIs. Conversely, recent clinical evidence highlights the significance of addressing pharmacodynamic interactions when administering the ALK-TKI ceritinib. This chapter focuses on some potential DDIs associated with ALK-TKIs in clinical settings, underscoring the need to evaluate these interactions in patients undergoing ALK-TKI treatment. In essence, a systematic understanding of pharmacological interactions, especially concerning drug absorption, elimination, transport, and metabolism, can contribute to averting adverse effects of medications.

Keywords

Administration · Pharmacodynamic · Pharmacokinetic · Pharmacology · Receptor antagonism · Therapies · Tyrosine kinase

1 Introduction

The phrase "drug-drug interaction" (DDI) typically refers to the situation where the effects of a medication, whether therapeutic or harmful, are altered by the simultaneous or prior use of other medically active substances (Nidhi 2012). A drug-drug interaction occurs when the response to the concurrent intake of two or more medications differs from what would be expected based on the known effects of each individual drug, or simply put, when the effects of drug A are affected by the presence of drug B (Tragni et al. 2008; Leone et al. 2012; Mozayani and Raymon 2004; Goldberg et al. 1996). These alterations may result in increased toxicity of one or more drugs or, conversely, a decrease in their therapeutic effectiveness, leading to a significant reduction or even complete loss of their intended benefits. An interaction is considered significant when the combined response differs from the sum of the individual pharmacological actions (Tragni et al. 2008). The occurrence of a pharmacological interaction depends on various factors related to patient characteristics (such as age and gender), drug administration methods (such as dosage and route of administration), and the clinical setting in which the drugs are prescribed (such as hospitals and medical offices) (May et al. 1977). Interactions are broadly classified into two main types: pharmacokinetic interactions (PKIs) and

Table 1 Classification of DDIs according to Micromedex [10]

Contraindicated	Concurrent use of the drugs is not recommended due to contraindications
Major	The interaction could pose a life-threatening risk and/or necessitate medical intervention to mitigate or prevent severe adverse effects
Moderate	The interaction could lead to a deterioration in the patient's condition and/or necessitate a modification of the therapy
Minor	The interaction is anticipated to result in minimal clinical effects

pharmacodynamic interactions (PDIs). PKIs involve interferences that occur during the processes of drug absorption, distribution, metabolism, and excretion (ADME). These processes naturally vary between individuals, making these interactions difficult to predict. The challenge lies in understanding the pharmacokinetic behavior of all drugs and the practical impossibility of determining their extent and clinical significance in advance. In contrast, pharmacodynamic interactions involve the effects resulting from the specific pharmacological actions of drugs and are generally more predictable (Zheng et al. 2018). Pharmacokinetic interactions involve the alteration, by drug A, of the ADME process of another drug B (Nidhi 2012). The most common pharmacokinetic interactions relate to drug metabolism, particularly affecting phase I reactions where cytochrome P-450 isoenzymes play a crucial role. Enzymatic inducers enhance metabolism, while inhibitors decrease it, with clinical consequences depending on the metabolite involved, considering that drugs can be metabolized into active, inactive, or toxic forms. Regarding the elimination process, certain drugs can affect the pH of the endotubular fluid, active transport systems, and renal blood flow, thereby influencing the excretion of other drugs. Pharmacodynamic interactions, related to mechanisms of action, result in synergistic phenomena leading to an increased pharmacological effect (for example, drowsiness induced by the simultaneous use of benzodiazepines and antihistamines) or antagonism, resulting in a decrease in the pharmacological effect. Antagonisms (competitive or noncompetitive) can be pharmacological, where an antagonist prevents the binding of an agonist drug to its receptor (for example, naloxone vs. morphine), or functional, when two drugs exhibit opposing effects by acting on different receptors (Nidhi 2012; Tragni et al. 2008). One widely accepted classification is provided by the Micromedex database, which categorizes interactions based on severity (refer to Table 1). It also assigns a level of documentation, ranging from excellent to unknown, based on available literature evidence (Micromedex 2022).

2 The Role of Intestinal Cytochrome P-450 (Cytochrome P-450, CYP-450) Enzymes

The intestinal CYP-450 enzymes play a crucial role in metabolizing a wide range of orally administered medications, aiding significantly in their removal from the body through what is known as the first-pass effect (Thelen and Dressman 2009). These enzymes, found both in the liver and the intestine, collectively participate in the intricate process of drug metabolism, facilitating their elimination. Notably, CYP3A, comprising CYP3A4 and CYP3A5, and CYP2C9 are key players in intestinal drug metabolism, representing approximately 80% and 14% of total CYP enzymes, respectively (Xie et al. 2016). This dominance highlights their significance in determining the fate of orally ingested pharmaceutical agents. Interestingly, CYP3A activity demonstrates both similarities and differences between hepatic and intestinal levels. For example, certain substances like rifampicin act as potent inducers of CYP3A in both the liver and the intestine, emphasizing its role in drug metabolism across various anatomical sites. Conversely, the influence of grapefruit juice appears primarily limited to intestinal CYP3A, emphasizing the complex interplay between dietary components and drug metabolism (Thelen and Dressman 2009). An intriguing aspect of intestinal drug metabolism involves the collaboration between intestinal CYP enzymes and P-glycoprotein (P-GP), a critical efflux transporter. These entities, coexisting in the intestine, interact in a manner akin to a coordinated defense mechanism against excessive drug absorption. In the absence of efflux transporters, orally administered drugs would accumulate excessively in the intestine, potentially overwhelming CYP enzymes within the enterocytes. This saturation scenario could result in decreased metabolite production and increased release of unchanged drug into the bloodstream (Thelen and Dressman 2009). However, the cooperation between intestinal CYP enzymes and P-GP serves as a strategic safeguard, ensuring efficient and well-regulated drug metabolism. Consequently, this interaction between intestinal CYP enzymes and P-GP holds significant implications for first-pass elimination. Many orally administered drugs undergo substantial metabolism by these intestinal enzymes before entering systemic circulation. Consequently, a considerable portion of these drugs is effectively eliminated at this early stage, influencing their overall bioavailability. Additionally, drugs acting as substrates for intestinal CYP enzymes often exhibit lower bioavailability levels and heightened susceptibility to drug-drug interactions (DDIs). Interactions may arise when these drugs encounter other substances affecting CYP activity, such as inhibitors or inducers. This intricate interplay can lead to alterations in pharmacokinetics and therapeutic outcomes, highlighting the clinical importance of understanding the dynamics of intestinal drug metabolism. Intestinal CYP-450 enzymes emerge as crucial contributors in the realm of drug metabolism, significantly influencing the clearance and bioavailability of orally administered drugs. The intricate coordination between these enzymes and other factors, like efflux transporters, provides a comprehensive understanding of how drugs undergo processing within the body. The interplay between intestinal CYP enzymes and P-GP, combined with their susceptibility to DDIs, underscores the complexity inherent in drug interactions and emphasizes the necessity for a holistic approach in drug development and clinical practice (Xie et al. 2016).

3 ALK Tyrosine Kinase Inhibitors (ALK-TKIs) and DDI

On a global scale, lung cancer emerges as one of the most prevalent and lethal types of cancer, with non-small cell lung cancer (NSCLC) being the predominant subtype. NSCLC has been identified as being primarily fueled by various activated oncogenes, initially associated with mutations in the epidermal growth factor receptor (EGFR) and now also linked to mutations in the anaplastic lymphoma kinase (*ALK*) gene. To combat this, a range of ALK tyrosine kinase inhibitors (ALK-TKIs) have been developed, including ceritinib, crizotinib, alectinib, lorlatinib, brigatinib, and entrectinib (Ricciardi et al. 2020). Classified into first, second, and third generations, these ALK-TKIs have become crucial components of clinical practice, improving patients' quality of life due to their excellent oral bioavailability. Upon oral administration, crizotinib, ceritinib, alectinib, and entrectinib typically reach their median peak plasma concentration (Cmax) within 4–6 h, while brigatinib and lorlatinib achieve theirs within 1–4 h and 1.2–2 h, respectively. Despite the undeniable benefits of oral administration, a potential drawback lies in the increased susceptibility to drug-drug interactions (DDIs), influenced by patient variability and the risk of heightened toxicity or reduced efficacy. The potential for DDIs is particularly pertinent in elderly patients with comorbidities (Ricciardi et al. 2020; Marcath et al. 2018). DDIs impacting absorption can lead to incomplete drug absorption, resulting in reduced bioavailability or the first-pass effect (Nidhi 2012). Cancer patients, often receiving treatments such as proton pump inhibitors (PPIs), histamine H2-receptor antagonists (H2RAs), and antacids to manage gastric acid hypersecretion, face challenges due to the elevated gastric pH. This change can affect the solubility, absorption, and effectiveness of pH-dependent drugs, including ALK tyrosine kinase inhibitors (ALK-TKIs) (Marcath et al. 2018). Despite studies indicating a considerable decrease in ALK-TKI solubility at a pH above 6.5, the reduction in the area under the curve (AUC) under these circumstances is clinically insignificant, typically around 10%, and does not necessitate dose adjustments. The metabolism of all ALK-TKIs involves enzymes from the CYP-450 family, with CYP3A4 being the primary isoform, but other isoforms also play significant roles (see Table 2). Notably, CYP inhibitors and inducers significantly affect ALK-TKIs, and these TKIs also impact the exposure to other drugs, as shown in the provided tables (see Table 3). Except for alectinib, potent CYP3A inhibitors or inducers should be avoided when concurrently using crizotinib, brigatinib, lorlatinib, ceritinib, and entrectinib. If unavoidable, dose adjustments may be necessary. Furthermore, as potent CYP3A inhibitors themselves, these ALK-TKIs can substantially influence midazolam exposure. Beyond hepatic CYP enzymes, intestinal isoforms also contribute to drug metabolism, and their inhibition or induction can alter drug absorption, adding another layer of complexity to the understanding of ALK-TKI interactions (Ricciardi et al. 2020; Marcath et al. 2018).

Table 2 Pharmacological characteristics of ALK-TKIs

	Metabolism	CYP3A4/5	CYP2B6	CYP2C9	UGT	Glycoprotein -P
Alectinib (Bedi et al. 2018)	CYP3A4	Weak inhibitor	Weak inductor	Weak inductor	Weak inductor	Weak inhibitor
Brigatinib (Hamilton et al. 2015)	CYP3A4 e CYP2C8	Strong inductor	Weak inductor	Weak inductor	Weak inductor	Weak inhibitor
Ceritinib (Ardini et al. 2016)	CYP3A4 e CYP2C9	Strong inhibitor	Weak inhibitor	Weak inhibitor	Weak inhibitor	Weak inhibitor
Crizotinib SCP (2022)	CYP3A4 e CYP3A5	Moderate inhibitor	Moderate inhibitor	Moderate inhibitor	Weak inhibitor	Strong inhibitor
Entrectinib (Tagalakis et al. 2007)	CYP3A4	Weak inhibitor	Moderate inhibitor	Moderate inhibitor	Moderate inhibitor	Moderate inhibitor
Lorlatinib SCP (2022)	CYP3A4 e UGT1A4	Moderate inhibitor	Weak inductor	Weak inductor	Weak inductor	Moderate inhibitor

UGT1A4, UDP-glucuronisyltransferase 1A4; UGT, uridine diphosphate-glucuronosyltransferase

Table 3 Effects of CYP inhibitors and inducers on ALK-TKIs

Drugs	CYP enzymes		CClinical relevance	Recommendations
	Inhibitor	Inductor		
Crizotinib Hamilton et al. 2015	Ketoconazole Itraconazole		++	Refrain from simultaneous administration of potent CYP3A inhibitors; if concurrent use is inevitable, decrease the crizotinib dosage to 250 mg/day
	Diltiazem/ verapamil	Rifampicin	+− +	Exercise caution when employing moderate CYP3A inhibitors. Steer clear of concurrent use with potent CYP3A inhibitors
Ceritinib Numico et al. 2005	Ketoconazoloe Fluconazole		+−	Refrain from simultaneous use of potent CYP3A inhibitors; if unavoidable, decrease the dose to one third
		Rifampicin Efavirenz	+−	Steer clear of concurrent use with potent inducers of CYP3A
Alectinib Ng et al. 2019	Posaconazole		−	No adjustments to the dose are necessary when alectinib is coadministered with CYP3A inhibitors or inducers
		Rifampicin	−	
Brigatinib Sorigue and Miljkovic 2019; FDA 2022a	Itraconazole		+	Refrain from simultaneous use of potent CYP3A inhibitors; if unavoidable, decrease the once-daily dose of brigatinib by approximately 50%
	Diltiazem/ Verapamil		+	Steer clear of coadministration with moderate CYP3A inhibitors; if unavoidable, reduce the once-daily dose of brigatinib by approximately 40%
	Gemfibrozil		−	No dose adjustment is necessary when brigatinib is coadministered with CYP2C8 inhibitors
		Rifampicin efavirenz	++	Avoid the simultaneous use of strong or moderate CYP3A inducers; if coadministration is unavoidable, adjust brigatinib as follows: increase the daily dose in 30 mg increments after

(continued)

Table 3 (continued)

				7 days of treatment, up to a maximum of two times the initial brigatinib dose
Loratinib Xu et al. 2015	Itraconazole		+	Refrain from coadministering strong CYP3A inhibitors; if simultaneous use is unavoidable, decrease the initial dose of lorlatinib from 100 mg to 75 mg, and further reduce it to 50 mg if adverse reactions occur at the 75 mg dose
		Rifampicin	+	Steer clear of coadministration with potent CYP3A inducers
Entrectinib Bedi et al. 2018	Itraconazole Erythromycin		+ +	For adults and pediatric patients aged 12 and older with a body surface area (BSA) exceeding 1.5 m2, it is advised to refrain from coadministering entrectinib with moderate or strong CYP3A inhibitors. If coadministration cannot be avoided, a recommended dosage of entrectinib is 100 mg for strong CYP3A4 inhibitors and 200 mg once daily for moderate CYP3A4 inhibitors For pediatric patients aged 12 and older with a body surface area (BSA) less than or equal to 1.5 m2, it is recommended to steer clear of coadministration with moderate or strong CYP3A inhibitors
		Rifampicin	+	Steer clear of coadministration with moderate or strong CYP3A inducers
		Efavirenz	+	Refrain from coadministration with moderate or strong CYP3A inducers

4 Focus: Interactions of ALK-TKIS with Direct Oral Anticoagulants (DOACS)

It is widely recognized that about one sixth of NSCLC patients are at increased risk of venous thromboembolism (VTE) and other thromboembolic complications, alongside a higher incidence of stroke and atrial fibrillation (Tagalakis et al. 2007; Numico et al. 2005; Ng et al. 2019; Puurunen et al. 2016; Sorigue and Miljkovic 2019). Therefore, preventing and managing thromboembolism is a significant clinical concern. Currently, direct oral anticoagulants (DOACs) are the standard treatment for VTE and for preventing thromboembolic complications in atrial fibrillation. DOACs, also referred to as "new" or "direct" oral anticoagulants, such as apixaban, edoxaban, rivaroxaban, and dabigatran, work by directly inhibiting factor Xa activation or the reversible activation of factor II. These agents offer efficacy, safety, and convenience compared to low molecular weight heparins (LMWHs) or vitamin K antagonists (VKAs). Unlike LMWHs and VKAs, which require daily subcutaneous injections or regular monitoring of the international normalized ratio, DOACs can be taken orally without the need for frequent monitoring (Sorigue and Miljkovic 2019). With the widespread use of DOACs in clinical practice, it is crucial to evaluate potential drug-drug interactions (DDIs) with other medications that patients with non-valvular atrial fibrillation (NVAF) might require, including ALK tyrosine kinase inhibitors (ALK-TKIs) in this context (see Table 4) (Tagalakis et al. 2007; Numico et al. 2005; Ng et al. 2019; Puurunen et al. 2016; Sorigue and Miljkovic 2019; FDA 2022a). Table 4 also includes potential DDIs with betrixaban, an FDA-approved drug for long-term thromboprophylaxis in patients with acute medical illnesses. Understanding these interactions is essential for ensuring the safe and effective coadministration of these medications in the complex therapeutic regimens of patients with NSCLC and associated thromboembolic risks.

5 Distribution

The distribution of a drug within the body is a crucial factor in determining its therapeutic effectiveness and potential interactions. This intricate process relies on two main elements: blood flow and the drug's affinity for plasma proteins. The latter is particularly significant in influencing a drug's ability to traverse cell membranes, permeate tissues, and exert its intended biological effects. In the case of anaplastic lymphoma kinase tyrosine kinase inhibitors (ALK-TKIs) like alectinib, crizotinib, brigatinib, ceritinib, and entrectinib, their interaction with plasma proteins plays a vital role in their distribution dynamics. These targeted therapies have a notable tendency to bind to various plasma proteins such as albumin, α1-acid lipoproteins, glycoproteins, and immunoglobulins. This binding is crucial in determining the fraction of the drug that remains free and unbound in the bloodstream, capable of traversing biological barriers and interacting with target tissues. An important phenomenon related to protein binding is the potential displacement of one drug by another from its binding site. This interaction can lead to changes in the

Table 4 Potential interactions of ALK-TKIs with DOACs [21][1]

	DOACs				
ALK-TKIs	Apixaban	Rivaroxaban	Betrixaban	Dabigatran	Edoxaban
Alectinib	Reduce the dose by 25%	Strongly contraindicated	Strongly contraindicated	Administer dabigatran 2 h before the dose of ALK-TKIs	Reduced interaction
Brigatinib	Strongly contraindicated				Strongly contraindicated
Ceritinib	Reduce the dose by 50%				Reduced interaction
Crizotinib	Reduce the dose by 25%				Reduced interaction
Entrectinib	Reduced interaction				Reduced interaction
Lorlatinib	Strongly contraindicated			Increase the dose of dabigatran by 200%	Reduced interaction

concentration of the displaced drug's unbound form, potentially influencing its distribution and apparent volume within the body. For highly protein-bound drugs like ALK-TKIs, interactions with similarly protein-bound drugs like phenytoin and warfarin are conceivable, potentially impacting their distribution characteristics (Xu et al. 2015; FDA 2022b; Hofman et al. 2019). However, the clinical relevance of these protein-binding site displacements is not always straightforward. While changes in protein binding can influence pharmacokinetics, the overall impact on exposure might be relatively minor. In practice, the potential for such interactions to significantly alter drug exposure is limited, despite the theoretical basis for these interactions. Furthermore, drug distribution within various tissues is regulated by transporters present on cell membranes. Alterations in the activity of these transporters can significantly influence the distribution patterns of drugs. For instance, P-glycoprotein (P-GP), a transporter that effluxes drugs out of cells, influences the distribution of crizotinib, contributing to its limited efficacy against brain metastases. However, concurrent administration of crizotinib with elacridar, a dual inhibitor of P-GP and breast cancer resistance protein (BCRP), has been shown to enhance the drug's accumulation within the brain. Similarly, the brain distribution of ceritinib, constrained by P-GP and BCRP, can be enhanced by coadministration with inhibitors of these transporters. In contrast, certain ALK-TKIs like lorlatinib, alectinib, and entrectinib are not substrates for P-GP and BCRP, allowing them to efficiently penetrate the blood-brain barrier (BBB) and target brain metastases associated with ALK-positive cancers. In summary, understanding the distribution intricacies of ALK-TKIs and their potential interactions is crucial for optimizing therapeutic outcomes and avoiding adverse effects. The interplay between protein binding, transporters, and the complex physiological environments of different tissues collectively contributes to the overall efficacy and safety profile of these targeted therapies (Hofman et al. 2019).

6 Drug Transporters

Transporters play a pivotal role in the membrane transport of various drugs, affecting processes like intestinal tissue distribution, hepatic absorption, and biliary and renal excretion. Their inhibition or induction can profoundly influence drug pharmacokinetics, causing changes in absorption, distribution, metabolism, and elimination. These transporters are widely distributed throughout the body, with a significant presence in the intestine, liver, kidneys, and the blood-brain barrier (BBB). They can be broadly categorized into two major families: ATP-binding cassette (ABC) transporters, named for their ATP-binding domain, and solute carrier transporters (SLCs). ABC transporters primarily function as drug efflux transporters, including P-glycoprotein (P-GP), multidrug resistance protein 2 (MRP2), and breast cancer resistance protein (BCRP). Conversely, SLC transporters act as drug influx transporters and include organic anion transporting peptides (OATPs), organic anion transporters (OATs), and organic cation transporters (OCTs). The potential for drug-drug interactions (DDIs) between drug transporters and ALK tyrosine

Table 5 The possible DDIs between drug transporters and ALK-TKIs

ALK-TKIs	Substrates	Recommendations
Crizotinib	P-GP, OATP1B1/3, OATP2B1, OCT2	Not available
Ceritinib	P-GP (MAJOR) BCRP (WEAK)	The European Medicines Agency (EMA) recommends exercising caution when concurrently using P-glycoprotein (P-GP) inhibitors and inducers
Alectinib	Not available	According to the European Medicines Agency (EMA), clinically significant drug-drug interactions (DDIs) with P-glycoprotein (P-GP) inhibitors and inducers are unlikely to occur frequently
Brigatinib	P-GP, BCRP	As per the guidance from the US Food and Drug Administration (FDA) and the European Medicines Agency (EMA), there is no need for dose adjustment for brigatinib when it is coadministered with P-glycoprotein (P-GP) and breast cancer resistance protein (BCRP) inhibitors
Lorlatinib	Not available	According to the European Medicines Agency (EMA), there is a low likelihood of clinically relevant drug-drug interactions (DDIs) occurring with P-glycoprotein (P-GP) and breast cancer resistance protein (BCRP) inhibitors or inducers
Entrectinib	Not available	Not available

kinase inhibitors (ALK-TKIs) is outlined in Table 5, while potential DDIs between ALK-TKIs and other transporter substrates are detailed in Table 6. Since hepatic elimination is the primary route for eliminating ALK-TKIs, the inhibition or induction of hepatic transporters and CYP enzymes can impact the excretion of the drugs involved, potentially leading to clinically relevant DDIs. Notably, alectinib and lorlatinib, being non-transporter substrates, are not expected to be significantly affected by coadministration with transporter inhibitors or inducers. Given that the liver and kidneys are the primary organs for drug elimination, renal or hepatic insufficiency can give rise to DDIs. Conditions such as renal or hepatic insufficiency can significantly impact the pharmacokinetics of drugs and lead to potential DDIs (EMA 2022a, b, c; Omote et al. 2018; FDA 2022c). Understanding these interactions is critical for ensuring the safe and effective coadministration of ALK-TKIs with other drugs, optimizing therapeutic outcomes and minimizing the risk of adverse effects.

7 Effects of Food on the Absorption of ALK-TKIS

Food-drug interactions can result in one of four pharmacokinetic effects on the absorption of an administered drug: increase, delay, decrease, or no effect, as highlighted by Koziolek et al. in 2019. These effects arise from various mechanisms, including alterations in gastrointestinal pH, bile salt secretion, gastric emptying time,

Table 6 The potential DDIs between ALK-TKIs and other transporter substrates

ALK-TKIs	Inhibitor	Recommendations
Crizotinib	P-GP, OCT1/2, OATP1B1/3, OATP2B1, OATP4C1, MATE1, MATE2-K	The European Medicines Agency (EMA) advises careful clinical surveillance when employing substances that are substrates for interactions, suggesting a cautious approach to monitoring in such cases
Ceritinib	P-GP, BCRP, OATP1B1/3, OAT1, OCT2	The European Medicines Agency (EMA) recommends exercising caution when using substrates concurrently, emphasizing careful consideration in such cases
Alectinib	P-GP, BCRP, BSEP	According to the European Medicines Agency (EMA), it is advisable to implement appropriate monitoring when coadministering with these substrates, emphasizing the importance of vigilant oversight in such situations
Brigatinib	P-GP, BCRP, OCT1, MATE1, MATE2-K	The European Medicines Agency (EMA) advises careful monitoring of patients when using substrates with a low therapeutic index concomitantly, highlighting the importance of vigilant observation in such cases
Lorlatinib	P-GP, OCT1, OAT3, MATE1, OATP1B1/3, BCRP	NA
Entrectinib	P-GP, BCRP, OATP1B1, and MATE1	According to New Drug Application (NDA) information, there is no need for dose adjustment of P-glycoprotein (P-GP) substrates when coadministered with entrectinib

Table 7 Effect of food on the absorption of ALK-TKIs

ALK-TKIs	BCS	Dose	Condition	Clinical relevance	Recommendations
Alectinib	4	600 mg single dose	Rich meal	No	Taking with or without food
Brigatinib	1	180 mg single dose	High-fat meal	No	Taking with or without food
Ceritinib	4	500 mg single dose	High-fat meal, Low-fat meal	Yes	Take in with food
		750 mg single dose	High-fat meal, Low-fat meal	Yes	Take in with food
		450 mg multiple dose	Low-fat meal	Yes	Take in with food
Crizotinib	4	250 mg single dose	High-fat meal	No	Taking with or without food
Entrectinib	2	600 mg single dose	High-fat meal	No	Taking with or without food
Lorlatinib	4	100 mg single dose	High-fat meal	No	Taking with or without food

BCS *Biopharmaceutics Classification System*

hepatic and gastrointestinal fluid flow, drug transporter activity, intestinal enzyme activity, and drug binding. The decision of whether to take a specific orally administered drug with or without food is influenced by these factors, presenting potential advantages and disadvantages in patients' daily lives. Table 7 delineates the primary effects of food on the absorption of ALK tyrosine kinase inhibitors (ALK-TKIs). Ceritinib and alectinib show significantly increased absorption when taken with meals, and it is recommended to administer them accordingly. On the other hand, crizotinib, brigatinib, lorlatinib, and entrectinib are believed to be minimally affected by food, and their administration is independent of meals. Specifically, ceritinib is recommended to be taken with food at a daily dose of 450 mg. In cases where patients cannot take ceritinib with food due to concurrent conditions, an alternative regimen with administration on an empty stomach is allowed. The dose should be adjusted accordingly, with an increase to 750 mg or 450 mg on an empty stomach for patients initially treated with 450 mg or 300 mg on a full stomach, respectively. If the initial treatment is 150 mg on a full stomach, the treatment should be suspended (Cho et al. 2017). Additionally, caution should be exercised to avoid the concurrent intake of grapefruit and/or grapefruit juice with ceritinib, as it can inhibit CYP3A in the intestinal wall, potentially increasing ceritinib bioavailability (Cholewka-Stafinska et al. 2017). Crizotinib, classified as a Biopharmaceutics Classification System (BCS) class 4 compound, can be taken independently of meals. Ceritinib, a BCS class 4 compound, shows increased absorption when taken with both high-fat and low-fat meals, with the recommended dose being 450 mg orally once a day with food (Tugnait et al. 2019; FDA 2022d; Otoukesh et al. 2019; EMA 2022d, e; FDA 2022e; Otten et al. 2022). Alectinib exhibits a substantial increase in AUC and Cmax when taken with a high-fat meal, highlighting the importance of considering food effects in its administration. Brigatinib, classified as a BCS class 1 compound, can be taken independently of meals, as its AUC and Cmax show minimal changes when administered with a high-fat meal (Tugnait et al. 2019; FDA 2022d; Otten et al. 2022). Lorlatinib, a BCS class 4 compound, is not significantly affected by food, allowing for independent administration (EMA 2022e; FDA 2022e; Otten et al. 2022). Entrectinib, classified as a BCS class 2 compound, shows no significant food effect on exposure, permitting administration without regard to food (Otten et al. 2022). Understanding these food-drug interactions is crucial for optimizing the therapeutic efficacy and safety of ALK-TKIs, providing valuable guidance to healthcare providers and patients in their daily management.

8 Pharmacodynamic Interactions

Recent clinical studies (Raedler 2015; Shaw et al. 2014; Hurtado et al. 2021; Santoro et al. 2022) consistently identify a significant prolongation of the QT interval as an adverse effect associated with ceritinib, a tyrosine kinase inhibitor widely used in targeted cancer therapy. This observation underscores the importance of exercising caution when administering ceritinib, particularly in patients with preexisting or potential risks of QT interval prolongation. The QT interval, reflecting the electrical depolarization and repolarization of the heart's ventricles, is a crucial parameter for evaluating cardiac rhythm. Prolongation of the QT interval can potentially lead to a life-threatening arrhythmia known as Torsades de Pointes. Given the clinical implications, special attention is warranted for patients concurrently using antiarrhythmic drugs due to the potential for pharmacodynamic interactions. Antiarrhythmic drugs are categorized into class I (e.g., quinidine, procainamide, and disopyramide) and class III (e.g., amiodarone, sotalol, dofetilide, and ibutilide) medications. Coadministration of ceritinib with these drugs requires careful monitoring and, when appropriate, dose adjustments to prevent excessive QT interval prolongation. The concern for potential interactions extends to other pharmaceutical agents identified as QT-prolonging, including domperidone, droperidol, chloroquine, halofantrine, clarithromycin, haloperidol, methadone, cisapride, and moxifloxacin. Combining ceritinib with any of these compounds heightens the risk of QT interval prolongation and associated cardiac complications. Therefore, a comprehensive assessment of the patient's medication profile is crucial before introducing ceritinib, especially when these agents are part of the treatment regimen. In cases where a combination of these medications is deemed necessary, close and vigilant monitoring of the QT interval is imperative. Regular electrocardiographic assessments should be conducted to promptly detect any abnormalities and mitigate potential cardiac complications. Collaborative efforts between oncologists, cardiologists, and other medical professionals are crucial to ensure the safe and effective use of ceritinib within the context of complex medication regimens. In conclusion, the emerging evidence from clinical studies underscores the significance of considering pharmacodynamic interactions when administering ceritinib. The potential for QT interval prolongation, especially in combination with antiarrhythmic drugs or other agents with QT-prolonging effects, necessitates a meticulous evaluation of the patient's medical history and medication regimen. This proactive approach, coupled with regular QT interval monitoring, is pivotal in minimizing the risks associated with cardiac arrhythmias and ensuring the well-being of patients undergoing ceritinib treatment (Snyder et al. 2012; Roskoski 2017; Morcos et al. 2017; Mao et al. 2013).

9 Conclusion

Article 32 of the Italian Constitution underscores health as a fundamental right of individuals and a matter of community interest. It places the responsibility on health authorities to ensure access to quality care, equitable service access, and efficient resource use. This involves the rational allocation of limited resources and the avoidance of wastage, particularly in drug use. A healthcare system prioritizing patient safety and efficient resource management must actively monitor prescriber adherence to quality criteria to prevent inappropriate drug use and mitigate undesirable consequences. A thorough understanding of pharmacological interactions, particularly in drug absorption, elimination, transport, and metabolism, is essential for averting adverse effects. Predicting pharmacodynamic interactions requires a profound understanding of the underlying mechanisms driving side effects, which is vital for enhancing patient safety and optimizing healthcare outcomes. The increasing prevalence of multiple drug use among older patients with multimorbidity underscores the importance of predicting pharmacokinetic interactions. Anaplastic lymphoma kinase tyrosine kinase inhibitors (ALK-TKIs) have become integral in oncological practice. Variations in the pharmacokinetics of crizotinib, ceritinib, alectinib, brigatinib, lorlatinib, and entrectinib highlight differences in absorption, metabolism, distribution, and excretion. Several clinically significant drug-drug interactions (DDIs) have been reported due to the inhibition or induction of hepatic CYP enzymes. Except for alectinib, CYP inhibitors and inducers can significantly impact the exposure of ALK-TKIs, leading to clinically relevant DDIs. Concomitant use of strong CYP3A inhibitors or inducers with crizotinib, ceritinib, brigatinib, lorlatinib, and entrectinib should be avoided, and dose adjustments are necessary if unavoidable. All six ALK-TKIs act as CYP3A inhibitors, with some, like crizotinib, ceritinib, brigatinib, and lorlatinib, influencing the exposure of midazolam. Clinical intervention is required when these ALK-TKIs are coadministered with other CYP3A substrates. Intestinal CYP enzymes are also involved in drug metabolism, and their inhibition or induction can alter drug absorption. For instance, grapefruit, acting as an intestinal CYP inhibitor, can increase the bioavailability of ALK-TKIs and should be avoided during treatment. In summary, pharmacokinetic DDIs can occur at every stage of drug-body interaction, and various agents can precipitate the onset of DDIs. The article emphasizes the importance of assessing DDIs in patients undergoing treatment with ALK-TKIs, and the adoption of electronic prescribing systems is recommended to inform users of possible interactions, providing support for clinicians and hospital pharmacists in choosing appropriate therapy and dosage, considering potential risks associated with poly-prescription.

Ethical Approval Not applicable.

Consent to Participate Not applicable.

Consent to Publish The authors consent to the publication of the chapter.

Authors' Contributions

FF Conceptualization, writing—original draft, methodology, supervision, validation
RL Writing—review and editing; MB: Supervision, validation
RP Supervision, validation
MZ Supervision, validation
GB Supervision, validation
GP Conceptualization, writing—original draft
AO Supervision, validation
MC Writing—review and editing; MB: Supervision, validation
AZ Writing—review and editing; MB: Supervision, validation

Availability of Data and Materials Full availability of data and materials. All stated data can be provided on request to the reader.

Code Availability Not applicable.

Declaration of Competing Interest The authors declare that they have no known competing financial interests or personal relationships that could have appeared to influence the work reported in this chapter.

The authors declare that the opinions expressed are of a personal nature and do not in any way commit the responsibility of the administrations to which they belong.

Funding No funding was received to conduct this study.

References

Ardini E, Menichincheri M, Banfi P, Bosotti R, De Ponti C, Pulci R et al (2016) Entrectinib, a Pan-TRK, ROS1, and ALK Inhibitor with Activity in Multiple Molecularly Defined Cancer Indications. Mol Cancer Ther 15(4):628–639

Bedi S, Khan SA, AbuKhader MM, Alam P, Siddiqui NA, Husain A (2018) A comprehensive review on Brigatinib – a wonder drug for targeted cancer therapy in non-small cell lung cancer. Saudi Pharm J 26(6):755–763

Cho BC, Kim DW, Bearz A, Laurie SA, McKeage M, Borra G et al (2017) ASCEND-8: a randomized phase 1 Study of Ceritinib, 450 mg or 600 mg, taken with a low-fat meal versus 750 mg in fasted state in patients with anaplastic lymphoma kinase (ALK)-Rearranged Metastatic Non-Small Cell Lung Cancer (NSCLC). J Thorac Oncol 12(9):1357–1367

Cholewka-Stafinska M, Polaniak R, Kardas M, Grajek M, Grochowska-Niedworok E (2017) Interaction of oral form anticancer drugs with grapefruit juice. Pol Merkur Lekarski 42(247): 30–33

European Medicines Agency EMA (2022a) Assessment report. Disponibile on line: https://www.ema.europa.eu/en/documents/assessment-report/alecensa-epar-public-assessment-report_en.pdf. Last access 9 Sept 2022

European Medicines Agency EMA (2022b) Multi-discipline review. Disponibile on line: https://www.accessdata.fda.gov/drugsatfda_docs/nda/2019/212725Orig1s000,%20212726Orig1s000MultidisciplineR.pdf. Last access 9 Sept 2022

European Medicines Agency EMA (2022c) Multi-discipline review. Disponibile on line: https://www.accessdata.fda.gov/drugsatfda_docs/nda/2018/210868Orig1s000MultidisciplineR.pdf. Last access 9 Sept 2022

European Medicines Agency EMA (2022d) Product information. Disponibile on line: https://www.ema.europa.eu/en/documents/product-information/xalkori-epar-product-information_en.pdf. Last access 9 Sept 2022

European Medicines Agency EMA (2022e) Product information. Disponibile on line: https://www.ema.europa.eu/en/documents/product-information/zykadia-epar-product-information_en.pdf. Last access 9 Sept 2022

Goldberg RM, Mabee J, Chan L, Wong S (1996) Drug-drug and drug disease interactions in ED: analysis of high risk population. Am J Emerg Med 14(5):450–477

Hamilton G, Rath B, Burghuber O (2015) Pharmacokinetics of crizotinib in NSCLC patients. Expert Opin Drug Metab Toxicol 11(5):835–842

Hofman J, Sorf A, Vagiannis D, Sucha S, Novotna E, Kammerer S, Küpper JH, Ceckova M, Staud F (2019) Interactions of Alectinib with Human ATP-Binding Cassette Drug Efflux Transporters and Cytochrome P450 Biotransformation Enzymes: Effect on Pharmacokinetic Multidrug Resistance. Drug Metab Dispos 47(7):699–709. https://doi.org/10.1124/dmd.119.086975

Hurtado FK, De Braud F, De Castro CJ, Luken MJ, Wang D et al (2021) Effect of ceritinib on the pharmacokinetics of coadministered CYP3A and 2C9 substrates: a phase I, multicenter, drug-

drug interaction study in patients with ALK + advanced tumors. Cancer Chemother Pharmacol 87:475–486

Koziolek M, Alcaro S, Augustijns P, Basit AW, Grimm M, Hens B et al (2019) The mechanisms of pharmacokinetic food-drug interactions – a perspective from the UNGAP group. Eur J Pharm Sci 134:31–59

Leone R, Magro L, De Salvia A (2012) Rilevanza clinica e aspetti medico-legali delle interazioni tra farmaci. Pratica Medica Aspetti Legali 6(2):43–50

Mao J, Johnson TR, Shen Z, Yamazaki S (2013) Prediction of crizotinib-midazolam interaction using the Simcyp population-based simulator: comparison of CYP3A time dependent inhibition between human liver microsomes versus hepatocytes. Drug Metab Dispos 41(2):343–352

Marcath LA, Coe TD, Hoylman EK, Redman BG, Hertz DL (2018) Prevalence of drug-drug interactions in oncology patients enrolled on National Clinical Trials Network oncology clinical trials. BMC Cancer 18:1155

May FE, Stewart RB, Cluff LE (1977) Drug interactions and multiple drug administration. Clin Pharmacol Ther 22:322–328

Micromedex® Healthcare Series. Thomson Reuters (Healthcare) Inc, Greenwood Village. Last access 9 Sept 2022

Morcos PN, Cleary Y, Guerini E, Dall G, Bogman K, De Petris L et al (2017) Clinical drug-drug interactions through cytochrome P450 3A (CYP3A) for the selective ALK inhibitor alectinib. Clin Pharmacol Drug Dev 6(3):280–291

Mozayani A, Raymon L (2004) Handbook of drug interactions: a clinical and forensic guide, 1st edn. Humana Press, Totowa

Ng TL, Smith DE, Mushtaq R, Patil T, Dimou A, Yang S et al (2019) ROS1 gene rearrangements are associated with an elevated risk of peridiagnosis thromboembolic events. J Thorac Oncol 14(4):596–605

Nidhi S (2012) Concept of drug interaction. Int Res J Pharm 3:120–122

Numico G, Garrone O, Dongiovanni V, Silvestris N, Colantonio I, Di Costanzo G et al (2005) Prospective evaluation of major vascular events in patients with nonsmall cell lung carcinoma treated with cisplatin and gemcitabine. Cancer 103(5):994–999

Omote S, Matsuoka N, Arakawa H, Nakanishi T, Tamai I (2018) Effect of tyrosine kinase inhibitors on renal handling of creatinine by MATE1. Sci Rep 8(1):9237

Otoukesh S, Sanchez T, Mirshahidi S, Wallace D, Mirshahidi H (2019) ASCEND-8- pharmacokinetic, safety, and efficacy data for ceritinib 450 mg with food in patients with anaplastic lymphoma kinase-positive non-small cell lung Cancer: a clinical perspective. Cancer Treat Res Commun 20:100149

Otten LS, Piet B, van den Heuvel M, Marzolini C, van Geel RM, Gulikers JL et al (2022) Practical recommendations to combine small-molecule inhibitors and direct oral anticoagulants in patients with nonsmall cell lung cancer. Eur Respir Rev 31:220004

Puurunen MK, Gona PN, Larson MG, Murabito JM, Magnani JW, O'Donnel CJ (2016) Epidemiology of venous thromboembolism in the Framingham Heart Study. Thromb Res 145:27–33

Raedler LA (2015) Zykadia (Ceritinib) approved for patients with crizotinib-resistant ALK-positive non small cell lung cancer. Am Health Drug Benefits 8:163–166

Ricciardi S, Cecere F, D'Andrea MR, D'Argento E, Gelibter JA, Giusti R et al (2020) Target therapies nel tumore al polmone ALK-positivo: gestione del trattamento nei centri di oncologia del Lazio Incontro di approfondimento e confronto sulla gestione dei pazienti e sulla strategia terapeutica nei carcinomi polmonari positivi al riarrangiamento di ALK. Recenti Prog Med 111(12):e63–e69

Roskoski R Jr (2017) Anaplastic lymphoma kinase (ALK) inhibitors in the treatment of ALK-driven lung cancers. Pharmacol Res 117:343–356

Santoro A, Su WC, Navarro A, Simonelli M, Yang JC, Ardizzoni A (2022) Phase Ib/II study of ceritinib in combination with ribociclib in patients with ALK-rearranged non–small cell lung cancer. Lung Cancer 166:170–177

Shaw AT, Kim D, Mehra R, Tan D, Felip E, Chow L et al (2014) Ceritinib in ALK-rearranged non small cell lung cancer. Am Health Drug Benefits 370:1189–1197

Snyder BD, Polasek TM, Doogue MP (2012) Drug interactions: principles and practice. Aust Prescr 35:85–88

Sorigue M, Miljkovic MD (2019) Atrial fibrillation and stroke risk in patients with cancer: a primer for oncologists. J Oncol Pract 15(12):641–650

Summary of Product Characteristics (SPC) – Lorlatinib. https://www.ema.europa.eu/en/documents/product-information/lorviqua-epar-product-information_it.pdf. Last access 9 Sept 2022

Tagalakis V, Levi D, Agulnik JS, Cohen V, Kasymjanova G, Small D (2007) High risk of deep vein thrombosis in patients with non-small cell lung cancer: a cohort study of 493 patients. J Thorac Oncol 2(8):729–734

Thelen K, Dressman JB (2009) Cytochrome P450-mediated metabolism in the human gut wall. J Pharm Pharmacol 61(5):541–558

Tragni E, Albrecht M, Favato G, Pieri V, Marcobelli A, Trotta MG et al (2008) Le potenziali interazioni tra farmaci: un indicatore di appropriatezza prescrittiva. GIFF 1(3):11–30

Tugnait M, Gupta N, Hanley MJ, Venkatakrishnan K, Sonnichsen D, Kertstein D et al (2019) The effect of a high-fat meal on the pharmacokinetics of brigatinib, an oral anaplastic lymphoma kinase inhibitor, in healthy volunteers. Clin Pharmacol Drug Dev 8(6):734–741

US Food and Drug Administration FDA (2022a). https://www.accessdata.fda.gov/drugsatfda_docs/label/2011/202570s000lbl.pdf. Last access 9 Sept 2022

US Food and Drug Administration FDA (2022b). https://www.accessdata.fda.gov/drugsatfda_docs/label/2019/205755s016lbl.pdf. Last access 9 Sept 2022

US Food and Drug Administration FDA (2022c). https://www.accessdata.fda.gov/drugsatfda_docs/label/2018/208772s004lbl.pdf. Last access 9 Sept 2022

US Food and Drug Administration FDA (2022d). https://www.accessdata.fda.gov/drugsatfda_docs/label/2018/210868s000lbl.pdf. Last access 9 Sept 2022

US Food and Drug Administration FDA (2022e). https://www.accessdata.fda.gov/drugsatfda_docs/label/2019/212725s000lbl.pdf. Last access 9 Sept 2022

Xie F, Ding X, Zhang QY (2016) An update on the role of intestinal cytochrome P450 enzymes in drug disposition. Acta Pharm Sin B 6(5):374–383

Xu H, O'Gorman M, Boutros T, Brega N, Kantaridis C, Tan W et al (2015) Evaluation of crizotinib absolute bioavailability, the bioequivalence of three oral formulations, and the effect of food on crizotinib pharmacokinetics in healthy subjects. J Clin Pharmacol 55(1):104–113

Zheng WY, Richardson LC, Li L, Westbrook JI, Baysari MT (2018) Drug-drug interactions and their harmful effects in hospitalised patients: a systematic review and meta-analysis. Eur J Clin Pharmacol 74:15–27

Potential Anticancer Activity of Novel Triazoles and Related Derivatives

José Aguirre-de Paz, Nancy Lara-Almazán, Alejandra Ancira-Cortez, and Brenda Gibbens-Bandala

Abstract

Due to their diverse pharmacological properties, triazoles are important tools in medicinal chemistry and may be involved in many cancer-related pathways. Structural modifications of this molecule can be useful in drug development. Although research efforts are directed toward the development of synthetic triazole analogs, much work needs to be done in this area of drug discovery. Medicinal chemists are interested in generating new triazole derivatives because of the potential therapeutic uses of these compounds. This chapter covers the general chemistry, methods of synthesis, and specific pharmacological actions of the triazole core. Data on commercially available clinical and investigational triazole compounds are also included. The purpose of this chapter is to increase recognition of the importance of these heterocycles through the design and synthesis of new triazole derivatives with advanced and unexplored pharmacological implications.

Keywords

Bioisostere · Cancer treatment · Pharmacological action · Triazole

J. Aguirre-de Paz
Departamento de Materiales Radiactivos, Instituto Nacional de Investigaciones Nucleares, Carretera México-Toluca S/N, Mexico

Departamento de Química Orgánica, Facultad de Química, Universidad Autónoma del Estado de México, Toluca, Estado de México, Mexico

N. Lara-Almazán · A. Ancira-Cortez · B. Gibbens-Bandala (✉)
Departamento de Materiales Radiactivos, Instituto Nacional de Investigaciones Nucleares, Carretera México-Toluca S/N, Mexico
e-mail: brenda.g.servicios@inin.gob.mx

Interdisciplinary Cancer Research, https://doi.org/10.1007/16833_2024_377
Published online: 13 October 2024

1 Introduction

Cancer is a disease that appears when abnormal cells grow uncontrollably, exceed their typical boundaries, and invade different organs (metastasis). Behind cardiovascular disease, cancer is the second cause of death worldwide. Despite the availability of effective anticancer treatments, the presence of side effects such as drug resistance and the inability to differentiate between cancerous and non-cancerous cells, coupled with the limitations of radiotherapy, has spurred the need to explore alternative and successful treatment options (Siegel et al. 2023; Alam 2022; Ferlay et al. 2021; Debela et al. 2021; Channabasappa et al. 2020).

Cancer is a major health challenge worldwide, requiring the continuous search for innovative therapeutic agents. Triazoles, nitrogen-containing heterocycles, are stable compounds with the ability to interact non-covalently with various biological targets through hydrogen bonding, hydrophobic interactions, dipole-dipole forces, and van der Waals. Therefore, they are an essential framework for drug discovery. Drugs containing triazole derivatives have been shown to have diverse pharmacological effects. These effects, in addition to their widely recognized antifungal properties, include anticancer, antituberculosis, antiviral, anti-inflammatory, anti-HIV, and antibacterial effects, among others (Siegel et al. 2023; Alam 2022; Dai et al. 2022; Bezerra Morais et al. 2022; Xu et al. 2019).

Triazoles could be classified into 1,2,4-triazole and 1,2,3-triazole with different pharmacokinetic and pharmacological properties. As a result, triazole hybrids could serve as potential models for identifying novel anticancer agents. The inhibition of several enzymes that contribute to the progression of this deadly disease is the basis for the anticancer activity of triazoles (Bezerra Morais et al. 2022; Channabasappa et al. 2020; Slavova et al. 2020).

This chapter provides a general description of triazoles and examines recent advances in the use of triazoles for cancer therapy, focusing on key trials, mechanisms of action, and potential applications.

2 Generalities of Triazoles

2.1 Chemistry of Triazoles

Triazoles are heterocyclic compounds that consist of a 5-membered heterocyclic ring with three nitrogen atoms and two carbon atoms, with the molecular formula $C_2H_3N_3$ (Dehaen and Bakulev 2015; Dixit et al. 2021). There are two possible positional arrangements of the nitrogen atoms in the five-membered ring, leading to the formation of two isomers, namely s-triazole or 1,2,4-triazole and ν-triazole or 1,2,3-triazole. Triazoles are divided into three main groups: triazole monocycles, benzotriazoles, and triazolium salts. There are three recognized subclasses of 1,2,3-triazole monocycles depending on the substituents positioned on the ring. It should be noted that although the 2H and 1H 1,2,3-triazoles are aromatic compounds, their 4H isomer is not an aromatic compound (Scheme 1) (Dai et al. 2022; Sermuksnyte

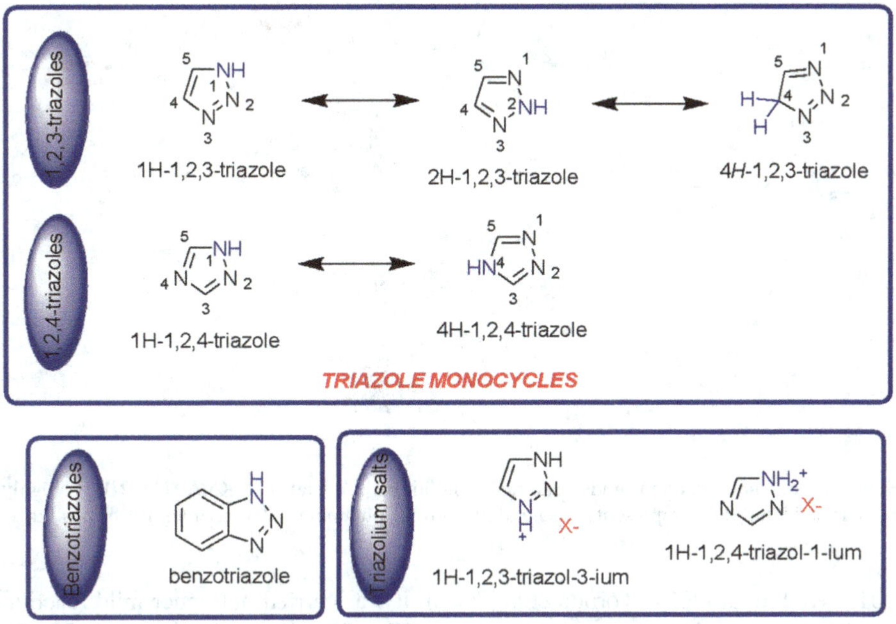

Scheme 1 Isomeric structures of the triazoles

et al. 2022; Rashdan and Shehadi 2022; Matin et al. 2022; Liang et al. 2021; Pinheiro et al. 2020).

2.2 Triazole Synthesis Routes

The synthesis of these compounds has been documented for over 100 years, with Silberrad being one of the pioneers. There are several methods for the synthesis of triazoles, some of which are described here. Since then, the number of reports on triazoles has steadily increased (Dai et al. 2022; Matin et al. 2022; Silberrad 1900).

2.2.1 Synthetic Approaches for 1,2,3-Triazole Analogs

Cu(I)-Catalyzed Azide–Alkyne Cycloaddition (CuAAC)

Copper-catalyzed alkyne azide cycloaddition (CuAAC) is a chemical reaction that occurs between an azide and a terminal alkyne, facilitated by a copper salt (Opsomer and Dehaen 2021). The CuAAC was discovered by Huisgen, who carried it out under conventional thermal conditions to give the mixture of 1,2,3-substituted triazoles in the 1,4- and 1,5- positions (Breugst and Reissig 2020; Huisgen 1963; Matin et al. 2022) (Scheme 2A). The reaction was optimized for 1,4-disubstituted-1,2,3-triazoles with excellent stereoselectivity, as shown by Meldal and Sharplees-Fokin. To this reaction, they attributed the concept of "click chemistry" (Garcia et al.

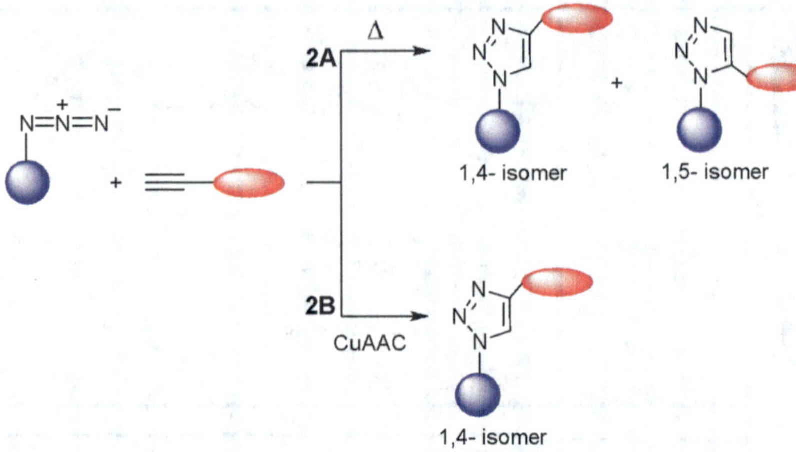

Scheme 2 Click reaction under thermal conditions **2A** and by "CuAAC" **2B** is highly regiospecific and today represents a general method for obtaining 1,2,3-triazoles-1,4-bisubstituted

2011; Kolb et al. 2001; Tornøe et al. 2002). It was carried out under mild reaction conditions at ambient temperature (Scheme 2B) (González-Lainez et al. 2022; Hu et al. 2022; Kolb et al. 2001). In particular, he was awarded the 2022 Nobel Prize for his contributions to click chemistry and cycloaddition reactions involving azide derivatives (Bertozzi 2023).

The corresponding copper acetylide is likely to be synthesized from the 1,3-dipolar cycloaddition between an azide and an alkyne reaction. (Gomes et al. 2019). According to the mechanism proposed by Fokin et al. in Scheme 3, based on theoretical investigations, the presence of a second copper atom facilitates the reaction. Furthermore, the isolation of proposed reaction intermediates based on several σ,π-bis(copper)alkynyl dinuclear species supports the mechanism (González-Lainez et al. 2022; Worrell et al. 2013).

Metal-Free Click Synthesis

The metal-free click synthesis is of great application in the 1,2,3-triazoles through green protocol because it allows for the evasion of heterocyclic product metal contamination (Ahmed et al. 2017).

This is a direct and selective reaction for the synthesis of 1,5-disubstituted-1,2,3-triazoles from three simple building blocks (Scheme 4). Fully functionalized and fused N-substituted heterocycles can also be synthesized using this methodology. The most effective conditions for obtaining yields above 90% involve the use of 30 mol% acetic acid as a catalyst when 4 Å molecular sieves are present. This should be carried out at 100 °C in a 1 M toluene solution (Ahmed et al. 2017; Matin et al. 2022; Opsomer and Dehaen 2021; Thomas et al. 2016).

On the other hand, the Dimroth synthesis for triazoles (Li and Corey 2011) (Scheme 5) involves the condensation of an azide with an activated ketone to

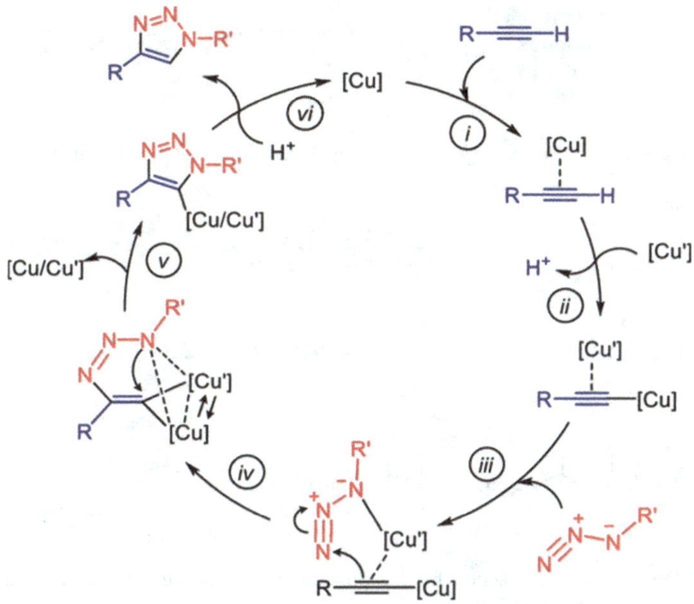

Scheme 3 Fokin mechanism. Catalytic cycle copper alkyne azide. (González-Lainez et al. 2022)

Scheme 4 Metal-free click synthesis. (Opsomer and Dehaen 2021)

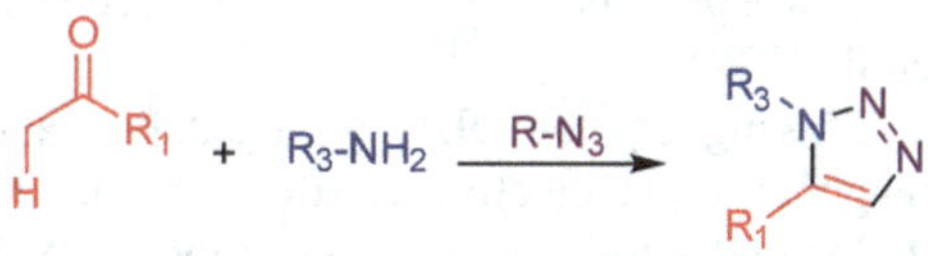

Scheme 5 Dimroth synthesis for triazoles

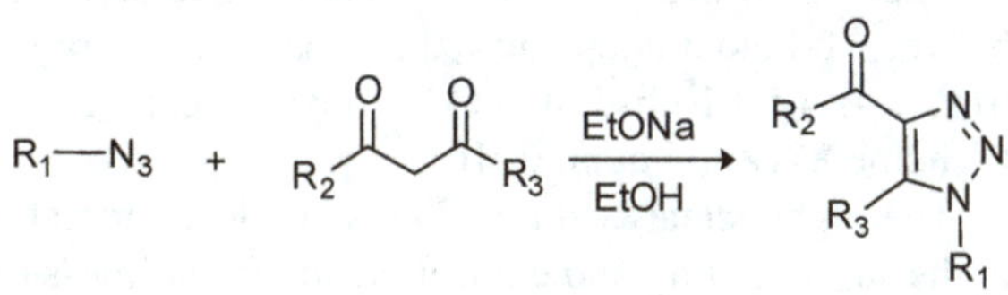

yield a derivative of 1,2,3-triazole. This reaction is typically carried out with an alkoxide and ethanol solvent at room temperature or reflux.

Organocatalytic 1,3-Dipolar Cycloaddition Reaction

OrgACC consists of (3 + 2)-cycloaddition and (3 + 2)-cycloaddition followed by hydrolysis, respectively, of nonhydrolyzed 1,2,3-triazoles and NH-1,2,3-triazoles. The use of this reaction has proven to be effective for the synthesis of these compounds (Scheme 6) (Jalani et al. 2016). The most efficient catalyst was found to be 1,8-diazabicyclo undec-7-ene (DBU), and several cyclic tertiary and aliphatic amines were investigated. In addition, chloroform and DMSO were identified as the

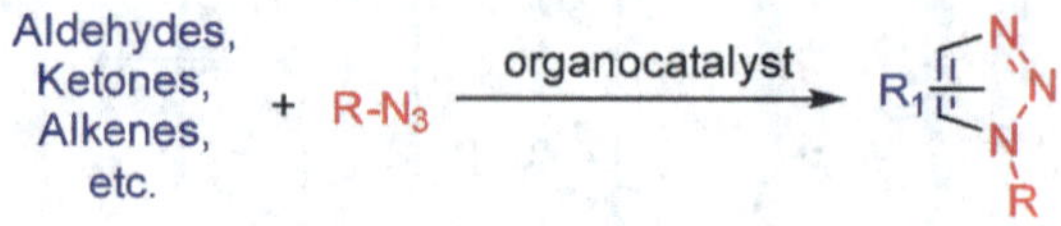

Scheme 6 General 1,3-Dipolar organocatalytic cycloaddition reaction. (Jalani et al. 2016)

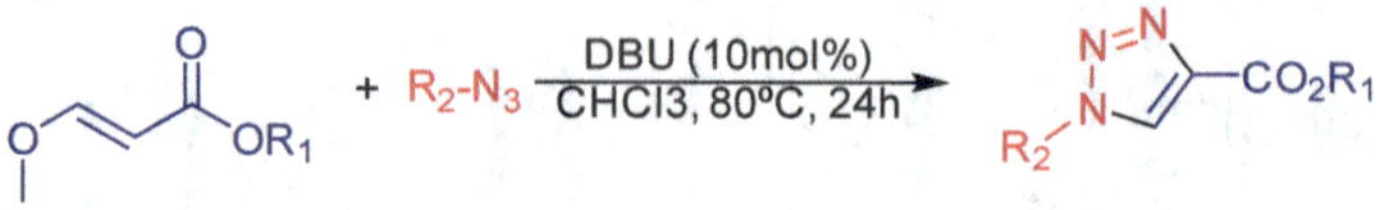

Scheme 7 Organocatalytic reaction to obtain 1,4-disubstituted-1,2,3-triazoles. (Li et al. 2015)

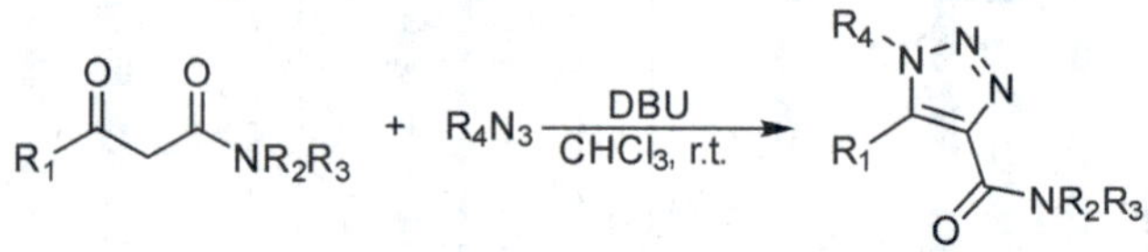

Scheme 8 Organocatalytic reaction for the preparation of 1,4,5-trisubstituted-1,2,3-triazole-4-carboxamide. (Zhou et al. 2016)

optimal solvents for the DBU-catalyzed 1,3-dipolar cycloaddition reaction (Matin et al. 2022).

Making use of DBU as a catalyst and azides and α,β-unsaturated esters as reagents, regioselective 1,4-disubstituted-1,2,3-triazole can be synthesized in high yields under the conditions described in Scheme 7 (Li et al. 2015).

The DBU organocatalytic enolate-mediated (3 + 2) cycloaddition reaction between β-ketoamides and azides leads to the preparation of the following 1,2,3-triazole-1,4,5-trisubstituted (4-carboxamides) with high regioselectivities and yields (Scheme 8) (Zhou et al. 2016).

The organocatalyzed reaction is an ideal alternative to metal-free cyclization due to the sustainability and environmental friendliness of the process and the absence of metals that can be toxic to biological systems. This preparation method produces diversely functionalized 1,2,3-triazoles (Jalani et al. 2016).

Ionic Liquid-Catalyzed Synthesis

Ionic liquids are typically described as compounds that have two primary characteristics in common: they are composed entirely of ions, and they have m.p. of less than 100 °C. (Nasrollahzadeh et al. 2021). They exhibit excellent high thermal stability, low vapor pressure, chemical stability, and conductivity (Chudasama et al. 2022; Zhao et al. 2021). Because of these properties, they have many applications in organic synthesis, including the regioselective synthesis of triazoles by cycloaddition (e.g., as catalysts and solvents). Other advantages of using ionic liquids for triazole synthesis include their low cost, greener designer liquids,

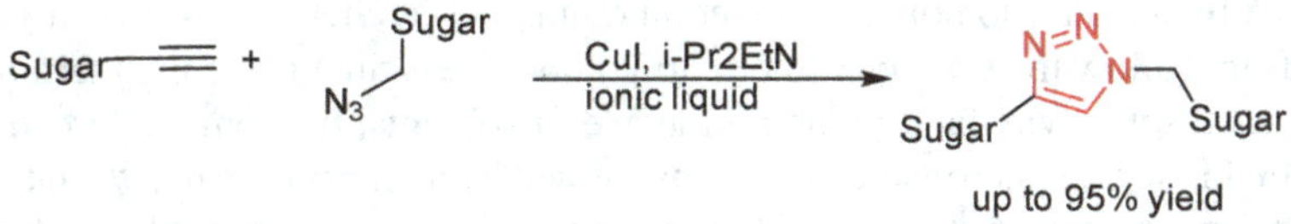

Scheme 9 Ionic liquid-catalyzed synthesis of 1–4 disubstituted triazole-linked C-disaccharide

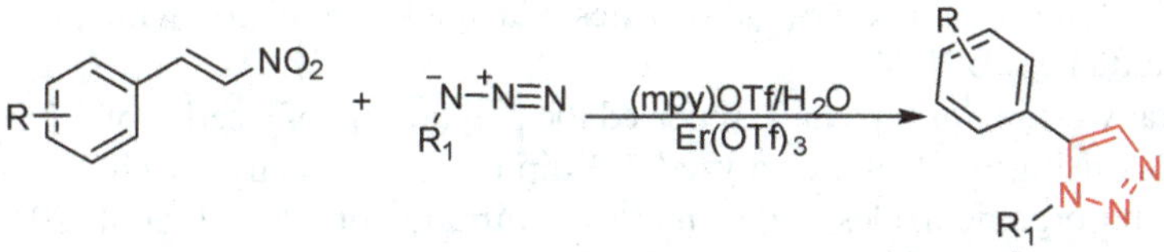

Scheme 10 Ionic liquid-catalyzed synthesis for the regioselective preparation of 1,5-disubstituted 1,2,3-triazoles. (Maiuolo et al. 2019).

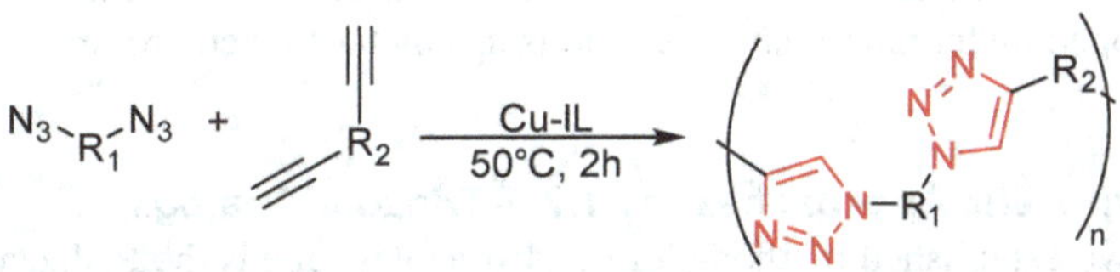

Scheme 11 Ionic liquid-catalyzed synthesis for click polymerization

recyclability, ease of operation, and potential for recovery (Chudasama et al. 2022; Daraie and Heravi 2019; Matin et al. 2022).

Marra et al. were among the first to study ionic liquids in the copper(I)-catalyzed azide-alkyne click reaction. A reaction of sugar acetylene with sugar azide was studied (CuI, i-Pr_2EtN, 80 °C) in an ionic liquid, resulting in a 1,4-disubstituted triazole-linked C-disaccharide with yields up to 95% (Scheme 9) (Marra et al. 2008). Since then, the study of triazole synthesis using ionic liquids has increased.

Maiuolu et al. used ionic liquids for the regioselective preparation of 1,5-disubstituted 1,2,3-triazoles via 1,3-dipolar cycloaddition. An environmentally friendly erbium (III) trifluoromethane sulfonate catalyst system facilitates this (Scheme 10). The reaction shows high regioselectivity, with the potential to reuse the catalytic system for up to six cycles and achieve satisfactory yields (Maiuolo et al. 2019).

Another example is the synthesis using copper-based ionic liquid (Cu-IL), which was easy to prepare. Under mild reaction conditions, it has been used to catalyze azide-alkyne click polymerization. PTA's with satisfactory molecular weights are readily synthesizable in high yields (up to 95%) (Scheme 11) (Li et al. 2020).

Microwave-Assisted Method

The triazoles described above are synthesized under thermal conditions that can last from several hours to days, and although reaction times and yields have been improved by the addition of catalytic compounds, researchers are now trying to find methods that allow the synthesis to be carried out in less time while maintaining high yields, good selectivity, and reducing the use of solvents, to promote "green chemistry." In this sense, microwave energy, harnessed by a microwave reactor laboratory with specific characteristics, is an alternative to synthetic routes that offer these advantages (Dharavath et al. 2020; Lidström et al. 2001; Strauss and Trainor 1995; Tiwari et al. 2023). It is worth noting that this technique has already been applied to the cycloaddition of alkynes and azides via click chemistry with good results (Appukkuttan et al. 2004).

Several working groups have reported the preparation of a series of 1,2,3-triazole derivatives using the Cu(I)-catalyzed 1,3-dipolar Cu(I)-catalyzed click reaction of alkynes and organic azides under microwave irradiation (Ashok et al. 2014, 2020; Dharavath et al. 2020; Nesaragi et al. 2021) and the results indicated higher yields in less time compared to conventional thermal conditions. It is also a simple method with minimal purification requirements and is cost-effective.

It should be noted that microwave-assisted syntheses of 1,2,3-triazoles have also been developed under microwave conditions in a metal-free environment (Garg et al. 2020).

2.2.2 Synthetic Approaches for 1,2,4-Triazole Analogs

There are two established methods for 1,2,4-triazoles: one is the Pellizzari reaction, and the other is Einhorn-Brunner (Atkinson and Polya 1952; Wang 2010) (Scheme 12).

In addition to the established methods, the acquisition of these compounds also includes the subsequent synthetic routes.

Cu-Catalyzed Synthesis

An example of copper-catalyzed synthesis was reported by Xu et al. Good yields of 1,2,4-triazole derivatives were obtained from one-pot reactions of two nitriles with

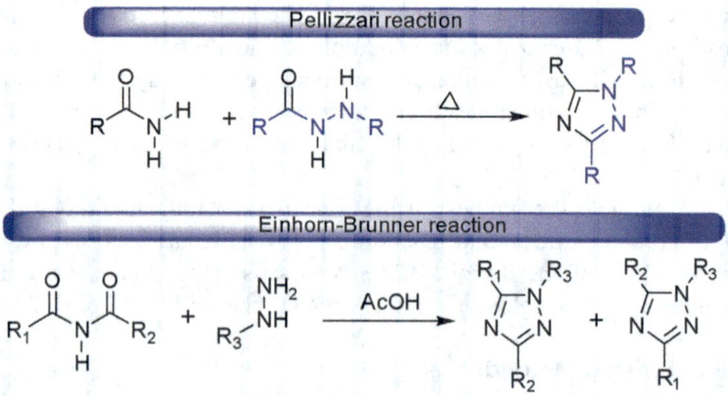

Scheme 12 Pellizzari and the Einhorn-Brunner reactions to obtain 1,2,4-triazoles

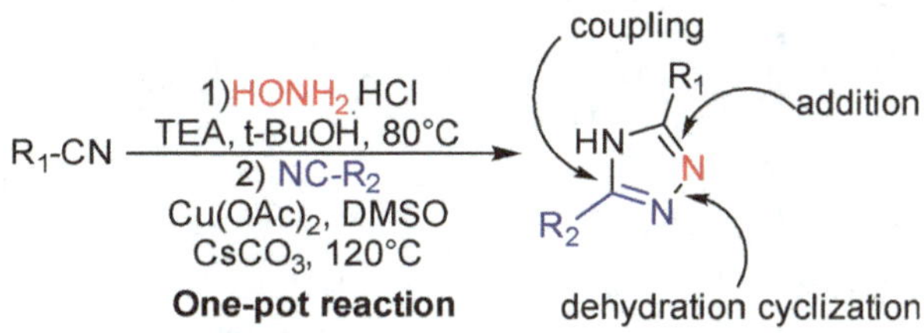

Scheme 13 Copper-catalyzed synthesis to obtain 1,2,4-triazoles derivatives. (Xu et al. 2015)

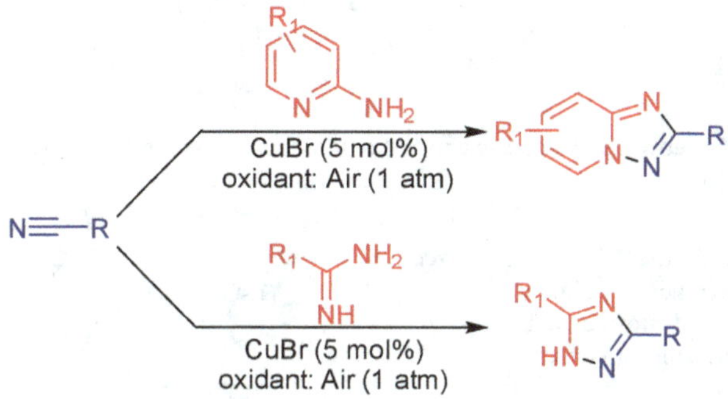

Scheme 14 Ueda and Nagasawa copper-catalyzed oxidative coupling reaction to obtain 1,2,4-triazole derivatives. (Ueda and Nagasawa 2009)

hydroxylamine using Cu(OAc)2. The reactions involve the sequential intermolecular addition of hydroxylamine to nitriles. The amidoxime is then treated with another nitrile in a copper-catalyzed reaction. Finally, intramolecular dehydration/cyclization takes place (Scheme 13) (Xu et al. 2015).

On the other hand, Ueda and Nagasawa also reported a facile one-step synthesis for the preparation of 1,2,4-triazole compounds via a copper-catalyzed oxidative coupling-type reaction in an air atmosphere (Scheme 14). Sequential copper-catalyzed oxidative coupling reactions are used in the process. N-C and N-N bonds are generated. The reaction has been described as being compatible with a broad range of chemical groups in order to achieve chemical diversification (Ueda and Nagasawa 2009).

The final example is two domino reactions for the synthesis of 3,5-diaryl-1,2,4-triazoles reported by Sudheendran et al. The first reaction is between two imidates and ammonium carbonate using $Cu(OTf)_2$ as the catalyst, with yields above 64% (Scheme 15A). The second reaction consists of the reaction between two amidines using $NaHCO_3$ as the base, $Cu(OTf)_2$ as the catalyst, 1,10-phenanthroline as an additive, and K3[Fe(CN)6]/air oxygen as an oxidizing agent to give 3,5-diaryl-1,2,4-triazoles in yields of up to 68% (Scheme 15B). The formation of three bonds in a single step characterizes this reaction (Sudheendran et al. 2014).

Base-Catalyzed Synthesis

Yeung et al. reported the synthesis of 3,5-disubstituted 1,2,4-triazoles in one step using hydrazide and nitrile condensing with a catalytic amount of K_2CO_3 in n-BuOH (Scheme 16). The process has been shown to have a broad scope by evaluating

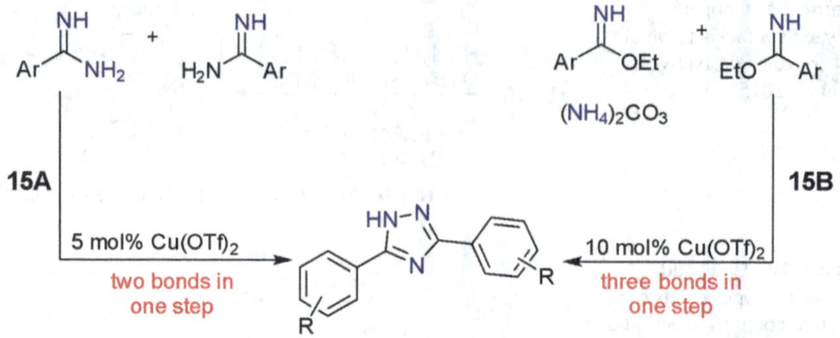

Scheme 15 Copper-catalyzed domino reactions for 3,5-diaryl-1,2,4-triazoles. (Sudheendran et al. 2014)

Scheme 16 Base-catalyzed synthesis to obtain 3,5-disubstituted 1,2,4-triazoles. (Yeung et al. 2005).

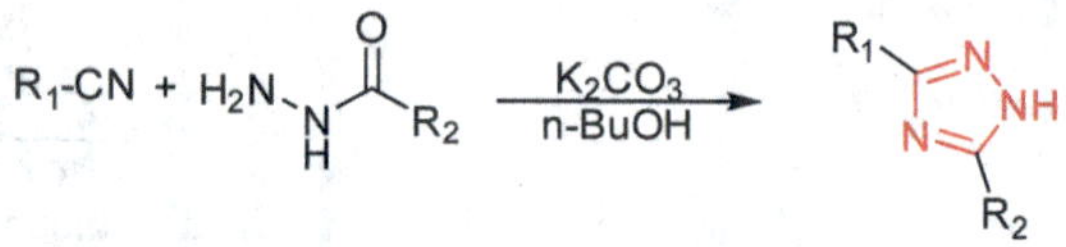

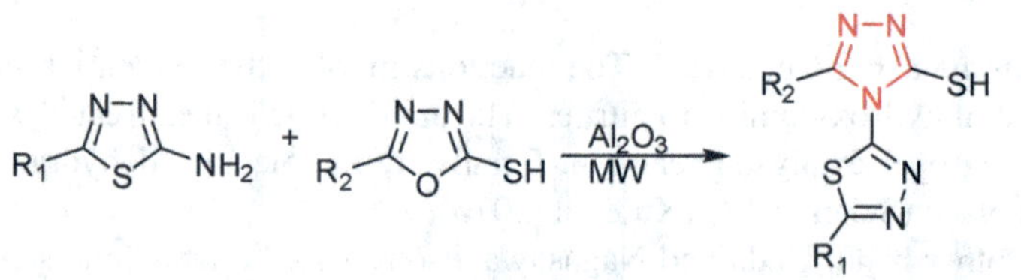

Scheme 17 Microwave-assisted synthesis of thiadiazolyl substituted triazoles. (Kidwai et al. 2000)

reaction partners with a range of electron-donor, electron-withdrawal, and heterocyclic compounds, all of which are well tolerated (Yeung et al. 2005).

Microwave-Assisted Method

Due to the advantages of microwave-assisted synthesis, several researchers have developed methods to optimize the synthesis of 1,2,4-triazoles and their derivatives (Xu et al. 2018; Ceylan et al. 2016; Sun et al. 2013; Kahveci et al. 2008a, b, 2015; Liu et al. 2014; Kidwai et al. 2001). For example, thiadiazolyl-substituted triazoles have been obtained by reacting 5-substituted-2-amino-1,3,4-thiadiazoles with 5-alkyl-2-mercapto-1,3,4-oxadiazoles, beginning from 1,3,4-thiadiazoles, by adsorption on acidic alumina under microwave irradiation on a solid alumina support. The reaction does not require organic solvents or corrosive or toxic mineral acids (Scheme 17). The process gives a fairly good yield of 77–93% and takes about 40–80 s (Kidwai et al. 2000).

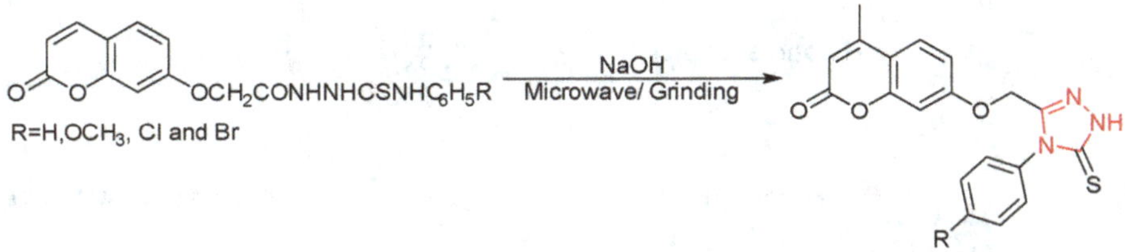

Scheme 18 Microwave-assisted synthesis of 3-mercapto-1, 2, 4-triazoles. (Reddy et al. 2014)

The reaction of substituted coumarins in the presence of NaOH and assisted by microwave and milling-accelerated heating allowed the preparation of 3-mercapto-1, 2, 4-triazoles (Scheme 18) (Reddy et al. 2014).

Vaithiyalingam et al. also reported the 3,5-disubstituted 1,2,4-triazole can be synthesized using a microwave-assisted process whereby a nitrile and a hydrazide undergo direct reaction under microwave irradiation without any base or solvent, allowing for a rapid synthesis (Vaithiyalingam et al. 2021).

The selection of the method depends on the specific starting materials, reaction conditions, and the desired triazole product. Triazole synthesis is a varied field, and researchers are trying to discover novel and effective strategies for the preparation of these compounds. In recent decades, the discovery of diverse biological properties of many triazole derivatives has accelerated the development of 1,2,3-triazole chemistry. This is an important aspect to consider (Bonandi et al. 2017; Zhou and Wang 2012; Kumar et al. 2021; Malik et al. 2020; Serafini et al. 2021; Zafar et al. 2021). The number of patented drugs and agrochemicals involving this type of derivative has grown significantly (Farooq 2021a). This has caused many researchers to seek to improve the methods of synthesis of triazole derivatives.

It's important to note that the choice of method will depend on the specific starting materials, the reaction conditions, and the desired triazole product. The field of triazole synthesis is a diverse one, and researchers continue to search for new and more efficient methods for the preparation of these compounds.

3 Triazoles: Biomimetics, Bioisostere, or Pharmacophore?

3.1 Biomimetics

Peptides are molecules found in many human organs and tissues. Their involvement in many biological processes makes them molecules of interest for medical strategies. They are nontoxic, highly specific, and have broad biological activity, giving them certain advantages as drugs (Albericio and Kruger 2012). However, their use in therapy is limited by low physical and chemical stability, variable solubility, low bioavailability, and susceptibility to in vivo enzymatic degradation, resulting in a short half-life. Therefore, peptides are modified to create innovative compounds, such as peptidomimetics, which mimic the biological properties of

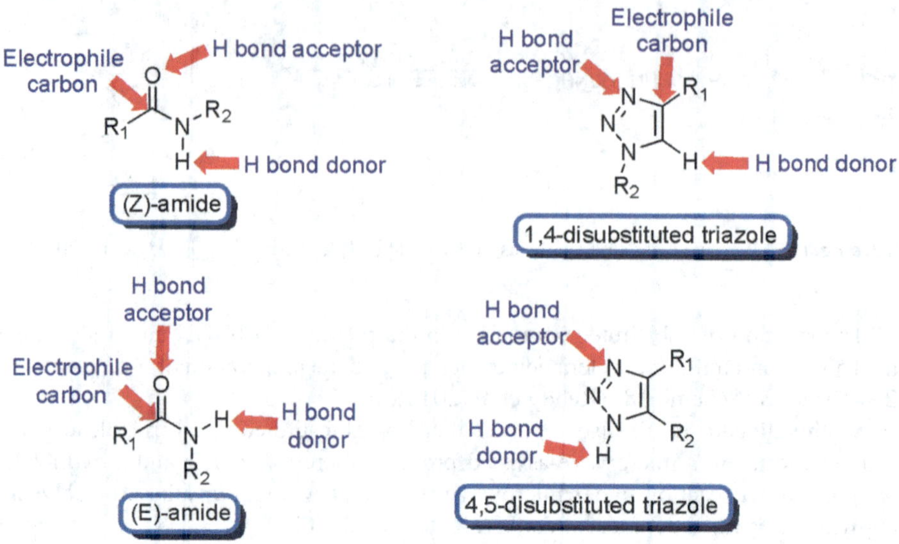

Diagram 1 1,2,3-triazoles electronically mimic amide moieties

peptides and can be used in pharmaceutical treatments. Peptidomimetics is a key medicinal chemistry technique used to design and explore therapeutic drugs (Agouram et al. 2021; Albericio and Kruger 2012; Marshall and Ballante 2017).

Replacing the amide with a heterocyclic, specifically the 1,2,3-triazole moiety, is an example of peptide mimicry. The structure of the 1,2,3-triazole, either in cis or in trans, suggests that this ring could mimic the peptide linkage. The 1,4-disubstituted triazole shows similarity to the trans conformation of the amide bond. The C (4) atom equals the amide carbonyl carbon electrically, while the nitrogen's lone pair resembles the amide's carbonyl oxygen. Also, the polarity of the C (5)-H bond resembles the N-H bond's hydrogen bond donor property. Optimal peptide mimicry is achieved due to the greater importance of the hydrogen bond donor/acceptor power, as well as the stronger dipolar moment of the triazole ring compared to the amide function. Differentiation between trans-peptide bond and the 1,4-disubstituted 1,2,3-triazole ring. (Diagram 1) (Agouram et al. 2021; Grob et al. 2021).

3.2 Bioisostere

Chemical substituents or groups known as bioisosteres are those that, in combination with other chemical or physical properties, confer substantially identical biological properties on a chemical molecule (Lengerli et al. 2022; Wermuth et al. 1998). In addition, their structural characteristics allow them to be both hydrogen bond donors (HBD) and acceptors (HBA), which in turn allows them to mimic different functional groups in terms of their properties. The potential of triazole rings as bioisosteres, with a focus on 1,2,3-triazoles and several examples to encourage

Table 1 Isosteres of triazoles

Isosteric effect	Examples	Applications in cancer	References
As an amide bond isosteres	Triazole-based analogues of Imatinib	Leukemia treatment	Bonandi et al. (2017), Gabba et al. (2017), Grob et al. (2021), Li et al. (2016) and Pirali et al. (2008)
	Triazole-based analogs of Vorinostat	Cutaneous T-cell lymphoma treatment	
	Triazole-based analogs of cryptophycin-52	Cytotoxic activity against multi-drug-resistant cancer cells	
	Triazole-based analogues of minigrastrin	Inhibition of cell migration of cancer cells	
	Triazole-based analogues of CCK2 receptor	Targeting of A431 cells	
As an ester bond isosteres	Triazole-based analogs of steganacin and podophyllotoxin	Activity against neuroblastoma cells	Bonandi et al. (2017)
As a carboxylic acid isosteres	Not yet described for cancer	No application in cancer	Giraudo et al. (2018) and Malik et al. (2020)
As an olefin rigid analog	Triazole-based analogues of combretastatin and cyanocombretatstin	Activity against cells of ovarian adenocarcinoma, SK-OV-3	Malik et al. (2020)

and guide their use in drug design. Among the examples included, amide bond replacement is the most common strategy, illustrating the adaptability of this isosteric effect. In addition, ester and carboxylic acid triazole isosteres are less commonly used than heterocyclic replacements (Bonandi et al. 2017; Farooq 2021b; Goetz et al. 2020). Table 1 summarizes the isosteric effect on the triazole ring.

3.3 Pharmacophore

The notion of a pharmacophore was first proposed by Ehrlich in 1909. His definition of a pharmacophore was "a molecular framework carrying (phoros) the essential features responsible for the biological activity of a drug (pharmacon)" (Ehrlich 1909). According to the very recent IUPAC definition, a pharmacophore model is "the array of electronic and steric characteristics required to provide the optimal supramolecular interfaces with a specific biological target to induce (or block) a biological response" (Wermuth et al. 1998). In this respect, the 1,2,3-triazole core offers a variety of pharmacophore properties, and hybrids containing or linked to a 1,2,3-triazole ring are most referred to as "lead compounds." As a result, the various biological functions, due to recent research interest in these molecules, and the properties of 1,2,3-triazole hybrids, conjugates, and related compounds are well known (Agalave et al. 2011; Bozorov et al. 2019).

4 Triazole Hybrids

The advantages of triazole hybrid molecules include the enhancement of drug-resistant cancers (Al-blewi et al. 2021) and the ability to interact with various molecular targets through hydrophobic interactions, hydrogen bonding, and van der Waals and dipolo-dipolo forces (Dheer et al. 2017). This molecule has the backbone of 1,2,3-triazoles and is divided into two types. Type I incorporates anticancer pharmacophores into its structure, whereas in type II, the triazole acts as a linking agent to bind two anticancer pharmacophores. The incorporation of pharmacophores into their structure results in numerous mechanisms of action (Scheme 19) (Liang et al. 2021; Xu et al. 2019).

4.1 Triazole-Hybrids: Type I

Many pharmacophores, including artemisinin, sugar coumarin/flavone, pyrimidine, indole/isatin, steroids, pyridine, azole, chalcone, quinazoline, quinone, and quinoline/quinolone have been discovered in recent years to potentially possess anticancer activity. Importantly, these assessments are objective and based on scientific evidence. Attaching these anticancer pharmacophores to the 1,2,3-triazole scaffold shows promising potential in developing novel anticancer candidates that effectively fight both drug-resistant and drug-sensitive cancers due to their individual action mechanisms (Rani et al. 2020; Xu et al. 2019).

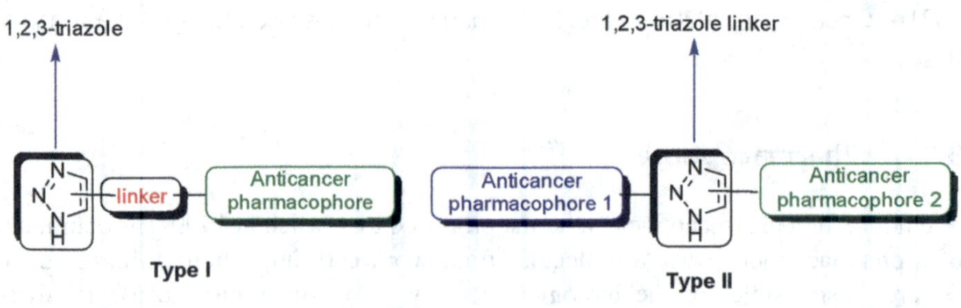

Scheme 19 Classification of 1,2,3 triazoles

4.1.1 1,2,3-Triazole Tethered 1,2,4-Trioxane Trimer (4 T)

Artemisinin (ART) has been used to treat a variety of cancer cells; iron-rich cancer cells are more sensitive to ART and its derivatives and conjugates (Kumar et al. 2019). The aim is to produce readily available synthetic 1,2,4-trioxanes with the same pharmacophore as ART (Image 1). 4 T treatment increased glutathione reductase and glucose-6-phosphate dehydrogenase activities in cancer cells compared to controls and decreased the reduced glutathione level in the treated cells. In addition, 4 T reduced OPN expression by approximately 0.5-fold in these cell lines. In addition, the key mitogen-activated protein kinase pathway proteins extracellular signal-regulated kinase 1/2 (~16-fold) and mitogen-activated protein kinase 1/2 (~1.8-fold) were also found to be activated by 4 T therapy. However, following 4 T therapy, these cancer cells showed a significant decrease in the amount of phosphorylated c-Jun, which is part of activator protein-1. They postulate that 4 T may help reduce the rate at which cancer spreads and becomes malignant (Khongsti et al. 2021; Pasupuleti et al. 2020; Wang et al. 2022).

4.1.2 Triazole-Chalcones

There is currently no effective chemotherapy for prostate cancer, the number one cause of death in men (Boettcher et al. 2019). The chemical preparation and in-vitro assessment of a new series of 2H-1,2,3-triazole nucleated chalcones with ring B targeting the PC-3 prostate cancer cell line were investigated (Image 2). Certain compounds showed good cytotoxicity when tested against the PC-3 cell line using the MTT assay. While the various hybrid α-methyl substituents are toxic, some compounds drastically reduced the viability of cells with IC50 values of 15.64, 28.55, 25.56, and μM (Pinheiro et al. 2020).

4.1.3 1,2,3-Triazole Thymine Derivatives

Breast cancer, including metastatic disease, remains incurable with current treatments and is the second leading cancer killer of women globally (Burguin et al. 2021). 1,2,3-Triazole analogs were tested in vitro against MDA-MB231 breast cancer cells. Results showed that hybrids had significant cytotoxic effects on MDA-MB231 cells (Image 3). Using human estrogen (Erα) 1X7R and 1A53 (homology models), docking studies were performed on the azido derivative (Vd) and 1,2,3-triazole analog (VIc), respectively. These studies indicated that

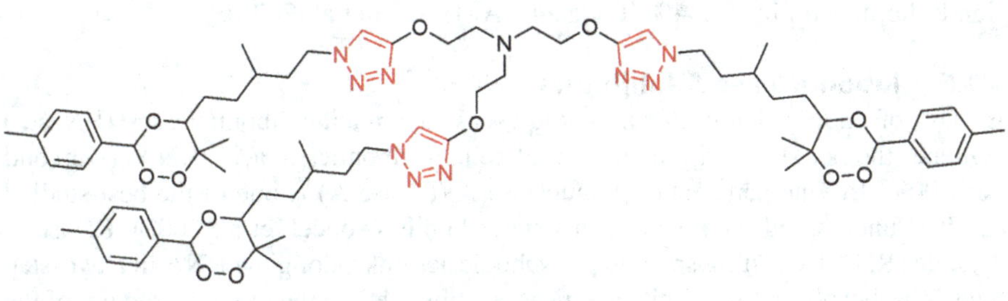

Image 1 1,2,3-triazole tethered 1,2,4-trioxane trimer

Image 2 Triazole-chalcone

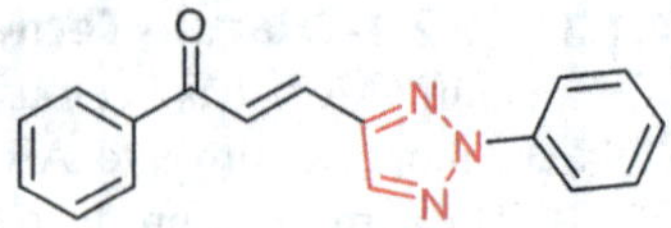

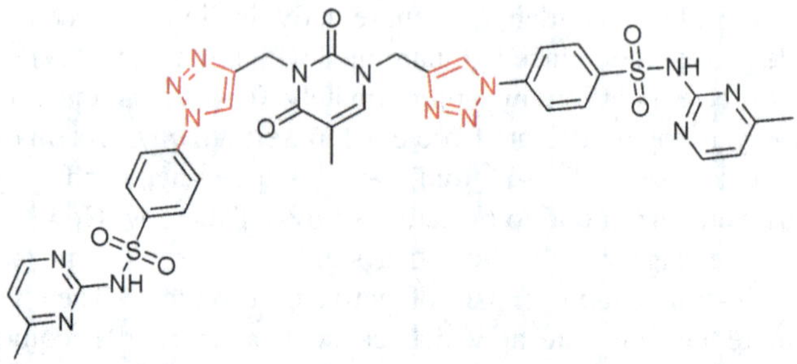

Image 3 Bis-1,2,3-Triazole Thymine Derivative

azido compounds (Vc-e) and 1,2,3-triazole analog (VIc) could potentially be used for the treatment of breast cancer (MDA-MB231) based on their potent cytotoxic activity (Almashal et al. 2020).

4.1.4 Alaninyl and Glycinyl Triazolyl-Oxazolidinones Against Kelly Neuroblastoma Cell Line

Of the children who die from cancer, 15% die from neuroblastoma (NB), the most common extracranial malignancy in children (Du and Yuan 2023). Clinical results show tumor recurrence rates of more than 50% and severe late side effects even with rigorous treatment in patients with high-risk NB. The most potent triazolyl-oxazolidinone was 5-nitrofuroylglycinyl containing a 4-methyltriazolyl group (PH-145), while the least potent was 5-nitrothiophenecarbonylalaninyl containing an L derivative (PH232L). These novel triazolyl-oxazolidinones significantly inhibited the proliferation of neuroblastoma Kelly cells. Tests of their potential to slow cancer progression showed that the 5-nitrothiophenecarbonyl-D-alaninyl containing derivative PH224D inhibited cell movement by 29.14%, and the 5-nitrofuroyl-D-alaninyl derivative PH-223D significantly reduced Kelly cell adhesion to fibronectin by 56.34% (Image 4) (Al-Hasawi et al. 2020).

4.1.5 Ribonuclease A Inhibitors

A class of endonuclease enzymes known as mammalian ribonucleases (RNases) regulates the post-transcriptional level of cellular ribonucleic acid (RNA) (Kim and Lee 2009). Bovine pancreatic ribonuclease A (RNase A) is one of the best-studied and best-understood members of this super-family (Souček et al. 2002). RNase A degrades RNA by cutting specific phosphodiester links along the RNA in a two-step transphosphorolytic-hydrolytic chemical reaction. Due to the overall structure of the modified nucleosides, the efficiency and type of inhibition depended on where the

Image 4 Triazol-linked 2-oxooxazolidinones

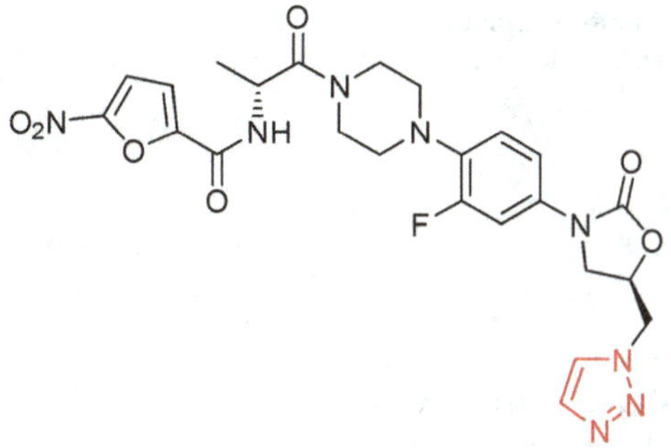

Image 5 Tetra-triazole linked to thymidine derivative

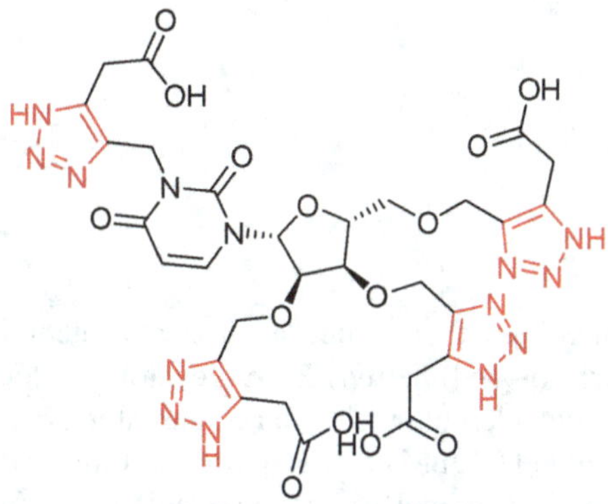

triazole ring was located in the molecule. The tris-triazolylated thymidine derivative has an inhibition constant of 2.3 ± 0.05 μM (T-3′, 5′, N-tris-CH2TzCH2COOH) was found to be the best inhibitor, whereas the tetra-triazolylated uridine (U-2′, 3′, 5′, N-tetrakis-CH2TzCH2COOH) was the least effective (Image 5) (Mondal et al. 2022).

4.2 1,2,3-Triazole as a Linker: Type II

1,2,3-triazoles have demonstrated the ability to mimic multiple functional groups, making them versatile molecules (Sahu et al. 2020). These molecules can act as carboxylic acid, amide, and ester-amide in various therapeutic approaches (Agouram et al. 2021). Synthesized using "click chemistry," the triazole acts as a central linker, often bridging two pharmacophores to create a variety of molecular architectures (Jiang et al. 2019). Type II triazoles are exemplified below:

4.2.1 Aconitine Derivatives-14 T

A promising therapeutic target is the molecular chaperone heat shock protein 90 (Hsp90) (Liang et al. 2016). One naturally occurring chemical that is a potential Hsp90 inhibitor is aconitine (Liang et al. 2016). The aconitine scaffold has been

Image 6 Linked triazole to azabicyclo octanone

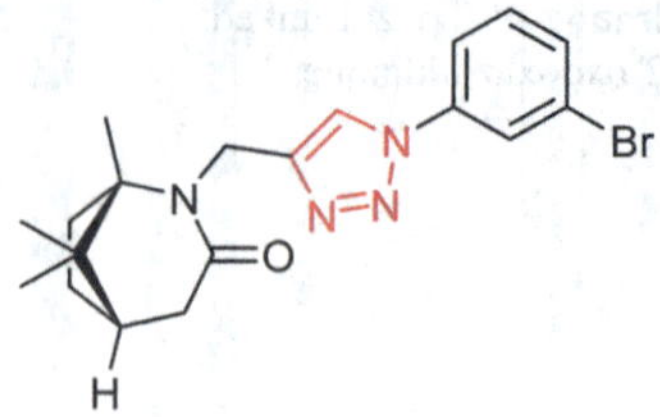

Image 7 1H-1,2,3-triazol-1-yl acetamide derivatives

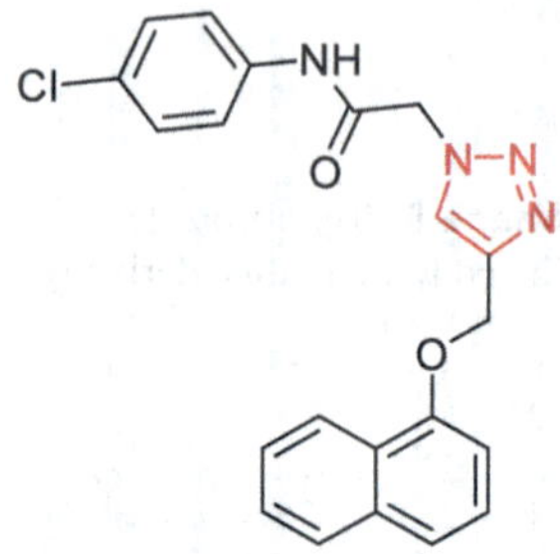

modified to produce a class of potent Hsp90 inhibitors, 2-((1-phenyl-1H-1,2,3-triazol-4-yl)methyl)-2-azabicyclo[3.2.1]octan-3-one derivatives. Among them, the molecule below showed remarkable Antiproliferative activity in LoVo cells (IC50 value0.02 mM) and Hsp90a inhibition (IC50 value 0.71 nM) (Image 6). A logical binding model of this molecule in complex with Hsp90a was obtained through molecular docking experiments (Zhang et al. 2021).

4.2.2 Triazoles Against CSCs

The primary culprits appear to be cancer stem cells (CSCs), which are involved in both tumor relapse and chemoresistance (Marzagalli et al. 2021; Rezayatmand et al. 2022). Four novel series of new chemical entities (NCEs) are the subject of the current study. To identify potential inhibitors of cancer stem cells (CSCs) in mammospheres (MDA-MB-231) and prostatospheres (PC-3), they screened hits using the sphere assay (Image 7) (Padhariya et al. 2021).

4.2.3 Tankyrase Inhibitor

Evidence suggests that glioblastoma (GBM) growth and resistance may be driven by a population of GSCs controlled by standard stem cell pathways, such as the WNT/catenin pathway (Shevchenko et al. 2019; Wang et al. 2021). Kierulf-Vieira et al. examine the impact of administering G007-LK, a small molecule inhibitor of tankyrase, on GSCs. Studies have shown G007-LK to be a potent Hippo and WNT/catenin pathway modulator in CRC (Image 8). This study was the first to evaluate the effect of a TNKS-specific inhibitor on primary GSC cultures. Results suggest that the WNT/catenin pathway may contribute to TMZ resistance. In vitro, G007-LK inhibited the proliferation of GSCs and reduced their sphere formation. Additionally, sphere formation but not proliferation was further reduced by

Image 8 4H-1,2,4-triazole condensed with 1,3,4-oxadiazol

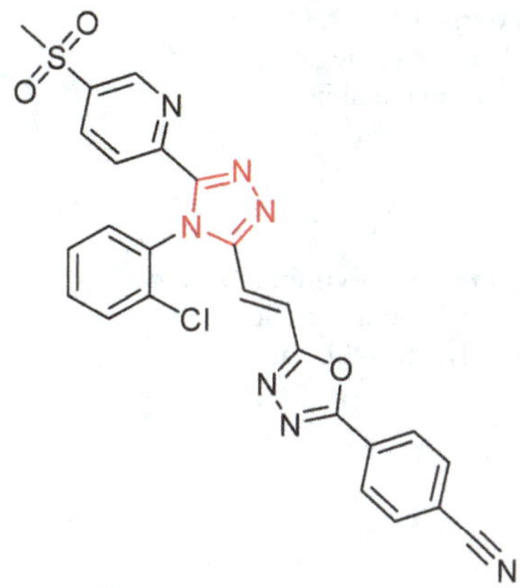

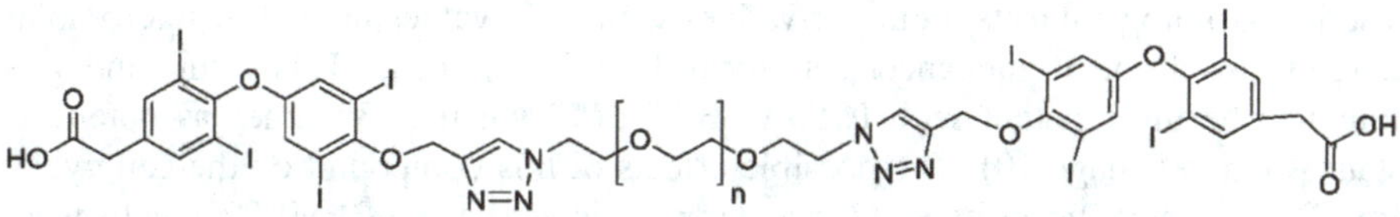

Image 9 P4000-bi-TAT and P1600-bi-TAT structures

co-treatment with TMZ. In all four cell cultures, G007-LK demonstrated TNKS inhibition by stabilizing TNKS1/2, AXIN1, and AMOT/AMOTL2. In addition, it reduced the expression of the common WNT/catenin and YAP/TAZ target genes (Kierulf-Vieira et al. 2020).

4.2.4 Mono and Bis-Triazole Tetraiodothyroacetic Acid Conjugated

Glioblastoma multiforme (GBM) is the deadliest brain cancer. Patients live on average only 12 months due to the severity of the disease, and the majority do not survive beyond two years (Grochans et al. 2022; Hanif et al. 2017). Conventional chemotherapy, radiation therapy, and surgery are standard treatments that can improve the five-year survival rate to between 5 and 8%. Godugu et al. found that the binding affinities of the three TAT integrin v ~ 3 antagonists to the v ~ 3 receptor did not differ significantly. In addition, the biological studies showed that there was no discernible difference in antitumor activity against glioblastoma between mono- and bi-TAT molecules with decreasing PEG linker sizes (Image 9) (Godugu et al. 2021).

4.2.5 PARP-1 Inhibition of 1,2,3-Triazole-Chalcone Conjugates

Leukemia is a potentially fatal non-epithelial malignancy characterized by uncontrolled proliferation of hematopoietic cells (Ci et al. 2022; Younes 2020). The current state of treatment for this malignancy is still lacking an effective and less harmful drug. At the National Cancer Institute, each synthetic chemical was tested

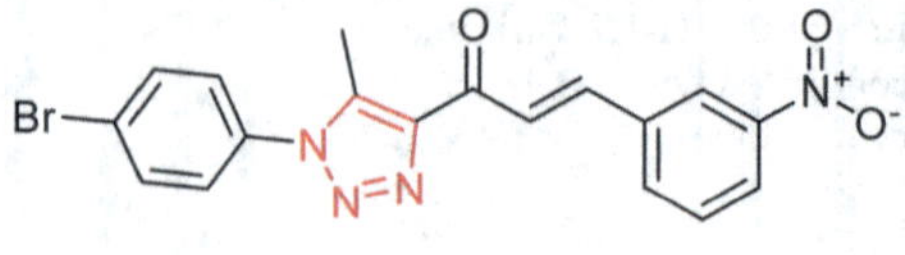

Image 10 1,2,3-Triazole chalcone conjugates, leukemia inhibitors

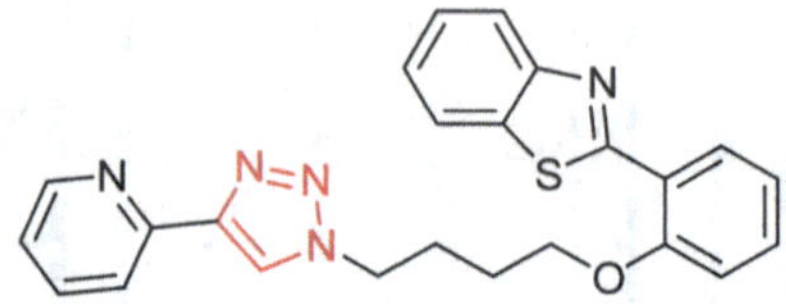

Image 11 Pyridin linked to 1H-1,2,3-triazole and phenylbenzothiazole

for cytotoxicity against sixty cancer cell lines. The most sensitive to the new chemicals were leukemia cancer cells. The most promising compounds underwent a series of biological tests. Four derivatives with IC50 values in the low micromolar range showed potent anticancer activity in RPMI-8226 cells. This compound was found to be most potent with IC50 of 3.17 μM, which is 32 times as potent as staurosporine (Image 10). The possible effects of this compound on the cell cycle, PARP-1, and specific anti-apoptotic and apoptotic markers in RPMI-8226 cells were further investigated. The results of these investigations showed that this molecule is capable of arresting the cell cycle in the S-phase and inducing apoptosis by upregulating BAX, caspase-3, and caspase-9 (Othman et al. 2022).

4.2.6 Pyridin-1,2,3-Triazol Based Ru(II)/Ir(III)/re(I) Complexes as Anticancer Agents

Using a normal cell line (HEK-293) as control, the cytotoxic activity of Ru(II)/Ir(III)/Re(I)-based 2-(2-(4-(4-(pyridin-2-yl)-1H-1,2,3-triazol-1-yl)butoxy) phenyl)benzo[d]thiazole complexes was assessed in different cancer cell lines (HeLa, MCF-7, and U87MG) (Image 11). Ru (IIa) and Re (IIb) complexes were significantly higher in cytotoxicity than Ir (IIIa) and Re (Ib) complexes. This complex inhibited both G2/M and S phase cell cycle arrest along with substantial ROS production and DNA intercalation, thereby inducing MCF-7 cell apoptosis (Thilak Babu and Paira 2023).

4.2.7 Curcumin-1,2,3-Triazole Versus the Mechanisms of Cancer Apoptosis

Neoplastic diseases are a major cause of death. To combat drug resistance, the clinical inadequacy of most anticancer drugs has led to extensive efforts to find new chemical entities with potent and safe antitumor profiles. The targeting of cancer cell apoptotic machinery has proven to be an effective strategy in this instance.

The next compound showed potency in the low micromolar range against the proliferation of T-cell acute lymphoblastic leukemia cells (Image 12). It carried a para-fluoro-phenyl moiety. Detailed biochemical studies showed that this analog had

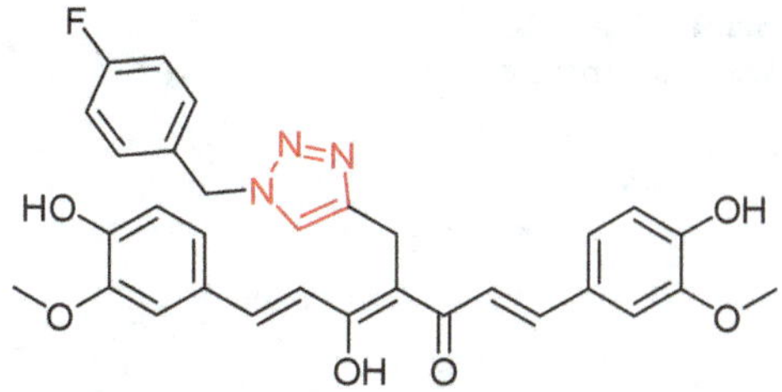

Image 12 Curcumin derivative linked to 1,2,3-triazole

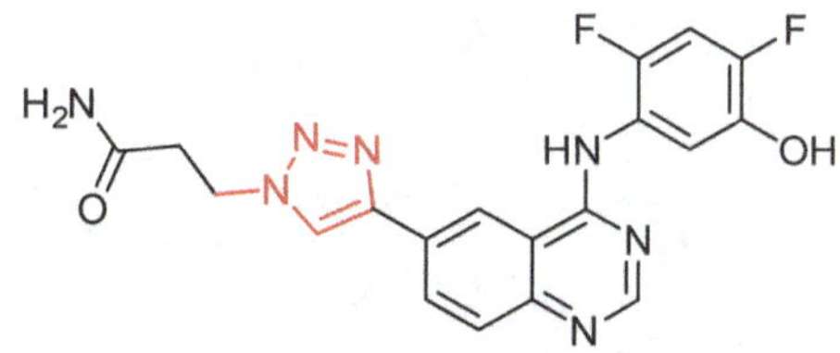

Image 13 1H-1,2,3-triazole-4-yl linked with quinazoline

cell death properties, being able to activate the mitochondrial apoptosis cascades and the receptor simultaneously. This unusual behavior has the potential to produce a more potent anticancer effect, in particular, a strong cytotoxic response (Seghetti et al. 2020).

4.2.8 4-(3-Hydroxyanilino)-6-(1H-1,2,3-Triazol-4-Yl) Quinazolines

The majority of approved kinase inhibitors are designed to target receptor tyrosine kinases, the most established being VEGFR (vascular endothelial growth factor receptor) kinases and EGFR (epidermal growth factor receptor). Cheng et al. have designed scaffold 9's 4-(3-hydroxyanilino)-6-(1H-1,2,3-triazol-4-yl)quinazolines, which are potent EGFR/VEGFR2 kinase inhibitors and selective B-Raf/B-RafV600E inhibitors (Image 13). The most potent and selective Raf kinase inhibitor, shown below, inhibited B-Raf/B-RafV600E at nanomolar concentrations (IC50: 50 and 57 nM) but was less effective against C-Raf (IC50: 1.0 μM). Regarding receptor tyrosine kinases, 9 m was inactive (IC50: >10 μM) against EGFRT790M and PDGFR-β but potent (IC50: 73 nM) against EGFR and VEGFR2. Cell proliferation was suppressed by this compound, which was associated with EGFR inhibition (Lee et al. 2021).

4.2.9 Azeliragon Triazole Analogs

Triple-negative breast cancer (TNBC) is the most serious form of breast cancer. Receptor for advanced glycation end-products (RAGE) signaling has been linked to tumor growth, metastasis, and relapse in breast cancer. This includes lymph node metastasis as well as TNBC arising from the primary tumor. The RAGE inhibitor azeliragon ($IC50 = 5.292 \pm 0.310$ μM) was shown to actively inhibit the TNBC cell line SUM149. Jizhao et al. prepared 26 azeliragon triazole analogs and screened them for anti-TNBC activity in vitro to develop a novel anti-TNBC agent. KC-10 was the most active molecule in Image 14, with an IC50 of 0.220 ± 0.034 μM (Xie et al. 2021).

Image 14 KC-10
Azeliragon triazole analog

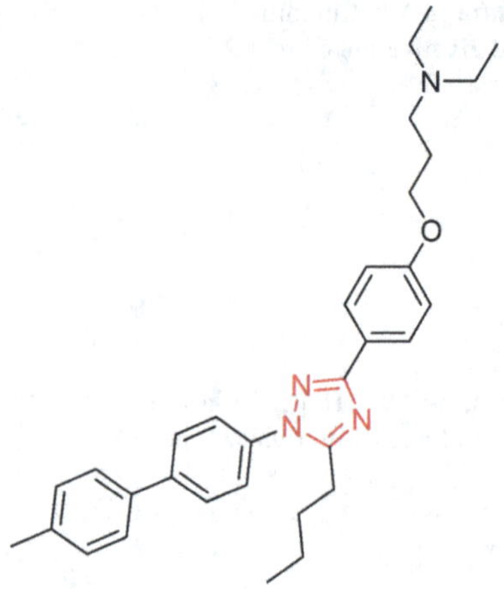

5 Therapeutic Application of Triazoles

Drugs containing triazole derivatives have been shown to have multiple pharmacological effects. These effects, in addition to their widely recognized antifungal properties, include anticancer (Lakkakula et al. 2019; Prachayasittikul et al. 2015; Ríos-Malváez et al. 2021), antitubercular, antiviral, anti-inflammatory, anti-HIV, and antibacterial effects, among others (Alam 2022; Bezerra Morais et al. 2022; Dai et al. 2022; Siegel et al. 2023; Xu et al. 2019) (Diagram 2).

5.1 Cancer Therapy

Triazoles have shown activity against a wide range of cancers. These include breast, lung, prostate, and colon cancer. The versatility of triazole derivatives allows the design of compounds with specific properties tailored to the characteristics of different cancers. Some triazoles have shown synergistic effects when used in combination with traditional chemotherapeutic agents, providing a potential avenue for improved treatment outcomes.

Understanding the mechanisms by which triazoles exert their anticancer effects is critical to their clinical development. These compounds have been shown to have diverse modes of action that affect different cellular processes.

One prominent mechanism is the inhibition of specific enzymes that are critical for cancer cell survival and proliferation. For example, triazole-based compounds have shown inhibitory activity against several kinases and enzymes involved in signaling pathways, thereby disrupting the uncontrolled growth of cancer cells.

Many of the triazoles utilized in cancer treatment specifically target breast cancer. In around 75% of diagnosed breast cancers, the tumors are estrogen receptor (ER) and/or progesterone receptor (PgR) receptor-positive, and estrogen serves as

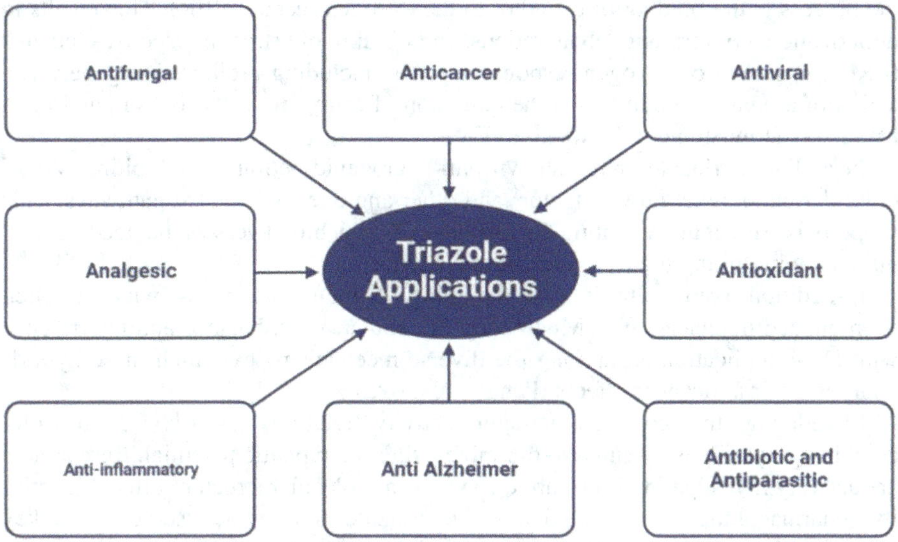

Diagram 2 The broad spectrum of the use of triazole rings

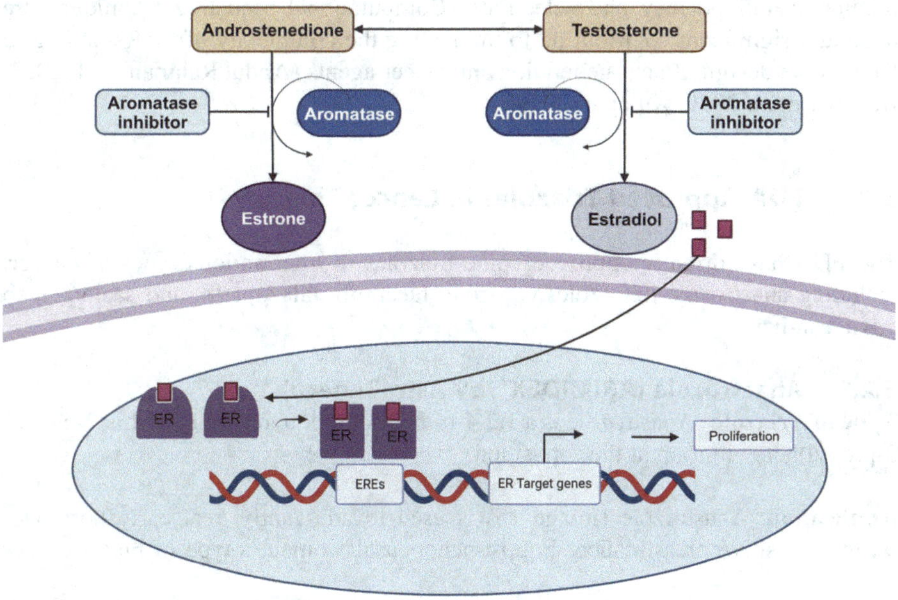

Diagram 3 Aromatase inhibitors mechanism

the primary stimulus for their growth and development. As such, aromatase inhibitors play a crucial role in treating breast cancer, as they work to suppress estrogen levels and elicit an endocrine response in ER-positive cancers. The mechanism of action of aromatase inhibitors is displayed in Diagram 3. The beginning of the process is the binding of estradiol to the estrogen receptor (ER). This results in dimerization, conformational alterations, and binding of estrogen response elements (EREs) upstream of estrogen-responsive genes, including proliferation genes. The action of aromatase inhibitors is the reduction of estrogen synthesis from androgen precursors (Johnston and Dowsett 2003).

In addition, triazoles have shown anti-angiogenic action by inhibiting VEGF (vascular endothelial growth factor) and other angiogenesis-related pathways. This property is critical in preventing the formation of new blood vessels that feed tumors, ultimately inhibiting their growth and metastasis.

In addition, some hybrids have the ability to induce apoptosis, which is often dysregulated in cancer cells. Modulation of cellular redox balance and interference with DNA replication are among the diverse mechanisms by which these hybrids manifest their anticancer effects (Peng et al. 2022).

Elucidating the complex structure-activity relationships of 1,2,3-triazole-containing hybrids is essential to optimizing their therapeutic potential. Researchers are actively investigating how subtle changes in molecular structure affect bioactivity, pharmacokinetics, and toxicity. The triazole ring, which serves as a key pharmacophore, is systematically modified to fine-tune interactions with target proteins or nucleic acids. The length and nature of the side chains, as well as the introduction of electron donating or withdrawing groups, play a key role in determining overall potency and selectivity. Computational modeling techniques are making a significant contribution to unraveling the complexity of SARs, aiding in the rational design of next-generation anticancer agents (Abdul Rahman et al. 2023; Bozorov et al. 2019; Xu et al. 2019).

5.2 FDA-Approved Triazoles in Cancer Therapy

The FDA has currently approved some triazoles to treat various types of cancer, including anastrozole, letrozole, vorozole, tucatinib, talazoparib, and sacituzumab govitecan-hziy.

5.2.1 Anastrozole (ARIMIDEX® by AstraZeneca)

Type of Triazole Anastrozole is a 1,2,4-triazole compound with a 3,5-bis(2-cyano-2-propyl)benzyl group at the 1-position.

Application Anastrozole (Image 15) is used to adjuvantly treat early hormone-receptor-positive breast cancer in postmenopausal women, a type of breast cancer

Image 15 Structure of anastrozole

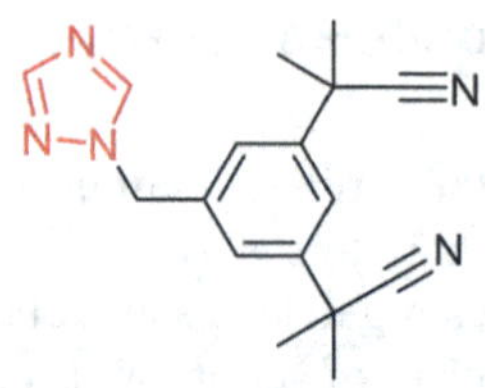

controlled by estrogen and/or progesterone. It is also used in the first-line treatment of locally advanced or metastatic hormone-receptor (HR)-positive or hormone-receptor-unknown breast cancer in postmenopausal women whose disease has progressed after they have received tamoxifen.

The most common type of gynecologic malignancy is endometrial cancer (EC), which is primarily treated with chemotherapy. However, a large number of malignant endometrial tumors express hormone receptors and may respond to hormone therapy. This makes hormonal therapy an attractive non-chemotherapeutic option by administering extended-release Onapris. Initial results in extensively pretreated patients with EC using onapristone extended release plus anastrozole for dual hormone blockade suggest that this combination is well tolerated and has promising activity.

Action Mechanism Aromatase inhibitor. Anastrozole is designed to deprive hormone receptor-positive breast cancer cells of the estrogen they require to grow by reducing estrogen levels in the body. This inhibition of estrogen synthesis may have a slowing or stopping effect on the progression of hormone receptor-positive breast cancer (Rashdan and Shehadi 2022).

5.2.2 Letrozole (Femara® by Novartis)

Type of Triazole Diphenylmethanes (1,2,4 triazole).

Application Letrozole (Image 16) is an aromatase inhibitor (AI) prescribed for the treatment of breast cancer patients (Biegon et al. 2020).

Adjuvant therapy is recommended in postmenopausal women with early HR-positive breast cancer, and for postmenopausal women who have already received standard adjuvant tamoxifen therapy, the extended adjuvant treatment is recommended. Postmenopausal women with HR-positive or unknown advanced breast cancer have first- and second-line options.

Action Mechanism Aromatase inhibitor. In reducing uterine weight, letrozole is as effective as ovariectomy in adult women with or without tumors, increasing serum LH and inducing regression of estrogen-dependent tumors. There is no significant effect on adrenal mineralocorticoid or glucocorticoid synthesis with this selective inhibitor of gonadal steroidogenesis. Letrozole inhibits estrogen biosynthesis in all tissues by competitive interaction with the heme group of the cytochrome P450

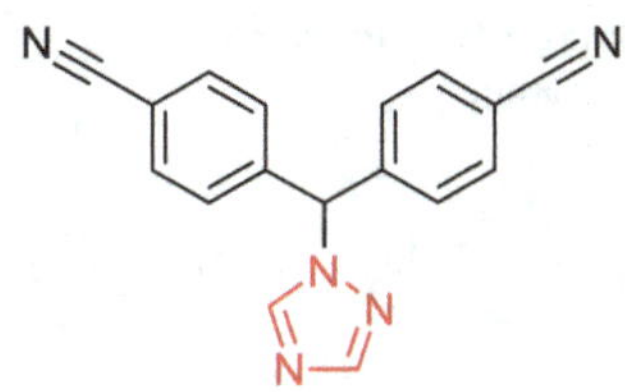

Image 16 Letrozole structure

subunit of the aromatase. The result is a decrease in estrogen levels (Malhotra et al. 2023; Rashdan and Shehadi 2022).

5.2.3 Vorozole (Rivizor®)

Type of Triazole *S*-vorozole (6-[(*S*)-(4-chlorophenyl)-1H-1,2,4-triazol-1-ylmethyl]-1-methyl-1H-benzotriazole).

Application Vorozole (Image 17) has proven effective in treating postmenopausal women with advanced breast cancer (Wiseman and Spencer 1997).

Action Mechanism Aromatase inhibitor. Vorozole binds to the cytochrome P450 moiety of aromatase, resulting in reversible inhibition of the enzyme. Originally developed as an antineoplastic drug, the compound undergoes significant liver metabolism and exhibits an elimination half-life of 8 h (Biegon et al. 2020; Rashdan and Shehadi 2022).

5.2.4 Tucatinib (TUKYSA®)

Type of Triazole 1,2,4-Triazole.

Application Tucatinib (Image 18), marketed by Seagen as Tukysa®, is an oral kinase inhibitor indicated for the treatment of advanced unresectable or metastatic HER2-positive breast cancer in adults. It is recommended in patients who have received one or more prior anti-HER2 therapies in the metastatic setting, including those with brain metastases, in combination with trastuzumab and capecitabine. Trastuzumab may be used in combination to treat adult patients with HER2-positive, RAS wild-type, metastatic, unresectable colorectal cancer that has progressed following treatment with chemotherapeutic agents, including oxaliplatin, fluoropyrimidine, and irinotecan.

Action Mechanism Tucatinib is a HER2 tyrosine kinase inhibitor. It inhibits the phosphorylation of HER3 and HER2 in vitro, resulting in the inhibition of AKT and

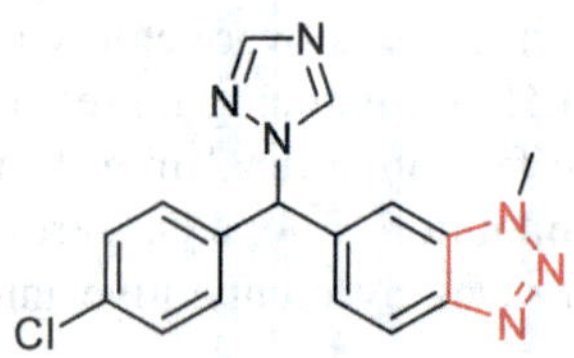

Image 17 Vorozole composition

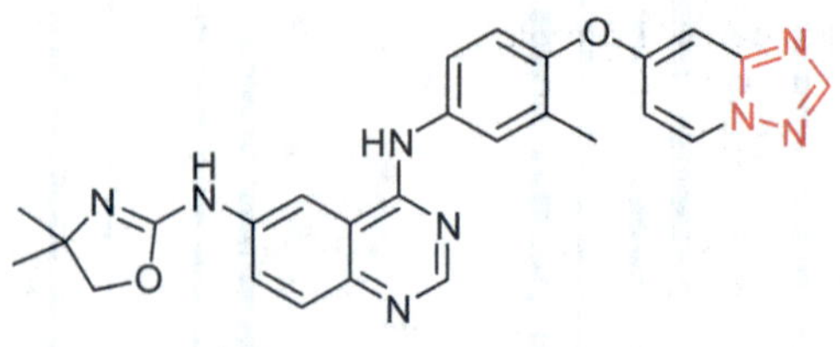

Image 18 Structure of Tucatinib

MAPK signaling, thereby inhibiting cell proliferation. Tucatinib demonstrated antitumor activity in HER2-expressing tumor cells in vivo. Tucatinib was effective in inhibiting the growth of HER2-expressing tumors in vivo. The combination of trastuzumab and tucatinib demonstrated enhanced antitumor activity both in vivo and in vitro when compared to either of the two drugs alone.

5.2.5 Talazoparib (TALZENNA®)

Type of Triazole Phenylquinoline (1*H*-1,2,4-triazole).

Application Talazoparib (Image 19) is an oral inhibitor of poly (ADP-ribose) polymerase (PARP) that is approved by the FDA and marketed by Pfizer under the trade name Talzenna ®. It is indicated as a single agent to treat adults with locally advanced or metastatic breast cancer who harbor HER2-negative germline BRCA mutations (gBRCAm). In 2023, the FDA approved talazoparib in combination with enzalutamide for the treatment of patients with metastatic castration-resistant prostate cancer harboring homologous recombination repair (HRR) mutations.

Action Mechanism Talazoparib is a PARP enzyme inhibitor that targets PARP1 and PARP2, both of which are involved in DNA repair. In vitro studies using cancer cells with mutations in DNA repair genes, like BRCA1 and BRCA2, have demonstrated that talazoparib-induced cytotoxicity could be due to its ability to inhibit PARP enzyme activity and promote the formation of PARP-DNA complexes. These processes lead to DNA damage, reduced cell proliferation, and apoptosis. Talazoparib has shown antitumor activity in patient-derived xenograft models of breast cancer that have mutations in BRCA1, mutations in BRCA2, or the wild-type BRCA1 and BRCA2.

5.2.6 Sacituzumab Govitecan-Hziy (TRODELVY®)

Type of Triazole Sacituzumab govitecan-hziy is an antibody-drug conjugate with linker 1.2,3 triazole presence.

Application Tecentriq sacituzumab govitecan-hziy (Image 20) is a Trop-2-directed antibody/topoisomerase inhibitor conjugate indicated for the treatment of locally advanced or metastatic breast cancer and urothelial cancer in adults. Locally advanced or metastatic breast cancer: This refers to unresectable triple-negative breast cancer treated with two or more prior lines of systemic therapy, including at least one line of therapy for metastatic disease. Patients with HR-positive,

Image 19 Talazoparib composition

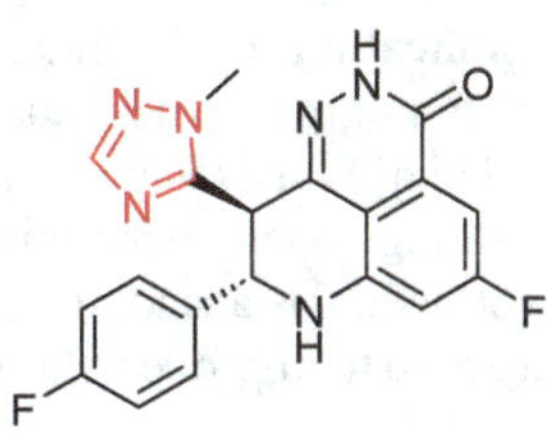

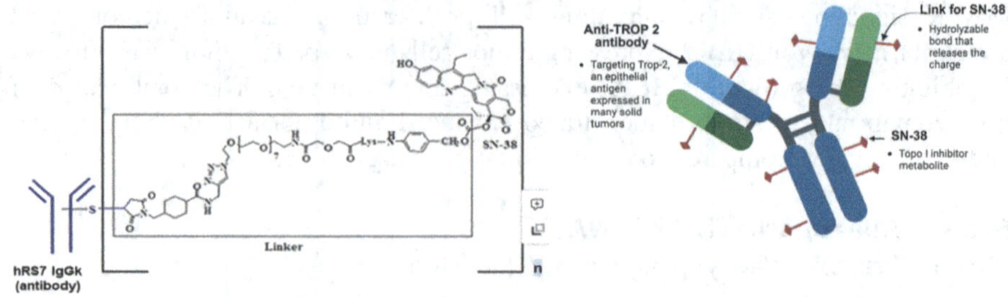

Image 20 Sacituzumab govitecan-hziy. (Rugo et al. 2020)

HER2-negative (IHC0, IHC1+, or IHC2+/ISH-) breast cancer that is locally advanced or metastatic may be diagnosed when unresectable and endocrine therapy and at least two prior systemic treatments for metastatic disease have been administered.

Locally advanced or metastatic urothelial cancer is also a potential diagnosis.

Patients with locally advanced or metastatic urothelial cancer (mUC) who have received platinum-based chemotherapy and treatment with a programmed death receptor 1 (PD-1) or programmed death ligand 1 (PD-L1) inhibitor.

Action Mechanism Sacituzumab govitecan-hziy is an antibody-drug conjugate. It is directed against Trop-2. This human antibody recognizing Trop-2 is linked via a linker to the topoisomerase I inhibitor SN-38. Pharmacological data show that sacituzumab govitecan-hziy binds to cancer cells expressing Trop-2. It is then internalized and releases SN-38 via linker hydrolysis. SN-38 interacts with topoisomerase I, preventing topoisomerase I-induced single-strand breaks, causing DNA damage, apoptosis, and cell death. In mouse xenograft models of triple-negative breast cancer, sacituzumab govitecan-hziy reduced tumor growth.

5.3 Triazoles in Clinical Trials

The importance of triazoles in medicinal chemistry is such that several molecules are already in clinical trials.

5.3.1 Carboxyamidotriazole (CAI)

Type of Triazole Bioactive molecules with 1,2,3-triazole core nucleus, 1,4,5-trisubstituted triazole.

Application CAI (Image 21) possesses antiangiogenic, antimetastatic, and antitumor properties due to its role in indirect involvement in Store-Operated Calcium Entry (Marzi et al. 2022).

Lung cancer, accounting for approximately 18.4% of all cancer-related deaths worldwide, is a leading cause of mortality. Various combinations of cytotoxic drugs are used to improve treatment response in patients with advanced non-small cell lung

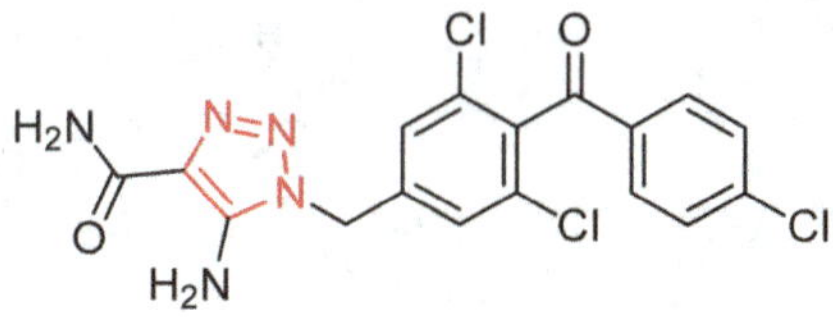

Image 21 Carboxyamidotriazole structure (CAI)

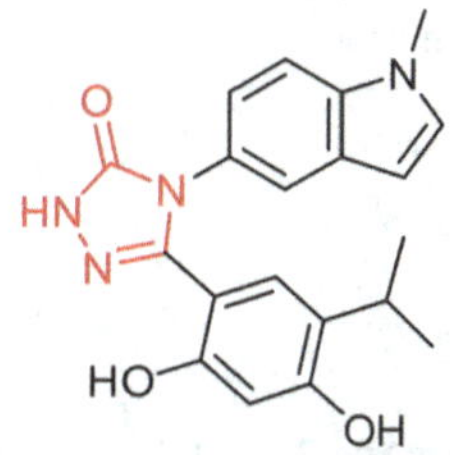

Image 22 Ganetespib composition

cancer (NSCLC). One such drug is carboxyamidotriazole (CAI), which inhibits non-voltage-dependent calcium channels that are involved in a variety of cellular signaling pathways. CAI blocks inositol trisphosphate (IP3) synthesis, nitric oxide (NO) production, and vascular endothelial growth factor-A (VEGF-A)-induced Ca^{2+}-dependent endothelial cell proliferation. Thus, CAI inhibits angiogenesis and abnormal growth of tumor cells by decreasing intracellular IP3 release, NO production, and Ca^{2+}-dependent VEGF-A production, as demonstrated in a randomized, double-blind, controlled Phase III trial of carboxyamidotriazole and chemotherapy in advanced non-small cell lung cancer (Alam 2022; Dai et al. 2022; Matin et al. 2022).

5.3.2 Ganetespib

In the initial Phase II trial of an Hsp90 inhibitor for colorectal cancer, ganetespib monotherapy demonstrated no efficacy in managing metastatic colorectal cancer unresponsive to chemotherapy. Further clinical studies are planned for Ganetespib (Image 22), a novel Hsp90 inhibitor, in combination with conventional cytotoxic treatments. This decision is based on promising preclinical evidence of the drug's combination activity and its safe profile. The study examines patients with refractory metastatic colorectal cancer, both KRAS mutated and wild type (Youssef et al. 2023).

5.4 Miscellaneous Triazoles for Oncology

5.4.1 TD139

Galectin (Gal)-3 has been implicated in the pathophysiology and exacerbation of idiopathic pulmonary fibrosis (IPF) and is a profibrotic beta-galactoside-binding lectin. A novel and potent small molecule inhibitor of Gal-3 is TD139 (Image 23).

Image 23 TD139 molecule

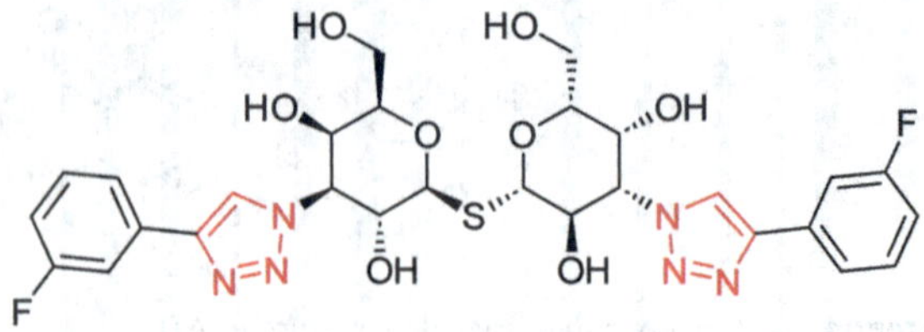

Image 24 The VT-464 molecule

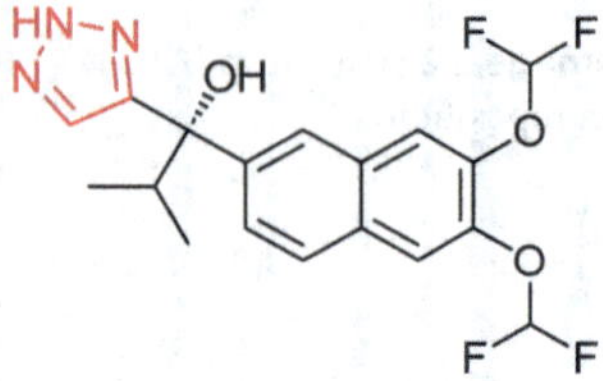

Image 25 ACT-777991 structure

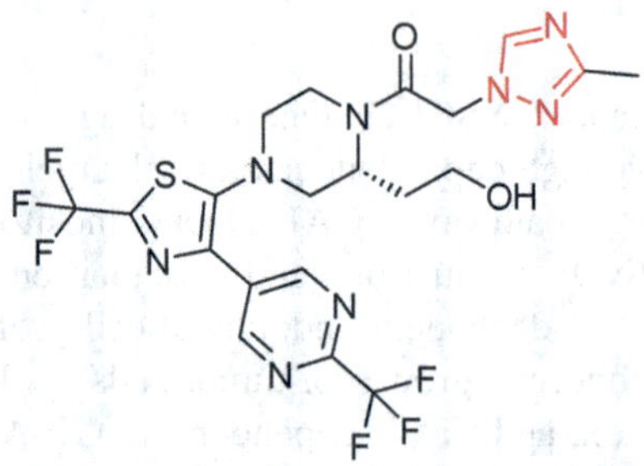

In both healthy volunteers and patients with IPF, it has been shown to be well tolerated. TD139 has been shown to reduce the expression of Gal-3 in bronchoalveolar lavage (BAL) macrophages and to coordinately reduce plasma biomarkers that are associated with the progression of IPF (Hirani et al. 2021).

5.4.2 VT-464

Abiraterone acetate (Image 24), an oral CYP17A1 inhibitor, is effective in treating prostate cancer because it reduces the biosynthesis of adrenal and intratumoral androgens. The oral drug, an exclusive class of CYP17 lyase-selective inhibitors, is currently in Phase 2 clinical trials for prostate cancer (Rafferty et al. 2014).

5.4.3 Act-777991

The G protein-coupled chemokine receptor CXCR3 is predominantly expressed on lymphoid lineage immune cells such as activated T cells. In the mouse model of acute pulmonary inflammation, the highly potent, unprecedentedly specific CXCR3 antagonist ACT-777991 (Image 25) showed dose-dependent activity and target engagement (Meyer et al. 2023).

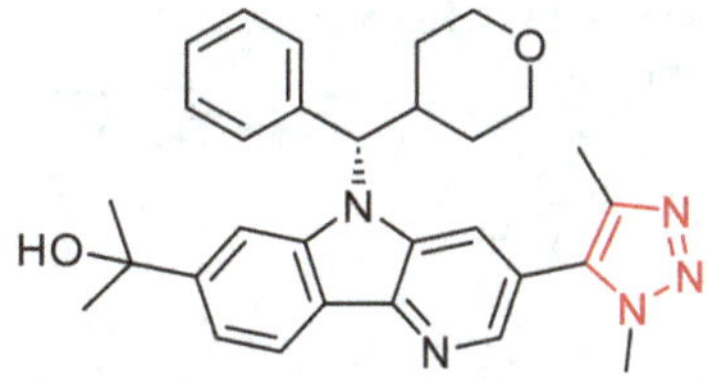

Image 26 BMS-986158 composition

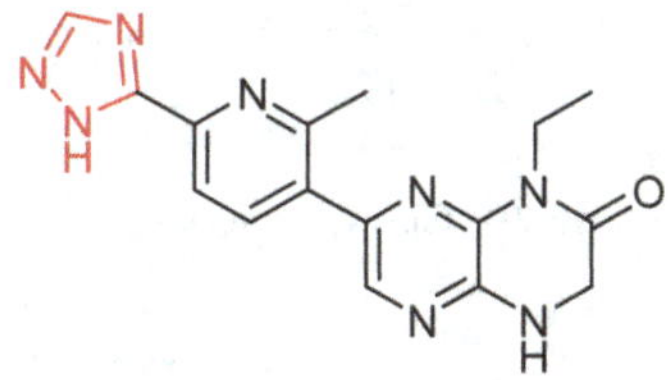

Image 27 CC-115 molecule

5.4.4 BMS-986158

The use of BET protein inhibitors as anticancer agents is justified by their involvement in the proliferation, survival, and oncogenic development of cancer cells. Both BET inhibition (BETi) and its combination with Janus kinase inhibition (JAKi) have been shown to reduce inflammatory signaling and ease disease burden in mouse models of myelofibrosis. For the treatment of patients with myelofibrosis, simultaneous inhibition of BET-mediated pathways and the JAK-STAT pathway has shown promise. BMS-986158, a selective oral compound (Image 26), is a small molecule BET inhibitor. It has demonstrated dose- and time-dependent regulation of BET target gene expression. It also exhibits a dose-proportio (Ayala et al. 2022).

5.4.5 CC-115

Effective molecularly targeted treatments for non-small cell lung cancer (NSCLC) are urgently needed. CC-115 (Image 27), a highly potent dual inhibitor of both mammalian targets of rapamycin (mTOR) and DNA-dependent protein kinase (DNA-PK), has been found to be efficacious when evaluated in multiple human NSCLC cells (Chen et al. 2022).

5.4.6 CKD-516

The leading cancer killer is lung cancer. For non-small cell lung cancer (NSCLC), docetaxel is used as a second- or third-line treatment. When NSCLC becomes resistant to tyrosine kinase inhibitors (TKIs) and epidermal growth factor receptor (EGFR), CKD-516, a vascular disrupting agent, can be combined with docetaxel for treatment. CKD-516's oral bioavailability (Image 28) was observed. It was determined that neither CKD-516 nor docetaxel had an effect on each other's pharmacokinetic properties or mean plasma concentration-time profile (Kim et al. 2023).

5.4.7 Cjoc42

Hepatoblastoma (HBL) and hepatocellular carcinoma (HCC) are cancers that are notoriously resistant to chemotherapy and associated with unfavorable outcomes. A

Image 28 CKD-516 structure

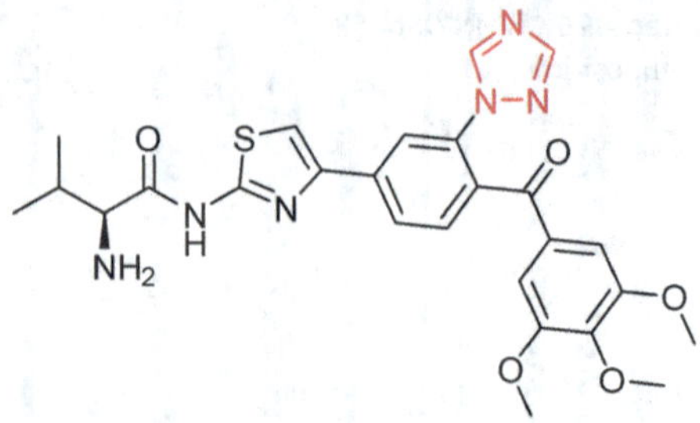

Image 29 Cjoc42 molecule

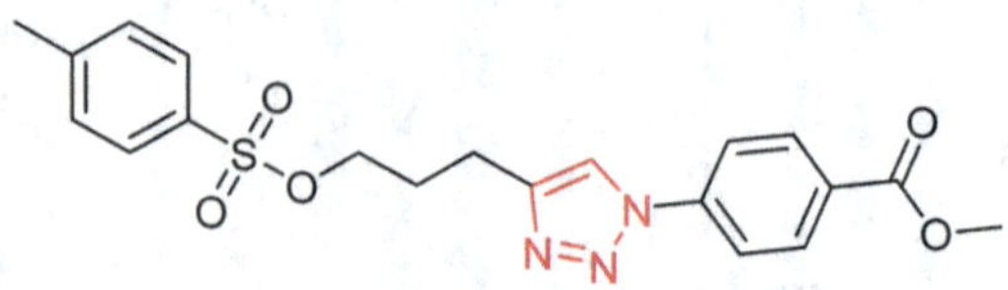

Image 30 HDAC3-IN-T326 molecule

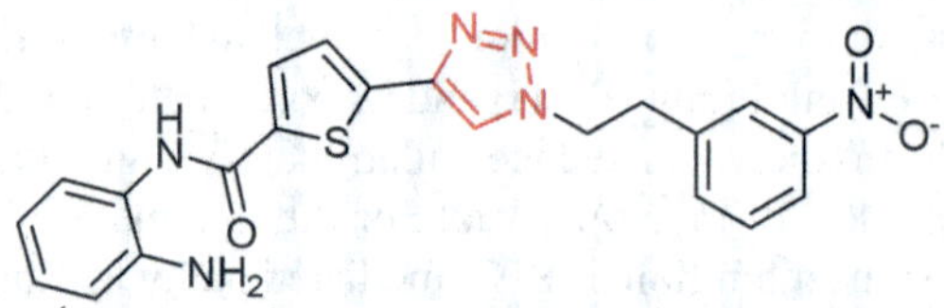

known oncogene called gankyrin, or Gank, is overexpressed in childhood liver cancer and is associated with chemoresistance. Given its ability to increase chemosensitivity, Cjoc42 (Image 29) shows promise as an adjuvant treatment for severe childhood liver cancer when combined with chemotherapy (D'Souza et al. 2021).

5.4.8 HDAC3-in-T326

Complexes of histone proteins bind to DNA to form chromatin, a higher-order structure. A nucleosome is formed when an octamer of histones is wrapped twice around approximately 150 base pairs of DNA. Histone-DNA and histone-nonhistone protein interactions can be altered by acetylating or deacetylating core histones with N-terminal tails that extend from the compact nucleosomal core particles. While they did not significantly inhibit other isozymes, HDAC3-IN-T326 exhibited robust HDAC3 inhibition with submicromolar IC50s. Also caused human colon cancer HCT116 (Image 30) cells to exhibit a dose-dependent selective increase in NF-κB acetylation, demonstrating the cells' preferential inhibition of HDAC3. In addition, these HDAC3-specific inhibitors stimulated HIV gene expression in quiescent HIV-positive cells and inhibited cancer cell proliferation (Suzuki et al. 2013).

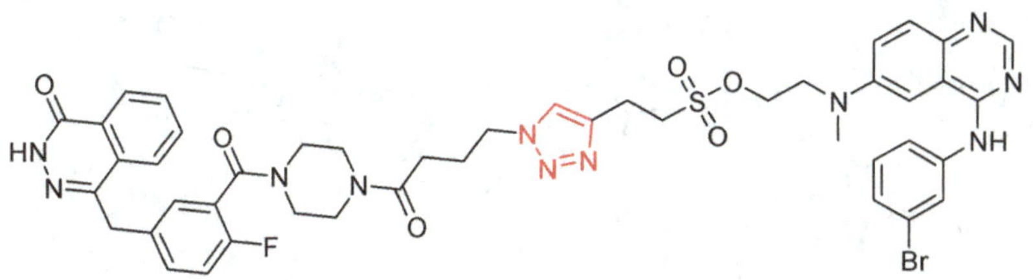

Image 31 JS230 composition

Image 32 OM-1700 structure

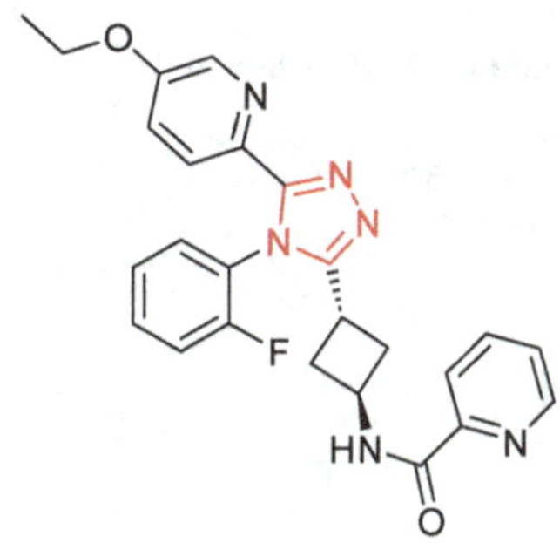

5.4.9 JS230

Several variables, including overexpression of epidermal growth factor receptor (EGFR) and DNA repair enzymes, can contribute to chemotherapy resistance in advanced malignancies. Therefore, most current standards of care combine multiple treatments. A novel linker allows the integration of multiple actions (including DNA lesioning, inhibition of EGFR phosphorylation, and inhibition of repair) into a single molecule. This led to the successful synthesis of JS230 (Image 31), a unique and potent combined molecule (Schmitt et al. 2020).

5.4.10 OM-1700

Many target proteins undergo post-translational modifications via poly-ADP ribosylation by tankyrase 1 and 2 (TNKS1/2). In addition, TNKS1/2 impacts the WNT/β-catenin and Hippo signaling pathways, both of which have been implicated in various human diseases, including cancer. OM-1700 (Image 32) demonstrates high selectivity for TNKS1/2, a clean off-target safety profile, improved permeability in Caco-2 cells, and microsomal stability. In addition, a mouse pharmacokinetic analysis shows a 15-fold increase in exposure, along with potent suppression of WNT/β-catenin signaling and proliferation in the COLO 320DM colon cancer cell line (Waaler et al. 2020).

5.4.11 PEN-866

SN-38, a small molecule that binds to HSP90, is combined with a cytotoxic payload in PEN-866 (Image 33). HSP90 is expressed at high levels in advanced malignant

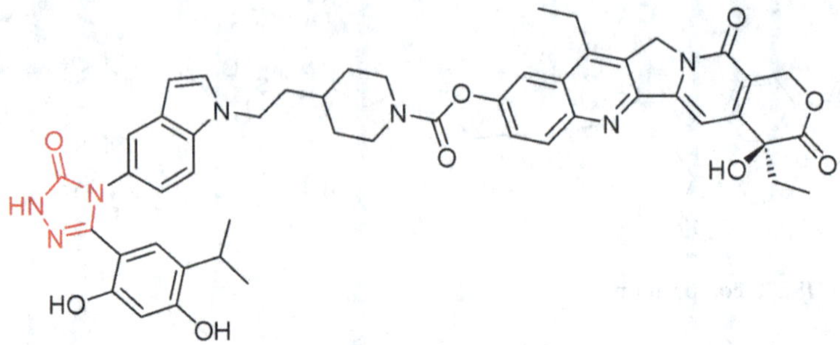

Image 33 PEN-866 molecule

Image 34 Selinexor molecule

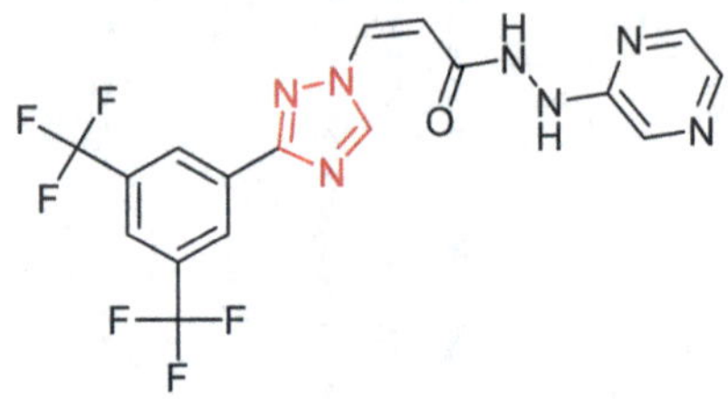

Image 35 SPS-7 structure

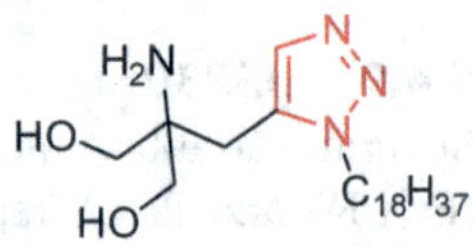

tumors. PEN-866 is designed to target and engage activated tumor HSP90 protein, resulting in the release of a cytotoxic payload and complete tumor regression in multiple xenograft models. The safety, tolerability, pharmacokinetics (PK), and preliminary efficacy of PEN-866 were evaluated in this first-in-human study (Falchook et al. 2020).

5.4.12 Selinexor

Selinexor (Image 34), often referred to as KPT-330 is a potent, selective, oral XPO1/CRM1 inhibitor. In patients with chronic lymphocytic leukemia, selinexor is used in combination with ibrutinib to treat acquired resistance. By reducing tumor formation, depleting anti-apoptotic proteins, and inducing apoptosis, selinexor enhances the anticancer activity of gemcitabine in human pancreatic cancer. Selinexor spares normal stem and progenitor cells but shows potent activity against early AML cells.

5.4.13 SPS-7

The most powerful derivative, SPS-7 (Image 35), exhibits greater anti-proliferative effects against hormone-refractory prostate cancer (HRPC) in humans than FTY720. It triggers the G1 cell cycle arrest Thymidine block-mediated synchronization model before apoptosis. The result was fortified by cyclin D1 expression decline and a substantial increase in p21 expression along with a corresponding RB phosphorylation reduction. Cyclin D1 levels were restored by overexpression of c-Myc, indicating its role in regulating the cell cycle. Efficient PI3K/Akt/mTOR signaling pathway-mediated translation control by 4EBP1 and p70S6K is critical for cell survival and proliferation. SPS-7 effectively impedes this translational process (Leu et al. 2016).

5.4.14 YQ456

Myoferlin (MYOF), a crucial protein for vesicular trafficking, has become a prominent cancer therapy target. The role of MYOF in colorectal cancer invasion, however, remains uncertain, and its efficacy as a targeted therapy has yet to be evaluated. Recently, the discovery of YQ456 (Image 36), a novel small molecule inhibitor of MYOF, has shown a remarkable ability to hinder invasion (IC50 = 110 nM) and strongly bind to MYOF (KD = 37 nM). YQ456 disrupts interactions between Ras-associated binding (Rab) proteins and MYOF at low nanomolar levels.

6 Future Prospects and Challenges

In this chapter, we have reviewed some 1,2,3- and 1,2,4-triazole methods, along with the importance of triazoles in the treatment of cancer. A summary of several important synthetic techniques using different nitrogen sources has been provided. Sodium azide, a highly toxic compound used in the synthesis of 1,2,3-triazole, is unsuitable for use as a nitrogen source on a large scale. Aryl/alkyl azide and azide-trimethylsilane are safer and more effective than sodium azide. Aminohydrazine, hydrazone, and diazo compounds are also primary nitrogen source components and have been documented in a wide range of literature. Amide, amidine, aryl diazonium salt, amidine hydrazone, and hydrazone are the main nitrogen sources used in 1,2,4-triazole synthesis. In recent years, excellent progress has been made in the synthesis of 1,2,4/1,2,3-triazole with low toxicity and good functional tolerance by copper-catalyzed cross-coupling. Copper-catalyzed click reaction is the most widely used type of metal catalysis. In addition, the advantages of performing the reaction in microwaves, which was the predominant option at that time, were considered. With the growth of the "green chemistry" movement, researchers are increasingly interested in metal-free catalytic synthesis techniques such as electrocatalysis and photocatalysis. Cycloaddition is also of great interest. It is expected that more

Image 36 YQ456 composition

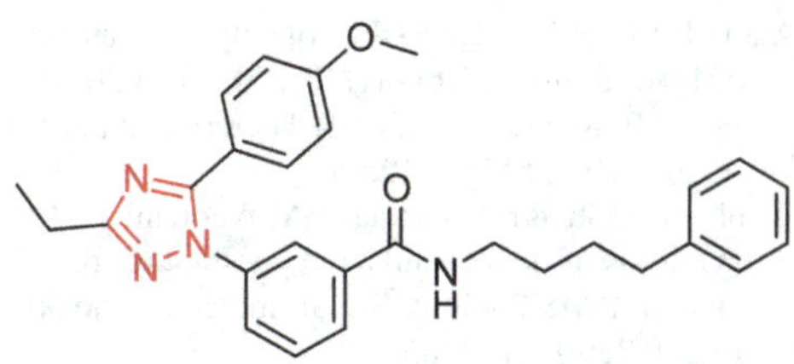

green economies and simple, mild synthetic techniques will emerge as a result of researchers' continued efforts.

The choice of a single synthetic route is impossible since it depends on the initial functional groups, neighboring groups, and labile groups present in the molecule; fortunately, as already observed, there are different synthetic routes that allow us to design and obtain triazoles in all their diversity.

While significant progress has been made in recent years in the use of triazoles in cancer therapy, challenges and opportunities remain. The development of triazole-based drugs faces hurdles such as bioavailability, toxicity, and off-target effects. Overcoming these challenges requires continued research efforts to optimize compound design and improve therapeutic efficacy.

In addition, exploring the potential of triazoles in combination therapies, either with traditional chemotherapeutic agents or other targeted therapies, holds promise for synergistic effects and improved treatment outcomes. As research in this area continues to evolve, the integration of triazoles into comprehensive cancer treatment strategies is likely to contribute to the growth of anticancer therapies.

7 Conclusion

Recent advances in triazole-based agents for cancer therapy underscore their potential as valuable additions to the oncologist's armamentarium. From their diverse mechanisms of action to their use in chemotherapy, targeted therapy, and immunotherapy, triazoles offer a multifaceted approach to fighting cancer. Further research and clinical trials will inevitably illuminate the complete therapeutic capabilities of triazoles, edging us closer to more personalized and efficient cancer treatments.

References

Abdul Rahman SM, Bhatti JS, Thareja S, Monga V (2023) Current development of 1,2,3-triazole derived potential antimalarial scaffolds: structure- activity relationship (SAR) and bioactive compounds. Eur J Med Chem 259:115699. https://doi.org/10.1016/j.ejmech.2023.115699

Agalave S, Maujan S, Pore V (2011) Click chemistry: 1,2,3-Triazoles as pharmacophores. Chem Asian J 6(10):2696–2718. https://doi.org/10.1002/asia.201100432

Agouram N, El Hadrami EM, Bentama A (2021) 1,2,3-Triazoles as biomimetics in peptide science. Molecules 26(10):2937. https://doi.org/10.3390/molecules26102937

Ahmed M, Razaq H, Faisal M, Siyal AN, Haider A (2017) Metal-free and azide-free synthesis of 1,2,3-triazoles derivatives. Synth Commun 47(13):1193–1200. https://doi.org/10.1080/00397911.2017.1303511

Alam MM (2022) 1,2,3-Triazole hybrids as anticancer agents: a review. Arch Pharm 355(1): e2100158. https://doi.org/10.1002/ardp.202100158

Albericio F, Kruger HG (2012) Therapeutic peptides. Future Med Chem 4(12):1527–1531. https://doi.org/10.4155/fmc.12.94

Al-blewi F, Shaikh SA, Naqvi A, Aljohani F, Aouad MR, Ihmaid S, Rezki N (2021) Design and synthesis of novel imidazole possessing triazole pharmacophore with anticancer activity and in silico ADMET with GSK-3β molecular docking studies. Int J Mol Sci 22(3):1162. https://doi.org/10.3390/ijms22031162

Al-Hasawi NA, Phillips OA, Al-Awadhi F, Sharaf LH, Amine SA, Novotny L (2020) Antiprogressive effects of a series of glycinyl and alaninyl triazolyl oxazolidinones on Kelly neuroblastoma cell line. Anticancer Res 40(9):5125–5140. https://doi.org/10.21873/anticanres.14516

Almashal FAK, Al-Hujaj HH, Jassem AM, Al-Masoudi NA (2020) A click synthesis, molecular docking, cytotoxicity on breast cancer (MDA-MB 231) and anti-HIV activities of new 1,4-Disubstituted-1,2,3-Triazole thymine derivatives. Russ J Bioorg Chem 46(3):360–370. https://doi.org/10.1134/S1068162020030024

Appukkuttan P, Dehaen W, Fokin VV, Van der Eycken E (2004) A microwave-assisted click chemistry synthesis of 1,4-Disubstituted 1,2,3-Triazoles via a copper(I)-catalyzed three-component reaction. Org Lett 6(23):4223–4225. https://doi.org/10.1021/ol048341v

Ashok D, Mohan Gandhi D, Srinivas G, Vikas Kumar A (2014) Microwave-assisted synthesis of novel 1,2,3-triazole derivatives and their antimicrobial activity. Med Chem Res 23(6): 3005–3018. https://doi.org/10.1007/s00044-013-0880-1

Ashok D, Reddy MR, Dharavath R, Ramakrishna K, Nagaraju N, Sarasija M (2020) Microwave-assisted synthesis of some new 1,2,3-triazole and their antimicrobial activity. J Chem Sci 132(1):47. https://doi.org/10.1007/s12039-020-1748-9

Atkinson MR, Polya JB (1952) 657. Triazoles. Part I. Unsymmetrical Einhorn–Brunner and related Pellizzari reactions. J Chem Soc 0(0):3418–3422. https://doi.org/10.1039/JR9520003418

Ayala R, Lopez N, Shacham Abulafia A, Alwan M, Yannakou CK, Raman I, Ribrag V, Fong CY, Volchek Y, Bonifacio M, Tucci A, Kiladjian J-J, Chang H, Das S, Wu B, Ravindran P, Shan V, Wang G, Esposito O et al (2022) BMS-986158, a potent BET inhibitor, as monotherapy and in combination with Ruxolitinib or Fedratinib in intermediate- or high-risk Myelofibrosis: first results from a phase 1/2 study. Blood 140(Supplement 1):9665–9667. https://doi.org/10.1182/blood-2022-159476

Bertozzi C (2023) A special virtual issue in celebrating the 2022 nobel prize, chemistry for the development of click chemistry and bioorthogonal chemistry. ACS Cent Sci 9(4):558–559. https://doi.org/10.1021/acscentsci.2c01430

Bezerra Morais PA, Javarini CL, Valim TC, Francisco CS, de Freitas Ferreira LC, Trancoso Bottocim RR, Neto ÁC, Júnior VL (2022) Triazole: a new perspective in medicinal chemistry and material science. Curr Org Chem 26(18):1691–1702. https://doi.org/10.2174/1385272827666221213145147

Biegon A, Shroyer KR, Franceschi D, Dhawan J, Tahmi M, Pareto D, Bonilla P, Airola K, Cohen J (2020) Initial studies with ^{11}C-vorozole PET detect overexpression of intratumoral aromatase in breast cancer. J Nucl Med 61(6):807–813. https://doi.org/10.2967/jnumed.119.231589

Boettcher A, Usman A, Morgans A, VanderWeele D, Sosman J, Wu J (2019) Past, present and future of immunotherapies for prostate cancer. Front Oncol 9:884. https://doi.org/10.3389/fonc.2019.00884

Bonandi E, Christodoulou M, Fumagalli G, Perdicchia D, Rastelli G, Passarella D (2017) The 1, 2, 3-triazole ring as a bioisostere in medicinal chemistry. Drug Discov Today 22(10):1572–1581. https://doi.org/10.1016/j.drudis.2017.05.014

Bozorov K, Zhao J, Aisa HA (2019) 1, 2, 3-Triazole-containing hybrids as leads in medicinal chemistry: a recent overview. Bioorg Med Chem 27(16):3511–3531. https://doi.org/10.1016/j.bmc.2019.07.005

Breugst M, Reissig H (2020) The Huisgen reaction: milestones of the 1, 3-dipolar cycloaddition. Angew Chem Int Ed 59(30):12293–12307. https://doi.org/10.1002/anie.202003115

Burguin A, Diorio C, Durocher F (2021) Breast cancer treatments: updates and new challenges. J Pers Med 11(8):808. https://doi.org/10.3390/jpm11080808

Ceylan S, Bayrak H, Basoglu Ozdemir S, Uygun Y, Mermer A, Demirbas N, Ulker S (2016) Microwave-assisted and conventional synthesis of novel antimicrobial 1,2,4-triazole derivatives containing nalidixic acid skeleton. Heterocycl Commun 22(4):229–237. https://doi.org/10.1515/hc-2016-0019

Channabasappa V, Kumar KA, Vagish CB, Sudeep P, Jayadevappa HP, Kumar A (2020) 1,2,4-triazoles: synthetic and medicinal perspectives. Int J Curr Res 12(8):12950–12960. https://doi.org/10.24941/ijcr.39386.08.2020

Chen F, Zhao H, Li C, Li P, Zhang Q (2022) An mTOR and DNA-PK dual inhibitor CC-115 hinders non-small cell lung cancer cell growth. Cell Death Discovery 8(1):293. https://doi.org/10.1038/s41420-022-01082-6

Chudasama SJ, Shah BJ, Patel KM, Dhameliya TM (2022) The spotlight review on ionic liquids catalyzed synthesis of aza- and oxa-heterocycles reported in 2021. J Mol Liq 361:119664. https://doi.org/10.1016/j.molliq.2022.119664

Ci T, Zhang W, Qiao Y, Li H, Zang J, Li H, Feng N, Gu Z (2022) Delivery strategies in treatments of leukemia. Chem Soc Rev 51(6):2121–2144. https://doi.org/10.1039/D1CS00755F

Dai J, Tian S, Yang X, Liu Z (2022) Synthesis methods of 1,2,3–/1,2,4-triazoles: a review. Front Chem 10:891484. https://doi.org/10.3389/fchem.2022.891484

Daraie M, Heravi MM (2019) A biocompatible chitosan-ionic liquid hybrid catalyst for regioselective synthesis of 1,2,3-triazols. Int J Biol Macromol 140:939–948. https://doi.org/10.1016/j.ijbiomac.2019.08.162

Debela D, Muzazu S, Heraro K, Ndalama M, Mesele B, Haile D, Kitui S, Manyazewal T (2021) New approaches and procedures in cancer treatment: current perspectives. SAGE Open Med 9:205031212110343. https://doi.org/10.1177/20503121211034366

Dehaen W, Bakulev V (2015) In: Dehaen W, Bakulev V (eds) Chemistry of 1,2,3-triazoles, vol 40. Springer International Publishing. https://doi.org/10.1007/978-3-319-07962-2

Dharavath R, Nagaraju N, Reddy M, Ashok D, Sarasija M, Vijjulatha M, Jyothi K, Prashanthi G (2020) Microwave-assisted synthesis, biological evaluation and molecular docking of novel coumarin-based 1, 2, 3-triazoles. RSC Adv 10(20):11615–11623. https://doi.org/10.1039/D0RA01052A

Dheer D, Singh V, Shankar R (2017) Medicinal attributes of 1,2,3-triazoles: current developments. Bioorg Chem 71:30–54. https://doi.org/10.1016/j.bioorg.2017.01.010

Dixit D, Verma PK, Marwaha RK (2021) A review on 'triazoles': their chemistry, synthesis and pharmacological potentials. J Iran Chem Soc 18(10):2535–2565. https://doi.org/10.1007/s13738-021-02231-x

D'Souza A, Cast A, Kumbaji M, Rivas M, Gulati R, Johnston M, Smithrud D, Geller J, Timchenko N (2021) The small molecule Cjoc42 improves chemosensitivity and increases levels of tumour suppressor proteins in hepatoblastoma cells and in mice by inhibiting the oncogene gankyrin. Front Pharmacol 12:580722. https://doi.org/10.3389/fphar.2021.580722

Du J, Yuan X (2023) Analysis of the incidence, characteristics, and risk factors of complications during induction chemotherapy in children with high-risk neuroblastoma. Eur J Pediatr 183:185. https://doi.org/10.1007/s00431-023-05273-w

Ehrlich P (1909) Über den jetzigen Stand der Chemotherapie. Ber Dtsch Chem Ges 42(1):17–47. https://doi.org/10.1002/cber.19090420105

Falchook GS, Bendell JC, Ulahannan SV, Sen S, Vilimas R, Kriksciukaite K, Mei L, Jerkovic G, Sarapa N, Bilodeau M, Bloss J, Thomas A (2020) Pen- 866, a miniature drug conjugate of a heat shock protein 90 (HSP 90) ligand linked to SN 38 for patients with advanced solid malignancies: phase I and expansion cohort results. J Clin Oncol 38(15_suppl):3515–3515. https://doi.org/10.1200/JCO.2020.38.15_suppl.3515

Farooq T (2021a) Advances in triazole chemistry. Elsevier. https://doi.org/10.1016/C2018-0-00687-8

Farooq T (2021b) Triazoles as bioisosteres in medicinal chemistry: a recent update. In: Advances in triazole chemistry. Elsevier, pp 31–47. https://doi.org/10.1016/B978-0-12-817113-4.00010-X

Ferlay J, Colombet M, Soerjomataram I, Piñeros M, Znaor A, Bray F (2021) Cancer statistics for 2020: an overview. Int J Cancer 149(4):778–789. https://doi.org/10.1002/ijc.33588

Gabba A, Robakiewicz S, Taciak B, Ulewicz K, Broggini G, Rastelli G, Krol M, Murphy PV, Passarella D (2017) Synthesis and biological evaluation of migrastatin macrotriazoles. Eur J Org Chem 2017(1):60–69. https://doi.org/10.1002/ejoc.201600988

Garcia MA, Rios ZG, Gonzalez J, Perez VM, Lara N, Fuentes A, Gonzalez C, Corona D, Cuevas-Yanez E (2011) The use of glucose as an alternative reducing agent in copper-catalyzed alkyne-azide cycloaddition. Lett Org Chem 8(10):701–706. https://doi.org/10.2174/157017811799304232

Garg A, Sarma D, Ali AA (2020) Microwave assisted metal-free approach to access 1,2,3-triazoles through multicomponent synthesis. Curr Res Green Sustainable Chem 3:100013. https://doi.org/10.1016/j.crgsc.2020.100013

Giraudo A, Krall J, Nielsen B, Sørensen TE, Kongstad KT, Rolando B, Boschi D, Frølund B, Lolli ML (2018) 4-Hydroxy-1,2,3-triazole moiety as bioisostere of the carboxylic acid function: a novel scaffold to probe the orthosteric γ-aminobutyric acid receptor binding site. Eur J Med Chem 158:311–321. https://doi.org/10.1016/j.ejmech.2018.08.094

Godugu K, Rajabi M, Mousa SA (2021) Anti-cancer activities of thyrointegrin αvβ3 antagonist mono- and bis-triazole tetraiodothyroacetic acid conjugated via polyethylene glycols in glioblastoma. Cancers 13(11):2780. https://doi.org/10.3390/cancers13112780

Goetz DB, Varney ML, Wiemer DF, Holstein SA (2020) Amides as bioisosteres of triazole-based geranylgeranyl diphosphate synthase inhibitors. Bioorg Med Chem 28(16):115604. https://doi.org/10.1016/j.bmc.2020.115604

Gomes RS, Jardim GAM, de Carvalho RL, Araujo MH, da Silva Júnior EN (2019) Beyond copper-catalyzed azide-alkyne 1,3-dipolar cycloaddition: synthesis and mechanism insights. Tetrahedron 75(27):3697–3712. https://doi.org/10.1016/j.tet.2019.05.046

González-Lainez M, Gallegos M, Munarriz J, Azpiroz R, Passarelli V, Jiménez MV, Pérez-Torrente JJ (2022) Copper-catalyzed Azide–Alkyne Cycloaddition (CuAAC) by functionalized NHC-based polynuclear catalysts: scope and mechanistic insights. Organometallics 41(15):2154–2169. https://doi.org/10.1021/acs.organomet.2c00246

Grob NM, Schibli R, Béhé M, Valverde IE, Mindt TL (2021) 1,5-Disubstituted 1,2,3-triazoles as amide bond Isosteres yield novel tumor-targeting minigastrin analogs. ACS Med Chem Lett 12(4):585–592. https://doi.org/10.1021/acsmedchemlett.0c00636

Grochans S, Cybulska AM, Simińska D, Korbecki J, Kojder K, Chlubek D, Baranowska-Bosiacka I (2022) Epidemiology of glioblastoma multiforme–literature review. Cancers 14(10):2412. https://doi.org/10.3390/cancers14102412

Hanif F, Muzaffar K, Perveen S, S. (2017) Glioblastoma multiforme: review of epidemiology and pathogenesis through clinical presentation and treatment. Asian Pac J Cancer Prev 18(1):3–9. https://doi.org/10.22034/APJCP.2017.18.1.3

Hirani N, MacKinnon AC, Nicol L, Ford P, Schambye H, Pedersen A, Nilsson UJ, Leffler H, Sethi T, Tantawi S, Gravelle L, Slack RJ, Mills R, Karmakar U, Humphries D, Zetterberg F, Keeling L, Paul L, Molyneaux PL et al (2021) Target inhibition of galectin-3 by inhaled TD139 in patients with idiopathic pulmonary fibrosis. Eur Respir J 57(5):2002559. https://doi.org/10.1183/13993003.02559-2020

Hu G, Chen J, Fan Y, Zhou H, Guo K, Fang Z, Xie L, Wang L, Wang Y (2022) A promoted Copper-catalysed Azide-Alkyne Cycloaddition (CuAAC) for broad spectrum peptide-engineered implants. Chem Eng J 427:130918. https://doi.org/10.1016/j.cej.2021.130918

Huisgen R (1963) 1, 3-dipolar cycloadditions. Past and future. Angew Chem Int Ed Engl 2(10):565–598. https://doi.org/10.1002/anie.196305651

Jalani H, Karagöz A, Tsogoeva S (2016) Synthesis of substituted 1,2,3-Triazoles via metal-free click cycloaddition reactions and alternative cyclization methods. Synthesis 49(01):29–41. https://doi.org/10.1055/s-0036-1588904

Jiang X, Hao X, Jing L, Wu G, Kang D, Liu X, Zhan P (2019) Recent applications of click-chemistry in drug discovery. Expert Opin Drug Discov 14(8):779–789. https://doi.org/10.1080/17460441.2019.1614910

Johnston SRD, Dowsett M (2003) Aromatase inhibitors for breast cancer: lessons from the lab. Nat Rev Cancer 3(11):821–831. https://doi.org/10.1038/nrc1211

Kahveci B, Özil M, Menteşe E, Buruk K (2008a) Microwave-assisted synthesis and antifungal activity of some new 1H-1, 2, 4-triazole derivatives. Russ J Org Chem 44(12):1816–1820. https://doi.org/10.1134/S1070428008120178

Kahveci B, Özil M, Serdar M (2008b) Microwave-assisted synthesis of some 1,2,4-triazol-5-one derivatives. Heteroat Chem 19(1):38–42. https://doi.org/10.1002/hc.20381

Kahveci B, Yılmaz F, Menteşe E, Ülker S (2015) Microwave-assisted synthesis of some new coumarin derivatives including 1,2,4-triazol-3-one and investigation of their biological activities. Chem Heterocycl Compd 51(5):447–456. https://doi.org/10.1007/s10593-015-1714-5

Khongsti K, Pasupuleti BG, Das B, Bez G (2021) 1,2,3-Triazole tethered 1,2,4-trioxane trimer induces apoptosis in metastatic cancer cells and inhibits proliferation, migration and invasion. Bioorg Chem 112:104952. https://doi.org/10.1016/j.bioorg.2021.104952

Kidwai M, Misra P, Bhushan KR, Dave B (2000) A novel route to 1,2,4-Triazoles. Synth Commun 30(16):3031–3040. https://doi.org/10.1080/00397910008087451

Kidwai M, Sapra P, Misra P, Saxena RK, Singh M (2001) Microwave assisted solid support synthesis of novel 1,2,4-triazolo[3,4-b]-1,3,4-thiadiazepines as potent antimicrobial agents. Bioorg Med Chem 9(2):217–220. https://doi.org/10.1016/S0968-0896(00)00245-5

Kierulf-Vieira K, Sandberg C, Waaler J, Lund K, Saberniak BM, Panagopoulos I, Brandal P, Krauss S, Langmoen IA, Vik-Mo EO (2020) Small molecule Tankyrase inhibitor reduces glioma stem cell proliferation and sphere formation. Cancers 12(6):1630. https://doi.org/10.3390/cancers12061630

Kim W-C, Lee CH (2009) The role of mammalian ribonucleases (RNases) in cancer. Biochim Biophys Acta Rev Cancer 1796(2):99–113. https://doi.org/10.1016/j.bbcan.2009.05.002

Kim SJ, Lee K, Park J, Park M, Kim UJ, Kim S, Ryu KH, Kang KW (2023) CKD-516 potentiates the anti-cancer activity of docetaxel against EGFR tyrosine kinase inhibitor-resistant lung cancer. Toxicol Res 39(1):61–69. https://doi.org/10.1007/s43188-022-00146-0

Kolb H, Finn M, Sharpless K (2001) Click-chemistry: diverse chemical function from a few good reactions. Angew Chem Int Ed Engl 40(11):2004–2021. https://doi.org/10.1002/1521-3773(20010601)40:11<2004::AID-ANIE2004>3.0.CO;2-5

Kumar M, Yadav T, Khair R, Peters G, Yergeri M (2019) Combination therapies of artemisinin and derivatives as a viable approach for future cancer treatment. Curr Pharm Des 25(31):3323–3338. https://doi.org/10.2174/1381612825666190902155957

Kumar S, Khokra SL, Yadav A (2021) Triazole analogues as potential pharmacological agents: a brief review. Future J Pharm Sci 7(1):106. https://doi.org/10.1186/s43094-021-00241-3

Lakkakula R, Roy A, Sridhar G (2019) Synthesis and anticancer activity of 1, 2, 3-triazole fused N-arylpyrazole derivatives. Russ J Gen Chem 89(4):831–835. https://doi.org/10.1134/S1070363219040315

Lee C-I, Liao C-B, Chen C-S, Cheng F-Y, Chung Y-H, Wang Y-C, Ciou S-Y, Hsueh W-Y, Lo T-H, Huang G-R, Huang H-Y, Tsai C-S, Lu Y-J, Chuang S-H, Huang J-J (2021) Design and synthesis of 4-anilinoquinazolines as Raf kinase inhibitors. Part 1. Selective B-Raf/B-RafV600E and potent EGFR/VEGFR2 inhibitory 4-(3-hydroxyanilino)-6-(1H-1,2,3-triazol-4-yl)quinazolines. Bioorg Chem 109:104715. https://doi.org/10.1016/j.bioorg.2021.104715

Lengerli D, Ibis K, Nural Y, Banoglu E (2022) The 1,2,3-triazole 'all-in-one' ring system in drug discovery: a good bioisostere, a good pharmacophore, a good linker, and a versatile synthetic tool. Expert Opin Drug Discov 17(11):1209–1236. https://doi.org/10.1080/17460441.2022.2129613

Leu W-J, Swain SP, Chan S-H, Hsu J-L, Liu S-P, Chan M-L, Yu C-C, Hsu L-C, Chou Y-L, Chang W-L, Hou D-R, Guh J-H (2016) Non-immunosuppressive triazole-based small molecule induces anticancer activity against human hormone-refractory prostate cancers: the role in inhibition of PI3K/AKT/mTOR and c-Myc signaling pathways. Oncotarget 7(47):76995–77009. https://doi.org/10.18632/oncotarget.12765

Li JJ, Corey EJ (2011) In: Li JJ, Corey EJ (eds) Name reactions in heterocyclic chemistry II. Wiley. https://doi.org/10.1002/9781118092828

Li W, Zhou X, Luan Y, Wang J (2015) Direct access to 1,4-disubstituted 1,2,3-triazoles through organocatalytic 1,3-dipolar cycloaddition reaction of α,β-unsaturated esters with azides. RSC Adv 5(108):88816–88820. https://doi.org/10.1039/C5RA19038J

Li Y-T, Wang J, Pan C, Meng F, Chu X, Ding Y, Qu W, Li H, Yang C, Zhang Q, Bai C, Chen Y (2016) SynthesIs and biological evaluation of 1, 2, 3-triazole and 1, 3, 4-oxadiazole derivatives of imatinib. Bioorg Med Chem Lett 26(5):1419–1427. https://doi.org/10.1016/j.bmcl.2016.01.068

Li B, Hu R, Qin A, Tang BZ (2020) Copper-based ionic liquid-catalyzed click polymerization of diazides and diynes toward functional polytriazoles for sensing applications. Polym Chem 11(12):2006–2014. https://doi.org/10.1039/C9PY01443H

Liang J, Zhang T, Li Z, Chen Z, Yan X, Meng F (2016) Predicting potential antitumor targets of aconitum alkaloids by molecular docking and protein–ligand interaction fingerprint. Med Chem Res 25(6):1115–1124. https://doi.org/10.1007/s00044-016-1553-7

Liang T, Sun X, Hou G, Gao F (2021) 1, 2, 3-Triazole containing compounds as anti-lung cancer agents: current developments, mechanisms of action, and structure-activity relationship. Front Pharmacol 12:661173. https://doi.org/10.3389/fphar.2021.661173

Lidström P, Tierney J, Wathey B, Westman J (2001) Microwave assisted organic synthesis—a review. Tetrahedron 57(45):9225–9283. https://doi.org/10.1016/S0040-4020(01)00906-1

Liu X-H, Weng J-Q, Wang B-L, Li Y-H, Tan C-X, Li Z-M (2014) Microwave-assisted synthesis of novel fluorinated 1,2,4-triazole derivatives, and study of their biological activity. Res Chem Intermed 40(8):2605–2612. https://doi.org/10.1007/s11164-013-1113-4

Maiuolo L, Russo B, Algieri V, Nardi M, Di Gioia ML, Tallarida MA, De Nino A (2019) Regioselective synthesis of 1,5-disubstituted 1,2,3-triazoles by 1,3-dipolar cycloaddition: role of Er(OTf)3, ionic liquid and water. Tetrahedron Lett 60(9):672–674. https://doi.org/10.1016/j.tetlet.2019.01.053

Malhotra A, Singh R, Acharya PC, Bansal R (2023) Hormones and antihormones in cancer chemotherapy. In: Medicinal chemistry of chemotherapeutic agents. Elsevier, pp 589–613. https://doi.org/10.1016/B978-0-323-90575-6.00004-1

Malik MS, Ahmed SA, Althagafi II, Ansari MA, Kamal A (2020) Application of triazoles as bioisosteres and linkers in the development of microtubule targeting agents. RSC Med Chem 11(3):327–348. https://doi.org/10.1039/C9MD00458K

Marra A, Vecchi A, Chiappe C, Melai B, Dondoni A (2008) Validation of the copper(I)-catalyzed azide−alkyne coupling in ionic liquids. Synthesis of a triazole-linked *C* -disaccharide as a case study. J Org Chem 73(6):2458–2461. https://doi.org/10.1021/jo7026454

Marshall GR, Ballante F (2017) Limiting assumptions in the design of peptidomimetics. Drug Dev Res 78(6):245–267. https://doi.org/10.1002/ddr.21406

Marzagalli M, Fontana F, Raimondi M, Limonta P (2021) Cancer stem cells—key players in tumor relapse. Cancers 13(3):376. https://doi.org/10.3390/cancers13030376

Marzi M, Farjam M, Kazeminejad Z, Shiroudi A, Kouhpayeh A, Zarenezhad E (2022) A recent overview of 1, 2, 3-Triazole-containing hybrids as novel antifungal agents: focusing on synthesis, mechanism of action, and Structure-Activity Relationship (SAR). J Chem 2022:1–50. https://doi.org/10.1155/2022/7884316

Matin MM, Matin P, Rahman MR, Ben Hadda T, Almalki FA, Mahmud S, Ghoneim MM, Alruwaily M, Alshehri S (2022) Triazoles and their derivatives: chemistry, synthesis, and therapeutic applications. Front Mol Biosci 9:864286. https://doi.org/10.3389/fmolb.2022.864286

Meyer EA, Äänismaa P, Ertel EA, Hühn E, Strasser DS, Rey M, Murphy MJ, Martinic MM, Pouzol L, Froidevaux S, Keller MP, Caroff E (2023) Discovery of clinical candidate ACT-777991, a potent CXCR3 antagonist for antigen-driven and inflammatory pathologies. J Med Chem 66(6):4179–4196. https://doi.org/10.1021/acs.jmedchem.3c00074

Mondal P, Dasgupta S, Pathak T (2022) Carboxymethyl tethered poly(disubstituted)triazoles built on nucleoside skeletons: a unique class of ribonuclease a inhibitors designed using chemical logic. Bioorg Med Chem 76:117065. https://doi.org/10.1016/j.bmc.2022.117065

Nasrollahzadeh M, Ghasemzadeh M, Gharoubi H, Nezafat Z (2021) Progresses in polysaccharide and lignin-based ionic liquids: catalytic applications and environmental remediation. J Mol Liq 342:117559. https://doi.org/10.1016/j.molliq.2021.117559

Nesaragi AR, Kamble RR, Bayannavar PK, Shaikh SKJ, Hoolageri SR, Kodasi B, Joshi SD, Kumbar VM (2021) Microwave-assisted regioselective syntheses of quinoline appended triazoles as potent antitubercular and antifungal agents via copper (I) catalyzed cycloaddition. Bioorg Med Chem Lett 41:127984. https://doi.org/10.1016/j.bmcl.2021.127984

Opsomer T, Dehaen W (2021) Metal-free syntheses of *N*-functionalized and *NH*-1,2,3-triazoles: an update on recent developments. Chem Commun 57(13):1568–1590. https://doi.org/10.1039/D0CC06654K

Othman EM, Fayed EA, Husseiny EM, Abulkhair HS (2022) Apoptosis induction, PARP-1 inhibition, and cell cycle analysis of leukemia cancer cells treated with novel synthetic 1,2,3-triazole-chalcone conjugates. Bioorg Chem 123:105762. https://doi.org/10.1016/j.bioorg.2022.105762

Padhariya KN, Athavale M, Srivastava S, Kharkar PS (2021) A novel series of substituted 1,2,3-triazoles as cancer stem cell inhibitors: synthesis and biological evaluation. Drug Dev Res 82(1): 68–85. https://doi.org/10.1002/ddr.21723

Pasupuleti BG, Khongsti K, Das B, Bez G (2020) 1,2,3-Triazole tethered 1,2,4-trioxanes: studies on their synthesis and effect on osteopontin expression in MDA-MB-435 breast cancer cells. Eur J Med Chem 186:111908. https://doi.org/10.1016/j.ejmech.2019.111908

Peng F, Liao M, Qin R, Zhu S, Peng C, Fu L, Chen Y, Han B (2022) Regulated cell death (RCD) in cancer: key pathways and targeted therapies. Signal Transduct Target Ther 7(1):286. https://doi.org/10.1038/s41392-022-01110-y

Pinheiro S, Pessôa JC, Pinheiro EMC, Muri EMF, Filho EV, Loureiro LB, Freitas MCR, Silva Junior CMD, Fiorot RG, Carneiro JWM, Rotamiro KM, Guimarães ARA, Rocha-Brito KJP, Greco SJ (2020) 2H-1,2,3-triazole-chalcones as novel cytotoxic agents against prostate cancer. Bioorg Med Chem Lett 30(19):127454. https://doi.org/10.1016/j.bmcl.2020.127454

Pirali T, Pagliai F, Boggio R, Canonico P, Sorba G, Tron G, Genazzani A (2008) Triazole modified histone deacetylase inhibitors as a rapid route to drug discovery. J Comb Chem 10(5):624–627. https://doi.org/10.1021/cc800061c

Prachayasittikul V, Pingaew R, Anuwongcharoen N, Worachartcheewan A, Nantasenamat C, Prachayasittikul S, Ruchirawat S, Prachayasittikul V (2015) Discovery of novel 1,2,3-triazole derivatives as anticancer agents using QSAR and in silico structural modification. Springerplus 4(1):571. https://doi.org/10.1186/s40064-015-1352-5

Rafferty SW, Eisner JR, Moore WR, Schotzinger RJ, Hoekstra WJ (2014) Highly-selective 4-(1,2,3-triazole)-based P450c17a 17,20-lyase inhibitors. Bioorg Med Chem Lett 24(11): 2444–2447. https://doi.org/10.1016/j.bmcl.2014.04.024

Rani A, Singh G, Maqbool U, Kaur G, Singh J (2020) CuAAC-ensembled 1,2,3-triazole-linked isosteres as pharmacophores in drug discovery: review. RSC Adv 10(10):5610–5635. https://doi.org/10.1039/C9RA09510A

Rashdan HRM, Shehadi IA (2022) Triazoles synthesis & applications as nonsteroidal aromatase inhibitors for hormone-dependent breast cancer treatment. Heteroat Chem 2022:1–16. https://doi.org/10.1155/2022/5349279

Reddy K, Mamatha R, Babu MS, Shiva K, Jayaveera K, Narayanaswamy G (2014) Synthesis and antimicrobial-activities of some triazole-, thiadiazole-, and oxadiazole-substituted coumarins. J Heterocyclic Chem 51(1):132–137. https://doi.org/10.1002/jhet.1745

Rezayatmand H, Razmkhah M, Razeghian I (2022) Drug resistance in cancer therapy: the pandora's box of cancer stem cells. Stem Cell Research Ther *13*(1):181. https://doi.org/10.1186/s13287-022-02856-6

Ríos-Malváez ZG, Cano-Herrera M-A, Dávila-Becerril JC, Mondragón-Solórzano G, Ramírez-Apan MT, Morales-Morales D, Barroso-Flores J, Santillán-Benítez JG, Unnamatla MVB, García-Eleno MA, González-Rivas N, Cuevas-Yañez E (2021) Synthesis, characterization and evaluation of cytotoxic activity of 4-(1, 2, 3-triazol-1-yl) salicylic acid derivatives. J Mol Struct 1225:129149. https://doi.org/10.1016/j.molstruc.2020.129149

Rugo HS, Bardia A, Tolaney SM, Arteaga C, Cortes J, Sohn J, Marmé F, Hong Q, Delaney RJ, Hafeez A, André F, Schmid P (2020) TROPiCS-02: A phase III study investigating sacituzumab govitecan in the treatment of HR+/HER2- metastatic breast cancer. Future Oncol 16(12): 705–715. https://doi.org/10.2217/fon-2020-0163

Sahu A, Sahu P, Agrawal R (2020) A recent review on drug modification using 1, 2, 3-triazole. Curr Chem Biol 14(2):71–87. https://doi.org/10.2174/2212796814999200807214519

Schmitt J, Huang S, Goodfellow E, Williams C, Jean-Claude BJ (2020) Design and synthesis of a tri-functional molecular system programmed to block EGFR tyrosine kinase, induce high levels of DNA damage, and inhibit the DNA repair enzyme (poly(ADPribose) polymerase) in prostate cancer cells. J Med Chem 63(11):5752–5762. https://doi.org/10.1021/acs.jmedchem.9b02008

Seghetti F, Di Martino RMC, Catanzaro E, Bisi A, Gobbi S, Rampa A, Canonico B, Montanari M, Krysko DV, Papa S, Fimognari C, Belluti F (2020) Curcumin-1,2,3-Triazole conjugation for targeting the cancer apoptosis machinery. Molecules 25(13):3066. https://doi.org/10.3390/molecules25133066

Serafini M, Pirali T, Tron GC (2021) Click 1, 2, 3-triazoles in drug discovery and development: from the flask to the clinic? pp 101–148. https://doi.org/10.1016/bs.aihch.2020.10.001

Sermuksnyte A, Kantminiene K, Jonuskiene I, Tumosiene I, Petrikaite V (2022) Effect of 1, 2, 4-triazole-3-thiol derivatives bearing hydrazone moiety on the cancer cell migration and growth of melanoma, breast, and pancreatic cancer spheroids. Pharmaceutics 15(8):1026. https://doi.org/10.3390/ph15081026

Shevchenko V, Arnotskaya N, Korneyko M, Zaytsev S, Khotimchenko Y, Sharma H, Bryukhovetskiy I (2019) Wnt pathway proteins as targets for regulation of CD133+ cancer stem cells in glioblastoma. Oncol Rep 41:3080. https://doi.org/10.3892/or.2019.7043

Siegel R, Miller K, Wagle N, Jemal A (2023) Cancer statistics, 2023. CA Cancer J Clin 73(1): 17–48. https://doi.org/10.3322/caac.21763

Silberrad O (1900) CX.—contributions to the chemistry of hydrotetrazines and triazoles. J Chem Soc Trans 77(0):1185–1191. https://doi.org/10.1039/CT9007701185

Slavova K, Todorov L, Belskaya N, Palafox M, Kostova I (2020) Developments in the use of 1, 2, 3-triazoles in the treatment of cancer. Recent Pat Anticancer Drug Discov 15(2):92–112. https://doi.org/10.2174/1574892815666200717164457

Souček J, Poučková P, Strohalm J, Plocová D, Hloušková D, Zadinová M, Ulbrich K (2002) Poly [N -(2-hydroxypropyl)methacrylamide] conjugates of bovine pancreatic ribonuclease (RNase A) inhibit growth of human melanoma in nude mice. J Drug Target 10(3):175–183. https://doi.org/10.1080/10611860290022606

Strauss C, Trainor R (1995) Developments in microwave-assisted organic chemistry. Aust J Chem 48(10):1665. https://doi.org/10.1071/CH9951665

Sudheendran K, Schmidt D, Frey W, Conrad J, Beifuss U (2014) Facile synthesis of 3,5-diaryl-1,2,4-triazoles via copper-catalyzed domino nucleophilic substitution/oxidative cyclization using amidines or imidates as substrates. Tetrahedron 70(8):1635–1645. https://doi.org/10.1016/j.tet.2014.01.019

Sun N-B, Fu J-Q, Weng J-Q, Jin J-Z, Tan C-X, Liu X-H (2013) Microwave assisted synthesis, antifungal activity and DFT theoretical study of some novel 1,2,4-Triazole derivatives containing the 1,2,3-Thiadiazole moiety. Molecules 18(10):12725–12739. https://doi.org/10.3390/molecules181012725

Suzuki T, Kasuya Y, Ota Y, Asamitsu K, Nakagawa H, Okamoto T (2013) Identification of highly selective and potent histone deacetylase-3 inhibitors using click chemistry -based combinatorial fragment assembly. PLoS ONE 8(7):e68669. https://doi.org/10.1371/journal.pone.0068669

Thilak Babu L, Paira P (2023) CuAAC "Click"-derived luminescent 2-(2-(4-(4-(Pyridin-2-yl)-1 *H* -1,2,3-triazol-1-yl)butoxy)phenyl)benzo[*d*]thiazole-based Ru(II)/Ir(III)/Re(I) complexes as anticancer agents. ACS Omega 8(36):32382–32395. https://doi.org/10.1021/acsomega.3c01639

Thomas J, Jana S, John J, Liekens S, Dehaen W (2016) ChemInform abstract: a general metal-free route towards the synthesis of 1,2,3-Triazoles from readily available primary amines and ketones. ChemInform 47(25). https://doi.org/10.1002/chin.201625146

Tiwari G, Khanna A, Mishra VK, Sagar R (2023) Recent developments on microwave-assisted organic synthesis of nitrogen- and oxygen-containing preferred heterocyclic scaffolds. RSC Adv 13(47):32858–32892. https://doi.org/10.1039/D3RA05986C

Tornøe C, Christensen C, Meldal M (2002) Peptidotriazoles on Solid Phase: 1, 2, 3-Triazoles via regiospecific copper (I)-catalyzed 1 ,3-dipolar cycloadditions of terminal alkynes to azides. J Org Chem 67(9):3057–3064. https://doi.org/10.1021/jo011148j

Ueda S, Nagasawa H (2009) Facile synthesis of 1,2,4-triazoles via a copper-catalyzed tandem addition–oxidative cyclization. J Am Chem Soc 131(42):15080–15081. https://doi.org/10.1021/ja905056z

Vaithiyalingam D, Nelson M, Chinnamadhaiyan M, Ayyanar S (2021) Microwave assisted synthesis of 3, 5-disubstituted 1, 2, 4-triazole based piperazine amide and urea derivatives. Trends J Sci Res 01(01):7–17. https://doi.org/10.31586/ojc.2021.010102

Waaler J, Leenders RGG, Sowa ST, Alam Brinch S, Lycke M, Nieczypor P, Aertssen S, Murthy S, Galera-Prat A, Damen E, Wegert A, Nazaré M, Lehtiö L, Krauss S (2020) Preclinical lead optimization of a 1,2,4-triazole based tankyrase inhibitor. J Med Chem 63(13):6834–6846. https://doi.org/10.1021/acs.jmedchem.0c00208

Wang Z (2010) Comprehensive organic name reactions and reagents. Wiley. https://doi.org/10.1002/9780470638859

Wang Z, Zhang H, Xu S, Liu Z, Cheng Q (2021) Adaptive transition of glioblastoma s cells and its implications for treatment. Signal Transduct Target Ther 6(1):124. https://doi.org/10.1038/s41392-021-00491-w

Wang Y, Ding R, Tai Z, Hou H, Gao F, Sun X (2022) Artemisinin-isatin hybrids with potential antiproliferative activity against breast cancer. Arab J Chem 15(3):103639. https://doi.org/10.1016/j.arabjc.2021.103639

Wermuth C, Ganellin C, Lindberg P, Mitscher L (1998) Glossary of terms used in medicinal chemistry. (IUPAC Recommendations 1998). Pure Appl Chem 70(5):1129–1143. https://doi.org/10.1351/pac199870051129

Wiseman L, Spencer C (1997) Vorozole. Drugs Aging 11(3):245–250. https://doi.org/10.2165/00002512-199711030-00007

Worrell B, Malik J, Fokin V (2013) Direct evidence of a di-nuclear copper intermediate in Cu(I)-catalyzed azide-alkyne cycloadditions. Science 340(6131):457–460. https://doi.org/10.1126/science.1229506

Xie J, Xu H, Xie Y, Lu X, Wang L (2021) Design, synthesis, and antiTNBC activity of Azeliragon triazole analogues. Bioorg Med Chem Lett 54:128444. https://doi.org/10.1016/j.bmcl.2021.128444

Xu H, Ma S, Xu Y, Bian L, Ding T, Fang X, Zhang W, Ren Y (2015) Copper-catalyzed one-pot synthesis of 1,2,4-Triazoles from nitriles and hydroxylamine. J Org Chem 80(3):1789–1794. https://doi.org/10.1021/jo502709t

Xu M, Zhu Y, Wang M, Khan I, Liu X-H, Weng J (2018) Microwave-assisted synthesis and antifungal activity of novel 1,2,4- Triazole Thioether derivatives containing pyrimidine moiety. Lett Drug Des Discovery 15(4):347–352. https://doi.org/10.2174/1570180814666170602082440

Xu Z, Zhao S, Liu Y (2019) 1, 2, 3-Triazole-containing hybrids as potential anticancer agents: current developments, action mechanisms and structure-activity relationships. Eur J Med Chem 183:111700. https://doi.org/10.1016/j.ejmech.2019.111700

Yeung K-S, Farkas ME, Kadow JF, Meanwell NA (2005) A base-catalyzed, direct synthesis of 3,5-disubstituted 1,2,4-triazoles from nitriles and hydrazides. Tetrahedron Lett 46(19):3429–3432. https://doi.org/10.1016/j.tetlet.2005.02.167

Younes S (2020) Anticancer activity of guggulsterone in human leukemic cells. Qatar University Digital Hub. Date 2020–06. https://qspace.qu.edu.qa/handle/10576/15222

Youssef ME, Cavalu S, Hasan AM, Yahya G, Abd-Eldayem MA, Saber S (2023) Role of Ganetespib, an HSP90 inhibitor, in cancer therapy: from molecular mechanisms to clinical practice. Int J Mol Sci 24(5):5014. https://doi.org/10.3390/ijms24055014

Zafar W, Sumrra SH, Chohan ZH (2021) A review: pharmacological aspects of metal based 1,2,4-triazole derived schiff bases. Eur J Med Chem 222:113602. https://doi.org/10.1016/j.ejmech.2021.113602

Zhang Y, Zhang T, Li X, Liang J, Tu S, Xu H, Xue W, Qian X, Zhang Z, Zhang X, Meng F (2021) 2-((1-phenyl-1H-1,2,3-triazol-4-yl)methyl)-2-azabicyclo[3.2.1]octan-3-one derivatives: simplification and modification of aconitine scaffold for the discovery of novel anticancer agents. Eur J Med Chem 210:112988. https://doi.org/10.1016/j.ejmech.2020.112988

Zhao Y, Han B, Liu Z (2021) Ionic-liquid-catalyzed approaches under metal-free conditions. Acc Chem Res 54(16):3172–3190. https://doi.org/10.1021/acs.accounts.1c00251

Zhou HC, Wang Y (2012) Recent researches in triazole compounds as medicinal drugs. Curr Med Chem 19(2):239–280. https://doi.org/10.2174/092986712803414213

Zhou X, Xu X, Liu K, Gao H, Wang W, Li W (2016) Organocatalytic 1,3-dipolar cycloaddition reaction of β-keto amides with azides—direct access to 1,4,5-trisubstituted 1,2,3-triazole-4-carboxamides. Eur J Org Chem 2016(10):1886–1890. https://doi.org/10.1002/ejoc.201600157

Anticancer Properties of Antipsychotic Drugs

Milica M. Borovcanin, Bojan Stojanovic, Milica Dimitrijevic Stojanovic, Bojana S. Stojanovic, Aleksandar Lazovic, and Marina Mitrovic

Abstract

Cancer has become a major public health threat and is responsible for over 20% of all deaths worldwide. In medical science, the treatment of cancer has always been a major challenge, with conventional methods such as surgery, chemotherapy, and radiotherapy forming the backbone of therapeutic strategies. Although these methods are central to the management and control of cancer, they are subject to significant limitations. The effectiveness of chemotherapy and radiotherapy is often hampered by the inherent resistance developed by cancer cells. Despite significant spending on cancer research and drug development, the proportion of approved therapies in oncology is low compared to various other indications, so new approaches are needed. An attractive approach in this area is drug repurposing, which involves finding new uses for known therapeutic drugs outside their original medical indications. The cooccurrence of mental health

M. M. Borovcanin (✉)
Department of Psychiatry, Faculty of Medical Sciences, University of Kragujevac, Kragujevac, Serbia
e-mail: milicaborovcanin@medf.kg.ac.rs

B. Stojanovic · A. Lazovic
Department of Surgery, Faculty of Medical Sciences, University of Kragujevac, Kragujevac, Serbia

M. Dimitrijevic Stojanovic
Department of Pathology, Faculty of Medical Sciences, University of Kragujevac, Kragujevac, Serbia

B. S. Stojanovic
Department of Pathophysiology, Faculty of Medical Sciences, University of Kragujevac, Kragujevac, Serbia

M. Mitrovic
Department of Biochemistry, Faculty of Medical Sciences, University of Kragujevac, Kragujevac, Serbia

Interdisciplinary Cancer Research, https://doi.org/10.1007/16833_2024_394
Published online: 20 September 2024

problems and cancer has received particular attention. In this context, the potential role of antipsychotic drugs in anticancer therapy represents a promising and interesting area of research. In recent years, research studies have found that antipsychotics reduced the incidence of certain types of cancer in patients with schizophrenia, suggesting that they may have anticancer potential. Antipsychotics, traditionally used to treat psychotic disorders, have shown a complex interplay of molecular mechanisms that go beyond neurotransmission theory. Some of these mechanisms intriguingly overlap with cancer pathways. This chapter explores the unconventional anticancer properties of antipsychotic drugs, focusing on their potential to modulate key molecular mechanisms overlapping with cancer pathways. Research has suggested that antipsychotics might offer new therapeutic avenues by affecting immune modulation, cell signalling, and apoptosis pathways. The chapter delves into preclinical studies on antipsychotics' effects on cancers, highlighting their immune system impact, potential to integrate into future treatment protocols, and the necessity for further exploration of their anticancer capabilities.

Keywords

Antipsychotic · Apoptosis · Autophagy · Cancer · Dopamine · Immune modulation

1 Introduction

Modern medicine seems to lack the integration of existing knowledge with technological and civilizational improvements. In most cases, a single line of research ends with the departure of the group leader, and there is no continuous longitudinal approach. In this context, it is essential to try to solve problems in an interdisciplinary way and on the basis of fundamental and not only topical and subspecialized points of view.

In clinical practice, psychiatric and neurological symptoms are often linked and treated together as neuropsychiatric conditions (Vesic et al. 2023). Sometimes drugs prescribed for one indication may have unexpected effects in resolving different symptoms that are not related to only one organ system, such as the central nervous system. Thus, for example, chlorpromazine (CPZ) was introduced in the treatment of patients with psychosis and in view of its efficacy in pulmonary pathology and the similarity observed with disorders of type 2 immunity (Borovcanin et al. 2013). In coronavirus disease 2019 (COVID-19), we have tried to improve the treatment by targeting all these molecules with potential effects on the respiratory system (Muric et al. 2020). From a much broader perspective, there are immunometabolic perturbances in various mental disorders, and only concomitant and systemic interventions could be of benefit (Borovcanin et al. 2023b).

The symptoms that remain with depression, such as fatigue, insomnia and even pain sensations, are often observed as concomitant symptoms with oncologic problems. In an attempt to efficiently address these problems in patients with cancer, we have already provided an overview of the current state-of-the-art in this field and proposed some new therapeutic targets (Borovcanin et al. 2023a). However, it seems that there are two different sides to this story. It is important to recognize the potential for immunologically targeted therapies in the treatment of mental health problems in oncology from an immunopsychiatric perspective. In addition, it should also be considered that psychotropic drugs may have anticancer properties through their unconventional mechanisms of action (Borovcanin and Vesic 2021).

Cancer has become a major threat to public health and is responsible for over 20% of all deaths worldwide (Mattiuzzi and Lippi 2019). This staggering statistic underlines the enormous challenge that cancer poses to medical science. The development of cancer is often associated with misrepaired or unrepaired cellular damage, which leads to genetic instability in normal cells and favours their transformation into malignant forms (Yao and Dai 2014). By 2030, it is predicted that without effective treatment, there will be 26 million new cancer diagnoses and 17 million cancer-related deaths each year (Thun et al. 2010). This alarming forecast highlights the urgent need for innovative treatment strategies.

In this context, the potential role of antipsychotic drugs in anticancer therapy represents a promising and interesting area of study. Antipsychotics, traditionally used to treat psychiatric disorders such as schizophrenia and bipolar disorder, have shown a complex interplay of molecular mechanisms. Some of these mechanisms overlap with cancer pathways in fascinating ways. Recent research has shown that antipsychotics are not only able to inhibit the proliferation of cancer cells by influencing various cellular signalling pathways, but can also enhance the efficacy of conventional anticancer agents (Hendouei et al. 2019). This multifaceted role of antipsychotics, which also has effects on a number of malignant tumours, including brain tumours, suggests that their use beyond psychiatric treatment needs to be re-evaluated and that they may have an important contribution to make in the fight against cancer (Lee et al. 2016).

In this chapter, we will present our current knowledge of the initial steps in exploring the anticancer properties of antipsychotic drugs in preclinical studies and the potential for integrating these facts into future treatment protocols. Different classes of antipsychotic drugs will be examined with regard to their effects on the immune system and specific target organs. New biomarkers are presented that link different networks of transmitters of the nervous system and the immune system, as well as those related to metabolism, and overall help us to improve cancer treatment.

2 Cooccurrence of Mental Problems and Cancer

In recent years, research studies have found that antipsychotics reduced the incidence of certain cancers in patients with schizophrenia (Fond et al. 2012), suggesting that they may have anticancer potential. This broader pharmacological profile suggests that the anticancer effects of antipsychotics may be mediated by mechanisms beyond their established psychiatric effects.

There are different explanations for the effects of antipsychotics on the development and treatment of cancer. Opposite to the previous notion, studies have shown that the risk of breast cancer is higher in patients receiving both first-generation antipsychotics and second-generation antipsychotics, either alone or in combination, regardless of the average dose of exposure (Wu Chou et al. 2017). Our previous study investigated the effects of long-acting injections of risperidone and paliperidone, which are known to increase prolactin levels, on patients with schizophrenia who were in remission (Borovcanin et al. 2018). This study found that these injections can lower alarmin interleukin (IL)-33 levels in the blood, which could have a balancing effect and possibly even anti-tumour properties. Based on our preclinical research, we have hypothesized a role for alarmins in the oncologic problems of patients with schizophrenia (Borovcanin and Vesic 2021). In this opinion paper, we discuss two clinically significant aspects of this hypothesis: the effects of antipsychotics on prolactin and dopamine levels.

Some antipsychotics have been found to cause an increase in prolactin levels, also known as "prolactin-raising" (Samperi et al. 2019) (Table 1). Some medical conditions such as idiopathic hyperprolactinaemia, prolactinomas, and Parkinson's disease (PD) have been linked with the potentially carcinogenic effects of prolactin. This is considered a risk factor for breast cancer, as it can promote carcinogenesis and the transition to invasive carcinoma. However, antipsychotic-induced hyperprolactinaemia has not been shown to be a fool proof adverse effect leading to carcinoma. Interestingly, there even may be a negative correlation between PD and neoplasms. Further research showed that patients with schizophrenia or PD who

Table 1 Antipsychotics grouping

Antipsychotics generation			
First		Second	Third
Loxapine	**HPRL**	Clozapine	Aripiprazole
Pimozide	<25% of patients	Sertindole	Brexpiprazole
Penfluridol		Asenapine	Cariprazine
Fluspirilene		Ziprasidone	
Droperidol		Quetiapine	
Haloperidol		Olanzapine	
Chlorpromazine (CPZ)		Lurasidone	
Levopromazine		Iloperidone	
Fluphenazine		Amisulpride	
Mesoridazine		Paliperidone	
Perphenazine		Risperidone	
Prochlorperazine			
Thioridazine			
Trifluoperazine (TFP)			
Thiothexene			
Flupentixol			
	>50% of patients		

HPRL hyperprolactinaemia

received antipsychotics had a lower risk of developing various types of cancer compared to the general population (Tacik et al. 2016; Gholipour et al. 2018).

The second aspect of the role of dopamine receptors in cancer is not yet clear and appears to be tumour-specific. The study of the correlation between antipsychotics, mainly as D2 receptor antagonists, and cancer began shortly after the approval of these drugs for psychiatric disorders. Initially, these were only isolated case reports of improved therapeutic response in cancer patients treated concomitantly with antipsychotics (Osterman 1961), and other studies have shown a clear association between antipsychotics as D2 receptor antagonists and antitumor effects (Strobl et al. 1990). The discovery that cancer patients taking antipsychotic drugs along with their antineoplastic therapy had better clinical outcomes initially reinforced the hypothesis that dopamine receptors may play an important role in tumour growth (Roney and Park 2018).

3 Anti-inflammatory Properties of Antipsychotics from the Clinical Perspective

Antipsychotics are drugs primarily used to treat schizophrenia, although the indications for their use are now broader and include psychopathology of speech and delusions, mood swings in bipolar disorder, and more severe forms of depressive disorder, while according to some guides they are also used for severe anxiety, delirium, dementia, insomnia, and impulsivity (Bjerre et al. 2018; van Schalkwyk et al. 2018). All available antipsychotics treat the positive symptoms of schizophrenia primarily by blocking D2 receptors, but also regulate serotonin and glutamate neurotransmission and are effective in treating cognitive and affective symptomatology (Miyamoto et al. 2005). A consensus has been reached that the classification of antipsychotics is based on the developmental stages of antipsychotics depending on their mechanism of action and receptor profile: the first generation of predominantly dopaminergic antagonists (low potency CPZ and levopromazine, and high potency haloperidol and fluphenazine), the second generation of antipsychotics with a broader receptor effect (with the exception of the D2 antagonism and the 5-hydroxytryptamine (5-HT)2A and 5-HT2C receptor antagonism of risperidone and paliperidone as well as the multi-target effect of clozapine, olanzapine, quetiapine, ziprasidone, asenapine, and iloperidone) and the third generation of new drugs (aripiprazole, brexpiprazole, and cariprazine) (Table 1).

However, antipsychotics not only affect the course of schizophrenia, but can also alter the immune response of treated patients. Abnormal cytokine levels can occur in acute exacerbations of schizophrenia independently of applied antipsychotics (Miller et al. 2011). These anti-inflammatory effects may also occur indirectly, through the resolution of acute psychological stress, which could lead to a decrease in pro-inflammatory cytokines such as IL-6, IL-1β, and tumour necrosis factor-alpha (TNF-α) (Mondelli et al. 2015).

In an in vitro study, the atypical antipsychotic risperidone was reported to reduce the production of pro-inflammatory cytokines by lipopolysaccharide-stimulated glial cells but had no effect on IL-10 (Obuchowicz et al. 2017) and paliperidone increased transforming growth factor beta (TGF-β) and IL-10 during acute stress and during prolonged chronic stress (MacDowell et al. 2016). From a much broader perspective, we have already discussed that certain atypical antipsychotics such as clozapine, risperidone, quetiapine, and olanzapine can significantly reduce the severity of experimental autoimmune encephalomyelitis, particularly in multiple sclerosis. This effect is achieved by downregulating the production of pro-inflammatory cytokines and chemokines and by attenuating T-cell infiltration, myeloid cell activation and upregulation of T-regulatory cells (Vesic et al. 2023), which may also be utilized in the treatment of carcinomas.

The anti-inflammatory effect of antipsychotics can be explained as a direct effect of the drugs by a decrease in pro-inflammatory and an increase in the level of circulating anti-inflammatory cytokines or by the inhibition of microglial activation (Kato et al. 2011). Most studies show that the systemic level of IL-6 decreases significantly and that there are favourable clinical outcomes following antipsychotic therapy (Borovcanin et al. 2017). Our results contributed to this notion that antipsychotic drugs should be considered as a confounding factor that upregulates the type 1 immune response and balances the overweighted type 2 immune response (Borovcanin et al. 2013). In the context of cognitive functioning and IL-17, we elaborate on the possibility that antipsychotics may improve cognitive functioning through adult hippocampal neurogenesis (Borovcanin et al. 2020).

Higher doses of prescribed risperidone may lead to an increase in Galectin-3 (Gal-3) levels and glycosylation of whole serum proteins following antipsychotic use (Telford et al. 2012; Minic Janicijevic et al. 2022). We have detailed these aspects of glycosylation considering the effects of antipsychotics (Borovcanin et al. 2021a, b). Studies in individuals suffering from schizophrenia revealed that typical antipsychotics have an impact on genes related to nuclear proteins, stress responses and phosphorylation. In contrast, atypical antipsychotics increased gene expression associated with the Golgi/endoplasmic reticulum and cytoplasmic transport. This indicates that atypical antipsychotics influence posttranslational modifications. In the group of typical antipsychotics, genes related to lipid metabolism were consistently downregulated compared to the group of atypical antipsychotics. Further evidence shows that antipsychotic treatment with olanzapine, risperidone and haloperidol can cause alterations in protein N-linked glycosylation in adipose tissue, which may contribute to dysregulated glycosylation in schizophrenia. Olanzapine has been found to upregulate insulin resistance, risperidone to upregulate fatty acid metabolism and haloperidol to upregulate nucleic acid metabolism.

We hypothesized that these anti-inflammatory effects of antipsychotics might occur indirectly via different cascades. We have wondered about the uricosuric effects of antipsychotic drugs, as they may cause a decrease in uric acid (UA) levels, with consequent anti-inflammatory or pro-inflammatory properties (Borovcanin et al. 2022). Antipsychotic drugs can increase UA levels, which is not desirable. We summarized that haloperidol treatment resulted in significantly lower plasma UA levels compared to healthy controls, which continued to decrease after haloperidol treatment was discontinued. Hyperuricemia was also found to be associated with the use of olanzapine and clozapine. However, in responders, risperidone treatment was found to normalize the decreased serum levels of UA, whereas this was not the case in non-responders.

Dopamine can modulate various immune functions such as proliferation, chemotaxis, antigen presentation, phagocytosis, cytokine secretion, and cell adhesion by affecting immune functions in cells expressing different amounts of D1 and D2-like receptors or other receptors that interact with dopamine, as detailed in the review by Channer et al. (2023). Many immune cells have receptors on their surface that interact with dopamine, which they can also take up by active transport. The uptake and release of dopamine can affect both the releasing cell and neighbouring cells and influence various functions. For example, dopamine can mediate the production of immunosuppressive factors such as TGF-β and IL-10 and activate B cells. It is likely that immune cells produce small amounts of dopamine themselves. These cells use dopamine to regulate themselves by activating dopamine receptors on neighbouring cells. Studies on macrophages show that dopamine can have both positive and negative effects on the immune system. It can influence the immune response by affecting phagocytosis and the production of nitric oxide (NO). In response to dopamine, stress response genes, activation of the nuclear factor kappa B pathway (NF-κB), and release of pro-inflammatory mediators increase. Dopamine has different effects on different immune cells. In microglia, activation of D1-like receptors inhibits NF-κB, while activation of D2-like receptors activates NF-κB. In neutrophils, dopamine increases extracellular loop formation and decreases NO production and transendothelial migration by acting on its receptors. However, dopamine has bidirectional effects on neutrophil phagocytosis. In eosinophils, dopamine influences the number of eosinophils. High doses of dopamine lead to eosinopenia, while low doses lead to eosinophilia. In mast cells, dopamine acting on D1-like receptors increases degranulation, while activation of D2-like receptors decreases cytokine production. The balance of dopamine receptors on dendritic cells has been found to influence T-cell differentiation. Increased expression of D1, D2, and D3 receptors on dendritic cells leads to the induction of a Th 1 phenotype in T cells. On the other hand, increased expression of D1 with low D2 expression leads to a Th 2 phenotype, while increased expression of D1, D3, and D5 together with low expression of D4 is associated with a Th 17 phenotype. When $CD4^+$ T cells are activated, dopamine stimulates the D1-like receptors, which in turn increases the production of IL-5 and IL-17. In addition, dopamine stimulates D2-like receptors, leading to reduced production of IL-2, IL-4, and interferon-gamma (IFN-γ). Dopamine has different effects on $CD8^+$ T cells depending on the type of receptor it acts on. Stimulation of D1-like receptors results in reduced cytotoxicity and immunosuppressive activity. On the other hand, dopamine increases the production of IL-10 and TNF-α by acting on D2-like receptors on resting $CD8^+$ T cells. It seems that dopamine mediates anti-inflammatory effects in inflammatory conditions and triggers inflammation in non-inflammatory conditions.

The immunomodulatory effects of antipsychotics in cancer therapy primarily relate to their influence on the immune system's ability to fight cancer cells. This includes increasing the activity of natural killer (NK) cells, which play a crucial role in the immune response against tumours. Antipsychotics can inhibit the proliferation of T-cells and stimulate the immune system, contributing to their potential anticancer effects. The modulation of immune pathways by antipsychotics therefore adds another layer to their therapeutic benefits and offers new approaches to cancer therapy that go beyond their traditional psychiatric applications.

4 Molecular Foundations for Anticancer Properties of Antipsychotics

The anticancer potential of antipsychotics is closely linked to their ability to modulate key intracellular signalling pathways, particularly the Akt/glycogen synthase kinase-3 (GSK-3) and Wnt pathways. These pathways are essential for cellular processes such as proliferation and survival, which are often dysregulated in cancer (Freyberg et al. 2010). By interfering with these pathways, antipsychotics may disrupt the cellular mechanisms that contribute to tumour growth and progression, highlighting their potential utility in cancer therapy.

In addition to interfering with these signalling pathways, antipsychotics can also interfere with cell cycle regulation, a crucial aspect of cancer cell biology. Precise control of the cell cycle is crucial for the prevention of tumorigenesis, and disruption of this process can lead to uncontrolled cell proliferation. Antipsychotics such as fluphenazine are known for their ability to regulate the cell cycle, potentially reducing cell proliferation and inducing apoptosis in cancer cells, which represents a new approach to cancer treatment (Vlachos et al. 2021).

Another significant aspect of the anticancer activity of antipsychotics is their potential to disrupt the efflux of chemotherapeutics from malignant cells. This mechanism is a common method of drug resistance in cancer cells, in which they expel chemotherapeutic agents, reducing their efficacy. By targeting these efflux pumps, antipsychotics could enhance the efficacy of chemotherapy, suggesting an additional pathway by which these drugs could exert anticancer effects (Vlachos et al. 2021).

4.1 Antipsychotics in Dopamine G-Protein-Coupled Receptors Dependent and Independent Signalling in Cancer Pathogenesis

Dopamine receptors are neurotransmitter receptors mainly expressed in the CNS (Grandy et al. 1989); however, the studies have confirmed that they are expressed at both messenger RNA (mRNA) and protein levels in various cancer cells in a cell type–specific manner, especially D2 receptors, including neuroblastoma (Deslauriers et al. 2011), glioma (Li et al. 2014), ovarian cancer (Moreno-Smith et al. 2011), breast cancer (Pornour et al. 2014), cervical cancer (Mao et al. 2015), and lung cancer (Hoeppner et al. 2015).

Dopamine receptors are G-protein-coupled receptors (GPCR) that are divided into two types: dopamine D1 and D2 receptors. D1 receptors, including D1 and D5 receptors, typically bind to the Gs/olf subunit and consequently activate adenylyl cyclase, induce the synthesis of cyclic adenosine monophosphate (cAMP), activate the protein kinase A (PKA) pathway and the transcription factor cAMP-response element binding protein (CREB), which is important for cell survival. D2 receptors such as D2, D3, and D4 receptors commonly interact with the Gi/o subunit and inhibit adenylyl cyclase, the cAMP/PKA pathway, voltage-activated Ca^{2+} channels and activate K^{+} channels (Beaulieu et al. 2015). Dopamine receptors have been studied in neurobiology mainly as key regulators of G-protein-dependent cellular processes. However, recent research has shown that dopamine receptors are able to exert some of their cellular functions via alternative signalling pathways that may or may not require cAMP (Beaulieu et al. 2015). There is compelling scientific evidence that dopamine receptors can communicate in vivo via pathways that are independent of cAMP/PKA and involve the multifunctional adaptor protein beta-arrestin 2 (Arr2) (Beaulieu et al. 2015). Arr2 can bind to phosphorylated and activated GPCR and induce their inactivation by clathrin-mediated endocytosis (Ferguson et al. 1996). Arr2 can also act as an anchor for kinases and phosphatases and subsequently form a signalling complex that activates various G-protein-independent pathway, including the Akt/GSK-3 pathway (Luttrell and Gesty-Palmer 2010).

Activation of the D2 receptor reduces cancer cell growth or promotes apoptosis in a variety of cancers (Roy et al. 2017). However, antagonism of dopamine D2 receptors by antipsychotics has shown anticancer effects in numerous cases, preferably in part through activation or inhibition of the cAMP/PKA pathway (Roy et al. 2017; Kline et al. 2018; Kang et al. 2017; Gil-Ad et al. 2006) or inhibition of the Akt/phosphoinositide 3-kinase (PI3K) pathway (Rho et al. 2011). In a recent study, the antitumor and antimetastatic effects of the antipsychotic thioridazine in hepatocellular carcinoma were shown to be due in part to dopamine D5 and D1 receptors (Lu et al. 2015). However, certain antipsychotic drugs, including pimozide, have shown good anticancer activity, mainly through an antagonistic effect on D2 receptors, although they can also bind to calmodulin, alpha receptors and 5HT7 serotonin receptors. Consequently, several antipsychotics whose anticancer effects have been demonstrated primarily through the dopamine receptors may also have a biological effect on other cellular targets, serotonin receptors, or other GPCR (Rosas-Cruz et al. 2021).

4.2 Antipsychotics and Akt Signalling Pathways in Cancer Pathogenesis

Antipsychotic drugs such as D2 receptor antagonists have been proposed as potential therapeutic targets for the phosphoinositide-3-kinases (PI3K)/Akt pathway, a crucial cell cycle regulator in cancer-related cells (Kang et al. 2012). The serine/threonine kinase Akt, also known as protein kinase B (PKB), is an important molecule in eukaryotic cells that plays an essential role in various intracellular functions. These functions include metabolism, cell stress response, cell cycle regulation, and processes that are critical for neuronal cell survival and brain function. The importance of Akt is also underlined by the fact that its deregulation plays a role in the pathogenesis of various diseases, including cancer, metabolic dysfunction, and mental disorders (Baudry et al. 2023).

Stimulation of receptor tyrosine kinases or GPCR at the plasma membrane by various survival signals, including growth factors and hormones, leads to activation of the Akt/PI3K pathway, which is initiated by the binding of Akt to phosphatidylinositol 3,4,5-triphosphate (PIP3), a lipid product of PI3K. Akt is then phosphorylated at two key residues, threonine (Thr308) and serine (Ser473), by intracellular kinases such as 3-phosphoinoitide-dependent protein kinase 1 (PDK1) and rictor-mTORC2 (mammalian target of rapamycin complex 2). Phosphorylation at Ser473 is particularly important as it stabilizes Akt and increases its activity (He et al. 2021). In cancer, the Akt signalling pathway is central as it controls the survival, proliferation, invasion, apoptosis, and angiogenesis of cancer cells. Dysregulation of the Akt signalling pathway is a major factor in cancer development, making it an important target for anticancer research (Rascio et al. 2021). In recent years, interest in the potential of antipsychotic drugs for cancer treatment has increased, particularly due to their ability to modulate cellular signalling pathways, including the PI3K/Akt/GSK-3β pathway (Hendouei et al. 2019). The influence of antipsychotics on these pathways may lead to changes in the cell cycle and affect survival and apoptosis in cancer cells, contributing to their potential anticancer effects.

4.3 Antipsychotics and Apoptotic Proteins of Akt Pathway in Cancer Pathogenesis

Akt may act in the cell by phosphorylating a number of downstream substrates, including key regulatory proteins of apoptosis such as proapoptotic Bcl-2-associated death promoter (BAD), caspase-9, forkhead box protein 1 (FOXO1), also called FKHR forkhead in rhabdomyosarcoma (FKHR), apoptosis signal-regulating kinase 1 (ASK1), CREB, mouse double minute 2 homolog (MDM2), Raf1, X-linked inhibitor of apoptosis (XIAP), etc. Akt phosphorylates the proapoptotic BAD protein and induces the dissociation of phosphorylated BAD from the BAD/BclXL or BAD/Bcl-2 complex, which in turn binds to the adaptor protein 14-3-3, causing the release of antiapoptotic Bcl-2 and the inhibition of Bax and caspase-3, thus enabling cell survival and inhibition of apoptosis (Braun et al. 2011; Nitulescu et al. 2018). As a result, several studies have shown that antipsychotics have an anticancer effect by inhibiting the Akt survival pathway and activating apoptosis, including ovarian cancer (Choi et al. 2008), breast cancer (Dakir et al. 2018), and pancreatic cancer (Chien et al. 2015). Akt can also inhibit apoptosis through direct phosphorylation and inhibition of caspase-9 activity. Some antipsychotics induce apoptosis by at least partially inhibiting Akt and directly activating caspase-9 (Xia et al. 2019). Similarly,

Akt phosphorylates the proapoptotic Bax at site S184, which inhibits the translocation of Bax into the mitochondria and the conformational activation of Bax and prevents apoptosis (Gardai et al. 2004). The antipsychotic flupentixol has antiproliferative and apoptotic effects in lung cancer cells by inhibiting the activation of Akt through decreasing the expression of antiapoptotic Bcl2 and increasing the activation of proapoptotic Bax (Dong et al. 2019).

4.4 Antipsychotics and Akt/Forkhead Box Protein Tumour Suppressor Regulation

In addition, Akt may phosphorylate and inactivate members of FKHRL1 such as the transcription factors FOXO1-3. FOXO is an important tumour suppressor protein that regulates the transcription of several genes involved in cell cycle regulation (Eijkelenboom and Burgering 2013), deoxyribonucleic acid (DNA) damage, response to stress and apoptosis (Greer and Brunet 2005), and cancer prevention (Jiang et al. 2013). In cancer cells, survival signals activate Akt/PI3K, which then phosphorylates FOXO1–3, causing it to bind to 14-3-3, remain in the cytosol and be inhibited, leading to tumorigenesis. Withdrawal of a survival factor or the administration of antitumor drugs promotes the dephosphorylation of FOXO1-3, its translocation to the nucleus and the regulation of certain genes. FOXO1-3 may promote apoptosis by increasing the expression of apoptosis-related genes such as TNFSF6, Fas ligand, Bim, bNip3, and Bcl-xL (Fu and Tindall 2008). A recent study has clearly demonstrated the antitumor effect of the antipsychotic drug trifluoperazine (TFP) in hepatocellular carcinoma by activating the FOXO1 pathway, decreasing Bcl-2, and increasing Bax expression (Jiang et al. 2017).

4.5 Antipsychotics and Akt-Mediated Regulation of p53 in Cancer Pathogenesis

Moreover, Akt plays a critical role in cell survival and death by regulating the activity of the E3 ubiquitin ligase MDM2, which is known to bind and negatively regulate the activity of the tumour suppressor p53. MDM2 is also phosphorylated by Akt at the Ser166 site, allowing it to enter the nucleus and target p53 for destruction (Parcellier et al. 2008). Nearly 50% of human tumours in cells are primarily caused by suppression of the tumour suppressor protein p53 as a result of its direct interaction with the MDM2 protein. One study showed that the antipsychotic drug fluspirilene caused significant inhibition of human colon carcinoma cell growth in a p53-dependent manner by suppressing the interaction between MDM2 and p53 (Patil et al. 2015). In another study, the antipsychotic drug pimozide showed an antitumor effect in breast cancer cells by increasing the expression of p53 through inhibition of the PI3K/Akt/MDM2 signalling pathway (Li et al. 2022). The most recent research has shown that the antihistamine cetirizine exhibits antitumor activity in human glioblastoma and neuroblastoma cell lines through activation of the p53 pathway and inhibition of MDM2 (Ghafoor and Yildiz 2023).

4.6 Antipsychotics and Akt/Calcium Signalling in Cancer Pathogenesis

Calcium (Ca^{2+}) signalling is associated with several key mechanisms that promote tumour growth. The primary endoplasmic reticulum (ER) Ca^{2+} release channel, the inositol 1,4,5-trisphosphate receptor (IP3R), is associated with Ca^{2+}-induced apoptotic death. Akt phosphorylates the IP3R by recognizing a consensus substrate motif common to all three IP3R isoforms (Khan et al. 2006). The IP3R plays a role in the mobilization of Ca^{2+} from intracellular storage, and IP3 binding mainly regulates channel function in this process. In addition, this receptor is involved in basic biological processes such as apoptosis, mitosis, and fertilization. The effects of various apoptotic stimuli are often correlated with Ca^{2+} outflow from the ER and Ca^{2+} accumulation in mitochondria (Pinton and Rizzuto 2006). Akt inhibits the release of Ca^{2+} from the IP3R and protects cells from apoptotic death induced by a number of Ca^{2+}-mediated apoptotic triggers (Szado et al. 2008). Shin et al. investigated the antitumor effect of clozapine on phosphatase and tensin homolog (PTEN)-negative U-87MG glioblastoma cells. Clozapine, an atypical antipsychotic, inhibited the uptake of Ca^{2+} via inotropic and voltage-dependent Ca^{2+} receptors and prevented IP3-dependent Ca^{2+} release. This resulted in inhibition of PI3K/Akt and Ca^{2+}/calmodulin pathways, which in turn led to cell cycle arrest and inhibited cell growth (Shin et al. 2006). A recent study showed that the antipsychotic drug TFP directly binds to the calmodulin/Ca^{2+} binding protein of IP3R, causing IP3R to irreversibly open and increase the release of Ca^{2+}. This effectively inhibited the growth, migration, and invasion of glioblastoma cells both in vitro and in vivo. Based on these results, TFP was proposed as a potential glioblastoma anticancer therapy (Kang et al. 2017).

An important component of the PI3K/Akt pathway is the activation of several downstream proteins, including NF-κB and mTOR (Khan et al. 2013). The PI3K/Akt/mTOR pathway plays a critical role in cell survival, growth and metabolism, and its modulation by antipsychotic drugs has been highlighted in cancer research (Shin et al. 2013). These drugs are thought to impact the pathway, possibly leading to significant alterations in cancer cell behaviour.

NF-κB, which is regulated by the PI3K/Akt pathway, plays a crucial role in transforming cyclin D1 expression and accelerating the cell cycle (Liu et al. 2020). NF-κB is located in the cytoplasm and is bound to the inhibitory protein IκB; its activation can occur in response to various stressors. Activation leads to phosphorylation and degradation of IκB, allowing NF-κB to enter the nucleus (Oeckinghaus and Ghosh 2009). Persistent activation of NF-κB is a common feature of solid tumours, and inhibition of this factor can make tumours more sensitive to chemotherapy and radiation. Overexpression of NF-κB suppresses apoptosis, suggesting that its inhibition may improve the efficacy of cancer therapies (Xia et al. 2014).

4.7 Antipsychotics and Mammalian Target of Rapamycin Complexes in Cancer Pathogenesis

Mammalian target of rapamycin (mTOR) is a large protein kinase that plays a crucial role in cellular functions and exists in cells in two different complexes: mTORC1 and mTORC2. These complexes, which include the components GβL, raptor (in mTORC1) and rector (in mTORC2), are essential for the regulation of various cellular processes (Zhou and Huang 2010). The raptor-containing mTORC1 complex is particularly sensitive to the immunosuppressive drug rapamycin. This complex interacts with raptor to form a nutrient-sensitive unit that signals for cell growth, indicating its significant role in cell metabolism and proliferation (Ganesh and Subathra Devi 2023).

CPZ, a well-known antipsychotic agent, has been shown to significantly affect these mTOR pathways. In particular, CPZ can induce G2/M phase arrest and apoptosis in cancer cells by regulating PI3K/Akt/mTOR-mediated autophagy pathways (Jhou et al. 2021). This mechanism highlights the potential of CPZ as a therapeutic agent in cancer treatment, where it acts on key regulatory pathways in cancer cells. By inhibiting the activity of the Akt/mTOR signalling pathway, CPZ contributes to the regulation of vital processes such as cell cycle progression and autophagy, which are critical for the survival and proliferation of cancer cells.

4.8 Antipsychotics and Kinase Pathways in Cancer Pathogenesis

GSK-3, an important protein kinase, plays an essential role in various cellular processes such as glucose metabolism, neurodevelopment, cellular differentiation, intracellular trafficking, apoptosis, regulation of gene transcription, and synaptic plasticity (Jaworski et al. 2019; Rayasam et al. 2009). The importance of GSK-3 for neurodevelopment and its potential involvement in neurodegenerative diseases such as Alzheimer's and in the development of cancer is particularly noteworthy (Lei et al. 2011). This kinase is regulated by inactivation through phosphorylation, a process that is essential for the maintenance of cellular homeostasis and function (Beurel et al. 2015).

A key regulatory mechanism of GSK-3 involves its inactivation by the Akt-PIP3 complex, a process critical for cellular signalling. Akt, which is activated in response to various stimuli, phosphorylates GSK-3 at specific serine residues, leading to its inactivation (Mayer and Arteaga 2016). This phosphorylation and subsequent inactivation of GSK-3 is critical for controlling its role in glycogen synthesis, which is regulated by the two subunits of GSK-3, α and β. Inhibition of these GSK-3 isoforms by Akt/PKB is crucial for the regulation of a variety of cellular processes, including those that are dysregulated in cancer (Beurel et al. 2015). Antipsychotics exert their effects in cancer therapy by modulating these kinase pathways. By affecting the Akt/GSK-3 axis, antipsychotic drugs can potentially disrupt the cellular mechanisms that contribute to cancer cell survival and proliferation (Freyberg et al. 2010). The modulation of cellular pathways by these drugs not only has implications for their primary psychiatric use, but also opens up possibilities for their use in oncology.

4.9 Antipsychotics and Akt/Wnt/β-Catenin Pathway in Cancer Pathogenesis

Akt/GSK3 signalling plays an important role in the regulation of the Wnt/β-catenin pathway (Freyberg et al. 2010). The Wnt/β-catenin pathway is nearly universal in all species and is involved in many important aspects of development, cell physiology and disease, including cancer (Nusse and Clevers 2017). β-catenin is activated by dephosphorylation, translocation to the nucleus and interaction with co-activators such as pygopus and Bcl-9 as well as T-cell factor/lymphoid enhancer factor (TCF/LEF) to activate Wnt target genes such as c-Myc, cyclin D1, and cyclin-dependent kinase inhibitor 1A (CDKN1A). These processes are mediated by the dopamine D2 receptor and lead to inactivation of GSK-3β through Akt phosphorylation. Numerous reports suggest that the antitumor effect of antipsychotics is mediated by inhibition of the Akt/GSK-3β/β-catenin pathway mediated by the D2 receptor. A study by Pulkoski-Gross et al. (2015) demonstrated the anti-metastatic activity of TFP by blocking D2 receptors, reducing the phosphorylation of Akt and β-catenin and thus inhibiting their action. In another study, the antipsychotic haloperidol was reported to inhibit the Wnt/β-catenin signalling cascade, thereby preventing the in vitro development of the hepatocellular carcinoma cell lines Hep3B and HepG2 (Fako et al. 2016). In addition, the antipsychotic drug thioridazine has an antitumor effect on glioma cells by inhibiting through the Wnt/β-catenin signalling pathway (Chu et al. 2019).

4.10 Antipsychotics and Cell Cycle and Cyclins in Cancer Pathogenesis

The cell cycle, a critical process of cell growth and division, is tightly regulated by a group of proteins called cyclins. These proteins activate cyclin-dependent kinases (CDKs), which are essential for the progression of the cell cycle (Ding et al. 2020). The regulation of the cell cycle is of utmost importance as alterations in the function of cyclins and CDKs are frequently associated with the development of cancer. Such alterations can lead to uncontrolled cell proliferation, which is a hallmark of cancerous growth (Casimiro et al. 2012).

CDK inhibitors have emerged as a promising therapeutic approach in cancer treatment. These inhibitors block the activity of CDKs, thereby regulating the cell cycle and preventing uncontrolled proliferation (Zhang et al. 2012). The research work of Balakrishnan et al. (2016) and Hydbring et al. (2016) underlines the potential of CDK inhibitors in cancer therapy. By targeting these key enzymes in the cell cycle pathway, CDK inhibitors can effectively halt the progression of the cycle and thus inhibit the growth and division of cancer cells.

Penfluridol, a first-generation diphenylpiperidine antipsychotic, is known for its indirect inhibition of CDKs (Tuan and Lee 2019). This property of penfluridol indicates its potential utility in cancer treatment and complements its known efficacy in psychiatric care. The ability of penfluridol and similar antipsychotic drugs to influence the cell cycle could open up new avenues in the treatment of cancer, particularly in cases where aberrant cell cycle progression is a key feature of the disease.

4.11 Antipsychotics and Apoptosis in Cancer Pathogenesis

The intricate signalling pathways governing cell apoptosis present critical targets for the development of anticancer drugs. Apoptosis, essentially a cellular self-destruction mechanism, is often dysregulated in cancerous cells. Apoptosis, characterized by features such as karyopyknosis, cytoplasmic blebbing, morphological alterations, DNA fragmentation by nucleases, and the eventual engulfment of apoptotic bodies by phagocytes, plays a pivotal role in cellular homeostasis (Pistritto et al. 2016).

Central to this process is the caspase family, in particular the initiator caspases such as caspase-2, 8, 9, 10, 11, and 12, which are closely linked to pro-apoptotic signals. Activation of these enzymes leads to the stimulation of downstream effector caspases, including caspase-3, 6, and 7, which induce apoptosis by cleaving specific aspartic acid residues in intracellular proteins (Parrish et al. 2013).

In addition, death receptors such as the Fas receptor and TNF receptors (DR3, DR4, and DR5) are involved in the apoptosis mechanism. Apoptosis is triggered by the binding of these receptors to their corresponding death ligands, which leads to the activation of caspase-8 and caspase-10 (Kantari et al. 2014). TNF-α and its receptor also initiate downstream signalling involving NF-κB and promote the expression of survival factors such as Bcl-2 and Fas-associated death domain-like IL-1β-converting enzyme-inhibitory protein (FLIP) (Hayden and Ghosh 2014). Inhibition of the NF-κB pathway is a sign of apoptosis.

Furthermore, mitochondria play an important role in mediating apoptosis. They release pro-apoptotic factors such as Smac/Diablo, apoptosis-inducing factor (AIF), Endo-G, cytochrome C, and the serine protease HtrA2/Omi, with cytochrome C playing a role in the activation of caspase-9 (Wang and Youle 2009). Mitochondrial regulation of apoptosis also involves Ca^{2+}-mediated signalling. Excessive Ca^{2+} accumulation in the mitochondria triggers apoptosis, with the Ca^{2+} balance between the endoplasmic reticulum and the mitochondria being controlled primarily by the Bcl-2 family. This family modulates the permeability of the mitochondrial membrane and is crucial for the regulation of apoptosis (Giorgi et al. 2012). According to a study by Qian et al. (2019), the antipsychotic drug thioridazine induced depolarization of mitochondrial membrane potential, activation of caspase-9, increased expression of Bax protein and decreased Bcl-2 protein, which in turn triggered mitochondrial-mediated apoptosis in lung and ovarian cancer cells.

The PI3K/Akt signalling pathway is of particular importance. PI3K, which is activated by various survival factors, subsequently activates Akt, which in turn inhibits pro-apoptotic members of the Bcl-2 family such as Bax, Bad, FOXO1, and GSK-3. The PI3K/Akt pathway also exerts anti-apoptotic effects by activating the NF-κB pathway, highlighting its vital role in antitumor strategies. According to one study, the antipsychotic drug penfluridol exerts the antitumor effect by inhibiting the Akt/GSK-3β/p70S6K pathway, activating protein phosphatase 2A and inducing apoptosis, resulting in increased expression of the proapoptotic proteins Puma, Bax, and Bim, and decreased expression of Bcl-2 (Chien et al. 2015).

Reactive oxygen species (ROS) play a dual role in cancer progression by affecting cell proliferation, survival, metastasis, and epithelial-mesenchymal transition through pathways such as mitogen-activated protein kinase (MAPK) and Ras-extracellular signal-regulated kinase (ERK). Although ROS can initiate various cell death pathways such as apoptosis, necrosis, and autophagy, they also support cancer cell survival and proliferation via the PI3K/Akt pathway. This dual nature emphasizes the need to develop cancer treatments based on both prooxidants and antioxidants.

4.12 Antipsychotics and Januse Kinase/Signal Transducer and Activator of Transcription Pathway in Cancer Pathogenesis

The family protein of signal transducer and activator of transcription (STAT) undergoes phosphorylation and activation by Januse kinase (JAK) in response to various cytokines and subsequently induces transcription of genes involved in cell survival and angiogenesis, including Bcl-2, Mcl-1, p53, survivin, and vascular endothelial growth factor (VEGF) (Bose et al. 2020). Dysregulation of the JAK/STAT signalling pathway promotes carcinogenesis, making them ideal targets for anticancer treatment approaches. STAT1, STAT3, and STAT5 have been shown to be overexpressed in numerous human cancer cells (Buettner et al. 2002). Several studies have unequivocally shown that several antipsychotics have anticancer effects on different types of cancer cells. The antipsychotic pimozide has been shown to have antitumor effects in a number of independent reports. These include inhibition of the STAT3 pathway in triple-negative breast cancer cells (Dees et al. 2020), induction of STAT3-mediated apoptosis in brain tumour cells (Ranjan et al. 2020), and inhibition of STAT5/cyclin D1 and STAT5/Bcl-xL signalling and induction of targeting TNF-related apoptosis-inducing ligand (TRAIL)/DR4-dependent apoptosis in peripheral T lymphomas (Xiao et al. 2021). In addition, the antipsychotic drug fluspirilene reduced the growth of glioma cells by inhibiting the STAT3 pathway (Dong et al. 2017). Aripoprazole also activated apoptosis and migration of gliomas by inhibiting Src-mediated activation of the Akt/STAT3 pathway (Kim et al. 2017).

4.13 Antipsychotics and Autophagy in Cancer Pathogenesis

Autophagy, a crucial self-degradation process, plays a significant role in maintaining cellular integrity by eliminating damaged organelles and improperly formed proteins generated during biosynthetic processes in lysosomes. This pathway is of fundamental importance for the self-preservation and degradation of cells (Chun and Kim 2018). It acts as a balancing force in cellular homeostasis, especially under stressful conditions, including the presence of cancer cells (Das et al. 2020).

One of the key pathways regulating autophagy is the Akt/m-TOR signalling pathway, which plays a central role in the study of cell growth, proliferation, and survival (Saxton and Sabatini 2017). Research by Koukourakis et al. (2016) and Yan et al. (2016) shed light on the intricate workings of this pathway in the context of autophagy (Jandrey et al. 2021). Activation or inhibition of this pathway can dramatically influence the process of autophagy, thereby impacting the survival and proliferation of cancer cells.

Antipsychotics are increasingly recognized for their potential anticancer properties in this context, in part due to their influence on autophagic pathways. By modulating the Akt/m-TOR signalling, these drugs can induce autophagy in cancer cells, leading to their self-degradation and subsequent reduction in tumour growth (Cui et al. 2021). This mechanism suggests a promising avenue for the use of antipsychotics as adjuncts in cancer therapy by harnessing their ability to trigger autophagic processes in cancer cells. Therefore, the study of autophagy, in particular its regulation through the Akt/m-TOR pathway, offers a new perspective for understanding how antipsychotics could contribute to cancer treatment.

4.14 Antipsychotics and Serotonergic Action in Cancer Pathogenesis

Serotonergic mechanisms of action have been primarily explored mainly in selective serotonin reuptake inhibitors, but the atypical profile and mechanisms of action of newer antipsychotics also include serotonin receptors and give these drugs additional valuable opportunities for resolving oncological problems. Sarrouilhe and Mesnil (2019) gave a critical insight into the linkage of serotonin and cancer. Recent studies have shown that serotonin plays a role in the spread of cancer cells, tumour angiogenesis, and migration, leading to carcinomas, gliomas, and carcinoids. Serotonin receptors involved in various stages of carcinogenesis, selective serotonin transporters (SERT), and serotonin synthesis pathways are potential targets for chemotherapy. Serotonin has an impact on MAPK and PI3K/Akt signalling, could activate MEK-ERK1/2, and JAK2-STAT3 signalling pathways, and be involved in a complex cross-talk between Wnt/β-catenin signalling and activation of mTOR downstream targets, activates Src/PI3K/Akt/mTOR/p70S6K phosphorylation signalling, and above all, targeting the serotonin system in cancer stem cells gives a rational for the treatment of resistant solid tumours.

5 Modern Approaches and Challenges in Cancer Treatment

The resistance is facilitated by the activation of cellular signal transduction pathways leading to increased expression of proteins that promote cellular survival, thereby reducing the efficacy of anticancer agents and ionizing radiation (Ouellette et al. 2022). In addition, the cytotoxic nature of oncological treatments poses another critical challenge—collateral damage to normal cells. This often results in severe side effects that affect the quality of life of patients undergoing these treatments (Baskar et al. 2012). For this reason, the medical community is constantly striving to refine and improve cancer treatment methods.

Recently, this pursuit has led to the introduction of innovative and more targeted therapeutic approaches. These include stem cell therapy, targeted therapy, ablation therapy, the use of nanoparticles and natural antioxidants, radionics, chemodynamic therapy, sonodynamic therapy and therapies based on the principle of ferroptosis (Debela et al. 2021). Each of these novel methods aims to overcome the shortcomings of traditional treatments by enabling a more targeted attack on cancer cells while minimizing damage to healthy tissue.

Additionally, the emergence of chimeric antigen receptor (CAR)-T cell therapy represents a groundbreaking development in the field of oncology. This therapy, which is particularly effective in certain types of B-cell leukaemia, exemplifies the shift towards more personalized and precise cancer treatment modalities (Wang et al. 2023).

The choice of treatment in oncology is highly individualized and takes into account factors such as the type of cancer, its stage, the available treatment options and the desired goals of the therapy. Often a combination of different treatments is used to optimize efficacy while reducing adverse effects. With advances in research, it is hoped that these novel treatments will not only increase the effectiveness of cancer therapy, but also improve the overall patient experience and outcomes.

Despite significant spending on cancer research and drug development, the proportion of approved therapies in oncology is low compared to various other indications, so new approaches are needed. One attractive approach in this area is drug repurposing, which involves finding new uses for known therapeutic drugs beyond their original medical indications. The advantages include lower development risk, a shorter timeframe and lower costs compared to completely new drug development approaches (Krouse et al. 2015; Sleire et al. 2017).

6 Conclusion

Psychotropic drugs and antipsychotics are interesting candidates for the repurposing of anticancer drugs. Although several in vitro and in vivo models have demonstrated the efficacy of this class of drugs in inhibiting cancer cell viability and tumour growth (Huang et al. 2018; Shaw et al. 2021; Zhuo et al. 2019), the pharmacological properties of antipsychotics remain elusive for potential clinical use in cancer therapy. As several epidemiological studies have found a lower incidence of cancer in patients undergoing long-term treatment with antipsychotics, this chapter focuses on the molecular basis of antipsychotic drugs in relation to their potential utility in anticancer therapy. These drugs, traditionally used for psychiatric conditions, show potential in modulating vital signalling pathways, regulating the cell cycle, and possibly overcoming chemotherapeutic resistance, thereby opening up innovative strategies in cancer management. Further research is essential to understand their pharmacological properties for clinical use in oncology, potentially positioning antipsychotics not only in psychiatric care, but also as a valuable component of comprehensive cancer therapy strategies.

Acknowledgements Thank Bojana Mircetic for the language editing. This research was supported by the Faculty of Medical Sciences, University of Kragujevac and the Ministry of Science, Technological Development and Innovation of the Republic of Serbia (Grant No. 451-03-65/2024-03/200111).

References

Balakrishnan A, Vyas A, Deshpande K, Vyas D (2016) Pharmacological cyclin dependent kinase inhibitors: implications for colorectal cancer. World J Gastroenterol 22(7):2159–2164. https://doi.org/10.3748/wjg.v22.i7.2159

Baskar R, Lee KA, Yeo R, Yeoh KW (2012) Cancer and radiation therapy: current advances and future directions. Int J Med Sci 9(3):193–199. https://doi.org/10.7150/ijms.3635

Baudry M, Su W, Bi X (2023) The Calpain proteolytic system. In: Bradshaw RA, Hart GW, Stahl PD (eds) Encyclopedia of cell biolog, 2nd edn. Academic, Oxford, pp 852–864

Beaulieu JM, Espinoza S, Gainetdinov RR (2015) Dopamine receptors – IUPHAR review 13. Br J Pharmacol 172(1):1–23. https://doi.org/10.1111/bph.12906

Beurel E, Grieco SF, Jope RS (2015) Glycogen synthase kinase-3 (GSK3): regulation, actions, and diseases. Pharmacol Ther 148:114–131. https://doi.org/10.1016/j.pharmthera.2014.11.016

Bjerre LM, Farrell B, Hogel M, Graham L, Lemay G, McCarthy L, Raman-Wilms L, Rojas-Fernandez C, Sinha S, Thompson W, Welch V, Wiens A (2018) Deprescribing antipsychotics for behavioural and psychological symptoms of dementia and insomnia: evidence-based clinical practice guideline. Can Fam Physician 64(1):17–27

Borovcanin MM, Vesic K (2021) Breast cancer in schizophrenia could be interleukin-33-mediated. World J Psychiatry 11(11):1065–1074. https://doi.org/10.5498/wjp.v11.i11.1065

Borovcanin M, Jovanovic I, Radosavljevic G, Djukic Dejanovic S, Stefanovic V, Arsenijevic N, Lukic ML (2013) Antipsychotics can modulate the cytokine profile in schizophrenia: attenuation of the type-2 inflammatory response. Schizophr Res 147(1):103–109. https://doi.org/10.1016/j.schres.2013.03.027

Borovcanin MM, Jovanovic I, Radosavljevic G, Pantic J, Minic Janicijevic S, Arsenijevic N, Lukic ML (2017) Interleukin-6 in schizophrenia-is there a therapeutic relevance? Front Psych 8:221. https://doi.org/10.3389/fpsyt.2017.00221

Borovcanin MM, Janicijevic SM, Jovanovic IP, Gajovic N, Arsenijevic NN, Lukic ML (2018) IL-33/ST2 pathway and Galectin-3 as a new Analytes in pathogenesis and Cardiometabolic risk evaluation in psychosis. Front Psych 9:271. https://doi.org/10.3389/fpsyt.2018.00271

Borovcanin MM, Minic Janicijevic S, Jovanovic IP, Gajovic NM, Jurisevic MM, Arsenijevic NN (2020) Type 17 immune response facilitates progression of inflammation and correlates with cognition in stable schizophrenia. Diagnostics (Basel) 10(11):926. https://doi.org/10.3390/diagnostics10110926

Borovcanin MM, Radosavljevic GD, Pantic J, Milovanovic J, Mijailovic NR, Arsenijevic AN, Arsenijevic NN (2021a) Contrasting roles of the Galectin-3 in the schizophrenia onset, clinical presentation, and somatic comorbidity. Curr Top Med Chem 21(16):1471–1487. https://doi.org/10.2174/1568026621666210611162420

Borovcanin MM, Vesic K, Jovanovic M, Mijailovic NR (2021b) Galectin-3 possible involvement in antipsychotic-induced metabolic changes of schizophrenia: a minireview. World J Diabetes 12(10):1731–1739. https://doi.org/10.4239/wjd.v12.i10.1731

Borovcanin MM, Janicijevic SM, Mijailovic NR, Jovanovic IP, Arsenijevic NN, Vesic K (2022) Uric acid potential role in systemic inflammation and negative symptoms after acute antipsychotic treatment in schizophrenia. Front Psych 12:822579. https://doi.org/10.3389/fpsyt.2021.822579

Borovcanin MM, Vesić K, Arsenijević D, Milojević-Rakić M, Mijailović NR, Jovanovic IP (2023a) Targeting underlying inflammation in carcinoma is essential for the resolution of depressiveness. Cells 12(5):710. https://doi.org/10.3390/cells12050710

Borovcanin MM, Vesic K, Petrovic I, Jovanovic IP, Mijailović NR (2023b) Diabetes mellitus type 2 as an underlying, comorbid or consequent state of mental disorders. World J Diabet 14(5): 481–493. https://doi.org/10.4239/wjd.v14.i5.481

Bose S, Banerjee S, Mondal A, Chakraborty U, Pumarol J, Croley CR, Bishayee A (2020) Targeting the JAK/STAT signaling pathway using Phytocompounds for cancer prevention and therapy. Cells 9(6):1451. https://doi.org/10.3390/cells9061451

Braun F, Bertin-Ciftci J, Gallouet AS, Millour J, Juin P (2011) Serum-nutrient starvation induces cell death mediated by Bax and puma that is counteracted by p21 and unmasked by Bcl-x(L) inhibition. PLoS One 6(8):e23577. https://doi.org/10.1371/journal.pone.0023577

Buettner R, Mora LB, Jove R (2002) Activated STAT signaling in human tumors provides novel molecular targets for therapeutic intervention. Clin Cancer Res 8(4):945–954

Casimiro MC, Crosariol M, Loro E, Li Z, Pestell RG (2012) Cyclins and cell cycle control in cancer and disease. Genes Cancer 3(11–12):649–657. https://doi.org/10.1177/1947601913479022

Channer B, Matt SM, Nickoloff-Bybel EA, Pappa V, Agarwal Y, Wickman J, Gaskill PJ (2023) Dopamine, immunity, and disease. Pharmacol Rev 75(1):62–158. https://doi.org/10.1124/pharmrev.122.000618

Chien W, Sun QY, Lee KL, Ding LW, Wuensche P, Torres-Fernandez LA, Tan SZ, Tokatly I, Zaiden N, Poellinger L, Mori S, Yang H, Tyner JW, Koeffler HP (2015) Activation of protein phosphatase 2A tumor suppressor as potential treatment of pancreatic cancer. Mol Oncol 9(4): 889–905. https://doi.org/10.1016/j.molonc.2015.01.002

Choi JH, Yang YR, Lee SK, Kim SH, Kim YH, Cha JY, Oh SW, Ha JR, Ryu SH, Suh PG (2008) Potential inhibition of PDK1/Akt signaling by phenothiazines suppresses cancer cell proliferation and survival. Ann N Y Acad Sci 1138:393–403. https://doi.org/10.1196/annals.1414.041

Chu CW, Ko HJ, Chou CH, Cheng TS, Cheng HW, Liang YH, Lai YL, Lin CY, Wang C, Loh JK, Cheng JT, Chiou SJ, Su CL, Huang CF, Hong YR (2019) Thioridazine enhances P62-mediated autophagy and apoptosis through Wnt/β-catenin signaling pathway in glioma cells. Int J Mol Sci 20(3):473. https://doi.org/10.3390/ijms20030473

Chun Y, Kim J (2018) Autophagy: an essential degradation program for cellular homeostasis and life. Cells 7(12):278. https://doi.org/10.3390/cells7120278

Cui F, Gu S, Gu Y, Yin J, Fang C, Liu L (2021) Alteration in the mRNA expression profile of the autophagy-related mTOR pathway in schizophrenia patients treated with olanzapine. BMC Psychiatry 21(1):388. https://doi.org/10.1186/s12888-021-03394-w

Dakir H, Pickard A, Srivastava K, McCrudden CM, Gross SR, Lloyd S, Zhang SD, Margariti A, Morgan R, Rudland PS, El-Tanani M (2018) The anti-psychotic drug pimozide is a novel chemotherapeutic for breast cancer. Oncotarget 9(79):34889–34910. https://doi.org/10.18632/oncotarget.26175

Das CK, Banerjee I, Mandal M (2020) Pro-survival autophagy: an emerging candidate of tumor progression through maintaining hallmarks of cancer. Semin Cancer Biol 66:59–74. https://doi.org/10.1016/j.semcancer.2019.08.020

Debela DT, Muzazu SG, Heraro KD, Ndalama MT, Mesele BW, Haile DC, Kitui SK, Manyazewal T (2021) New approaches and procedures for cancer treatment: current perspectives. SAGE Open Med 9:20503121211034366. https://doi.org/10.1177/20503121211034366

Dees S, Pontiggia L, Jasmin JF, Mercier I (2020) Phosphorylated STAT3 (Tyr705) as a biomarker of response to pimozide treatment in triple-negative breast cancer. Cancer Biol Ther 21(6): 506–521. https://doi.org/10.1080/15384047.2020.1726718

Deslauriers J, Lefrançois M, Larouche A, Sarret P, Grignon S (2011) Antipsychotic-induced DRD2 upregulation and its prevention by α-lipoic acid in SH-SY5Y neuroblastoma cells. Synapse 65(4):321–331. https://doi.org/10.1002/syn.20851

Ding L, Cao J, Lin W, Chen H, Xiong X, Ao H, Yu M, Lin J, Cui Q (2020) The roles of cyclin-dependent kinases in cell-cycle progression and therapeutic strategies in human breast cancer. Int J Mol Sci 21(6):1960. https://doi.org/10.3390/ijms21061960

Dong Y, Furuta T, Sabit H, Kitabayashi T, Jiapaer S, Kobayashi M, Ino Y, Todo T, Teng L, Hirao A, Zhao SG, Nakada M (2017) Identification of antipsychotic drug fluspirilene as a potential anti-glioma stem cell drug. Oncotarget 8(67):111728–111741. https://doi.org/10.18632/oncotarget.22904

Dong C, Chen Y, Li H, Yang Y, Zhang H, Ke K, Shi XN, Liu X, Li L, Ma J, Kung HF, Chen C, Lin MC (2019) The antipsychotic agent flupentixol is a new PI3K inhibitor and potential anticancer drug for lung cancer. Int J Biol Sci 15(7):1523–1532. https://doi.org/10.7150/ijbs.32625

Eijkelenboom A, Burgering BM (2013) FOXOs: signalling integrators for homeostasis maintenance. Nat Rev Mol Cell Biol 14(2):83–97. https://doi.org/10.1038/nrm3507

Fako V, Yu Z, Henrich CJ, Ransom T, Budhu AS, Wang XW (2016) Inhibition of wnt/β-catenin signaling in hepatocellular carcinoma by an antipsychotic drug Pimozide. Int J Biol Sci 12(7): 768–775. https://doi.org/10.7150/ijbs.14718

Ferguson SS, Downey WE 3rd, Colapietro AM, Barak LS, Ménard L, Caron MG (1996) Role of beta-arrestin in mediating agonist-promoted G protein-coupled receptor internalization. Science 271(5247):363–366. https://doi.org/10.1126/science.271.5247.363

Fond G, Macgregor A, Attal J, Larue A, Brittner M, Ducasse D, Capdevielle D (2012) Antipsychotic drugs: pro-cancer or anti-cancer? A systematic review. Med Hypotheses 79(1):38–42. https://doi.org/10.1016/j.mehy.2012.03.026

Freyberg Z, Ferrando SJ, Javitch JA (2010) Roles of the Akt/GSK-3 and Wnt signaling pathways in schizophrenia and antipsychotic drug action. Am J Psychiatry 167(4):388–396. https://doi.org/10.1176/appi.ajp.2009.08121873

Fu Z, Tindall DJ (2008) FOXOs, cancer and regulation of apoptosis. Oncogene 27(16):2312–2319. https://doi.org/10.1038/onc.2008.24

Ganesh SK, Subathra Devi C (2023) Molecular and therapeutic insights of rapamycin: a multi-faceted drug from Streptomyces hygroscopicus. Mol Biol Rep 50(4):3815–3833. https://doi.org/10.1007/s11033-023-08283-x

Gardai SJ, Hildeman DA, Frankel SK, Whitlock BB, Frasch SC, Borregaard N, Marrack P, Bratton DL, Henson PM (2004) Phosphorylation of Bax Ser184 by Akt regulates its activity and apoptosis in neutrophils. J Biol Chem 279(20):21085–21095. https://doi.org/10.1074/jbc.M400063200

Ghafoor NA, Yildiz A (2023) Targeting MDM2-p53 Axis through drug repurposing for cancer therapy: a multidisciplinary approach. ACS Omega 8(38):34583–34596. https://doi.org/10.1021/acsomega.3c03471

Gholipour N, Ohradanova-Repic A, Ahangari G (2018) A novel report of MiR-4301 induces cell apoptosis by negatively regulating DRD2 expression in human breast cancer cells. J Cell Biochem 119(8):6408–6417. https://doi.org/10.1002/jcb.26577

Gil-Ad I, Shtaif B, Levkovitz Y, Nordenberg J, Taler M, Korov I, Weizman A (2006) Phenothiazines induce apoptosis in a B16 mouse melanoma cell line and attenuate in vivo melanoma tumor growth. Oncol Rep 15(1):107–112

Giorgi C, Baldassari F, Bononi A, Bonora M, De Marchi E, Marchi S, Missiroli S, Patergnani S, Rimessi A, Suski JM, Wieckowski MR, Pinton P (2012) Mitochondrial Ca(2+) and apoptosis. Cell Calcium 52(1):36–43. https://doi.org/10.1016/j.ceca.2012.02.008

Grandy DK, Litt M, Allen L, Bunzow JR, Marchionni M, Makam H, Reed L, Magenis RE, Civelli O (1989) The human dopamine D2 receptor gene is located on chromosome 11 at q22-q23 and identifies a TaqI RFLP. Am J Hum Genet 45(5):778–785

Greer EL, Brunet A (2005) FOXO transcription factors at the interface between longevity and tumor suppression. Oncogene 24(50):7410–7425. https://doi.org/10.1038/sj.onc.1209086

Hayden MS, Ghosh S (2014) Regulation of NF-κB by TNF family cytokines. Semin Immunol 26(3):253–266. https://doi.org/10.1016/j.smim.2014.05.004

He Y, Sun MM, Zhang GG, Yang J, Chen KS, Xu WW, Li B (2021) Targeting PI3K/Akt signal transduction for cancer therapy. Signal Transduct Target Ther 6(1):425. https://doi.org/10.1038/s41392-021-00828-5

Hendouei N, Saghafi F, Shadfar F, Hosseinimehr SJ (2019) Molecular mechanisms of anti-psychotic drugs for improvement of cancer treatment. Eur J Pharmacol 856:172402. https://doi.org/10.1016/j.ejphar.2019.05.031

Hoeppner LH, Wang Y, Sharma A, Javeed N, Van Keulen VP, Wang E, Yang P, Roden AC, Peikert T, Molina JR, Mukhopadhyay D (2015) Dopamine D2 receptor agonists inhibit lung cancer progression by reducing angiogenesis and tumor infiltrating myeloid derived suppressor cells. Mol Oncol 9(1):270–281. https://doi.org/10.1016/j.molonc.2014.08.008

Huang J, Zhao D, Liu Z, Liu F (2018) Repurposing psychiatric drugs as anti-cancer agents. Cancer Lett 419:257–265. https://doi.org/10.1016/j.canlet.2018.01.058

Hydbring P, Malumbres M, Sicinski P (2016) Non-canonical functions of cell cycle cyclins and cyclin-dependent kinases. Nat Rev Mol Cell Biol 17(5):280–292. https://doi.org/10.1038/nrm.2016.27

Jandrey EHF, Bezerra M, Inoue LT, Furnari FB, Camargo AA, Costa ÉT (2021) A key pathway to cancer resilience: the role of autophagy in glioblastomas. Front Oncol 11:652133. https://doi.org/10.3389/fonc.2021.652133

Jaworski T, Banach-Kasper E, Gralec K (2019) GSK-3β at the intersection of neuronal plasticity and neurodegeneration. Neural Plast 2019:4209475. https://doi.org/10.1155/2019/4209475

Jhou AJ, Chang HC, Hung CC, Lin HC, Lee YC, Liu WT, Han KF, Lai YW, Lin MY, Lee CH (2021) Chlorpromazine, an antipsychotic agent, induces G2/M phase arrest and apoptosis via regulation of the PI3K/AKT/mTOR-mediated autophagy pathways in human oral cancer. Biochem Pharmacol 184:114403. https://doi.org/10.1016/j.bcp.2020.114403

Jiang Y, Zou L, Lu WQ, Zhang Y, Shen AG (2013) Foxo3a expression is a prognostic marker in breast cancer. PLoS One 8(8):e70746. https://doi.org/10.1371/journal.pone.0070746

Jiang J, Huang Z, Chen X, Luo R, Cai H, Wang H, Zhang H, Sun T, Zhang Y (2017) Trifluoperazine activates FOXO1-related signals to inhibit tumor growth in hepatocellular carcinoma. DNA Cell Biol 36(10):813–821. https://doi.org/10.1089/dna.2017.3790. Erratum in: DNA Cell Biol 36(12):1178

Kang S, Dong SM, Kim BR, Park MS, Trink B, Byun HJ, Rho SB (2012) Thioridazine induces apoptosis by targeting the PI3K/Akt/mTOR pathway in cervical and endometrial cancer cells. Apoptosis 17(9):989–997. https://doi.org/10.1007/s10495-012-0717-2

Kang S, Hong J, Lee JM, Moon HE, Jeon B, Choi J, Yoon NA, Paek SH, Roh EJ, Lee CJ, Kang SS (2017) Trifluoperazine, a well-known antipsychotic, inhibits glioblastoma invasion by binding to Calmodulin and disinhibiting calcium Release Channel IP3R. Mol Cancer Ther 16(1):217–227. https://doi.org/10.1158/1535-7163.MCT-16-0169-T

Kantari C, Lafont E, Walczak H (2014) Death receptor-induced apoptotic and nonapoptotic signaling. In: McManus LM, Mitchell RN (eds) Pathobiology of human disease. Academic, San Diego, pp 131–144

Kato TA, Monji A, Mizoguchi Y, Hashioka S, Horikawa H, Seki Y, Kasai M, Utsumi H, Kanba S (2011) Anti-inflammatory properties of antipsychotics via microglia modulations: are antipsychotics a 'fire extinguisher' in the brain of schizophrenia? Mini Rev Med Chem 11(7):565–574. https://doi.org/10.2174/138955711795906941

Khan MT, Wagner L 2nd, Yule DI, Bhanumathy C, Joseph SK (2006) Akt kinase phosphorylation of inositol 1,4,5-trisphosphate receptors. J Biol Chem 281(6):3731–3737. https://doi.org/10.1074/jbc.M509262200

Khan KH, Yap TA, Yan L, Cunningham D (2013) Targeting the PI3K-AKT-mTOR signaling network in cancer. Chin J Cancer 32(5):253–265. https://doi.org/10.5732/cjc.013.10057

Kim MS, Yoo BC, Yang WS, Han SY, Jeong D, Song JM, Kim KH, Aravinthan A, Kim JH, Kim JH, Kim SC, Cho JY (2017) Src is the primary target of aripiprazole, an atypical antipsychotic drug, in its anti-tumor action. Oncotarget 9(5):5979–5992. https://doi.org/10.18632/oncotarget.23192

Kline CLB, Ralff MD, Lulla AR, Wagner JM, Abbosh PH, Dicker DT, Allen JE, El-Deiry WS (2018) Role of dopamine receptors in the anticancer activity of ONC201. Neoplasia 20(1):80–91. https://doi.org/10.1016/j.neo.2017.10.002

Koukourakis MI, Mitrakas AG, Giatromanolaki A (2016) Therapeutic interactions of autophagy with radiation and temozolomide in glioblastoma: evidence and issues to resolve. Br J Cancer 114(5):485-496. https://doi.org/10.1038/bjc.2016.19. PMID: 26889975; PMCID: PMC4782209

Krouse AJ, Gray L, Macdonald T, McCray J (2015) Repurposing and rescuing of Mibefradil, an antihypertensive, for cancer: a case study. Assay Drug Dev Technol 13(10):650–653. https://doi.org/10.1089/adt.2015.29014.ajkdrr

Lee JK, Nam DH, Lee J (2016) Repurposing antipsychotics as glioblastoma therapeutics: potentials and challenges. Oncol Lett:1281–1286. https://doi.org/10.3892/ol.2016.4074

Lei P, Ayton S, Bush AI, Adlard PA (2011) GSK-3 in Neurodegenerative Diseases. Int J Alzheimers Dis 2011:189246. https://doi.org/10.4061/2011/189246

Li J, Zhu S, Kozono D, Ng K, Futalan D, Shen Y, Akers JC, Steed T, Kushwaha D, Schlabach M, Carter BS, Kwon CH, Furnari F, Cavenee W, Elledge S, Chen CC (2014) Genome-wide shRNA screen revealed integrated mitogenic signaling between dopamine receptor D2 (DRD2) and epidermal growth factor receptor (EGFR) in glioblastoma. Oncotarget 5(4):882–893. https://doi.org/10.18632/oncotarget.1801

Li J, Qu P, Zhou XZ, Ji YX, Yuan S, Liu SP, Zhang QG (2022) Pimozide inhibits the growth of breast cancer cells by alleviating the Warburg effect through the P53 signaling pathway. Biomed Pharmacother 150:113063. https://doi.org/10.1016/j.biopha.2022.113063

Liu X, Shao Y, Zhou J, Qian G, Ma Z (2020) Nuclear factor κB signaling and its related non-coding RNAs in cancer therapy. Mol Ther Nucleic Acids 19:208–217. https://doi.org/10.1016/j.omtn.2019.11.007

Lu M, Li J, Luo Z, Zhang S, Xue S, Wang K, Shi Y, Zhang C, Chen H, Li Z (2015) Roles of dopamine receptors and their antagonist thioridazine in hepatoma metastasis. Onco Targets Ther 8:1543–1552. https://doi.org/10.2147/OTT.S77373

Luttrell LM, Gesty-Palmer D (2010) Beyond desensitization: physiological relevance of arrestin-dependent signaling. Pharmacol Rev 62(2):305–330. https://doi.org/10.1124/pr.109.002436. Erratum in: Pharmacol Rev 62(3):564

MacDowell KS, Caso JR, Martín-Hernández D, Moreno BM, Madrigal JLM, Micó JA, Leza JC, García-Bueno B (2016) The atypical antipsychotic Paliperidone regulates endogenous antioxidant/anti-inflammatory pathways in rat models of acute and chronic restraint stress. Neurotherapeutics 13(4):833–843. https://doi.org/10.1007/s13311-016-0438-2

Mao M, Yu T, Hu J, Hu L (2015) Dopamine D2 receptor blocker thioridazine induces cell death in human uterine cervical carcinoma cell line SiHa. J Obstet Gynaecol Res 41(8):1240–1245. https://doi.org/10.1111/jog.12691

Mattiuzzi C, Lippi G (2019) Current cancer epidemiology. J Epidemiol Glob Health 9(4):217–222. https://doi.org/10.2991/jegh.k.191008.001

Mayer IA, Arteaga CL (2016) The PI3K/AKT pathway as a target for cancer treatment. Annu Rev Med 67:11–28. https://doi.org/10.1146/annurev-med-062913-051343

Miller BJ, Buckley P, Seabolt W, Mellor A, Kirkpatrick B (2011) Meta-analysis of cytokine alterations in schizophrenia: clinical status and antipsychotic effects. Biol Psychiatry 70(7):663–671. https://doi.org/10.1016/j.biopsych.2011.04.013

Minic Janicijevic S, Jovanovic IP, Gajovic NM, Jurisevic MM, Debnath M, Arsenijevic NN, Borovcanin MM (2022) Galectin-3 mediated risk of inflammation in stable schizophrenia, with only possible secondary consequences for cognition. World J Psychiatry 12(9): 1183–1193. https://doi.org/10.5498/wjp.v12.i9.1183

Miyamoto S, Duncan GE, Marx CE, Lieberman JA (2005) Treatments for schizophrenia: a critical review of pharmacology and mechanisms of action of antipsychotic drugs. Mol Psychiatry 10(1):79–104. https://doi.org/10.1038/sj.mp.4001556

Mondelli V, Ciufolini S, Belvederi Murri M, Bonaccorso S, Di Forti M, Giordano A, Marques TR, Zunszain PA, Morgan C, Murray RM, Pariante CM, Dazzan P (2015) Cortisol and inflammatory biomarkers predict poor treatment response in first episode psychosis. Schizophr Bull 41(5): 1162–1170. https://doi.org/10.1093/schbul/sbv028

Moreno-Smith M, Lu C, Shahzad MM, Pena GN, Allen JK, Stone RL, Mangala LS, Han HD, Kim HS, Farley D, Berestein GL, Cole SW, Lutgendorf SK, Sood AK (2011) Dopamine blocks stress-mediated ovarian carcinoma growth. Clin Cancer Res 17(11):3649–3659. https://doi.org/10.1158/1078-0432.CCR-10-2441

Muric NN, Arsenijevic NN, Borovcanin MM (2020) Chlorpromazine as a potential antipsychotic choice in COVID-19 treatment. Front Psych 11:612347. https://doi.org/10.3389/fpsyt.2020.612347

Nitulescu GM, Van De Venter M, Nitulescu G, Ungurianu A, Juzenas P, Peng Q, Olaru OT, Grădinaru D, Tsatsakis A, Tsoukalas D, Spandidos DA, Margina D (2018) The Akt pathway in oncology therapy and beyond (review). Int J Oncol 53(6):2319–2331. https://doi.org/10.3892/ijo.2018.4597

Nusse R, Clevers H (2017) Wnt/β-catenin signaling, disease, and emerging therapeutic modalities. Cell 169(6):985–999. https://doi.org/10.1016/j.cell.2017.05.016

Obuchowicz E, Bielecka-Wajdman AM, Paul-Samojedny M, Nowacka M (2017) Different influence of antipsychotics on the balance between pro- and anti-inflammatory cytokines depends on glia activation: an in vitro study. Cytokine 94:37–44. https://doi.org/10.1016/j.cyto.2017.04.004

Oeckinghaus A, Ghosh S (2009) The NF-kappaB family of transcription factors and its regulation. Cold Spring Harb Perspect Biol 1(4):a000034. https://doi.org/10.1101/cshperspect.a000034

Osterman E (1961) Has chlorpromazine a cytostatic effect? A few reflections in connection with a case and the modern literature. Nord Psykiatr Tidsskr 15:154–159. https://doi.org/10.3109/08039486109167943

Ouellette MM, Zhou S, Yan Y (2022) Cell signaling pathways that promote Radioresistance of cancer cells. Diagnostics (Basel) 12(3):656. https://doi.org/10.3390/diagnostics12030656

Parcellier A, Tintignac LA, Zhuravleva E, Hemmings BA (2008) PKB and the mitochondria: AKTing on apoptosis. Cell Signal 20(1):21–30. https://doi.org/10.1016/j.cellsig.2007.07.010

Parrish AB, Freel CD, Kornbluth S (2013) Cellular mechanisms controlling caspase activation and function. Cold Spring Harb Perspect Biol 5(6):a008672. https://doi.org/10.1101/cshperspect.a008672

Patil SP, Pacitti MF, Gilroy KS, Ruggiero JC, Griffin JD, Butera JJ, Notarfrancesco JM, Tran S, Stoddart JW (2015) Identification of antipsychotic drug fluspirilene as a potential p53-MDM2 inhibitor: a combined computational and experimental study. J Comput Aided Mol Des 29(2): 155–163. https://doi.org/10.1007/s10822-014-9811-6

Pinton P, Rizzuto R (2006) Bcl-2 and Ca2+ homeostasis in the endoplasmic reticulum. Cell Death Differ 13(8):1409–1418. https://doi.org/10.1038/sj.cdd.4401960

Pistritto G, Trisciuoglio D, Ceci C, Garufi A, D'Orazi G (2016) Apoptosis as anticancer mechanism: function and dysfunction of its modulators and targeted therapeutic strategies. Aging (Albany NY) 8(4):603–619. https://doi.org/10.18632/aging.100934

Pornour M, Ahangari G, Hejazi SH, Ahmadkhaniha HR, Akbari ME (2014) Dopamine receptor gene (DRD1-DRD5) expression changes as stress factors associated with breast cancer. Asian Pac J Cancer Prev 15(23):10339–10343. https://doi.org/10.7314/apjcp.2014.15.23.10339

Pulkoski-Gross A, Li J, Zheng C, Li Y, Ouyang N, Rigas B, Zucker S, Cao J (2015) Repurposing the antipsychotic trifluoperazine as an antimetastasis agent. Mol Pharmacol 87(3):501–512. https://doi.org/10.1124/mol.114.096941

Qian G, Dai L, Yu T (2019) Thioridazine sensitizes cisplatin against Chemoresistant human lung and ovary cancer cells. DNA Cell Biol 38(7):718–724. https://doi.org/10.1089/dna.2019.4715

Ranjan A, Kaushik I, Srivastava SK (2020) Pimozide suppresses the growth of brain tumors by targeting STAT3-mediated autophagy. Cells 9(9):2141. https://doi.org/10.3390/cells9092141

Rascio F, Spadaccino F, Rocchetti MT, Castellano G, Stallone G, Netti GS, Ranieri E (2021) The pathogenic role of PI3K/AKT pathway in cancer onset and drug resistance: an updated review. Cancers (Basel) 13(16):3949. https://doi.org/10.3390/cancers13163949

Rayasam GV, Tulasi VK, Sodhi R, Davis JA, Ray A (2009) Glycogen synthase kinase 3: more than a namesake. Br J Pharmacol 156(6):885–898. https://doi.org/10.1111/j.1476-5381.2008.00085.x

Rho SB, Kim BR, Kang S (2011) A gene signature-based approach identifies thioridazine as an inhibitor of phosphatidylinositol-3′-kinase (PI3K)/AKT pathway in ovarian cancer cells. Gynecol Oncol 120(1):121–127. https://doi.org/10.1016/j.ygyno.2010.10.003

Roney MSI, Park SK (2018) Antipsychotic dopamine receptor antagonists, cancer, and cancer stem cells. Arch Pharm Res 41(4):384–408. https://doi.org/10.1007/s12272-018-1017-3

Rosas-Cruz A, Salinas-Jazmín N, Velázquez MAV (2021) Dopamine receptors in cancer: are they valid therapeutic targets? Technol Cancer Res Treat 20:15330338211027913. https://doi.org/10.1177/15330338211027913

Roy S, Lu K, Nayak MK, Bhuniya A, Ghosh T, Kundu S, Ghosh S, Baral R, Dasgupta PS, Basu S (2017) Activation of D2 dopamine receptors in CD133+ve cancer stem cells in non-small cell lung carcinoma inhibits proliferation, Clonogenic ability, and invasiveness of these cells. J Biol Chem 292(2):435–445. https://doi.org/10.1074/jbc.M116.748970

Samperi I, Lithgow K, Karavitaki N (2019) Hyperprolactinaemia. J Clin Med 8(12):2203. https://doi.org/10.3390/jcm8122203. PMID: 31847209; PMCID: PMC6947286

Sarrouilhe D, Mesnil M (2019) Serotonin and human cancer: a critical view. Biochimie 161:46–50. https://doi.org/10.1016/j.biochi.2018.06.016

Saxton RA, Sabatini DM (2017) mTOR signaling in growth, metabolism, and disease. Cell 168(6):960–976. https://doi.org/10.1016/j.cell.2017.02.004. Erratum in: Cell 169(2):361–371

Shaw V, Srivastava S, Srivastava SK (2021) Repurposing antipsychotics of the diphenylbutylpiperidine class for cancer therapy. Semin Cancer Biol 68:75–83. https://doi.org/10.1016/j.semcancer.2019.10.007

Shin SY, Choi BH, Ko J, Kim SH, Kim YS, Lee YH (2006) Clozapine, a neuroleptic agent, inhibits Akt by counteracting Ca2+/calmodulin in PTEN-negative U-87MG human glioblastoma cells. Cell Signal 18(11):1876–1886. https://doi.org/10.1016/j.cellsig.2006.02.004

Shin SY, Lee KS, Choi YK, Lim HJ, Lee HG, Lim Y, Lee YH (2013) The antipsychotic agent chlorpromazine induces autophagic cell death by inhibiting the Akt/mTOR pathway in human U-87MG glioma cells. Carcinogenesis 34(9):2080–2089. https://doi.org/10.1093/carcin/bgt169

Sleire L, Førde HE, Netland IA, Leiss L, Skeie BS, Enger PØ (2017) Drug repurposing in cancer. Pharmacol Res 124:74–91. https://doi.org/10.1016/j.phrs.2017.07.013

Strobl JS, Kirkwood KL, Lantz TK, Lewine MA, Peterson VA, Worley JF (1990) Inhibition of human breast cancer cell proliferation in tissue culture by the neuroleptic agents pimozide and thioridazine. Cancer Res 50(17):5399–5405

Szado T, Vanderheyden V, Parys JB, De Smedt H, Rietdorf K, Kotelevets L, Chastre E, Khan F, Landegren U, Söderberg O, Bootman MD, Roderick HL (2008) Phosphorylation of inositol 1,4,5-trisphosphate receptors by protein kinase B/Akt inhibits Ca2+ release and apoptosis. Proc Natl Acad Sci USA 105(7):2427–2432. https://doi.org/10.1073/pnas.0711324105

Tacik P, Curry S, Fujioka S, Strongosky A, Uitti RJ, van Gerpen JA, Diehl NN, Heckman MG, Wszolek ZK (2016) Cancer in Parkinson's disease. Parkinsonism Relat Disord 31:28–33. https://doi.org/10.1016/j.parkreldis.2016.06.014

Telford JE, Bones J, McManus C, Saldova R, Manning G, Doherty M, Leweke FM, Rothermundt M, Guest PC, Rahmoune H, Bahn S, Rudd PM (2012) Antipsychotic treatment of acute paranoid schizophrenia patients with olanzapine results in altered glycosylation of serum glycoproteins. J Proteome Res 11(7):3743–3752. https://doi.org/10.1021/pr300218h

Thun MJ, DeLancey JO, Center MM, Jemal A, Ward EM (2010) The global burden of cancer: priorities for prevention. Carcinogenesis 31(1):100–110. https://doi.org/10.1093/carcin/bgp263

Tuan NM, Lee CH (2019) Penfluridol as a candidate of drug repurposing for anticancer agent. Molecules 24(20):3659. https://doi.org/10.3390/molecules24203659

van Schalkwyk GI, Beyer C, Johnson J, Deal M, Bloch MH (2018) Antipsychotics for aggression in adults: a meta-analysis. Prog Neuro-Psychopharmacol Biol Psychiatry 81:452–458. https://doi.org/10.1016/j.pnpbp.2017.07.019

Vesic K, Gavrilovic A, Mijailović NR, Borovcanin MM (2023) Neuroimmune, clinical and treatment challenges in multiple sclerosis-related psychoses. World J Psychiatr 13(4): 161–170. https://doi.org/10.5498/wjp.v13.i4.161

Vlachos N, Lampros M, Voulgaris S, Alexiou GA (2021) Repurposing antipsychotics for cancer treatment. Biomedicines 9(12):1785. https://doi.org/10.3390/biomedicines9121785

Wang C, Youle RJ (2009) The role of mitochondria in apoptosis. Annu Rev Genet 43:95–118. https://doi.org/10.1146/annurev-genet-102108-134850

Wang C, Wang J, Che S, Zhao H (2023) CAR-T cell therapy for hematological malignancies: history, status and promise. Heliyon 9(11):e21776. https://doi.org/10.1016/j.heliyon.2023.e21776

Wu Chou AI, Wang YC, Lin CL, Kao CH (2017) Female schizophrenia patients and risk of breast cancer: a population-based cohort study. Schizophr Res 188:165–171. https://doi.org/10.1016/j.schres.2017.01.019

Xia Y, Shen S, Verma IM (2014) NF-κB, an active player in human cancers. Cancer Immunol Res 2(9):823–830. https://doi.org/10.1158/2326-6066.CIR-14-0112

Xia Y, Jia C, Xue Q, Jiang J, Xie Y, Wang R, Ran Z, Xu F, Zhang Y, Ye T (2019) Antipsychotic drug Trifluoperazine suppresses colorectal cancer by inducing G0/G1 arrest and apoptosis. Front Pharmacol 10:1029. https://doi.org/10.3389/fphar.2019.01029

Xiao Z, Liang J, Deng Q, Song C, Yang X, Liu Z, Shao Z, Zhang K, Wang X, Li Z (2021) Pimozide augments bromocriptine lethality in prolactinoma cells and in a xenograft model via the STAT5/cyclin D1 and STAT5/Bcl xL signaling pathways. Int J Mol Med 47(1):113–124. https://doi.org/10.3892/ijmm.2020.4784

Yan Y, Jiang K, Liu P, Zhang X, Dong X, Gao J, Liu Q, Barr MP, Zhang Q, Hou X, Meng S, Gong P (2016) Bafilomycin A1 induces caspase-independent cell death in hepatocellular carcinoma cells via targeting of autophagy and MAPK pathways. Sci Rep 6:37052. https://doi.org/10.1038/srep37052. PMID: 27845389; PMCID: PMC5109251

Yao Y, Dai W (2014) Genomic instability and cancer. J Carcinog Mutagen 5:1000165. https://doi.org/10.4172/2157-2518.1000165

Zhang M, Zhang L, Hei R, Li X, Cai H, Wu X, Zheng Q, Cai C (2012) CDK inhibitors in cancer therapy, an overview of recent development. Am J Cancer Res 11(5):1913–1935

Zhou H, Huang S (2010) The complexes of mammalian target of rapamycin. Curr Protein Pept Sci 11(6):409–424. https://doi.org/10.2174/138920310791824093

Zhuo C, Xun Z, Hou W, Ji F, Lin X, Tian H, Zheng W, Chen M, Liu C, Wang W, Chen C (2019) Surprising anticancer activities of psychiatric medications: old drugs offer new hope for patients with brain cancer. Front Pharmacol 10:1262. https://doi.org/10.3389/fphar.2019.01262

S-(de)-Nitrosylation of Caspases: The Achilles Heel in the Expanding Sea of Cancer Treatment Regimens

Surupa Chakraborty, Ankita Choudhuri, Akansha Mishra, Anirban Ray, Kumar Sachin, Nirmalya Dey, and Rajib Sengupta

Abstract

Protein S-nitrosylation, or S-nitrosylation, in general, is a redox-regulated posttranslational mechanism that has gained momentum over the years as a double-edged sword with unprecedented versatility in playing crucial roles in multiple debilitating disorders or disease conditions, including cancer. The prominence of this reversible redox modification upon the covalent attachment of NO/NO moiety (N_2O_3; autoxidation of NO)/NO bearing compounds (nitrous acid, metal nitrosyl complexes, NO donors, and peroxynitrite) to sulfhydryl (thiol) groups is highlighted by the fine-tuning of the S-nitrosylation and S-denitrosylation-based redox switch, which markedly hints toward its cellular prudence in basal and stimulus-induced (in the presence of nitrosative stressors) conditions, thus extending the credibility of NO-based research in dodging abrogated redox equilibrium in disease states.

S-nitrosylation of specific endogenous caspase-like cysteine proteases (mainly, caspases 3, 8, and 9) leads to the dysregulation or inhibition of their proteolytic activity and further downstream signaling cascade leading to apoptosis per se, which can differentially influence oncogenic potential and/or cancer prevention, depending on the specificity of the targeted substrate protein and NO transport machinery/delivery system in healthy and cancer cells; reversibility or S-denitrosylation of caspases is efficiently ensured by two ubiquitous redox checkpoint systems, thioredoxin and lipoic acid, that aid in counteracting any nitro-oxidative shift in caspase thiol status.

S. Chakraborty · A. Choudhuri · A. Mishra · A. Ray · N. Dey · R. Sengupta (✉)
Amity Institute of Biotechnology Kolkata, Amity University Kolkata, Kolkata, West Bengal, India
e-mail: rsengupta@kol.amity.edu

K. Sachin
Himalayan School of Biosciences, Swami Rama Himalayan University, Dehradun, India

Interdisciplinary Cancer Research, https://doi.org/10.1007/16833_2024_296
Published online: 04 July 2024

Knowledge and understanding of these redox-based protein posttranslational mechanisms regulating apoptotic signaling cascades may pave the way for strategizing novel redox-based therapeutic regimens to jeopardize cellular homeostasis, cell growth, and survivability in cancer cells.

Keywords

Antioxidant therapy · Cancer · Caspases · Glutathione · Lipoic acid · Redox regulation · S-denitrosylation · S-nitrosylation · Thioredoxin

Abbreviations

AO	antioxidant
CASP-SNO	S-nitrosocaspase
DHLA	dihydrolipoic acid
Grx	glutaredoxin
GSH	glutathione
GSNO	S-nitrosoglutathione
H_2O_2	hydrogen peroxide
HOCl	hypochlorous acid
LA	lipoic acid
LD	lipoamide dehydrogenase
LMW	low molecular weight
MAP3K	mitogen-activated protein kinase kinase kinase
MDR	multidrug resistance
NO	nitric oxide
NO_2	nitrogen dioxide
NO_2^-	nitrite
NO_3^-	nitrate
NOS	nitric oxide synthases
$O_2^{\bullet -}$	superoxide radical
$OH^{\bullet}$	hydroxyl radical
$ONOO^-$	peroxynitrite
PSNO	S-nitrosoprotein
RNS	reactive nitrogen species
ROS	reactive oxygen species
RSNO	S-nitrosothiol
Shc	Src homologous and collagen
TME	tumor microenvironment
TNF	tumor necrosis factor
TRP14	Thioredoxin-related protein of 14 kDa
Trx	thioredoxin
TrxR	thioredoxin reductase
TXNIP	thioredoxin interacting protein

1 Introduction

Reactive oxygen species (ROS) and reactive nitrogen species (RNS) such as superoxide ($O_2^{\bullet -}$), hydroxyl radical ($OH^{\bullet}$), hydrogen peroxide (H_2O_2), hypochlorous acid (HOCl), nitric oxide ($NO^{\bullet}$), nitrogen dioxide ($NO_2^{\bullet}$), nitrite (NO_2^-), nitrate (NO_3^-), peroxynitrite ($ONOO^-$), and other H_xNO_y forms are the putative free radical/non-radical players in the premonition of several disease pathologies, including cancer, owing to their highly reactive nature, high responsiveness, and short half-life span that can cause exclusively damaging effects in favor of the development of oxidative/nitrosative stress (Di Meo et al. 2016). Interestingly, beyond the well-established recognition as "Molecule of the Year, 1992" and "Nobel Prize, 1998", due to its involvement as an endogenous, small, lipophilic, inorganic secondary messenger and regulatory molecule with pleiotropic effects in a plethora of functional significances such as vasodilation, neurotransmission, and immunological processes, nitric oxide free radical or nitric oxide-related isoforms (NO_x, H_xNO_y) are recognized as potential cellular oxidants that contribute to nitro-oxidative stress (Xu and Liu 1998). Upon the abrogation of the redox equilibrium between the intracellular production of pro-oxidants/oxidants, their localization, and scavenging pathways for these intracellular stressors, the steady-state NO levels varying from low (20 nM) to high (500 nM) leads to nitro-oxidative stress that eventually results in mitochondrial dysfunction, disruption in energy metabolism and ion channel function, cellular and cell membrane damage, collateral damage to major biomolecules, including lipids, proteins, and nucleic acids, protein posttranslational modifications, inactivation of functional enzymes and signaling pathways and further apoptosis-, autophagy-, ferroptosis-, or pyroptosis-mediated cell death (Lancaster Jr 2006). The sustenance of RNS and ROS in in vivo biological systems is kinetically well characterized, but the intrinsic challenges in delineating the individual contributions of these reactants and the hinge of considering the biochemical reactions mitigated by them as "quantitively minor" processes are still a concern. Nonetheless, a growing body of scientific literature over the last few decades has warranted further research utilizing the correlation with such cellular stressors in the hope of a reversal of protein posttranslational modifications, attenuation of carcinogenesis, genotoxicity, and cytotoxicity, or at least a substantial improvement of the clinical phenotypes/outcomes in different types of cancers (Lancaster Jr 2006; Hirst and Robson 2007; Karwowska and Kononiuk 2020).

In an attempt to generalize the utilization of nitric oxide in chemo- and radio-sensitizing tumors and cancer cells, it is crucial to understand that nitric oxide and its reaction products act as a "double-aged sword" in reaping the clinical benefits, either as an inducer or inhibitor of apoptosis. Thus, what looks like a "scientific eureka" might be just a case of wishful thinking, unless the threshold concentration serving pro-apoptotic or anti-apoptotic effects is attained (Li and Wogan 2005; Kim et al. 1999). There is irrefutable scientific evidence that a vast repertoire of thiol-bearing proteins such as those belonging to the TNF-superfamily, MAPK family, NF-kB signaling pathway, majority of the caspases, cathepsins, VCAM-1, TRAP1, TP53, GRIN2A, CBFB, CALR, EGFR, cFLIP, C-Src, H-Ras, COX2, H1F1α, Galectin-1,

BCL-2, Prx-2, Rac1/2, STAT1/3, PFKM, ERK1/2, Keap1, LTBP1, androgen receptor, integrin α6, RB, and caveolin-1 participate in S-nitrosoprotein (PSNO) and S-nitrosothiol (RSNO) formation, in response to higher than physiological concentrations of NO and several other intermediates in augmented nitrosative stress conditions, demonstrated in different types of cancers (Wang 2012; Li et al. 1997; Bhattacharyya et al. 2022; Li et al. 2013; Papaleo et al. 2023; Kaliyaperumal et al. 2015; Plenchette 2015; Muntané and Bonavida 2015; Tan et al. 2019; Sharma et al. 2021; Koning et al. 2023). Given this abundance of literature, it is however, crucial to pinpoint the selective protein candidates such as caspases, that can render the most significant benefits in their native (active) forms by directly triggering the chances of programmed cell death or apoptosis in cancer cells, thus adding credibility to research lying at the intersection of S-nitrosylation and its reversibility utilizing cellular reductases or antioxidants and caspase-dependent apoptosis. As a cumulative proof-of-concept for strategizing a therapeutic regimen based on this approach, we demonstrate convincing arguments for the properties of endogenous S-denitrosylases or nitric oxide synthase (NOS) scavengers in inhibiting caspase-S-nitrosylation and/or NO signaling, formulating the rationale for combinatorial antioxidant therapy in dodging cancer and the degree of malignancy and metastasis.

2 Caspases and Cancer

The perspective on most of the cellular pathways responsible for maintaining the cellular integrity lacks the spatio-temporal clarity on the presence of conflicting molecules within the same niche. The dynamicity of these pathways in responding differentially to the local stimuli is fundamental for comprehending the underlying complexity of the mechanisms that further influence cellular fate. This necessarily adds an impetus to identify and understand the transient or permanent interactions occurring in a carefully orchestrated manner, thus pushing the limits of deciphering more precise and effective interventions for cell fate modulation. With functionally discordant or compatible biomolecules forming the basis of the interactions that provide the cell its consequentiality, introducing any deviation or disruption in these reaction cascades, coupled with the establishment of a state of chronic nitro-oxidative stress, results in the clinical manifestations of a plethora of diseases and disorders. The contrasting existence of both the pro-apoptotic and anti-apoptotic machinery within our cells resembles the two ends of a homeostatic "seesaw", with both sides executing a counteracting force or overload on the other side to maintain the finely tuned balance of apoptotic processes in normal physiological conditions. This pivotal balance that the cell is attuned to maintain constitutes the coherently functioning environment that is capable of recognizing and responding to both intracellular (mitochondrial pathway/mitochondrial stimulus-dependent) and extracellular (death receptor stimulus-dependent) cues. In the instance of the well-characterized caspase-dependent apoptosis, the origin of these "cues" plays a decisive role in defining the pathway of apoptosis adopted by the apoptotic caspases (Group II caspases), which in turn triggers a cascade of reactions following the conformational changes induced upon the initiator caspases. Subsequently, the latter proteolytically cleaves the effector caspases that dismantle the coordinated network of cellular machinery (Olsson and Zhivotovsky 2011).

However, despite the vast spectrum of caspases, which often overlap in their functionality to maintain the "caspase cascade", they are rendered ineffective in cancer cells, leading to the onset of several types of cancer. This inherent property of cancer cells to subdue caspases and thereby prevent apoptosis is in part a function of the opposing biomolecules that interfere in the processing of caspases, effectively overcoming the barrier of cell death and introducing aberrations in the cellular repertoire. While normal cellular programming majorly encompasses a series of intricate morphological and biochemical events, levels and actions of caspases and caspase inhibitors, and a cautious balance between the pro-apoptotic and anti-apoptotic proteins regulating the downstream signaling pathways that determine cellular fate, any disruption in the balance caused by the preferential favor of anti-apoptotic components or the functional impairment of the pro-apoptotic machinery is responsible for the altered pathophysiology linked with the onset of cancer (Boice and Bouchier-Hayes 2020; Wong 2011).

Dissecting the multiple layers in the conundrum that involves the induction or evasion of apoptosis reveals yet another aspect: the regulation of caspases by distinct biological entities that are strictly not confined to the niche of inducing cellular death. The intrinsic nature of these entities ensures that the posttranslational modifications of a vast array of cellular proteins allow multiple signaling cascades to progress in a synchronized manner. These modifications, as well as the crosstalk between the major and supporting players of complementary signaling pathways, intertwine their corresponding functionality to influence the cellular fate of apoptosis, senescence, or evasion, further rationalizing their dynamic (patho)physiological relevance. In the context of caspases, posttranslational modifications have been inextricably linked to influencing cell death (Zamaraev et al. 2017), highlighting the governance of several factors when it comes to exploring the dormant existence of caspases in a cancer cell. S-nitrosylation is one of the posttranslational modifications that deepens the intricacies of dormant caspases, particularly because of the labile, reactive nature of the NO moiety, which turns into a relatively stable modification when it becomes associated with a thiol in a protein, only capable of being removed by S-denitrosylating systems that exhibit the specificity for it. With this concept of an inactive caspase being associated with S-nitrosylation, the perspective of caspases and cancer clarified to an extent might open avenues to explore the same under the spectrum of redox biochemistry.

3 S-Nitrosylation of Caspases

Caspases are master-class proteases involved in apoptosis, belonging to a family of C14 proteases (Barret and Rawling's classification) that bear an Asp residue in the P1 pocket of the scissile bond (Barrett 1997). The members of the caspase gene family can be divided into three groups; caspases 1, 4, and 5 are involved in the inflammatory response, and the two other groups consisting of 2, 3, 7, and 6, 8, 9, 10 carry out the apoptotic pathways (extrinsic and intrinsic) in cells. The catalytic site of caspases consists of a cysteine-histidine dyad, which carries out their proteolytic activity by cleaving the Asp residue. Nitric oxide (NO) is a profound gaseous signaling molecule that takes part in an array of cellular pathways. Under normal conditions, NO is produced by the enzymatic oxidation of L-arginine to L-citrulline and can thereby regulate the biological activity directly *via* the posttranslational modifications of its cognate protein substrates. Depending on the redox state of the cell and oxygen concentration, NO can act in deleterious ways, forming higher oxidative species like sulfenic and sulfenic acids or regulating other protein activities by S-nitrosylation (Zech et al. 1999).

It has been previously established that the presence of excess NO or low molecular weight (LMW) dithiols in the system can modify the cysteine (SH) residue of caspases 3, 8, and 9 and can undergo S-nitrosylation, thereby inhibiting its activity (Mannick et al. 1999, 2001; Sengupta et al. 2009, 2010; Chakraborty et al. 2023) (Table 1). The S-nitrosylated form of caspases, whose proapoptotic ability is inhibited by NO, has been reportedly detected in untreated non-tumorigenic cells as well as in cancer cells, and their further accumulation was ensured after TrxR knockdown or exposure to Trx/TrxR inhibitors (Stoyanovsky et al. 2005; Sengupta et al. 2007, 2009, 2010; Benhar et al. 2008; Chakraborty et al. 2023). However, it remains a pondering question how caspases present at nanomolar level concentrations (< 50 nM) behold susceptibility to S-nitrosylation in cancer cells, even in the presence of comparatively higher (micromolar to millimolar) levels of endogenous and ubiquitous cellular S-denitrosylases such as Trx/TrxR system (mainly cytosolic Trx1) and glutathione (GSH); what distinguishes the cellular fate of caspase-induced apoptosis in normal or non-cancerous cells and safeguarding of caspase-SNOs in cancer cells or tumor microenvironment (TME) is yet to be known. The plausible hypotheses to address this scientific riddle could be: (i) the reduced efficiency of the two major enzyme systems that are capable of performing the biochemistry of S-denitrosylation, thus affecting the dynamic turnover of the S-NO group from caspases; (ii) increased caspase-SNO accumulation in proportion to Trx/TrxR inhibition in the face of nitrosative stress in cancer cells; (iii)opposing activities of the nitric oxide synthases (NOS) and Trx system, thus abrogating the redox switch maintaining the S-nitrosylation/S-denitrosylation homeostatic balance to a point of no return; (iv) downregulation of antioxidant (Trx, SOD, GR, etc.) genes due to transcriptional repression in the face of nitrosative stress; (v) nuclear translocation of Trx1 in response to oxidative stress, NF-κB activation, UV-B irradiation, or TNF-α treatment; (vi) the intracellular milieu (pH imbalance, steric hindrance from other LMW RSNOs generated, neighboring groups, and/or proximal protein residues) surrounding the caspase-SNO functional group may antagonize the S-denitrosylase activity of the Trx system and GSH in TME. Regardless, the idea of encouraging a fail-safe exogenous supplementation of S-denitrosylases/antioxidants in the reversal of caspase-SNO modifications in cancer cells could elucidate their apoptotic functions. This is only to be contrasted with the conventional approaches bearing a higher concentration of NO delivery to tumor cells, which invites the

Table 1 Summarization of major intracellular thiol proteases (caspases) involved in apoptotic signaling cascades, perturbation of which leads to debilitating diseases, like cancer

Parameters	Caspase 8	Caspase 9	Caspase 3
Type	Initiator caspase Involved in the extrinsic or receptor-mediated pathway (Elmore 2007)	Initiator caspase Involved in intrinsic or mitochondrial-mediated apoptotic pathway (Elmore 2007)	Effector caspase Involved in terminal or execution pathway of apoptosis (CPP32 subfamily) (Elmore 2007, Fernandes-Alnemri et al. 1994)
Molecular weight Length	55.391 kDa 479 amino acids	46.281 kDa 416 amino acids	31.608 kDa 277 amino acids
Subcellular localization	Cytoplasm, nucleus	Cytosolic region, mitochondria, nucleus, protein-containing complex	Cytoplasm and mitochondrial intermembrane space
Gene name	CASP8 (Uniprot ID: Q14790)	CASP9 (Uniprot ID: P55211)	CASP3 (Uniprot ID: P42574)
Amino acid residues for protease activation	Catalytic triad consisting of Cys360, His317 and the backbone carbonyl oxygen atom of Arg258 (Watt et al. 1999)	Cys285, His237, Trp340, Arg341, and Arg179 (Renatus et al. 2001)	N-terminal region pro-domain (31–37 amino acid sequence) (Pelletier et al. 2004)
Susceptible Cys residue(s) for S-nitrosylation	Only catalytic thiol (Kim et al. 2000)	Catalytic Cys325 (in the conserved sequence QACGG) (Zhang et al. 2016)	Catalytic Cys163 (in the conserved sequence QACRG) (Tewari et al. 1995), active site Cys285 (p17), and poly-S-nitrosylation in $(p12/p17)_2$ tetramer (Zech et al. 1999)
Functional significance upon NO (donor) treatment	Inhibition of caspase activity *via* S-nitrosylation, activation of caspases 9 and 3; 1.7 mol of bound NO/mol of enzyme (Sengupta et al. 2010, Kim et al. 2000)	Inhibition of activation and proteolytic activity of caspase *via* S-nitrosylation of procaspase and inhibition of cyt c release; 0.064 μmol NO/mg protein (Chakraborty et al. 2023, Török et al. 2002, Zhang et al. 2016, Kim and Tannenbaum 2004)	Concentration-dependent decrease of catalytic activity; 1–3 mol of RSNOs/ mol of enzyme (Li et al. 1997, Zech et al. 1999)

(continued)

Table 1 (continued)

Parameters	Caspase 8	Caspase 9	Caspase 3
Pathophysiological relevance	Suppresses TNF-α-induced hepatocyte apoptosis *via* inhibition of bid cleavage and mitochondrial cyt c release Inhibits propagation of apoptotic signaling cascade (antiapoptotic effect) Resistance to anticancer drug and Fas antibody apoptosis upon caspase 8 deficiency	Dysregulates mitochondrial apoptotic pathway Promotes carcinogenesis in the background of chronic inflammation Suggestive of chemopreventive strategies Resistance to apoptosis and substitution of p53 loss in oncogenic transformation upon caspase 9 deletion in embryonic stem cells and Myc-expressing cells, respectively	Modulates elevation of protease activity at relatively low concentration Inhibition of spontaneous TNF-α-induced apoptosis in hepatocytes through induction of HSP 70 at higher NO concentrations Direct (S-nitrosylation-based) or indirect (cGMP-dependent) inhibition of activity Prevents PARP degradation and intranucleosomal DNA fragmentation, representing a leap toward malignant transformation

downsides of cytostatic effects, with an implicated cellular cytotoxicity if delivered to the wrong site or normal cells (Cook et al. 2004; Reddy et al. 2023; Melino et al. 1997; Mannick et al. 1999, 2001; Kim et al. 2002; Shen et al. 2016; Stanford et al. 2001; Kim et al. 2017; Ren et al. 2016; Salvatori et al. 2023; Hirota et al. 1999).

4 S-Denitrosylation of S-Nitrosylated Caspases (GSH and Redoxins-Mediated)

The property of S-denitrosylation, or reversible S-nitrosylation, renders the endogenous cellular S-denitrosylases beneficial for maintaining the free thiol/S-nitrosylated thiol balance under basal, stimulus-coupled, and/or nitrosative stress conditions (Chakraborty et al. 2022). The baffling realization of the existence and discovery of several isoforms belonging to the thioredoxin superfamily as well as enzymes or compounds other than the ubiquitous and well-established thioredoxin/thioredoxin reductase (Trx/TrxR) system, bearing close structural resemblances with shared redox potencies and enzymatic activities, has boosted intense research in the development of LMW thiol-bearing compounds like DHLA/LA system-based drug designing (Stoyanovsky et al. 2005). The time- and concentration-dependent S-denitrosylation of S-nitrosocaspases (CASP-SNO) in the presence of physiologically relevant concentrations of potential cellular reductants or S-denitrosylases like 5–10 mM GSH, 5–50 μM reduced thioredoxin (Trx-$(SH)_2$) alone, or the complete Trx system (Trx/TrxR/NADPH), 50–100 μM lipoic acid (LA) system (LA/lipoamide dehydrogenase (LD)/NADH), or dihydrolipoic acid (DHLA) alone, cater to the appreciation of Nature's tricky way of retaining the cellular homeostatic balance between endogenous NO donors like S-nitrosothiols (RSNOs) and target substrate proteins (S-nitrosoproteins or PSNOs) to the extent whereby a reductive cellular milieu is preferentially favored for conserving the structural and functional implications of the reduced (native) caspases in distinct cellular processes (Table 2; Fig. 1).

Li et al. (1997), in their early pioneering works on NO-mediated regulation and control of caspases and further, apoptosis, succeeded in establishing consistency in the enzymatic behavior of seven members of the caspase family (caspases 1, 2, 3, 4, 6, 7, and 8) due to S-nitrosylation of the active site cysteine thiol(s) upon exogenous supplementation of NO donors or intracellular iNOS-mediated NO release (Li et al. 1997). The SNAP/NO donor-induced caspase inhibition was completely reversed in the presence of 5 mM DTT, a synthetic reductant that mirrors the activity of endogenous cellular reductants, such as GSH. Despite the early promise of the NO molecule in catalyzing the proteolytic activity of most caspases, its application in beholding theranostic values in oncogenic conditions might require the consideration of only caspases 8, 9, and 3, which are the major contributors of the TNF-α/Act. D/Fas antibody/transforming growth factor β1, and cycloheximide-based immunostimulated apoptosis (Li et al. 1997; Kim et al. 1997; Sengupta et al. 2007; Sengupta et al. 2009; Sengupta et al. 2010; Chakraborty et al. 2023; Woo et al. 1998). S-nitrosylated caspase 3 zymogen (32 kDa) can be S-denitrosylated by Fas stimulation, rendering its cleavage and further, intracellular proteolytic and apoptotic activity (Mannick et al. 1999). Intriguingly, it has been reported that caspase 3, unlike other caspases, renders susceptibility to undergo poly-S-nitrosylation at multiple sites other than the catalytic site, with an average stoichiometry of 2 mol of bound NO molecules per mole of the tetrameric enzyme (1–3 mol of bound NO to each of the p12 and p17 subunits). The reversibility of this transient reaction mechanism by a concomitant reduction of S-nitrosylated caspase 3 (CASP 3-SNO) to its reduced, native counterpart, CASP 3-SH, is conditional on the target S-nitrosylated cysteine residue, owing to the possibility of S-denitrosylation of all SNOs in its p12 and p17 subunits, except for a single p17 SNO group (Zech et al. 1999). This inherent stability of the active site Cys 285 in the presence of physiological GSH levels is possibly attributed to its higher nucleophilicity as compared with the other cysteine residues; however, Trx system or DTT-catalyzed S-denitrosylation efficiently restored the enzyme's catalytic activity, suggesting (i) stringency or specificity of caspase 3 toward the choice of S-denitrosylases, (ii) ability of the complete Trx system at physiologically relevant concentrations, in fully reconstituting caspase 3 activity, and (iii) the integral cellular highlight of safeguarding the apoptotic control of caspase 3, which behaves as a fulcrum, adjoining the fate of both the extrinsic and intrinsic pathways of apoptosis. Sengupta et al. (2009) confirmed the speculations of DHLA and LA/LD/NADH system's

Table 2 Putative redox players in reversing S-nitrosylation of endogenous caspases

Reported caspase(s)	Considerable evidence in S-denitrosylation of caspases			References
	Model system(s)	S-denitrosylases involved	Physiological effect	
Caspase 8-SNO	Wild-type and TrxR-deficient HepG2 cells	DTT LMM compounds with vicinal dithiols (DHLA/LA system) Trx system Grx system (unknown) GSH (unknown)	Reactivation of caspase 8 activity Direct S-NO reduction/S-S functions in caspase 8-S-NO or an equilibrium shift between caspase 8, caspase 8-SNO, GSNO, and GSH (unknown)	Sengupta et al. (2010)
Caspase 9-SNO	Recombinant pure protein, wild-type and TrxR-deficient HepG2 cells, 293 T cells, HT-29 cells, in vivo system	DHLA/LA system Trx system DTT Grx system (unknown) GSH (unknown) NOS inhibitors (indirect S-denitrosylase activity)	Time-dependent reactivation of caspase 9 activity Cleavage of procaspase 9 and subsequent apoptosis	Chakraborty et al. (2023), Zech et al. (1999), Zhang et al. (2016)
Caspase 3-SNO	Recombinant pure protein, wild-type and TrxR-deficient HepG2 cells, Jurkat cells, 10C9 cells, HeLa cells, HEK cells, BJAB, HAEC, rat tissues, in vivo systems	Trx2 system majorly (upon Fas stimulation) Trx1 system TRP14 DHLA/LA system DTT GSH (conditional* and mostly no S-denitrosylation activity) Grx1 system (coupled with DTT or GSH)	*S-denitrosylation of all S-NO groups by GSH in its p12 subunit except one (active site cysteine) Activation of catalytic site cysteine and reconstitution of enzyme activity Promotes apoptotic signaling Dissociation of ASM (acid sphingomyelinase) from a second Cys-SNO	Stoyanovsky et al. (2005), Sengupta et al. (2007), Sengupta et al. (2009), Mannick et al. (1999), Kim and Tannenbaum (2004), Benhar et al. (2008), Ren et al. (2019), Pader et al. (2014)

behavior in catalyzing the S-denitrosylation of CASP 3-SNO alone, or alongside the Trx system, thereby underpinning reasonable questions of such remarkable versatility of caspase 3 as a double-edged sword, in the face of nitro-oxidative stress under basal and pathological settings (Sengupta et al. 2009). In marked contrast to caspase 3, the other caspases including the indispensable caspases 8 and 9, have the susceptibility to S-nitrosylation at their catalytic cysteine residues and are further catabolized by the GSH, LA system, and Trx system with moderate to high catalytic efficiency, which makes the biological and clinical relevance of redox (S-nitrosylation and S-denitrosylation)-mediated apoptotic modulation (suppression or stimulation) to cancer progressively clear (Li et al. 1997; Sengupta et al. 2007, 2009, 2010; Chakraborty et al. 2023; Benhar et al. 2008).

In response to the fluctuations in reduced free thiol or protein (caspase) thiol state and further attenuation of their proteolytic activities, a therapeutic application of S-denitrosylases stands promising to reverse the cysteine thiol modification, i.e., S-nitrosylation, thereby inducing apoptosis *via* activation of endogenous caspases. The additional immunogenic privileges provided by these antioxidants, or S-denitrosylases, include the least possibility of triggering an immunogenic response or any adverse side effects, which is otherwise predictable for novel, synthetic drugs unknown to the body's cells, tissues, and organs. However, skepticism and some puzzling questions still remain unanswered to reap the clinical benefits of NO in cancer therapeutics, given the fact that (i) drug development with NO donors/ scavengers, NOS inhibitors, antioxidant (AO) therapy, or the use of pro-drugs is still in its infancy; (ii) combinatorial therapeutic approaches with cancer cell-targeted AO or drug delivery might expectedly increase the sensitization of specific cells toward conventional chemotherapies, as well as dodge the therapy-insensitive tumors/ cancers toward the widely acclaimed anticancer drugs; (iii) amplifying the need of translational medical research from core research in the field of nitric oxide, antioxidants, and cellular denitrosylases as possible drug candidates, to entering clinical trials, requires attention and approval in record time for testing the possibilities of efficacy/cellular responses in co-implementing these drugs with first-line therapies or even as standalone drugs that can trigger target-specific apoptosis; (iv) modulation of the S-(de)nitrosylation based regulational control on apoptotic pathways might reshape our understanding of the hallmarks of cancer from a novel point of view; (v) assessing the cumulative outcomes of our hypothesized therapeutic intervention in all possible types of cancer cell lines and in vivo models is a necessary pre-requisite to bridge the knowledge gap concerning the effect of these LMW drugs and antioxidants on the localized tumor microenvironment and on its respective cellular decision to enter senescence, trigger a concomitant apoptosis or rather survive; and finally, (vi) cancer is a multifactorial debilitating disease and the acceleration of potentially acceptable, novel anticancer or tumor-suppressive drugs over the decades have majorly failed to reach the hands of masses, owing to the requirement of certified clearance at multiple levels, thus adding to futile and arduous search for more. Instead of enlarging the spectrum of more novel drugs to dodge cancer in multiple mechanisms, utilizing LMW compounds and mimetics having well-regarded, high (patho)physiological implications, as drugs, with more research standardization on dosages or time of intake, depending on the need of the situation (including the type of cancer, stage of cancer, size of the tumor, age of patients, toxicity effects if any, contradictory cellular outcomes, if any, improved drug delivery methods like intravenous or nebulizer based, etc.) would cut short the time of drug designing and development, and also maximize the therapeutic window by a universal drug/drug combination that can fine-tune the plethora of major key players in triggering cancer cell death.

5 Antioxidant Therapy for Cancer

The formidable challenges in the conventional cancer therapeutic regimens, like the risk of developing multidrug resistance (MDR) and the lack of efficiency and specificity in targeting cancer cells, have prompted scientists to shift their focus to novel drug designing and development of anticancer treatments based on diverse cytotoxic or apoptotic approaches that can directly trigger the activation of the key elements of apoptosis, otherwise dormant in cancer cells (Kolenko et al. 2000; Davis et al. 2003; Debatin 2004; Liu et al. 2010; Rahmanian et al. 2016; Boice and Bouchier-Hayes 2020; Kim et al. 2001; Mueller et al. 2003; Hasenjäger et al. 2004). The single-handed dependency on caspase-induced cancer cell death in the context of apoptosis resistance is yet to be fully understood. More significantly, the mechanisms underlying the activation of caspases must be tightly regulated based on the local concentration, spatiotemporal control of endogenous S-denitrosylases, other vital parameters, and the theranostic potentials of delivery of caspase activators/inducers to specific tissues, as well as the extent of caspase activation based on patients' responses or individual cancer subtypes, remain an open-ended question. Owing to the multifunctional spectrum and omnipotent versatility of NO in contributing to cancer cell differentiation, tumorigenesis, angiogenesis, MDR, regulation of gain or loss of functional mutation, apoptosis, and protein posttranslational modifications such as S-nitrosylation, targeted NO inducers or NO scavengers' delivery has garnered sufficient attention in cancer therapeutics, depending on the need of the situation (Vong and Nagasaki 2020; Wu et al. 2023; Jin et al. 2017; Bao et al. 2023; Kim et al. 2017; Alimoradi et al. 2019; Reddy et al. 2023).

The exploration of S-denitrosylases or antioxidants for their translational potential to reverse the S-nitrosylation of endogenous major caspases (caspases 3/8/9) might demonstrate a therapeutic strategy based on the PSNO (here, caspase-SNO) degradation pathway and the reciprocal relationship of NO in rescuing or promoting cancer cells to programmed cell death (apoptosis) (Fig. 2). Based on our understanding of experimental evidence, it is comprehensible that the Trx1/Trx system can be regarded as a positive or negative regulator of apoptosis, via preconditioning of apoptotic S-nitrosoproteins into their active counterparts, or by mitigating nitro-oxidative stress by binding to its inhibitor, TXNIP (thioredoxin interacting protein, also referred to as thioredoxin binding protein 2 or Vitamin-D3-upregulated protein) that releases pro-apoptotic proteins such as ASK1, a mitogen-activated protein kinase kinase kinase (MAP3K) from the Trx(1/2)-ASK1 interaction, thereby activating it. Consequently, ASK1 further activates c-Jun N-terminal kinase and p38 MAP kinase pathways, required for tumor necrosis factor (TNF)-α-induced apoptosis (Li et al. 2013; Lu and Holmgren 2012; Saitoh et al. 1998; Yoshihara et al. 2010; Saxena et al. 2010). Mitochondrial Trx2 and GSH present in high levels can also impart cellular protection against apoptosis in lower stress conditions by reducing disulfide bonds that allow the reversal of the dimer-tetramer transition of $p66^{Shc}$ (Shc: Src homologous and collagen); alkaline mitochondrial pH enhances the thiol sensitivity toward oxidation, thus favoring the active, tetrameric structure of $p66^{Shc}$ which can concurrently release apoptotic factors under conditions of ROS overload and excessive oxidative stress (Gertz et al. 2008). Similarly, the glutaredoxin (Grx) system coupled with GSH, belonging to the Trx superfamily of thiol–disulfide oxidoreductases, exhibits its antioxidant properties as a major cellular disulfide reductant along with its roles as S-denitrosylase and S-deglutathionylase, which impart sustenance of redox homeostasis in tandem with the Trx system (Holmgren 2000; Lillig and Holmgren 2007; Chakraborty et al. 2022; Ren et al. 2019; Chakraborty et al. 2023). Despite the fact that there are reports claiming the expression, subcellular localization, and translocation of several cancer-specific Grx isoforms (Grx2a, Grx2b, and Grx2c) and their probable mechanistic roles involving tumorigenesis and cellular protection from apoptosis by the attenuation of oxidative stress, the dosage-dependent, site-specific supplementation of Grx and/or lipoic acid, glutathione, etc. can increase the rate of Trx-catalyzed S-denitrosylation of caspases in cancer cells, owing to the faster reduction of oxidized Trx (Lundberg et al. 2001; Nakamura et al. 2000; Lönn et al. 2008; Enoksson et al. 2005; Lu and Holmgren 2012; Zhang et al. 2014; Li et al. 2014; Ho et al. 2000). The attenuation of S-nitroso modification of caspases in cancer cells, together with the redox-based translational induction of caspase-dependent apoptosis by the supplementation of antioxidants, antagonize the anti-apoptotic effects of Trx and Grx, conditional on the concentration and redox status of the active site cysteines of these antioxidants (Enoksson et al. 2005; Lillig et al. 2004; Anathy et al. 2009; Wu et al. 2010; Wu et al. 2011; Lei et al. 2016; Wen et al. 2020; Song and Lee 2003). However, the S-denitrosylase activity of Grx independently and Grx coupled with GSH or other antioxidants like LA on caspases remains yet to be fully established as a proof-of-concept. Ren et al. (2019) first identified S-nitrosylated caspase 3 as susceptible to Grxs-catalyzed S-denitrosylation, thus giving credence to the theory (Ren et al. 2019).

The overarching goal of exploring the therapeutic potential of antioxidants in the posttranslational regulation of apoptotic machinery is to understand their connecting link in redox-driven biological and molecular mechanisms in the context of debilitating disorders like cancer, with particular emphasis on the contribution of S-denitrosylation of caspases 3/8/9 toward apoptosis and harness their efficiency in the development of new diagnostic and theranostic approaches. Whether the contribution of S-denitrosylation-mediated activation of caspases in the face of nitrosative/nitro-oxidative stress is aided by the influx/exogenous supplementation of antioxidant enzymes, gene delivery methods for the expression of major cellular oxidoreductases behaving as "antioxidants", or viral delivery of antioxidant enzyme genes to specific cancer tissues targeting cytosolic/compartmentalized caspases, intracellular reduction of Trx supplemented by LA, Grx, GSH, catalase, antioxidants, etc. (Holmgren 2000; Nakamura et al. 2009; Agrawal et al. 2006; Agrawal et al. 2012; Ridet et al. 2006; Kamezaki et al. 2008; Anestål et al. 2008; Arlt et al. 2013; Bai and Cederbaum 2000; Chen et al. 2003; Finley et al. 2011; Goodman et al. 2011; Lippman et al. 2009), or conjugated delivery of such with caspase-specific immunogenic stimulators, seem to rely majorly on the nature, concentration, and duration of the apoptotic inducers chosen for the redox-based antioxidant therapies as well as the localization of the substrates for S-denitrosylases (here, caspases) that can further reason for the differential outcomes in several cancer phenotypes. Thus, the quest for designing reliable cancer therapeutics supported by the pieces of evidence highlighted previously necessitates further research to optimize the specificity of the drug target within the cancer cells, or TME, stage of cancer concerned, dosage, and mode of antioxidant drug delivery strategies that are designed with relevance to their inhibitory efficiencies in cancer cell proliferation and the threshold concentration ideally suited to perform their S-denitrosylase activities.

6 Conclusion

The cornerstone assumption in the relentless search for designing novel cancer therapeutic regimens has been an inherent need to specifically target a universal signaling pathway, such as apoptosis, that is shared by all types of tumors and malignancies. Instigating cell-specific apoptotic reprogramming of cancers and more specifically, tinkering with the proteolytic activities of cysteinyl proteases (caspases), which are established as primary or key inducers of apoptosis, provides a solid benchmark idea or notion that can be a potential trailblazer in the field of human cancer and cure. The inhibition of caspase activity, mainly, the activity of major initiator and executioner caspases, has been attributed to the S-nitrosylation of critical cysteine residues and thus correlated with the loss of redox-regulated apoptotic control. A comprehensive discussion concerning possible treatment modalities aimed at redox-regulated caspase-induced cell death in cancer-specific cells requires the following considerations: (i) endogenous dosage measurement of NO; accumulation of toxic NO levels upon exogenous and excess levels of NO/NO donors would lead to a forced paradigm shift in the anti-apoptotic versus pro-apoptotic behavior of NO, though questioning the relevance in an in vivo situation; (ii) cellular susceptibility of survival is largely dependent on their respective antioxidant levels; (iii) S-denitrosylation of caspases leads to a reconstitution of their proteolytic activity, further triggering downstream apoptotic cascades, the results being consistent with in vitro and in vivo experiments; (iv) cell- or tissue-specific administration of NOS inhibitors or NO scavengers would prevent S-nitrosylation mediated inhibition of caspases; (v) inhibition of apoptosis by NO might be substantiated by several parameters, including stimuli-like growth factors, TNF, Fas ligand, cGMP-mediated, and S-nitrosylation-mediated, however S-nitrosylation mediated inhibition gains a new high with results implicating consistency in both upstream and downstream caspases (caspases 8, 9, and 3); (vi) a minute and detailed insight into the scientific literature also suggests that abrogation of endogenous caspase activity under physiological concentrations of NO/NO donor (s), is primarily attributed to S-nitrosylation reaction mechanisms, though other mechanisms at several other steps of the apoptotic cascade have also been suggested;

the reversibility of such processes ensured by endogenous antioxidants or cellular S-denitrosylase systems like Trx and LA/DHLA, or enhancing their potential by exogenous administration might bolster the possibility of an active caspase, available for triggering the apoptotic signaling cascade in cancer cells or tumors, and finally, vii) an efficient drug delivery system for NO donors or NO scavengers, or NOS inhibitors (Fig. 1). Nonetheless, the fact that NO can now be acclaimed as a universal caspase inhibitor, beholding the capacity to halt apoptosis by inhibiting caspases and other cognate substrates of apoptosis, also raises its biological implications and contribution in safeguarding cellular integrity by mediating cellular rescue even after the activation of caspases has been triggered (Li et al. 1997; Kim et al. 1997, 2000; Sengupta et al. 2007, 2009, 2010; Chakraborty et al. 2023; Benhar et al. 2008; Török et al. 2002; Zeigler et al. 2003; Jiang et al. 2009).

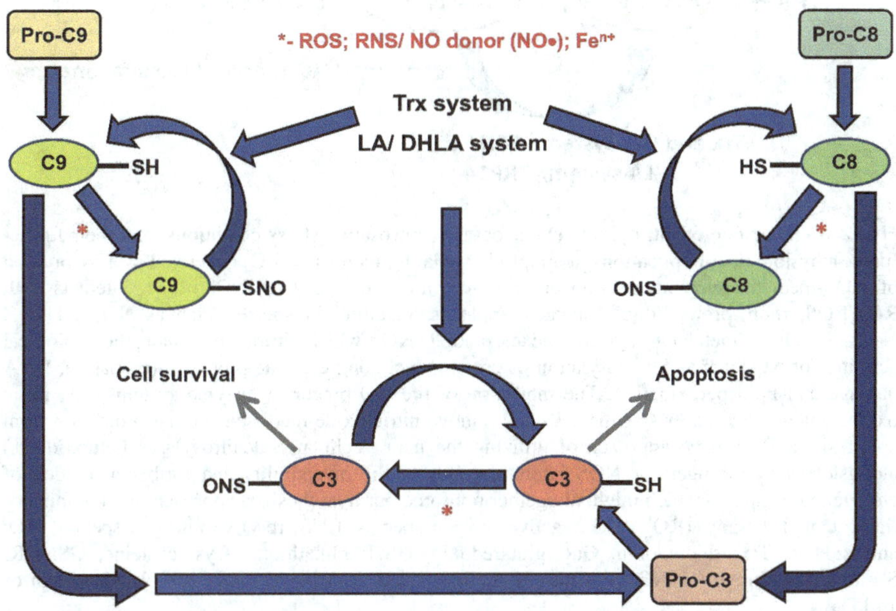

Fig. 1 A figurative representation illustrating the interdependence of caspases and their proteolytic activity on S-(de)-nitrosylation and further cellular survivability or subjection to caspase-induced apoptotic cell death, upon modulating the redox equilibrium. S-nitrosylation of the active site cysteines of both upstream and downstream caspases in the original zymogen or active form aids in cautiously evading apoptosis in cancer cells. The endogenous, ubiquitous cellular dithiols, such as Trx and LA system/DHLA cater to the catabolism of S-nitrosocaspase(s) as a function of their cellular compartmentalization and tissue distribution, thus restoring their catalytic activities and further increasing the cellular susceptibility to apoptosis

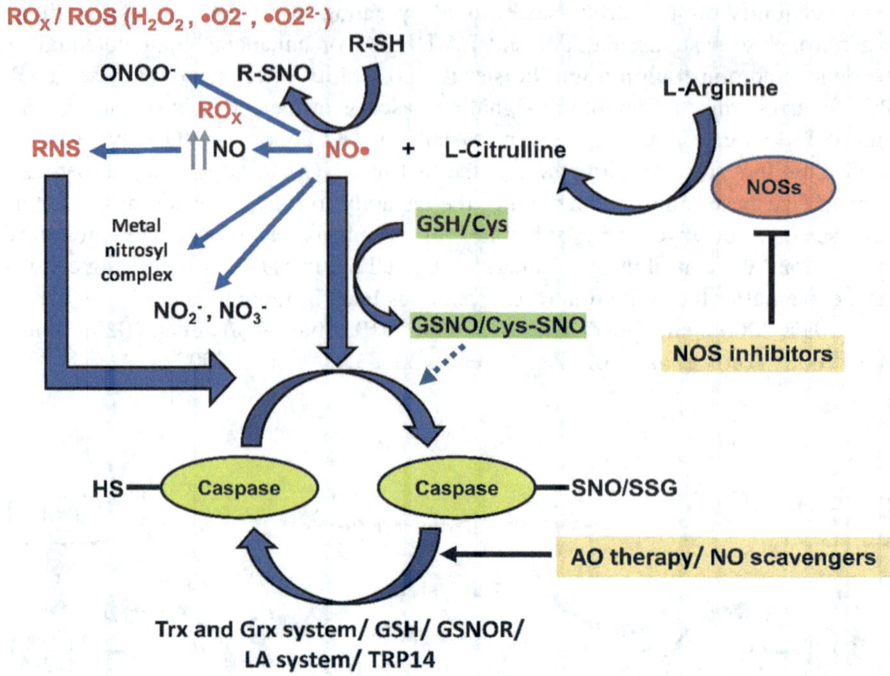

Fig. 2 Cellular fate of nitric oxide under basal or nitrosative stress conditions, and their further (patho)physiological implications in apoptotic signaling pathways. NO, generated as a by-product of NOS-mediated enzymatic turnover of L-Arginine (substrate) to L-Citrulline, interacts with ROx/ROS, (non)-protein thiols, metal complexes, resulting in species such as NO_2^-, NO_3^-, N_2O_3, $ONOO^-$, metal nitrosyl complexes, and RSNOs which further modulate the biological activities of NO such as S-nitrosylation of proteins including cysteine proteases (caspases), DNA damage and lipid peroxidation. The inhibition of the NO precursor enzyme systems, i.e., nitric oxide synthases in cancer-specific cells can remove nitric oxide-mediated cellular protection from apoptosis; a synergistic approach of utilizing the major cellular S-denitrosylases (antioxidants) alongside NO scavengers or NOS inhibitors, aids in the reversibility and further activation of endogenous caspases which might altogether reinforce our hypothesized approach of a combinatorial potential therapy. (RO_x/ROS: reactive oxygen species, RNS: reactive nitrogen species, AO: antioxidants, Trx: thioredoxin, Grx: glutaredoxin, GSH: glutathione, Cys: cysteine, GSNOR: S-nitrosoglutathione (GSNO) reductase, LA: lipoic acid, TRP14: Thioredoxin-related protein of 14 kDa)

Acknowledgments This work is dedicated to the memories of Prof. Arne Holmgren and Prof. Detcho Stoyanovsky. We are grateful to Prof. Holmgren and Prof. Stoyanovsky for their motivation, help, and support.

Conflict of Interest Disclosure The authors of this manuscript declare no conflict of interest. The authors have no financial or proprietary interests in any material discussed in this article.

References

Agrawal L, Louboutin JP, Reyes BA, Van Bockstaele EJ, Strayer DS (2006) Antioxidant enzyme gene delivery to protect from HIV-1 gp120-induced neuronal apoptosis. Gene Ther 13:1645–1656. https://doi.org/10.1038/sj.gt.3302821

Agrawal L, Louboutin JP, Reyes BA, Van Bockstaele EJ, Strayer DS (2012) HIV-1 tat neurotoxicity: a model of acute and chronic exposure, and neuroprotection by gene delivery of antioxidant enzymes. Neurobiol Dis 45:657–670. https://doi.org/10.1016/j.nbd.2011.10.005

Alimoradi H, Greish K, Gamble AB, Giles GI (2019) Controlled delivery of nitric oxide for cancer therapy. Pharm Nanotechnol 7:279–303. https://doi.org/10.2174/2211738507666190429111306

Anathy V, Aesif SW, Guala AS, Havermans M, Reynaert NL, Ho YS, Budd RC, Janssen-Heininger YM (2009) Redox amplification of apoptosis by caspase-dependent cleavage of glutaredoxin 1 and S-glutathionylation of Fas. J Cell Biol 184:241–252. https://doi.org/10.1083/jcb.200807019

Anestål K, Prast-Nielsen S, Cenas N, Arnér ES (2008) Cell death by SecTRAPs: thioredoxin reductase as a prooxidant killer of cells. PLoS One 3:e1846. https://doi.org/10.1371/journal.pone.0001846

Arlt A, Sebens S, Krebs S, Geismann C, Grossmann M, Kruse ML, Schreiber S, Schäfer H (2013) Inhibition of the Nrf2 transcription factor by the alkaloid trigonelline renders pancreatic cancer cells more susceptible to apoptosis through decreased proteasomal gene expression and proteasome activity. Oncogene 32:4825–4835. https://doi.org/10.1038/onc.2012.493

Bai J, Cederbaum AI (2000) Overexpression of catalase in the mitochondrial or cytosolic compartment increases sensitivity of HepG2 cells to tumor necrosis factor-alpha-induced apoptosis. J Biol Chem 275:19241–19249. https://doi.org/10.1074/jbc.M000438200

Bao Y, Ge Y, Wu M, Mao Z, Ye J, Tong W (2023) Record-high ultrasound-sensitive NO nanogenerators for cascade tumor Pyroptosis and immunotherapy. Adv Sci (Weinh) 10:e2302278. https://doi.org/10.1002/advs.202302278

Barrett AJ (1997) Nomenclature Committee of the International Union of biochemistry and molecular biology (NC-IUBMB). Enzyme nomenclature. Recommendations 1992. Supplement 4: corrections and additions. Eur J Biochem 250:1–6. https://doi.org/10.1111/j.1432-1033.1997.001_1.x

Benhar M, Forrester MT, Hess DT, Stamler JS (2008) Regulated protein denitrosylation by cytosolic and mitochondrial thioredoxins. Science 320:1050–1054. https://doi.org/10.1126/science.1158265

Bhattacharyya C, Chakraborty S, Sengupta R (2022) NO news: S-(de)nitrosylation of cathepsins and their relationship with cancer. Anal Biochem 655:114872. https://doi.org/10.1016/j.ab.2022.114872

Boice A, Bouchier-Hayes L (2020) Targeting apoptotic caspases in cancer. Biochim Biophys Acta, Mol Cell Res 1867:118688. https://doi.org/10.1016/j.bbamcr.2020.118688

Chakraborty S, Sircar E, Bhattacharyya C, Choudhuri A, Mishra A, Dutta S, Bhatta S, Sachin K, Sengupta R (2022) S-Denitrosylation: a crosstalk between glutathione and redoxin systems. Antioxidants (Basel) 11:1921. https://doi.org/10.3390/antiox11101921

Chakraborty S, Choudhuri A, Mishra A, Bhattacharyya C, Billiar TR, Stoyanovsky DA, Sengupta R (2023) Nitric oxide and thioredoxin modulate the activity of caspase 9 in HepG2 cells. Biochim Biophys Acta Gen Subj 1867:130452. https://doi.org/10.1016/j.bbagen.2023.130452

Chen X, Mele J, Giese H, Van Remmen H, Dollé ME, Steinhelper M, Richardson A, Vijg J (2003) A strategy for the ubiquitous overexpression of human catalase and CuZn superoxide dismutase genes in transgenic mice. Mech Ageing Dev 124:219–227. https://doi.org/10.1016/s0047-6374(02)00161-6

Cook T, Wang Z, Alber S, Liu K, Watkins SC, Vodovotz Y, Billiar TR, Blumberg D (2004) Nitric oxide and ionizing radiation synergistically promote apoptosis and growth inhibition of cancer by activating p53. Cancer Res 64:8015–8021. https://doi.org/10.1158/0008-5472.CAN-04-2212

Davis R, Jia D, Cinar B, Sikka SC, Moparty K, Zhau HE, Chung LW, Agrawal KC, Abdel-Mageed AB (2003) Functional androgen receptor confers sensitization of androgen-independent prostate cancer cells to anticancer therapy via caspase activation. Biochem Biophys Res Commun 309: 937–945. https://doi.org/10.1016/j.bbrc.2003.08.096

Debatin KM (2004) Apoptosis pathways in cancer and cancer therapy. Cancer Immunol Immunother 53:153–159. https://doi.org/10.1007/s00262-003-0474-8

Di Meo S, Reed TT, Venditti P, Victor VM (2016) Role of ROS and RNS sources in physiological and pathological conditions. Oxidative Med Cell Longev 2016:1245049. https://doi.org/10.1155/2016/1245049

Elmore S (2007) Apoptosis: a review of programmed cell death. Toxicol Pathol 35:495–516. https://doi.org/10.1080/01926230701320337

Enoksson M, Fernandes AP, Prast S, Lillig CH, Holmgren A, Orrenius S (2005) Overexpression of glutaredoxin 2 attenuates apoptosis by preventing cytochrome c release. Biochem Biophys Res Commun 327:774–779. https://doi.org/10.1016/j.bbrc.2004.12.067

Fernandes-Alnemri T, Litwack G, Alnemri ES (1994) CPP32, a novel human apoptotic protein with homology to Caenorhabditis elegans cell death protein Ced-3 and mammalian interleukin-1 beta-converting enzyme. J Biol Chem 269:30761–30764

Finley JW, Kong AN, Hintze KJ, Jeffery EH, Ji LL, Lei XG (2011) Antioxidants in foods: state of the science important to the food industry. J Agric Food Chem 59:6837–6846. https://doi.org/10.1021/jf2013875

Gertz M, Fischer F, Wolters D, Steegborn C (2008) Activation of the lifespan regulator p66Shc through reversible disulfide bond formation. Proc Natl Acad Sci USA 105:5705–5709. https://doi.org/10.1073/pnas.0800691105

Goodman M, Bostick RM, Kucuk O, Jones DP (2011) Clinical trials of antioxidants as cancer prevention agents: past, present, and future. Free Radic Biol Med 51:1068–1084. https://doi.org/10.1016/j.freeradbiomed.2011.05.018

Hasenjäger A, Gillissen B, Müller A, Normand G, Hemmati PG, Schuler M, Dörken B, Daniel PT (2004) Smac induces cytochrome c release and apoptosis independently from Bax/Bcl-x(L) in a strictly caspase-3-dependent manner in human carcinoma cells. Oncogene 23:4523–4535. https://doi.org/10.1038/sj.onc.1207594

Hirota K, Murata M, Sachi Y, Nakamura H, Takeuchi J, Mori K, Yodoi J (1999) Distinct roles of thioredoxin in the cytoplasm and in the nucleus. A two-step mechanism of redox regulation of transcription factor NF-kappaB. J Biol Chem 274:27891–27897. https://doi.org/10.1074/jbc.274.39.27891

Hirst DG, Robson T (2007) Nitrosative stress in cancer therapy. Front Biosci 12:3406–3418. https://doi.org/10.2741/2322

Ho FM, Liu SH, Liau CS, Huang PJ, Lin-Shiau SY (2000) High glucose-induced apoptosis in human endothelial cells is mediated by sequential activations of c-Jun NH(2)-terminal kinase and caspase-3. Circulation 101:2618–2624. https://doi.org/10.1161/01.cir.101.22.2618

Holmgren A (2000) Antioxidant function of thioredoxin and glutaredoxin systems. Antioxid Redox Signal 2:811–820. https://doi.org/10.1089/ars.2000.2.4-811

Jiang ZL, Fletcher NM, Diamond MP, Abu-Soud HM, Saed GM (2009) S-nitrosylation of caspase-3 is the mechanism by which adhesion fibroblasts manifest lower apoptosis. Wound Repair Regen 17:224–229. https://doi.org/10.1111/j.1524-475X.2009.00459.x

Jin Z, Wen Y, Hu Y, Chen W, Zheng X, Guo W, Wang T, Qian Z, Su BL, He Q (2017) MRI-guided and ultrasound-triggered release of NO by advanced nanomedicine. Nanoscale 9:3637–3645. https://doi.org/10.1039/c7nr00231a

Kaliyaperumal K, Sharma AK, McDonald DG, Dhindsa JS, Yount C, Singh AK, Won JS, Singh I (2015) S-Nitrosoglutathione-mediated STAT3 regulation in efficacy of radiotherapy and cisplatin therapy in head and neck squamous cell carcinoma. Redox Biol 6:41–50. https://doi.org/10.1016/j.redox.2015.07.001

Kamezaki F, Tasaki H, Yamashita K, Tsutsui M, Koide S, Nakata S, Tanimoto A, Okazaki M, Sasaguri Y, Adachi T, Otsuji Y (2008) Gene transfer of extracellular superoxide dismutase ameliorates pulmonary hypertension in rats. Am J Respir Crit Care Med 177:219–226. https://doi.org/10.1164/rccm.200702-264OC

Karwowska M, Kononiuk A (2020) Nitrates/nitrites in food-risk for Nitrosative stress and benefits. Antioxidants (Basel) 9:241. https://doi.org/10.3390/antiox9030241

Kim JE, Tannenbaum SR (2004) S-Nitrosation regulates the activation of endogenous procaspase-9 in HT-29 human colon carcinoma cells. J Biol Chem 279:9758–9764. https://doi.org/10.1074/jbc.M312722200

Kim YM, Talanian RV, Billiar TR (1997) Nitric oxide inhibits apoptosis by preventing increases in caspase-3-like activity via two distinct mechanisms. J Biol Chem 272:31138–31148. https://doi.org/10.1074/jbc.272.49.31138

Kim YM, Bombeck CA, Billiar TR (1999) Nitric oxide as a bifunctional regulator of apoptosis. Circ Res 84:253–256. https://doi.org/10.1161/01.res.84.3.253

Kim YM, Kim TH, Chung HT, Talanian RV, Yin XM, Billiar TR (2000) Nitric oxide prevents tumor necrosis factor alpha-induced rat hepatocyte apoptosis by the interruption of mitochondrial apoptotic signaling through S-nitrosylation of caspase-8. Hepatology 32:770–778. https://doi.org/10.1053/jhep.2000.18291

Kim PK, Mahidhara R, Seol DW (2001) The role of caspase-8 in resistance to cancer chemotherapy. Drug Resist Updat 4:293–296. https://doi.org/10.1054/drup.2001.0223

Kim PK, Kwon YG, Chung HT, Kim YM (2002) Regulation of caspases by nitric oxide. Ann N Y Acad Sci 962:42–52. https://doi.org/10.1111/j.1749-6632.2002.tb04054.x

Kim J, Yung BC, Kim WJ, Chen X (2017) Combination of nitric oxide and drug delivery systems: tools for overcoming drug resistance in chemotherapy. J Control Release 263:223–230. https://doi.org/10.1016/j.jconrel.2016.12.026

Kolenko VM, Uzzo RG, Bukowski R, Finke JH (2000) Caspase-dependent and -independent death pathways in cancer therapy. Apoptosis 5:17–20. https://doi.org/10.1023/a:1009677307458

Koning T, Cordova F, Aguilar G, Sarmiento J, Mardones GA, Boric M, Varas-Godoy M, Lladser A, Duran WN, Ehrenfeld P, Sanchez FA (2023) S-Nitrosylation in endothelial cells contributes to tumor cell adhesion and extravasation during breast cancer metastasis. Biol Res 56:51. https://doi.org/10.1186/s40659-023-00461-2

Lancaster JR Jr (2006) Nitroxidative, nitrosative, and nitrative stress: kinetic predictions of reactive nitrogen species chemistry under biological conditions. Chem Res Toxicol 19:1160–1174. https://doi.org/10.1021/tx060061w

Lei XG, Zhu JH, Cheng WH, Bao Y, Ho YS, Reddi AR, Holmgren A, Arnér ES (2016) Paradoxical roles of antioxidant enzymes: basic mechanisms and health implications. Physiol Rev 96:307–364. https://doi.org/10.1152/physrev.00010.2014

Li CQ, Wogan GN (2005) Nitric oxide as a modulator of apoptosis. Cancer Lett 226:1–15. https://doi.org/10.1016/j.canlet.2004.10.021

Li J, Billiar TR, Talanian RV, Kim YM (1997) Nitric oxide reversibly inhibits seven members of the caspase family via S-nitrosylation. Biochem Biophys Res Commun 240:419–424. https://doi.org/10.1006/bbrc.1997.7672

Li H, Wan A, Xu G, Ye D (2013) Small changes huge impact: the role of thioredoxin 1 in the regulation of apoptosis by S-nitrosylation. Acta Biochim Biophys Sin Shanghai 45:153–161. https://doi.org/10.1093/abbs/gms103

Li S, Sun Y, Qi X, Shi Y, Gao H, Wu Q, Liu X, Yu H, Zhang C (2014) Protective effect and mechanism of glutaredoxin 1 on coronary arteries endothelial cells damage induced by high glucose. Biomed Mater Eng 24:3897–3903. https://doi.org/10.3233/BME-141221

Lillig CH, Holmgren A (2007) Thioredoxin and related molecules – from biology to health and disease. Antioxid Redox Signal 9:25–47. https://doi.org/10.1089/ars.2007.9.25

Lillig CH, Lönn ME, Enoksson M, Fernandes AP, Holmgren A (2004) Short interfering RNA-mediated silencing of glutaredoxin 2 increases the sensitivity of HeLa cells toward doxorubicin and phenylarsine oxide. Proc Natl Acad Sci USA 101:13227–13232. https://doi.org/10.1073/pnas.0401896101

Lippman SM, Klein EA, Goodman PJ, Lucia MS, Thompson IM, Ford LG, Parnes HL, Minasian LM, Gaziano JM, Hartline JA, Parsons JK, Bearden JD 3rd, Crawford ED, Goodman GE, Claudio J, Winquist E, Cook ED, Karp DD, Walther P, Lieber MM, Kristal AR, Darke AK, Arnold KB, Ganz PA, Santella RM, Albanes D, Taylor PR, Probstfield JL, Jagpal TJ, Crowley JJ, Meyskens FL Jr, Baker LH, Coltman CA Jr (2009) Effect of selenium and vitamin E on risk of prostate cancer and other cancers: the selenium and vitamin E cancer prevention trial (SELECT). JAMA 301:39–51. https://doi.org/10.1001/jama.2008.864

Liu T, Wu LY, Choi JK, Berkman CE (2010) Targeted photodynamic therapy for prostate cancer: inducing apoptosis via activation of the caspase-8/-3 cascade pathway. Int J Oncol 36:777–784. https://doi.org/10.3892/ijo_00000553

Lönn ME, Hudemann C, Berndt C, Cherkasov V, Capani F, Holmgren A, Lillig CH (2008) Expression pattern of human glutaredoxin 2 isoforms: identification and characterization of two testis/cancer cell-specific isoforms. Antioxid Redox Signal 10:547–557. https://doi.org/10.1089/ars.2007.1821

Lu J, Holmgren A (2012) Thioredoxin system in cell death progression. Antioxid Redox Signal 17: 1738–1747. https://doi.org/10.1089/ars.2012.4650

Lundberg M, Johansson C, Chandra J, Enoksson M, Jacobsson G, Ljung J, Johansson M, Holmgren A (2001) Cloning and expression of a novel human glutaredoxin (Grx2) with mitochondrial and nuclear isoforms. J Biol Chem 276:26269–26275. https://doi.org/10.1074/jbc.M011605200

Mannick JB, Hausladen A, Liu L, Hess DT, Zeng M, Miao QX, Kane LS, Gow AJ, Stamler JS (1999) Fas-induced caspase denitrosylation. Science 284:651–654. https://doi.org/10.1126/science.284.5414.651

Mannick JB, Schonhoff C, Papeta N, Ghafourifar P, Szibor M, Fang K, Gaston B (2001) S-Nitrosylation of mitochondrial caspases. J Cell Biol 154:1111–1116. https://doi.org/10.1083/jcb.200104008

Melino G, Bernassola F, Knight RA, Corasaniti MT, Nistico G, Finazzi-Agro A (1997) S-nitrosylation regulates apoptosis. Nature 388:432–433. https://doi.org/10.1038/41237

Mueller T, Voigt W, Simon H, Fruehauf A, Bulankin A, Grothey A, Schmoll HJ (2003) Failure of activation of caspase-9 induces a higher threshold for apoptosis and cisplatin resistance in testicular cancer. Cancer Res 63:513–521

Muntané J, Bonavida B (2015) Special collection: nitric oxide in cancer. Redox Biol 6:505–506. https://doi.org/10.1016/j.redox.2015.09.038

Nakamura H, Bai J, Nishinaka Y, Ueda S, Sasada T, Ohshio G, Imamura M, Takabayashi A, Yamaoka Y, Yodoi J (2000) Expression of thioredoxin and glutaredoxin, redox-regulating proteins, in pancreatic cancer. Cancer Detect Prev 24:53–60

Nakamura H, Hoshino Y, Okuyama H, Matsuo Y, Yodoi J (2009) Thioredoxin 1 delivery as new therapeutics. Adv Drug Deliv Rev 61:303–309. https://doi.org/10.1016/j.addr.2009.01.003

Olsson M, Zhivotovsky B (2011) Caspases and cancer. Cell Death Differ 18:1441–1449. https://doi.org/10.1038/cdd.2011.30

Pader I, Sengupta R, Cebula M, Xu J, Lundberg JO, Holmgren A, Johansson K, Arnér ES (2014) Thioredoxin-related protein of 14 kDa is an efficient L-cystine reductase and S-denitrosylase. Proc Natl Acad Sci USA 111:6964–6969. https://doi.org/10.1073/pnas.1317320111

Papaleo E, Tiberti M, Arnaudi M, Pecorari C, Faienza F, Cantwell L, Degn K, Pacello F, Battistoni A, Lambrughi M, Filomeni G (2023) TRAP1 S-nitrosylation as a model of population-shift mechanism to study the effects of nitric oxide on redox-sensitive oncoproteins. Cell Death Dis 14:284. https://doi.org/10.1038/s41419-023-05780-6

Pelletier M, Cartron PF, Delaval F, Meflah K, Vallette FM, Oliver L (2004) Caspase 3 activation is controlled by a sequence located in the N-terminus of its large subunit. Biochem Biophys Res Commun 316:93–99. https://doi.org/10.1016/j.bbrc.2004.02.021

Plenchette S (2015) Role of S-Nitrosylation in the extrinsic apoptotic signalling pathway in cancer. Redox Biol 5:415. https://doi.org/10.1016/j.redox.2015.09.017

Rahmanian N, Hosseinimehr SJ, Khalaj A (2016) The paradox role of caspase cascade in ionizing radiation therapy. J Biomed Sci 23:88. https://doi.org/10.1186/s12929-016-0306-8

Reddy TP, Glynn SA, Billiar TR, Wink DA, Chang JC (2023) Targeting nitric oxide: say NO to metastasis. Clin Cancer Res 29:1855–1868. https://doi.org/10.1158/1078-0432.CCR-22-2791

Ren Z, Gu X, Lu B, Chen Y, Chen G, Feng J, Lin J, Zhang Y, Peng H (2016) Anticancer efficacy of a nitric oxide-modified derivative of bifendate against multidrug-resistant cancer cells. J Cell Mol Med 20:1095–1105. https://doi.org/10.1111/jcmm.12796

Ren X, Sengupta R, Lu J, Lundberg JO, Holmgren A (2019) Characterization of mammalian glutaredoxin isoforms as S-denitrosylases. FEBS Lett 593:1799–1806. https://doi.org/10.1002/1873-3468.13454

Renatus M, Stennicke HR, Scott FL, Liddington RC, Salvesen GS (2001) Dimer formation drives the activation of the cell death protease caspase 9. Proc Natl Acad Sci USA 98:14250–14255. https://doi.org/10.1073/pnas.231465798

Ridet JL, Bensadoun JC, Déglon N, Aebischer P, Zurn AD (2006) Lentivirus-mediated expression of glutathione peroxidase: neuroprotection in murine models of Parkinson's disease. Neurobiol Dis 21:29–34. https://doi.org/10.1016/j.nbd.2005.06.003

Saitoh M, Nishitoh H, Fujii M, Takeda K, Tobiume K, Sawada Y, Kawabata M, Miyazono K, Ichijo H (1998) Mammalian thioredoxin is a direct inhibitor of apoptosis signal-regulating kinase (ASK) 1. EMBO J 17:2596–2606. https://doi.org/10.1093/emboj/17.9.2596

Salvatori L, Malatesta S, Illi B, Somma MP, Fionda C, Stabile H, Fontanella RA, Gaetano C (2023) Nitric oxide prevents glioblastoma stem cells' expansion and induces temozolomide sensitization. Int J Mol Sci 24:11286. https://doi.org/10.3390/ijms241411286

Saxena G, Chen J, Shalev A (2010) Intracellular shuttling and mitochondrial function of thioredoxin-interacting protein. J Biol Chem 285:3997–4005. https://doi.org/10.1074/jbc.M109.034421

Sengupta R, Ryter SW, Zuckerbraun BS, Tzeng E, Billiar TR, Stoyanovsky DA (2007) Thioredoxin catalyzes the denitrosation of low-molecular mass and protein S-nitrosothiols. Biochemistry 46:8472–8483. https://doi.org/10.1021/bi700449x

Sengupta R, Billiar TR, Atkins JL, Kagan VE, Stoyanovsky DA (2009) Nitric oxide and dihydrolipoic acid modulate the activity of caspase 3 in HepG2 cells. FEBS Lett 583:3525–3230. https://doi.org/10.1016/j.febslet.2009.10.016

Sengupta R, Billiar TR, Kagan VE, Stoyanovsky DA (2010) Nitric oxide and thioredoxin type 1 modulate the activity of caspase 8 in HepG2 cells. Biochem Biophys Res Commun 391:1127–1130. https://doi.org/10.1016/j.bbrc.2009.12.036

Sharma V, Fernando V, Letson J, Walia Y, Zheng X, Fackelman D, Furuta S (2021) S-Nitrosylation in tumor microenvironment. Int J Mol Sci 22:4600. https://doi.org/10.3390/ijms22094600

Shen X, Burguillos MA, Osman AM, Frijhoff J, Carrillo-Jiménez A, Kanatani S, Augsten M, Saidi D, Rodhe J, Kavanagh E, Rongvaux A, Rraklli V, Nyman U, Holmberg J, Östman A, Flavell RA, Barragan A, Venero JL, Blomgren K, Joseph B (2016) Glioma-induced inhibition of caspase-3 in microglia promotes a tumor-supportive phenotype. Nat Immunol 17:1282–1290. https://doi.org/10.1038/ni.3545

Song JJ, Lee YJ (2003) Differential role of glutaredoxin and thioredoxin in metabolic oxidative stress-induced activation of apoptosis signal-regulating kinase 1. Biochem J 373:845–853. https://doi.org/10.1042/BJ20030275

Stanford A, Chen Y, Zhang XR, Hoffman R, Zamora R, Ford HR (2001) Nitric oxide mediates dendritic cell apoptosis by downregulating inhibitors of apoptosis proteins and upregulating effector caspase activity. Surgery 130:326–332. https://doi.org/10.1067/msy.2001.116411

Stoyanovsky DA, Tyurina YY, Tyurin VA, Anand D, Mandavia DN, Gius D, Ivanova J, Pitt B, Billiar TR, Kagan VE (2005) Thioredoxin and lipoic acid catalyze the denitrosation of low molecular weight and protein S-nitrosothiols. J Am Chem Soc 127:15815–15823. https://doi.org/10.1021/ja0529135

Tan C, Li Y, Huang X, Wei M, Huang Y, Tang Z, Huang H, Zhou W, Wang Y, Hu J (2019) Extensive protein S-nitrosylation associated with human pancreatic ductal adenocarcinoma pathogenesis. Cell Death Dis 10:914. https://doi.org/10.1038/s41419-019-2144-6

Tewari M, Quan LT, O'Rourke K, Desnoyers S, Zeng Z, Beidler DR, Poirier GG, Salvesen GS, Dixit VM (1995) Yama/CPP32 beta, a mammalian homolog of CED-3, is a CrmA-inhibitable protease that cleaves the death substrate poly(ADP-ribose) polymerase. Cell 81:801–809. https://doi.org/10.1016/0092-8674(95)90541-3

Török NJ, Higuchi H, Bronk S, Gores GJ (2002) Nitric oxide inhibits apoptosis downstream of cytochrome C release by nitrosylating caspase 9. Cancer Res 62:1648–1653

Vong LB, Nagasaki Y (2020) Nitric oxide Nano-delivery systems for cancer therapeutics: advances and challenges. Antioxidants (Basel) 9:791. https://doi.org/10.3390/antiox9090791

Wang Z (2012) Protein S-nitrosylation and cancer. Cancer Lett 320:123–129. https://doi.org/10.1016/j.canlet.2012.03.009

Watt W, Koeplinger KA, Mildner AM, Heinrikson RL, Tomasselli AG, Watenpaugh KD (1999) The atomic-resolution structure of human caspase-8, a key activator of apoptosis. Structure 7:1135–1143. https://doi.org/10.1016/s0969-2126(99)80180-4

Wen J, Li X, Zheng S, Xiao Y (2020) Upregulation of Glutaredoxin 2 alleviates oxygen-glucose deprivation/reoxygenation-induced apoptosis and ROS production in neurons by enhancing Nrf2 signaling via modulation of GSK-3β. Brain Res 1745:146946. https://doi.org/10.1016/j.brainres.2020.146946

Wong RS (2011) Apoptosis in cancer: from pathogenesis to treatment. J Exp Clin Cancer Res 30:87. https://doi.org/10.1186/1756-9966-30-87

Woo M, Hakem R, Soengas MS, Duncan GS, Shahinian A, Kägi D, Hakem A, McCurrach M, Khoo W, Kaufman SA, Senaldi G, Howard T, Lowe SW, Mak TW (1998) Essential contribution of caspase 3/CPP32 to apoptosis and its associated nuclear changes. Genes Dev 12:806–819. https://doi.org/10.1101/gad.12.6.806

Wu H, Xing K, Lou MF (2010) Glutaredoxin 2 prevents H(2)O(2)-induced cell apoptosis by protecting complex I activity in the mitochondria. Biochim Biophys Acta 1797:1705–1715. https://doi.org/10.1016/j.bbabio.2010.06.003

Wu H, Lin L, Giblin F, Ho YS, Lou MF (2011) Glutaredoxin 2 knockout increases sensitivity to oxidative stress in mouse lens epithelial cells. Free Radic Biol Med 51:2108–2117. https://doi.org/10.1016/j.freeradbiomed.2011.09.011

Wu Y, Xie H, Li Y, Bao X, Lu GL, Wen J, Gao Y, Li Y, Zhang Z (2023) Nitric oxide-loaded bioinspired lipoprotein normalizes tumor vessels to improve intratumor delivery and chemotherapy of albumin-bound paclitaxel nanoparticles. Nano Lett 23:939–947. https://doi.org/10.1021/acs.nanolett.2c04312

Xu WM, Liu LZ (1998) Nitric oxide: from a mysterious labile factor to the molecule of the Nobel Prize. Recent progress in nitric oxide research. Cell Res 8:251–258. https://doi.org/10.1038/cr.1998.25

Yoshihara E, Chen Z, Matsuo Y, Masutani H, Yodoi J (2010) Thiol redox transitions by thioredoxin and thioredoxin-binding protein-2 in cell signaling. Methods Enzymol 474:67–82. https://doi.org/10.1016/S0076-6879(10)74005-2

Zamaraev AV, Kopeina GS, Prokhorova EA, Zhivotovsky B, Lavrik IN (2017) Post-translational modification of caspases: the other side of apoptosis regulation. Trends Cell Biol 27:322–339. https://doi.org/10.1016/j.tcb.2017.01.003

Zech B, Wilm M, van Eldik R, Brüne B (1999) Mass spectrometric analysis of nitric oxide-modified caspase-3. J Biol Chem 274:20931–20936. https://doi.org/10.1074/jbc.274.30.20931

Zeigler MM, Doseff AI, Galloway MF, Opalek JM, Nowicki PT, Zweier JL, Sen CK, Marsh CB (2003) Presentation of nitric oxide regulates monocyte survival through effects on caspase-9 and caspase-3 activation. J Biol Chem 278:12894–12902. https://doi.org/10.1074/jbc.M213125200

Zhang H, Du Y, Zhang X, Lu J, Holmgren A (2014) Glutaredoxin 2 reduces both thioredoxin 2 and thioredoxin 1 and protects cells from apoptosis induced by auranofin and 4-hydroxynonenal. Antioxid Redox Signal 21(5):669–681. https://doi.org/10.1089/ars.2013.5499

Zhang D, Zhao N, Ma B, Wang Y, Zhang G, Yan X, Hu S, Xu T (2016) Procaspase-9 induces its cleavage by transnitrosylating XIAP via the Thioredoxin system during cerebral ischemia-reperfusion in rats. Sci Rep 6:24203. https://doi.org/10.1038/srep24203

Microbial-Based Therapies in Cancer Treatment Under the One Health Initiative

Charalampos Filippou, Yiannis Panayiotou, Sophia C. Themistocleous, Christina A. Kousparou, Timo Fischer, Giorgos Marangos, Andreas Matheou, Christoforos Rozario, Stephanos Christodoulides, Zoi-Dorothea Pana, Stylianos Kakoullis, Christos D. Argyropoulos, Elizabeth O. Johnson, Constantinos Tsioutis, and Andreas Yiallouris

Abstract

Microbial-based therapies have emerged as a promising frontier in cancer treatment. Traditional therapies often lack specificity and cause harmful side effects, necessitating more targeted approaches. Microorganisms naturally exhibit tumor-targeting properties and complex interactions with the tumor microenvironment. They can exert direct antitumor effects or serve as delivery vehicles for therapeutic payloads.

This comprehensive chapter explores the potential applications of microbes in cancer management under the One Health initiative framework.

Bacteria demonstrate direct anticancer activities through secretion of cytotoxic elements and antiproliferative effects. Certain species preferentially colonize hypoxic tumor niches. Genetic engineering enables tumor-specific targeting and delivery of cytotoxic genes, prodrug-activating enzymes, and immunomodulators. Oncolytic viruses selectively replicate within and lyse cancer cells, releasing tumor antigens to stimulate antitumor immunity. Viruses are engineered for enhanced targeting, replication, and immune stimulation. Fungi and protozoa also show promise, with β-glucan modulating the tumor microenvironment. Probiotics and prebiotics impact cancer prevention, progression, and treatment response through modulation of inflammation and immunity. Microbial therapies face challenges including balancing virulence reduction without compromising antitumor effects.

C. Filippou · S. C. Themistocleous · C. A. Kousparou · S. Christodoulides · Z.-D. Pana · E. O. Johnson · A. Yiallouris (✉)
School of Medicine, European University Cyprus, Nicosia, Cyprus

Medical Innovation Centre (MEDIC), School of Medicine, European University, Nicosia, Cyprus
e-mail: a.yiallouris@euc.ac.cy

Y. Panayiotou · T. Fischer · G. Marangos · A. Matheou · C. Rozario · S. Kakoullis · C. D. Argyropoulos · C. Tsioutis
School of Medicine, European University Cyprus, Nicosia, Cyprus

Interdisciplinary Cancer Research, https://doi.org/10.1007/16833_2024_262
Published online: 29 June 2024

Achieving full tumor eradication requires attention to tumor heterogeneity and resistance mechanisms. Optimization of delivery methods is crucial to disseminate therapies systemically. Combination therapies integrating microbes with chemotherapy, radiation, or immunotherapy show enhanced efficacy and reduced toxicity.

The One Health initiative recognizes the interconnectivity between human, animal, and environmental health factors impacting cancer risk. It emphasizes multidisciplinary collaboration to address challenges like antimicrobial resistance through prudent antimicrobial use. Continued advancements in genetic engineering, delivery methods, and characterization of combinatorial regimens hold the potential to further optimize microbial cancer treatments. Rigorous clinical evaluation is imperative. Microbial therapies represent a significant stride in cancer management by focusing on targeted delivery coupled with activation of innate and adaptive antitumor immunity. With ongoing developments, these innovative approaches offer hope for more effective and less toxic personalized therapies.

Keywords

Genetic engineering of microbes · Immunomodulation · Microbial-based cancer therapy · Microbiome in cancer · One Health initiative

1 Introduction

With tens of millions of deaths being recorded worldwide every year due to cancer, the disease is one of the leading causes of death worldwide. Hence, cancer presents a significant global health challenge, with current treatment options often being limited by lack of specificity, harmful side effects, and diminishing effectiveness over time due to drug resistance. The necessity for targeted, personalized, and multifaceted approaches to cancer management, which are more effective, is increasingly evident (Lee et al. 2018). In this landscape, the innovative use of microorganisms in cancer therapy has emerged as a promising new frontier, offering hope for more effective and targeted treatments (Ma and Yu 2006).

Microorganisms, including bacteria, viruses, and protozoans, exhibit complex interactions with the tumor microenvironment (TME), influencing cancer development and progression in various ways. Their diverse roles range from direct antitumor agents to immune activators and vectors in antitumor therapy. Bacteria, for instance, can induce apoptosis, modify cell proliferation, and exert anti-angiogenic effects while simultaneously activating antitumor immunity (Jiang et al. 2022). Certain bacterial species possess innate antitumor properties derived from secreted elements such as toxins, enzymes, biosurfactants, or secondary metabolites, which exert a cytotoxic impact on cancer cells. Moreover, the concept of tumor-targeted microbial replication and "bactofection" involves the utilization of a bacterium's natural or enhanced tumor affinity to transport anticancer payloads (Sedighi et al. 2019). Probiotic bacterial and gut microbiota modulation are also known for their role in enhancing cancer prevention and treatment, chiefly by modulating inflammation and immune responses within the tumor microenvironment. These bacteria can also be genetically engineered to serve as tumor-targeting vectors, delivering therapeutic agents like cytotoxic genes, prodrug-activating enzymes, and immunoregulatory molecules directly to tumor sites (Allemailem 2021). However, the success of bacterial-based cancer drugs in clinical trials is ambiguous, primarily due to the challenges of overcoming host immunity and achieving tumor specificity (Omer et al. 2022).

Combining microbiota-based therapies with conventional treatments has shown potential in enhancing efficacy while reducing the toxicity associated with traditional therapies. Despite existing challenges, the promise of engineered microbes as sophisticated drug delivery systems for advanced microbial anticancer therapies remains resilient (Ma et al. 2019). Obligate or facultative anaerobic bacteria, including *Bifidobacterium*, *Clostridium*, *Salmonella*, and *Escherichia coli*, can leverage metabolic advantages in low-oxygen environments and serve as immunotherapeutic agents, inducing inflammatory responses, releasing heat shock proteins, and activating dendritic cells to foster antitumor T cell and antibody responses (Zhao et al. 2023). Their derivatives demonstrate direct anticancer activities, manifesting cytotoxic, antiproliferative, or pro-apoptotic effects on cancer cells. Engineered bacteria expressing cytotoxic polypeptides such as FasL, TNFs, or tumor necrosis factor–related apoptosis-inducing ligand (TRAIL) are designed to induce apoptosis in cancer cells upon tumor colonization. Tumor-targeting bacteria can also express prodrug-activating enzymes, converting nontoxic prodrugs into effective chemotherapy drugs locally within tumors. Additionally, biofilm-forming bacteria are currently explored for controlled drug delivery, imaging, and restricting tumor metastasis through tumor capsule formation (Divyashree et al. 2022; Ikryannikova et al. 2023).

The challenges in this field include balancing the reduction of bacterial virulence without diminishing antitumor effects, ensuring tumor localization over normal tissues, and addressing the neutralization of host immunity. Combination therapies are being investigated to overcome limitations like incomplete tumor eradication by bacteria alone, aiming to enhance multimodal treatment regimens (Rommasi 2022). Embracing a more holistic approach toward cancer treatment, leveraging the unique properties of microorganisms, represents a significant stride in the ongoing battle against cancer. Similarly, viruses modified for selective anticancer properties, known as oncolytic viruses, represent a clinically approved approach demonstrating minimal side effects (Jhawar et al. 2017). Additionally, microbial therapy advantages include tumor-targeting coupled with activating both innate and adaptive antitumor immunity. While such approaches hold promise, challenges remain in balancing microbial virulence with antitumor potency. Additional key obstacles include achieving full tumor eradication, overcoming host immunity, addressing tissue specificity issues, and mitigating the risk of resistance development. Innovations like bacterial-mediated delivery of immunomodulators and combining microbial therapies with radiation or chemotherapy seek to help surmount these limitations (Jhawar et al. 2017).

Going forward, continued advancements in genetic engineering, delivery methods, and combinatorial strategies hold potential to further optimize microbial cancer treatments (Ma et al. 2019). This comprehensive review delves into their potential applications in cancer therapy under the One Health initiative.

2 The Mechanisms of Microbial Therapy

2.1 Direct Oncolysis and Tumor Microenvironment

A diverse and dynamic approach is adopted in the field of cancer, focusing on the intricate and personalized nature of therapeutic options. Treatment is currently customized based on multiple critical factors, as is the stage, the environment and microenvironment of the cancer, alongside the patient's age, any comorbidities and history of past treatments. Cancers in their early stage respond more effectively to treatment compared to those in advanced or metastatic stages. Additionally, the molecular or immunohistochemical subtypes of cancer, such as those seen in breast cancer (BC) (like luminal, HER2-enriched, basal-like, or triple-negative), significantly guide the design of the treatment plan (Agostinetto et al. 2022).

Conventional methods broadly applied include surgery, radiotherapy, and chemotherapy; however, these are subject to limitations such as nonspecific cytotoxicity that results in damage of normal cells and instigate undesirable host side effects. This cytotoxicity limits the "safe" dosage that can be safely administered, reducing their overall effectiveness. Unfortunately, these treatments are rendered ineffective due to the development of drug or radio-resistance in cancer cells. In this context, gene therapy emerges as an innovative alternative, involving the direct delivery of functional genes into tumor tissues using either biological or non-biological vectors (Rodrigues and Sanatani 2012). Available vectors include viral or bacterial vectors, where both are instrumental in protecting and shielding the genes as they transport the genes to the tumor and facilitate their entry into cells ensuring their expression within the tumor. The introduced genes may inhibit processes essential for cancer survival, such as cell proliferation, angiogenesis, and metastasis. Use of vectors may hinder formation of blood vessels through the expression of genes like endostatin that inhibits angiogenesis. While, the immunotherapy approach focuses on modifying the cancer immune response, utilizing cytokines like IL-18, expressed by bacteria like *Salmonella*, to reactivate immune cells and suppress tumor-secreted immunosuppressive cytokines.

These genes may also involve suicide genes or tumor suppressor genes, targeting the tumor directly or immunotherapy genes modulating the immune response within the tumor microenvironment. These processes present a targeted and potentially more effective approach to cancer treatment. Delving into the specifics, nonviral vectors, like cationic lipids and polymers, can be utilized as vectors but are less efficient compared to viral vectors. Viral vectors are highly effective due to their natural ability to elicit immune responses. Oncolytic viruses (OVs), such as T-VEC approved for melanoma treatment, can directly destroy tumors and stimulate immunity by releasing tumor antigens. Adenoviruses are noted for their high transduction efficiency and selectively target tumors, while retroviruses offer stable gene integration but come with safety concerns. Other viruses like vaccinia and measles are also under study (Bashor et al. 2022; Howarth et al. 2010). Furthermore, the potential of viral vector–dendritic cell (DC) vaccines is highlighted. These vaccines utilize DC transduced with viral vectors to enhance antigen presentation and activate T cells at tumor sites. Adenoviral vectors, in particular, are shown to be effective for immunotherapy applications (Lee et al. 2023).

Innovative therapeutic approaches also encompass a range of strategies, including cell-based and tumor protein/peptide vaccines, aimed at triggering a robust immune response against cancer cells. The use of heat shock proteins, DNA vaccines, and recombinant viral or bacterial vectors is explored to enhance vaccine immunogenicity, thereby improving the effectiveness of the immune response against cancer cells (Kaczmarek et al. 2023). The oncolytic approach, employing replication-competent bacteria or viruses like certain strains of *Salmonella*, *Clostridium*, herpes, and vaccinia viruses, is a cornerstone of this discussion. These agents are uniquely adapted to the tumor microenvironment, characterized by low oxygen levels, and are capable of infecting and replicating within tumor tissues, leading to the direct destruction of cancer cells. Additional examples include diphtheria and pseudomonas toxins, and TRAIL, which specifically target cancer cells (https://www.ncbi.nlm.nih.gov/pmc/articles/PMC4968310/). Whereas *Listeria monocytogenes* stands out for its efficiency in gene delivery to the cytosol (Paterson et al. 2010). This comprehensive overview underscores the synergy of biotechnology and immunotherapy in cancer treatment, reflecting the individualized nature of therapy based on a variety of factors and pointing toward more targeted and potentially effective treatment modalities (Li et al. 2018).

2.2 Immunotherapy and Microbial Interactions

Immunotherapy is emerging as a significant treatment option for various blood and solid cancers. Bacterial metabolites can disturb the activities of local immune cells, by altering immunoglobulin secretion, encouraging lymphocyte differentiation into regulatory T cells and T helper 17 cells, producing immunomodulatory cytokines, and impacting the epigenetic regulation of histone deacetylase enzymes. Regarding the link between human microbiota and BC, several metabolites have been identified as potential risk factors or protective agents. These include compounds like estrogens, active phytoestrogens, short-chain fatty acids, lithocholic acid, and cadaverine. The gut microbiota's role in estrogen production, primarily through β-glucuronidase enzyme activity in certain intestinal bacteria, can lead to increased systemic estrogen reabsorption, thus potentially heightening hormone-dependent BC risk in women. On the other hand, metabolites like phytoestrogens, lithocholic acid, and cadaverine are noted for their protective effects against BC development. Chronic inflammation induced by gut bacteria, linked to cancer formation, involves pathogen-associated molecular patterns that stimulate Toll-like receptors (TLR) and activate NF-κB, a key inflammation and cancer regulator. Activation of NF-κB triggers the release of cytokines like IL-6, IL-12, IL-17, IL-18, and tumor necrosis factor-alpha, fostering persistent inflammation in the tumor microenvironment. Intestinal bacteria's secondary metabolites and pro-inflammatory molecules, transferred to the liver via the portal vein, may also contribute to cancer development. For example, butyrate, a microbial metabolite, can enhance antitumor CD8 T cell response by influencing the ID2-dependent IL-12 signaling pathway. The microorganisms that constitute the gut microbiome play a pivotal role in emitting bioactive low molecular weight substances, such as folates, short-chain fatty acids, and biotin, that alter methylation substrates or affect the activity of epigenetic enzymes (Alpuim Costa et al. 2021; Laborda-Illanes et al. 2020).

Immune checkpoint inhibitors, a class of therapies activating the immune system against tumors by blocking inhibitory T lymphocyte interactions with malignant cell ligands, show promise in BC treatment, especially in the triple-negative subtype. Although BC is not typically as immunogenic as other cancers like lung cancer or melanoma, recent studies indicate immunotherapy benefits, particularly in triple-negative cases. Clinical trials have yielded varied response rates to different immunotherapies, used alone or in combination with chemotherapy. The KEYNOTE-012 trial, assessing pembrolizumab monotherapy in previously treated triple-negative BC, reported an overall response rate (ORR) of 18.5% and a median response time of 17.9 weeks. The KEYNOTE-086 trial, using pembrolizumab as a first-line metastatic triple-negative BC, achieved an ORR of 23%. Other trials like NCT01375842 and JAVELIN, evaluating atezolizumab and avelumab, observed ORRs of 10% and 5.2%, respectively.

Combining immunotherapy with chemotherapy has also been explored, with atezolizumab and nab-paclitaxel achieving a 67% ORR in first-line treatment. The IMpassion 130 trial, evaluating the outcomes of this combination in untreated metastatic triple-negative BC, showed progression-free survival benefits. The ENHANCE-1/KEYNOTE-150 trial, evaluating eribulin with pembrolizumab, indicated higher ORR in PD-L1-positive BC patients. The KEYNOTE-355 trial combined pembrolizumab with chemotherapy, demonstrating significant progression-free survival benefits in high PD-L1 patients. These findings collectively suggest the potential of immune checkpoint inhibitors in improving outcomes for triple-negative BC, especially those with high PD-L1 expression (Adams et al. 2019; Nanda et al. 2016).

3 Microbial Agents in Cancer Therapy

3.1 Bacterial-Based Cancer Therapies

Bacterial-based cancer therapy, alternatively termed bacterial oncolysis, is a cutting-edge approach leveraging the capacity of bacteria to survive the hypoxic settings of a tumor, offering a significant advantage over traditional cancer treatments. The overall concept of bacterial oncolysis is that bacterial infections can stimulate an inflammatory response in patients that potentially leads to tumor regression (Sedighi et al. 2019). This was first observed in 1867 by German physician Wilhelm Busch, who noted a rapid tumor regression in a cancer patient infected with *Streptococcus pyogenes* (Oelschlaeger 2010). Similar observations were made in New York by surgeon William B. Coley in sarcoma patients. Tumor regression was observed in these patients following bacterial infections, and it was hypothesized that the immune response activated for shielding the body against bacterial toxins also targeted the tumor cells.

The process involves introducing a bacterium systemically that will then be able to breach the tumor microenvironment through either active or passive targeting mechanisms. Inflammation frequently occurs in tumors that increase the repression of TNF-α in tumor vessels subsequently enhancing permeability of blood vessels allowing bacteria to penetrate the tumor; this is known as passive targeting (Duong et al. 2019). Active targeting, on the other hand, involves the interaction of ligands and antigen-presenting cells expressed on the surface of bacteria to interact with the tumor-infecting dendritic cells, macrophages, and other antigen-presenting cells like myeloid-derived suppressor cells (MDSCs) (Gabrilovich and Nagaraj 2009). Further to this, apoptotic tumor cells emanate specific chemical signals drawing in bacteria via chemotactic movement aiding their penetration into the tumor and augment their efficacy. Mathematical models, such as the cylindroid model for *Salmonella* Typhimurium (*S.* Typhimurium), are instrumental in understanding the balance between chemotaxis and bacterial proliferation within tumors. Bacterial-mediated cancer therapy is especially favorable due to the ability of bacteria to penetrate the hypoxic tumor tissue, delivering direct antitumor outcomes, activate immunomodulatory effects or source genomic engineering plasticity. For example, a bacterial vector has been designed from an attenuated *S.* Typhimurium strain to secrete *Vibrio vulnificus* flagellin B, inspiring immunotherapy that can act in synergy with radiotherapy (Liu et al. 2023). The same vector passing proapoptotic cytokine Fas ligand achieves antitumor activity in both breast and colon carcinoma in mice models (Loeffler et al. 2008). Additionally, *E. coli* can engulf solid tumors and facilitate the clearance of tumor cells through infectious defense mechanisms similarly to *Bifidobacterium* and *Clostridium* that proliferate deep into solid tumors, not accessible to drugs, where they activate antitumor immunity. Cancer immunotherapy often involves triggering a specific immune response, enabling immune cells, particularly CD8+ and CD4+ T lymphocytes, to attack cancer cells. Bacterial infections in cancer patients lead to the release of heat shock proteins, like Hsp70, from necrotic cells. These proteins mature dendritic cells and generate effective antigen-specific immune responses (Lou et al. 2021).

Antimicrobial proteins produced by bacteria, as are bacteriocins, establish pores in cell membranes, by interfering with the arrangement of phospholipids, influencing the influx/efflux of ions that destabilizes the cell membrane subsequently expressing antitumor and anti-metastatic effects. This disruption to the ion homeostasis also obstructs the cell cycle of tumor cells (Rommasi 2022). Lipopolysaccharides (LPS) are expressed on the outer membrane of gram-negative bacteria, and in high concentrations, they can be toxic to the human body resulting in multiple pathologies such as sepsis or even death. Therefore, LPS-based vaccines, that also exhibit anticancer properties through multiple pathways, require a slight modification prior to use where the bacteria is attenuated (Sawant et al. 2020). Also produced by multiple gram-negative bacteria is the cytolethal distending toxin (CDT). CDTs arrest the cell cycle and cell-cycle inhibiting factors (Cifs) can block mitosis and lymphocyte expansion. Specific toxins like *Corynebacterium diphtheriae*–produced diphtheria toxin (DT) and *Clostridium perfringens* enterotoxin (CPE) target tumor-specific receptors and antigens, inhibiting tumor growth. DT has been modified for selective binding to cancer cells and shows cytotoxic effects against various cancer cell lines. CPE toxins rapidly induce cytolysis by binding to receptors upregulated in tumor cells, showing potential in breast cancer therapy. Other toxins, like exotoxin T from *Pseudomonas aeruginosa*, have shown cytotoxicity against a wide range of cancer cell lines. Immunotoxins, which link toxins to antibodies or cytokines, target cancer cells specifically and are a promising area in cancer therapy research. The ongoing challenge is to find suitable protein molecules for immunotoxins that have minimal immunogenicity and high potency in killing cancer cells (Divyashree et al. 2022; Sawant et al. 2020).

The process of bactofection is a genetic engineering technique where DNA, RNA, or proteins are introduced into host cells with the purpose of delivering favorable therapeutic proteins directly into the tumor cells or in the tumor microenvironment. Genetically modifying bacteria to express tumor-specific ligands or engineered to target tumor-associated antigens to treat cancer patients is also known as bacterial-mediated cancer therapy (BMCT). Proceeding with bacterial-based therapies requires a focus on bacterial attenuation, improvement of tumor targeting, and the development of vector strategies for delivering anticancer cargo on bioengineered bacteria (Baban et al. 2010). For example, a *Salmonella* strain SHJ2037, engineered to express an arginine-glycine-aspartate (RGD) peptide on the bacterial surface, expresses high tumor specificity and enhanced tumor activity in MDA-MB-231 breast cancer cells and MDA-MB-435 melanoma xenografts due to its affinity for $\alpha v\beta 3$ integrin (Park et al. 2016). Alternatively, *Pseudomonas aeruginosa* has been programmed to carry antitumor drugs to the tumor microenvironment and will be released once exposed to near-infrared light as the bacterium transitions from biofilm to lysis state (Fu et al. 2023). An exciting approach to therapeutics is the induction of apoptotic ligands such as TNF-α, FasL, and TRAILs. Several studies have shown the anticancer potential of engineered bacteria that express these death inducers; however, factors such as toxicity and short circulation half-life after systemic administration limit this approach. Following intravenous administration of an attenuated *S.* Typhimurium proved effective and expressed antitumor effects against murine breast, CT-26 colon, and a form of lung metastases, with minimal toxic effects (Loeffler et al. 2008). Similar results were observed in *S.* Typhimurium delivering FasL in B16 melanoma tumors (Loeffler et al., 2008).

3.2 Oncolytic Viruses in Cancer Treatment

Oncolytic viruses (OVs) are engineered to specifically target and destroy cancer cells as they hijack cellular processes, offering a dual approach to cancer treatment: direct cell lysis and immune system activation. These viruses are uniquely capable of replicating within cancer cells while sparing normal cells, leading to the shutoff of host mRNA and protein synthesis. Genetic modifications enable viral replication to occur exclusively in cancer cells by deleting viral genes essential for replication in normal cells but redundant in cancer cells due to cellular mutations (Rahman and McFadden 2021). Additionally, tumor-specific viral promoters are employed to induce replication exclusively within cancer cells overexpressing certain signaling proteins. Another strategy leverages the reliance on tumor-specific deregulated intracellular pathways, such as elevated Ras signaling commonly found in cancer cells, to initiate viral replication. Oncolytic paramyxoviruses and myxoma viruses selectively replicate in cells exhibiting activated Ras signaling. Upon infecting cancer cells, OVs replicate efficiently via these mechanisms, leading to the selective destruction of cancer cells from within. Some viruses also encode genes that induce cancer cell death directly, such as apoptotic ligands. The resultant cell lysis releases thousands of new viral progeny over several days, causing the bystander killing of neighboring tumor cells (Rahman and McFadden 2021).

As cancer cells undergo lysis, they release tumor-associated antigens along with new viral progeny. These antigens are taken up by antigen-presenting cells like dendritic cells, which then stimulate the immune system activating CD8+ T cell responses against viral and tumor epitopes presented on MHC-I, CD4+ T cell help for both humoral and cytotoxic responses, and the production of neutralizing and tumor-specific antibodies. This immune activation leads to the development of long-term memory T cell responses, which are instrumental in eliminating distant metastatic tumors and enhancing the therapeutic effect of OVs beyond the local tumor site (Del Prete et al. 2023). Antibodies contribute to complement-dependent cytotoxicity and antibody-dependent cellular cytotoxicity of cancer cells. Cytokines like IFNγ, produced during immune stimulation, inhibit tumor growth and metastasis. Memory CD8+ T cells specific to tumor antigens provide long-term immunity against recurrence and metastasis (Lin et al. 2023).

Selective replication mechanisms in OVs include the incorporation of tumor-specific microRNA binding sites, allowing replication only in tumor cells overexpressing specific miRNAs. The combination of OVs with checkpoint inhibitors further enhances T cell infiltration and the antitumor immunity unleashed by the viruses. Enhanced effectiveness is achieved by engineering viruses to express immune-stimulatory molecules like granulocyte-macrophage-colony-stimulating factor (GM-CSF) or tumor-associated antigens, thereby broadening antitumor T cell responses. Many OVs can be injected directly into accessible tumors while systemic delivery may involve conjugating viruses to ligands that target tumor vasculature or cancer cells (Lin et al. 2023). Nanocarriers and fusogenic lipids can encapsulate viruses to improve biodistribution.

Adenoviruses and herpes simplex viruses are engineered for selective replication in specific tumor types. Bystander cytotoxic mechanisms are also employed for improved tumor killing. Monitoring and detection of OVs involve molecular imaging techniques for tracking viral spread and replication in tumors over time, complemented by routine tumor biopsies to assess changes in tumor gene expression and immune cell infiltration. Future directions include improving systemic delivery methods, tumor targeting, overcoming challenges like neutralizing antibodies and immunosuppression, and combining OVs with other immunotherapies like checkpoint inhibitors, oncolytic bacteria, and adoptive T cell therapies. Additional preclinical studies are necessary to investigate mechanisms of action and optimize dosing for clinical use. In summary, OVs combine direct oncolytic effects with stimulation of robust tumor-specific adaptive and innate immunity for effective cancer treatment (Fang et al. 2023).

3.3 Cancer Treatment Involving Fungi and Protozoa

β-glucan, a prevalent polysaccharide found in the cell walls of bacteria and fungi, plays a crucial role in cancer therapy due to its interaction with the tumor microenvironment (TME). In fungi, β-glucan consists of D-glucopyranose polymers linked by a β(1,3) backbone and a β(1,6) side chain, all in a β anomeric configuration. This complex structure enables β-glucan to bind to pathogen recognition receptors (PRRs), activating adaptive immunity. Additionally, β-glucan interacts with the C3 receptor (CR3) on antigen-presenting cells and natural killer cells, pivotal in innate immunity activation. When soluble β-glucan and iC3b bind to the CR3 receptor, it triggers the receptor, leading to the destruction of iC3b-coated tumor cells through CR3-dependent cellular cytotoxicity (DCC). Another critical aspect of β-glucan's anticancer properties is its influence on macrophage polarization, a significant factor in tumorigenesis. β-glucan exposure has been linked to increased glycolysis levels and reduced oxidative phosphorylation in macrophages. M1 macrophages, known for their pro-inflammatory and anti-tumorigenic traits, are characterized by glycolytic metabolism. In contrast, M2 macrophages, or tumor-associated macrophages (TAMs), are identified by their oxidative phosphorylation. Therefore, β-glucan exposure can shift the balance toward more M1 macrophages and fewer M2 macrophages in the TME, promoting cancer cell death (Shanmugam and Abirami 2019; Ullah et al. 2019).

Despite these promising effects, the clinical effectiveness of β-glucan in cancer therapy is still limited, with only a small percentage of patients experiencing a full response. This limitation is partly due to the immunosuppressive nature of the TME, which can lead to resistance to various anticancer medications. However, β-glucan is safe and non-immunogenic, making it an attractive adjunct to traditional cancer therapies. In preclinical models, combining fungal β-glucan with chemotherapeutic drugs has shown significant antitumor effects compared to chemotherapy alone. This combination has led to increased hematopoiesis in advanced-stage cancer patients. Microbial polysaccharides (MPs) like β-glucan play vital roles in immune response modulation and signal transduction. Glycans and MPs derived from Basidiomycetes, such as krestin, schizophyllan, and lentinan, exhibit anticancer properties through immunostimulation, downregulation of NF-κB responses, and induction of tumor cell apoptosis. Polysaccharide peptides from the mushroom YunZhi (*Coriolus versicolor/Trametes versicolor*) have been used in Asia for decades alongside chemotherapy to treat breast cancer (BC) patients. These peptides, known for their antiproliferative properties, significantly reduce BC cell proliferation by upregulating the *p21* gene expression. Meta-analyses have concluded that *Coriolus versicolor* can increase survival rates in cancer patients, including those with BC (Chow et al. 2003; L.Y. Eliza et al. 2012).

Other beneficial MPs include Levan, which induces apoptotic cell death in MCF-7 BC cells, and the proteoglucan D-fraction from *Grifola frondosa*, known to reduce mammary tumor cell migration and lung metastases. A clinical trial on D-fraction in breast and lung cancer patients (stages II–IV) demonstrated its ability to hinder cancer progression and metastasis while increasing NK cell activity. This evidence highlights the potential of MPs in enhancing antitumor immunity in BC patients without significant toxicities. However, further clinical trials are necessary to evaluate D-fraction's efficacy in combination with chemotherapy in a broader patient population. The integration of MPs like β-glucan in cancer treatment regimens could potentially revolutionize cancer therapy, offering more effective and less toxic alternatives to current treatments.

Toxoplasma lysate antigen (TLA) has been a focus for many researchers. A uracil auxotrophic carbamoyl phosphate synthase (CPS) mutant of *Toxoplasma gondii* has been employed in the treatment of various cancers including pancreatic, melanoma, ovarian, and lung cancers. Utilizing these strains led to a notable rise in IL-12 levels, a cytokine that mediates inflammation and activates immune cells. Mouse model studies have shown that using the *T. gondii* auxotrophic CPS strain can provide sustained cancer protection. Additionally, a protein from *Plasmodium falciparum*, VAR2CSA, linked with diphtheria toxin, has been experimented against tumor cell lines and mouse models in vivo. These experiments, both in vitro and in vivo, revealed a significant presence of chondroitin sulfate in melanoma cells (Sanders et al. 2015).

3.4 Probiotics and Prebiotics in Cancer

The term "probiotics" is used to describe a mixture of live microorganisms which includes yeasts and mostly gram-positive bacteria that are given to improve the flora of the gut microbiome. The gut microbiota, composed of trillions of bacteria and other microorganisms, plays a very important role in maintaining the normal physiology of a healthy individual as they influence the metabolism of complex carbohydrates such as cellulose or increase the half-life of certain drugs such as contraceptives. It is crucial to note that although they support many essential functions of the organism, they have been shown to be involved or implicated in certain types of cancers. Studies have shown that specific probiotic strains of

Lactobacillus fermentum and *Enterococcus faecium* RM11 were associated with anti-tumorigenic activity in the colon (Ghanavati et al. 2020).

In addition, current scientific investigations have demonstrated the potent growth-inhibitory, pro-apoptotic, and antiproliferative characteristics of live *Lactobacillus casei* (*L. casei*) ATCC393 and its components. As demonstrated by in vitro studies on CT26 and HT29 colon cancer cells, *L. casei* primarily functions by suppressing the expression of survivin and increasing the expression of tumor necrosis TRAIL (Tiptiri-Kourpeti et al. 2016). Increased expression of survival is associated with poorer clinical outcomes and more aggressive illness, while it also inhibits apoptosis proteins in various cancers (Jaiswal et al. 2015). While TRAIL has been correlated with apoptosis induction in different types of cancers through activation of death receptors (DR4 and DR5) (van der Sloot et al. 2006).

Despite many studies demonstrating the effectiveness of live probiotics, some studies show that dead probiotics may even confer an even greater benefit to the host. In a study conducted by Lee H. A et al., utilizing dead *Lactobacillus plantarum* (*L. plantarum*) with nano-sized inhibits azoxymethane/dextran sulfate sodium-induced (AOM/DSS) CAC in mice better than live bacterium. Dead *L. Plantarum* mainly functions by increasing IgA secretion, reducing inflammation and apoptosis (Lee et al. 2015).

4 One Health Approach in Cancer Ecology

The One Health approach represents a transformative paradigm in modern healthcare, advocating for a transdisciplinary and multisectoral collaboration that interlinks the health of humans, animals, and the environment. This holistic framework, rooted in the acknowledgement of shared ecosystems and interconnected health dynamics, has become increasingly relevant in addressing complex health challenges like infectious diseases, zoonoses, and notably, cancer. Central to the One Health concept is the understanding of the intricate relationship between microbiota and cancer. Research has illuminated the profound influence of microbiomes on cancer development, progression, and even treatment response. The human microbiome, in particular, not only serves as a potential biomarker for various cancers but also offers a novel avenue for therapeutic intervention. Manipulating the microbiome, for instance, through dietary changes or microbial transplants, opens doors to more personalized, effective, and holistic cancer treatments. These interventions are promising not only in their efficacy but also in their potential to reduce side effects and improve the mental well-being of patients who often seek treatments that extend beyond conventional pharmaceutical approaches (Kleber et al. 2022; Dujon et al. 2021; "One Health" n.d.).

The One Health approach also emphasizes the importance of recognizing and mitigating the risk factors shared between humans and animals. This includes exposure to environmental carcinogens, lifestyle choices, and notably, antimicrobial resistance (AMR), which has emerged as a critical concern in both human and veterinary medicine. The misuse of antibiotics, especially in agricultural settings for growth promotion in livestock, has contributed significantly to the rise of AMR. This practice, although increasingly regulated, continues in some regions, posing a serious threat not only to animal health but also to human health and cancer therapy. In the context of cancer, AMR complicates the emerging field of microbial cancer therapy, which involves using genetically modified bacteria to combat cancer cells. For example, the use of non-typhoidal Salmonella (NTS) in microbial cancer therapy is challenged by the existence of antibiotic-resistant strains, which can be transferred from animals to humans through the consumption of contaminated food and will run through food chains. Such resistant strains could jeopardize the efficacy of microbial cancer treatments, compounding the challenges faced by patients undergoing these therapies. Furthermore, the One Health approach recognizes the potential transmissibility of cancers between animals, and perhaps, between animals and humans. This understanding is crucial in monitoring and potentially preventing outbreaks and pandemics of transmissible cancers, which are emerging threats to biodiversity and human health. Moreover, the study of cancer in animals, particularly how their immune systems combat neoplasms, provides valuable insights for human cancer research, offering new therapeutic targets and treatment strategies. Environmental factors, ranging from pollutants to dietary habits, play a significant role in shaping the microbiota of both humans and animals. These factors, in turn, have far-reaching implications for health and disease, including cancer. For instance, agricultural practices like the use of fertilizers can alter the microbiota of crops, which, when consumed, impacts the human gut microbiota. This interaction underscores the bidirectional relationship between the environment and health, necessitating a comprehensive understanding and management of these factors under the One Health umbrella. The One Health approach also advocates for rigorous surveillance and detection strategies that span across human medicine, veterinary medicine, and environmental science. By monitoring and analyzing patterns in cancer and microbiota behavior, early detection of environmental carcinogens and emerging health threats can be achieved. This surveillance is further enhanced by leveraging technologies like artificial intelligence and machine learning, which can integrate and analyze vast datasets from diverse sources, leading to more precise and timely interventions (Dujon et al. 2020; Epstein et al. 2016; Kerr et al. 2015).

Addressing AMR within the One Health framework involves not only curbing the inappropriate use of antimicrobials in human and animal medicine but also improving the living conditions of animals to reduce the need for such interventions. This strategy aligns with the broader goals of One Health, which include promoting health, preventing disease, and maintaining ecosystem balance. Ethical considerations are integral to the One Health approach, ensuring that interventions in human and animal health, as well as environmental management, adhere to ethical standards. This includes humane treatment of animals, equitable access to healthcare, and responsible use of medical and environmental resources. One Health initiative, with its emphasis on the interconnectivity of human, animal, and environmental health, offers a comprehensive framework for understanding and addressing health challenges, particularly in the realm of cancer. By focusing on the role of microbiota in cancer and the implications of factors like antimicrobial resistance, the One Health approach not only advances our understanding of cancer but also opens new avenues for effective and holistic treatments. It calls for collaborative efforts across disciplines, integrating insights from human and veterinary medicine, environmental science, and beyond, to foster a healthier, more sustainable world (Pesavento et al. 2018; Sepp et al. 2019; White et al. 2023).

5 Challenges and Limitations

The everlasting challenges posed by conventional anticancer therapies, such as systemic toxicity, poor tumor infiltration, and resistance development, reinforced the efforts in developing improved therapeutic strategies. However, the use of microbial agents, as promising as it stands, brings its own challenges and limitations.

5.1 Safety Concerns and Side Effects

As the agents used aim to modulate immune responses in the tumor microenvironment, an important task is balancing the microbial-induced immune stimulation, attenuation, and immune evasion, with some immunity-driven side effects seeming inevitable. In the case of oncolytic viruses, these vary depending on the virus used, but usually include mild flu-like symptoms and local reactions at the injection site (Chhabra and Kennedy 2022). However, more severe adverse effects such as neurotoxicity and systemic inflammatory responses have been reported in major vector candidates (Dold et al. 2016; Nakashima et al. 2018). Microbial-induced toxicity is the central factor to consider when developing these tools, particularly since the target group often endures compromised immune defenses and increased susceptibility to opportunistic infections. Balancing toxicity with the dose required for an acceptable efficacy is perhaps the most challenging aspect of microbial-based therapies.

When dealing with replicating entities, both intra-host and inter-host spreading are considered. The concern of an oncolytic virus disseminating from a patient and regaining its pathogenic potential has been lessened by the lack of any report of person-to-person transmission (Chhabra and Kennedy 2022). Nevertheless, a loosely controlled microbial replication inside the host could lead to unintended spread and infection of nontarget tissues (Din et al. 2016). Importantly, even otherwise harmless microbial derivatives could lead to a systemic infection, as they would bypass inherent immune defenses when administered directly in the blood (Vähä-Koskela et al. 2007). Efforts to limit these risks include the engineering of attenuated or compartmentalized microbial agents which are unable to replicate on their own. However, a significant number of deaths was demonstrated in animal models even following the deletion of virulence factor genes, highlighting the need for careful examination of each specific therapeutic candidate (Dang et al. 2001).

Another safety concern is the risk of microbial genomic integration into the host genome, which, in the case of oncolytic viruses can be viewed as a double-edged sword. Whereas this process is utilized in methods using retroviral vectors, it is also circumvented using viruses replicating in the cytoplasm such as vaccinia (Broyles 2003; Logg et al. 2012). Whatever the case, incidents of viral genomic integration leading to alterations in immune cell populations infiltrating tumors, as well as the activation of oncogenes, highlighted the need for tight control of microbial genetic material use (Hacein-Bey-Abina et al. 2003; Nienhuis et al. 2006).

5.2 Genetic Modifications and Their Ethical Implications

Genetic engineering of microbes has been a central component of this therapeutic strategy, with *E. coli* and *S.* Typhimurium being among the most frequently investigated bacteria due to their easily modifiable genome.

Most importantly, modifications have been implicated to attenuate microbes so as to limit the risk of virulence and toxicity to the host. Examples include genetic alterations that impact the synthesis or structure of bacterial toxins such as LPS, which can in turn significantly reduce the induction of proinflammatory mediators in the host (Low et al. 1999, 2004). However, achieving sufficient attenuation while retaining the beneficial properties of the bacteria is a challenging task, considering that some virulence factors are responsible for their antitumoral activity (Duong et al. 2019). This was reflected by phase I trials using attenuated strains indicating poor tumor specificity and insufficient efficacy when bacteria were used on their own (Toso et al. 2002).

Besides attenuation, genetic manipulation has been used to enhance the mechanisms underlying tumor suppression by these microbes, by improving migration, tumor specificity, or the immune cell populations that infiltrate the tumor microenvironment. *E. coli* strains were engineered to specifically target tumors and release antagonist molecules for CD47, which is commonly expressed in multiple cancer types (Chowdhury et al. 2019). Furthermore, genetically engineered *Salmonella* strains were shown to increase tumor infiltration of proinflammatory M1-like macrophages, CD4, and CD8 T cells, while suppressing the activities of M2-like anti-inflammatory macrophages (Xu et al. 2022). Engineered bacteria were shown to increase the expression of a range of immunostimulatory molecules such as IL-2, IFN-γ, TNF-α, and CXCL16, leading to enhanced tumor infiltration of T cells (Duong et al. 2019; Savage et al. 2023). Beneficial effects of bacterial genetic manipulation were demonstrated in phase I clinical trials, where there was a significant IL-2-induced increase in circulating NK and NKT cell numbers in cancer patients (Gniadek et al. 2020).

In the case of oncolytic viruses, genetic modification has been heavily employed to improve each of the different stages of tumor growth regulation: targeting, intratumoral replication, cell lysis, and orchestration of the immune response. The profound ability of viruses to specifically target surface receptors has been utilized to manipulate their capsid proteins, respectively, such as in the cases of *adenovirus* and *lentivirus* delivery systems (Morizono et al. 2005). On the other hand, several modifications exploiting promoters driving the uncontrolled proliferation in tumor cells have been engineered, for the enhanced proliferation and activity of *adenoviruses* in tumor sites (Post et al. 2007; Ramesh et al. 2006). Besides the heavily studied *adenovirus* vector, other viruses modified genetically for enhanced replication and killing ability include *herpes simplex virus*, *vesicular stomatitis virus,* and *reovirus* (Cristi et al. 2022).

It is becoming apparent that genetic modifications are an essential component of microbial-based anticancer therapy. However, they also raise ethical considerations that need careful examination. First, any manipulation of microbial genetic material raises the question of creating pathogenic strains which are released outside the laboratory setting. Any potential long-term effects on human health and the environment need to be assessed and longitudinally monitored closely. It is essential that any human trials conducted with genetically modified microbes necessitate informed consent, with participants fully understanding the modifications taking place, as well as their benefits and potential risks involved. Finally, as these engineered tools move through the clinical development and market approval ladder, it is vital to establish the transparent patenting and ownership of these genetically modified microbes, as well as open access to these therapies for the public (Cook-Deegan and Heaney 2010).

5.3 Resistant Tumor Populations

Due to their nature, microbial-based methods are viewed as promising solutions for tackling the issue of drug resistance faced in conventional anticancer therapy. For example, the hypoxic environment in tumors often underlies resistance to traditional treatment, but at the same time, engineered bacteria such as *Bifidobacterium, Bacillus, Clostridium, Salmonella, Mycobacterium,* and *Listeria* can easily grow and operate under these conditions (Bernardes et al. 2010). Whatever the case, the proneness of tumor cells to mutation could underlie the development of resistance to any given therapy, leading to a significant loss of therapeutic efficacy (Bernardes et al. 2010). To date, tumor resistance has not been a substantial issue in systems using bacterial components; however, this is not the case with oncolytic viruses.

Viral entry into tumor cells triggers a differential gene expression by default, leading to changes in the regulation of tumor cell morphology, surface proteins, cell growth, development, proliferation, and signaling (Song et al. 2012). Therefore, these transcriptional changes can lead to resistance of tumor cells at several stages in the lifecycle of oncolytic viruses: binding and infiltration, transcription, translation, or spreading. Resistance mechanisms identified against viral treatments predominantly include tumor-cell-dependent interferon signaling but also other mechanisms such as epigenetic modifications, barriers to viral entry and spread, and hypoxia-mediated inhibition (Bhatt et al. 2021). For instance, the downregulation of enzymes regulating the density of the extracellular matrix was shown to prevent tumor infiltration and attachment of *adenovirus* vectors (Watanabe et al. 2010). Beyond interferon signaling, molecular signaling pathways regulating cell survival in tumor populations can protect cells from viral infection and viral-induced lysis, thus limiting the effect of oncolytic viruses. For example, the activation of the tumor protein p53 was shown to restrict infectivity and replication of *vesicular stomatitis virus* and *adenovirus* vectors in pancreatic tumor models (Sunamura et al. 2004).

Resistance has been documented in several different cancer types and against a wide range of different viruses, with *vesicular stomatitis virus, herpes simplex virus*, and *adenovirus* vectors being the most studied in resistance mechanisms (Bhatt et al. 2021). An important factor to consider is tumor heterogeneity, as the differences between tumor types could determine the effectiveness of any specific treatment. It is apparent that although systems using engineered microbes with enhanced adjuvant effect can significantly limit the growth of some tumors, other tumors can be completely resistant to this therapy or might be simply growing at a slower rate (Felgner et al. 2016). Therefore, beyond safety and efficacy, tumor specificity is a vital component to investigate while developing microbial systems, with combinatorial drug therapy perhaps required for achieving the optimum effect in each specific tumor environment.

5.4 Delivery and Specificity Challenges

Optimizing the delivery of microbial systems to the tumor microenvironment is one of the greatest tasks faced, with the multiple delivery methods investigated primarily categorized into local and systemic. As tumors have a much more complicated vasculature and larger intercapillary distances compared to healthy tissues, direct intratumoral delivery of therapeutic agents is sometimes necessary for the targeting of distal cells (Jain 1998). This method is the commonest used for the delivery of oncolytic viruses, as it avoids the dilution of the therapeutic agent into circulation and any unwanted sequestration in non-targeted, healthy tissues (Goradel et al. 2022). However, local delivery has insufficient efficacy on distant metastases and can be problematic in deep, inaccessible, or mechanically injured tumors (Harrington et al. 2019). Therefore, in some cases, systemic delivery is the only viable option but can be hindered by neutralizing antibodies, complement activation, and poor virus escape from the vascular system. Notably, intraperitoneal delivery has been used as an alternative route to intravenous delivery of oncolytic viruses, demonstrating lower toxicity (Kulu et al. 2009).

Overall, bacterial vectors can be introduced intratumorally and are more motile augmenting distribution and tumor specificity compared to viral vectors. An obvious obstacle in delivering microbial components to the required tissue is the host immune response as it is programmed to defend against foreign pathogenic entities. Therefore, intratumoral introduction of the microbial agent permits it to circumvent the hosts' immune defenses. However, this can also be achieved by camouflaging the delivering agent, as in the case of oncolytic viruses transported in carrier cells or by modified *Listeria* systems (Roy and Bell 2013). *Listeria* naturally infect antigen-presenting cells, but also myeloid-derived suppressor cells (MDSCs), which can directly deliver them to the tumor microenvironment, protecting them from the host immune response (Chandra et al. 2013). Even so, an immune response trigger following initial delivery is inevitable, as evident from studies showing a TNF-α-induced blood influx to the tumor site following *Salmonella* accumulation (Leschner et al. 2009). Alarmingly, this indicates the dependence on an immune response for targeted delivery, but at the same time an underlying cause of unwanted bacterial toxicity (Leschner et al. 2009).

Besides the delivery of microbials themselves, bacteria such as *Clostridia, Bifidobacteria*, and *Salmonella* have been thoroughly investigated as vectors for the targeted delivery of other therapeutic molecules into the tumor microenvironment. These biological vectors are more stable and programmable compared to chemically synthesized particles and can be used for the delivery of cytokines, cytotoxins, prodrug-converting enzymes, nucleic acid peptides immune-modulators, and suicide genes (Cao and Liu 2020; Patyar et al. 2010; Sawant et al. 2020). However, it is important to note that in many cases, the delivery of these molecules across bacterial membranes needs further optimization due to inefficient delivery to the site of interest (Felgner et al. 2016). It is most likely that bacteria release these molecules passively upon lysis, and further investigation is required to determine whether their therapeutic effect is sufficient following delivery in the periphery or whether specific tumor targeting is required (Goradel et al. 2022). In any way, the control of microbial gene expression is critical for ensuring the specificity of delivery to tumor cells. In the case of certain bacteria, this can be achieved by inserting the expression of therapeutic molecules under promoters induced by factors such as hypoxia, low pH, or radiation (Sawant et al. 2020). However, the effectiveness of such promoters in vivo requires further investigation. The optimization of hypoxia-dependent tumor specificity is particularly important for facultative anaerobic bacteria such as *Salmonella, Listeria,* and *Escherichia*, as these can also proliferate in oxygenated, healthy tissues causing unwanted damage (Shen et al. 2022).

6 Diet, Gut Microbiota, and Cancer Risk

Cancer, a multifaceted disease affecting 20.2% of the global population, represents a significant public health challenge due to its complex etiopathogenesis. This condition arises from a multitude of factors, including genetic and epigenetic changes, environmental influences, and crucially, lifestyle factors such as diet. The intricate link between diet and cancer risk has been a subject of extensive research over the decades (Mattiuzzi and Lippi 2019; Pope et al. 2017; Tanaka et al. 2021).

The recent advancements in metagenomic analysis have opened new avenues in understanding the role of gut microbiota in cancer development. The human gut is a hub of microbial activity, with bacterial concentrations reaching 10^{11}–10^{12} cells per gram of luminal content. This microbial population is vast, outnumbering human cells by nearly tenfold. Among the over 3,000 bacterial taxa identified in human feces, an average individual harbors around 200 taxa within the gut. Significantly, about 30% of these constitute the "core" microbiota, present in almost every individual (Li et al. 2014; Qin et al. 2010; Salonen et al. 2012; Zhao and Yu 2016).

Dietary habits play a pivotal role in determining the composition and functionality of the gut microbiota. Foods that are not digested and absorbed in the small intestine reach the colon, where they serve as substrates for the gut microbiota. Even short-term dietary changes can induce notable shifts in the microbial composition. These changes can be direct, affecting the microbiota itself, or indirect, through modifications in colonic transit time or luminal pH. The extent of these alterations is proportional to the magnitude of dietary change. Researchers have therefore tried to define the microbial component in a more simplistic way. A study conducted by Arumugam et al. analyzed the gut microbial communities of individuals from four countries and suggested the existence of just three predominant clusters (enterotypes), dominated by *Prevotella*, *Bacteroides*, and *Ruminococcus*. However, due to the wide inter-individual variability in people's diet and colonic physiology, the three "enterotypes" story has been proved as overly optimistic (Arumugam et al. 2011; Camilleri 2018).

The gut microbiota carries out several key functions that promote health. These functions include breaking down ingested food into absorbable nutrients, stimulating the immune system, preventing the growth of pathogenic bacteria, and producing a range of biologically significant compounds like short-chain fatty acids (SCFAs) and neuromodulatory substances. There is a dynamic and reciprocal interaction between the gut microbiota and the host, yet the specific mechanisms of communication are not fully understood (Boeckxstaens et al. 2016; Zhao and Yu 2016).

Emerging research suggests that gut microbiota composition alterations, or "dysbiosis," might play a role in cancer pathogenesis (Pope et al. 2017). This is hypothesized to involve immune response mechanisms triggered by the recognition of gut microbiota by the host's innate immune system. Preliminary data indicate a connection between abnormal gut microbiota composition and cancer development. However, the exact functional role of these microbial alterations in cancer remains elusive. Research in this field has been constrained by studies with limited sample sizes and durations. The identification of specific microbial signatures correlated with cancer could provide valuable insights for both diagnosis and therapy. Yet, no precise microbial signature indicative of certain bacterial taxa in the gut microbiome of cancer patients has been conclusively established (Fang and Ragin 2020; Kipanyula et al. 2013; Pevsner-Fischer et al. 2016; Sinha et al. 2018).

Notably, cancer patients have been observed to exhibit lower concentrations of the "beneficial" enterotype *Prevotella* and higher concentrations of the "pathogenic" enterotype *Bacteroides*. This observation was supported by a study by Ou et al., which compared the gut microbiota of African Americans on a high-fat Western diet (a high-colon cancer risk group) with rural native Africans on a high-fiber diet (a low-colon cancer risk group). The study revealed stark differences in gut microbiota composition and metabolites between the two groups. African Americans predominantly had *Bacteroides*, while rural native Africans had a predominance of *Prevotella*. Additionally, rural native Africans exhibited higher levels of SCFAs, particularly butyrate, known for its protective anti-tumorigenic effects in animal models. In contrast, the African American samples showed higher levels of microbial genes encoding for secondary bile acid synthesis, which has been linked to pro-inflammatory and pro-tumorigenic effects.

Determining whether the observed alterations in gut microbiota composition are a cause or a consequence of cancer poses a significant challenge in this research area. Current findings indicate an association between diet, gut microbiota, and cancer risk. Diets high in fiber are linked with a dominance of *Prevotella* and a lower cancer risk. In contrast, high-fat Western diets correlate with a dominance of *Bacteroides* and an increased cancer risk. However, these findings need further validation through robust, large-scale, and longer-duration interventional studies to establish causality (Cao et al. 2014; Horvath et al. 2022; Ou et al. 2013; Zeng et al. 2019).

Therefore, the interplay between diet, gut microbiota, and cancer risk is a complex and multifaceted topic that requires further exploration. Understanding the underlying mechanisms is essential for translating this knowledge into effective personalized healthcare treatments. The potential for diet to influence cancer risk through the modulation of gut microbiota offers a promising area for future research and possible intervention strategies. However, the challenge remains in distinguishing between cause and effect in the intricate relationship among diet, gut microbiota, and cancer.

7 Recent Advancements

7.1 Advances in Genetic Engineering to Improve Specificity

The utilization of bacteria in cancer treatment presents unique challenges and opportunities. The primary concern is the potential pathogenicity and toxicity of bacteria to human cells and organs. This risk is balanced by the advantageous genetic modifiability of bacteria, enabling their engineering into versatile platforms for cancer therapy through synthetic biology techniques. This process typically involves introducing various plasmids into bacterial cells to enable the expression of therapeutic proteins, anticancer agents, or tumor-specific antigens, thus enhancing antitumor activity while reducing systemic toxicity. Such advancements have been documented in various studies (Jiang et al. 2010; Lee 2012; Zhou et al. 2018). To counteract the inherent pathogenicity of bacteria like *E. coli*, *Salmonella*, *Listeria*, and *Clostridium*, strategies often involve deleting genes responsible for virulence factors. For instance, Low et al. (1999) showed that the disruption of the *msbB* gene in *Salmonella* and *E. coli*, which affects the myristoylation of lipid A, reduces the expression of tumor necrosis factor α. This genetic modification also leads to a decrease in the lipopolysaccharide content of *Salmonella*, thereby enhancing its safety profile, as demonstrated in phase I clinical trials (Toso et al. 2002). In another example, Quintero et al. (2016) engineered the *Salmonella* strain VNP20009 to express *Pseudomonas* exotoxin A, targeting epidermal growth factor receptors, and showing significant antitumor activity against receptor-positive tumor cells. However, a critical consideration in using bacteria for cancer therapy is the need for precise control over the expression of therapeutic genes. Upon entry into the body, bacteria may temporarily localize in normal organs, posing risks of healthy tissue toxicity due to the continuous expression of cytotoxic drugs. This necessitates controlling the expression of therapeutic genes at specific times and locations, enhancing drug concentration in solid tumors while reducing systemic toxicity (Din et al. 2016). Advances in this area include designing expression systems sensitive to endogenous or exogenous stimuli, such as using hypoxia in the tumor microenvironment (TME) to design inducible promoters for expressing anticancer peptides, gene fragments, and proteins in bacteria, ensuring specific delivery to tumors. Zhao et al. (2005) developed an auxotrophic *Salmonella* strain that preferentially colonizes tumor tissue, owing to the abundant leucine and arginine in the tumor environment.

In addition to bacterial therapy, oncolytic virotherapy represents another frontier in cancer treatment. Despite chemotherapy and radiotherapy being standard treatments, they are often accompanied by significant side effects. Oncolytic virotherapy, in contrast, has shown minimal side effects in clinical trials. However, this approach is not without its challenges. The complexity and heterogeneity of cancers mean that a single class of oncolytic viruses may not be universally effective (Yun et al. 2022). Cancers can confer resistance to specific types of viruses, posing a significant challenge in identifying suitable viral applicants. The only oncolytic virus approved for therapy by the European Commission is a genetically engineered herpes simplex virus, Talimogene Laherparepvec (T-VEC). T-VEC is constructed by removing the ICP34.5 and replacing it with two copies of the human granulocyte-macrophage-colony-stimulating factor (*GM-CSF*) gene. This modification is crucial as ICP34.5 dephosphorylates eIF2, preventing interruption of protein synthesis caused by PKR, which is implicated in tumorigenesis. The deletion of ICP47 increases viral replication by halting the immune system's destructive action and increasing the expression of MHC1 on the surface of cancer cells. Consequently, this genetically modified virus can replicate in cancer cells and cause abortive infection (auto-destruction before the virus can replicate) in normal cells. Moreover, the activation of T cells by dendritic cells is enhanced by the GM-CSF, leading to the activation of the immune system (Bommareddy et al. 2017; Ferrucci et al. 2021). The fields of bacterial therapy and oncolytic virotherapy are evolving, offering new approaches to cancer treatment. These strategies leverage the genetic modifiability of bacteria and the specific targeting abilities of viruses to enhance the effectiveness of cancer treatments while aiming to minimize side effects. Despite the challenges, including the need for precise control and the complexity of cancer resistance mechanisms, these approaches represent promising avenues for improving cancer therapies. Continued research and development in these areas are essential to fully harness their potential for more effective and targeted cancer treatments.

7.2 Combination Therapies Using Microbes and Traditional Treatments

The integration of bacteriotherapy with conventional cancer treatments, such as chemotherapy and radiotherapy, represents a promising frontier in oncology. This approach aims to enhance the efficacy of traditional treatments while minimizing their adverse effects. In chemotherapy, the use of bacteriotherapy can target hypoxic tumors, which are often resistant to conventional treatments, thereby increasing the efficiency of chemotherapy. Genetically modified bacteria offer selective tumor targeting and can be used as vehicles for drug or gene delivery. They can directly destroy tumors or be utilized in bacterial-based cancer vaccines, such as the use of genetically engineered *Salmonella* bacteria that replicate within tumors and express effector genes. Moreover, bacterial endotoxins combined with chemotherapy can also combat cancer effectively. The role of bacteriotherapy in mitigating chemotherapy-induced toxicity, particularly gastrointestinal side effects, is also significant. Probiotic formulas like VSL-3 have shown effectiveness in reducing complications in animal models, while specific strains like *Streptococcus thermophilus* and *Lactobacillus rhamnosus* GG have been beneficial in alleviating chemotherapy-related complications in humans. Additionally, certain probiotics have demonstrated the potential in controlling chemotherapy complications in advanced breast cancer patients and reducing tumor resistance to radiotherapy in head and neck cancer patients (Sedighi et al. 2019).

In radiotherapy, the use of bacteriotherapy exploits the presence of hypoxic zones within solid tumors, typically resistant to radiation. Facultative or obligate anaerobic bacteria can selectively replicate in these zones, potentially allowing lower doses of radiation to be used, thereby sparing healthy tissues. Engineered strains, like the ΔppGpp strain of *Salmonella*, can carry genes for cytotoxic proteins and facilitate optical imaging, thus enhancing radiotherapy. Combining radiotherapy with bacterial therapy using engineered strains has been shown to reduce tumor growth more effectively than bacterial therapy alone. Furthermore, bacterial flagellin and its derivatives have been found to protect against radiation syndromes affecting the gastrointestinal and hematopoietic systems. Studies have shown that combining X-rays with *Salmonella* can produce supra-additive antitumor effects. Researchers are also exploring the synergy between radiotherapy and bacteriotherapy using different bacterial strains, observing significant therapeutic effects and, in some cases, long-term remission. However, high doses of radiation combined with bacteriotherapy might pose toxicity risks for certain organs (Bettegowda et al. 2003; Sedighi et al. 2019).

Clostridium acetobutylicum has indicated that radiation-inducible genes can be activated at specific doses, suggesting that fractionated radiotherapy could trigger enhanced protein expression, potentially increasing TNFa production in recombinant clostridia following irradiation. The combination of bacteriotherapy with conventional cancer treatments is still in its nascent stages and faces challenges, including potential toxicity and the need for extensive research to fully understand and optimize these approaches (Sedighi et al. 2019; Zhou et al. 2018). The preliminary results are promising, offering hope for more effective and targeted cancer therapies that could improve patient outcomes and reduce side effects. Moreover, bacteriotherapy has shown potential in conjunction with OVs, both exhibiting tumor-selective replication after systemic administration. Viral-mediated oncolysis is emerging as a more effective and less toxic approach compared to other treatment methods. By combining different microorganisms, like vesicular stomatitis virus and non-pathogenic *E. coli*, researchers have demonstrated improved therapeutic outcomes in animal models. This approach underscores the evolving landscape of cancer treatment, where combining different biological agents can lead to more effective and less harmful therapies. The integration of bacteriotherapy with traditional cancer treatments like chemotherapy and radiotherapy offers a novel and potentially effective strategy for cancer treatment. While it is still a developing field requiring further research and refinement, the initial findings suggest a promising future for this interdisciplinary approach in oncology (Ghasemi Darestani et al. 2023).

7.3 Bacteriobot as a Novel Drug Delivery System in Cancer Therapy

To enhance the efficacy of cancer drug delivery, researchers have explored an innovative drug delivery system (DDS) known as "microbot," which utilizes biodegradable and biocompatible materials. This cutting-edge method employs bacterial-based fabrication techniques for cancer treatment, where bacteria serve as both microactuators and microsensors, guiding microstructures directly to tumors. A pivotal study introduced "bacteriobot," a creation that synergizes strong therapeutic bacteria (*Salmonella* Typhimurium) with Cy5.5-coated polystyrene microbeads. Extensive in vitro and in vivo examinations in a mouse model demonstrated that these bacteriobots exhibit a higher migration velocity toward tumor cell lysates or spheroids compared to normal cells, suggesting a targeted approach in cancer treatment. Building on this concept, Park et al. developed a microbot therapy by encapsulating therapeutic bacteria (*S.* Typhimurium) within alginate microbeads. This bacterial-encapsulated system offers protection against the immune system, presenting a safer alternative to the direct inoculation of bacteria into tumor cells. Such targeted prodrug therapy in cancer treatment shows promise due to its diverse target selection, tumor specificity, systemic safety, and efficacy. The recombinant CD95L-based prodrug is highlighted as a versatile and multifunctional drug, analogous to a Swiss army knife, offering effective cancer treatment with minimal side effects. The application of bacteria in cancer therapy is complex, akin to a double-edged sword. While the use of bacteria for cancer treatment is feasible and their potential in treating solid tumors has been recognized for decades, the clinical application has been hindered by the risk of uncontrollable adverse side effects. Recent advancements have identified and studied certain attenuated species of bacteria capable of treating cancer with minimal or no side effects, marking a significant step forward in safe cancer therapy applications. However, bacteria alone may not fully realize their therapeutic potential; their modification as antitumor agents, anti-oncogenes, or immunogenic antigens, coupled with other therapeutic processes, is expected to enhance their efficacy in cancer treatment. The field of using bacteria as anticancer agents is relatively nascent, necessitating further studies to fully understand and validate their clinical significance in cancer therapy. The findings from various studies underscore the potential of bacterial-based cancer therapy, but also highlight the need for optimization and further development of this promising treatment approach (Kassahn et al. 2007; Park et al. 2015).

7.4 Microbiomes as Cancer Diagnostics

Extensive research has established a clear connection between microbiota and cancer, with various studies providing insights into this relationship. For instance, studies using gnotobiological mice with compromised immune systems have shown that microbiota plays a significant role in cancer development. An IL-10 knockout mouse study demonstrated that these mice developed spontaneous colitis, which worsened in a specific pathogen-free environment, leading to adenocarcinoma in older mice due to an unregulated Th1 response. Similarly, STAT3-conditional animals developed chronic colitis from macrophages and neutrophils, likely due to disrupted IL-10 and active Th1 response. Research on Toll-like receptor (TLR) signaling in mice has furthered our understanding of the link between microorganisms and cancer. Mice lacking TLR-4 were found to be less susceptible to colitis-related cancers, indicating that local microbiota can induce overwhelming immunological reactions if critical immune tolerance components are disrupted. In germ-free IL-10 knockout mice, colitis does not develop, nor is there any abnormal immune stimulation. However, colonization by the NC101 *E. coli* strain leads to rapid tumor formation, likely due to increased DNA damage. Pathogenic bacteria, including *E. coli*, *Streptococcus bovis*, *Helicobacter pylori*, *Bacteroides fragilis*, *Enterococcus* spp., and some Enterobacteriaceae family members, are implicated in several diseases, including colorectal cancer (CRC). These organisms can attach to epithelial layers, leading to hyperplasia, and produce toxins that compromise epithelial barrier functionality, harm endothelial cells, and induce inflammation. *E. coli*, for example, can stimulate tumor growth through attachment to colonic epithelial cells and exhibit pro-tumorigenic activities by degrading DNA or the mucous layer/epithelia. The polyketide synthase (PKS) complex in *E. coli* is a significant source of cytotoxicity, promoting colon cancer development in IL-10−/−murine models. The human microbiome influences various biological pathways, including hormonal and metabolic processes, triggering cancer initiation, proliferation, and/or genetic instability or inducing apoptosis. The effect of gut microbiota dysbiosis on development, progression, and prognosis is evident in breast cancer (BC), through direct and indirect signaling pathways. Treating BC through microbial therapy involves managing microbiota to target the immune response. Studies have identified *Propionibacterium* and *Staphylococcus* in abundance in healthy, high-risk, and tumor-adjacent normal tissues, but less so in tumor tissue. The *Staphylococcus* genus is negatively associated with the expression of the oncogene *TRAF4*, while *Propionibacterium* expression is positively correlated with the activation of T cells. Normal breast tissue is characterized by an enriched presence of bacteria like *Lactobacillus*, associated with a progesterone receptor (PR)-positive status. Tumor tissues show a significant decrease in these bacteria. *Lactobacillus acidophilus*, for instance, increases cytokine expression, promoting antitumor immunity and has anti-angiogenic effects. *Micrococcus luteus* in in vivo models hinders tumor growth, potentially by upregulating M1-macrophage-related genes. Similarly, *Sphingomonas yanoikuyae* affects the immune response through the proliferation of invariant NKT cells. *E. coli* produces antimicrobial peptides that affect cell survival through cell cycle arrest and DNAse activity. Colicin A, for example, increases apoptosis in multiple breast cancer cell lines. Focus on *Bifidobacterium* is due to their anaerobic status, making them ideal for delivering therapeutic genetic material to tumor necrotic centers. They also metabolize lapachol, synthesizing cytotoxic metabolites against BC. The histologic grade of breast tumors is associated with distinct microbial profiles, with certain bacteria found in non-tumor tissues inhibiting invasion or promoting antitumor activity. Modifying or eliminating certain microbial communities can reverse the environmental conditions favoring cancer and trigger apoptosis. Complementary to traditional BC therapies, restoring breast microbiota to their natural concentrations not only ensures a functional immune response but also prevents interference with cancer drugs administered or their metabolites (Bernardo et al. 2023; Hidaka et al. 2007; Roy and Trinchieri 2017; Urbaniak et al. 2016).

8 Conclusion

It is evident that the future of cancer treatment could be significantly advanced through the development of therapies that employ agents involved in multiple human biological reactions, such as the immune response and metabolism. These therapies are promising not only in terms of their efficacy but also in their potential to reduce the adverse side effects commonly associated with traditional cancer treatments. The novel approach of using microbial-based therapies offers a multifaceted strategy for enhancing cancer treatment, characterized by selective tumor targeting, activation of both innate and adaptive antitumor immunity, and the ability to overcome drug resistance mechanisms (Table 1). The integration of these innovative treatments with traditional methods could potentially diminish drug resistance, a significant hurdle in current cancer therapy. This can be partly achieved through a microbiome screen test, which identifies potential targets that may improve patient prognosis and help avert drug resistance. Establishing standardized protocols and clinical guidelines is crucial for ensuring the efficient and safe application of these therapies. It is essential to have a uniform system in place for the collection of evidence related to the efficacy and safety of these treatments.

The connection between the gut and breast microbiome colonies and their impact on the immune system needs to be thoroughly investigated. This understanding is critical for the design of new drugs that operate by modifying the gut microbiota or

Table 1 Overview of microbial-based therapies and their clinical trials in cancer treatment

Therapeutic microbe	Clinical status	Type of cancer	Study objective	References
(Lactobacillus acidophilus, lactobacillus plantarum, lactobacillus casei, and lactobacillus bulgaricus) & (Bifidobacterium breve, Bifidobacterium longum, Bifidobacterium infantis) & Streptococcus thermophilus	N/A	Gastrointestinal cancer	NCT03704727: Probiotic formulated by a mixture of lactobacilli and Bifidum strains and *Streptococcus thermophilus* will be evaluated to determine its ability to reduce gastrointestinal permeability following chemotherapy. This may improve patient outcome	Andersen (2019)
Bacteroides	Observational	Colorectal cancer	NCT06091137: Determine whether patients undergoing an appendectomy due to colorectal will present a dysbiosis of microbes such as *Bacteroides fragilis*	Yu (2023)
Bacteroides	Phase 2	Weight loss in breast cancer patients	NCT04499950: Compare how the ratio between *Bacteroides* and firmicutes microbiome affect weight loss in breast cancer patients	Sidney Kimmel Comprehensive Cancer Center at Johns Hopkins (2023)
Bacteroides	Observational	Esophageal cancer	NCT05967910: Study the effects of gut microbiome on chronic stress and how the microbiome affects immune checkpoint inhibitor efficacy in cancer treatment	Wu (2023)
Bifidobacteria	Phase 1 Phase 2	Liver cancer patients	NCT05620004: Liver cancer patients undergoing immunotherapy will be treated with the microbe to determine its safety and efficacy as a therapeutic	Xie (2022)
Bifidobacteria	N/A	Metastatic colorectal cancer patients	NCT04131803: Evaluate the outcomes of combining standard chemotherapy with probiotics composed of *Bifidobacterium trifidum* live powder	Second Affiliated Hospital, School of Medicine, Zhejiang University (2021)

Bifidobacteria	N/A	Liver cancer	NCT05032014: Will enhancing the concentration of probiotics, such as *Bifidobacterium*, in liver cancer improve PD-1 inhibitor activity?	Xu (2021a)
Bifidobacteria	N/A	Acute lymphocytic leukemia—pediatric patients	NCT01600781: Place children diagnosed with acute lymphoblastic leukemia on a dietary supplement enriched with fiber and measure the quality of life of patients and whether immune response is enhanced	Children's Cancer Hospital Egypt 57357 (2015)
Bifidobacterium & lactobacillus	N/A	Non-small cell lung cancer patients	NCT05094167: Do these microbiota improve the efficacy of immune checkpoint inhibitor, Carilizumab, in combination with platinum?	Xu (2021b)
Clostridium novyi	Phase 1	Advanced solid tumors	NCT03435952: Determine tolerable dose that can be prescribed in combination with pembrolizumab. Any effects of the spores on the disease will also be evaluated	M.D. Anderson Cancer Center (2023a)
Clostridium novyi	Phase 1	Solid tumors	NCT01924689: Intratumoral injection of *C. Novyi*-NT expressed manageable toxicities and antitumoral activities	BioMed Valley Discoveries, Inc (2019)
Coriolus versicolor/ Trametes versicolor	Phase 1	Breast cancer	NCT00680667: To determine the side effect and effective dose at which the mushroom extract, *Coriolus versicolor*, is effective in treating women with breast cancer between stages I-III following radiation therapy	Masonic Cancer Center, University of Minnesota (2017)
Coriolus versicolor/ Trametes versicolor	Phase 3	Thoracic cancer	NCT04871412: Directing thoracic cancer patients to include certain dietary (*Coriolus versicolor* among them) supplements pre- and post-operation to potentially prolong overall survival and decrease adverse effects	Ottawa Hospital Research Institute (2023)
Coriolus versicolor/ Trametes versicolor	N/A	Cervical cancer prevention	NCT04624568: Avert progression of HPV to cervical cancer by prescribing Papilocare®, a vaginal gel that improves uterine cervical epithelial lining	Centre Hospitalier Régional d'Orléans (2023)
Coriolus versicolor/ Trametes versicolor	N/A	Lung neoplasms and breast carcinoma	NCT02603016: Patients will be given Maitake mushrooms (*Grifola frondosa*) extract to evaluate treatment	Wu (2017)

(continued)

Table 1 (continued)

Therapeutic microbe	Clinical status	Type of cancer	Study objective	References
Coriolus versicolor/ Trametes versicolor	N/A	Prevent cervical cancer	NCT04210336: Papilocare® has shown therapeutic outcomes against low-grade cervical lesions linked with HPV and illustrates positive results with increasing HPV clearance following 6-month treatment period. *Coriolus versicolor* is a Papilocare® ingredient	Serrano et al. (2021)
EO2040	Phase 2	Colorectal cancer	NCT05350501: Evaluate the therapeutic properties of a microbiome-derived vaccine (EO2040) when administered in interaction with nivolumab	Enterome (2023a)
EO2463	Phase 1 phase 2	Non-Hodgkin lymphoma	NCT04669171: Measure tolerability, safety, immunogenicity and efficacy of EO2463 during treatment with lenalidomide and/or rituximab	Enterome (2023b)
EO4010	Phase 1 Phase 2	Metastatic colorectal carcinoma	NCT05589597: Assess the safety immunogenicity and efficacy of a microbial-derived therapeutic vaccine (EO4010) combined with ICI	Enterome (2023c)
Fecal microbiota transplantation (FMT)	Early phase 1	Pancreatic ductal adenocarcinoma	NCT04975217: Investigate gut microbiome of PDAC patients and assess tolerability and safety of treatments with FMT	M.D. Anderson Cancer Center (2023b)
FMT	Phase 2	Non-small cell lung cancer and melanoma	NCT04951583: Record the changes that occur to tumor microenvironment following treatment with immune checkpoint inhibitors (ICI) and FMT. Additionally, this study will identify the effects of FMT on overall survivor of patients	Centre hospitalier de l'Université de Montréal (CHUM) (2023)
GB104	Phase 1	Colorectal cancer	NCT05943041: Measure changes that may occur to immune status of the body and/or any changes in LARS	GI biome, Inc. (2023)
Inosine (restored by *lactobacillus reuteri*)	Phase 2 Phase 3	Advanced, recurrent or metastatic solid tumors	Inosine administered in synergy with ICI and presence or absence of chemotherapy to determine efficacy of this gut microbial metabolite	He et al. (2016)

Lacticaseibacillus	N/A	Acute lymphoblastic leukemia	NCT05939791: Evaluate the effect of *lactobacillus casei* (dairy probiotics) in children diagnosed with acute lymphoblastic leukemia	Comenius University (2023)
Lactobacillus	Observational	Oesophageal cancer	NCT05967910: Study the effects of gut microbiome on chronic stress and how the microbiome affects immune checkpoint inhibitor efficacy in cancer treatment	Wu (2023)
Lactobacillus	N/A	Liver cancer patients	NCT05032014: Do probiotics enhance PD-1 inhibitor treatment	Xu (2021a)
Listeria	Phase 1	Carcinoma and liver metastases	NCT00327652: The maximum planned *listeria* dose is tolerated in patients with carcinoma and liver metastases. Immune activity was increased in cancer patients	Le et al. (2012)
Listeria	Phase 1	Metastatic castration-resistant prostate cancer	NCT02625857: No significant differences were recorded in immune response	Janssen Research & Development, LLC (2019)
Listeria	Phase 2	Metastatic pancreatic cancer	NCT01417000: Recorded safety and efficacy of prescribed live-attenuated *listeria monocytogenes* vaccine (CRS-207) in pancreatic ductal adenocarcinoma patients	Aduro biotech, Inc. (2018a)
Listeria	Phase 2	Metastatic pancreatic adenocarcinoma	NCT02004262: Evaluate the safety and immune response in patients treated with GVAX in synergy with CRS-207 or CRS-207 alone all in comparison to chemotherapy. Results recorded increased overall survival and resulted in more tolerable side effects	Aduro biotech, Inc. (2018b)
Listeria	Phase 1	Grade III/IV astrocytomas	NCT01967758: Phase I study that would record safety, immunogenicity, and tolerability of another live-attenuated listeria monocytogenes. Vaccine (ADU-623). No results found	Providence Health & Services (2018)
Listeria	Phase 1	Unresectable malignant pleural mesothelioma	NCT01675765: Tumor size decreased in patients following administration of CRS-207 whereas combining CRS-207 with chemotherapy significantly altered tumor microenvironment and patient response to treatment	Aduro biotech, Inc. (2020)

(continued)

Table 1 (continued)

Therapeutic microbe	Clinical status	Type of cancer	Study objective	References
Listeria	Phase 2	Persistent or recurrent cervical cancer	NCT01266460:Phase II trial indicated that a live-attenuated listeria monocytogenes cancer vaccine ADXS11–001 increased overall survival in women with progressive cervical cancer	Huh et al. (2020)
Listeria	Phase 2	HPV-positive oropharyngeal squamous cell carcinoma	NCT02002182: Administration of ADXS 11–001 increased HPV-specific T cell activity more than twofold	Sikora (2022)
MET-4 bacterial strains	N/A	Locoregionally advanced oropharyngeal squamous cell carcinoma 2	NCT03838601: MET-4 administered in combination with chemoradiotherapy. An oral dose of MET4 will be used to determine its toxicity, engraftment, and safety	Watson et al. (2021)
Microbial ecosystem therapeutics	Phase 2 Phase 3	Incurable local advanced or metastatic solid malignancy	NCT03686202 microbial ecosystem therapeutics (MET) involves treatment with bacteria isolated from the stool of a healthy donor. This study will administer MET in synergy with immune checkpoint inhibitors and determine MET safety, tolerability, and engraftment	University Health Network, Toronto (2023)
Mix vaccine with a microbial-based therapy	Phase 1 Phase 2	Prostate cancer	NCT02338700: Measure safety and effectiveness of prescribing the mix vaccine to patients undergoing standard treatment. Immunology index and progression-free survival will also be recorded	Fuda Cancer Hospital, Guangzhou (2015a)
Mix vaccine with a microbial-based therapy	Phase 1 Phase 2	Pancreatic	NCT02338752: Patients undergoing cancer standard treatment will be administered the mix vaccine to determine safety, outcome, progression-free survival and immunology index compared to controls	Fuda Cancer Hospital, Guangzhou (2019)

Mix vaccine with a microbial-based therapy	Phase 1 Phase 2	Breast cancer	NCT02338804: Breast cancer patients undergoing treatment according to National Comprehensive Cancer Network (NCCN) will be injected with a mix vaccine to determine its effects, if any on cancer progression and safety of the vaccine. Immunology index and other parameters will be assessed	Fuda Cancer Hospital, Guangzhou (2015b)
Mix vaccine with a microbial-based therapy	Phase 1 Phase 2	Hepatocyte carcinoma	NCT02338778: A group of patients undergoing treatment according to NCCN will also receive a mix vaccine injection to determine safeness and effectiveness of the vaccine in drug progression. Will also measure other parameters such as immunology index and hematology	Fuda Cancer Hospital, Guangzhou (2015c)
MV-s-NAP	Phase I	HER2-positive breast cancer	NCT04521764: Study investigating the side effects and therapeutic dose of MV-s-NAP (modified measles virus) on breast cancer. Laboratory work has shown that the virus abolishes breast cancer cells	Mayo Clinic (2023)
Salmonella	Observational	Acute colitis and early identification of patients requiring diagnostic colonoscopy	NCT02709213: Evaluate the role of *salmonella* spp. as a cancer or colitis biomarker	Meyer (2020)
Salmonella	Phase I	Advanced and/or metastatic	NCT00004988: Phase I trial: *Salmonella typhimurium* (VNP20009) administered to nonresponsive metastatic melanoma or renal cell carcinoma patients. Observed tumor colonization with no antitumor effects	National Cancer Institute (NCI) (2008)
Salmonella	Phase I	Unresectable hepatic metastasis	Evaluating the efficacy of a modified *salmonella typhimurium* in treatments of patients with unresectable hepatic metastases from solid tumor cancer	Masonic Cancer Center, University of Minnesota (2020)
Salmonella	Phase I	Advanced solid tumors	NCT00006254: Does *salmonella typhimurium* express antitumor effects against advanced solid tumors	Vion Pharmaceuticals (2013)

(continued)

Table 1 (continued)

Therapeutic microbe	Clinical status	Type of cancer	Study objective	References
Salmonella	Phase I	Multiple myeloma	NCT03762291: Determine the safe dose of the *Salmonella*-derived cancer vaccine, TXSVN in patients diagnosed with multiple myeloma	Lulla (2023)
Salmonella	Phase 1 Phase 2	Advanced solid tumor	NCT05038150: Phase I/II study in patients with advanced solid tumors to determine safety, tolerability, and efficacy of *salmonella typhimurium* SGN1	Guangzhou Sinogen Pharmaceutical Co., Ltd (2023a)
Salmonella	Phase 2	Metastatic pancreatic cancer	NCT04589234: Assess the effect of *salmonella typhimurium* together with standard chemotherapy in metastatic pancreatic cancer patients	Salspera LLC (2022)
Salmonella	Phase I	Advanced or metastatic solid tumor	NCT00004216: Phase I study on the effectiveness of a genetically modified *salmonella typhimurium* (VNP20009). No effective results on cancer growth	Heimann and Rosenberg (2003)
Salmonella	Phase 1 Phase 2	Advanced solid tumor	NCT05103345: Evaluate the safety, maximum tolerated dose, optimal biological dose, and tolerability of modified *salmonella typhimurium* SGN1 administered through injection intratumorally	Guangzhou Sinogen Pharmaceutical Co., Ltd (2023b)
Salmonella	Early phase 1	Neuroblastoma	NCT04049864: Investigate the immunogenicity and safety of a DNA vaccine strategy administered in synergy with *salmonella enterica*	Meleshko (2022)
Salmonella	Observational	Biliary tract cancers	NCT00339560: Determine whether concentrations of *Salmonella typhi* or other bacterial antibodies affect the risk of developing biliary tract cancers	National Cancer Institute (NCI) (2020)
Shigella	Observational	Acute colitis and early identification of patients requiring diagnostic colonoscopy	NCT02709213: Evaluate the role of *Shigella* spp. as a cancer or colitis biomarker	Meyer (2020)

Streptococcus pyogenes	Phase 1	Invasive bladder cancer	NCT05085990: Investigate the toxicity and safety of TARA-002 (a lyophilized biological preparation of *streptococcus pyogenes*). Further to the safety results above, this study evaluates the antitumor effects of TARA-002 in high-grade invasive bladder cancer	Protara Therapeutics (2024)
Streptococcus pyogenes	Phase 1 Phase 2	Invasive bladder cancer	NCT05951179: Investigate the toxicity and safety of TARA-002 (a lyophilized biological preparation of *streptococcus pyogenes*). Further to the safety results above, this study evaluates the antitumor effects of TARA-002 in high-grade invasive bladder cancer	Protara Therapeutics (2023)
Streptococcus pyogenes	Phase 1	Invasive bladder cancer	NCT05085977: Investigate the toxicity and safety of TARA-002 (a lyophilized biological preparation of *streptococcus pyogenes*). Further to the safety results above, this study evaluates the antitumor effects of TARA-002 in high-grade invasive bladder cancer	Protara Therapeutics (2024)
Vibrio	Observational	Acute colitis and early identification of patients requiring diagnostic colonoscopy	NCT02709213: Expose the role of *vibrio* sp. as a cancer or colitis biomarker	Meyer (2020)

This table summarizes the therapeutic use of various microbes in oncology, detailing their clinical status, specific cancer types targeted, and study objectives employing microbiota transport vectors introduced peritumorally. Understanding and leveraging the relationship between different microbiomes and cancer cells could open new avenues for targeted treatment strategies. In the realm of microbial-based therapies, significant progress has been made in recent decades, yet numerous challenges remain. The field of genetic engineering presents opportunities for precise control over microbial behavior and enhanced tumor specificity. However, a balance must be struck to reduce virulence without compromising the natural antitumor properties of microorganisms while ensuring host safety. One of the key challenges in achieving full tumor eradication is the inherent heterogeneity of tumors and their mechanisms of immune evasion. Moreover, the development of resistance against microbial therapies necessitates a multi-layered treatment approach. The optimization of delivery methods is another crucial aspect, as it is challenging to disseminate these therapies throughout solid tumors and metastatic sites. Techniques such as intratumoral injections, systemic administration, and the use of novel carriers and targeting ligands are being explored to overcome these barriers. The combination of microbial therapies with chemotherapy, radiotherapy, or immunotherapy is a promising strategy that seeks to enhance the efficacy of treatment while minimizing toxicity. However, the synergistic effects and safety profiles of these combinations require thorough investigation and characterization.

For the effective translation of these promising approaches into clinical solutions, several avenues of future research are critical. The continuous refinement of genetic tools will enable more precise control over microbial behavior, potentially leading to the development of "smart" microbes that respond to specific tumor cues for targeted colonization. Understanding microbial interactions within diverse tumor microenvironments is key to optimizing personalized therapies. This may include studying colonization factors, immune modulation, and metabolic influences on distinct cancer subtypes. Furthermore, the exploration of combination regimens is pivotal. Defining optimal synergies between microbial therapies and other treatment modalities could maximize the benefits of multimodal treatment strategies. This will require dose scheduling, vector engineering, and evaluation in advanced preclinical models. Rigorous clinical evaluation through well-designed trials, including longitudinal immune monitoring, biomarker analyses, and assessment of patient-reported outcomes, is essential to elucidate the true therapeutic impacts of these treatments.

In conclusion, while the full clinical translation of microbial-based cancer treatments presents major scientific and logistical challenges, the promise of these therapies remains strong. Continued advancements in engineering precision, systems-level understanding of tumors, and structured clinical testing are positioning these therapies at an inflection point in cancer management. With ongoing research support and multidisciplinary collaborations, microbial approaches have the potential to revolutionize cancer treatment, offering hope for more effective and less toxic therapies in the future.

Compliance with Ethical Standards All authors declare they have no conflict of interest.

References

Adams S, Schmid P, Rugo HS, Winer EP, Loirat D, Awada A, Cescon DW, Iwata H, Campone M, Nanda R, Hui R, Curigliano G, Toppmeyer D, O'Shaughnessy J, Loi S, Paluch-Shimon S, Tan AR, Card D, Zhao J, Karantza V, Cortés J (2019) Pembrolizumab monotherapy for previously treated metastatic triple-negative breast cancer: cohort a of the phase II KEYNOTE-086 study. Ann Oncol 30:397–404

Aduro Biotech, Inc (2018a) A phase 2, randomized, multicenter, open-label study of the efficacy and immune response of the sequential administration of GVAX pancreas vaccine alone or followed by CRS-207 in adults with metastatic pancreatic adenocarcinoma (Clinical trial registration No. NCT01417000). clinicaltrials.gov

Aduro Biotech, Inc (2018b) A phase 2B, randomized, controlled, multicenter, open-label study of the efficacy and immune response of GVAX pancreas vaccine (with cyclophosphamide) and CRS 207 compared to chemotherapy or to CRS-207 alone in adults with previously-treated metastatic pancreatic adenocarcinoma (Clinical trial registration No. NCT02004262). clinicaltrials.gov

Aduro Biotech, Inc (2020) A phase 1B study to evaluate the safety and induction of immune response of CRS-207 in combination with pemetrexed and cisplatin as front-line therapy in adults with malignant pleural mesothelioma (Clinical trial registration No. NCT01675765). clinicaltrials.gov

Agostinetto E, Gligorov J, Piccart M (2022) Systemic therapy for early-stage breast cancer: learning from the past to build the future. Nat Rev Clin Oncol 19:763–774

Allemailem KS (2021) Innovative approaches of engineering tumor-targeting bacteria with different therapeutic payloads to fight cancer: a smart strategy of disease management. Int J Nanomedicine 16:8159–8184

Alpuim Costa D, Nobre JG, Batista MV, Ribeiro C, Calle C, Cortes A, Marhold M, Negreiros I, Borralho P, Brito M, Cortes J, Braga SA, Costa L (2021) Human microbiota and breast cancer—is there any relevant link?—a literature review and new horizons toward personalised medicine. Front Microbiol 12:584332

Andersen JR (2019) The Effects of probiotics on intestinal permeability in gastrointestinal cancer patients in chemotherapy (Clinical trial registration No. NCT03704727). clinicaltrials.gov

Arumugam M, Raes J, Pelletier E, Le Paslier D, Yamada T, Mende DR, Fernandes GR, Tap J, Bruls T, Batto J-M, Bertalan M, Borruel N, Casellas F, Fernandez L, Gautier L, Hansen T, Hattori M, Hayashi T, Kleerebezem M, Kurokawa K, Leclerc M, Levenez F, Manichanh C, Nielsen HB, Nielsen T, Pons N, Poulain J, Qin J, Sicheritz-Ponten T, Tims S, Torrents D, Ugarte E, Zoetendal EG, Wang J, Guarner F, Pedersen O, de Vos WM, Brunak S, Doré J, Weissenbach J, Ehrlich SD, Bork P (2011) Enterotypes of the human gut microbiome. Nature 473:174–180

Baban CK, Cronin M, O'Hanlon D, O'Sullivan GC, Tangney M (2010) Bacteria as vectors for gene therapy of cancer. Bioeng Bugs 1:385–394

Bashor CJ, Hilton IB, Bandukwala H, Smith DM, Veiseh O (2022) Engineering the next generation of cell-based therapeutics. Nat Rev Drug Discov 21:655–675

Bernardes N, Seruca R, Chakrabarty AM, Fialho AM (2010) Microbial-based therapy of cancer. Bioeng Bugs 1:178–190

Bernardo G, Le Noci V, Ottaviano E, De Cecco L, Camisaschi C, Guglielmetti S, Di Modica M, Gargari G, Bianchi F, Indino S, Sartori P, Borghi E, Sommariva M, Tagliabue E, Triulzi T, Sfondrini L (2023) Reduction of *Staphylococcus epidermidis* in the mammary tumor microbiota induces antitumor immunity and decreases breast cancer aggressiveness. Cancer Lett 555: 216041

Bettegowda C, Dang LH, Abrams R, Huso DL, Dillehay L, Cheong I, Agrawal N, Borzillary S, McCaffery JM, Watson EL, Lin K-S, Bunz F, Baidoo K, Pomper MG, Kinzler KW, Vogelstein B, Zhou S (2003) Overcoming the hypoxic barrier to radiation therapy with anaerobic bacteria. Proc Natl Acad Sci USA 100:15083–15088

Bhatt DK, Chammas R, Daemen T (2021) Resistance mechanisms influencing oncolytic Virotherapy, a systematic analysis. Vaccine 9:1166

BioMed Valley Discoveries, Inc (2019) Phase I safety study of intratumoral injection of *Clostridium novyi*-NT spores in patients with treatment-refractory solid tumor malignancies (Clinical trial registration No. NCT01924689). clinicaltrials.gov

Boeckxstaens G, Camilleri M, Sifrim D, Houghton LA, Elsenbruch S, Lindberg G, Azpiroz F, Parkman HP (2016) Fundamentals of Neurogastroenterology: physiology/motility—sensation. Gastroenterology S0016-5085(16):00221–00223

Bommareddy PK, Patel A, Hossain S, Kaufman HL (2017) Talimogene Laherparepvec (T-VEC) and other oncolytic viruses for the treatment of melanoma. Am J Clin Dermatol 18:1–15

Broyles SS (2003) Vaccinia virus transcription. J Gen Virol 84:2293–2303

Camilleri M (2018) Cannabinoids and gastrointestinal motility: pharmacology, clinical effects, and potential therapeutics in humans. Neurogastroenterol Motil 30:e13370

Cao Z, Liu J (2020) Bacteria and bacterial derivatives as drug carriers for cancer therapy. J Control Release 326:396–407

Cao H, Luo S, Xu M, Zhang Y, Song S, Wang S, Kong X, He N, Cao X, Yan F, Wang B (2014) The secondary bile acid, deoxycholate accelerates intestinal adenoma–adenocarcinoma sequence in Apcmin/+ mice through enhancing Wnt signaling. Fam Cancer 13:563–571

Centre hospitalier de l'Université de Montréal (CHUM) (2023) Phase II trial of fecal microbial transplantation in patients with advanced non-small cell lung cancer and melanoma treated with immune checkpoint inhibitors. (Clinical trial registration No. NCT04951583). clinicaltrials.gov

Centre Hospitalier Régional d'Orléans (2023) Papilocare®: effects on regression of histologically confirmed cervical intraepithelial lesions 1 and tolerance. (Clinical trial registration No. NCT04624568). clinicaltrials.gov

Chandra D, Jahangir A, Quispe-Tintaya W, Einstein MH, Gravekamp C (2013) Myeloid-derived suppressor cells have a central role in attenuated *Listeria monocytogenes*-based immunotherapy against metastatic breast cancer in young and old mice. Br J Cancer 108:2281–2290

Chhabra N, Kennedy J (2022) A review of cancer immunotherapy toxicity II: adoptive cellular therapies, kinase inhibitors, monoclonal antibodies, and oncolytic viruses. J Med Toxicol 18: 43–55

Children's Cancer Hospital Egypt 57357 (2015) Effect of oral supplementation with a fibre enriched paediatric sip feed on the nutritional status, gut microbiota and quality of life of children with acute lymphocytic leukemia: an Egyptian pilot study (Clinical trial registration No. NCT01600781). clinicaltrials.gov

Chow LWC, Lo CSY, Loo WTY, Hu X, Sham JST (2003) Polysaccharide peptide mediates apoptosis by up-regulating p21 gene and down-regulating cyclin D_1 gene. Am J Chin Med 31:1–9

Chowdhury S, Castro S, Coker C, Hinchliffe TE, Arpaia N, Danino T (2019) Programmable bacteria induce durable tumor regression and systemic antitumor immunity. Nat Med 25: 1057–1063

Comenius University (2023) The effect of physical exercise and dairy probiotics (*Lactobacillus casei*) on Gut microbiome in childhood cancer survivors (Clinical trial registration No. NCT05939791). clinicaltrials.gov

Cook-Deegan R, Heaney C (2010) Patents in genomics and human genetics. Annu Rev Genomics Hum Genet 11:383–425

Cristi F, Gutiérrez T, Hitt MM, Shmulevitz M (2022) Genetic modifications that expand oncolytic virus potency. Front Mol Biosci 9

Dang LH, Bettegowda C, Huso DL, Kinzler KW, Vogelstein B (2001) Combination bacteriolytic therapy for the treatment of experimental tumors. Proc Natl Acad Sci 98:15155–15160

Del Prete A, Salvi V, Soriani A, Laffranchi M, Sozio F, Bosisio D, Sozzani S (2023) Dendritic cell subsets in cancer immunity and tumor antigen sensing. Cell Mol Immunol 20:432–447

Din MO, Danino T, Prindle A, Skalak M, Selimkhanov J, Allen K, Julio E, Atolia E, Tsimring LS, Bhatia SN, Hasty J (2016) Synchronized cycles of bacterial lysis for in vivo delivery. Nature 536:81–85

Divyashree M, Prakash SK, Aditya V, Aljabali AA, Alzahrani KJ, Azevedo V, Góes-Neto A, Tambuwala MM, Barh D (2022) Bugs as drugs: neglected but a promising future therapeutic strategy in cancer. Future Oncol 18:1609–1626

Dold C, Rodriguez Urbiola C, Wollmann G, Egerer L, Muik A, Bellmann L, Fiegl H, Marth C, Kimpel J, von Laer D (2016) Application of interferon modulators to overcome partial resistance of human ovarian cancers to VSV-GP oncolytic viral therapy. Mol Ther Oncolytics 3:16021

Dujon AM, Gatenby RA, Bramwell G, MacDonald N, Dohrmann E, Raven N, Schultz A, Hamede R, Gérard A-L, Giraudeau M, Thomas F, Ujvari B (2020) Transmissible cancers in an evolutionary perspective. iScience 23:101269

Dujon AM, Brown JS, Destoumieux-Garzón D, Vittecoq M, Hamede R, Tasiemski A, Boutry J, Tissot S, Alix-Panabieres C, Pujol P, Renaud F (2021) On the need for integrating cancer into the one health perspective. Evol Appl 14:2571–2575

Duong MT-Q, Qin Y, You S-H, Min J-J (2019) Bacteria-cancer interactions: bacteria-based cancer therapy. Exp Mol Med 51:152

Enterome (2023a) A phase 2 trial of EO2040, a miCrobiaL-derived peptide therApeUtic vaccine, in combination with nivolumab, for treatment of patients with circulating tumor DNA-dEfined minimal residual disease of colorectal cancer stage II, III, or IV after completion of curative therapy (the “CLAUDE” Study) (Clinical trial registration No. NCT05350501). clinicaltrials.gov

Enterome (2023b) A global multicenter phase 1/2 trial of EO2463, a novel microbial-derived peptide therapeutic vaccine, as monotherapy, and in combination with lenalidomide and rituximab, for treatment of patients with indolent non-Hodgkin’s lymphoma (Clinical trial registration No. NCT04669171). clinicaltrials.gov

Enterome (2023c) A global multicenter phase 1/2 trial of EO4010, a novel microbial derived peptide therapeutic vaccine, in combination with nivolumab, for treatment of patients with previously treated metastatic colorectal carcinoma (Clinical trial registration No. NCT05589597). clinicaltrials.gov

Epstein B, Jones M, Hamede R, Hendricks S, McCallum H, Murchison EP, Schönfeld B, Wiench C, Hohenlohe P, Storfer A (2016) Rapid evolutionary response to a transmissible cancer in Tasmanian devils. Nat Commun 7:12684

Fang CY, Ragin CC (2020) Addressing disparities in cancer screening among U.S. immigrants: progress and opportunities. Cancer Prev Res (Phila) 13:253–260

Fang C, Xiao G, Wang T, Song L, Peng B, Xu B, Zhang K (2023) Emerging Nano-/biotechnology drives oncolytic virus-activated and combined cancer immunotherapy. Research (Wash D C) 6:0108

Felgner S, Kocijancic D, Frahm M, Weiss S (2016) Bacteria in cancer therapy: renaissance of an old concept. Int J Microbiol 2016:1

Ferrucci PF, Pala L, Conforti F, Cocorocchio E (2021) Talimogene Laherparepvec (T-VEC): an Intralesional cancer immunotherapy for advanced melanoma. Cancers (Basel) 13:1383

Fu S, Zhang R, Gao Y, Xiong J, Li Y, Pu L, Xia A, Jin F (2023) Programming the lifestyles of engineered bacteria for cancer therapy. Natl Sci Rev 10:nwad031

Fuda Cancer Hospital, Guangzhou (2015a) Safety issue and efficacy study of combining mix vaccine and standard therapy in the treatment of prostate carcinoma patient (Clinical trial registration No. NCT02338700). clinicaltrials.gov

Fuda Cancer Hospital, Guangzhou (2015b) Safety issue and efficacy study of combining mix vaccine and standard therapy in the treatment of breast carcinoma patient (Clinical trial registration No. NCT02338804). clinicaltrials.gov

Fuda Cancer Hospital, Guangzhou (2015c) Safety issue and efficacy study of combining mix vaccine and standard therapy in the treatment of hepatocyte carcinoma patient (Clinical trial registration No. NCT02338778). clinicaltrials.gov

Fuda Cancer Hospital, Guangzhou (2019) Safety issue and efficacy study of combining mix vaccine and standard therapy in the treatment of pancreatic carcinoma patient (Clinical trial registration No. NCT02338752). clinicaltrials.gov

Gabrilovich DI, Nagaraj S (2009) Myeloid-derived-suppressor cells as regulators of the immune system. Nat Rev Immunol 9:162–174

Ghanavati R, Asadollahi P, Shapourabadi MB, Razavi S, Talebi M, Rohani M (2020) Inhibitory effects of lactobacilli cocktail on HT-29 colon carcinoma cells growth and modulation of the notch and Wnt/β-catenin signaling pathways. Microb Pathog 139:103829

Ghasemi Darestani N, Gilmanova AI, Al-Gazally ME, Zekiy AO, Ansari MJ, Zabibah RS, Jawad MA, Al-Shalah SAJ, Rizaev JA, Alnassar YS, Mohammed NM, Mustafa YF, Darvishi M, Akhavan-Sigari R (2023) Mesenchymal stem cell-released oncolytic virus: an innovative strategy for cancer treatment. Cell Commun Signal 21:43

GI Biome, Inc (2023) Open-label, single-center, dose-escalation phase 1 clinical study to evaluate the safety and tolerability of GB104, and explore gut microbial composition in patients who completed curative colectomy and planned therapy of colorectal cancer (Clinical trial registration No. NCT05943041). clinicaltrials.gov

Gniadek TJ, Augustin L, Schottel J, Leonard A, Saltzman D, Greeno E, Batist G (2020) A phase I, dose escalation, single dose trial of Oral attenuated *Salmonella Typhimurium* containing human IL-2 in patients with metastatic gastrointestinal cancers. J Immunother 43:217

Goradel NH, Alizadeh A, Hosseinzadeh S, Taghipour M, Ghesmati Z, Arashkia A, Negahdari B (2022) Oncolytic virotherapy as promising immunotherapy against cancer: mechanisms of resistance to oncolytic viruses. Future Oncol 18:245–259

Guangzhou Sinogen Pharmaceutical Co., Ltd (2023a) Phase I/IIa, open-label study to evaluate safety, tolerability and preliminary efficacy of modified *Salmonella* Typhimurium SGN1 in patients with advanced solid tumor (Clinical trial registration No. NCT05038150). clinicaltrials.gov

Guangzhou Sinogen Pharmaceutical Co., Ltd (2023b) A phase I/IIa, open-label, dose escalation and dose-expansion study to evaluate the safety and tolerability of modified *Salmonella* Typhimurium SGN1 administered via intratumoral injection in patients with advanced solid tumors (Clinical trial registration No. NCT05103345). clinicaltrials.gov

Hacein-Bey-Abina S, Von Kalle C, Schmidt M, McCormack MP, Wulffraat N, Leboulch P, Lim A, Osborne CS, Pawliuk R, Morillon E, Sorensen R, Forster A, Fraser P, Cohen JI, de Saint Basile G, Alexander I, Wintergerst U, Frebourg T, Aurias A, Stoppa-Lyonnet D, Romana S, Radford-Weiss I, Gross F, Valensi F, Delabesse E, Macintyre E, Sigaux F, Soulier J, Leiva LE, Wissler M, Prinz C, Rabbitts TH, Le Deist F, Fischer A, Cavazzana-Calvo M (2003) LMO2-associated clonal T cell proliferation in two patients after gene therapy for SCID-X1. Science 302:415–419

Harrington K, Freeman DJ, Kelly B, Harper J, Soria J-C (2019) Optimizing oncolytic virotherapy in cancer treatment. Nat Rev Drug Discov 18:689–706

He B, Hoang TK, Wang T, Ferris M, Taylor CM, Tian X, Luo M, Tran DQ, Zhou J, Tatevian N, Luo F, Molina JG, Blackburn MR, Gomez TH, Roos S, Rhoads JM, Liu Y (2016) Resetting microbiota by *Lactobacillus reuteri* inhibits T reg deficiency–induced autoimmunity via adenosine A2A receptors. J Exp Med 214:107–123

Heimann DM, Rosenberg SA (2003) Continuous intravenous administration of live genetically modified *Salmonella Typhimurium* in patients with metastatic melanoma. J Immunother 26: 179–180

Hidaka A, Hamaji Y, Sasaki T, Taniguchi S, Fujimori M (2007) Exogeneous cytosine deaminase gene expression in *Bifidobacterium breve* I-53-8w for tumor-targeting enzyme/prodrug therapy. Biosci Biotechnol Biochem 71:2921–2926

Horvath TD, Ihekweazu FD, Haidacher SJ, Ruan W, Engevik KA, Fultz R, Hoch KM, Luna RA, Oezguen N, Spinler JK, Haag AM, Versalovic J, Engevik MA (2022) *Bacteroides ovatus* colonization influences the abundance of intestinal short chain fatty acids and neurotransmitters. iScience 25:104158

Howarth JL, Lee YB, Uney JB (2010) Using viral vectors as gene transfer tools (cell biology and toxicology special issue: ETCS-UK 1 day meeting on genetic manipulation of cells). Cell Biol Toxicol 26:1–20

Huh WK, Brady WE, Fracasso PM, Dizon DS, Powell MA, Monk BJ, Leath CA, Landrum LM, Tanner EJ, Crane EK, Ueda S, McHale MT, Aghajanian C (2020) Phase II study of axalimogene filolisbac (ADXS-HPV) for platinum-refractory cervical carcinoma: an NRG oncology/gynecologic oncology group study. Gynecol Oncol 158:562–569

Ikryannikova LN, Gorokhovets NV, Belykh DA, Kurbatov LK, Zamyatnin AA (2023) Bacterial therapy of cancer: a way to the dustbin of history or to the medicine of the future? Int J Mol Sci 24:9726

Jain RK (1998) The next frontier of molecular medicine: delivery of therapeutics. Nat Med 4: 655–657

Jaiswal PK, Goel A, Mittal RD (2015) Survivin: a molecular biomarker in cancer. Indian J Med Res 141:389–397

Janssen Research & Development, LLC (2019) An open-label, phase 1 study of the safety and immunogenicity of JNJ-64041809, a live attenuated *Listeria monocytogenes* immunotherapy, in subjects with metastatic castration-resistant prostate cancer (Clinical trial registration No. NCT02625857). clinicaltrials.gov

Jhawar SR, Thandoni A, Bommareddy PK, Hassan S, Kohlhapp FJ, Goyal S, Schenkel JM, Silk AW, Zloza A (2017) Oncolytic viruses—natural and genetically engineered cancer immunotherapies. Front Oncol 7:202

Jiang S-N, Phan TX, Nam T-K, Nguyen VH, Kim H-S, Bom H-S, Choy HE, Hong Y, Min J-J (2010) Inhibition of tumor growth and metastasis by a combination of *Escherichia coli*–mediated Cytolytic therapy and radiotherapy. Mol Ther 18:635–642

Jiang T, Yang T, Chen Y, Miao Y, Xu Y, Jiang H, Yang M, Mao C (2022) Emulating interactions between microorganisms and tumor microenvironment to develop cancer theranostics. Theranostics 12:2833–2859

Kaczmarek M, Poznańska J, Fechner F, Michalska N, Paszkowska S, Napierała A, Mackiewicz A (2023) Cancer vaccine therapeutics: limitations and effectiveness—a literature review. Cells 12:2159

Kassahn D, Nachbur U, Brunner T (2007) CD95L pro-drug: a novel Swiss Army knife in cancer therapy? Cell Death Differ 14:393–394

Kerr P, Liu J, Cattadori I, Ghedin E, Read A, Holmes E (2015) Myxoma virus and the Leporipoxviruses: an evolutionary paradigm. Viruses 7:1020–1061

Kipanyula MJ, Seke Etet PF, Vecchio L, Farahna M, Nukenine EN, Nwabo Kamdje AH (2013) Signaling pathways bridging microbial-triggered inflammation and cancer. Cell Signal 25: 403–416

Kleber KT, Iranpur KR, Perry LM, Cruz SM, Razmara AM, Culp WTN, Kent MS, Eisen JA, Rebhun RB, Canter RJ (2022) Using the canine microbiome to bridge translation of cancer immunotherapy from pre-clinical murine models to human clinical trials. Front Immunol 13: 983344

Kulu Y, Dorfman JD, Kuruppu D, Fuchs BC, Goodwin JM, Fujii T, Kuroda T, Lanuti M, Tanabe KK (2009) Comparison of intravenous versus intraperitoneal administration of oncolytic herpes simplex virus 1 for peritoneal carcinomatosis in mice. Cancer Gene Ther 16:291–297

Laborda-Illanes A, Sanchez-Alcoholado L, Dominguez-Recio ME, Jimenez-Rodriguez B, Lavado R, Comino-Méndez I, Alba E, Queipo-Ortuño MI (2020) Breast and gut microbiota action mechanisms in breast cancer pathogenesis and treatment. Cancers 12:2465

Le DT, Brockstedt DG, Nir-Paz R, Hampl J, Mathur S, Nemunaitis J, Sterman DH, Hassan R, Lutz E, Moyer B, Giedlin M, Louis J-L, Sugar EA, Pons A, Cox AL, Levine J, Murphy AL, Illei P, Dubensky TW Jr, Eiden JE, Jaffee EM, Laheru DA (2012) A live-attenuated listeria vaccine (ANZ-100) and a live-attenuated listeria vaccine expressing Mesothelin (CRS-207) for advanced cancers: phase I studies of safety and immune induction. Clin Cancer Res 18:858–868

Lee C-H (2012) Engineering bacteria toward tumor targeting for cancer treatment: current state and perspectives. Appl Microbiol Biotechnol 93:517–523

Lee HA, Kim H, Lee K-W, Park K-Y (2015) Dead Nano-sized *Lactobacillus plantarum* inhibits Azoxymethane/dextran sulfate sodium-induced colon cancer in Balb/c Mice. J Med Food 18: 1400–1405

Lee YT, Tan YJ, Oon CE (2018) Molecular targeted therapy: treating cancer with specificity. Eur J Pharmacol 834:188–196

Lee K-W, Yam JWP, Mao X (2023) Dendritic cell vaccines: a shift from conventional approach to new generations. Cells 12:2147

Leschner S, Westphal K, Dietrich N, Viegas N, Jablonska J, Lyszkiewicz M, Lienenklaus S, Falk W, Gekara N, Loessner H, Weiss S (2009) Tumor invasion of *Salmonella enterica* Serovar typhimurium is accompanied by strong hemorrhage promoted by TNF-α. PLoS One 4:e6692

Li J, Jia H, Cai X, Zhong H, Feng Q, Sunagawa S, Arumugam M, Kultima JR, Prifti E, Nielsen T, Juncker AS, Manichanh C, Chen B, Zhang W, Levenez F, Wang J, Xu X, Xiao L, Liang S, Zhang D, Zhang Z, Chen W, Zhao H, Al-Aama JY, Edris S, Yang H, Wang J, Hansen T, Nielsen HB, Brunak S, Kristiansen K, Guarner F, Pedersen O, Doré J, Ehrlich SD, Bork P, Wang J (2014) An integrated catalog of reference genes in the human gut microbiome. Nat Biotechnol 32:834–841

Li T, Kang G, Wang T, Huang H (2018) Tumor angiogenesis and anti-angiogenic gene therapy for cancer. Oncol Lett 16:687–702

Lin D, Shen Y, Liang T (2023) Oncolytic virotherapy: basic principles, recent advances and future directions. Sig Transduct Target Ther 8:1–29

Liu Z, Lim S-H, Min J-J, Jung S (2023) Synergistic antitumor effect of combined radiotherapy and engineered *Salmonella Typhimurium* in an intracranial sarcoma mouse model. Vaccine 11:1275

Loeffler M, Le'Negrate G, Krajewska M, Reed JC (2008) Inhibition of tumor growth using *Salmonella* expressing Fas ligand. JNCI J Natl Cancer Inst 100:1113–1116

Logg CR, Robbins JM, Jolly DJ, Gruber HE, Kasahara N (2012) Chapter eleven—retroviral replicating vectors in cancer. In: Friedmann T (ed) Methods in enzymology, gene transfer vectors for clinical application. Academic Press, pp 199–228

Lou X, Chen Z, He Z, Sun M, Sun J (2021) Bacteria-mediated synergistic cancer therapy: small microbiome has a big Hope. Nanomicro Lett 13:37

Low KB, Ittensohn M, Le T, Platt J, Sodi S, Amoss M, Ash O, Carmichael E, Chakraborty A, Fischer J, Lin SL, Luo X, Miller SI, Zheng L, King I, Pawelek JM, Bermudes D (1999) Lipid a mutant salmonella with suppressed virulence and TNFα induction retain tumor-targeting in vivo. Nat Biotechnol 17:37–41

Low KB, Ittensohn M, Luo X, Zheng L-M, King I, Pawelek JM, Bermudes D (2004) Construction of VNP20009. In: Springer CJ (ed) Suicide gene therapy: methods and reviews, methods in molecular medicine™. Humana Press, Totowa, pp 47–59

Lulla P (2023) Multiple myeloma trial of orally administered salmonella based Survivin Vaccine (Clinical trial registration No. NCT03762291). clinicaltrials.gov

LY Eliza W, Fai CK, Chung LP (2012) Efficacy of Yun Zhi (Coriolus versicolor) on survival in cancer patients: systematic review and meta-analysis. IAD 6:78–87

M.D. Anderson Cancer Center (2023a) A phase Ib investigation of pembrolizumab in combination with intratumoral injection of *Clostridium novyi*-NT in patients with treatment-refractory solid tumors (Clinical trial registration No. NCT03435952). clinicaltrials.gov

M.D. Anderson Cancer Center (2023b) Pilot study using fecal microbial transplants in patients with pancreatic cancer (Clinical trial registration No. NCT04975217). clinicaltrials.gov

Ma X, Yu H (2006) Global burden of cancer. Yale J Biol Med 79:85–94

Ma W, Mao Q, Xia W, Dong G, Yu C, Jiang F (2019) Gut microbiota shapes the efficiency of cancer therapy. Front Microbiol 10:1050

Masonic Cancer Center, University of Minnesota (2017) Phase I clinical trial of *Trametes versicolor* in women with breast cancer (Clinical trial registration No. NCT00680667). clinicaltrials.gov

Masonic Cancer Center, University of Minnesota (2020) A phase 1 study of an IL-2 expressing, attenuated *Salmonella* typhimurium in patients with unresectable hepatic spread from any non-hematologic primary (Clinical trial registration No. NCT01099631). clinicaltrials.gov

Mattiuzzi C, Lippi G (2019) Current cancer epidemiology. J Epidemiol Glob Health 9:217–222

Mayo Clinic (2023) Phase I trial of intratumoral administration of a measles virus derivative expressing the *Helicobacter pylori* neutrophil-activating protein (NAP) (MV-s-NAP) in patients with metastatic breast cancer (Clinical trial registration No. NCT04521764). clinicaltrials.gov

Meleshko A (2022) Pilot clinical study of DNA vaccination against neuroblastoma (Clinical trial registration No. NCT04049864). clinicaltrials.gov

Meyer J (2020) Colitis prospective cohort study: determining the aetiologies of acute colitis and developing a diagnostic score to identify patients requiring specific investigations (Clinical trial registration No. NCT02709213). clinicaltrials.gov

Morizono K, Xie Y, Ringpis G-E, Johnson M, Nassanian H, Lee B, Wu L, Chen ISY (2005) Lentiviral vector retargeting to P-glycoprotein on metastatic melanoma through intravenous injection. Nat Med 11:346–352

Nakashima H, Nguyen T, Kasai K, Passaro C, Ito H, Goins WF, Shaikh I, Erdelyi R, Nishihara R, Nakano I, Reardon DA, Anderson AC, Kuchroo V, Chiocca EA (2018) Toxicity and efficacy of a novel GADD34-expressing oncolytic HSV-1 for the treatment of experimental glioblastoma. Clin Cancer Res 24:2574–2584

Nanda R, Chow LQM, Dees EC, Berger R, Gupta S, Geva R, Pusztai L, Pathiraja K, Aktan G, Cheng JD, Karantza V, Buisseret L (2016) Pembrolizumab in patients with advanced triple-negative breast cancer: phase Ib KEYNOTE-012 study. J Clin Oncol 34:2460–2467

National Cancer Institute (NCI) (2008) A phase I trial of a live, genetically modified *Salmonella typhimurium* (VNP20009) for the treatment of cancer by intravenous administration (Clinical trial registration No. NCT00004988). clinicaltrials.gov

National Cancer Institute (NCI) (2020) A population-based case-control study of biliary tract cancers in Shanghai, China (Clinical trial registration No. NCT00339560). clinicaltrials.gov

Nienhuis AW, Dunbar CE, Sorrentino BP (2006) Genotoxicity of retroviral integration in hematopoietic cells. Mol Ther 13:1031–1049

Oelschlaeger TA (2010) Bacteria as tumor therapeutics? Bioeng Bugs 1:146–147

Omer R, Mohsin MZ, Mohsin A, Mushtaq BS, Huang X, Guo M, Zhuang Y, Huang J (2022) Engineered bacteria-based living materials for biotherapeutic applications. Front Bioeng Biotechnol 10:870675

One Health [WWW Document] (n.d.). https://www.who.int/news-room/questions-and-answers/item/one-health. Accessed 11 July 2023

Ottawa Hospital Research Institute (2023) Pioneering pre- and post-operative integrative care to improve thoracic cancer quality of care—the thoracic peri-operative integrative surgical care evaluation (POISE) Trial—Stage II (Clinical trial registration No. NCT04871412). clinicaltrials.gov

Ou J, Carbonero F, Zoetendal EG, DeLany JP, Wang M, Newton K, Gaskins HR, O'Keefe SJD (2013) Diet, microbiota, and microbial metabolites in colon cancer risk in rural Africans and African Americans. Am J Clin Nutr 98:111–120

Park SJ, Lee YK, Cho S, Uthaman S, Park I-K, Min J-J, Ko SY, Park J-O, Park S (2015) Effect of chitosan coating on a bacteria-based alginate microrobot. Biotechnol Bioeng 112:769–776

Park S-H, Zheng JH, Nguyen VH, Jiang S-N, Kim D-Y, Szardenings M, Min JH, Hong Y, Choy HE, Min J-J (2016) RGD peptide cell-surface display enhances the targeting and therapeutic efficacy of attenuated salmonella-mediated cancer therapy. Theranostics 6:1672–1682

Paterson Y, Guirnalda PD, Wood LM (2010) Listeria and salmonella bacterial vectors of tumor-associated antigens for cancer immunotherapy. Semin Immunol 22:183–189

Patyar S, Joshi R, Byrav DP, Prakash A, Medhi B, Das B (2010) Bacteria in cancer therapy: a novel experimental strategy. J Biomed Sci 17:21

Pesavento PA, Agnew D, Keel MK, Woolard KD (2018) Cancer in wildlife: patterns of emergence. Nat Rev Cancer 18:646–661

Pevsner-Fischer M, Tuganbaev T, Meijer M, Zhang S-H, Zeng Z-R, Chen M-H, Elinav E (2016) Role of the microbiome in non-gastrointestinal cancers. World J Clin Oncol 7:200–213

Pope JL, Tomkovich S, Yang Y, Jobin C (2017) Microbiota as a mediator of cancer progression and therapy. Transl Res 179:139–154

Post DE, Sandberg EM, Kyle MM, Devi NS, Brat DJ, Xu Z, Tighiouart M, Van Meir EG (2007) Targeted cancer gene therapy using a hypoxia inducible factor–dependent oncolytic adenovirus armed with interleukin-4. Cancer Res 67:6872–6881

Protara Therapeutics (2023) A phase 1b/2, dose expansion, open-label study to evaluate safety and anti-tumor activity, of intravesical instillation of TARA-002 in Adults with high-grade non-muscle invasive bladder cancer (Clinical trial registration No. NCT05951179). clinicaltrials.gov

Protara Therapeutics (2024) A phase 1a/b dose finding, open-label study to evaluate safety and toxicity of intravesical instillation of TARA-002 in adults with high-grade non-muscle invasive bladder cancer (Clinical trial registration No. NCT05085990). clinicaltrials.gov

Providence Health & Services (2018) Phase I study of safety and immunogenicity of ADU-623, a live-attenuated *Listeria monocytogenes* Strain (ΔactA/ΔinlB) expressing the EGFRvIII-NY-ESO-1 vaccine, in patients with treated and recurrent WHO Grade III/IV Astrocytomas (Clinical trial registration No. NCT01967758). clinicaltrials.gov

Qin J, Li R, Raes J, Arumugam M, Burgdorf KS, Manichanh C, Nielsen T, Pons N, Levenez F, Yamada T, Mende DR, Li J, Xu J, Li S, Li D, Cao J, Wang B, Liang H, Zheng H, Xie Y, Tap J, Lepage P, Bertalan M, Batto J-M, Hansen T, Le Paslier D, Linneberg A, Nielsen HB, Pelletier E, Renault P, Sicheritz-Ponten T, Turner K, Zhu H, Yu C, Li S, Jian M, Zhou Y, Li Y, Zhang X, Li S, Qin N, Yang H, Wang J, Brunak S, Doré J, Guarner F, Kristiansen K, Pedersen O, Parkhill J, Weissenbach J, Bork P, Ehrlich SD, Wang J (2010) A human gut microbial gene catalogue established by metagenomic sequencing. Nature 464:59–65

Quintero D, Carrafa J, Vincent L, Bermudes D (2016) EGFR-targeted Chimeras of Pseudomonas ToxA released into the extracellular milieu by attenuated Salmonella selectively kill tumor cells. Biotechnol Bioeng 113(12):2698–2711. https://doi.org/10.1002/bit.26026. Epub 2016 Jul 8. PMID: 27260220; PMCID: PMC5083144

Rahman MM, McFadden G (2021) Oncolytic viruses: newest frontier for cancer immunotherapy. Cancers (Basel) 13:5452

Ramesh N, Ge Y, Ennist DL, Zhu M, Mina M, Ganesh S, Reddy PS, Yu D-C (2006) CG0070, a conditionally replicating granulocyte macrophage Colony-stimulating factor–armed oncolytic adenovirus for the treatment of bladder cancer. Clin Cancer Res 12:305–313

Rodrigues G, Sanatani M (2012) Age and comorbidity considerations related to radiotherapy and chemotherapy administration. Semin Radiat Oncol 22:277–283

Rommasi F (2022) Bacterial-based methods for cancer treatment: what we know and where we are. Oncol Ther 10:23–54

Roy DG, Bell JC (2013) Cell carriers for oncolytic viruses: current challenges and future directions. OV 2:47–56

Roy S, Trinchieri G (2017) Microbiota: a key orchestrator of cancer therapy. Nat Rev Cancer 17: 271–285

Salonen A, Salojärvi J, Lahti L, de Vos WM (2012) The adult intestinal core microbiota is determined by analysis depth and health status. Clin Microbiol Infect 18(Suppl 4):16–20

Salspera LLC (2022) A phase 2 study of Saltikva (attenuated *Salmonella typhimurium* containing the human gene for interleukin-2) in patients with metastatic pancreatic cancer (Clinical trial registration No. NCT04589234). clinicaltrials.gov

Sanders KL, Fox BA, Bzik DJ (2015) Attenuated *Toxoplasma gondii* therapy of disseminated pancreatic cancer generates long-lasting immunity to pancreatic cancer. Onco Targets Ther 5: e1104447

Savage TM, Vincent RL, Rae SS, Huang LH, Ahn A, Pu K, Li F, de los Santos-Alexis K, Coker C, Danino T, Arpaia N (2023) Chemokines expressed by engineered bacteria recruit and orchestrate antitumor immunity. Sci Adv 9:eadc9436

Sawant SS, Patil SM, Gupta V, Kunda NK (2020) Microbes as medicines: harnessing the power of bacteria in advancing cancer treatment. Int J Mol Sci 21:7575

Second Affiliated Hospital, School of Medicine, Zhejiang University (2021) Efficacy and safety of probiotics combined with standard chemotherapy plus targeted therapy in patients with metastatic colorectal cancer: a prospective, open-label, randomized, multi-center clinical trial (Clinical trial registration No. NCT04131803). clinicaltrials.gov

Sedighi M, Zahedi Bialvaei A, Hamblin MR, Ohadi E, Asadi A, Halajzadeh M, Lohrasbi V, Mohammadzadeh N, Amiriani T, Krutova M, Amini A, Kouhsari E (2019) Therapeutic bacteria to combat cancer; current advances, challenges, and opportunities. Cancer Med 8:3167–3181

Sepp T, Ujvari B, Ewald PW, Thomas F, Giraudeau M (2019) Urban environment and cancer in wildlife: available evidence and future research avenues. Proc R Soc B 286:20182434

Serrano L, López AC, González SP, Palacios S, Dexeus D, Centeno-Mediavilla C, Coronado P, de la Fuente J, López JA, Vanrell C, Cortés J (2021) Efficacy of a *Coriolus versicolor*–based vaginal gel in women with human papillomavirus–dependent cervical lesions: the PALOMA study. J Low Genit Tract Dis 25:130

Shanmugam M, Abirami RG (2019) Microbial polysaccharides—chemistry and applications. J Biol Act Prod Nat 9:73–78

Shen H, Aggarwal N, Wun KS, Lee YS, Hwang IY, Chang MW (2022) Engineered microbial systems for advanced drug delivery. Adv Drug Deliv Rev 187:114364

Sidney Kimmel Comprehensive Cancer Center at Johns Hopkins (2023) A phase II single arm adaptive weight loss study in women with early stage breast cancer (Clinical trial registration No. NCT04499950). clinicaltrials.gov

Sikora A (2022) Window of opportunity trial of Neoadjuvant ADXS 11–001 vaccination prior to robot -assisted resection of HPV-positive oropharyngeal squamous cell carcinoma (Clinical trial registration No. NCT02002182). clinicaltrials.gov

Sinha R, Ahsan H, Blaser M, Caporaso JG, Carmical JR, Chan AT, Fodor A, Gail MH, Harris CC, Helzlsouer K, Huttenhower C, Knight R, Kong HH, Lai GY, Hutchinson DLS, Le Marchand L, Li H, Orlich MJ, Shi J, Truelove A, Verma M, Vogtmann E, White O, Willett W, Zheng W, Mahabir S, Abnet C (2018) Next steps in studying the human microbiome and health in prospective studies, Bethesda, MD, may 16–17, 2017. Microbiome 6:210

Song T-J, Haddad D, Adusumilli P, Kim T, Stiles B, Hezel M, Socci ND, Gönen M, Fong Y (2012) Molecular network pathways and functional analysis of tumor signatures associated with development of resistance to viral gene therapy. Cancer Gene Ther 19:38–48

Sunamura M, Hamada H, Motoi F, Oonuma M, Abe H, Saitoh Y, Hoshida T, Ottomo S, Omura N, Matsuno S (2004) Oncolytic Virotherapy as a novel strategy for pancreatic cancer. Pancreas 28:326

Tanaka Y, Shimizu S, Shirotani M, Yorozu K, Kitamura K, Oehorumu M, Kawai Y, Fukuzawa Y (2021) Nutrition and cancer risk from the viewpoint of the intestinal microbiome. Nutrients 13:3326

Tiptiri-Kourpeti A, Spyridopoulou K, Santarmaki V, Aindelis G, Tompoulidou E, Lamprianidou EE, Saxami G, Ypsilantis P, Lampri ES, Simopoulos C, Kotsianidis I, Galanis A, Kourkoutas Y, Dimitrellou D, Chlichlia K (2016) Lactobacillus casei exerts anti-proliferative effects accompanied by apoptotic cell death and up-regulation of TRAIL in colon carcinoma cells. PLoS One 11:e0147960

Toso JF, Gill VJ, Hwu P, Marincola FM, Restifo NP, Schwartzentruber DJ, Sherry RM, Topalian SL, Yang JC, Stock F, Freezer LJ, Morton KE, Seipp C, Haworth L, Mavroukakis S, White D, MacDonald S, Mao J, Sznol M, Rosenberg SA (2002) Phase I study of the intravenous administration of attenuated *Salmonella typhimurium* to patients with metastatic melanoma. J Clin Oncol 20:142–152

Ullah S, Khalil AA, Shaukat F, Song Y (2019) Sources, extraction and biomedical properties of polysaccharides. Food Secur 8:304

University Health Network, Toronto (2023) Feasibility study of microbial ecosystem therapeutics (MET-4) to evaluate effects of fecal microbiome in patients on immunotherapy (MET4-IO) (Clinical trial registration No. NCT03686202). clinicaltrials.gov

Urbaniak C, Gloor GB, Brackstone M, Scott L, Tangney M, Reid G (2016) The microbiota of breast tissue and its association with breast cancer. Appl Environ Microbiol 82:5039–5048

Vähä-Koskela MJV, Heikkilä JE, Hinkkanen AE (2007) Oncolytic viruses in cancer therapy. Cancer Lett 254:178–216

van der Sloot AM, Tur V, Szegezdi E, Mullally MM, Cool RH, Samali A, Serrano L, Quax WJ (2006) Designed tumor necrosis factor-related apoptosis-inducing ligand variants initiating apoptosis exclusively via the DR5 receptor. Proc Natl Acad Sci 103:8634–8639

Vion Pharmaceuticals (2013) A phase I trial of a live, genetically modified *Salmonella typhimurium* (VNP20009) for the treatment of cancer by intravenous administration (Clinical trial registration No. NCT00006254). clinicaltrials.gov

Watanabe Y, Kojima T, Kagawa S, Uno F, Hashimoto Y, Kyo S, Mizuguchi H, Tanaka N, Kawamura H, Ichimaru D, Urata Y, Fujiwara T (2010) A novel translational approach for human malignant pleural mesothelioma: heparanase-assisted dual virotherapy. Oncogene 29: 1145–1154

Watson GA, Heirali A, Oliva Bernal M, Cochrane K, Allen-Vercoe E, Eliason A, Jennings S, Taylor R, Hosni A, Hope A, Bratman SV, Chepeha DB, Weinreb I, Perez-Ordonez B, Waldron J, Xu W, Hansen AR, Siu LL, Coburn B, Spreafico A (2021) Prospective manipulation of the gut microbiome with microbial ecosystem therapeutic 4 (MET4) in locoregionally advanced oropharyngeal squamous cell carcinoma (LA-OPSCC) undergoing primary chemoradiation (ROMA2). J Clin Oncol 39:6059–6059

White J, Amato KR, Decaestecker E, McKenzie VJ (2023) Editorial: impact of anthropogenic environmental changes on animal microbiomes. Front Ecol Evol 11:1204035

Wu Z (2017) Phase 1 study of clinical nutrition that research safety and efficacy in lung neoplasms and breast carcinoma (Clinical trial registration No. NCT02603016). clinicaltrials.gov

Wu F (2023) The effect of chronic stress on efficacy of immune checkpoint inhibitors in patients with newly diagnosed esophageal cancer (Clinical trial registration No. NCT05967910). clinicaltrials.gov

Xie C (2022) Safety and efficacy of bifidobacterium therapy in patients with advanced liver cancer receiving immunotherapy: a randomized controlled, single-center clinical Trial (Clinical trial registration No. NCT05620004). clinicaltrials.gov

Xu Q (2021a) Probiotics enhance the treatment of PD-1 inhibitors in patients with liver cancer (Clinical trial registration No. NCT05032014). clinicaltrials.gov

Xu Q (2021b) The mechanism of probiotic lactobacillus bifidobacterium V9(Kex02)improving the efficacy of carilizumab combined with platinum in non-small cell lung cancer patients (Clinical trial registration No. NCT05094167). clinicaltrials.gov

Xu H, Piao L, Wu Y, Liu X (2022) IFN-γ enhances the antitumor activity of attenuated *Salmonella-mediated* cancer immunotherapy by increasing M1 macrophage and CD4 and CD8 T cell counts and decreasing neutrophil counts. Front Bioeng Biotechnol 10

Yu J (2023) Altered Gut microbiome composition by appendectomy contributes to colorectal cancer (Clinical trial registration No. NCT06091137). clinicaltrials.gov

Yun C-O, Hong J, Yoon A-R (2022) Current clinical landscape of oncolytic viruses as novel cancer immunotherapeutic and recent preclinical advancements. Front Immunol 13:953410

Zeng H, Umar S, Rust B, Lazarova D, Bordonaro M (2019) Secondary bile acids and short chain fatty acids in the colon: a focus on colonic microbiome, cell proliferation, inflammation, and cancer. Int J Mol Sci 20:1214

Zhao Y, Yu Y-B (2016) Intestinal microbiota and chronic constipation. Springerplus 5:1130

Zhao M, Yang M, Li X-M, Jiang P, Baranov E, Li S, Xu M, Penman S, Hoffman RM (2005) Tumor-targeting bacterial therapy with amino acid auxotrophs of GFP-expressing *Salmonella typhimurium*. Proc Natl Acad Sci USA 102:755–760

Zhao X, Xie N, Zhang H, Zhou W, Ding J (2023) Bacterial drug delivery Systems for cancer therapy: "why" and "how.". Pharmaceutics 15:2214

Zhou S, Gravekamp C, Bermudes D, Liu K (2018) Tumour-targeting bacteria engineered to fight cancer. Nat Rev Cancer 18:727–743

Bacteria-Based Approach to Cancer Therapy

Duy Binh Tran, Radka Bokorova, and Tohru Yamada

Abstract

Currently, surgery, radiation therapy, and chemotherapy alone or in combination are the most common methods for cancer treatment. However, conventional therapies often lack cancer selectivity, which can result in severe adverse effects. Although many efforts have been made, effective and targeted approaches to cancer treatment are still needed. One promising avenue involves harnessing the potential of bacteria for cancer therapy. In this chapter, we summarize recent advancements and future perspectives on bacteria-based strategies for cancer treatment. Central to the success of such strategies is the critical role played by genetic engineering and bacterial modification in ensuring safety and precision in the complex in vivo environment. Moreover, we review the potential for synergistic combination therapies, which integrate bacterial approaches with conventional treatments like chemo-, immuno-, and radiation therapy. This chapter also sheds light on the current status of research and development in the field, spanning preclinical investigations, animal models, and the transition to clinical trials and human applications, as well as future directions and remaining challenges will also be discussed.

D. B. Tran · R. Bokorova
Department of Surgery, Division of Surgical Oncology, University of Illinois College of Medicine, Chicago, IL, USA
e-mail: tdbinh22@uic.edu

T. Yamada (✉)
Department of Surgery, Division of Surgical Oncology, University of Illinois College of Medicine, Chicago, IL, USA

Richard & Loan Hill Department of Biomedical Engineering, University of Illinois College of Engineering, Chicago, IL, USA
e-mail: tohru@uic.edu

Interdisciplinary Cancer Research, https://doi.org/10.1007/16833_2024_337
Published online: 21 August 2024

Keywords

Anticancer · Bacterial interventions · Cancer therapy · Combination therapies · Engineered bacteria · Hypoxia · Probiotics · Tumor microenvironment · Tumor targeting

1 Introduction

Cancer is a heterogeneous disease that presents substantial difficulties in terms of diagnosis, therapy, and prevention. Despite the advances in conventional therapies, such as chemotherapy, radiation, and immunotherapy, many types of cancers remain incurable or relapse after treatment (Miller et al. 2022; Zhang et al. 2022a, b; Anand et al. 2023). Moreover, the current obstacles in cancer therapeutics, including heightened toxicity to normal cells, limited efficacy in treating deep tumor tissue, and the potential for developing drug resistances in cancer cells, have sparked the investigation of alternative methods (Gyanani et al. 2021; Anand et al. 2023). One of the major challenges in drug resistance arises from insufficient blood flow and oxygen supply in tumors, specifically within the hypoxic tumor microenvironment. This leads to decreased sensitivity in most tumors, resulting in poor therapeutic effects and increased resistance and metastasis (Chen et al. 2023). Hence, there is a medical need for novel and innovative approaches to combat cancer.

A prime example of earlier studies into the potential use of bacteria for cancer therapy dates back to as early as the nineteenth century, Dr. William Coley conducted injections of *Streptococcus pyogenes* and *S. marcescens* into patients with inoperable bone and soft tissue sarcomas. This treatment approach resulted in remission of the patients' cancer (Coley 1910; McCarthy 2006). In addition, the findings of several bacterial strains, including *Bifidobacteria*, *Clostridium*, *Escherichia*, *Listeria*, and *Salmonella* species, reveal the capability to naturally target tumors with easy penetration and rapid proliferation in the hypoxic tumor site (Vivarelli et al. 2019; Fan et al. 2022). They can selectively colonize tumors, change the immune system, break down the tumor microenvironment, and deliver therapeutic molecules (Cavarretta et al. 2017; Dean et al. 2020; Chen et al. 2021; Jiang et al. 2023; Kreitz et al. 2023; Ma et al. 2023) that are difficult to do with traditional therapies. In recent years, a significant amount of studies have been conducted on the design and evaluation of bacterial-mediated cancer therapy, aiming to develop therapeutic approaches that are both safe and effective. Therefore, a new strategy for the treatment of cancer with engineered bacteria has emerged, primarily focusing on delivering anticancer agents to tumor sites through the use of bacteria as carriers (Liu et al. 2022; Rommasi 2022; Zhao et al. 2023).

Engineered bacteria, genetically modified to serve as delivery vectors and therapeutic agents, possess the ability to transport a variety of therapeutic agents—such as cytotoxic agents, cytokines, prodrug-converting enzymes, therapeutic peptides/proteins, and immunomodulators—to the tumor site. This strategy enhances the accumulation of anticancer tumor payloads at the tumor sites and enables accurate timing of drug delivery. Simultaneously, it helps reduce systemic toxicity to the host by regulating bacterial gene expression (Yin et al. 2018; Leventhal et al. 2020; Hosseini-Giv et al. 2021; Yang et al. 2021). In particular, engineered bacteria appear to have the ability to differentiate between tumors and normal tissues with reduced toxicity (Nguyen et al. 2010; Yang et al. 2021).

In this article, we will provide a comprehensive overview of the mechanisms, engineering, and current applications of engineered bacterial approaches for cancer therapy. We will also discuss the current research and developments in this field, as well as the future directions and challenges.

2 Mechanisms of Bacterial Action in Cancer Therapy

2.1 Tumor-Targeting Properties

Bacteria employ various strategies, such as utilizing their innate motility, the ability to generate inflammatory reactions to elude the immune system, and chemotaxis, to target and enter tumors (Kang et al. 2022; Palma et al. 2022; Baer et al. 2023; Zhou et al. 2023a, b). Motility is an essential characteristic that enables bacteria to penetrate tumor tissue more deeply. A study by Forbes et al. revealed that *Salmonella* cells rapidly multiplied within tumors, forming colonies that swiftly spread throughout the entire tumor tissue region within a mere 3 days after being injected intravenously (Ganai et al. 2011). It is evident that the host immune response plays a significant role in shaping the distribution of bacteria within tumor tissue. Moreover, *Listeria* spp. selectively targets tumors by engaging in intracellular infection of tumor-infiltrating myeloid-derived suppressor cells, inducing their migration to the immunosuppressive tumor microenvironment (Chandra et al. 2013; Quispe-Tintaya et al. 2013). The transported *Listeria* subsequently undergoes transmission from myeloid-derived suppressor cells to cancer cells via a distinctive cell-cell spread mechanism (Chandra et al. 2013). Tumor microenvironments are characterized by low oxygen concentrations in hypoxic tumors, making them potentially attractive to obligate anaerobes. It's not surprising to discover that *C. novyi*-NT and *C. butyricum* are found to endure and thrive in oxygen-depleted environments within tumors (Roberts et al. 2014; Staedtke et al. 2016). Additionally, several studies have indicated that *S. typhimurium* has a chemotactic affinity toward and sustained residence within tumors, facilitated by the presence of metabolites released by dormant cancer cells in the tumor microenvironment (Kasinskas and Forbes 2006; Kasinskas and Forbes 2007). Song et al. demonstrated that *E. coli* was attracted by specific biochemical molecules, including clusterin, serglycin, and transforming growth factor-β2, which are secreted by carcinoma cells. As a result, they preferentially colonized and proliferated lung cancer cells (Song et al. 2018a, b). Meanwhile, our previous study showed a significantly higher level of circulating *Pseudomonas aeruginosa*-secreted azurin in the sera of cystic fibrosis patients. In response to this event, human cancer cells increased the secretion of aldolase A (Choi et al. 2023), also known as fructose-bisphosphate aldolase. This glycolytic enzyme is widely conserved in bacteria, archaea, and eukaryotic species (Jewett and Sibley 2003; Tunio et al. 2010; Diaz et al. 2016). It is intriguing that this activity played a role in the colonization of *P. aeruginosa* in cancer cells. In addition, our research uncovered a correlation between the presence of *P. aeruginosa* and azurin in tumors and improved overall survival rates in cancer patients. Taken together, our findings reveal the bidirectional regulation of bacterial-cancer communication, suggesting the possibility of azurin in inhibiting tumor growth (Choi et al. 2023).

After successfully colonizing and penetrating tumors, living bacteria proliferate within the tumor microenvironment (Duong et al. 2019). Some of those bacteria can alter cancer cells proliferation by causing necrosis, apoptosis, or by releasing toxins, enzymes, and bacterial metabolites (Fig. 1) (Patyar et al. 2010; Stachowiak et al. 2012; Aganja et al. 2022). Interestingly, distinct mechanisms are displayed by different strains of bacteria to suppress tumors in tumor microenvironments. For example, *C. perfringens* can produce enterotoxin that can damage the DNA or membranes of cancer cells (Pahle et al. 2017). Meanwhile, *Listeria* spp. kills cancer cells by activating $NADP^+$ oxidase and elevating intracellular calcium levels, thereby initiating reactive oxygen species (ROS) production (Kim et al. 2009). In the case of *Salmonella*, upon entering the tumor, *S. typhimurium* continues to proliferate and eliminate cancer cells directly by initiating apoptosis, necrosis, and cell rupture (Ganai et al. 2011; Zheng et al. 2017). In a previous study, we

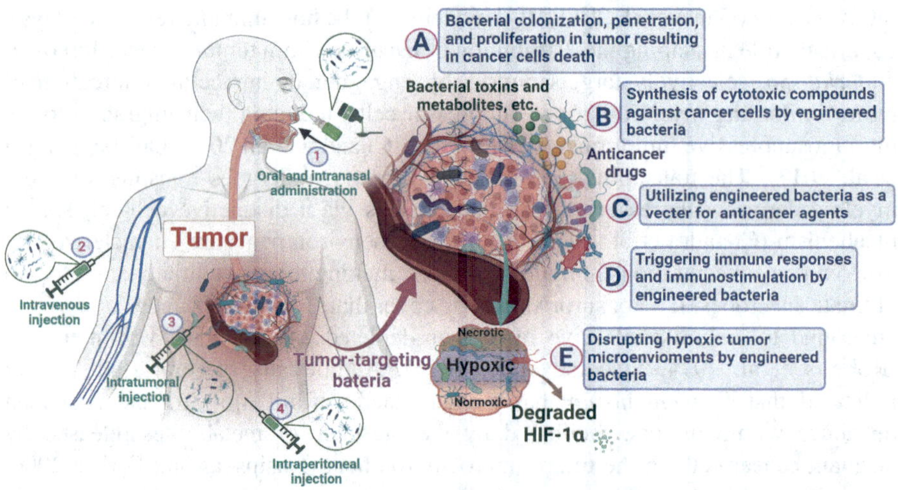

Fig. 1 Bacterial effects in tumor. Engineered bacteria are delivered through systemic administration such as ① oral and intranasal administration, ② intravenous, ③ intratumoral, and ④ intraperitoneal injection. Such bacteria can colonize, penetrate, and proliferate within the tumor microenvironment (**a**). Bacterial toxins and metabolites can kill tumor cells by inducing apoptosis or autophagy (**b**). Anticancer agents can be transported by engineered bacteria to enhance their specificity (**c**). Engineered bacteria that have colonized the tumor microenvironment can stimulate immune cells to eradicate tumors (**d**). Engineered bacteria can regulate the tumor microenvironment by reducing hypoxia (**e**)

demonstrated that the administration of *P. aeruginosa*-secreted azurin to transgenic mice that spontaneously develop mammary tumors resulted in reduced tumor growth (Choi et al. 2023). The mice were intraperitoneally injected with either PBS control or 2.5 mg/kg of azurin three times per week for 60 days. The results showed that the azurin group not only significantly reduced tumor volume but also improved survival rates compared to the control group (Choi et al. 2023).

A plethora of studies indicate that bacteria can regulate the tumor microenvironment by degrading the extracellular matrix, disrupting the blood supply, alleviating hypoxia, and adjusting to pH levels (Singhal and Shah 2020; Yuan et al. 2023). For instance, *C. histolyticum* degrades the extracellular matrix, which includes collagen and hyaluronic acid, through the secretion of collagenases (Shi et al. 2010), while *S. enterica* causes vascular injury and hemorrhage, which reduces blood flow and oxygen delivery to tumors (Leschner et al. 2009). It has also been reported that *E. coli* generates hydrogen peroxide, which serves to elevate oxygen levels and lowers the pH within tumors (Kumar and Imlay 2013). It is evident that the capacity of such bacteria to specifically target, penetrate, and proliferate within tumors presents a promising advantage, addressing some issues in existing therapies. However, more research is required to fully understand why these bacteria target and grow in tumors and their associated benefits.

2.2 Immune Activation Properties

Tumor hypoxia refers to a biological state marked by inadequate oxygen supply to tissues, leading to a compromise in normal biological functioning. Further, the abnormal tumor proliferation increases their vulnerability to hypoxia, particularly in malignant solid tumors. Hypoxia in the tumor microenvironment also contributes to the suppressive activity of local immune cells (Chouaib et al. 2017; Roy et al. 2020). During the progression of tumors, the uncontrolled development of cancer cells leads to the depletion of oxygen and nutrients that are necessary for immune cells (Zhang and Romero 2018; Zhao et al. 2021). The immune cells therefore become exhausted, adopt a suppressive phenotype characterized by the secretion of pro-cancer cytokines and chemokines, and exhibit a diminished responsiveness to anticancer signals. Bacterial components such as peptidoglycan, lipopolysaccharides, flagellin, CpG motifs, and lipoteichoic acid (Silhavy et al. 2010; Vendeville et al. 2011; Matsuura 2013) can activate the immune system by stimulating innate immune cells such as macrophages, dendritic cells, natural killer cells, and neutrophils, to produce pro-inflammatory cytokines and chemokines. These signaling molecules, in turn, can recruit and activate adaptive immune cells, such as T cells and B cells (Häcker et al. 2002; Sukhithasri et al. 2013; D'Orazio 2019; Zhang et al. 2022a, b; Yin et al. 2023; Zhou et al. 2023a, b). For instance, flagellin from *S. typhimurium* has been observed to elicit an antitumor response from $CD8^+$ T cells and natural killer cells, while simultaneously reducing the frequency of regulatory T cells (Tregs) (Hajam et al. 2017; Zhou et al. 2018). In addition to enhancing immunity against tumors by encouraging the release of immune-stimulating agents, Saccheri et al. demonstrated that *Salmonella* spp. induces an increased production of connexin-43 in melanoma cells (Saccheri et al. 2010). This protein reduces the production of the immunosuppressive enzyme indoleamine 2,3-dioxygenase (IDO) and enhances the cross-presentation and transfer of processed tumor antigenic peptides between dendritic cells and cancer cells (Saccheri et al. 2010; Lin et al. 2017). Specifically, a dual mechanism involving direct death of cancer cells via *Listeria* infection and a cytotoxic T cell response targeting *Listeria* antigens is responsible for the reduction in tumor size caused by *Listeria* spp. (Kim et al. 2009; Stavru et al. 2011). Also, *Listeria* species induce an immune-stimulating phenotype in a portion of myeloid-derived suppressor cells infected with *Listeria*, resulting in the production of the cytokine interleukin-12 (IL-12), a cytokine linked to increased responses from T and NK cells (Chandra et al. 2013). *E. coli* can express antigens that can induce targeted antibody or T cell responses against tumors (Bennek et al. 2019; Uchida et al. 2020; de Alwis et al. 2021). Meanwhile, *Lactobacillus* exhibits the ability to inhibit the activity or expression of immunosuppressive factors, including regulatory T cells, myeloid-derived suppressor cells, or programmed death-ligand 1 (Winnie et al. 2023). Also, the oral administration of *L. rhamnosus* GG resulted in an augmentation of tumor-infiltrating dendritic cells and facilitated the recruitment of $CD8^+$ T cells via the type I interferon (IFN) signaling pathway (Si et al. 2022). In sum, it is postulated that some bacterial infections have a substantial influence on tumor regression by rousing a wide range of immune cells within the tumor microenvironment, in addition to its inherent anticancer effects. Despite variations in primary mechanisms, it appears that some bacteria employ an immunotherapy strategy, which shows potential through the use of advanced genetic engineering techniques on bacterial strains.

3 Genetic Engineering of Bacteria

3.1 Engineering Bacteria for Safety

One of the primary challenges associated with utilizing bacteria as therapeutic agents lies in ensuring their safety. This implies that engineered bacteria should not harm the host cells or cause unwanted side effects. It should be noted that certain bacterial products contribute to their inherent antitumor activity (Hiraoka et al. 2004; Yamada et al. 2004; Hong et al. 2006; Taylor et al. 2009). Therefore, attenuation strategies should be precisely tuned to ensure a reduction in virulence without compromising their antitumor efficacy. *S. typhimurium* VNP20009 has been engineered to attenuate its virulence or toxicity by deleting *msbB* and *purI* genes involved in pathogenicity and metabolism. This strain has been thoroughly tested in mice with tumors, showing promising specificity in tumor-targeting and growth-inhibiting effects (Cunningham and Nemunaitis 2001; Toso et al. 2002). In another study, genes associated with endotoxin were either suppressed or rendered less functional in order to modify a *Salmonella* strain with diminished detrimental effects. *Salmonella* strains with mutations in *relA* and *spoT*, which play a crucial role in the production of ppGpp, a signaling molecule linked to the expression of toxin genes, showed minimal toxicity (Fujimori 2006). Remarkably, the elimination of the *phoP* and *phoQ* genes in *Salmonella* not only preserved its capacity to combat cancer, but also resulted in a reduction of its harm to healthy tissues (Cheng et al. 2014). As a result, these mutated strains have been employed for both vaccine manufacturing and as a means of transporting tumor treatments (Matsui et al. 2015; Shprung et al. 2021).

3.2 Engineering Bacteria to Enhance Therapeutic Effectiveness

3.2.1 Enhancing Tumor-Targeting Ability

It is important for therapeutic agents to have a tumor-targeting ability, as it not only determines the therapeutic efficacy but also ensures the elimination of off-target damage. Ensuring survival of the engineered bacteria in tumor sites while preventing it in normal tissues is of utmost importance in enhancing tumor targeting. *L. monocytogenes* was effectively facilitated by antibodies or ligands that bind to tumor-specific receptors, thereby significantly increasing their affinity for tumor cells. This particular strain has the ability to effectively target and infiltrate various tumor cell lines, including the human cancer cell lines (SK-BR-3, SKOV-3), the murine 4 T1 tumor cell line, and the isogenic 4 T1-HER2 cell line (Heisig et al. 2011). It is well documented that the $\alpha_v\beta_3$ integrin is overexpressed on cancer cells (Brooks et al. 1994, 1995; Friedlander et al. 1995; Gladson 1996; Liu et al. 2008a, b). *S. typhimurium* strain SHJ203, a ppGpp-deficient strain, was genetically engineered to target tumors by displaying the integrin-binding peptide Arg-Gly-Asp on the bacterial surface. The resulting strain demonstrated enhanced tumor selectivity and significantly higher anticancer activity in xenografts of MDA-MB-435 melanoma and MDA-MB-231 breast cancer cells (Park et al. 2016). In addition, developing auxotrophic mutants is a deliberate strategy to enhance the targeting abilities of bacteria. By leveraging the differences in nutrient composition between normal tissues and tumor sites, bacteria can be precisely engineered to colonize and proliferate exclusively within the tumor tissue. For instance, *Salmonella* A1, an auxotrophic strain for leucine and arginine, and *Salmonella* SF104, with a mutated *aroA* gene requiring aromatic amino acids, was designed to prevent proliferation in normal tissues while specifically colonizing in tumor sites due to their requirement for aromatic amino acids (Zhao et al. 2005; Felgner et al. 2016). Similarly, *E. coli* Nissle was engineered by Leventhal et al. with the deletion of two auxotrophies (*thyA* and *dapA*), rendering it unable to survive outside the tumor microenvironment (Leventhal et al. 2020). Through the inactivation of the *dal/dat* locus, an *L. monocytogenes* strain was engineered to be auxotrophic for the cell wall component D-alanine. This resulted in a mutant strain that was significantly attenuated virulence yet retained the capability of inducing cytotoxic T cells (Thompson et al. 1998; Zheng et al. 2017).

3.2.2 Enhancing Evasiveness and Controlling Proliferation

In addition to engineering tumor targeting, enhancing the escape abilities of bacteria from the host immune system is also crucial to improving therapeutic effectiveness. Currently, *Listeria* serves as a vaccine strain primarily utilized for expressing tumor antigens (Flickinger et al. 2018; Oladejo et al. 2021; Su et al. 2021). The attenuation of virulence is achieved through the deletion of the *prfA* gene. However, these engineered strains face challenges in evading host innate immune cells, including macrophages, neutrophils, and dendritic cells. This limitation impedes their ability to carry tumor antigens effectively, thereby reducing therapeutic effectiveness. To address this issue, such engineered bacteria were genetically modified to reduce the levels of PrfA and *Listeria* hemolysin O, aiming to reduce immune responses in the host. It suggests that the advanced strain can significantly enhance the expression of tumor antigens, indicating they may hold great potential for the delivery of other therapeutic drugs (Wood and Paterson 2014). Another challenge is the vigorous proliferation of bacteria in the host cells. Therefore, the genetically engineered bacteria must aim to regulate and maintain the stability of the microecology. In nature, when the bacterial population reaches a critical density, the lysis factor derived from the bacteriophage is released (Hibbing et al. 2010; Tasaki et al. 2017). It diffuses to surrounding cells and induces lysis. Based on this, Din et al. devised a synchronized lysis circuit (SLC) that integrates the phage φX174 cleavage gene E to regulate bacterial proliferation in vivo. As expected, the bacterial populations can be controlled, allowing surviving bacteria to continue regenerating and maintaining the dynamic balance of local bacterial populations in vivo (Din et al. 2016).

3.2.3 Enhancing Cytotoxic Agents

Bacteria can carry cytotoxic or cytostatic agents with intrinsic antitumor activity (Song et al. 2018a, b; Zhou et al. 2018; Ebrahimzadeh et al. 2021). To enhance the efficiency of cancer therapy, bacteria will be genetically engineered using inducible promoters to augment the expression of cytotoxic agents. Our previous studies have demonstrated that cupredoxin protein azurin, which is secreted by an opportunistic pathogen *P. aeruginosa,* triggers apoptosis in various types of cancer cells (Yamada et al. 2002a, b; Punj et al. 2004; Yamada et al. 2005; Choi et al. 2023; Taglialegna 2023). Site-directed mutants of azurin improved the p53 stabilization ability, enhancing apoptotic cell death (Hu et al. 2023). A fusion protein of azurin with cationic elastin-like protein showed a significantly higher anti-proliferative effect as compared to azurin alone (Bhardwaj and Mishra 2023). In other studies, *S. typhimurium* and *E. coli* have been genetically modified to produce Cytolysin A, a 34 kDa protein that forms pores and causes hemolysis. This modification is facilitated by either a constitutive promoter or inducible promoters activated by arabinose or doxycycline. These engineered bacteria have exhibited remarkable antitumor activity (Jiang et al. 2010; Jiang et al. 2013). TNF-α, TRAIL, and the Fas ligand, acting as cytotoxic agents, can induce apoptosis in tumor cells. However, due to their short half-life and potential hepatotoxicity, their therapeutic application faces challenges (Ganai et al. 2009; Nagakura et al. 2009; Cao et al. 2010; Yoon et al. 2011). An engineered *S. Typhimurium* strain, developed by Ganai et al., was designed to express murine TRAIL under the regulation of the radiation-inducible *recA* promoter. TRAIL was gradually released by irradiation, resulting in significantly reduced mammary tumor growth and an improvement in the survival rate (Ganai et al. 2009).

3.2.4 Enhancing Immunomodulatory Capabilities

Bacteria that have been genetically modified can be altered to carry or express exogenous immunotherapeutic agents, which not only makes them more effective against tumors but also enhances their immune regulatory effects (Poorebrahim et al. 2020; Ma et al. 2023). To enhance the anticancer immune response, bacteria have been genetically engineered to express cytokines, chemokines, and tumor antigens, and/or facilitate the recruitment of immune cells to approach the tumor site (Gurbatri et al. 2022; Savage et al. 2023). Many studies have highlighted the notable progress of attenuated *S. typhimurium* in expressing interleukin-2 (IL-2), a development that underwent evaluation in mouse, veterinary canine, and human clinical trials (NCT01099631) (Ha et al. 2012; Fritz et al. 2016; Zhou et al. 2018). A study within this context involved the utilization of attenuated *S. typhimurium* to secrete *Vibrio vulnificus* flagellin B into the tumor microenvironment (Zheng et al. 2017). The presence of this antigen demonstrated a capacity to enhance the polarization of macrophages from M2-type (anti-inflammatory) to M1-type (pro-inflammatory). Moreover, it led to an augmentation of macrophage secretion of antitumor cytokines, specifically interleukin-1β (IL-1β) and tumor necrosis factor-alpha (TNF-α) (Zheng et al. 2017). Also, improving the immune systems in mice and preventing them from developing intestinal infections can be accomplished by orally administering a mutant strain of *S. typhimurium* that does not produce the ZnuABC zinc transport system (Zhang et al. 2016). In addition, attenuated *S. typhimurium* for the synthesis of interleukin-18 showed the enhanced infiltration of $DX5^+$ NK cells and $CD3^+/CD4^+$ T cells within the tumor microenvironment (Loeffler et al. 2008). Important cytokines, such as interleukin-1β (IL-1β), tumor necrosis factor-alpha (TNF-α), interferon-gamma (IFN-γ), and granulocyte-macrophage colony-stimulating factor (GM-CSF), were consequently overexpressed. This orchestrated immune response culminated in the manifestation of a discernible antitumor effect (Loeffler et al. 2008).

3.3 Engineering Bacteria for Prodrug-Converting Enzymes

Many studies demonstrated that prodrug-converting enzymes can convert prodrugs into cytotoxic agents targeting tumors (Malekshah et al. 2016; Sheikh et al. 2021). Bacteria have the capacity to synthesize and transport various prodrug-converting enzymes (Cheng et al. 2008; Friedlos et al. 2008; Weibel et al. 2008; Tang et al. 2009). To optimize this capability of bacteria, the genetic modifications have been conducted. For example, 5-Aziridinyl-2,4-dinitrobenzamide (CB1954) is a monofunctional DNA-alkylating agent that is activated by nitroreductase (Knox et al. 1988; Djeha et al. 2001; Palmer et al. 2003; Theys et al. 2006). The engineered *C. sporogenes*, encoding nitroreductase, convert the prodrug CB1954 into a highly toxic bifunctional DNA-alkylating agent, resulting in the formation of multiple DNA cross-links (Heap et al. 2014). Likewise, the enzyme cytosine deaminase (CD) serves as a noteworthy example of this approach, as it facilitates the conversion of the non-toxic prodrug 5-fluorocytosine (5-FC) into the cytotoxic chemotherapeutic agent 5-fluorouracil (5-FU) (Dresselaers et al. 2003). In preclinical studies, natural tumor-targeting bacteria, including *S. typhimurium*, *Clostridium* spp., and the probiotic bacterium *B. longum*, have been genetically modified to express CD. This modification enables the synthesis of 5-FU, resulting in significant antitumor effects (King et al. 2002; Liu et al. 2002; Barbé et al. 2005; Sasaki et al. 2006; Liu et al. 2008a, b). In addition to the aforementioned engineered bacteria, *E. coli* DH5α expressing β-glucuronidase has also been developed as a distinct prodrug-converting enzyme delivery strain. This strain can hydrolyze the 9-aminocamptothecin glucuronide (9ACG) prodrug, converting it into the topoisomerase I inhibitor 9-aminocamptothecin (9 AC), thereby efficiently inhibiting tumor growth (Zhou et al. 2018).

3.4 Engineering Bacteria for Payload Delivery

In order to achieve drug loading within bacterial cells, drugs can be introduced into bacterial cells either by direct incorporation or by loading them into bacteria in the form of nucleic acids utilizing gene-editing technology (Zhao et al. 2023). Xie et al. loaded 5-fluorouracil (5-FU) and zoledronic acid into *E. coli,* then proceeded to modify the surface of *E. coli* with Au nanorods whereas Zoaby et al. aimed to deliver doxorubicin liposomes to *S. typhimurium* (Zoaby et al. 2017; Xie et al. 2021). On the other hand, gene editing in bacteria involves the transfection of DNA fragments expressing anticancer substances in the form of plasmids. This manipulation enables the regulation of bacteria, ensuring the continuous production of anticancer-related substances such as cytotoxic agents, tumor antigens, immune factors, and other bioactive compounds. Consequently, this approach facilitates the sustained and prolonged delivery of therapeutic effects within the tumor. An attenuated strain of *S. typhimurium* has the ability to produce cytolysin A when the L-arabinose promoter is activated. Upon reaching the tumor site, the introduction of L-arabinose activates the promoter, allowing the bacteria to express cytolysin A (Nguyen et al. 2010). This targeted activation mechanism enables the bacteria to selectively eliminate tumor cells while minimizing damage to normal tissue.

4 Engineered Bacteria in Synergistic Cancer Therapy

In recent years, many studies have indicated that the combination of traditional cancer treatments—chemotherapy, photodynamic and photothermal therapy, radiotherapy, and immunotherapy—with engineered bacteria has promising potential in

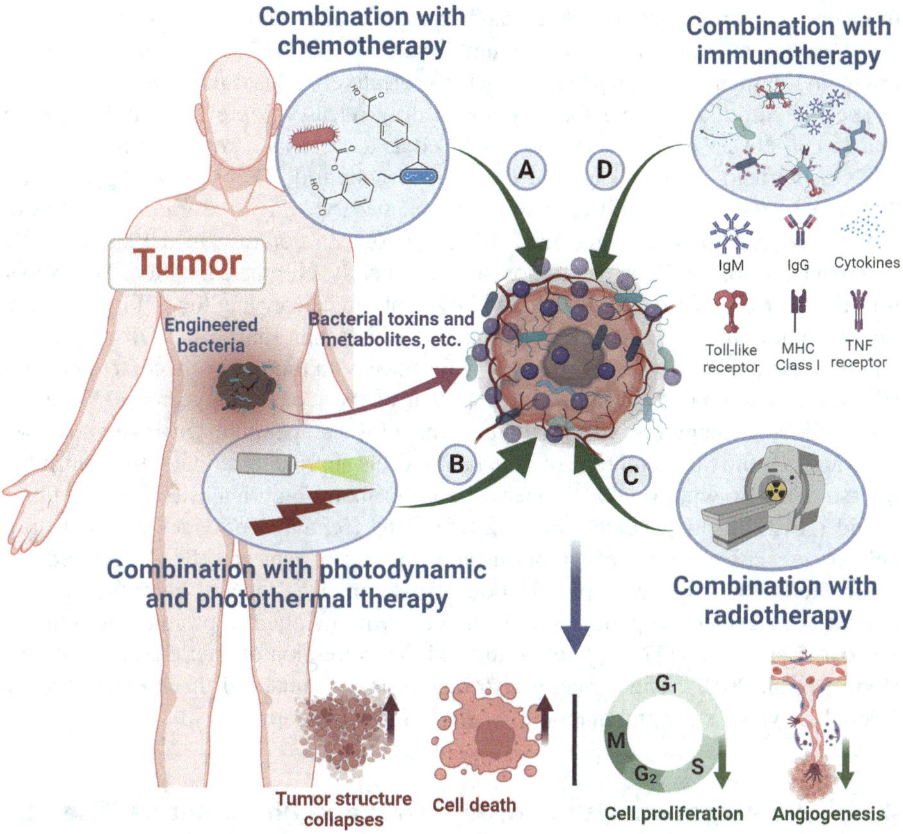

Fig. 2 Engineered bacteria in combination therapy. Engineered bacterial therapy in combination with traditional cancer treatments such as chemotherapy (**a**), photodynamic and photothermal therapy (**b**), radiotherapy (**c**), and immunotherapy (**d**)

cancer treatment (Fig. 2). In this section, we summarize recent strategies on bacteria in combination with traditional cancer treatments.

4.1 Combination with Chemotherapy

Despite recent advancements in drug delivery systems, chemotherapy continues to face challenges such as off-target effects and restricted intratumoral delivery (Yadav et al. 2021). As previously mentioned, leveraging the tumor-colonizing characteristics of bacteria and their ability to penetrate deeply into hypoxic intratumoral regions, bacterial-mediated chemotherapy has successfully addressed the aforementioned challenges, thereby enhancing the therapeutic efficacy of chemotherapeutics (Duong et al. 2019). Engineered bacteria have been designed to form conjugates with anticancer drugs through stimulus-responsive linkers. Upon intravenous administration, bacteria-carrying drugs show a preference for translocating to the tumor interstitium (Wang et al. 2022a, b). In the tumor microenvironments, the drug-loaded bacteria selectively release the drugs in response to specific stimuli, allowing for on-demand drug release. A previous study showed that *E. coli* Nissle 1917 (EcN) was employed as a bacterial carrier for immobilizing DOX using acid-labile linkages of cis-aconitic anhydride (EcN-ca-Dox) (Xie et al. 2017). After the injection of EcN-ca-Dox conjugates for 3 days, the amount of DOX in tumors reached approximately 5.0% ID g^{-1} tissue. In contrast, in the single DOX treatment group, DOX at the tumor site was nearly eliminated. After 30 days of injection of EcN-ca-Dox conjugate and DOX into mice carrying the 4 T1 tumor, the tumor volume in the EcN-ca-Dox group was lower than that in the Dox group. In addition, the median survival time at 50% for mice with tumors that were treated with EcN-ca-Dox was nearly 50% longer than that of the Dox therapy group (Xie et al. 2017). Ektate et al. pioneered a method in which low-temperature-sensitive liposomes were loaded onto the membrane of *Salmonella*. This approach facilitates the controlled release of DOX within colon cancer cells by utilizing high-intensity focused ultrasound (HIFU) heating (Ektate et al. 2018). This technique provides efficient drug delivery, reaching both the cytoplasm and nucleus of cancer cells. Moreover, the engineered strain induced a polarization of macrophages toward the antitumor M1 phenotype, elevated the population of Th1 cells with heightened production of tumor necrosis factor-alpha (TNF-α), and mitigated the expression of interleukin-10 (IL-10) (Ektate et al. 2018). This strategy also demonstrates enhanced therapeutic efficacy through a synergistic combination of chemo-immunotherapy.

4.2 Combination with Photodynamic and Photothermal Therapy

To date, several studies have shown that bacteria can be used as carriers to deliver therapeutic agents for photodynamic and photothermal therapy. *Salmonella* was engineered to express fluorogenic-activated protein (FAP), activated by a specific laser photosensitizer. FAP inhibits tumor growth by generating ROS (He et al. 2016). The combination of this engineered *Salmonella* and photodynamic therapy effectively suppresses the proliferation of cancer cells, improving animal survival rates in colon cancer models. The intratumoral injection of engineered *Salmonella* penetrated in the vascular system, giving rise to thrombus formation that darkens the tumor site, thereby facilitating enhanced near-infrared (NIR) absorption (Guo et al. 2022). Simultaneously, the targeted laser activation of photosensitizers induced the production of ROS, leading to cell lysis and the subsequent release of antigens that trigger the activation of immune cells. Furthermore, this synergistic impact not only enhanced the immune response triggered by bacteria against the tumor but also mitigated the potential negative side effects linked to bacterial therapy (Guo et al. 2022).

In photothermal therapy, photosensitizers that absorb light in the NIR spectrum are employed to convert light energy into heat, capable of selectively eliminating specific cells. Photosensitizers have been loaded onto the surface of bacteria during bacterial-mediated photothermal therapy, resulting in the development of a bacteria-driven photosensitizer delivery system. Irradiation of bacteria loaded with photosensitizers using a near-infrared laser led to the elimination of solid tumors (Luo et al. 2022). This combination shows great potential for effectively and safely treating solid malignancies (Nam et al. 2018). In a noteworthy study, Chen et al. loaded indocyanine green (ICG)-containing photosensitizers, known as iron oxide nanoparticles (INPs), onto the surface of *S. typhimurium* YB1 via amide bonds. This process resulted in the development of a biotic and abiotic complex designated as YB1-INPs for the delivery of anticancer drugs. The YB1-INPs exhibited a remarkable ability to specifically target tumors, effectively inhibiting tumor growth in mice when exposed to NIR laser irradiation. Additionally, they demonstrated their potential in fluorescence imaging (Chen et al. 2019a, b). C57BL/6 mice with transplanted MB49 bladder tumors were intravenously injected with either INPs or YB1-INPs. After 12 h of injection, mice were subjected to radiation. The temperature of the tumor in the INPs treatment reached only 43 °C, which was not high enough to completely eliminate the tumor. In contrast, the temperature of the tumor in the YB1-INPs treatment reached up to 63 °C. After 28 days of YB1-INPs treatment, the tumor was completely eradicated, leading to a 100% survival rate (Chen et al. 2019a, b). It is evident that melanin, known for its ability to convert 99.9% of absorbed light energy into heat, is effective in photothermal therapy for antitumor efficacy. To leverage this property, Gujrati et al. developed engineered outer membrane vesicles encapsulating melanin (OMV_{Mel}) for the specific targeting of tumor tissue, serving both diagnostic and ablative purposes (Gujrati et al. 2019).

4.3 Combination with Radiotherapy

Bacterial approach in combination with radiotherapy is emerging as an innovative option for tumor treatment. Although a few studies have been conducted on the application of bacteria to enhance radiotherapy, this approach remains a promising avenue in the field of therapeutic radiation oncology. In a colon cancer model exposed to 21 Gy of radiation, the synergistic treatment method on irradiation with *E. coli* demonstrated a considerable tumor reduction and the production of cytolysin A from *E. coli* (Jiang et al. 2010). Another approach involved the use of attenuated *Salmonella* VNP20009 loaded with antigen-adsorbing cationic polymer nanoparticles, combined with irradiation. This combination significantly enhanced the activation of dendritic cells and triggered a robust systemic antitumor response (Wang et al. 2022a, b). In a recent study, engineered *E. coli* and Bi_2S_3 nanoparticles were used to create a comprehensive nanosystem that improved radiation sensitivity (Algethami et al. 2015; Galain et al. 2022). *E. coli* was engineered to infiltrate tumor sites and enhance the expression of cytolysin A protein, triggering a shift in the cell cycle from a state of resistance to radiation to a state of sensitivity to radiation. At the same time, the Bi_2S_3 nanoparticles demonstrated the ability to increase radiation sensitivity by inducing DNA damage and stimulating intracellular ROS production

(Pan et al. 2022). Overall, bacteria-mediated radioimmunotherapy represents a promising and adaptable combination antitumor strategy.

4.4 Combination with Immunotherapy

Cancer immunotherapy in combination with bacterial approach appears to have enormous potential. Some bacteria can activate the immune system and play a role in synthesizing or delivering anticancer drugs, thereby enhancing the overall antitumor effect (Zhou et al. 2023a, b). As described earlier, bacteria have been genetically engineered to serve as a means of delivering antigens for cancer treatment. After systemic administration (Fig. 1), engineered bacteria that secrete antigens colonize tumor tissue, subsequently triggering the infiltration of immune cells. The invading bacteria release antigens that, in turn, stimulate intratumoral T cells, initiating an immune response against tumor cells (Yang et al. 2021). For instance, *E. coli* TOP10 demonstrated a notable decrease in tumors in a mouse model of colon carcinoma. This was achieved by promoting the generation of $CD8^+$ T and $CD4^+$ cells that specifically target the tumors. $CD8^+$ T cells were the primary effectors in immunological responses against tumors throughout this event (Stern et al. 2015). Attenuated *S. typhimurium* strains have been utilized to secrete a diverse array of tumor antigens, such as CEA-scFv, HPV16-E7, and *V. vulnificus* flagellin B, which serve to trigger the immune response (Zheng et al. 2017). Also, engineered probiotics have the potential to act as carriers for delivering checkpoint-blocking nanobodies, that include programmed cell death–ligand 1 (PD-L1) and cytotoxic T lymphocyte–associated protein-4 (CTLA-4), hence boosting antitumor efficacy (Gurbatri et al. 2020). A recent study showed that systematically administered bacterial outer membrane vesicles could stimulate the production of antitumor cytokines, such as interferon-γ and C-X-C motif chemokine ligand 10 (CXCL10), thereby activating a potent antitumor response (Kim et al. 2017). Specifically, Chen et al. developed polymeric micelles (ORFT) loaded with Tegafur (FT) and coated with outer membrane vesicles. The micelles were further surface-modified using phospholipid polyethylene glycol RGD. Remarkably, the ORFT group treatment demonstrated a significantly higher presence of effector memory T cells, along with a significant increase in both interferon-gamma (IFN-γ) and interleukin-12 (IL-12) levels compared to the FT group. Therefore, the tumor volumes in the ORFT group decreased by 50% compared to those in the FT group (Chen et al. 2019a, b).

5 Clinical Trials of Engineered Bacteria-Based Therapeutics

Dr. William Coley suggested the treatment of cancer using the live agent erysipelas (*S. pyogenes*) (Coley 1910). Since then, various types of bacteria including *Mycobacterium bovis*, *Bifidobacterium* spp., *S. typhimurium*, *L. monocytogenes*, and *C. novyi* have been genetically modified to help deliver therapeutics to solid tumors such as bladder, liver, colon, breast, and brain cancer (Staedtke et al. 2015; Liu et al.

2016; Galain et al. 2022; Song et al. 2023; Vajari et al. 2023). To date, engineered bacterial strains, which have demonstrated promising results in preclinical studies, have undergone clinical testing in humans to evaluate both their therapeutic efficacy and safety. Currently, clinicaltrials.gov lists over 76 clinical trials involving live bacteria for cancer therapy. Among these studies, 35 clinical trials focus on applied engineered bacteria. Table 1 shows representative completed and ongoing clinical studies.

Several engineered bacterial strains, which demonstrate promising results in preclinical studies, have undergone clinical testing in humans to evaluate their therapeutic efficacy and safety. For example, widely employed in clinical practice, a live vaccine comprises an attenuated suspension of bovine tuberculosis (Kulchavenya et al. 2013; Tran et al. 2014; Lenis et al. 2020). The attenuated *S. typhimurium* VNP20009 strain was the first *Salmonella* strain to undergo phase I human clinical trials. Developed by Vion Pharmaceuticals, Inc. in 1999, its efficacy was evaluated in 45 patients with metastatic melanoma and one patient with metastatic renal carcinoma (Sznol 1999). The study involved escalating doses (1×10^6—1×10^9 CFU/m^2 administered via intravenous injection), revealing a maximum-tolerated dose of 3.0×10^8 CFU/m^2. It showed that several patients elevated the levels of interleukin-1 (IL-1), tumor necrosis factor-alpha (TNF-α), interleukin-6 (IL-6), and interleukin-12 (IL-12), in addition to tumor colonization in their bodies. Despite this, there was no evidence of objective tumor regression, not even in patients whose malignancies had already colonized (Chen et al. 1998; Low et al. 1999; Toso et al. 2002). One notable example involves the co-administration of attenuated *S. typhimurium* VNP20009 expressing CD and 5-FC in patients with refractory head and neck, as well as esophageal cancer (Nemunaitis et al. 2003). Bacterial colonization and 5-FU production in the tumor were observed in only two out of the three patients. In addition, in a completed phase I clinical trial, investigators explored the efficacy and safety of attenuated *S. typhimurium* χ4550 expressing interleukin-2 (IL-2) in patients with liver cancer (Cunningham and Nemunaitis 2001).

Listeria vaccine strains have exhibited highly promising outcomes (Kang et al. 2022). Such strains were evaluated in phase II (NCT02004262) and phase III (NCT02853604) clinical trials. The studies showed the involvement of *Listeria* CRS-207, engineered to express mesothelin, in a series of clinical trials targeting diverse tumors, including pancreatic cancer, mesothelioma, lung cancer, and ovarian cancer (Le et al. 2012; Le et al. 2015; Hassan et al. 2019; Tsujikawa et al. 2020). The results of a phase II trial, which included 303 patients, indicated that the combination of Cyclophosphamide (Cy)/GVAX Pancreas vaccine and CRS-207 was well-tolerated by cancer patients and led to extended survival time for those with metastatic pancreatic cancer (Le et al. 2015). In a subsequent phase III trial involving patients with pancreatic cancer, the Cy/GVAX + CRS-207 group did not exhibit a prolonged survival advantage compared to the chemotherapy group. However, the findings indicated that the survival rate with CRS-207 alone closely approached that of the chemotherapy group (Le et al. 2019). Despite this, the encouraging outcomes have motivated researchers to pursue further development of bacterial products for

Table 1 Clinical trials with engineered bacteria-based cancer therapy

Trial no.	Title	Status	Conditions	Phases	Number of enrolled patients	Start year	Completed year/ Ongoing
NCT04589234	Saltikva for metastatic pancreatic cancer	Recruiting	Metastatic pancreatic cancer	II	60	2020	Ongoing
NCT05651022	DECOY20 study in patients with advanced solid tumors	Recruiting	Solid tumor	I	35	2023	Ongoing
NCT05677113	A study of QBECO versus placebo in the treatment of colorectal cancer that has spread to the liver	Recruiting	Colorectal cancer, liver metastases	II	115	2023	Ongoing
NCT05120596	First in human study of T3P-Y058-739 (T3P)	Recruiting	Advanced solid tumor	I II	100	2022	Ongoing
NCT06019312	*L. plantarum* 299v and gut microbiome, diarrhea, and *C. difficile* infection in colorectal cancer patients	Recruiting	Colorectal cancer, *Clostridioides difficile* infection	N/A	60	2023	Ongoing
NCT05383703	Clinical study of MNC-168 enteric-coated capsule in the treatment of advanced intestinal solid tumor	Not yet recruiting	Advanced malignant solid tumors	I	24	2022	Ongoing
NCT03838601	Role of microbiome as a biomarker in locoregionally-advanced oropharyngeal squamous cell carcinoma 2	Active, not recruiting	Head and neck squamous cell carcinoma	N/A	30	2019	Ongoing
NCT04193904	A study of live biotherapeutic product MRx0518 with hypofractionated radiation therapy in resectable pancreatic cancer	Terminated	Pancreatic cancer	I	13	2019	2023
NCT03637803	Live biotherapeutic product MRx0518 and pembrolizumab combination study in solid tumors	Terminated	Solid tumor, non-small cell lung cancer, renal cell carcinoma, melanoma, bladder cancer	I II	63	2019	2023

NCT03934827	MRx0518 in patients with solid tumors waiting for surgical removal of the tumor	Active, not recruiting	Melanoma, breast cancer, uterine cancer, ovarian cancer, prostate cancer, bladder cancer, renal cancer, lung cancer, head and neck cancer	I	120	2019	2022
NCT04025307	Phase I trial of bacTRL-IL-12 in adult subjects with advanced, treatment-refractory solid tumors	Terminated	Cancer, solid tumors	I	5	2019	2020
NCT04910698	Efficacy of antibiotic short course for bloodstream infections in acute myeloid leukemia patients with febrile neutropenia	Completed	Acute myeloid leukemia, febrile neutropenia, bloodstream infection	N/A	104	2020	2020
NCT03234465	Efficacy, safety and tolerability of AG013 in oral mucositis compared to placebo when administered three times per day	Terminated	Oral mucositis	II	200	2017	2020
NCT03358511	Engineering gut microbiome to target breast cancer	Completed	Breast cancer	N/A	7	2017	2020
NCT02766699	A study to evaluate the safety, tolerability and immunogenicity of EGFR(V)-EDV-Dox in subjects with recurrent glioblastoma multiforme (GBM)	Unknown status	Glioblastoma, astrocytoma, Grade IV	I	20	2016	2020
NCT02544685	Prevention of febrile neutropenia by synbiotics in pediatric cancer patients	Unknown status	Febrile neutropenia, neutropenia, infection in an immunocompromised host, cancer	II	120	2010	2019
NCT02853604	Study of ADXS11-001 in participants with high risk locally advanced cervical cancer	Terminated	High risk cervical cancer, advanced cervical cancer	III	110	2015	2019

(continued)

Table 1 (continued)

Trial no.	Title	Status	Conditions	Phases	Number of enrolled patients	Start year	Completed year/ Ongoing
NCT01266460	Vaccine therapy in treating patients with persistent or recurrent cervical cancer	Completed	Cervical adenocarcinoma, cervical adenosquamous carcinoma	II	54	2011	2018
NCT01675765	Safety and efficacy of listeria in combination with chemotherapy as front-line treatment for malignant pleural mesothelioma	Completed	Malignant pleural mesothelioma	I	60	2014	2019
NCT02625857	Safety and immunogenicity of JNJ-64041809, a live attenuated double-deleted *Listeria* immunotherapy, in participants with metastatic castration-resistant prostate cancer	Completed	Prostatic neoplasms, castration-resistant	I	26	2015	2018
NCT01967758	Phase I study of safety and immunogenicity of ADU-623	Completed	Astrocytic tumors, glioblastoma multiforme, anaplastic astrocytoma, brain tumor	I	11	2014	2018
NCT02015104	Study of Bacillus Calmette-Guerin (BCG) combined with PANVAC versus BCG alone in adults with high grade non-muscle invasive bladder cancer who failed at least 1 course of BCG	Completed	Bladder cancer	II	32	2013	2018
NCT02966457	A study of DEcolonization in patients with HAematological Malignancies (DEHAM)	Completed	Hematological infection	IV	62	2017	2017

NCT02751736	The effect of probiotics on bowel function restoration after ileostomy closure in patients with rectal cancer	Unknown status	Rectal cancer	N/A	40	2016	2017
NCT02010203	A phase I/II study of HS-410 in patients with non-muscle invasive bladder cancer after TURBT	Terminated	Bladder cancer	I II	104	2013	2018
NCT01924689	Safety study of intratumoral injection of *C. novyi*-NT spores to treat patients with solid tumors that have not responded to standard therapies	Completed	Solid tumor malignancies	I	24	2013	2017
NCT01417000	Safety and efficacy of combination *Listeria*/GVAX immunotherapy in pancreatic cancer	Completed	Metastatic pancreatic cancer	II	93	2011	2016
NCT02004262	Safety and efficacy of combination *Listeria*/GVAX pancreas vaccine in the pancreatic cancer setting (ECLIPSE)	Completed	2nd-, 3rd-line and greater metastatic pancreatic cancer	II	303	2014	2016
NCT01099631	IL-2 expressing, attenuated *S. typhimurium* in unresectable hepatic spread	Completed	Liver cancer, hepatoma, liver neoplasms, biliary cancer	I	22	2010	2014
NCT01118819	Safety study of *C. novyi*-NT spores to treat patients with solid tumors that have not responded to standard therapies	Terminated	Solid tumor malignancies	I	5	2011	2013
NCT00358397	One time injection of bacteria to treat solid tumors that have not responded to standard therapy	Terminated	Tumors	I	2	2006	2008
NCT00327652	Study of safety and tolerability of intravenous CRS-100 in adults with carcinoma and liver metastases	Completed	Neoplasm metastasis, liver neoplasms, carcinoma	I	9	2006	2008

(continued)

Table 1 (continued)

Trial no.	Title	Status	Conditions	Phases	Number of enrolled patients	Start year	Completed year/ Ongoing
NCT00004216	VNP20009 in treating patients with advanced or metastatic solid tumors that have not responded to previous therapy	Completed	Unspecified adult solid tumor, protocol specific	I		1999	2008
NCT00006254	VNP20009 in treating patients with advanced solid tumors	Completed	Unspecified adult solid tumor, protocol specific	I		2000	2008
NCT00004988	Treatment of patients with cancer with genetically modified *S. typhimurium* bacteria	Completed	Cancer, neoplasm, neoplasm metastasis	I	45	2000	2002

N/A not applicable

tumor treatment. A phase III (NCT02853604) clinical trial evaluated the therapeutic efficacy of this immunotherapy in patients with cervical cancer. In a cohort of 110 patients with platinum-refractory cervical carcinoma, the results demonstrated the tolerability of engineered *L. monocytogenes* (ADXS-11–001) immunotherapy.

In the ongoing clinical trial involving 30 patients (NCT03838601) (Spreafico 2023), these engineered bacteria selectively colonize solid tumor tissues, delivering plasmid DNA encoding the pro-inflammatory transgene Interleukin-12 (IL-12) to the tumor microenvironment. Consequently, interleukin-12 (IL-12) is expressed, stimulating both local and systemic antitumor immune responses. Likewise, the impact of *L. plantarum* 299v in combination with inulin on the gut microbiome was evaluated (Kaźmierczak-Siedlecka 2023). The objective of the study is to reduce chemotherapy and radiotherapy-induced diarrhea and prevent the infection of *C. difficile* in 60 colorectal cancer patients (NCT06019312).

6 Conclusion and Future Perspectives

6.1 General Challenges of Bacteria-Based Approaches

Even though many studies on bacteria-based therapy have found promising results in preclinical models, there are still limitations. Firstly, safety is a primary concern owing to the infectious characteristics of the bacteria. The utilization of bacteria is a deliberate strategy aimed at converting tumor tissue into a localized infection with the capacity to eliminate tumors. However, this approach carries serious consequences if the infection spreads throughout the entire body. Controlling bacterial toxicity necessitates timely antibiotic intervention, effective therapeutic infection management, and the careful selection of safe bacterial strains (Toso et al. 2002; Tang et al. 2022). Moreover, the use of live bacteria carrying antibiotic-resistance genes, which have the potential to cause severe infections, is generally not suitable for clinical applications (Imperial and Ibana 2016). Secondly, the challenge in inhibiting the anticancer effectiveness of bacteria lies in the limited efficiency of drug loading. In theory, overloading the bacterial surface with drugs has the potential to decrease bacterial activity and motility. Likewise, bacteria cannot take up drugs, as an excessive uptake of drugs into bacterial cells can lead to bacterial death (Zhao et al. 2023). Thirdly, the quality control for live bacteria is more complex than small molecule agents, in general. For example, to ensure the quality of the finished products, strict aseptic protocols must be followed during the production of live bacteria (Abla and Mehanna 2022).

6.2 Future Perspectives

Bacteria, as a nascent drug delivery system, can efficiently penetrate tumor tissues, facilitating precise delivery. They possess the ability to trigger a cascade of immune responses against tumors, resulting in the inhibition of tumor growth and migration.

Bacterial carriers exhibit improved tumor-targeting capabilities and increased safety profiles as a result of genetic interventions. Engineered bacteria have the inherent ability to autonomously generate anticancer agents, ensuring sustained therapeutic effects. Moreover, the offspring of these bacteria can retain the capacity to produce targeted substances. These distinctive biological characteristics of bacterial carriers make them particularly advantageous for cancer treatment, providing benefits that are typically absent in conventional delivery methods such as liposomes, micelles, and nanoparticles. Therefore, the bacteria-based approaches have significant promise for a wide range of applications in the field of cancer treatment.

Acknowledgments The figures were generated by BioRender. This work was supported by NIH/National Cancer Institute (R01CA272564 and R21CA280814) to TY.

Conflict of Interest There is no conflict of interest declared by the authors.

References

Abla KK, Mehanna MM (2022) Freeze-drying: a flourishing strategy to fabricate stable pharmaceutical and biological products. Int J Pharm 628:122233. https://doi.org/10.1016/j.ijpharm.2022.122233

Aganja RP, Sivasankar C, Senevirathne A, Lee JH (2022) *Salmonella* as a promising curative tool against cancer. Pharmaceutics 14:2100. https://doi.org/10.3390/pharmaceutics14102100

Algethami M, Geso M, Piva T, Blencowe A et al (2015) Radiation dose enhancement using Bi_2S_3 nanoparticles in cultured mouse PC3 prostate and B16 melanoma cells. NanoWorld J 1:99–104. https://doi.org/10.17756/nwj.2015-013

Anand U, Dey A, Chandel AKS, Sanyal R et al (2023) Cancer chemotherapy and beyond: current status, drug candidates, associated risks and progress in targeted therapeutics. Genes Dis 10: 1367–1401. https://doi.org/10.1016/j.gendis.2022.02.007

Baer HM, Sandilya S, Steiner TS (2023) Evading the toll booth: how “silent” flagellins may bind yet fail to activate TLR5. Sci Immunol 8:eadf0244. https://doi.org/10.1126/sciimmunol.adf0244

Barbé S, Van ML, Theys J, Geukens N et al (2005) Secretory production of biologically active rat Interleukin-2 by *Clostridium acetobutylicum* DSM792 as a tool for anti-tumor treatment. FEMS Microbiol Lett 246:67–73. https://doi.org/10.1016/j.femsle.2005.03.037

Bennek E, Mandić AD, Verdier J, Roubrocks S et al (2019) Subcellular antigen localization in commensal *E. coli* is critical for T cell activation and induction of specific tolerance. Mucosal Immunol 12:97–107. https://doi.org/10.1038/s41385-018-0061-0

Bhardwaj R, Mishra P (2023) Multiresponsive nanoscale self-assembly of Azurin-Elastin-like polypeptide fusion protein for enhanced prostate cancer therapy. Biomacromolecules 25:508. https://doi.org/10.1021/acs.biomac.3c01125

Brooks PC, Montgomery AM, Rosenfeld M, Reisfeld RA et al (1994) Integrin $\alpha_v\beta_3$ antagonists promote tumor regression by inducing apoptosis of angiogenic blood vessels. Cell 79:1157–1164. https://doi.org/10.1016/0092-8674(94)90007-8

Brooks PC, Strömblad S, Klemke R, Visscher D et al (1995) Antiintegrin *alpha* v *beta* 3 blocks human breast cancer growth and angiogenesis in human skin. J Clin Invest 96:1815–1822. https://doi.org/10.1172/JCI118227

Cao HD, Yang YX, Lü L, Liu SN et al (2010) Attenuated *Salmonella typhimurium* carrying TRAIL and VP3 genes inhibits the growth of gastric cancer cells *in vitro* and *in vivo*. Tumori 96:296–303. https://doi.org/10.1177/030089161009600218

Cavarretta I, Ferrarese R, Cazzaniga W, Saita D et al (2017) The microbiome of the prostate tumor microenvironment. Eur Urol 72:625–631. https://doi.org/10.1016/j.eururo.2017.03.029

Chandra D, Jahangir A, Quispe-Tintaya W, Einstein M, Gravekamp C (2013) Myeloid-derived suppressor cells have a central role in attenuated *Listeria monocytogenes*-based immunotherapy against metastatic breast cancer in young and old mice. Br J Cancer 108:2281–2290. https://doi.org/10.1038/bjc.2013.206

Chen JJ, Sun Y, Nabel GJ (1998) Regulation of the proinflammatory effects of Fas ligand (CD95L). Science 282:1714–1717. https://doi.org/10.1126/science.282.5394.1714

Chen F, Zang Z, Chen Z, Cui L et al (2019a) Nanophotosensitizer-engineered *Salmonella* bacteria with hypoxia targeting and photothermal-assisted mutual bioaccumulation for solid tumor therapy. Biomaterials 214:119226. https://doi.org/10.1016/j.biomaterials.2019.119226

Chen Q, Bai H, Wu W, Huang G, Li Y, Wu M, Tang G, Ping Y (2019b) Bioengineering bacterial vesicle-coated polymeric nanomedicine for enhanced cancer immunotherapy and metastasis prevention. Nano Lett 20:11–21. https://doi.org/10.1021/acs.nanolett.9b02182

Chen J, Qiao Y, Chen G, Chang C, Dong H, Tang B, Cheng X, Liu X, Hua Z (2021) *Salmonella* flagella confer anti-tumor immunological effect via activating Flagellin/TLR5 signaling within tumor microenvironment. Acta Pharm Sin B 11:3165–3177. https://doi.org/10.1016/j.apsb.2021.04.019

Chen Z, Han F, Du Y, Shi H, Zhou W (2023) Hypoxic microenvironment in cancer: molecular mechanisms and therapeutic interventions. Signal Transduct Target Ther 8:70. https://doi.org/10.1038/s41392-023-01332-8

Cheng C, Lu Y, Chuang K, Hung W, Shiea J, Su Y, Kao C, Chen B, Roffler S, Cheng T (2008) Tumor-targeting prodrug-activating bacteria for cancer therapy. Cancer Gene Ther 15:393–401. https://doi.org/10.1038/cgt.2008.10

Cheng X, Zhang X, Zhou Y, Zhang C, Hua ZC (2014) A *Salmonella Typhimurium* mutant strain capable of RNAi delivery: higher tumor-targeting and lower toxicity. Cancer Biol Ther 15: 1068–1076. https://doi.org/10.4161/cbt.29185

Choi JK, Naffouje SA, Goto M, Wang J, Christov K, Rademacher DJ, Green A, Stecenko AA, Chakrabarty AM, Das Gupta TK, Yamada T (2023) Cross-talk between cancer and *Pseudomonas aeruginosa* mediates tumor suppression. Commun Biol 6:16. https://doi.org/10.1038/s42003-022-04395-5

Chouaib S, Noman M, Kosmatopoulos K, Curran M (2017) Hypoxic stress: obstacles and opportunities for innovative immunotherapy of cancer. Oncogene 36:439–445. https://doi.org/10.1038/onc.2016.225

Coley WB (1910) The treatment of inoperable sarcoma by bacterial toxins (the mixed toxins of the *Streptococcus erysipelas* and the *Bacillus prodigiosus*). Proc R Soc Med 3:1–48

Cunningham C, Nemunaitis J (2001) A phase I trial of genetically modified *Salmonella typhimurium* expressing cytosine deaminase (TAPET-CD, VNP20029) administered by intratumoral injection in combination with 5-fluorocytosine for patients with advanced or metastatic cancer. Protocol no: CL-017. Version: April 9, 2001. Hum Gene Ther 12:1594–1596

D'Orazio SEF (2019) Innate and adaptive immune responses during *Listeria monocytogenes* infection. Microbiol Spectr 7. https://doi.org/10.1128/microbiolspec.GPP3-0065-2019

de Alwis R, Liang L, Taghavian O, Werner E, The HC, Thu TNH, Duong VT, Davies DH, Felgner PL, Baker S (2021) The identification of novel immunogenic antigens as potential *Shigella* vaccine components. Genome Med 13:8. https://doi.org/10.1186/s13073-020-00824-4

Dean SN, Rimmer MA, Turner KB, Phillips DA, Caruana JC, Hervey WJT, Leary DH, Walper SA (2020) *Lactobacillus acidophilus* membrane vesicles as a vehicle of bacteriocin delivery. Front Microbiol 11:710. https://doi.org/10.3389/fmicb.2020.00710

Diaz SA, Martin SR, Howell SA, Grainger M, Moon RW, Green JL, Holder AA (2016) The binding of *Plasmodium falciparum* adhesions and erythrocyte invasion proteins to aldolase is enhanced by phosphorylation. PLoS One 11:e0161850. https://doi.org/10.1371/journal.pone.0161850

Din MO, Danino T, Prindle A, Skalak M et al (2016) Synchronized cycles of bacterial lysis for *in vivo* delivery. Nature 536:81–85. https://doi.org/10.1038/nature18930

Djeha AH, Thomson TA, Leung H, Searle PF, Young LS, Kerr DJ, Harris PA, Mountain A, Wrighton CJ (2001) Combined adenovirus-mediated nitroreductase gene delivery and CB1954 treatment: a well-tolerated therapy for established solid tumors. Mol Ther 3:233–240. https://doi.org/10.1006/mthe.2000.0250

Dresselaers T, Theys J, Nuyts S, Wouters B, de Bruijn E, Anné J, Lambin P, Van Hecke P, Landuyt W (2003) Non-invasive 19F MR spectroscopy of 5-fluorocytosine to 5-fluorouracil conversion by recombinant *Salmonella* in tumours. Br J Cancer 89:1796–1801. https://doi.org/10.1038/sj.bjc.6601345

Duong MTQ, Qin Y, You SH, Min JJ (2019) Bacteria-cancer interactions: bacteria-based cancer therapy. Exp Mol Med 51:1–15. https://doi.org/10.1038/s12276-019-0297-0

Ebrahimzadeh S, Ahangari H, Soleimanian A, Hosseini K, Ebrahimi V, Ghasemnejad T, Soofiyani SR, Tarhriz V, Eyvazi S (2021) Colorectal cancer treatment using bacteria: focus on molecular mechanisms. BMC Microbiol 21:1–12. https://doi.org/10.1186/s12866-021-02274-3

Ektate K, Munteanu MC, Ashar H, Malayer J, Ranjan A (2018) Chemo-immunotherapy of colon cancer with focused ultrasound and *Salmonella*-laden temperature sensitive liposomes (thermobots). Sci Rep 8:13062. https://doi.org/10.1038/s41598-018-30106-4

Fan JY, Huang Y, Li Y, Muluh TA, Fu SZ, Wu JB (2022) Bacteria in cancer therapy: a new generation of weapons. Cancer Med 11:4457–4468. https://doi.org/10.1002/cam4.4799

Felgner S, Frahm M, Kocijancic D, Rohde M, Eckweiler D, Bielecka A, Bueno E, Cava F, Abraham W-R, Curtiss R III (2016) *aroA*-deficient *Salmonella enterica* serovar Typhimurium is more than a metabolically attenuated mutant. MBio 7:e01220–e01216. https://doi.org/10.1128/mbio.01220-01216

Flickinger JC, Rodeck U, Snook AE (2018) Listeria monocytogenes as a vector for cancer immunotherapy: current understanding and progress. Vaccines (Basel) 6:48. https://doi.org/10.3390/vaccines6030048

Friedlander M, Brooks PC, Shaffer RW, Kincaid CM, Varner JA, Cheresh DA (1995) Definition of two angiogenic pathways by distinct α_v integrins. Science 270:1500–1502. https://doi.org/10.1126/science.270.5241.1500

Friedlos F, Lehouritis P, Ogilvie L, Hedley D, Davies L, Bermudes D, King I, Martin J, Marais R, Springer CJ (2008) Attenuated *Salmonella* targets prodrug activating enzyme carboxypeptidase G2 to mouse melanoma and human breast and colon carcinomas for effective suicide gene therapy. Clin Cancer Res 14:4259–4266. https://doi.org/10.1158/1078-0432.CCR-07-4800

Fritz SE, Henson MS, Greengard E, Winter AL et al (2016) A phase I clinical study to evaluate safety of orally administered, genetically engineered *Salmonella enterica* serovar Typhimurium for canine osteosarcoma. Vet Med Sci 2:179–190. https://doi.org/10.1002/vms3.32

Fujimori M (2006) Genetically engineered *Bifidobacterium* as a drug delivery system for systemic therapy of metastatic breast cancer patients. Breast Cancer 13:27–31. https://doi.org/10.2325/jbcs.13.27

Galain I, Cardoso M, Tejería E, Mourglia-Ettlin G, Arbildi P, Terán M, Pérez Barthaburu M, Aguiar I (2022) Enhancement of radiation response of breast cancer cells through the incorporation of Bi_2S_3 nanorods. J Nanopart Res 24:68. https://doi.org/10.1007/s11051-022-05455-x

Ganai S, Arenas R, Forbes N (2009) Tumor-targeted delivery of TRAIL using *Salmonella typhimurium* enhances breast cancer survival in mice. Br J Cancer 101:1683–1691. https://doi.org/10.1038/sj.bjc.6605403

Ganai S, Arenas RB, Sauer JP, Bentley B, Forbes NS (2011) In tumors *Salmonella* migrate away from vasculature toward the transition zone and induce apoptosis. Cancer Gene Ther 18:457–466. https://doi.org/10.1038/cgt.2011.10

Gladson CL (1996) Expression of integrin *alpha* v *beta* 3 in small blood vessels of glioblastoma tumors. J Neuropathol Exp Neurol 55:1143–1149. https://doi.org/10.1097/00005072-199611000-00005

Gujrati V, Prakash J, Malekzadeh-Najafabadi J, Stiel A (2019) Bioengineered bacterial vesicles as biological nano-heaters for optoacoustic imaging. Nat Commun 10:1114. https://doi.org/10.1038/s41467-019-09034-y

Guo Y, Song M, Liu X, Chen Y, Xun Z, Sun Y, Tan W, He J, Zheng JH (2022) Photodynamic therapy-improved oncolytic bacterial immunotherapy with FAP-encoding *S. typhimurium*. J Control Release 351:860–871. https://doi.org/10.1016/j.jconrel.2022.09.050

Gurbatri CR, Lia I, Vincent R, Coker C, Castro S, Treuting PM, Hinchliffe TE, Arpaia N, Danino T (2020) Engineered probiotics for local tumor delivery of checkpoint blockade nanobodies. Sci Transl Med 12:eaax0876. https://doi.org/10.1126/scitranslmed.aax0876

Gurbatri CR, Arpaia N, Danino T (2022) Engineering bacteria as interactive cancer therapies. Science 378:858–864. https://doi.org/10.1126/science.add9667

Gyanani V, Haley JC, Goswami R (2021) Challenges of current anticancer treatment approaches with focus on liposomal drug delivery systems. Pharmaceuticals (Basel) 14:835. https://doi.org/10.3390/ph14090835

Ha X-q, Yin Q, Zhao H-b, Hui L, Wang M-l, Peng J-h, Dong J-z, Deng Z-y, Zhao Y, Zhang Y-y (2012) Inhibitory effects of the attenuated *Salmonella typhimurium* containing the IL-2 gene on hepatic tumors in mice. J Biomed Biotechnol 2012:1. https://doi.org/10.1155/2012/946139

Häcker G, Redecke V, Häcker H (2002) Activation of the immune system by bacterial CpG-DNA. Immunology 105:245–251. https://doi.org/10.1046/j.0019-2805.2001.01350.x

Hajam IA, Dar PA, Shahnawaz I, Jaume JC, Lee JH (2017) Bacterial flagellin-a potent immunomodulatory agent. Exp Mol Med 49:e373–e373. https://doi.org/10.1038/emm.2017.172

Hassan R, Alley E, Kindler H, Antonia S, Jahan T, Honarmand S, Nair N, Whiting CC, Enstrom A, Lemmens E (2019) Clinical response of live-attenuated, *Listeria monocytogenes* expressing mesothelin (CRS-207) with chemotherapy in patients with malignant pleural mesothelioma. Clin Cancer Res 25:5787–5798. https://doi.org/10.1158/1078-0432.CCR-19-0070

He J, Wang Y, Missinato MA, Onuoha E et al (2016) A genetically targetable near-infrared photosensitizer. Nat Methods 13:263–268. https://doi.org/10.1038/nmeth.3735

Heap JT, Theys J, Ehsaan M, Kubiak AM, Dubois L, Paesmans K, Van Mellaert L, Knox R, Kuehne SA, Lambin P (2014) Spores of *Clostridium* engineered for clinical efficacy and safety cause regression and cure of tumors *in vivo*. Oncotarget 5:1761. https://doi.org/10.18632/oncotarget.1761

Heisig M, Frentzen A, Bergmann B, Galmbacher K, Gentschev I, Hotz C, Schoen C, Stritzker J, Fensterle J, Rapp UR, Goebel W (2011) Specific antibody-receptor interactions trigger InlAB-independent uptake of *Listeria monocytogenes* into tumor cell lines. BMC Microbiol 11:163. https://doi.org/10.1186/1471-2180-11-163

Hibbing ME, Fuqua C, Parsek MR, Peterson SB (2010) Bacterial competition: surviving and thriving in the microbial jungle. Nat Rev Microbiol 8:15–25. https://doi.org/10.1038/nrmicro2259

Hiraoka Y, Yamada T, Goto M, Das Gupta TK, Chakrabarty AM (2004) Modulation of mammalian cell growth and death by prokaryotic and eukaryotic cytochrome c. Proc Natl Acad Sci USA 101:6427–6432. https://doi.org/10.1073/pnas.0401631101

Hong CS, Yamada T, Fialho AM, Gupta TKD, Chakrabarty AM (2006) Disrupting the entry barrier and attacking brain tumors: the role of the Neisseria H.8 epitope and the Laz protein. Cell Cycle 5:1633–1641. https://doi.org/10.4161/cc.5.15.2991

Hosseini-Giv N, Bahrami AR, Matin MM (2021) Application of bacterial directed enzyme prodrug therapy as a targeted chemotherapy approach in a mouse model of breast cancer. Int J Pharm 606:120931. https://doi.org/10.1016/j.ijpharm.2021.120931

Hu J, Jiang W, Zuo J, Shi D, Chen X, Yang X, Zhang W, Ma L, Liu Z, Xing Q (2023) Structural basis of bacterial effector protein azurin targeting tumor suppressor p53 and inhibiting its ubiquitination. Commun Biol 6:59. https://doi.org/10.1038/s42003-023-04458-1

Imperial IC, Ibana JA (2016) Addressing the antibiotic resistance problem with probiotics: reducing the risk of its double-edged sword effect. Front Microbiol 7:1983. https://doi.org/10.3389/fmicb.2016.01983

Jewett TJ, Sibley LD (2003) Aldolase forms a bridge between cell surface adhesions and the actin cytoskeleton in apicomplexan parasites. Mol Cell 11:885–894. https://doi.org/10.1016/s1097-2765(03)00113-8

Jiang SN, Phan TX, Nam TK, Nguyen VH, Kim HS, Bom HS, Choy HE, Hong Y, Min JJ (2010) Inhibition of tumor growth and metastasis by a combination of *Escherichia coli*–mediated cytolytic therapy and radiotherapy. Mol Ther 18:635–642. https://doi.org/10.1038/mt.2009.295

Jiang SN, Park SH, Lee HJ, Zheng JH, Kim HS, Bom HS, Hong Y, Szardenings M, Shin MG, Kim SC, Ntziachristos V, Choy HE, Min JJ (2013) Engineering of bacteria for the visualization of targeted delivery of a cytolytic anticancer agent. Mol Ther 21:1985–1995. https://doi.org/10.1038/mt.2013.183

Jiang M, Yang Z, Dai J, Wu T, Jiao Z, Yu Y, Ning K, Chen W, Yang A (2023) Intratumor microbiome: selective colonization in the tumor microenvironment and a vital regulator of tumor biology. MedComm 4:e376. https://doi.org/10.1002/mco2.376

Kang SR, Nguyen DH, Yoo SW, Min JJ (2022) Bacteria and bacterial derivatives as delivery carriers for immunotherapy. Adv Drug Deliv Rev 181:114085. https://doi.org/10.1016/j.addr.2021.114085

Kasinskas RW, Forbes NS (2006) *Salmonella typhimurium* specifically chemotax and proliferate in heterogeneous tumor tissue *in vitro*. Biotechnol Bioeng 94:710–721. https://doi.org/10.1002/bit.20883

Kasinskas RW, Forbes NS (2007) *Salmonella typhimurium* lacking ribose chemoreceptors localize in tumor quiescence and induce apoptosis. Cancer Res 67:3201–3209. https://doi.org/10.1158/0008-5472.CAN-06-2618

Kaźmierczak-Siedlecka K (2023) The impact of *Lactobacillus plantarum* 299v in combination with inulin on gut microbiome, chemotherapy and radiotherapy-induced diarrhoea, and *Clostridioides difficile* infection in colorectal cancer patients in periooperative period. Clinicaltrials.gov. https://clinicaltrials.gov/study/NCT06019312. Accessed 20 Dec 2023

Kim SH, Castro F, Paterson Y, Gravekamp C (2009) High efficacy of a *Listeria*-based vaccine against metastatic breast cancer reveals a dual mode of action. Cancer Res 69:5860–5866. https://doi.org/10.1158/0008-5472.CAN-08-4855

Kim OY, Park HT, Dinh NTH, Choi SJ, Lee J, Kim JH, Lee SW, Gho YS (2017) Bacterial outer membrane vesicles suppress tumor by interferon-γ-mediated antitumor response. Nat Commun 8:626. https://doi.org/10.1038/s41467-017-00729-8

King I, Bermudes D, Lin S, Belcourt M, Pike J, Troy K, Le T, Ittensohn M, Mao J, Lang W (2002) Tumor-targeted *Salmonella* expressing cytosine deaminase as an anticancer agent. Hum Gene Ther 13:1225–1233. https://doi.org/10.1089/104303402320139005

Knox RJ, Friedlos F, Jarman M, Roberts JJ (1988) A new cytotoxic, DNA interstrand crosslinking agent, 5-(aziridin-1-yl)-4-hydroxylamino-2-nitrobenzamide, is formed from 5-(aziridin-1-yl)-2,4-dinitrobenzamide (CB 1954) by a nitroreductase enzyme in Walker carcinoma cells. Biochem Pharmacol 37:4661–4669. https://doi.org/10.1016/0006-2952(88)90335-8

Kreitz J, Friedrich MJ, Guru A, Lash B, Saito M, Macrae RK, Zhang F (2023) Programmable protein delivery with a bacterial contractile injection system. Nature 616:357–364. https://doi.org/10.1038/s41586-023-05870-7

Kulchavenya E, Kholtobin D, Filimonov P (2013) *Mycobacterium tuberculosis* and *bovis* as causes for shrinking bladder. J Case Rep Pr 3:57–61

Kumar SR, Imlay JA (2013) How *Escherichia coli* tolerates profuse hydrogen peroxide formation by a catabolic pathway. J Bacteriol 195:4569–4579. https://doi.org/10.1128/JB.00737-13

Le DT, Brockstedt DG, Nir-Paz R, Hampl J et al (2012) A live-attenuated *Listeria* vaccine (ANZ-100) and a live-attenuated *Listeria* vaccine expressing mesothelin (CRS-207) for advanced cancers: phase I studies of safety and immune induction. Clin Cancer Res 18:858–868. https://doi.org/10.1158/1078-0432.CCR-11-2121

Le DT, Wang-Gillam A, Picozzi V, Greten TF, Crocenzi T, Springett G, Morse M, Zeh H, Cohen D, Fine RL (2015) Safety and survival with GVAX pancreas prime and *Listeria monocytogenes*–expressing mesothelin (CRS-207) boost vaccines for metastatic pancreatic cancer. J Clin Oncol 33:1325. https://doi.org/10.1200/JCO.2014.57.4244

Le DT, Picozzi VJ, Ko AH, Wainberg ZA et al (2019) Results from a phase IIb, randomized, multicenter study of GVAX pancreas and CRS-207 compared with chemotherapy in adults with previously treated metastatic pancreatic adenocarcinoma (ECLIPSE study). Clin Cancer Res 25:5493–5502. https://doi.org/10.1158/1078-0432.CCR-18-2992

Lenis AT, Lec PM, Chamie K (2020) Bladder cancer: a review. JAMA 324:1980–1991. https://doi.org/10.1001/jama.2020.17598

Leschner S, Westphal K, Dietrich N, Viegas N, Jablonska J, Lyszkiewicz M, Lienenklaus S, Falk W, Gekara N, Loessner H, Weiss S (2009) Tumor invasion of *Salmonella enterica* Serovar Typhimurium is accompanied by strong hemorrhage promoted by TNF-α. PLoS One 4:e6692. https://doi.org/10.1371/journal.pone.0006692

Leventhal DS, Sokolovska A, Li N, Plescia C, Kolodziej SA et al (2020) Immunotherapy with engineered bacteria by targeting the STING pathway for anti-tumor immunity. Nat Commun 11:2739. https://doi.org/10.1038/s41467-020-16602-0

Lin HC, Yang CJ, Kuan YD, Wang WK, Chang WW, Lee CH (2017) The inhibition of indoleamine 2, 3-dioxygenase 1 by connexin 43. Int J Med Sci 14:1181. https://doi.org/10.7150/ijms.20661

Liu S, Minton N, Giaccia A, Brown J (2002) Anticancer efficacy of systemically delivered anaerobic bacteria as gene therapy vectors targeting tumor hypoxia/necrosis. Gene Ther 9:291–296. https://doi.org/10.1038/sj.gt.3301659

Liu SC, Ahn GO, Kioi M, Dorie MJ, Patterson AV, Brown JM (2008a) Optimized clostridium-directed enzyme prodrug therapy improves the antitumor activity of the novel DNA cross-linking agent PR-104. Cancer Res 68:7995–8003. https://doi.org/10.1158/0008-5472.CAN-08-1698

Liu Z, Wang F, Chen X (2008b) Integrin $\alpha_v\beta_3$-targeted cancer therapy. Drug Dev Res 69:329–339. https://doi.org/10.1002/ddr.20265

Liu X, Jiang S, Piao L, Yuan F (2016) Radiotherapy combined with an engineered *Salmonella typhimurium* inhibits tumor growth in a mouse model of colon cancer. Exp Anim 65:413–418. https://doi.org/10.1538/expanim.16-0033

Liu Y, Feng J, Pan H, Zhang X, Zhang Y (2022) Genetically engineered bacterium: principles, practices, and prospects. Front Microbiol 13. https://doi.org/10.3389/fmicb.2022.997587

Loeffler M, Le'Negrate G, Krajewska M, Reed JC (2008) IL-18-producing *Salmonella* inhibit tumor growth. Cancer Gene Ther 15:787–794. https://doi.org/10.1038/cgt.2008.48

Low KB, Ittensohn M, Le T, Platt J, Sodi S, Amoss M, Ash O, Carmichael E, Chakraborty A, Fischer J, Lin SL, Luo X, Miller SI, Zheng L, King I, Pawelek JM, Bermudes D (1999) Lipid a mutant *Salmonella* with suppressed virulence and TNFα induction retain tumor-targeting *in vivo*. Nat Biotechnol 17:37–41. https://doi.org/10.1038/5205

Luo M, Chen X, Gao H, Yang F, Chen J, Qiao Y (2022) Bacteria-mediated cancer therapy: a versatile bio-sapper with translational potential. Front Oncol 12:980111. https://doi.org/10.3389/fonc.2022.980111

Ma X, Liang X, Li Y, Feng Q, Cheng K, Ma N, Zhu F, Guo X, Yue Y, Liu G, Zhang T, Liang J, Ren L, Zhao X, Nie G (2023) Modular-designed engineered bacteria for precision tumor immunotherapy via spatiotemporal manipulation by magnetic field. Nat Commun 14:4607. https://doi.org/10.1038/s41467-023-39906-3

Malekshah OM, Chen X, Nomani A, Sarkar S, Hatefi A (2016) Enzyme/prodrug systems for cancer gene therapy. Curr Pharmacolo Rep 2:299–308. https://doi.org/10.1007/s40495-016-0073-y

Matsui H, Isshiki Y, Eguchi M, Ogawa Y, Shimoji Y (2015) Evaluation of the live vaccine efficacy of virulence plasmid-cured, and *phoP*- or *aroA*-deficient *Salmonella enterica* serovar Typhimurium in mice. J Vet Med Sci 77:181–186. https://doi.org/10.1292/jvms.14-0013

Matsuura M (2013) Structural modifications of bacterial lipopolysaccharide that facilitate gram-negative bacteria evasion of host innate immunity. Front Immunol 4:109. https://doi.org/10.3389/fimmu.2013.00109

McCarthy EF (2006) The toxins of William B. Coley and the treatment of bone and soft-tissue sarcomas. Iowa Orthop J 26:154–158

Miller KD, Nogueira L, Devasia T, Mariotto AB, Yabroff KR, Jemal A, Kramer J, Siegel RL (2022) Cancer treatment and survivorship statistics, 2022. CA Cancer J Clin 72:409–436. https://doi.org/10.3322/caac.21731

Nagakura C, Hayashi K, Zhao M, Yamauchi K, Yamamoto N, Tsuchiya H, Tomita K, Bouvet M, Hoffman RM (2009) Efficacy of a genetically-modified *Salmonella typhimurium* in an orthotopic human pancreatic cancer in nude mice. Anticancer Res 29:1873–1878

Nam J, Son S, Ochyl LJ, Kuai R, Schwendeman A, Moon J (2018) Chemo-photothermal therapy combination elicits anti-tumor immunity against advanced metastatic cancer. Nat Commun 9:1074. https://doi.org/10.1038/s41467-018-03473-9

Nemunaitis J, Cunningham C, Senzer N, Kuhn J, Cramm J, Litz C, Cavagnolo R, Cahill A, Clairmont C, Sznol M (2003) Pilot trial of genetically modified, attenuated *Salmonella* expressing the *E. coli* cytosine deaminase gene in refractory cancer patients. Cancer Gene Ther 10:737–744. https://doi.org/10.1038/sj.cgt.7700634

Nguyen VH, Kim HS, Ha JM, Hong Y, Choy HE, Min JJ (2010) Genetically engineered *Salmonella typhimurium* as an imageable therapeutic probe for cancer. Cancer Res 70:18–23. https://doi.org/10.1158/0008-5472.CAN-09-3453

Oladejo M, Paterson Y, Wood LM (2021) Clinical experience and recent advances in the development of listeria-based tumor immunotherapies. Front Immunol 12:642316. https://doi.org/10.3389/fimmu.2021.642316

Pahle J, Menzel L, Niesler N, Kobelt D, Aumann J, Rivera M, Walther W (2017) Rapid eradication of colon carcinoma by *Clostridium perfringens* enterotoxin suicidal gene therapy. BMC Cancer 17:129. https://doi.org/10.1186/s12885-017-3123-x

Palma V, Gutiérrez MS, Vargas O, Parthasarathy R, Navarrete P (2022) Methods to evaluate bacterial motility and its role in bacterial-host interactions. Microorganisms 10:563. https://doi.org/10.3390/microorganisms10030563

Palmer D, Milner A, Kerr D, Young L (2003) Mechanism of cell death induced by the novel enzyme-prodrug combination, nitroreductase/CB1954, and identification of synergism with 5-fluorouracil. Br J Cancer 89:944–950. https://doi.org/10.1038/sj.bjc.6601211

Pan P, Dong X, Chen Y, Zeng X, Zhang XZ (2022) Engineered bacteria for enhanced radiotherapy against breast carcinoma. ACS Nano 16:801–812. https://doi.org/10.1021/acsnano.1c08350

Park SH, Zheng JH, Nguyen VH, Jiang SN, Kim DY, Szardenings M, Min JH, Hong Y, Choy HE, Min JJ (2016) RGD peptide cell-surface display enhances the targeting and therapeutic efficacy of attenuated *Salmonella*-mediated cancer therapy. Theranostics 6:1672–1682. https://doi.org/10.7150/thno.16135

Patyar S, Joshi R, Byrav DSP, Prakash A, Medhi B, Das BK (2010) Bacteria in cancer therapy: a novel experimental strategy. J Biomed Sci 17:21. https://doi.org/10.1186/1423-0127-17-21

Poorebrahim M, Abazari MF, Sadeghi S, Mahmoudi R, Kheirollahi A, Askari H, Wickström SL, Poortahmasebi V, Lundqvist A, Kiessling R, Cid-Arregui A (2020) Genetically modified immune cells targeting tumor antigens. Pharmacol Ther 214:107603. https://doi.org/10.1016/j.pharmthera.2020.107603

Punj V, Bhattacharyya S, Saint-Dic D, Vasu C, Cunningham EA, Graves J, Yamada T, Constantinou AI, Christov K, White B, Li G, Majumdar D, Chakrabarty AM, Das Gupta TK (2004) Bacterial cupredoxin azurin as an inducer of apoptosis and regression in human breast cancer. Oncogene 23:2367–2378. https://doi.org/10.1038/sj.onc.1207376

Quispe-Tintaya W, Chandra D, Jahangir A, Harris M, Casadevall A, Dadachova E, Gravekamp C (2013) Nontoxic radioactive *Listeria*(at) is a highly effective therapy against metastatic pancreatic cancer. Proc Natl Acad Sci USA 110:8668–8673. https://doi.org/10.1073/pnas.1211287110

Roberts NJ, Zhang L, Janku F, Collins A et al (2014) Intratumoral injection of *Clostridium novyi*-NT spores induces antitumor responses. Sci Transl Med 6:249ra111. https://doi.org/10.1126/scitranslmed.3008982

Rommasi F (2022) Bacterial-based methods for cancer treatment: what we know and where we are. Oncol Ther 10:23–54. https://doi.org/10.1007/s40487-021-00177-x

Roy S, Kumaravel S, Sharma A, Duran CL, Bayless KJ, Chakraborty S (2020) Hypoxic tumor microenvironment: implications for cancer therapy. Exp Biol Med (Maywood) 245: 1073–1086. https://doi.org/10.1177/1535370220934038

Saccheri F, Pozzi C, Avogadri F, Barozzi S, Faretta M, Fusi P, Rescigno M (2010) Bacteria-induced gap junctions in tumors favor antigen cross-presentation and antitumor immunity. Sci Transl Med 2:44ra57. https://doi.org/10.1126/scitranslmed.3000739

Sasaki T, Fujimori M, Hamaji Y, Hama Y, Ki I, Amano J, Taniguchi S (2006) Genetically engineered *Bifidobacterium longum* for tumor-targeting enzyme-prodrug therapy of autochthonous mammary tumors in rats. Cancer Sci 97:649–657. https://doi.org/10.1111/j.1349-7006.2006.00221.x

Savage TM, Vincent RL, Rae SS, Huang LH, Ahn A et al (2023) Chemokines expressed by engineered bacteria recruit and orchestrate antitumor immunity. Sci Adv 9:eadc9436. https://doi.org/10.1126/sciadv.adc9436

Sheikh S, Ernst D, Keating A (2021) Prodrugs and prodrug-activated systems in gene therapy. Mol Ther 29:1716–1728. https://doi.org/10.1016/j.ymthe.2021.04.006

Shi L, Ermis R, Garcia A, Telgenhoff D, Aust D (2010) Degradation of human collagen isoforms by *Clostridium collagenase* and the effects of degradation products on cell migration. Int Wound J 7:87–95. https://doi.org/10.1111/j.1742-481X.2010.00659.x

Shprung T, Wani NA, Wilmes M, Mangoni ML, Bitler A, Shimoni E, Sahl HG, Shai Y (2021) Opposing effects of PhoPQ and PmrAB on the properties of *Salmonella enterica* serovar Typhimurium: implications on resistance to antimicrobial peptides. Biochemistry 60:2943–2955. https://doi.org/10.1021/acs.biochem.1c00287

Si W, Liang H, Bugno J, Xu Q, Ding X, Yang K, Fu Y, Weichselbaum RR, Zhao X, Wang L (2022) *Lactobacillus rhamnosus* GG induces cGAS/STING-dependent type I interferon and improves response to immune checkpoint blockade. Gut 71:521–533. https://doi.org/10.1136/gutjnl-2020-323426

Silhavy TJ, Kahne D, Walker S (2010) The bacterial cell envelope. Cold Spring Harb Perspect Biol 2:a000414. https://doi.org/10.1101/cshperspect.a000414

Singhal R, Shah YM (2020) Oxygen battle in the gut: hypoxia and hypoxia-inducible factors in metabolic and inflammatory responses in the intestine. J Biol Chem 295:10493–10505. https://doi.org/10.1074/jbc.REV120.011188

Song J, Zhang Y, Zhang C, Du X, Guo Z, Kuang Y, Wang Y, Wu P, Zou K, Zou L, Lv J, Wang Q (2018a) A microfluidic device for studying chemotaxis mechanism of bacterial cancer targeting. Sci Rep 8:6394. https://doi.org/10.1038/s41598-018-24748-7

Song S, Vuai MS, Zhong M (2018b) The role of bacteria in cancer therapy—enemies in the past, but allies at present. Infect Agent Cancer 13:9. https://doi.org/10.1186/s13027-018-0180-y

Song Q, Zhang X, Liu W, Wei H, Liang W, Zhou Y, Ding Y, Ji F, Ho-Kwan Cheung A, Wong N, Yu J (2023) *Bifidobacterium pseudolongum*-generated acetate suppresses non-alcoholic fatty liver disease-associated hepatocellular carcinoma. J Hepatol 79:1352–1365. https://doi.org/10.1016/j.jhep.2023.07.005

Spreafico A (2023) Role of microbiome as a biomarkers in locoregionally-advanced oropharyngeal squamous cell carcinoma 2. Clinicaltrials.gov. https://clinicaltrials.gov/study/NCT03838601. Accessed 20 Dec 2023

Stachowiak R, Lyzniak M, Budziszewska BK, Roeske K, Bielecki J, Hoser G, Kawiak J (2012) Cytotoxicity of bacterial metabolic products, including Listeriolysin O, on leukocyte targets. J Biomed Biotechnol 2012:954375. https://doi.org/10.1155/2012/954375

Staedtke V, Bai R-Y, Sun W, Huang J, Kibler KK, Tyler BM, Gallia GL, Kinzler K, Vogelstein B, Zhou S, Riggins GJ (2015) *Clostridium novyi*-NT can cause regression of orthotopically implanted glioblastomas in rats. Oncotarget 6:5536–5546. https://doi.org/10.18632/oncotarget.3627

Staedtke V, Roberts NJ, Bai R-Y, Zhou S (2016) *Clostridium novyi*-NT in cancer therapy. Genes Dis 3:144–152. https://doi.org/10.1016/j.gendis.2016.01.003

Stavru F, Archambaud C, Cossart P (2011) Cell biology and immunology of *Listeria monocytogenes* infections: novel insights. Immunol Rev 240:160–184. https://doi.org/10.1111/j.1600-065X.2010.00993.x

Stern C, Kasnitz N, Kocijancic D, Trittel S, Riese P, Guzman CA, Leschner S, Weiss S (2015) Induction of $CD4^+$ and $CD8^+$ anti-tumor effector T cell responses by bacteria mediated tumor therapy. Int J Cancer 137:2019–2028. https://doi.org/10.1002/ijc.29567

Su L, Zhang Y, Zhang X, Liu T, Liu S, Li Y, Jiang M, Tang T, Shen H, Wang C (2021) Combination immunotherapy with two attenuated *Listeria* strains carrying shuffled HPV-16 E6E7 protein causes tumor regression in a mouse tumor model. Sci Rep 11:13404. https://doi.org/10.1038/s41598-021-92875-9

Sukhithasri V, Nisha N, Biswas L, Anil Kumar V, Biswas R (2013) Innate immune recognition of microbial cell wall components and microbial strategies to evade such recognitions. Microbiol Res 168:396–406. https://doi.org/10.1016/j.micres.2013.02.005

Sznol M (1999) A phase I trial of a live, genetically modified *Salmonella Typhimurium* (VNP20009) for the treatment of cancer by intratumoral injection. Clinicaltrials.gov. https://clinicaltrials.gov/study/NCT00004216. Accessed 20 Dec 2023

Taglialegna A (2023) *Pseudomonas* against cancer. Nat Rev Microbiol 21:131–131. https://doi.org/10.1038/s41579-023-00856-8

Tang W, He Y, Zhou S, Ma Y, Liu G (2009) A novel *Bifidobacterium infantis*-mediated TK/GCV suicide gene therapy system exhibits antitumor activity in a rat model of bladder cancer. J Exp Clin Cancer Res 28:155. https://doi.org/10.1186/1756-9966-28-155

Tang Q, Peng X, Xu B, Zhou X, Chen J, Cheng L (2022) Current status and future directions of bacteria-based immunotherapy. Front Immunol 13:911783. https://doi.org/10.3389/fimmu.2022.911783

Tasaki S, Nakayama M, Shoji W (2017) Self-organization of bacterial communities against environmental pH variation: controlled chemotactic motility arranges cell population structures in biofilms. PLoS One 12:e0173195. https://doi.org/10.1371/journal.pone.0173195

Taylor BN, Mehta RR, Yamada T, Lekmine F, Christov K, Chakrabarty AM, Green A, Bratescu L, Shilkaitis A, Beattie CW, Das Gupta TK (2009) Noncationic peptides obtained from azurin preferentially enter cancer cells. Cancer Res 69:537–546. https://doi.org/10.1158/0008-5472.CAN-08-2932

Theys J, Pennington O, Dubois L, Anlezark G, Vaughan T, Mengesha A, Landuyt W, Anné J, Burke P, Dûrre P (2006) Repeated cycles of *Clostridium*-directed enzyme prodrug therapy result in sustained antitumour effects *in vivo*. Br J Cancer 95:1212–1219. https://doi.org/10.1038/sj.bjc.6603367

Thompson RJ, Bouwer HA, Portnoy DA, Frankel FR (1998) Pathogenicity and immunogenicity of a *Listeria monocytogenes* strain that requires D-alanine for growth. Infect Immun 66:3552–3561. https://doi.org/10.1128/IAI.66.8.3552-3561.1998

Toso JF, Gill VJ, Hwu P, Marincola FM, Restifo NP (2002) Phase I study of the intravenous administration of attenuated salmonella typhimurium to patients with metastatic melanoma. J Clin Oncol 20:142–152. https://doi.org/10.1200/JCO.2002.20.1.142

Tran V, Liu J, Behr MA (2014) BCG Vaccines. Microbiol Spectr 2:MGM2-0028-2013. https://doi.org/10.1128/microbiolspec.MGM2-0028-2013

Tsujikawa T, Crocenzi T, Durham JN, Sugar EA et al (2020) Evaluation of cyclophosphamide/GVAX pancreas followed by listeria-mesothelin (CRS-207) with or without Nivolumab in patients with pancreatic cancer. Clin Cancer Res 26:3578–3588. https://doi.org/10.1158/1078-0432.CCR-19-3978

Tunio SA, Oldfield NJ, Berry A, Ala'Aldeen DA, Wooldridge KG, Turner DP (2010) The moonlighting protein fructose-1, 6-bisphosphate aldolase of *Neisseria meningitidis*: surface localization and role in host cell adhesion. Mol Microbiol 76:605–615

Uchida AM, Boden EK, James EA, Shows DM, Konecny AJ, Lord JD (2020) *Escherichia coli*-specific $CD4^+$ T cells have public T-cell receptors and low interleukin 10 production in Crohn's disease. Cell Mol Gastroenterol Hepatol 10:507–526. https://doi.org/10.1016/j.jcmgh.2020.04.013

Vajari MK, Sanaei M-J, Salari S, Rezvani A, Ravari MS, Bashash D (2023) Breast cancer vaccination: latest advances with an analytical focus on clinical trials. Int Immunopharmacol 123:110696. https://doi.org/10.1016/j.intimp.2023.110696

Vendeville A, Larivière D, Fourmentin E (2011) An inventory of the bacterial macromolecular components and their spatial organization. FEMS Microbiol Rev 35:395–414. https://doi.org/10.1111/j.1574-6976.2010.00254.x

Vivarelli S, Salemi R, Candido S, Falzone L, Santagati M, Stefani S, Torino F, Banna GL, Tonini G, Libra M (2019) Microbiota and cancer: from pathogenesis to therapy. Cancers (Basel) 11:38. https://doi.org/10.3390/cancers11010038

Wang J, Guo N, Hou W, Qin H (2022a) Coating bacteria for anti-tumor therapy. Front Bioeng Biotechnol 10:1020020. https://doi.org/10.3389/fbioe.2022.1020020

Wang W, Xu H, Ye Q, Tao F, Wheeldon I, Yuan A, Hu Y, Wu J (2022b) Systemic immune responses to irradiated tumors via the transport of antigens to the tumor periphery by injected flagellate bacteria. Nat Biomed Eng 6:44–53. https://doi.org/10.1038/s41551-021-00834-6

Weibel S, Stritzker J, Eck M, Goebel W, Szalay AA (2008) Colonization of experimental murine breast tumors by *Escherichia coli* K-12 significantly alters the tumor microenvironment. Cell Microbiol 10:1235–1248. https://doi.org/10.1111/j.1462-5822.2008.01122.x

Winnie F, Qing L, Fenfen J, Wei L, Harry Cheuk Hay L, Xing K, Weixin L, Kenneth Kin-Wah T, Zhong Z, Xiaoxing L, Xiang Z, Joseph JYS, Jun Y (2023) *Lactobacillus gallinarum*-derived metabolites boost anti-PD1 efficacy in colorectal cancer by inhibiting regulatory T cells through modulating IDO1/Kyn/AHR axis. Gut 72:2272. https://doi.org/10.1136/gutjnl-2023-329543

Wood LM, Paterson Y (2014) Attenuated *Listeria monocytogenes*: a powerful and versatile vector for the future of tumor immunotherapy. Front Cell Infect Microbiol 4:51. https://doi.org/10.3389/fcimb.2014.00051

Xie S, Zhao L, Song X, Tang M, Mo C, Li X (2017) Doxorubicin-conjugated *Escherichia coli* Nissle 1917 swimmers to achieve tumor targeting and responsive drug release. J Control Release 268:390–399. https://doi.org/10.1016/j.jconrel.2017.10.041

Xie S, Zhang P, Zhang Z, Liu Y, Chen M, Li S, Li X (2021) Bacterial navigation for tumor targeting and photothermally-triggered bacterial ghost transformation for spatiotemporal drug release. Acta Biomater 131:172–184. https://doi.org/10.1016/j.actbio.2021.06.030

Yadav A, Singh S, Sohi H, Dang S (2021) Advances in delivery of chemotherapeutic agents for cancer treatment. AAPS PharmSciTech 23:25. https://doi.org/10.1208/s12249-021-02174-9

Yamada T, Goto M, Punj V, Zaborina O, Chen ML, Kimbara K, Majumdar D, Cunningham E, Das Gupta TK, Chakrabarty AM (2002a) Bacterial redox protein azurin, tumor suppressor protein p53, and regression of cancer. Proc Natl Acad Sci USA 99:14098–14103. https://doi.org/10.1073/pnas.222539699

Yamada T, Goto M, Punj V, Zaborina O, Kimbara K, Gupta TKD, Chakrabarty AM (2002b) The bacterial redox protein azurin induces apoptosis in J774 macrophages through complex formation and stabilization of the tumor suppressor protein p53. Infect Immun 70:7054–7062. https://doi.org/10.1128/IAI.70.12.7054-7062.2002

Yamada T, Hiraoka Y, Gupta TKD, Chakrabarty AM (2004) Rusticyanin, a bacterial electron transfer protein, causes G1 arrest in J774 and apoptosis in human cancer cells. Cell Cycle 3:1182–1187

Yamada T, Fialho AM, Punj V, Bratescu L, Gupta TKD, Chakrabarty AM (2005) Internalization of bacterial redox protein azurin in mammalian cells: entry domain and specificity. Cell Microbiol 7:1418–1431. https://doi.org/10.1111/j.1462-5822.2005.00567.x

Yang M, Yang F, Chen W, Liu S, Qiu L, Chen J (2021) Bacteria-mediated cancer therapies: opportunities and challenges. Biomater Sci 9:5732–5744. https://doi.org/10.1039/d1bm00634g

Yin L, Meng Z, Zhang Y, Hu K, Chen W, Han K, Wu B-Y, You R, Li C-H, Jin Y, Guan Y-Q (2018) *Bacillus* spore-based oral carriers loading curcumin for the therapy of colon cancer. J Control Release 271:31–44. https://doi.org/10.1016/j.jconrel.2017.12.013

Yin R, Wang T, Dai H, Han J, Sun J, Liu N, Dong W, Zhong J, Liu H (2023) Immunogenic molecules associated with gut bacterial cell walls: chemical structures, immune-modulating functions, and mechanisms. Protein Cell 14:776–785. https://doi.org/10.1093/procel/pwad016

Yoon WS, Chae YS, Hong J, Park YK (2011) Antitumor therapeutic effects of a genetically engineered *Salmonella typhimurium* harboring TNF-α in mice. Appl Microbiol Biotechnol 89:1807–1819. https://doi.org/10.1007/s00253-010-3006-4

Yuan Z, Li Y, Zhang S, Wang X, Dou H, Yu X, Zhang Z, Yang S, Xiao M (2023) Extracellular matrix remodeling in tumor progression and immune escape: from mechanisms to treatments. Mol Cancer 22:48. https://doi.org/10.1186/s12943-023-01744-8

Zhang L, Romero P (2018) Metabolic control of $CD8^+$ T cell fate decisions and antitumor immunity. Trends Mol Med 24:30–48. https://doi.org/10.1016/j.molmed.2017.11.005

Zhang X, Cheng X, Lai Y, Zhou Y, Cao W, Hua ZC (2016) *Salmonella* VNP20009-mediated RNA interference of ABCB5 moderated chemoresistance of melanoma stem cell and suppressed tumor growth more potently. Oncotarget 7:14940. https://doi.org/10.18632/oncotarget.7496

Zhang T, Tamman H, Coppieters't Wallant K, Kurata T et al (2022a) Direct activation of a bacterial innate immune system by a viral capsid protein. Nature 612:132–140. https://doi.org/10.1038/s41586-022-05444-z

Zhang Z, Liu X, Chen D, Yu J (2022b) Radiotherapy combined with immunotherapy: the dawn of cancer treatment. Signal Transduct Target Ther 7:258. https://doi.org/10.1038/s41392-022-01102-y

Zhao M, Yang M, Li X-M, Jiang P, Baranov E, Li S, Xu M, Penman S, Hoffman RM (2005) Tumor-targeting bacterial therapy with amino acid auxotrophs of GFP-expressing *Salmonella typhimurium*. Proc Natl Acad Sci USA 102:755–760. https://doi.org/10.1073/pnas.0408422102

Zhao H, Wu L, Yan G, Chen Y, Zhou M, Wu Y, Li Y (2021) Inflammation and tumor progression: signaling pathways and targeted intervention. Signal Transduct Target Ther 6:263. https://doi.org/10.1038/s41392-021-00658-5

Zhao X, Xie N, Zhang H, Zhou W, Ding J (2023) Bacterial drug delivery systems for cancer therapy: "why" and "how". Pharmaceutics 15:2214. https://doi.org/10.3390/pharmaceutics15092214

Zheng JH, Nguyen VH, Jiang SN, Park SH, Tan W, Hong SH, Shin MG, Chung IJ, Hong Y, Bom HS (2017) Two-step enhanced cancer immunotherapy with engineered *Salmonella typhimurium* secreting heterologous flagellin. Sci Transl Med 9:eaak9537. https://doi.org/10.1126/scitranslmed.aak9537

Zhou S, Gravekamp C, Bermudes D, Liu K (2018) Tumor-targeting bacteria engineered to fight cancer. Nat Rev Cancer 18:727–743. https://doi.org/10.1038/s41568-018-0070-z

Zhou B, Szymanski CM, Baylink A (2023a) Bacterial chemotaxis in human diseases. Trends Microbiol 31:453–467. https://doi.org/10.1016/j.tim.2022.10.007

Zhou M, Tang Y, Xu W, Hao X, Li Y, Huang S, Xiang D, Wu J (2023b) Bacteria-based immunotherapy for cancer: a systematic review of preclinical studies. Front Immunol 14: 1140463. https://doi.org/10.3389/fimmu.2023.1140463

Zoaby N, Shainsky-Roitman J, Badarneh S, Abumanhal H, Leshansky A, Yaron S, Schroeder A (2017) Autonomous bacterial nanoswimmers target cancer. J Control Release 257:68–75. https://doi.org/10.1016/j.jconrel.2016.10.006

Index

N. Rezaei (ed.), *Cancer Treatment Modalities: An Interdisciplinary Approach*, Interdisciplinary Cancer Research 24, https://doi.org/10.1007/978-3-032-03866-1